HANDBOOK OF NONPRESCRIPTION DRUGS

9TH EDITION

Edward G. Feldmann, Ph.D.
Project Director and Managing Editor

William L. Blockstein, Ph.D.
Pharmaceutical Editor

Linda L. Young
Editorial Coordinator and Copyeditor

James V. McGinnis
Manager of Art and Production

Vicki L. Meade
Editorial Projects Manager

Laura C. Lawson
Director of Publications Management

Anatomical Drawings: Walter Hilmers, Jr., and Judith M. Guenther, with Alexa L. Chun

Copyediting: Lois W. Sierra

Drug Product Tables: Prepared and produced by Facts and Comparisons, Inc.

Proofreading: Elisabeth C. Griffin, Ann Henderson, Kathleen Nash, and Alisa D. Williams

Indexing: Winfield Swanson

Typesetting: Applied Graphics Technologies

Printing: Arcata Graphics Company

Library of Congress Catalog Number 86-640099
ISSN 0889-7816
ISBN 0-917330-60-9

Trademarks/Trade names: With regard to registered trademarks and/or trade names, the convention followed in this
Handbook is to use an initial capital letter when giving the names of pharmaceutical entities, products, or devices that are
identified in the text by a protected trademark or trade name.

Nonproprietary, generic, or common names of articles are cited without initial capitalization.

HANDBOOK OF NONPRESCRIPTION DRUGS

9TH EDITION

Published by

AMERICAN PHARMACEUTICAL ASSOCIATION

The National Professional Society of Pharmacists
2215 Constitution Avenue, N.W.
Washington, DC 20037

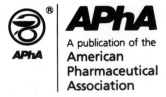

CONTENTS

ADVISORY PANEL

The American Pharmaceutical Association wishes to gratefully acknowledge the helpful guidance and useful suggestions provided by a newly constituted body for the Ninth Edition; this select group of participants, designated the "Advisory Panel," consisted of the following four individuals:

Timothy R. Covington, Pharm.D.
Bruno Professor of Pharmacy and Chairman, Department of Pharmacy Practice, School of Pharmacy, Samford University, Birmingham, Alabama

Janet P. Engle, Pharm.D.
Clinical Assistant Professor and Clinical Pharmacy Coordinator, College of Pharmacy, The University of Illinois, Chicago, Illinois

Daniel A. Hussar, Ph.D.
Remington Professor of Pharmacy, Philadelphia College of Pharmacy and Science, Philadelphia, Pennsylvania

Margaret Yarborough, M.S.
Director, Diabetes Care Center, Cary, North Carolina

AUTHORS & REVIEWERS

1 THE SELF-CARE MOVEMENT

AUTHORS

Gary A. Holt, Ph.D.
Assistant Professor, School of Pharmacy, University of Wyoming, Laramie, Wyoming

Edwin L. Hall, Ph.D.
Professor of Pharmacy, Pharmacy Administration, School of Pharmacy, Samford University, Birmingham, Alabama

REVIEWERS

Wesley G. Byerly, Pharm.D.
Director, Drug Information Services, Department of Pharmacy, North Carolina Baptist Hospital, Winston-Salem, North Carolina

Jere E. Goyan, Ph.D.
Dean and Professor, School of Pharmacy, University of California, San Francisco, California

Joseph L. Kanig, Ph.D.
President, Kanig Consulting & Research Associates, Danbury, Connecticut

Peter P. Lamy, Ph.D., Sc.D.
Director, The Center for the Study of Pharmacy and Therapeutics for the Elderly; Assistant Dean and Professor, School of Pharmacy, University of Maryland, Baltimore, Maryland

Richard P. Penna, Pharm.D.
Associate Executive Director, American Association of Colleges of Pharmacy, Alexandria, Virginia

Alexander M. Schmidt, M.D.
Director, Technology Advancement Center, University Hospital Consortium, Inc., Oakbrook Terrace, Illinois

Dorothy L. Smith, Pharm.D.
President, Consumer Health Information Corporation, McLean, Virginia

John T. Walden, B.A.
Senior Vice President and Director of Public Affairs, Nonprescription Drug Manufacturers Association, Washington, D.C.

2   PATIENT ASSESSMENT AND CONSULTATION

AUTHORS

Wendy Klein-Schwartz, Pharm.D.
Associate Professor, School of Pharmacy, University of Maryland, Baltimore, Maryland

John M. Hoopes, Pharm.D.
Executive Vice President, Drug Counter Pharmacies, Gaithersburg, Maryland

REVIEWERS

Danial E. Baker, Pharm.D.
Associate Professor and Director, Drug Information, College of Pharmacy, Washington State University-Spokane, Spokane, Washington

William C. Gong, Pharm.D.
Associate Professor of Clinical Pharmacy, School of Pharmacy, University of Southern California, Los Angeles, California

Daniel A. Hussar, Ph.D.
Remington Professor of Pharmacy, Philadelphia College of Pharmacy and Science, Philadelphia, Pennsylvania

Michael E. Montagne, Ph.D.
Associate Professor, College of Pharmacy and Allied Health, Northeastern University, Boston, Massachusetts

Judith M. Ozbun, M.S.
Associate Professor, College of Pharmacy, North Dakota State University, Fargo, North Dakota

Robert L. Snively, B.S. (Pharmacy)
Consultant, Stockley Center, Georgetown, Delaware; Clinical Instructor, Philadelphia College of Pharmacy and Science, Philadelphia, Pennsylvania

Gilbert N. Weise, B.S. (Pharmacy)
Pharmacist and President, Weise Pharmacy, Jacksonville, Florida

3   THE FDA'S OTC DRUG REVIEW

AUTHOR

William E. Gilbertson, Pharm.D.
Director, Division of OTC Drug Evaluation, Food and Drug Administration, Rockville, Maryland

REVIEWERS

David B. Brushwood, J.D.
Professor, College of Pharmacy, University of Florida, Gainesville, Florida

Joseph L. Fink III, J.D.
Associate Vice Chancellor of Academic Affairs, University of Kentucky, Lexington, Kentucky

Carl Roberts, Esquire
Hanson, O'Brien, Birney & Butler, Rockville, Maryland

Larry M. Simonsmeier, J.D.
Associate Dean and Professor, College of Pharmacy, Washington State University, Pullman, Washington

Gary L. Yingling, Esquire
McKenna, Conner & Cuneo, Washington, D.C.

4 IN-HOME DIAGNOSTIC PRODUCTS

AUTHOR

Susan Pawlak Meyer, Ph.D.
Director of Academic Affairs, American Association of Colleges of Pharmacy, Alexandria, Virginia

REVIEWERS

Wesley G. Byerly, Pharm.D.
Director, Drug Information Services, Department of Pharmacy, North Carolina Baptist Hospital, Winston-Salem, North Carolina

Stephen M. Caiola, M.S.
Associate Professor and Vice Chairman, Division of Pharmacy Practice, and Director, Pharmacy Area Health Education Centers Program, School of Pharmacy, The University of North Carolina, Chapel Hill, North Carolina

Betsy A. Carlisle, Pharm.D.
Clinical Assistant Professor, College of Pharmacy, The University of Illinois, Chicago, Illinois

Louise S. Parent, Pharm.D.
Clinical Assistant Professor, College of Pharmacy, The University of Illinois, Chicago, Illinois

Wynn W. Waite, Pharm.D.
Clinical Coordinator of Pharmacy Services, Presbyterian Hospital, Albuquerque, New Mexico

5 INTERNAL ANALGESIC PRODUCTS

AUTHOR

W. Kent Van Tyle, Ph.D.
Professor of Pharmacology, College of Pharmacy, Butler University, Indianapolis, Indiana

REVIEWERS

Joseph Greensher, M.D., F.A.A.P.
Medical Director, Winthrop-University Hospital, Mineola, New York

Arthur G. Lipman, Pharm.D.
Professor of Clinical Pharmacy, College of Pharmacy, University of Utah, Salt Lake City, Utah

James K. Marttila, Pharm.D.
Pharmacy Director, Mayo Clinic, Rochester, Minnesota

Joel Owerbach, Pharm.D.
Associate Director of Pharmacy for Clinical and Educational Services, Rochester Medical Group Associates, P.C., Rochester, New York

Leslie A. Shimp, Pharm.D., M.S.
Associate Professor, College of Pharmacy, The University of Michigan, Ann Arbor, Michigan

Anthony J. Silvagni, D.O., M.Sc.
Associate Professor of Family Practice and Clinical Pharmacology, University of Osteopathic Medicine and Health Sciences, Des Moines, Iowa

William E. Wade, Pharm.D.
Assistant Professor, College of Pharmacy, The University of Georgia, Athens, Georgia

6 ANTIPYRETIC DRUG PRODUCTS

AUTHOR

Thomas E. Lackner, Pharm.D.
Chief Clinical Pharmacist, Pharmacy Corporation of America, Fridley, Minnesota

REVIEWERS

Neta A. Hodge, Pharm.D.[†]
Clinical Pharmacist, Philadelphia, Pennsylvania

Gary A. Holt, Ph.D.
Assistant Professor, School of Pharmacy, University of Wyoming, Laramie, Wyoming

Daniel A. Hussar, Ph.D.
Remington Professor of Pharmacy, Philadelphia College of Pharmacy and Science, Philadelphia, Pennsylvania

Robert L. Snively, B.S. (Pharmacy)
Consultant, Stockley Center, Georgetown, Delaware; Clinical Instructor, Philadelphia College of Pharmacy and Science, Philadelphia, Pennsylvania

W. Kent Van Tyle, Ph.D.
Professor of Pharmacology, College of Pharmacy, Butler University, Indianapolis, Indiana

Thomas Wiser, Pharm.D.
Professor, School of Pharmacy, Campbell University, Buies Creek, North Carolina

[†] *Deceased*

7 MENSTRUAL PRODUCTS

AUTHORS

Catherine Angell Sohn, Pharm.D.
Clinical Associate Professor of Pharmacy, Philadelphia College of Pharmacy and Science, Philadelphia, Pennsylvania

Barbara H. Korberly, Pharm.D.
Director, Medical Affairs, McNeil Consumer Products Company, Fort Washington, Pennsylvania

REVIEWERS

Rinaldo A. Brusadin, M.S.
Pharmacist and Owner, The Apothecary, Inc., Worthington, Ohio

Charma A. Konnor, B.S. (Pharmacy)
Regulatory Affairs Pharmacist, Vienna, Virginia

Rosalie Sagraves, Pharm.D.
Associate Professor, College of Pharmacy, The University of Oklahoma, Oklahoma City, Oklahoma

Leslie A. Shimp, Pharm.D., M.S.
Associate Professor, College of Pharmacy, The University of Michigan, Ann Arbor, Michigan

Kenneth A. Skau, Ph.D.
Associate Professor of Pharmacology, University of Cincinnati, College of Pharmacy, Cincinnati, Ohio

Geralynn B. Smith, M.S.
Assistant Professor, College of Pharmacy and Allied Health Professions, Wayne State University, Detroit, Michigan

Karam F. A. Soliman, Ph.D.
Professor and Chairman, Division of Basic Pharmaceutical Sciences, College of Pharmacy, Florida A & M University, Tallahassee, Florida

8 COLD AND ALLERGY PRODUCTS

AUTHORS

Bobby G. Bryant, Pharm.D.
Associate Professor, Albany College of Pharmacy, Union University, Albany, New York

Thomas P. Lombardi, Pharm.D.
Clinical Pharmacy Coordinator, Department of Pharmacy, St. Peter's Hospital, Albany, New York

REVIEWERS

Darrell F. Bennett, B.S. (Pharmacy)
Pharmacist in Charge, Student Health Service, California Polytechnic Health Center, San Luis Obispo, California

Thomas D. DeCillis, B.S. (Pharmacy)
Retired Officer, U.S. Public Health Service, North Port, Florida

Alex Gringauz, Ph.D.
Professor of Medicinal Chemistry, Arnold and Marie Schwartz College of Pharmacy and Health Sciences, Long Island University, Brooklyn, New York

H. Won Jun, Ph.D.
Professor of Pharmaceutics, School of Pharmacy, University of Georgia, Athens, Georgia

Raymond W. Roberts, Pharm.D.
Corporate Director, Pharmacy Services, Kimberly Quality Care, Atlanta, Georgia

D. Barry Smith, Pharm.D.
President, Medical Dental Pharmacy, Inc., Fresno, California

Karen J. Tietze, Pharm.D.
Associate Professor of Clinical Pharmacy, Philadelphia College of Pharmacy and Science, Philadelphia, Pennsylvania

9 ASTHMA PRODUCTS

AUTHORS

H. William Kelly, Pharm.D.
Associate Professor of Pharmacy, College of Pharmacy, and Associate Professor of Pediatrics, School of Medicine, University of New Mexico, Albuquerque, New Mexico

Celeste Lindley, Pharm.D.
Assistant Professor, School of Pharmacy and Medicine, University of North Carolina, Chapel Hill, North Carolina

REVIEWERS

Darrell F. Bennett, B.S. (Pharmacy)
Pharmacist in Charge, Student Health Service, California Polytechnic Health Center, San Luis Obispo, California

Sandra M. Gawchik, D.O.
Co-Director, Allergy and Clinical Immunology, Crozer-Chester Medical Center, Division of Allergy and Clinical Immunology, Chester, Pennsylvania

Kenneth R. Keefner, Ph.D.
Vice President, Parenteral Division, Home Health Care Equipment Services, Inc., St. Louis, Missouri

Pamela A. Simon, Pharm.D.
Clinical Assistant Professor, College of Pharmacy, The University of Illinois, Chicago, Illinois

Gary D. Smith, Pharm.D.
Contracts and Pricing Administrator, Partners National Health Plans, Minneapolis, Minnesota

Craig Stern, Pharm.D.
Director of Operations, Northridge Pharmacy, Northridge, California

10 SLEEP AID AND STIMULANT PRODUCTS

AUTHORS

James P. Caro, B.S. (Pharmacy), M.B.A.
Director, Special Projects Division, Professional Services Development Group, American Society of Hospital Pharmacists, Bethesda, Maryland

Susan R. Dombrowski, M.S.
Senior Editor, Special Projects Division, American Society of Hospital Pharmacists, Bethesda, Maryland

REVIEWERS

Kenneth A. Bachmann, Ph.D.
Professor of Pharmacology, College of Pharmacy, The University of Toledo, Toledo, Ohio

Patricia A. Camazzola, Pharm.D.
Director, Department of Pharmacy, Huron Valley Hospital, Milford, Massachusetts

M. Lynn Crismon, Pharm.D.
Associate Professor and Head, The Clinical Division at Austin, The University of Texas, Austin, Texas

Charma A. Konnor, B.S. (Pharmacy)
Regulatory Affairs Pharmacist, Vienna, Virginia

Arthur J. McBay, Ph.D.
Consultant, Forensics Toxicology; Professor Emeritus, School of Pharmacy, and Adjunct Professor of Pathology, University of North Carolina, Chapel Hill, North Carolina

James K. Marttila, Pharm.D.
Pharmacy Director, Mayo Clinic, Rochester, Minnesota

Michael Z. Wincor, Pharm.D.
Assistant Professor of Clinical Pharmacy, School of Pharmacy, University of Southern California, Los Angeles, California

11 ANTACID PRODUCTS

AUTHOR

William R. Garnett, Pharm.D.
Professor, School of Pharmacy, Virginia Commonwealth University, Richmond, Virginia

REVIEWERS

Stephen M. Caiola, M.S.
Associate Professor and Vice Chairman, Division of Pharmacy Practice, and Director, Pharmacy Area Health Education Centers Program, School of Pharmacy, The University of North Carolina, Chapel Hill, North Carolina

Thomas E. Lackner, Pharm.D.
Chief Clinical Pharmacist, Pharmacy Corporation of America, Fridley, Minnesota

Buford T. Lively, Ph.D.
Assistant Dean for Administrative and External Affairs, Professor of Pharmacy and Health Care Administration, The University of Toledo, College of Pharmacy, Toledo, Ohio

Robert S. Mosser, M.D., F.A.C.P.
Adjunct Professor of Medicine, University of California at Los Angeles, Bakersfield, California

Roy C. Parish, Jr., Pharm.D.
Assistant Professor, College of Pharmacy, The University of Georgia, Athens, Georgia

Pamela A. Simon, Pharm.D.
Clinical Assistant Professor, College of Pharmacy, The University of Illinois, Chicago, Illinois

C. Wayne Weart, Pharm.D.
Professor and Director, Pharmacy Education in Family Medicine, Medical University of South Carolina, Charleston, South Carolina

12 EMETIC AND ANTIEMETIC PRODUCTS

AUTHORS

Gary M. Oderda, Pharm.D., M.P.H.
Director, Maryland Poison Center; Professor, School of Pharmacy, University of Maryland, Baltimore, Maryland

Barbara H. Korberly, Pharm.D.
Director, Medical Affairs, McNeil Consumer Products Company, Fort Washington, Pennsylvania

REVIEWERS

Betsy A. Carlisle, Pharm.D.
Clinical Assistant Professor, College of Pharmacy, The University of Illinois, Chicago, Illinois

Metta Lou Henderson, Ph.D.
Professor of Pharmacy, Raabe College of Pharmacy, Ohio Northern University, Ada, Ohio

Gary A. Holt, Ph.D.
Assistant Professor, School of Pharmacy, University of Wyoming, Laramie, Wyoming

Alan H. Lau, Pharm.D.
Associate Professor of Pharmacy Practice, College of Pharmacy, University of Illinois, Chicago, Illinois

Anthony J. Silvagni, D.O., Pharm.D.
Chairman, Department of Physiology and Pharmacology, University of Osteopathic Medicine and Health Sciences, Des Moines, Iowa

Anthony R. Temple, M.D.
Director, Regulatory and Medical Affairs, McNeil Consumer Products Company, Fort Washington, Pennsylvania

13 ANTIDIARRHEAL AND OTHER GASTROINTESTINAL PRODUCTS

AUTHOR

R. Leon Longe, Pharm.D.
Professor of Pharmacy Practice, College of Pharmacy, University of Georgia, Athens, Georgia

REVIEWERS

Timothy R. Covington, Pharm.D.
Bruno Professor of Pharmacy and Chairman, Department of Pharmacy Practice, School of Pharmacy, Samford University, Birmingham, Alabama

Joseph T. DiPiro, Pharm.D.
Associate Professor, Medical College of Georgia, Augusta, Georgia

Herbert L. DuPont, M.D.
Mary W. Kelsey Professor and Director, Division of Infectious Diseases, The University of Texas Medical School, Houston, Texas

Stuart Feldman, Ph.D.
Professor and Chairman of Pharmaceutics, College of Pharmacy, University of Houston, Houston, Texas

Walter D. Hadley, B.S. (Pharmacy)
Community Practitioner, Corner Drug Store, Noblesville, Indiana

Wayne A. Kradjan, Pharm.D.
Professor of Pharmacy Practice, School of Pharmacy, University of Washington, Seattle, Washington

Richard K. Ogden, D.O.
Chairman, Department of General Practice, Lakeside Hospital, Kansas City, Missouri

Thomas S. Sisca, Pharm.D.
Assistant Director, Clinical Pharmacy Services and Drug Information, Memorial Hospital, Easton, Maryland

14   ANTHELMINTIC PRODUCTS

AUTHOR

John M. Kinsella, Ph.D.
Instructor, School of Pharmacy and Allied Health Sciences, University of Montana, Missoula, Montana

REVIEWERS

J. Fred Bennes, B.S. (Pharmacy)
Clinical Assistant Professor, School of Pharmacy, State University of New York, Buffalo, New York

Kathryn K. Bucci, Pharm.D.
Assistant Professor of Pharmacy Practice, Campbell University, Durham, North Carolina

Donald O. Fedder, B.S. (Pharmacy), Dr. P.H.
Associate Professor and Director, Community Pharmacy Programs, School of Pharmacy, University of Maryland, Baltimore, Maryland

Susan Pawlak Meyer, Ph.D.
Director of Academic Affairs, American Association of Colleges of Pharmacy, Alexandria, Virginia

David E. Stewart, Pharm.D.
Pharmacist and Vice President, Stewart's Pharmacy; Assistant Professor, Pharmacy Practice, College of Pharmacy, University of Tennessee, McMinnville, Tennessee

William E. Wade, Pharm.D.
Assistant Professor, College of Pharmacy, The University of Georgia, Athens, Georgia

15   LAXATIVE PRODUCTS

AUTHORS

Clarence E. Curry, Jr., Pharm.D.
Associate Professor of Pharmacy Practice, College of Pharmacy, Howard University, Washington, D.C.

Demetris Tatum-Butler, Pharm.D.
Assistant Professor, College of Pharmacy, Howard University, Washington, D.C.

REVIEWERS

R. Randolph Beckner, Pharm.D.
Assistant Director, Department of Pharmacy, Barnes Hospital, St. Louis, Missouri

Eddie L. Boyd, Pharm.D.
Associate Professor, College of Pharmacy, University of Michigan, Ann Arbor, Michigan

Anthony T. Buatti, B.S. (Pharmacy), M.B.A.
Assistant Professor of Health Care Administration, College of Pharmacy and Allied Health Professions, St. John's University, Jamaica, New York

Janice A. Gaska, Pharm.D.
Associate Professor of Clinical Pharmacy and Director, Pharmacy Continuing Education, Philadelphia College of Pharmacy and Science, Philadelphia, Pennsylvania

James K. Marttila, Pharm.D.
Pharmacy Director, Mayo Clinic, Rochester, Minnesota

Katheryn Russi, M.P.A.
Associate Professor and Director, Division of Pharmacy Practice, College of Pharmacy and Health Sciences, Drake University, Des Moines, Iowa

16 DIABETES CARE PRODUCTS

AUTHORS

L. M. Evenson-St. Amand, Pharm.D.
Assistant Professor of Pharmacy Practice, College of Pharmacy, Washington State University, Pullman, Washington

R. Keith Campbell, M.B.A.
Associate Dean and Professor of Pharmacy Practice, Certified Diabetes Educator, College of Pharmacy, Washington State University, Pullman, Washington

REVIEWERS

Charles Y. McCall, Pharm.D.
Associate Professor of Pharmacy Practice, College of Pharmacy, University of Georgia, Athens, Georgia

Charles D. Ponte, Pharm.D.
Professor of Clinical Pharmacy and Family Medicine, Schools of Pharmacy and Medicine, West Virginia University Health Sciences Center, Morgantown, West Virginia

David A. Sclar, Ph.D.
Assistant Professor of Pharmacy, School of Pharmacy, University of Southern California, Los Angeles, California

Kenneth A. Skau, Ph.D.
Associate Professor, College of Pharmacy, University of Cincinnati Medical Center, Cincinnati, Ohio

Michael S. Torre, B.S. (Pharmacy), M.S.
Clinical Professor and Chairman, Department of Clinical Pharmacy Practice, College of Pharmacy and Allied Health Professions, St. John's University, Jamaica, New York

Thomas Wiser, Pharm.D.
Professor of Pharmacy Practice, School of Pharmacy, Campbell University, Buies Creek, North Carolina

17 NUTRITIONAL SUPPLEMENT, MINERAL, AND VITAMIN PRODUCTS

AUTHORS

Marianne Ivey, Pharm.D.
Director, Department of Pharmacy Services, University of Cincinnati Medical Center, Cincinnati, Ohio

Gary Elmer, Ph.D.
Associate Professor, Medicinal Chemistry, School of Pharmacy, University of Washington, Seattle, Washington

REVIEWERS

Lester G. Bruns, Ph.D.
Professor of Biochemistry and Nutritional Biochemistry, St. Louis College of Pharmacy, St. Louis, Missouri

Donald R. Gronewold, B.S. (Pharmacy)
President, Don's Pharmacy, Washington, Illinois

Carl J. Malanga, Ph.D.
Professor and Chairman, Basic Pharmaceutical Sciences, School of Pharmacy, West Virginia University Health Sciences Center, Morgantown, West Virginia

William A. Miller, Pharm.D.
Professor and Chairman, Department of Hospital Pharmacy Practice, College of Pharmacy, Medical University of South Carolina, Charleston, South Carolina

Merlin V. Nelson, Pharm.D.
Assistant Professor, College of Pharmacy and Allied Health Professions, Wayne State University, Detroit, Michigan

Gail H. Rosen, Pharm.D.
Director, Nutritional Support Services, University of Maryland Medical System, Department of Pharmacy Services, Baltimore, Maryland

J. Ken Walters, Jr., Pharm.D.
Assistant Director of Pharmacy, Francis Scott Key Medical Center, Baltimore, Maryland

18   INFANT FORMULA PRODUCTS

AUTHORS

Michael W. McKenzie, Ph.D.
Associate Dean for Student Affairs and Professor, University of Florida, College of Pharmacy, Gainesville, Florida

Kenneth J. Bender, Pharm.D.
Director of Pharmacy Services, Truckee Meadows Hospital, Reno, Nevada

A. Jeanece Seals, M.S., R.D.
Director, Maternal and Child Health, Tennessee Department of Health and Environment, Nashville, Tennessee

REVIEWERS

Tery L. Baskin, B.S. (Pharmacy), P.D.
Director, Arkansas Pharmacists Services Company; Owner, McCain Pharmacy, Little Rock, Arkansas

F. James Grogan, Pharm.D.
Associate Professor of Clinical Pharmacy, St. Louis State College of Pharmacy, St. Louis, Missouri

Cynthia Kirman, Pharm.D.
Drug Information Center, Sinai Hospital of Detroit, Detroit, Michigan

Howard C. Mofenson, M.D.
Director, Long Island Regional Poison Control Center, Nassau County Medical Center, East Meadow, New York

Rosalie Sagraves, Pharm.D.
Associate Professor, College of Pharmacy, The University of Oklahoma City, Oklahoma City, Oklahoma

Paul C. Walker, Pharm.D.
Director of Pharmacy, Michigan Department of Mental Health, Lafayette Clinic; Adjunct Assistant Professor, College of Pharmacy and Allied Health Professions, Wayne State University, Detroit, Michigan

19 WEIGHT CONTROL PRODUCTS

AUTHOR

Glenn D. Appelt, Ph.D.
Professor of Pharmacology, School of Pharmacy, University of Colorado, Boulder, Colorado

REVIEWERS

Robert L. Beamer, Ph.D.
Professor of Medicinal Chemistry and Biochemistry, College of Pharmacy, University of South Carolina, Columbia, South Carolina

Patricia A. Camazzola, Pharm.D.
Director, Department of Pharmacy, Huron Valley Hospital, Milford, Massachusetts

William S. Lackey, B.S. (Pharmacy), M.B.A.
Retired Pharmacist; Past President, Fellow American College of Apothecaries, Tucson, Arizona

William A. Parker, Pharm.D., M.B.A.
Pharmacist Associate, Shoppers Drug Mart, Fenwick Medical Centre, Halifax; Sessional Lecturer, Dalhousie University, Nova Scotia, Canada

Leon Shargel, Ph.D.
Associate Professor, Pharmacy and Pharmacology, Massachusetts College of Pharmacy and Allied Health Sciences, Boston, Massachusetts

Alan M. Siegal, M.D.
Professor of Medicine, Interim Director of Division of Gerontology, University of Alabama, Birmingham, Alabama

20 OPHTHALMIC PRODUCTS

AUTHOR

Dick R. Gourley, Pharm.D.
Professor of Clinical Pharmacy and Dean, College of Pharmacy, University of Tennessee, Memphis, Tennessee

REVIEWERS

Chris Bapatla, Ph.D.
Assistant Director, Research and Development Stability, Alcon Laboratories, Inc., Fort Worth, Texas

Jimmy D. Bartlett, O.D.
Associate Professor, School of Optometry, University of Alabama, Birmingham, Alabama

Alexander F. Demetro, Pharm.D.
Pharmacist, Westwood Prescriptionists, San Jose, California

Eugene I. Isaacson, Ph.D.
Professor of Pharmaceutical Chemistry, College of Pharmacy, Idaho State University, Pocatello, Idaho

Ralph W. Trottier, Ph.D., J.D.
Professor and Attorney at Law, Department of Pharmacology, Morehouse School of Medicine, Atlanta, Georgia

John R. Yuen, Pharm.D.
Clinical Pharmacy Fellow in Ocular Pharmacy, School of Pharmacy, University of Southern California, Los Angeles, California

21 CONTACT LENSES AND LENS CARE PRODUCTS

AUTHORS

Thomas A. Gossel, Ph.D.
Professor of Pharmacology and Chairman, Department of Pharmacology and Biomedical Sciences, College of Pharmacy, Ohio Northern University, Ada, Ohio

J. Richard Wuest, Pharm.D.
Professor of Clinical Pharmacy, College of Pharmacy, University of Cincinnati Medical Center, Cincinnati, Ohio

REVIEWERS

Chris Bapatla, Ph.D.
Assistant Director, Research and Development Stability, Alcon Laboratories, Inc., Fort Worth, Texas

Byron A. Barnes, Ph.D.
Dean Emeritus, St. Louis College of Pharmacy, St. Louis, Missouri

William J. Benjamin, O.D., Ph.D.
Associate Professor, School of Optometry, University of Alabama, Birmingham, Alabama

Janet P. Engle, Pharm.D.
Clinical Assistant Professor and Clinical Pharmacy Coordinator, College of Pharmacy, The University of Illinois, Chicago, Illinois

Susan C. Miller, Ph.D.
Senior Staff Researcher, Syntex Research, Palo Alto, California

Thomas F. Patton, Ph.D.
Vice President, Operations, Oread Laboratories, Inc., Lawrence, Kansas

James Socks, O.D., M.B.A.
Director of International Marketing for Contact Lens Care, Alcon Laboratories, Inc., Fort Worth, Texas

Jerry Stein, Ph.D.
Assistant Director of Clinical Sciences, Alcon Laboratories, Inc., Fort Worth, Texas

Wynn W. Waite, Pharm.D.
Clinical Coordinator of Pharmacy Services, Presbyterian Hospital, Albuquerque, New Mexico

John R. Yuen, Pharm.D.
Clinical Pharmacy Fellow in Ocular Pharmacy, School of Pharmacy, University of Southern California, Los Angeles, California

22 OTIC PRODUCTS

AUTHOR

Keith O. Miller, Pharm.D.
Quality Assurance Coordinator, Marymount Hospital, Garfield Heights, Ohio

REVIEWERS

Carl F. Emswiller, Jr., B.S. (Pharmacy)
Pharmacist, Emswiller Pharmacy, Leesburg, Virginia

Janet P. Engle, Pharm.D.
Clinical Assistant Professor and Clinical Pharmacy Coordinator, College of Pharmacy, The University of Illinois, Chicago, Illinois

Jerry D. Karbeling, B.S. (Pharmacy)
Karbeling Pharmacy Services Inc., Big Creek Pharmacy, Polk City, Iowa

Michael S. Maddux, Pharm.D.
Associate Professor, College of Pharmacy, University of Illinois, Chicago, Illinois

Dennis Richmond, M.D., P.C.
Family Practitioner in Private Practice, Lafayette, Indiana

Ralph W. Trottier, Ph.D., J.D.
Professor and Attorney at Law, Department of Pharmacology, Morehouse School of Medicine, Atlanta, Georgia

23   ORAL HEALTH PRODUCTS

AUTHOR

Karen A. Baker, B.S. (Pharmacy), M.S.
Assistant Professor, College of Dentistry, and Adjunct Assistant Professor, College of Pharmacy, University of Iowa, Iowa City, Iowa

REVIEWERS

Thomas D. DeCillis, B.S. (Pharmacy)
Retired Officer, U.S. Public Health Service, North Port, Florida

Lowell S. Lakritz, D.D.S.
Private Practitioner, Family Dentistry, Madison, Wisconsin

Thomas D. McGregor, B.S. (Pharmacy), M.B.A.
Adjunct Assistant Professor, School of Pharmacy, University of Wisconsin-Madison, Madison, Wisconsin; Pharmacist, Moreland Plaza Pharmacy, Waukesha, Wisconsin

Roger H. Scholle, D.D.S.
Private Practitioner, General Dentistry; Assistant Professor, Northwestern University Dental School, Chicago, Illinois; Editor, Journal of the Illinois State Dental Society, Springfield, Illinois

Carl Stone, M.A., D.D.S.
Associate Professor, School of Dentistry, University of Detroit, Detroit, Michigan

Kenneth W. Witte, Pharm.D.
Clinical Assistant Professor, University of Illinois, College of Pharmacy, Chicago, Illinois

24   OSTOMY CARE PRODUCTS

AUTHORS

Michael L. Kleinberg, M.S.
Director, Professional Services, Immunex Corporation, Seattle, Washington; Associate Clinical Professor, School of Pharmacy, University of California, San Francisco, California

Melba C. Connors, R.N., C.E.T.N.
Enterostomal Therapist, San Diego, California

REVIEWERS

George B. Browning, B.S. (Pharmacy)
Pharmacist and Owner, Medical Arts Building Pharmacy, Melbourne, Florida

Theodore Eisenstat, M.D.
Associate Professor of Surgery, Department of Surgery, Robert Wood Johnson School of Medicine, New Brunswick, New Jersey

K. Richard Knoll, Pharm.D.
Associate Professor, College of Pharmacy, University of Arkansas Medical Center, Little Rock, Arkansas

Mary M. Losey, M.S.
Director, Office of Student Services, School of Pharmacy and Pharmacal Sciences, Purdue University, West Lafayette, Indiana

Gary R. Schmidt, B.S. (Pharmacy)
Clinical Instructor, In-Patient Pharmacy, William Middleton Veterans' Administration Hospital, Madison, Wisconsin

Joan Lerner Selekof, R.N., B.S.N., C.E.T.N.
Enterostomal Therapy Nurse, Medical–Surgical II Division, University of Maryland Medical System, Baltimore, Maryland

25 CONTRACEPTIVE METHODS AND PRODUCTS

AUTHOR

Roberta S. Carrier, Pharm.D.
Assistant Professor of Pharmacy and Coordinator, Community Pharmacy Practice (Externship), School of Pharmacy, University of Wisconsin-Madison, Madison, Wisconsin

REVIEWERS

Emily C. Bennett, R.N.C., M.S.
Clinical Assistant Professor, Department of Obstetrics and Gynecology, Medical College of Virginia, Virginia Commonwealth University, Richmond, Virginia

Sandra H. Hak, Pharm.D.
President, ProPharma, Ltd., Chapel Hill, North Carolina

Peter P. Lamy, Ph.D., Sc.D.
Director, The Center for the Study of Pharmacy and Therapeutics for the Elderly; Assistant Dean and Professor, School of Pharmacy, University of Maryland, Baltimore, Maryland

David M. Margulies, M.D.
Private Practitioner, Obstetrics and Gynecology, Bethesda, Maryland

Timothy D. Moore, M.S.
Senior Director, Department of Pharmacy, The Ohio State University Hospitals, Columbus, Ohio

Louise S. Parent, Pharm.D.
Clinical Assistant Professor, College of Pharmacy, The University of Illinois, Chicago, Illinois

26 HEMORRHOIDAL PRODUCTS

AUTHOR

Benjamin Hodes, Ph.D.
Professor of Pharmaceutics and University Director, Division of Continuing Education, Duquesne University, Pittsburgh, Pennsylvania

REVIEWERS

Thomas D. DeCillis, B.S. (Pharmacy)
Retired Officer, U.S. Public Health Service, North Port, Florida

Ross L. Egger, M.D.
Medical Director, Blue Cross and Blue Shield of Indiana, Indianapolis, Indiana

Sidney Fish, B.S. (Pharmacy)
Owner and Pharmacist, Northtown Pharmacy, Amherst, New York

Anthony Palmieri III, Ph.D.
Manager, Patient Liaison, The Upjohn Company, Kalamazoo, Michigan

Lee E. Smith, M.D.
Professor of Surgery, George Washington University Medical Center, Washington, D.C.

Quentin M. Srnka, Pharm.D., M.B.A.
Professor, College of Pharmacy, University of Tennessee, Memphis, Tennessee

27 PERSONAL CARE PRODUCTS

AUTHORS

Donald R. Miller, Pharm.D.
Associate Professor of Pharmacy, College of Pharmacy, North Dakota State University, Fargo, North Dakota

Mary Kuzel, Pharm.D.
Assistant Professor of Pharmacy Practice, College of Pharmacy, North Dakota State University, Fargo, North Dakota

REVIEWERS

George M. Hocking, Ph.D.
Professor Emeritus, School of Pharmacy, Auburn University, Auburn, Alabama

Linda Hogan, M.S.
Manager of Licensing, Marion Laboratories, Inc., Kansas City, Missouri

Alan W. Hopefl, Pharm.D.
Associate Professor of Clinical Pharmacy, St. Louis College of Pharmacy, St. Louis, Missouri

Lawrence A. Lemchen, B.S. (Pharmacy)
Clinical Consultant Pharmacist, Pharmacy Corporation of America, Division of Beverly Enterprises, Tukwila, Washington

Reid A. Nishikawa, Pharm.D.
Senior Pharmacist, University of California at Davis Medical Center, Sacramento, California

Geralynn B. Smith, M.S.
Assistant Professor, College of Pharmacy and Allied Health Professions, Wayne State University, Detroit, Michigan

Linda Gore Sutherland, B.S. (Pharmacy), M.B.A.
Pharmacist and Director, Drug Information Services, School of Pharmacy, University of Wyoming, Laramie, Wyoming

28 TOPICAL ANTI-INFECTIVE PRODUCTS

AUTHORS

Michael R. Jacobs, Pharm.D.
Associate Professor of Clinical Pharmacy, School of Pharmacy, Temple University, Health Sciences Center, Philadelphia, Pennsylvania

Paul Zanowiak, Ph.D.
Professor of Pharmaceutics, School of Pharmacy, Temple University, Philadelphia, Pennsylvania

REVIEWERS

Miriam P. Calhoun, B.S.
Interdisciplinary Scientist, Food and Drug Administration (Retired); Consultant, Pharmaceutical Regulatory Affairs, Potomac, Maryland

Robert J. Cluxton, Jr., Pharm.D.
Associate Professor of Clinical Pharmacy, College of Pharmacy, University of Cincinnati, Cincinnati, Ohio

Howard L. Maibach, M.D.
Professor of Dermatology, University of California Medical School, San Francisco, California

Stewart B. Siskin, Pharm.D.
Associate Director, Clinical Research, Bristol-Myers Company, Buffalo, New York

Marilyn Speedie, Ph.D.
Associate Professor and Chairman, Department of Biomedicinal Chemistry, School of Pharmacy, University of Maryland, Baltimore, Maryland

29   ACNE PRODUCTS

AUTHOR

Joye Anne Billow, Ph.D.
Professor of Pharmacy and Head, Department of Pharmacy Practice, South Dakota State University, Brookings, South Dakota

REVIEWERS

Darrell F. Bennett, B.S. (Pharmacy)
Pharmacist in Charge, Student Health Service, California Polytechnic Health Center, San Luis Obispo, California

Angele C. D'Angelo, M.S.
Editorial Director, U.S. Pharmacist, Jobson Publishing Corporation, New York, New York

Henry A. Palmer, Ph.D.
Clinical Professor and Associate Dean for Professional Affairs, School of Pharmacy, University of Connecticut, Storrs, Connecticut

Charles D. Ponte, Pharm.D.
Professor of Clinical Pharmacy and Family Medicine, Schools of Pharmacy and Medicine, West Virginia University Health Sciences Center, Morgantown, West Virginia

J. Richard Wuest, Pharm.D.
Professor of Clinical Pharmacy, College of Pharmacy, University of Cincinnati Medical Center, Cincinnati, Ohio

30   DERMATITIS, DRY SKIN, DANDRUFF, SEBORRHEIC DERMATITIS, AND PSORIASIS PRODUCTS

AUTHOR

Joseph R. Robinson, Ph.D.
Professor of Pharmacy, University of Wisconsin, Center for Health Sciences, Madison, Wisconsin

REVIEWERS

J. Fred Bennes, B.S. (Pharmacy)
Clinical Assistant Professor, School of Pharmacy, State University of New York at Buffalo, Buffalo, New York

Emery W. Brunett, Ph.D.
Associate Professor of Pharmacy, School of Pharmacy, University of Wyoming, Laramie, Wyoming

Peter J. Cascella, Ph.D.
Pharmacokinetics Reviewer, Department of Biopharmaceutics, Food and Drug Administration, Rockville, Maryland

George E. Francisco, Pharm.D.
Associate Dean and Associate Professor, College of Pharmacy, University of Georgia, Athens, Georgia

Joseph L. Kanig, Ph.D.
President, Kanig Consulting & Research Associates, Danbury, Connecticut

Anthony J. Lamonica, B.S. (Pharmacy)
President and Pharmacist, Prescription Shoppe, Inc., Everett, Massachusetts

31 DIAPER RASH AND PRICKLY HEAT PRODUCTS

AUTHOR

Gary H. Smith, Pharm.D.
Professor and Director, Drug Information Services and Division of Clinical Pharmacy, School of Pharmacy, University of Arizona, Tucson, Arizona

REVIEWERS

Timothy Boehmer, B.S. (Pharmacy)
Maternity Center Pharmacist, Providence Hospital, Anchorage, Alaska

John A. Bosso, Pharm.D.
Professor of Clinical Pharmacy, College of Pharmacy, University of Houston, Houston, Texas

Miriam P. Calhoun, B.S.
Interdisciplinary Scientist, Food and Drug Administration (Retired); Consultant, Pharmaceutical Regulatory Affairs, Potomac, Maryland

Dennis P. Hays, Pharm.D.
Director of Pharmacy, Cook County Hospital, Chicago, Illinois

Debra Ricciatti-Sibbald, M.S.
President, Debary Dermatologicals, Mississaugua, Ontario, Canada

Paul C. Walker, Pharm.D.
Director of Pharmacy, Michigan Department of Mental Health, Lafayette Clinic; Adjunct Assistant Professor, Department of Pharmacy Practice, College of Pharmacy and Allied Health Professions, Wayne State University, Detroit, Michigan

32 EXTERNAL ANALGESIC PRODUCTS

AUTHOR

Arthur I. Jacknowitz, Pharm.D.
Professor and Chairman, Department of Clinical Pharmacy, West Virginia University Health Sciences Center, Morgantown, West Virginia

REVIEWERS

Thomas A. Gossel, Ph.D.
Professor of Pharmacology and Chairman, Department of Pharmacology and Biomedical Sciences, College of Pharmacy, Ohio Northern University, Ada, Ohio

Neta A. Hodge, Pharm.D.[†]
Clinical Pharmacist, Philadelphia, Pennsylvania

Roy C. Parish, Jr., Pharm.D.
Assistant Professor, College of Pharmacy, The University of Georgia, Athens, Georgia

Craig Stern, Pharm.D.
Director of Operations, Northridge Pharmacy, Northridge, California

Randall L. Vanderveen, Ph.D.
Assistant Dean and Associate Professor, College of Pharmacy, Oregon State University, Corvallis, Oregon

J. Richard Wuest, Pharm.D.
Professor of Clinical Pharmacy, College of Pharmacy, University of Cincinnati Medical Center, Cincinnati, Ohio

[†] *Deceased*

33 BURN AND SUNBURN PRODUCTS

AUTHOR

Chester A. (CAB) Bond, Pharm.D.
Professor and Associate Dean, School of Pharmacy, University of Wisconsin, Madison, Wisconsin

REVIEWERS

Robert W. Bennett, M.S.
Associate Professor of Clinical Pharmacy and Associate Director of Continuing Education, Purdue University, School of Pharmacy and Pharmacal Sciences, West Lafayette, Indiana

Julie Rivkin Berman, Pharm.D.
Clinical Pharmacy Specialist–Surgery, Detroit Receiving Hospital and University Health Center, Detroit, Michigan

Miriam P. Calhoun, B.S.
Interdisciplinary Scientist, Food and Drug Administration (Retired); Consultant, Pharmaceutical Regulatory Affairs, Potomac, Maryland

Walter T. Gloor, Ph.D.
Professor, School of Pharmacy and Allied Health Professions, Creighton University, Omaha, Nebraska

Ray E. Marcrom, Pharm.D.
Owner and Pharmacist, Marcrom's Pharmacy, P.C., Manchester, Tennessee

Katheryn Russi, M.P.A.
Associate Professor and Director, Division of Pharmacy Practice, College of Pharmacy and Health Sciences, Drake University, Des Moines, Iowa

34 SUNSCREEN AND SUNTAN PRODUCTS

AUTHOR

Edward M. DeSimone II, Ph.D.
Associate Professor of Pharmacy and Assistant Dean for Academic Affairs, School of Pharmacy and Allied Health Professions, Creighton University, Omaha, Nebraska

REVIEWERS

Julie Rivkin Berman, Pharm.D.
Clinical Pharmacy Specialist–Surgery, Detroit Receiving Hospital and University Health Center, Detroit, Michigan

Martin J. Jinks, Pharm.D.
Professor and Director, Professional Practice Unit, College of Pharmacy, Washington State University, Pullman, Washington

Linda K. McCoy, Pharm.D.
Manager of Clinical Pharmacy Services, Good Samaritan Regional Medical Center, Phoenix, Arizona

Shirley P. McKee, B.S. (Pharmacy)
Pharmacist, Houston, Texas

Katheryn Russi, M.P.A.
Associate Professor and Director, Division of Pharmacy Practice, College of Pharmacy and Health Sciences, Drake University, Des Moines, Iowa

J. Allen Scoggin, Pharm.D.
Associate Professor of Pharmacy Administration, College of Pharmacy, University of Tennessee, Memphis, Tennessee

Stewart B. Siskin, Pharm.D.
Associate Director, Clinical Research, Bristol-Myers Company, Buffalo, New York

35 POISON IVY AND POISON OAK PRODUCTS

AUTHOR

Henry Wormser, Ph.D.
Professor of Pharmaceutical Chemistry, Wayne State University, College of Pharmacy and Allied Health Professions, Detroit, Michigan

REVIEWERS

Andrew J. Bartilucci, Ph.D.
Vice President for Health Professions, Clinical Services and Research, St. John's University, Jamaica, New York

David C. Beck, M.D.
Dermatologist, West Lafayette, Indiana

Thomas A. Gossel, Ph.D.
Professor of Pharmacology and Chairman, Department of Pharmacology and Biomedical Sciences, Ohio Northern University, College of Pharmacy, Ada, Ohio

Jerry D. Karbeling, B.S. (Pharmacy)
Karbeling Pharmacy Services Inc., Big Creek Pharmacy, Polk City, Iowa

Robert B. Sause, Ph.D.
Associate Professor, Department of Pharmacy and Administrative Sciences, College of Pharmacy and Allied Health Professions, St. John's University, Jamaica, New York

Joel L. Zatz, Ph.D.
Professor and Chair, Department of Pharmaceutics, College of Pharmacy, Rutgers University, The State University of New Jersey, Piscataway, New Jersey

36 INSECT STING AND BITE PRODUCTS

AUTHORS

Farid Sadik, Ph.D.
Professor and Associate Dean, College of Pharmacy, University of South Carolina, Columbia, South Carolina

Jeffrey C. Delafuente, M.S.
Associate Professor of Pharmacy and Medicine, College of Pharmacy, University of Florida, J. Hillis Miller Health Center, Gainesville, Florida

REVIEWERS

Michael R. DeLucia, B.S. (Pharmacy)
Associate Director, Clinical Services, and Director, Drug Information, Crozer-Chester Medical Center, Chester, Pennsylvania

Douglas W. Johnson, Ph.D.
Associate Extension Professor, Department of Entomology, University of Kentucky, Lexington, Kentucky

JoAnn T. Johnson, B.S. (Pharmacy)
Freelance Pharmacist, Princeton, Kentucky; Member, Scientific Advisory Board, National Pediculosis Association, Newton, Massachusetts

Abdul A. Khan, Ph.D.
Research Entomologist, San Francisco, California

Howard L. Maibach, M.D.
Professor of Dermatology, University of California Medical School, San Francisco, California

James R. Morse, M.S.
Assistant Professor, The University of Arizona, College of Pharmacy, Tucson, Arizona

Bernard P. Romano, B.S. (Pharmacy)
Owner and Pharmacist, Pacific Pharmacy, San Francisco, California

37   FOOT CARE PRODUCTS

AUTHOR

Nicholas G. Popovich, Ph.D.
Professor of Pharmacy Practice, Purdue University, School of Pharmacy and Pharmacal Sciences, West Lafayette, Indiana

REVIEWERS

Donald O. Fedder, B.S. (Pharmacy), Dr. P.H.
Associate Professor and Director, Community Pharmacy Programs, School of Pharmacy, University of Maryland, Baltimore, Maryland

Sandra M. Gawchik, D.O.
Co-Director, Allergy and Clinical Immunology, Crozer-Chester Medical Center, Chester, Pennsylvania

Thomas J. Holmes, Jr., Ph.D.
Associate Professor, School of Pharmacy, Campbell University, Buies Creek, North Carolina

Edward R. Hommel, D.P.M.
Private Practitioner, Podiatry, Madison, Wisconsin

Damien Howell, M.S. (Physical Therapy)
Damien Howell Physical Therapy, Richmond, Virginia

Brian R. Wright, D.P.M.
President, Fan-Laburnum Podiatry, Ltd., Richmond, Virginia

A   NONPRESCRIPTION DRUGS AND THE ELDERLY
(MINICHAPTER)

AUTHOR

Peter P. Lamy, Ph.D., Sc.D.
Director, The Center for the Study of Pharmacy and Therapeutics for the Elderly; Assistant Dean and Professor, School of Pharmacy, University of Maryland, Baltimore, Maryland

B   NONPRESCRIPTION DRUG USE IN CHILDREN
(MINICHAPTER)

AUTHORS

Mark W. Veerman, Pharm.D.
Pediatric Clinical Specialist, Shands Hospital; Clinical Assistant Professor, College of Pharmacy, University of Florida, Gainesville, Florida

Miriam L. Marcadis, Pharm.D.
Clinical Associate, College of Pharmacy, University of Illinois, Chicago, Illinois

COLOR ILLUSTRATION CONTRIBUTORS

Jean A. Borger, B.A.
Manager of Special Services (Retired), Bureau of Communications, American Dental Association, Buffalo Grove, Illinois

Richard C. Childers, M.D., P.A.
Diplomate, American Board of Dermatology; Private Practice of Dermatology, Gainesville, Florida

Stanley Cullen, M.D.
Diplomate, American Board of Dermatology; Fellow, American Academy of Dermatology; Private Practice of Dermatology, Gainesville, Florida

Alfred C. Griffin, D.D.S.[†]
Private Practice of Dentistry, Falls Church, Virginia; Board Member, Children's National Medical Center, Georgetown University, Washington, D.C.

Harold L. Hammond, D.D.S., M.S.
Diplomate, American Board of Oral Pathology; Professor of Oral Pathology and Diagnosis, and Director, Surgical Oral Pathology Laboratory, College of Dentistry, University of Iowa, Iowa City, Iowa

R. Gary Sibbald, M.D., F.R.C.P.(C), (Med), F.R.C.P.(C), (Dermatology), M.A.C.P.
Diplomate, American Board of Dermatology; Private Practice of Dermatology, Toronto, Ontario, Canada

[†] *Deceased*

PREFACE

"The mission of the American Pharmaceutical Association . . . is to serve its members, enabling them to advance the practice and science of pharmacy."

This quote is from the preamble of a new mission statement for APhA, which is currently being carefully crafted and widely debated.

Service to its members and contributing to the advancement of health care have been the leading hallmarks of this Association ever since it was founded in 1852. Therefore, this central mission has remained constant, even though its specific application has continually changed and evolved to meet contemporary needs.

Unquestionably, APhA's *Handbook of Nonprescription Drugs* constitutes one of the foremost examples of the Association's program to fulfill its mission. In developing the *Handbook*, and then continuing to revise and update it, APhA serves its members—as well as all pharmacists, pharmacy students, fellow health care practitioners, and consumers—by making available a comprehensive, convenient, and easy-to-use compilation of information on nonprescription drugs and drug products.

Furthermore, through use of this information resource, APhA members and their professional colleagues are in the position of being able to significantly advance pharmacy in particular and health care in general.

Self-care, self-medication, and nonprescription drug use are no longer just ancillary to achieving or maintaining good health. Today they constitute an integral part of the drug use process. Recognition of this major development has prompted APhA to include an entirely new chapter on this subject as the introductory chapter of this ninth edition.

Moreover, maturation of the widespread public trend toward nonprescription drug use has been due, in no small part, to the greater availability of safe and effective nonprescription drug products. In turn, the nonprescription drug industry and the U.S. Food and Drug Administration have been key participants in transforming the image of nostrums of dubious value into a broad-based spectrum of beneficial and efficacious drug products. Furthermore, both the nonprescription drug industry and the FDA have contributed valuable information and professional assistance in helping APhA to prepare this new edition.

However, the so-called "bottom line" is how well this new compendium of drug information will advance the course of patient care and good health. Through the years, the past eight editions of the *Handbook* have enjoyed very widespread use as texts in schools of pharmacy and as information resources in pharmacy practice.

APhA takes great pride in this achievement, and we are confident that this new edition will further promote the good health and well-being of patients everywhere.

John A. Gans, Pharm.D.
Executive Vice President
American Pharmaceutical Association

INTRODUCTION

AN ONGOING COMMITMENT

A quarter of a century ago, in 1965, the American Pharmaceutical Association initially set the wheels in motion that led to the publication of the first edition of a modest, thin reference book bravely titled the *Handbook of Nonprescription Drugs*. By today's standards, that volume was miniscule in its breadth of subject matter as well as its depth of coverage, but it met with immediate, enthusiastic response from both pharmacy practitioners and pharmacy educators. The principal reason was simple enough: There just was no other source available for meaningful information regarding nonprescription drugs.

Now in 1990, the Association proudly presents its Ninth Edition in this highly acclaimed series. Each new edition has built upon its predecessor, broadening the scope of its coverage as well as increasing the depth of information for the drug classes previously discussed.

Each successive past edition of the *Handbook* has been characterized by a continuing evolution of the book's fundamental scope, thrust, and character. The present edition continues this long-standing tradition, and it reflects APhA's ongoing commitment to pharmacy, the health care community, and the well-being of the general public.

DRUG RECLASSIFICATION

Ever since the Prescription Legend or Durham–Humphrey Amendments to the Federal Food, Drug, and Cosmetic Act were enacted on the federal level, on infrequent occasions, various drug entities have been moved from prescription to nonprescription status, or vice versa. Such reclassifications have been informally referred to as drug "switches," and often as "Rx-to-OTC switching."

This phenomenon has increased dramatically in recent years, and knowledgeable observers forecast that it will continue to grow as more and more medications are reclassified from prescription to nonprescription status. In 1987, the APhA House of Delegates adopted a statement supporting the term "transition class of drugs" to describe drugs in the reclassification process from prescription to nonprescription status.

At least one market research firm has predicted that "switches of pharmaceuticals to OTC drugs [are] seen as redefining the industry in the 1990's." In another report, that same market research firm also forecasts that "increased self medication, [coupled with] no cure for the common cold, signals growth in OTC medications." The trends seen by this firm and other similar market observers all point toward enormous expansion and growth in nonprescription drug demand and use.

Finally, a leading pharmacy trade journal carried a feature article in mid-1989 entitled "The Rx-to-OTC Revolution," with extensive data, drug listings, and quotes from prominent government and industry officials to support the thesis that the drug reclassification phenomenon is even accelerating in its intensity.

Hence, not only is the scope of the field covered in this *Handbook* continuing to grow, but the crucial importance of having a comprehensive reference source of information in this subject field is expanding as well.

THE PHARMACIST'S ROLE

Pharmacist Joseph D. Williams, the board chairman and CEO of Warner-Lambert Company, one of the largest U.S. pharmaceutical companies, was interviewed in early 1990 as to his thoughts on today's practice of pharmacy. In specifically addressing the pharmacist's role in nonprescription drug therapy, this former chairman of the Pharmaceutical Manufacturers Association proclaimed, "Pharmacists make a valuable contribution by helping patients select OTC products, and particularly in easing the transition from prescription medications to OTCs by guiding correct use."

And in the "Rx-to-OTC Revolution" article cited

above, the report concluded with the observation: "By emphasizing the Rx-only origins of so many newly approved OTC products, the pharmacist can change the way people think about those products, and about OTC products in general. The pharmacist can drive home the message that all drugs, OTC as well as Rx, are *drugs*; the difference is a difference of degree, not of kind." Clearly, therefore, the role of the pharmacist, the authority of the pharmacist, and the responsibility of the pharmacist are all increasing dramatically in the realm of nonprescription drug counseling and use. In order to fulfill these expanded roles, the pharmacist—or other participating health care practitioners—need a reliable, comprehensive base of information. And it is that function which the *Handbook* is intended to serve.

Indeed, the *Standards of Practice of the Profession of Pharmacy* contains a section subtitled "Standards of Practice for Pharmacists Serving the Self-Medicating Patient," with a series of ten individual duties described under that heading. In order to be able to fulfill most of those functions, the pharmacist must have detailed information readily at hand covering identification of symptoms, proper medication dosage, recommended dosage frequency, preferred method of administration, potential for drug-related adverse reactions, and similar health condition vis-à-vis drug therapy interrelationships. And, again, it is that expansive spectrum of facts and information concerning nonprescription therapeutic agents and the drug products in which they are formulated that the *Handbook* attempts to cover.

SCOPE OF NINTH EDITION

Continuing Features

This new edition attempts to retain all those features that were accorded high acclaim from users of past editions. These include, among others, the general information chapter on patient assessment and consultation, questions to ask the patient or consumer that appear at the beginning of each chapter, expanded clinical information, color plates of special conditions, relevant anatomical drawings, full product tables, and a comprehensive index.

Moreover, the general organization of chapter content, as well as the review process followed in the preparation and revision of the chapters—both of which proved to be so effective and workable for the last several editions—remain essentially the same.

Quoting from the last edition (as to chapter organization): "The authors were appointed on the basis of their expertise in the specific subject matters. To help

standardize the content of each chapter, detailed guidelines were provided to each author. Each chapter contains the following basic information:

- Description of the conditions considered for self-medication in the chapter;
- Anatomy and physiology of the affected systems;
- Etiology of the conditions;
- Pathophysiology of the affected systems;
- Signs and symptoms that patients could present;
- Assessment criteria;
- Primary pharmacologic agents contained in nonprescription products;
- Secondary formulation ingredients and specialized dosage forms;
- Rationale for label warnings on products;
- Considerations in product selection;
- Practical patient advice;
- Summary and conclusions."

And, quoting again (as to the review process): "The review process was expanded and every chapter was reviewed by a panel of approximately 6 to 10 experts. Every chapter was also reviewed by at least two pharmacists who specialized in the subject area, a pharmacy educator, and a physician, dentist, podiatrist, and/or dietitian whenever appropriate. To ensure that the information was pertinent to the practice situation, every chapter was reviewed by a community pharmacy practitioner and a hospital pharmacy practitioner. In total, there were 168 reviewers for the Eighth Edition. [For this Ninth Edition there were 195 reviewers.]

"The reviewers were requested to review the manuscripts from the standpoint of accuracy, completeness, and practicality of the information. The initial comments were reviewed by a senior reviewer and/or the author(s). The revised second drafts of the manuscripts (for new chapters) were reviewed again by the review panels to provide acceptable manuscripts that reflected a consensus of scientific thought."

The so-called "bottom line" of this extensive editorial effort is the development of a compendium of information that represents a consensus view of a group of relative experts on each class of therapeutic agents or health care agents. This is in contrast to virtually every other information source which, no matter how "expert" the particular author or authors may be, still presents the viewpoint or thinking of a single individual on each given subject. It is this *authoritativeness* that makes the *Handbook of Nonprescription Drugs* an especially reliable and valuable reference work.

New Features

In the past, each new edition of the *Handbook* has proven to be doubly valuable to the reader; specifically, (a) the dynamic state of the nonprescription drug marketplace has resulted in literally thousands of product or product-related changes each year—hence the need for a comprehensive updating of previous content in order to keep it current and accurate; and (b) as the scope of nonprescription drug therapy has expanded, entirely new chapters have been added to discuss these broad new areas.

And, in both respects—updating of previous content and addition of entirely new areas of coverage—this Ninth Edition matches, and probably exceeds, any of its predecessors.

Within the latter category, i.e., entirely new features, the following constitute several of the more notable major additions:

- Two entirely new, full-length chapters are included; these cover the subjects of "The Self-Care Movement" and "In-Home Diagnostic Products," respectively. Both are timely subjects and serve to round out the *Handbook's* coverage of its subject field.

- Two entirely new "minichapters" are also introduced to the reader for the first time; these differ from regular chapters in that they deal with classes of patients, rather than classes of products. In particular, these minichapters discuss the special considerations involving nonprescription drug use in the elderly and in children, respectively.

- An extensive listing of company names, addresses, telephone numbers, and (if available) toll-free telephone numbers of the major nonprescription drug manufactures is provided for the first time. This appears as a self-standing appendix beginning on page 1033. This listing should prove to be useful to *Handbook* users in ordering products as well as in obtaining specialized information concerning specific drug products.

- Two other chapter-related appendices have been newly added to existing chapters. These are a listing of major poison control centers (with their emergency telephone numbers) at the end of the chapter on "Emetic and Antiemetic Products," and a listing of major sources of information on AIDS disease at the end of the chapter on "Contraceptive Methods and Products."

- Comprehensive cross-referencing between chapters was made a major objective of the editors in revising every chapter. In previous editions, each chapter dealt with its subject matter in somewhat of a vacuum with only occasional referrals to other chapters discussing related considerations. However, in this edition, readers will find liberal cross-references to related information in other chapters.

Major Changes

Beyond these "new features," there have been many instances of new treatment of former information, of significant new information or standards related to existing products, and of shifting emphasis to reflect contemporary concerns and developments. These changes are simply too numerous to detail here, but some of the more notable major changes need to be mentioned if only to indicate the broad scope and considerable significance of those changes.

Hence, the following examples provide an overview of the more substantial, newly introduced changes:

- Updating of all drug product tables has been capably handled by Facts and Comparisons, Inc. (F&C), of St. Louis, Missouri. For all previous editions, this task was performed by the *Handbook* staff. However, the increasing number of changes relating to drug products, the frequency of such changes, and the difficulty in keeping abreast of those changes presented a greater challenge than ever before. This situation, coupled with the experience and extensive database at F&C, made it highly attractive for APhA to enter into a joint venture for them to update the product tables for this edition.

- Actions finalized by the Food and Drug Administration as part of its "OTC Drug Review" during the 4 years since the completion of the previous edition of the *Handbook* have required enormous changes and revisions throughout the book. Such revisions have been due to reclassification of some drugs from prescription to nonprescription status, classification of various ingredients as unsafe or ineffective, or modifications in dosage of formulated products.

- Other regulatory or standards-related actions by the FDA, the National Research Council (NRC), and the United States Pharmacopeia (USP) made it necessary or desirable to incorporate other changes or new information. For example, the FDA established a voluntary labeling program for classifying sunglasses, as well as absorbency standards for tampons; and the NRC issued revised Recommended Dietary (Daily) Allowances (RDA) for human nutrition. Each of these developments involved commensurate changes in the *Handbook* content.

- The presentation of information in the *Handbook* underwent a total overhaul. This is most evident in the complete reorganization of the order of individual chapters. The objective is to present the various drug product categories in a more logical anatomical order.

- Miscellaneous major public health concerns of new or growing significance necessitated the inclusion of new or expanded information on subjects such as Lyme disease, AIDS, and tryptophan-induced eosinophilia–myalgia syndrome.

ACKNOWLEDGMENTS

Any undertaking that is as massive as the development of a new edition of the *Handbook of Nonprescription Drugs* requires the active participation, efforts, and contributions of a small army of people. Because several hundred people have made highly valuable and significant contributions, it is impossible to acknowledge those people other than by including their names in the lists of authors, coauthors, reviewers, contributors of illustrations, production staff, editorial staff, and consultants. And even in so doing, many others who have assisted still go unnamed; for example, the hundreds of people at the various pharmaceutical firms who have supplied product data and other information.

Consequently, we are limited to being able to say that we thank them all—individually and collectively—for truly, each of these several hundred people made valuable contributions that, taken together, made possible this monumental new edition. Thank you, all!

In expressing our gratitude, and that of APhA as the publisher, it is particularly appropriate to stress the extensive contributions that are made by the authors and reviewers. These people devote many hours to the unsung task of writing, rewriting, updating, reviewing, and critiquing the individual chapters. Their only compensation is the personal satisfaction that they derive from making such a meaningful contribution to their profession and to the public. Pharmacy and the allied health professions are blessed to have this rich resource of generous and talented volunteers.

As noted above, under the heading of "Major Changes," the huge task of updating the product tables was assumed by an outside firm for the first time in the *Handbook's* long history. The people at Facts and Comparisons, Inc., who took on this chore, and who met the tight schedule involved, deserve special mention. They are C. Sue Sewester, President; Bernie R. Olin, Pharm. D., Editor-in-Chief; Mary K. Hulbert, Coordinating Editor; and Charles E. Dombek, B.S. (Pharmacy), M.A., Assistant Editor.

Two other people, at two other outside organizations, made key contributions that enormously advanced the project of preparing this new edition. They are, respectively, William E. Gilbertson and John T. (Jack) Walden. Dr. Gilbertson is the continuing author of the present chapter 3 dealing with FDA's OTC Drug Review; but in his capacity as Director of the FDA's Division of OTC Drug Evaluation, he and his associate, Melvin Lessing, also provided the *Handbook* office with updated information on FDA actions on nonprescription drugs that helped to assure the timeliness and accuracy of the entire content. Mr. Walden served on the review panel of the new chapter 1 on The Self-Care Movement; but in his capacity as Senior Vice President and Director of Public Affairs of the Nonprescription Drug Manufacturers Association (formerly, the Proprietary Association), he also functioned effectively as an informal and unofficial ombudsman between the *Handbook* staff and the nonprescription drug industry.

The entire APhA staff also dedicated itself to assisting the *Handbook* staff in "getting the job done." Again, although our desire is to name them all, that is impractical. But the continuous support provided by John A. Gans, Joan S. Zaro, and Laura C. Lawson, plus the welcome assistance of James V. McGinnis and Vicki L. Meade, pulled the project through on many occasions.

Finally, the central, full-time task of managing the project was, for the first time, a really shared responsibility. In fact, it closely resembled a "troika," and it proved to be a very effective and efficient operation.

The Project Director had the direct, on-site, full-time assistance of a skilled and highly motivated assistant, Linda L. Young, whose formal title is Editorial Coordinator and Copyeditor, but who functioned as the "communications nerve-center" during the production of the new edition.

Secondly, the Project Director had the tremendous benefit of an off-site, part-time professional colleague, William L. Blockstein, whose personal knowledge of the field of nonprescription drug therapy coupled with his firsthand acquaintance with virtually every "expert" in the field, made him an invaluable asset within the triumvirate in helping oversee preparation of this edition.

The Project Director is especially pleased to be able to acknowledge the dedicated work of Ms. Young and Dr. Blockstein, and publicly expresses his deep gratitude and appreciation to both of them.

Edward G. Feldmann, Ph.D.
Project Director and
Managing Editor

Gary A. Holt and Edwin L. Hall

THE SELF-CARE MOVEMENT

A CULTURAL PERSPECTIVE

Americans are increasingly interested in self-care and self-medication. Health care professionals have a corresponding interest in understanding this important trend. Understanding self-care and self-medication involves a consideration of the self-care movement within the context of the American culture.

Self-Care Decision Making

One might postulate an illness experience model that considers the options available to the patient (Table 1). Assume that a person concludes that something is wrong (e.g., pain or discomfort). Having reached this conclusion, the person adopts a sick role for which certain options become available. The patient can tolerate the problem or turn to one of the structural domains of health care in our society: popular domain, folk domain, or professional domain. Each domain has its own system, social role, interaction setting, and institutions. The popular domain (i.e., self-care) is the most common option involved in initial response to illness episodes. Even when a decision is eventually made to enter the folk or professional domains, decisions still occur in the popular domain, usually within the context of the family.

Sick role options often result in negotiations and transactions between the patient and health care providers. These transactions generally involve honest differences in belief systems, attitudes, values, expectations, and goals. When practitioners and patients disagree, clinical management and patient counseling can become more difficult (1). For example, parents often ask pharmacists to recommend cold products that are inappropriate for infants or small children. Even

though the pharmacist insists that this therapy is inappropriate, the parents may insist on using these products. (See Minichapter B, *Nonprescription Drug Use in Children.*)

Various social and economic factors also influence the choice of and response to an option (1). For example, people who have grown up in rural cultures where medical care is relatively inaccessible may have a much greater tolerance for pain, discomfort, and illness in general.

Self-Care

Self-care has been defined as a process in which individuals function effectively on their own behalf in health promotion, in health decision making, and in disease prevention, detection, and treatment. This definition emphasizes that the individual—as the *subject* of health care decision action, rather than an *object* of it (2)—actively participates in the decision-making process. As such, the individual serves as a primary health resource in the health care system (2, 3).

Self-care practices can include anything that individuals do in their own behalf to promote or improve their health status. For example, the "Breslow 7" are common self-care activities (Table 2). Self-care practices can include health maintenance activities, disease prevention, both traditional and nontraditional medical practices, folk or popular remedies, and care of self in illness.

The self-care movement includes both consumers and health professionals and encourages consumers to develop skills and knowledge in both illness and wellness orientations. Furthermore, self-care involves more than just those things that people do for themselves; it also includes the things that people do for each other. This social network can include family and friends, as well as self-help groups of various kinds (3). Self-care practices, including self-medication, are not viewed as a substitute for supervised medical treatment when professional intervention is indicated (4).

Self-Medication

Self-medication is defined as the act of properly and responsibly treating oneself with nonprescription medications (5, 6). Although self-medication is always viewed as a self-care practice, not all self-care involves self-medication. Nonprescription products do not require a physician's prescription and are usually used without medical supervision. However, consultations with health professionals are often involved.

Self-medication provides freedom to choose from the myriad products approved for nonprescription sale in order to assist in the management of easily recognizable conditions that can be safely treated without professional help (7, 8). Americans have an ample supply of nonprescription drug products from which to choose; however, it is not known how many nonprescription products actually exist because products are sometimes made available without the approval of the Food and Drug Administration (FDA). Estimates have ranged from 300,000 to 500,000 products (300,000 is the figure quoted most often). These products are manufactured by 12,000 firms and involve 700–800 active ingredients (8–11). (See Chapter 3, *The FDA's OTC Drug Review*.)

Generally speaking, products approved for self-medication should be safe and effective within a wide range of dosages and should act in a clearly recognizable fashion, demonstrably, and quickly. Nonprescription drugs should be relatively stable, even under less than optimal storage conditions, should be designed for use for a limited number of clearly identifiable and related conditions, and should not contain unnecessary ingredients (12).

Research consistently indicates that self-medication and self-care practices are widespread. Studies indicate that the average American experiences one potentially self-treatable health problem every 3 days. These problems tend to be mild complaints; consumers simply tolerate them, or they may attempt some kind of self-care practice (13, 14). About 90% of people are reported to be "a little under the weather" at some time during each month (Tables 3 and 4) (15). A study of college-age students identified 81 illnesses for which self-treatment was mentioned as a primary source of care. These illnesses included colds, sore throats, headaches, labor

pains, cancer, bronchitis, and high blood pressure (16). People appear more likely to resort to self-treatment when they perceive their illness to be not serious or not amenable to professional medical intervention (16).

TABLE 1	An illness experience model that considers self-care options

Problem is perceived by the patient
Illness experience options
  Do not treat
  Treat
    Popular domain (self, family, social network)
      Self-treatment:
        Home remedy (e.g., alcoholic beverages, honey, lemon, baking soda, onions, hot or cold water)
        Nonprescription products
        Prescription medications already at home
    Folk domain (nonprofessional healers)
      Naturopathic healers
      Herbalists
      Acupressure therapists
    Professional domain
      Traditional medical care
Outcome

Adapted from "Health Care Practices and Perceptions—A Consumer Survey of Self-Medication," prepared for The Proprietary Association by Harry Heller Research Corp. (HHR#72792), Washington, D.C., 1984; F. D. Wolinsky, "The Sociology of Health, Principles, Professions, and Issues," Little, Brown and Co., Boston, Mass., 1980; and A. Kleinman, *Ann. Intern. Med., 88* (2), 251–258 (1978).

TABLE 2	Seven basic practices that correlate to physical well-being and lifespan

1. Sleeping 7 to 8 hours each night
2. Eating three meals a day at regular times with little snacking
3. Eating breakfast every day
4. Maintaining desired body weight
5. Avoiding excessive alcohol consumption
6. Getting regular exercise
7. Not smoking

Adapted from E. P. Eckholm, in "The Nation's Health," P. R. Lee et al., Eds., Boyd and Fraser, San Francisco, Calif., 1981. (Assembled by N. E. Belloc and L. Breslow after studying the lives of 7,000 men and women in California.)

Self-medication practices are learned early and extend throughout life. One study found that 75% of children under 2 years of age had been given a nonprescription drug at least once (17); another study indicated that among ambulatory elderly, 70% of females and 58% of males took at least one nonprescription drug (18). Furthermore, many people supplement prescribed medications with self-prescribed products (12, 19, 20).

Nonprescription Drugs

Nonprescription drugs are also known as over-the-counter (OTC) or nonlegend products. Historically, they have also been referred to as "patent medicines" or as "proprietary medicines." Both of these terms are considered to be obsolete because of the regulations that now govern the sale of nonprescription products and because of the negative connotations associated with the patent medicines of the late 1800s and early 1900s. The term "proprietary medicines" has also been questioned because consumers are no longer the sole

TABLE 4	Incidence of seven categories of health problems*
Problem category	**% reporting problems**
Skin	67
Pain	57
General well-being	53
Respiratory	49
Eye, ear, and mouth	44
Digestive system	40
Feminine	27

*Reported by 1,459 adults during the 2 weeks before the study.
Adapted from "Health Care Practices and Perceptions—A Consumer Survey of Self-Medication," prepared for The Proprietary Association by Harry Heller Research Corp. (HHR#72792), Washington, D.C., 1984.

target audience of these products. Some nonprescription products are promoted to physicians and other health professionals more heavily than to the public (21).

Historically, nonprescription medications have proven useful for the treatment of symptoms of minor, self-limiting conditions (e.g., headaches and colds) (8, 22, 23). Many contemporary nonprescription products are also capable of curing or preventing diseases (e.g., motion sickness products) and can be used to manage chronic conditions once a diagnosis has been made by a health professional (e.g., aspirin therapy for arthritis) (8, 24). Still other products exist as urgently needed drugs for potentially life-threatening conditions for which the patient needs ready access (e.g., insulin) (25).

TABLE 3	The most common health problems reported by adults in two studies during the previous year	
Problem	**% reporting the problem**	
	STUDY 1	STUDY 2
Aches and pains	—	72
Back problems	—	40
Bruises	32	—
Common cold	60	47
Constipation	26	—
Cough	—	33
Cuts and scratches (minor)	46	57
Diarrhea	31	—
Headaches	29	71
Insect stings and bites	30	37
Muscle aches and pains	37	—
Overindulgence in food	32	—
Overweight	—	29
Sinus problems	29	43
Sore throat *not* associated with a cold	25	—
Sunburn	25	—
Upset stomach and indigestion	59	43
Virus and influenza	27	—

Adapted from "Health Care Practices and Perceptions—A Consumer Survey of Self-Medication," prepared for The Proprietary Association by Harry Heller Research Corp. (HHR#72792), Washington, D.C., 1984; and C. H. Kline, in "Self-Care, Self-Medication in America's Future—A Symposium," The Proprietary Association, Washington, D.C., 1980.

CULTURAL TRENDS— FACTORS THAT INFLUENCE SELF-CARE AND SELF-MEDICATION

Many factors influence self-care and self-medication. Table 5 summarizes factors proposed by various health scholars and writers. Self-care can be significantly affected by changes in any of these factors, which can influence both attitudinal and policy changes. Because these factors reflect belief systems of both consumers and health professionals involved in the self-care movement, consideration of them helps in understanding self-care, self-medication, and realistic clinical roles for nonprescription drug products.

TABLE 5 Factors likely to influence the pattern and extent of self-medicating and self-care attitudes and practices

Consumer attitudes and beliefs
Perceived seriousness of disease
Levels of acceptance by health professionals and consumers
Changing values
Growing beliefs in prevention and planning for health and health care
Increased emphasis on overall health and fitness
Individual acceptance of a personal responsibility for health
Growing public frustrations with, and suspicions of, the medical industry and its institutions, and estrangement from health care providers

Consumer education/sophistication
Educational level and sophistication of the public
Quality and quantity of information and communication available to consumers
Quality and quantity of communication between patients and health professionals
Availability of pharmacists and other health professionals with useful, free information
Educational materials available to the consumer through the lay press, media, and other sources
Patterns, quality, and types of advertising
Language and information provided on package labeling and package inserts

Demographic characteristics
Aging population
Gender differences

Accessibility/availability considerations
Distribution and availability of health care professionals and health services (including home health services)

Products
Range and types of products permitted for nonprescription sale
Development and availability of new products and new technology, including those designed to meet new needs
Competition
Packaging
Safety
Efficacy

Economy
Increasing health care costs
Standards of living and the economy
Convenience

Alternate approaches to health
Acceptance and acknowledgment of self-care as a response to disease
Alternate health care approaches (e.g., naturalism, herbalism, holism)

Consumer Attitudes and Beliefs

Consumer beliefs and attitudes can also become important considerations. It has been shown that distance from health care services can affect willingness to travel to those services. However, these same studies also indicate that willingness to travel is affected by the patient's perceived seriousness of the illness involved (16, 26). Perceived seriousness can affect not only patient decisions regarding the types of health care used (e.g., popular domain versus professional domain) but also how the patient reacts to the illness (18, 27, 28). Other variables affecting consumer willingness or desire for self-care products include changing values, growing beliefs in prevention, overall health and fitness, and individual acceptance of a personal responsibility for health (11, 21, 29).

Some social scientists have said that self-care practices could actually weaken trust in health professionals by reducing demand for high-quality health care or the efforts to improve and expand needed professional health services. For example, self-medication may be used as an excuse for not providing professional services to the poor or other groups (30).

Yet demands for self-medication products appear to be deeply rooted in the American culture. Threats to cherished cultural values such as independence and freedom of action are deeply resented. Consumers often lament that health care providers have too much control, thus restricting access to desired medications and related products. In reality, health care professionals have a legitimate and ethical obligation to act to help ensure consumer health.

American consumers know they are an integral component of the U.S. health care system and continue to look for self-care opportunities, including self-medication (31). Self-medication may be increasing in importance because of a greater social emphasis on personal responsibility for health and because of social trends that discourage dependence on professional intervention (e.g., the general consumer movement, itself) (24, 29, 32–35).

Consumers may self-medicate in an effort to avoid problems with health professionals. Many consumers believe that their health care needs are not being met, question the ability of the health care industry to satisfy all of these needs, and are becoming less satisfied with the care that they receive (1, 4, 9, 29, 30, 36–38).

There is evidence that some consumer fears, anxieties, and suspicions may be justified. Various health authorities, writers, and studies have questioned the safety and efficacy of certain traditional health care practices, raised concerns about the competency of some practitioners, expressed concerns about iatrogenesis, and reflected social frustrations with the traditional health care system (27, 39–44).

Other sources of anxiety may exist as well. Patients may be embarrassed about examinations by health professionals or about discussing personal matters. This is also a concern for pharmacists because counseling often occurs in places where conversations can be overheard by other patrons (e.g., the dispensing counter or in product aisles). (See Chapter 2, *Patient Assessment and Consultation*.) Still other patients may fear what they might be told by a health professional. For example, children are often afraid they will be given an injection. Adults may fear the diagnosis or therapy or that normal lifestyles will be disrupted (45, 46).

Regardless of the reason, self-medication allows the consumer to avoid certain anxieties, suspicions, and frustrations. While this can represent a naive or even hazardous viewpoint, it is a component of consumer belief systems.

Consumer Education/Sophistication

It appears that many consumers are taking a more active role in their own health care, particularly through self-education efforts. As of 1979, an estimated 5,000 self-help books were available to the American public, which attests to the popularity of independent study regarding health matters (30). Although some of the literature available to the public is of questionable accuracy, consumer interest in health education appears to be very real. Many consumers are now more knowledgeable about health and about handling everyday health problems. As a result, they are more willing to take responsibility for their own health, more willing to acknowledge the limitations of self-care, and more willing to make appropriate lifestyle changes (8, 13, 24, 34, 47–51).

Even though many consumers are well informed, other consumers harbor misinformation and inaccurate beliefs regarding medications, therapy, and health care (45). Historically, consumers have tended to gather bits and pieces of information from health professionals,

advertisements, friends, relatives, books, magazines, and a variety of other sources (13, 50, 52–54). The accuracy of much of this information is questionable at best.

One study of 1,233 Americans indicated that 35% use the *Physicians' Desk Reference* (PDR) for information (52). Even though the PDR is not written for consumers, it can be found in most major bookstores. It is important to realize, however, that being *informed* does not necessarily mean being *enlightened*. People can have information without having understanding. Information without understanding (e.g., consumer use of physician references) can often lead to poor self-medication decisions.

Self-Diagnosis

Similarly, consumers may make inaccurate clinical assessments (45). The majority of consumers lack an adequate background to accurately diagnose most clinical conditions. Instead, people want causes that are simple and easy to comprehend and about which they can do something (55). This can cause consumers to choose more pleasing explanations instead of complicated or serious ones. Because one disease can mimic another, the layperson may misdiagnose potentially serious conditions (12). Consumers must understand the limits of their ability to self-diagnose and self-medicate, as well as the risks of exceeding those limits (5, 25, 56).

Self-diagnosis is affected by numerous factors, including previous experience with the disease; previous experience with health professionals or the health care system; availability of health care professionals and services; a tolerance of the symptoms involved; perceptions of the seriousness of the disease; input from friends, family, peers, and fellow workers; gender; and age (16, 45, 57).

The risks of self-diagnosis are also influenced by the tendency of consumers to view symptoms as temporary. Thus, they may delay seeking professional help to see how the condition evolves (57). Similarly, the use of nonprescription products can mask symptoms that would normally be good diagnostic indicators (58).

Misinformation and inaccurate beliefs can result in unrealistic expectations. For example, consumers may expect cold products to completely eliminate cold symptoms, and many people believe that a daily bowel movement is required for good health. Unrealistic expectations result in disappointments, frustrations, and health care problems as the health care system and its practitioners fail to satisfy these expectations. Guided by unrealistic expectations, consumers may make inappropriate nonprescription purchases. Thus, health professionals must strive to educate consumers so that they will adopt beliefs and expectations for reasonable outcomes of medications and therapy.

Accurate diagnosis and therapy can require the services of a health professional who can think and act objectively on behalf of the individual. It is important for health professionals to recognize factors that affect self-diagnosis because self-medication is an issue not only of the availability of safe and effective drug products but also of whether these products will be used for an appropriate indication.

Inappropriate Usage

Because consumers may be misinformed about diseases, drug products, and therapy, they may select inappropriate products for their needs, or they may not wisely use products that have been selected (32, 59). All medications, including nonprescription drugs, can be misused or abused. The term "abuse" most correctly denotes "misuse" that is associated with social disapproval. Even so, the terms are used inconsistently and often interchangeably, depending on the situations involved. Either situation warrants patient counseling efforts on the part of health professionals.

Misuse and abuse can involve unrealistic expectations about what these products can be expected to accomplish and inadvertent medication errors such as taking a dose too often or not often enough, taking too much or too little at each dose, dosage omissions, premature discontinuation of therapy, and improper storage of the product in the home (60). It can also involve deliberate recklessness, attempts to derive pleasurable sensations, or use when another product, or no product at all, is indicated (12).

The degree of consumer sophistication, the level of education, and the ability to interpet and use labeling information are important factors in determining the appropriateness of self-medication. Studies have indicated that consumer groups of differing educational levels have different behavioral patterns regarding health care utilization and self-medication practices (13, 26). Less-educated people are more likely to treat problems, more likely to contact a professional, and more likely to take prescription medications in the home. Well-educated individuals are more likely to purchase the brands recommended by a pharmacist (61). However, well-educated people tend to be younger, so nonprescription utilization trends may also be influenced by factors such as age and income (13).

Demographic Characteristics

Age

Older Americans tend to use more medications of all types, including nonprescription drugs (35, 62). However, a recent survey conducted by Medical Eco-nomics Company indicates that the frequency of self-medication drops off after age 60 (63). The number of elderly has been increasing since 1900, and this trend is expected to continue (26). Depending on the age used to define elderly, this group comprises about 12–17% of the population but consumes 30% of all medications. By the year 2000, the elderly may consume as much as 50% of all medications. Elderly patients account for 39% of all hospitalizations and 51% of deaths from drug reactions. They are also more likely to experience adverse drug reactions and drug interactions. Mismedication is thought to be a significant problem with this population (62, 64). (See Minichapter A, *Nonprescription Drugs and the Elderly.*)

The commonly reported health problems vary with increasing age. Younger adults (under 55 years of age) are more likely to report minor cuts and scratches, colds, sinus problems, acne, lip problems, and dental problems. Older Americans (over 55 years of age) are more likely to report arthritis and rheumatism, back problems, ear problems, sleeping problems, and feet problems (13).

Gender

Historically, women have been more likely to make medication purchases, contact health professionals, and use nonprescription products (13, 19, 20, 35). This role may change as more women enter the workforce because then women, like men, may have less time to attend to these activities. Additionally, changes in the careers and traditional roles for women can affect educational and income levels, both of which affect health care behaviors (26, 65).

Men and women report different problems for which self-medication may be used. Women are more likely to report suffering from overweight, anxiety, stomach problems, indigestion, headaches, fatigue, sleeping problems, arthritis, lip problems, and skin problems. Men are more likely to report muscle aches and pains, minor cuts and scratches, colds, and dental problems (13).

Accessibility/Availability Considerations

The availability of health services affects health care utilization (16). For example, studies have shown that people are less willing to travel to a health care service facility as the distance to that facility increases (26). This reflects not only a proximity consideration but also a personnel availability issue. The American public does not have unlimited access to professional care, especially for minor problems. Consumer demands far exceed the health care industry's resources to satisfy them. If only a small percentage of self-medicating consumers were to suddenly seek professional care, the patient load would overwhelm the medical services and resources that are currently available (4, 6, 11, 21, 31, 66, 67). Self-care has been described as being "far more generous, flexible, available, safe, acceptable and less costly . . . than any organized professional system could undertake, finance, or conceptually tolerate" (30). Self-medication is thought to encourage optimal use of medical resources by promoting their effective and efficient use and by conserving manpower resources for those individuals for whom professional care is essential (4, 33, 68, 69). This latter characteristic could actually increase professional satisfaction because professionals are freed to address health problems that require greater knowledge and skills and that are more professionally rewarding (8, 65, 70). Thus, self-medication is seen as a means for reducing the need for professional services and is considered to be an essential component of any workable health care system (8, 34, 48, 69, 71).

TABLE 6 The fastest growing categories of nonprescription drug products as projected in 1986 (in unit growth %/yr)	
Category	**Unit growth (%/yr)**
Home diagnostic test kits	9.0%
Contact lens solutions	7.8%
Eye care products	4.4%
Prepared infant formulas	4.0%
Arthritic pain relievers	4.0%
General pain relievers	4.0%
Contraceptives	3.5%
Asthma medications	3.0%
Menstrual relief products	3.0%
Average of 31 other categories	1.3%
All 40 categories	2.6%

Adapted from C. H. Kline, in "Self-Medication—Making It Work Better for More People," Proceedings of the World Federation of Proprietary Medicine Manufacturers 8th General Assembly, The Proprietary Association, Washington, D.C., 1986.

The Nature and Availability of Nonprescription Products

Obviously, the availability of products will influence self-medication practices. For example, when certain categories of products first become available, consumers can be expected to use them. Or if certain products within a category are removed from the market, consumer use of the overall category will decline. Promotion, marketing, and advertising also influence consumer behaviors regarding purchase and use.

The fastest growing categories of nonprescription products (as projected in 1986) are listed in Table 6.

A significant factor involved in the availability of nonprescription products is consumer safety. Nonprescription drugs are defined as drugs that are recognized by experts to be safe and effective for consumers to use by following the required label directions and warnings (32, 72). Although designed to be safe and effective for self-medication, the potential for harm always exists. In reality, no drug can be considered to be absolutely safe (48). Drug products can cause significant adverse reactions; mask the existence of potentially serious conditions; interact with foods, other drugs, and even laboratory tests in harmful ways; or result in other health hazards (45, 70, 73). (See Chapter 3, *The FDA's OTC Drug Review*.)

Nonprescription drug products are considered to be relatively safe. This means that these products can be used safely without professional supervision as long as labeled directions are followed (23). The majority of consumers who use these products as directed should

not experience significant problems. Side effects should be minor and predictable so that appropriate adaptations and lifestyle changes can be made.

In addition to the consideration of safety, there is the matter of efficacy. To varying degrees, nonprescription products have always been effective for many conditions (45). Even poorly formulated products can be expected to achieve successes in the treatment of self-limiting conditions. As a result of the FDA review process, the reclassification of some prescription drugs as nonprescription, and changes in federal regulations over the years, nonprescription products have become increasingly effective for their intended and promoted uses. Studies indicate that many consumers are able to self-medicate with a high degree of success, both in terms of choosing appropriate products and of being satisfied with the products selected (13, 59).

In part, successful nonprescription therapy occurs as a result of the nature of the conditions being treated. It has been suggested that more than 75% of all illness episodes are self-limiting or have no specific remedies (39, 57). Of those patients being seen by physicians, many have minor ailments while others have chronic disorders. Neither minor nor chronic disorders are often amenable to energetic or dramatic therapeutic efforts, so a significant percent of patients being seen by practitioners probably could benefit from varying degrees of self-medication.

Successful nonprescription therapy can also be explained in terms of the nature of health care. Rene Dubos, David Mechanic, and other health scholars have suggested that the true purpose of medicine has never been to produce health. Rather, its tasks involve the recognition and treatment of both symptoms and diseases, disease prevention, and health promotion (74, 75). Dubos has proposed that "to heal does not necessarily imply to cure. It can simply mean helping people to achieve a way of life compatible with their individual aspirations—to restore their freedom to make choices —even in the presence of continuing disease" (76). Thus, curing disease is only seen as one aspect of medical care. Alleviating the manifestations of disease is often a more important role (77). Often this involves making a distinction between *disease* (abnormalities in the structure and function of body organs and systems) and *illness* (the human experience of sickness) (1, 36). A cure orientation on the part of either consumers or health professionals is often unrealistic and unattainable. A more achievable objective may be one of relieving the discomforts of illness (37, 78). Certainly, nonprescription products can function in this capacity.

The Economy

The advantage cited most often as a rationale for self-medication is that it is a less expensive form of health care. Health professionals and prescription medications are considered to be more expensive, which directly encourages self-medication (6–9, 11, 15, 21, 24, 48). Hospital charges, physician fees, and costs of other health-related products and services have risen significantly and have contributed to consumer demands for low-cost alternatives, including self-medication (12, 37, 79–83).

Four times as many health problems are treated with nonprescription drugs than are taken to physicians (13, 32), and 60–95% of all illness episodes are initially treated with some form of self-care, including self-medication (6, 9, 11, 31, 57, 60, 68, 84–86). Total sales of the major groups of nonprescription drugs in 1985 were $7.6 billion, or about $30 per capita (21). The Nonprescription Drug Manufacturers Association reports that in 1987 the total sales of all nonprescription drugs (including vitamins) reached $13.3 billion. The estimated growth in nonprescription product sales is about 2% a year, and sales may reach $38 billion by the year 2000 (47). Although 60% of medications purchased by American consumers are nonprescription, these purchases account for less than 2% of the U.S. health care dollar. This suggests that self-medication is a significant, but cost-effective, component of the U.S. health care system (8).

Ironically, prescription drugs are often reimbursed in third-party programs, while nonprescription drugs are not (87). Thus, proposed cost savings can vary depending on the situation involved or the manner in which studies are conducted. For example, research

estimates suggest that Americans would have spent $10.5 billion more in 1987 for health care if nonprescription products were not available. This figure could rise to $34.1 billion by the year 2000. These estimates include time lost from work, medical fees, prescription costs, insurance services, and travel (32).

Cost concerns are complicated by the fact that people expect to live longer and better lives, and that health care costs tend to increase with advancing age. As the average age of the population increases and health care becomes less affordable, self-medicating may become more attractive (15, 48). (See Minichapter A, *Nonprescription Drugs and the Elderly*.)

In addition to monetary costs, self-medication is considered to be cost-effective in terms of time savings. Traditional health care involves time lost from work, time for physician visits, and time required to obtain prescriptions from a pharmacy. Self-medication can reduce many of these time losses (15, 47, 57, 58, 79).

Finally, the decision to self-medicate may be largely a matter of convenience (6, 12, 32, 45, 48, 58). Nonprescription products can be purchased at many locations, including nonpharmacy outlets such as convenience stores or grocery stores, and can be purchased when the consumer is going to these locations for other reasons. Even when barriers exist to professional health care services, nonprescription products are readily available.

Alternatives in Health Care

With increasing education, consumers may become more aware of alternatives in health care. Movements such as the holistic movement have emphasized that individual health does not necessarily require the services of traditional health care professionals and institutions (49). Consumers recognize that medical and health information and services are not restricted to a select group. Furthermore, the attainment of health is not absolutely dependent on the services of health care professionals. Thus, public suspicions and frustrations may not always reflect a suspicion of health professionals as much as they reflect a growing awareness of alternate opportunities for self-care (88).

THE PHARMACIST'S ROLE IN SELF-CARE

It is generally agreed that the pharmacist can have an enormously expanded role in providing information, advice, and counseling and that pharmacies can become information and education centers in the community

(11, 89, 90). Functioning in the midst of an extraordinary information network, the pharmacist is able to keep up with and disseminate current information on all drug products. This role can serve the public well by promoting safe and effective products and self-care practices (10, 85, 89). Studies indicate considerable consumer support for pharmacist information services, a high level of consumer confidence in information provided by pharmacists, and consumers' desire for more personalized services and consultation on the drugs they take (9, 11, 53, 54, 61, 91).

Ironically, studies also indicate that consumers do not always have access to information when they want it. In a study of 221 adults who wanted information, 61.1% could not or did not find anyone to ask. More than 74% of these individuals decided not to purchase a nonprescription product because they were not certain which product to buy and/or they did not know how to use the product being considered (91).

Informational services also include emphasizing and explaining label instructions at the time of purchase, especially regarding indications, directions, and warnings. This is particularly important for people who may not understand label information or for individuals who may have difficulty reading labels because of small print. From an educational perspective, it is important not only to emphasize what labels say but also to explain *why* the information is there. When consumers understand why particular information exists, they are more likely to remember and comply with therapy (10, 92, 93). (See Chapter 2, *Patient Assessment and Consultation*.)

REFERENCES

1   A. Kleinman, *Ann. Intern. Med., 88 (2)*, 251–258 (1978).
2   C. Lough and B. Stewart, in "The Nation's Health," P. R. Lee et al., Eds., Boyd & Fraser, San Francisco, Calif., 1981, pp. 445–453.
3   T. Ferguson, *Am. Pharm., NS20 (6)*, 12–18 (1980).
4   "Self-Medication in Health Care—An International Perspective," World Federation of Proprietary Medicine Manufacturers (reproduced by the Proprietary Association), Washington, D.C., 1985, pp. 1–2.
5   "Self-Medication," FDA Consumer Memo, U.S. Department of Health, Education, and Welfare, Public Health Service, Food and Drug Administration (FDA), DHEW Pub. No. FDA 73–3025, Washington, D.C.

6   *Am. Drug., 185 (5)*, 56 (1982).
7   P. Godfrey, in "New Resources in Self-Medication—A Symposium," The Proprietary Association, Washington, D.C., 1982, pp. 1–2.
8   F. E. Young, in "Self-Care, Self-Medication in America's Future—A Symposium," The Proprietary Association in cooperation with the FDA, Washington, D.C., 1988, pp. 4–10.
9   J. B. Esmay and A. I. Wertheimer, *J. Commun. Health, 5 (1)*, 54–66 (1979).
10   W. E. Gilbertson, *Pharm. Times, 47*, 22–27 (1981).
11   T. A. Gossel and J. R. Wuest, *U.S. Pharmacist, 6 (8)*, 14 (1981).
12   Council of Europe, European Public Health Community, *Drug Intell. Clin. Pharm., 10 (1)*, 16–33 (1976).
13   "Health Care Practices and Perceptions—A Consumer Survey of Self-Medication," prepared for the Proprietary Association by Harry Heller Research Corp. (HHR#72792), Washington, D.C., 1984, pp. 5–95.
14   D. M. Vickery, in "Rx-OTC: New Resources in Self-Medication—A Symposium," The Proprietary Association, Washington, D.C., 1982, pp. 29–32.
15   B. S. Gelb, in "Self-Medication—Making It Work Better for More People," Proceedings of the World Federation of Proprietary Medicine Manufacturers 8th General Assembly, The Proprietary Association, Washington, D.C., 1986, pp. 54–58.
16   F. D. Wolinsky, "The Sociology of Health: Principles, Professions and Issues," Little, Brown and Co., Boston, Mass., 1980, pp. 122–160.
17   L. Maiman et al., *J. Commun. Health, 10 (3)*, (1985).
18   B. S. Siegel, "Love, Medicine & Miracles," Harper and Row, New York, N.Y., 1988, pp. 11–63.
19   A. Leibowitz, *Med. Care, 27 (1)*, 85–93 (1989).
20   G. A. Holt et al., oral presentation at the 40th Annual Conference of The National Council of Aging, Washington, D.C., April 1990.
21   C. H. Kline, in "Self-Medication—Making It Work Better for More People," Proceedings of the World Federation of Proprietary Medicine Manufacturers 8th General Assembly, The Proprietary Association, Washington, D.C., 1986, pp. 13–18.
22   A. H. Hayes, in "Self-Medication—Making It Work Better for More People," Proceedings of the World Federation of Proprietary Medicine Manufacturers 8th General Assembly, The Proprietary Association, Washington, D.C., 1986, pp. 8–13.
23   W. S. Pray, *U.S. Pharmacist, 14 (9)*, 19–23 (1989).
24   W. I. Bergman, in "Self-Care, Self-Medication in America's Future—A Symposium," The Proprietary Association in cooperation with the FDA, Washington, D.C., 1988, pp. 51–54.
25   E. W. Rosenberg, in "New Resources in Self-Medication—A Symposium," The Proprietary Association, Washington, D.C., 1982, pp. 13–15.
26   A. Donabedian et al., "Medical Care Chartbook," Health Administration Press, Ann Arbor, Mich., 1986, pp. 3, 6, 45–108.
27   N. Cousins, in "Anatomy of an Illness—As Perceived by the Patient," Bantam Books, New York, N.Y., 1979, pp. 27–107.
28   L. Dossey, "Space, Time & Medicine," Shambhala Publications, Boulder, Colo., 1982, pp. 3–15.
29   A. H. White, in "Self-Care, Self-Medication in America's Future—A Symposium," The Proprietary Association in cooperation with the FDA, Washington, D.C., 1988, pp. 19–23.
30   L. S. Levin, in "Self-Medication, The New Era—A Symposium," The Proprietary Association, Washington, D.C., 1980, pp. 44–57.
31   G. E. Davy, *Am. Drug., 182 (1)*, 71–72 (1980).
32   F. E. Young, *FDA Consumer, 22 (10)*, 6–7 (Dec. 1988–Jan. 1989).
33   E. Fefer, in "Self-Medication—Making It Work Better for More People," Proceedings of the World Federation of Proprietary Medicine Manufacturers 8th General Assembly, Washington, D.C. The Proprietary Association, Washington, D.C., 1986, pp. 6–8.
34   F. E. Samuel, Jr., in "Self-Care, Self-Medication in America's Future—A Symposium," The Proprietary Association in cooperation with the FDA, Washington, D.C., 1988, pp. 47–50.

35 M. Montagne and B. A. Bleidt, *U.S. Pharmacist, 14 (6)*, 53–60 (1989).

36 A. Kleinman, in "The Nation's Health," P. R. Lee et al., Eds., Boyd and Fraser, San Francisco, Calif., 1981, pp. 18–20.

37 J. Fry, in "Self-Medication, The New Era—A Symposium," The Proprietary Association, Washington, D.C., 1980, pp. 2–6.

38 F. E. Young, in "Self-Care, Self-Medication in America's Future—A Symposium," The Proprietary Association in cooperation with the FDA, Washington, D.C., 1988, p. 57.

39 F. J. Ingelfinger, in "The Nation's Health," P. R. Lee, et al., Eds., Boyd and Fraser, San Francisco, Calif., 1981, pp. 478–484.

40 R. Dubos, "Mirage of Health," Harper Torchbook, New York, N.Y., 1980.

41 I. Illich, in "The Nation's Health," P. R. Lee et al., Eds., Boyd & Fraser, San Francisco, Calif., 1981, pp. 75–83.

42 E. P. Eckholm, in "The Nation's Health," P. R. Lee et al., Eds., Boyd and Fraser, San Francisco, Calif., 1981, pp. 501–509.

43 R. L. Kane in "The Nation's Health," P. R. Lee et al., Eds., Boyd and Fraser, San Francisco, Calif., 1981, pp. 326–332.

44 M. Silverman and P. R. Lee, in "The Nation's Health," P. R. Lee et al., Eds., Boyd and Fraser, San Francisco, Calif., 1981, pp. 320–325.

45 G. A. Holt and E. L. Hall, *J. Pharm. Technol.*, 213–218 (1986).

46 Council of Europe Public Health Community, *Drug Intell. Clin. Pharm., 10*, 172–178 (1976).

47 C. H. Kline, in "Self-Care, Self-Medication in America's Future—A Symposium," The Proprietary Association in cooperation with the FDA, Washington, D.C., 1988, pp. 15–18.

48 I. Rosenfeld, in "Self-Care, Self-Medication in America's Future—A Symposium," The Proprietary Association, Washington, D.C., 1988, pp. 36–40.

49 G. A. Holt, *Am. Pharm., NS23 (1)*, 38 (1983).

50 T. G. Harris, in "Self-Care, Self-Medication in America's Future—A Symposium," The Proprietary Association in cooperation with the FDA, Washington, D.C., 1988, pp. 43–46.

51 C. Pergola, *Am. Drug., 189 (6)*, 102 (1984).

52 "A Study of Attitudes, Concerns and Information Needs for Prescription Drugs and Related Illnesses," The CBS Consumer Model, CBS Television Network, New York, 1984, p. 8.

53 M. Glaser, *Drug Topics, 124 (17)*, 42–45 (1980).

54 H. J. Baldwin et al., *Commun. Quart., 35 (1)*, 84–102, (1987).

55 L. Thomas in "The Nation's Health," P. R. Lee et al., Eds., Boyd and Fraser, San Francisco, Calif., 1981, pp. 68–71.

56 J. T. Doluisio, "New Resources in Self-Medication—A Symposium," The Proprietary Association, Washington, D.C., 1982, pp. 11–13.

57 A. G. Hartzema, *Pharm. Internat., 3 (2)*, 57–59 (1982).

58 S. Rottenberg, in "Self-Medication, The New Era—A Symposium," The Proprietary Association, Washington, D.C., 1980, pp. 30–38.

59 "Self-Medication in Health Care—An International Perspective," World Federation of Proprietary Medicine Manufacturers (reproduced by the Proprietary Association), Washington, D.C., 1985, pp. 11–12.

60 "Talk About Prescriptions Month," National Council on Patient Information and Education, Washington, D.C., 1988, p. 1.

61 R. Laverty, *Drug Topics, 128 (10)*, 54–60 (1984).

62 "Priorities and Approaches for Improving Prescription Medicine Use by Older Americans," A Report of the National Council on Patient Information and Education, Washington, D.C., 1987, pp. 1–9.

63 *Drug Topics, 134 (3)*, 34 (1990).

64 "31 Medicine Moments for Talk About Prescriptions Month, October, 1989," National Council on Patient Information and Education, Washington, D.C., 1989, pp. 1–5.

65 R. F. Laverty, *Drug Topics, 128 (9)*, 38–45 (1984).

66 D. Helm, in "Self-Medication—Making It Work Better for More People," Proceedings of the World Federation of Proprietary Medicine Manufacturers 8th General Assembly, The Proprietary Association, Washington, D.C., 1986, pp. 86–87.

67 J. L. Kanig, in "Self-Medication—Making It Work Better for More People," Proceedings of the World Federation of Proprietary Medicine Manufacturers 8th General Assembly, The Proprietary Association, Washington, D.C., 1986, pp. 67–70.

68 L. S. Levin, in "Self-Medication—Making It Work Better for More People," Proceedings of the World Federation of Proprietary Medicine Manufacturers 8th General Assembly, The Proprietary Association, Washington, D.C., 1986, pp. 81–83.

69 J. T. Fay, in "Self-Care, Self-Medication in America's Future—A Symposium," The Proprietary Association in cooperation with the FDA, Washington, D.C., 1988, pp. 41–42.

70 P. B. Hutt, in "New Resources in Self-Medication—A Symposium," The Proprietary Association, Washington, D.C., 1982, pp. 34–39.

71 G. E. Davy, in "Self-Medication—Making It Work Better for More People," Proceedings of the World Federation of Proprietary Medicine Manufacturers 8th General Assembly, The Proprietary Association, Washington, D.C., 1986, pp. 93–96.

72 "Pharmacy Law Digest," J. L. Fink et al., Eds., Facts and Comparisons Division, J. B. Lippincott, St. Louis, Mo., 1987, pp. 8, 15.

73 A. Kaplan, in "New Resources in Self-Medication—A Symposium," The Proprietary Association, Washington, D.C., 1982, pp. 4–6.

74 J. S. Chapman, in "The Nation's Health," P. R. Lee et al., Eds., Boyd and Fraser, San Francisco, Calif., 1981, pp. 14–17.

75 R. J. Haggerty, in "The Nation's Health," P. R. Lee et al., Eds., Boyd and Fraser, San Francisco, Calif., 1981, pp. 21–26.

76 R. Dubos, in "The Nation's Health," P. R. Lee et al., Eds., Boyd and Fraser, San Francisco, Calif., 1981, pp. 6–13.

77 R. Dubos, in "Anatomy of Illness as Perceived by the Patient," Bantam Books, New York, N.Y. (1979), pp. 11–23.

78 A. M. Schmidt, in "Self-Medication, The New Era—A Symposium," The Proprietary Association, Washington, D.C., 1980, pp. 1–2.

79 Martha Glaser, *Drug Topics, 124*, 31–34 (1980).

80 *Am. Drug., 178 (11)*, 18 (1979).

81 R. B. Helms, in "New Resources in Self-Medication—A Symposium," The Proprietary Association, Washington, D.C., 1982, pp. 23–25.

82 D. G. Vidt, in "New Resources in Self-Medication—A Symposium," The Proprietary Association, Washington, D.C., 1982, pp. 22–23.

83 H. A. Waxman, in "Self-Care, Self-Medication in America's Future—A Symposium," The Proprietary Association in cooperation with the FDA, Washington, D.C., 1988, pp. 29–32.

84 J. D. Cope, in "Self-Care, Self-Medication in America's Future—A Symposium," The Proprietary Association in cooperation with the FDA, Washington, D.C. 1988, pp. 1–2.

85 J. T. Doluisio, *Am. Pharm., NS23 (1)*, 26–28 (1983).

86 *Pharm. Times, 50 (4)*, 36–39 (1984).

87 E. W. Rosenberg, in "Self-Medication—Making It Work Better for More People," Proceedings of the World Federation of Proprietary Medicine Manufacturers 8th General Assembly, The Proprietary Association, Washington, D.C., 1986, pp. 83–85.

88 D. C. Oppenheimer, *U.S. Pharmacist, 4 (10)*, 10 (1979).

89 T. G. Harris, in "Self-Care, Self-Medication in America's Future—A Symposium," The Proprietary Association in cooperation with the FDA, Washington, D.C., 1988, pp. 55–56.

90 P. Temin, in "New Resources in Self-Medication—A Symposium," The Proprietary Association, Washington, D.C., 1982, p. 27.

91 E. L. Hall et al., *Calif. Pharm., XXX (12)*, 20 (1983).

92 G. A. Holt, *Am. Pharm., NS21 (7)*, 46 (1981).

93 J. R. Kidd, "How Adults Learn," Association Press, New York, N.Y., 1977, pp. 268–291.

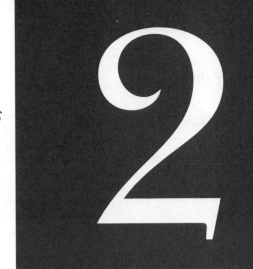

Wendy Klein-Schwartz and John M. Hoopes

PATIENT ASSESSMENT AND CONSULTATION

Self-care, self-diagnosis, and self-medication are important components of the health care system in the United States. Many people do not seek the attention of a physician, but self-diagnose and treat their symptoms with nonprescription drugs and home remedies. A number of factors, including age (e.g., over 75 years of age), sex (e.g., female), socioeconomic status (e.g., income under $6,000 per year), and symptomatology (e.g., the number of distinct and separate symptoms), increase the incidence of self-medication (1). The present trend of reclassifying ("switching") prescription drugs as nonprescription is another factor contributing to the increase in self-medication.

In 1988, over $9 billion were spent on nonprescription drugs. Compared to 1987 figures, dollar sales of nonprescription drugs in pharmacies increased 9.5% (2). Of the total sales, 46.8% of expenditures for nonprescription drugs were made in pharmacies. The remaining expenditures were made in food stores and mass merchandising outlets.

Nonprescription drugs allow the individual to manage relatively minor medical problems rapidly, inexpensively, and conveniently without unnecessary visits to a physician. (See Chapter 1, *The Self-Care Movement.*) However, appropriate use of these products, like any other drug, requires certain restrictions and limitations. Although warnings are required on the labels of nonprescription drug products, labeling alone may be inadequate; the consumer often needs assistance in selecting and properly using nonprescription drugs.

Many consumers do not appreciate or are not aware of the need for professional assistance in the selection of nonprescription drugs. This attitude has recently become more evident by the large number of nonprescription products that are purchased in nonpharmacy outlets, such as supermarkets and local convenience stores (2, 3). Table 1 gives a general indication of the percentage of nonprescription products purchased in such outlets. Some investigators have said "The only thing that differentiates the nonprescription department in a pharmacy from a similar department in a food store is the pharmacist" (3). Similarly, it is inappropriate for nonprofessional pharmacy personnel, such as technicians or clerks, to provide advice on nonprescription products. Inappropriate nonprofessional advice may also expose the pharmacist to the risk of liability if an adverse event should occur. These inquiries should always be referred to the pharmacist. It is essential to increase the consumer's awareness of the importance of consulting the pharmacist, especially when considering a drug for the first time. Just as the pharmaceutical industry promotes a product, pharmacists must emphasize the value of their guidance in purchasing a nonprescription drug.

A consumer's choice of nonprescription product is usually based on prior use; advice from pharmacists, neighbors, and/or relatives; and exposure to commercial advertisements. Even though consumers usually first hear about a new nonprescription drug from several of these sources, the pharmacist's advice is mentioned most frequently as the most important factor in their choice of products (4).

THE PROFESSIONAL OPPORTUNITY

One study showed that consumers chose a particular pharmacist because the pharmacist discussed instructions for using a nonprescription drug with them, gave advice on health problems, and recommended cer-

TABLE 1   Expenditures for nonprescription drugs: 1984 (in thousands)[a]

Category	Total Expenditures ($)	Expenditures in Pharmacies ($)	Expenditures in Pharmacies (%)
Internal analgesics	1,676,445	866,680	52
Cough & cold	1,589,695	888,608	56
Vitamins	1,365,637	842,711	62
Antacids	805,905	404,334	50
Baby medicaments	413,885	126,390	31
Eye care	388,763	225,717	58
Laxatives	383,583	259,393	68
Suntan lotions and screens	304,214	145,346	48
First aid	290,759	210,600	72
Appetite suppressants	264,264	166,486	63
External analgesics	181,447	119,308	66
Acne preparations	159,765	113,433	71
Hemorrhoidal preparations	140,405	109,516	78
Antidiarrheals	121,806	66,993	55
Feminine hygiene	115,447	57,403	50
Contraceptives[b]	67,062	53,213	79
Other OTCs	262,341	187,064	71
Total	8,531,423	4,843,195	57

[a]Does not include dental products, skin lotions, baby formulas.
[b]Does not include condoms or vaginal sponges.
Compiled from *Drug Topics*, *129*, 34 (1985).

tain nonprescription drugs for minor health problems. Friendliness, courtesy, and neatness were also cited by consumers as factors influencing their choice of a pharmacist. In 95% of the cases, consumers used the recommended medication, and 92% of the consumers said that they were satisfied with the purchase. Eighty-seven percent either had bought the item again or said they would. Sixty-nine percent of the consumers said their pharmacists supplied information and advice when they requested them, and 9 out of 10 consumers said they would follow a pharmacist's advice, particularly if the pharmacist advised seeking medical help for a possibly serious medical disorder (5).

According to the 1979 Schering report, the friendliness of the pharmacist was more important than the atmosphere of the pharmacy (6). However, only 34% of the consumers surveyed thought that pharmacists were easy to approach. Even though a pharmacist's advice is frequently followed, over one-half the consumers do not seek their pharmacists' advice regularly (5). An analysis of consumer use of nondispensing pharmacy services found that while consumers had not used most of

the services available, the majority had obtained advice on nonprescription medication and on minor health problems from their pharmacists. The majority of consumers considered pharmacists to be competent and to have professional dispositions toward their patients (7).

Pharmacists are increasingly aware of the importance of patient counseling as a professional function. Pharmacists report that giving consultations to patients on nonprescription drugs, including recommending a particular preparation, is a vital pharmacy service (8). In a survey sent to 228 pharmacies, 98% of the responding pharmacists indicated they counsel patients on the use of nonprescription and prescription drugs (9). They reported that this activity generally took 1–3 minutes and was usually initiated by the pharmacist. Of 394 independent and chain pharmacists surveyed, 79% indicated they are having more discussions on nonprescription drugs with patients (10). According to 63% of the pharmacists, patients frequently come to them instead of consulting a physician, and 49% of the pharmacists indicated they are frequently consulted until a medical appointment can be arranged. Patients most frequently ask about dosage/use and product safety/side effects; product efficacy followed by price and product ingredients are other frequently asked questions.

Not all evaluations of pharmacists' counseling, however, are positive or encouraging. Interviews with patients reveal low estimates of pharmacists' counseling activity (11). While pharmacists rank second behind physicians as a source of drug information and are highly visible to consumers, the quality of information provided by pharmacists has been considered marginal (12). Consumers have indicated that community pharmacists make themselves available to answer drug-related questions, but generally do not voluntarily provide counseling (13).

Significant impediments to providing counseling are the pharmacist's self-perception of competence and willingness to counsel patients. A significant relationship has been demonstrated between the pharmacist's self-confidence and willingness to provide expanded services in community pharmacies and the actual provision of such services (14).

Advising patients on self-medication is an important part of pharmacy practice and provides the pharmacist an opportunity to act in a primary care role. Additionally, in this role the pharmacist can perform a triage function (15). Potential exists for community pharmacists to become more active as referral sources. If pharmacists deter healthy people from using more costly health care services or products and refer more ill patients to physicians, health care delivery in the United States would be improved. The pharmacist can play an important role in helping patients assume the "sick role" (i.e., patients recognizing that they are sick and require care) (16). Because the pharmacist is frequently the patient's first contact with the health care system, the pharmacist is in a position to assess the situation and recommend a course of action. The course of action may include recommending a nonprescription drug, dissuading the patient from buying a nonprescription drug when drug therapy is not indicated, recommending a nondrug modality of treatment, or referring the person to another health care practitioner. If self-medication is warranted, the pharmacist must select the most appropriate product as well as give the patient specific recommendations for its correct use. To successfully educate a patient to self-medicate safely, the pharmacist must have effective communication and counseling skills.

COMMUNICATING

Communication Skills

Establishing a positive pharmacist–patient relationship is important and can be furthered by knowing those factors that facilitate or inhibit communication (9, 17). Poor communication often exists between patients and health care professionals, resulting in frustration for both and, in part, for poor compliance by the patient (18, 19). As the role of pharmacists in patient care expands, they will be expected to communicate even more extensively with patients and other health professionals. Because communication is part of everyday interaction, it is often assumed to be effective. However, factors such as the patient's personality and perception of pharmacists can markedly affect communication and ultimately patient care.

As information is exchanged, the participants change roles as senders and receivers. Effective communication is achieved when what the sender wishes to communicate matches what is received. What is received is influenced by the content of the message, as well as by the process used to convey the message. Communication, therefore, may be improved by paying attention to both what is said and how it is said. The sender can be certain of the message sent by obtaining feedback from the receiver. Certain skills can be developed to improve communication, which when combined with an understanding of the physical and psychologic barriers in the pharmacy, will optimize the patient–pharmacist interaction.

An effective pharmacist–patient relationship can only be established if pharmacists seem to be capable,

empathetic sources of information, and if patients feel they need the information. Patients' past experiences with pharmacists may influence their attitudes toward pharmacists as information sources (2, 15). Patients' past use of pharmacists' counseling and perception of pharmacists as providers of these services are important factors in their intention to use a pharmacist again (7).

A pharmacist should feel confident in the role of counselor and should put patients at ease. Because patients will resent being told what they already know, the pharmacist should first determine what they know and then fill in the gaps (5). When counseling patients, the pharmacist should use words that a lay person can understand and avoid using complex medical terminology (15, 20).

Verbal Communication

Knowing the factors that inhibit positive communication and trying to eliminate them should improve the pharmacist–patient interaction (16). The pharmacist's underlying attitude toward the patient will influence the quality of communication (21). The effective pharmacist must eliminate psychosocial barriers by avoiding biases toward a patient's level of education, socioeconomic or cultural background, interests, or attitude. Listening is an important component of communication. After asking a question, the pharmacist should be alert and receptive to the patient's response.

Listening requires that the patient be allowed to state the problem completely and receive the pharmacist's undivided attention. The pharmacist must respond with empathy and clarify the details of the patient's problem. Empathy is conveyed by paraphrasing the patient's words or by reflecting on what was said in terms of the pharmacist's own experience. For instance, after listening to a complaint of pain from a patient, the pharmacist should describe the pain just told by the patient ending with a statement such as "That must be very uncomfortable." This tells the patient that more was heard than just the details of the complaint. Interrupting or expressing disinterest or disapproval may inhibit the patient's expression of problems and concerns. Alternatively, encouraging the patient to talk, exploring the patient's comments, and expressing understanding will facilitate communication. The pharmacist should reinforce correct decisions the patient has made, while being nonjudgmental, and communicate warmth, feeling, and interest in the patient's concerns.

Every effort should be made to ask questions carefully. The patient should feel that the pharmacist's questions convey a genuine desire to be of assistance. A patient may refuse to cooperate if the questions indicate only superficial curiosity. To prevent a negative initial reaction, the pharmacist should explain the reason for asking personal questions. An explanation such as "For me to select a product for your specific problem, I need some additional information," may be helpful in obtaining the consumer's cooperation.

Two types of questions are generally asked. Open-ended questions are useful in gathering information regarding the medical problem. An example of an open-ended question is "Can you tell me more about the symptoms you have?" Open-ended questions allow more flexibility and provide more information than questions that can be answered with yes or no. Using open-ended questions, however, may cause the conversation to stray from the subject. The pharmacist must keep the conversation focused. Summarizing the conversation with its important points or redirecting it with a question specific to the subject may be used in such circumstances. Closed-ended questions are useful when information is needed about a specific item. An example of a closed-ended question is "How long have you had this pain?" It is important to ask one question at a time. The use of two questions in rapid succession or multiple choice questions will only cause confusion and restrict communication.

Nonverbal Communication

Nonverbal communication skills are also important in counseling patients on nonprescription drugs (22, 23). Because body language is as important as what is said, the pharmacist must be aware of nonverbal behavior (22). Posture, body orientation, and distance from the patient influences the effectiveness with which the pharmacist conveys a message. The pharmacist's interpretation of the patient's nonverbal communication is also important.

Physical barriers to communication should be removed. High counters, glass separators, and elevated platforms inhibit communication; the pharmacist should try to be at the same eye-level as the patient (22). Discussions between the patient and pharmacist should be as private and uninterrupted as possible (15). If the pharmacist anticipates or perceives that a patient is embarrassed or uncomfortable discussing the problem, a quiet or private counseling area should be used. Ideally, a specific relatively private area of the pharmacy should be designated for patient consultation. Information obtained from a patient should remain confidential.

Communication Facilitators

Special communication techniques may be required with some patients (24, 25). Writing down the information may be necessary if the patient is deaf or is hearing-impaired. However, it should be kept in mind that up to 20% of Americans are functionally illiterate (26). If the patient has poor hearing or is deaf but reads lips, the pharmacist should be physically close to and directly in front of the patient. A quiet, well-lighted environment is essential because background noise can markedly diminish the hearing-impaired individual's ability to communicate. Visual cues will greatly facilitate communication with these individuals. The pharmacist should face the patient at all times, speak directly to the patient, and maintain eye contact while speaking. In addition, the pharmacist should speak slowly and distinctly in a low-pitched, moderately toned voice. Yelling only serves to further distort the sound.

When counseling blind patients, pharmacists should first identify themselves as a pharmacist. Because a blind patient cannot be aware of visual nonverbal communication, the pharmacist should depend on tone of voice as well as verbal feedback to convey empathy and interest in the patient's problem. If touching seems appropriate, the pharmacist should ask the blind person if it would be acceptable.

A patient's response can be used to assess the effectiveness of the pharmacist's advice and communication skills. Acceptance of the pharmacist's advice and other positive verbal and nonverbal feedback will indicate a patient's respect for the pharmacist and satisfaction with the advice given.

The discussion should be concluded with encouragement for follow-up with a statement such as "Please let me know whether you feel better in a couple of days," or "If your cough is not better in a few days, you should see your physician. Be sure to tell your physician that you have been taking this medicine." A patient will sense caring on the part of the pharmacist. The pharmacist's concern for the correct use of the nonprescription drugs will also reinforce that these products are drugs and must be used carefully. In addition, follow-up provides feedback that allows pharmacists to assess whether their communication skills require modification and whether they have provided useful information.

If an effective pharmacist–patient relationship is established, the patient will probably return to that particular pharmacist for further self-medication advice and for the dispensing of any needed prescriptions. In other words, an effective patient counseling service for nonprescription drugs can contribute to increased demand for other professional services.

PATIENT INTERVIEW

Self-medication counseling is a primary care activity that carries with it a great professional responsibility.

The initial interaction between the patient and the pharmacist is frequently initiated by the patient (Figure 1). The patient may approach the pharmacist with a symptom, often in the form of a question such as "What do you recommend for . . . ?" On the other hand, the patient may ask a product-related question such as "Which of these two products do you recommend?" The pharmacist should also assist a patient who is deliberating over nonprescription products and intervene when a patient selects a product that is contraindicated or has significant potential for causing problems.

Historical Data

The pharmacist must concentrate on the patient's medical history and accumulate a subjective data base from which an assessment can be made. The patient history is a very powerful tool available to the pharmacist in assessing the clinical condition presented by a given patient. The community pharmacist is limited almost exclusively to the patient history; therefore, the pharmacist must develop good history-taking skills.

When evaluating the problem, the pharmacist must view the patient and the disease as a whole, rather than keying in only on the drug therapy aspects. This enables the pharmacist to make the most appropriate recommendation, which may or may not include a drug.

The second step in the decision-making process is identifying the condition that the patient seeks to treat. Patients may initially present incomplete and vague information. By asking specific questions, the pharmacist can determine the patient's real needs and obtain a problem-oriented and patient-oriented history. The objective is to determine what the specific symptoms are and whether they are amenable to self-medication.

The pharmacist can determine the specific symptoms by asking the following questions:

- Onset—When did the symptom start?

- Duration—How long does it last? Does it come and go, or is it continuous?

- Severity—How severe is the symptom?

- Description—Can you describe the symptom?

- Acute versus chronic—Is this a new problem or the recurrence or continuation of an old one?

- Associated symptoms—Are there other symptoms that occur concurrently?

- Precipitating or exacerbating factors—Does any food, drug, or physical activity make the symptom worse?

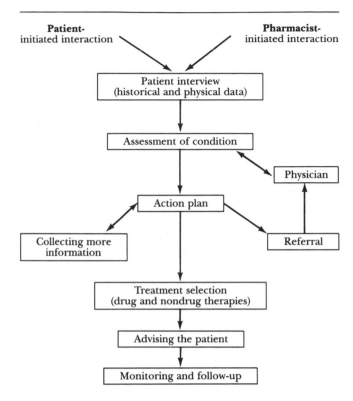

FIGURE 1   Patient–pharmacist consultation process.

- Relief factors—Does anything relieve the symptom? What has relieved it in the past?

- Previous therapy—What has been done so far to treat the symptom?

The next step is to gather patient-related data. The pharmacist must consider the patient's characteristics before assessing the condition. The pharmacist should therefore selectively elicit the following information:

- Patient—Is the consumer or someone else the patient?

- Age—How old is the patient? Is the patient an infant, a child, or an elderly person?

- Sex—Is the patient male or female? If the patient is female, is she pregnant or breast-feeding?

- Other illnesses—Does the patient have any other diseases that may alter the expected effects of a given nonprescription drug or be aggravated by the drug's effects? Is the complaint related to chronic disease?

- Special diets and nutritional requirements—Is the patient on a special diet? Does the patient have any special nutritional requirements?

- Other drugs—Is the patient on any prescription, nonprescription, or social drugs (e.g., vitamins or food supplements, caffeine, nicotine, alcohol, or marijuana)?

- Allergies—Does the patient have any allergies?

- Adverse drug reactions—Has the patient experienced adverse drug reactions in the past?

After taking the patient history, the pharmacist should determine if the drug being considered for recommendation has any absolute or relative contraindications. In addition, the pharmacist should ascertain if the patient is in a high-risk group because of age, other illnesses, or pregnancy. Similarly, the pharmacist should determine whether the patient has confused the condition, done any harm by waiting to seek advice, or worsened the condition by previous self-treatment.

The pharmacist must ask questions to obtain enough information to identify and assess the problem before a plan for self-treatment or physician referral can be formulated. Obviously, the pharmacist must do this within certain time constraints by approaching the problem logically and keeping questioning direct and to the point. The pharmacist must decide which of the given questions are appropriate to the patient's condition. With experience, the pharmacist should be able to acquire the necessary information to assess a particular condition within a few minutes.

Observed Physical Data

In addition to the historical data, physical data are extremely helpful in assessing the medical problem. Physical data include information such as pulse rate, heart sounds, respiration rate, age, and weight. Depending on the training and skill of the health care practitioner, physical data are collected by all or some of the following techniques: observation or inspection, palpation or manipulations, percussion, and auscultation. The importance of each in the process of data collection depends upon the system involved. For example, the skin is easily assessed by inspection and palpation. The lung requires percussion and auscultation. All four skills are essential in examining the abdomen.

Some physical data may be collected easily by the pharmacist. Physical data have been collected by pharmacists routinely for years, and some pharmacists have acquired additional skills, which, in appropriate settings, have greatly expanded their ability to assess and monitor patients' medical conditions. However, the majority of pharmacists obtains physical data exclusively through observational skills.

Observational skills can be extremely valuable. Many clues to a patient's overall health and the seriousness of a condition can come from simply observing the patient. The degree of discomfort caused by pain may be judged from facial expressions or lack of use of a particular limb. Toxicity from an infection may be manifested by lethargy and pallor. Many errors have been made because such data were ignored. Inspection of the skin in a patient with a dermatologic condition is very useful, especially with hydrocortisone available as a nonprescription drug. Skin rashes, for example, may result from a simple contact phenomenon or may indicate systemic disease. If a serious disease is suspected, the pharmacist should immediately refer the patient to a physician for diagnosis.

Assessment of Condition

Assessment is the evaluation of all the data (historical and physical) collected from the patient to determine the etiology and severity of the medical condition. Etiology refers to the cause of the condition. Determining this may assist in selecting a particular type of therapy. Severity refers to the relative significance of the condition.

Assessment of severity will vary depending upon the condition. Conditions may be considered severe only when they accumulate to a certain level, such as diabetics with hyperglycemia or polyuria. The higher the level, the more severe the problem is, and the potential for referral is greater. (See Chapter 16, *Diabetes Care Products*.) Some conditions may be considered severe only when they become symptomatic or when the symptoms begin to impair the functional activity of the patient. For instance, the pharmacist may elect not to recommend a cough suppressant for a patient with an intermittent cough, although the cough should be treated if it is keeping the patient awake at night. However, certain conditions should be considered severe whenever they are present. Such is the case when ketonuria is noted by a diabetic or when an insulin-dependent diabetic is unable to take in calories because of vomiting.

Determining etiology and severity is essential to making appropriate conclusions about treatment and the need for referral. Many times the determination is not conclusive because certain data may not be accessible. Action may be required in such situations because the information suggests that a certain etiology is responsible or that the condition is particularly severe. For example, an acutely inflamed joint that is swollen, warm to the touch, tender, and painful may be caused by trauma, bacterial infection, gout, or rheumatoid arthritis. This may require examination of the joint fluid; the patient should be referred immediately to a physician. Finally, certain groups of patients are at greater risk of complications and require more careful evaluation. These groups include the elderly; infants and children; those with certain chronic diseases, such as diabetes or renal or heart disease; those with multiple medical conditions; those taking multiple medications; those recently hospitalized; and those being treated by several physicians.

- Obtaining data on preexisting medical conditions to determine whether self-treatment is appropriate;

- Seeking the physician's assistance in evaluating the problem;

- Determining if the physician wants to see the patient or if the patient should go to the emergency room;

- Determining if the physician wants to deal with the problem over the phone with the patient;

- Providing information on the reason for referral.

ACTION PLAN

After collecting all the available information and assessing the patient's condition, the pharmacist must quickly formulate an action plan. Many times the pharmacist must do this without having all the desired information. Areas of uncertainty will always exist, but a well-considered plan can ensure proper management of the patient.

A sound action plan requires careful attention to four specific areas:

- Collecting more information;

- Physician referral;

- Selecting treatment;

- Advising the patient on self-treatment.

Collecting More Information

The pharmacist may need more information to properly assess the patient's condition. This may require specific action such as talking to a parent or another adult or calling a physician. If enough information is available to assess the condition, the pharmacist then must decide whether to refer the patient to a physician or to advise self-treatment.

The pharmacist may need to contact the patient's physician for additional information to use in assessing the patient's condition. The pharmacist may also want to contact the physician to make a direct referral. Communication between pharmacists and physicians is often desirable to avoid conflict in the overall management of the patient and to overcome the problem of overlapping responsibilities.

Situations in which communication between the pharmacist and physician may be necessary include:

Physician Referral

If the plan involves physician referral, the pharmacist must consider the type of treatment center to which the patient will be referred (physician's office or emergency care facility) as well as the urgency for treatment. Some conditions do not require the immediate attention or extensive evaluation of emergency care treatment. A proper referral will reflect consideration of these two factors.

When advising a patient to see a physician, the pharmacist should use tact and firmness so that the patient is not frightened unnecessarily, but is convinced of the value of the advice. When making a referral, the pharmacist should tell the patient to whom and why the referral is being made.

The pharmacist should refer a patient to a physician in any of the following situations:

- The symptoms are too severe to be endured by the patient without definitive diagnosis and treatment.

- The symptoms are minor but have persisted and do not appear to be due to some easily identifiable cause.

- The symptoms have returned repeatedly for no readily recognizable cause.

- The pharmacist is in doubt about the patient's medical condition.

Selecting Treatment

When advising self-treatment, the pharmacist must consider several factors. One factor is identifying a therapeutic objective based on a consideration of the condition and the patient. The objective should be measurable and achievable. As a result of this decision, a therapeutic modality, either drug or nondrug, may be recommended. Final selection of a specific modality requires reviewing drug variables (dosage forms, ingredients, side effects, adverse reactions, relative effectiveness, and price) and matching them with patient variables (age, sex, drug history, other physiologic problems, and ability to pay).

Self-treatment with a nondrug modality may be indicated. Selection of the nondrug modality will be modified based on patient variables. For example, the pharmacist may recommend that a patient with vomiting and diarrhea only drink fluids for a 24-hour period to provide bowel rest. However, if the patient is an insulin-dependent diabetic, the pharmacist must modify this recommendation because diabetics must maintain specific caloric intake. Communicating with the physician is a must in this situation.

Selection of monitoring indices is influenced by the therapeutic objective, the toxic or adverse effects of the selected treatment, the nature of the condition, and the ability of the patient to understand the condition and its treatment. The objective in treating sinusitis with decongestants, for example, is to facilitate drainage and relieve symptoms such as headache. The first objective can be measured by observing or asking about the nature of nasal discharge (quantity, color, and viscosity), the second by simply asking about the headache. Indices of toxicity are those symptoms indicative of too high dosing or of an untoward reaction. Finally, indices that indicate the disease may be worsening and may require special attention should be identified.

Advising the Patient on Self-Treatment

The final step in the action plan is the pharmacist advising the patient on self-treatment; good communication is vital in this step. The primary purpose is to educate the patient and gain the patient's acceptance of the plan. Specifically, advice should be given in the following areas:

- Reasons for self-treatment;

- Description of the drug and/or treatment;

- Administration guidelines;

- Side effects and precautions;

- General treatment guidelines.

Advising the patient about the suggested treatment plan should involve a summary of the condition and the reasons for treatment. The meaning of the patient's symptoms should be explained along with their significance. Available alternate treatments, along with their relative merits, should be presented at this point. The therapeutic objective(s) should be explained clearly.

At this point, the nonprescription drug(s) selected by the pharmacist should be discussed. The therapeutic action of the ingredients (e.g., decongestants, antihistamines, laxatives) should be briefly described in lay terms. The patient should be told how the product will affect the symptoms as well as the condition. Patients need to know the role the drug will play in achieving the therapeutic objective(s). Finally, the patient should be told about the available dosage forms of the product (tablet, capsule, liquid) and the availability of a generic product.

Administration guidelines should be explained clearly and concisely. Some thought should be given to deciding what is most important for the patient to remember because many patients may remember only part of the information. Covering a few of the most important points is better than overwhelming patients with information.

Patients will remember dosage instructions better if the instructions are tied to specific times of the day, rather than just being told to take the medication three times daily. Having patients review their normal daily activities will help them establish the best times to take their medication. The length of treatment is vital information to include.

Telling the patient about the most common side effects or adverse reactions associated with a drug is very important. Instructions on how to manage the reactions should be included. Special warnings about activities, other drugs, foods, or beverages that should be avoided and medical conditions that may be complicated by use of the drug should also be discussed.

Finally, general treatment guidelines helpful in managing the condition should be offered to the patient. The guidelines might include lifestyle changes, additional products or services, and information sources. The treatment guidelines should also include a list of signs and symptoms that indicates whether the drug is working or causing adverse effects and when a physician's advice is needed. The patient should be encouraged to check back if the condition does not improve within a specific period of time or if problems with the medication develop.

To determine if the patient has understood the dosage instructions and the treatment guidelines, the pharmacist should ask the patient to repeat them.

Follow-up of a patient's problem is critical and may take many forms. Simply advising patients to call or return if symptoms fail to resolve is a method of ensuring follow-up in responsible patients. Other medical conditions or situations may require a telephone call, a letter, or monitoring by a third party. The length of time between follow-up intervals should be considered in the final recommendation. The interval would be influenced by both the type of medical condition and the patient involved.

HIGH-RISK AND SPECIAL GROUPS

Generalizing about patients is difficult and often misleading, particularly with regard to any predictable response to therapy. Therapy for every patient must be individualized. This includes assessing the particular variables of the drug used that may predispose the patient to adverse effects.

Four groups of patients (the elderly, the very young, pregnant patients, and nursing mothers) often experience a higher incidence of adverse drug effects. Because adverse effects may have dire consequences in some of these high-risk patients, they require special attention. Awareness of the physiologic state, the existence of pathologic conditions, and the special social context of these patients is necessary for proper assessment of their medical conditions and recommendation of treatment.

Geriatric and Pediatric Patients

In many respects geriatric and pediatric patients require surprisingly similar considerations. Both groups share a need for different drug dosages than other age groups because of altered pharmacokinetic parameters; a decreased ability to cope with illness or drug side effects because of physiologic changes associated with either normal aging or child development; patterns of impaired judgment because of either altered sensory function or immaturity; different drug effects unique to their age groups; adverse effects unique to their age groups; and a need for special consideration in administering medications. Because each group is heterogeneous, it is important to consider these factors individually.

Normal, or physiologic aging, is associated with physiologic changes that alter the pharmacokinetics of certain drugs (27–29). These changes include documented significant increases in proportion of body fat and decreases in renal function, total body water, lean body mass, concentration of plasma albumin, organ perfusion, and hepatic microsomal enzyme activity. This may lead to altered absorption, distribution, metabolism, and elimination of certain drugs. The result is

often an unexpected accumulation of the drug to toxic levels. Thus, continuous caution in dosing the elderly is required. (See Minichapter A, *Nonprescription Drugs and the Elderly*.)

The pediatric patient is in a continuous state of development of body and organ functions. Data on pharmacokinetics in neonates, infants, and children have been more exclusively studied for prescription drugs than for nonprescription. In the neonate, factors such as decreased gastric acidity, prolonged gastric emptying, irregular peristalsis, immature biliary function, and altered intestinal enzyme systems are responsible for alterations in the oral absorption of drugs (30–32). Continuous changes in body weight and relative body composition (lipid content and body water compartments) as well as differences in protein binding account for distribution differences of drugs in the body. Drug metabolism is usually slower in the neonate and young infant than in older infants and children. Similarly, renal drug elimination is impaired in the neonate and young infant, but improves rapidly over the first year of life. (See Minichapter B, *Nonprescription Drug Use in Children*.)

Physiologic State

Illness in children and the elderly is potentially more serious because their physiologic states are less tolerant of changes. Both are very susceptible to fluid loss; therefore, fever, vomiting, or diarrhea represent greater potential risks to them. Pulmonary function is decreased in the elderly, which predisposes them to the complications of respiratory tract infections. Although similar changes are found in the body systems of all elderly people, the changes may be quite varied among individuals, making the elderly a very heterogeneous group. The common cold can be serious in the first few years of life because children are more susceptible to infections such as otitis media and pneumonia. These examples demonstrate the need for treatment plans that differ according to the age of the patient, as well as the need for closer monitoring of the very young and the elderly.

Assessment of pediatric and elderly patients requires recognition that patient judgment may be altered. In the young, immaturity requires that others provide information and carry out parts of the plan. The elderly may require special consideration when an organic brain syndrome has developed. Subtle changes in mental status, such as confusion, should be anticipated in elderly patients where an illness has caused them anxiety over their overall state of health. Additionally, central nervous system (CNS) depressants should be anticipated to have more effect on judgment in the elderly adult than in the nonelderly adult.

Drugs may have unusual yet predictable effects in

the elderly and in children. Antihistamines and CNS depressants may cause excitation. Paradoxical reactions of this type are rare in nonelderly adults.

Certain adverse effects are more often seen in the young and the elderly. Elderly patients frequently have altered urinary bladder function and must make a conscious effort to maintain good bladder control. Incontinence may be precipitated in such patients by administration of antihistamines, which have sedative properties that may reduce bladder control (33).

Diseases

Children have different diseases than adults or frequently have different causes for similar conditions. For example, rashes in children are frequently the result of common viral illnesses such as measles or chickenpox, which are rarely causes of rashes in adults. Other conditions such as otitis media and febrile seizures occur more frequently in children. Certain symptoms have particular significance in children. Fever in any infant less than 6 weeks of age is a very serious sign and requires immediate attention because of the increased risk of a serious infection such as bacterial septicemia.

The elderly also differ from other age groups in several ways. They tend to have serious and multiple diseases such as coronary artery disease, chronic renal failure or congestive heart failure, and other similar conditions. These conditions can be aggravated by concurrent therapy for other acute problems. Also, their nutritional status is often marginal, making them more susceptible to illness. Social supports to supply the aid required by an illness are often lacking for the elderly. Lastly, physiologic changes associated with aging may alter the presentation of certain illnesses and confuse their assessment. For example, the elderly do not mount fevers to the same degree as younger patients and have altered pain perception, which may cause them to overlook a serious condition.

Special dosage considerations may be necessary for children and the elderly. Because of memory lapses, some elderly patients may require unique drug delivery systems to aid them in adhering to their daily dosage regimen. Also, elderly patients with cognitive impairment are less likely to read and interpret labels and to differentiate colors correctly (34), which further emphasize their need for special dosage considerations. Because infants and children are unable to swallow tablets and capsules, chewable tablets and liquid preparations are required. This may apply to some elderly patients as well. To assist in accurate delivery of liquid preparations, devices such as calibrated droppers and spoons are needed. Parents may need instructions on using these devices to measure dosages accurately, as well as advice on giving medications to reluctant or struggling children.

The Pregnant Patient

Pregnancy introduces a very important variable in drug therapy. Because most drugs cross the placenta to some extent, a drug taken by the mother can expose the fetus to the drug. Drug therapy during pregnancy may be necessary to treat preexisting medical conditions or may be considered for the management of common complaints of pregnancy such as vomiting or constipation. The desire to ease the mother's discomfort must be balanced with concern for the developing fetus.

Unequivocal evidence of teratogenesis is available for some drugs such as thalidomide, androgens, cancer chemotherapeutic agents, tetracyclines, hydantoins, and oral anticoagulants (35). Many more drugs are suspect, and each year additional drugs are shown to be potentially harmful if used during pregnancy. A major problem faced by the pregnant patient, her physician, and her pharmacist is the lack of readily available information on the teratogenic effects of various drugs. This lack of information on prescription drugs has been partly remedied by the FDA's labeling revision program, which places all prescription drugs into one of five categories (A, B, C, D, X) according to the level of risk to the fetus (36, 37). Although this categorization may increase the amount of information readily available on prescription drugs, a paucity of data on nonprescription drugs still exists. Therefore, knowing the potential danger many nonprescription drugs pose to pregnant women is essential in preventing unnecessary exposure of unborn children to drugs.

Potential Problems

Animal studies and epidemiologic human studies are the methods used in determining potential teratogens. Interpreting data from these types of studies is difficult. Although data from animal studies can be useful, the data must be evaluated cautiously because the animal may be more or less susceptible than a human to the teratogenic effect of a drug. For example, rats and mice are relatively insensitive to thalidomide, the prototype human teratogen. On the other hand, meclizine, an antiemetic available both with and without a prescription, is teratogenic in some strains of mice and rats, but appears to be safe for humans (38–40). Retrospective human studies are often inaccurate because of differences in the mothers' abilities to recall drug use during pregnancy. Data from prospective studies are difficult to interpret because of the need to follow a very large number of subjects.

Drug use during pregnancy is very common. A prospective study of 186 women found that the average number of drug products used during pregnancy was 11.0 (41). Another study of drug use in the last trimester of pregnancy found that each woman took an average of 8.7 drugs (42). An average of 6.9 (80%) of these were taken without the supervision or knowledge of a physician. The drugs most commonly taken by the women were prenatal vitamins (86%), aspirin (69%), and antacids (60%). Although recent data from the United States are lacking, surveys from other countries indicate a substantial decline in drug use during pregnancy over the last two decades (43).

Management of the Pregnant Patient

Several factors are important in determining whether a drug taken by a pregnant woman will produce an adverse effect in the fetus (40). The ability of the drug to pass from maternal circulation via the placenta to fetal circulation and the stage of pregnancy are important factors in determining teratogenic susceptibility. The first trimester, when organogenesis occurs, is the period of greatest teratogenic susceptibility for the embryo and is the critical period for induction of major anatomical malformations. However, exposure at other periods of gestation may be no less important because the exact critical period is dependent upon the specific drug in question.

Generally, it is prudent to avoid the use of any drug during pregnancy. Evidence of teratogenicity has even implicated products such as aspirin. Aspirin is available in a variety of prescription and nonprescription drugs and is frequently taken during pregnancy. Conflicting data are available on the teratogenicity of aspirin (40, 44). Although animal studies and retrospective studies in humans have found aspirin to be teratogenic, prospective human studies have not found a difference in malformation rates between infants exposed to aspirin in utero and those not exposed. Similarly, there are conflicting reports on the relationship between prenatal use of aspirin and the incidence of stillbirths, neonatal deaths, or reduced birth weight. Use of aspirin late in the pregnancy has been associated with increases in the length of gestation and in the duration of labor (45). These effects are related to inhibition of prostaglandin synthesis by aspirin. In addition, because of aspirin's effect on platelet function, perinatal aspirin ingestion has been found to increase the incidence of hemorrhage in both the pregnant woman and the newborn during and following delivery (45–48). Therefore, aspirin should be avoided, if possible, during the last trimester. Because acetaminophen is generally considered safe for use in pregnancy, it is the nonprescription drug of choice for antipyresis and analgesia, when taken in standard therapeutic doses (49). (See Chapter 5, *Internal Analgesic Products.*)

Although caffeine has been implicated as a potential teratogen in animals (50–53), studies in humans have not found caffeine to be teratogenic (54, 55). Although pregnant women do not necessarily need to eliminate caffeine from their diets, they might be wise to moderate their caffeine intake. Caffeine is found in coffee, tea, cola drinks, some other soft drinks, cocoa, and chocolate. Caffeine is also in many nonprescription drugs such as headache, cold, allergy, and stimulant drugs, as well as in prescription drugs. (See Chapter 10, *Sleep Aid and Stimulant Products.*)

A possible link between the use of nonprescription vaginal spermicides and the birth of infants with congenital disorders has been reported (56). However, weaknesses in these studies, as well as subsequent negative reports, seem to suggest that teratogenicity is not caused by these spermicides (57, 58). (See Chapter 25, *Contraceptive Methods and Products.*) Cigarette smoking and alcohol have also been associated with increased risk to the fetus and congenital abnormalities (59–62).

A variety of widely used agents that were not considered teratogenic in the past has the potential to adversely affect the fetus. The decision to suggest a drug must be based on an up-to-date knowledge of the literature and a very critical risk-to-benefit evaluation of both the mother and the fetus.

The assessment and management of the pregnant patient require observation of the following principles:

- Be alert to the possibility of pregnancy in women of child-bearing age who have certain key symptoms of early pregnancy, such as nausea, vomiting, and frequent urination. Any woman of child-bearing age could be pregnant. If so, she should be warned "Don't take this drug if you're pregnant."

- Advise the pregnant patient to avoid using drugs, in general, at any stage of pregnancy.

- Advise the pregnant patient to increase her reliance on nondrug modalities as treatment alternatives.

For example, the first approach to nausea and vomiting should be eating small, frequent meals and avoiding foods, smells, or situations that cause vomiting (63). Next, taking an effervescent glucose or buffered carbohydrate solution may be effective. (See Chapter 12, *Emetic and Antiemetic Products.*) Only if these measures are ineffective should an antihistamine or antiemetic be considered. The patient should be referred to a physician for certain problems that carry increased risk of poor outcomes in pregnancy (e.g., high blood pressure, vaginal bleeding, urinary tract infections, rapid weight gain, or edema).

The pharmacist can aid the self-medicating woman in deciding which drug or nondrug modalities to consider and when self-medication may be harmful to her or her unborn child.

The Nursing Mother

Drug use while breast-feeding could cause an adverse effect in the infant. The concentration of a drug in the milk depends on a number of factors, including the concentration of the drug in the mother's blood; the drug's molecular weight, lipid solubility, degree of ionization, and degree of binding to plasma and milk proteins; and the active secretion of the drug into the milk. Other important considerations include the relationship between the time of taking a drug and the time of a breast-feeding, as well as the drug's potential for causing toxicity in infants.

When taken in therapeutic dosages, most drugs are not present in breast milk in sufficient amounts to significantly harm the infant. However, a number of drugs are contraindicated for use while breast-feeding. A number of other drugs should be used cautiously by nursing mothers.

When advising a nursing mother on self-medication, the pharmacist should decide if the drug is really necessary, recommend the safest drug (e.g., acetaminophen instead of aspirin), and advise the mother to take the medication just after a breast-feeding or just before the infant's lengthy sleep periods (64). For drugs that present a risk to the infant (e.g., aspirin), the blood concentration of the drug in the nursing infant should be measured, if possible.

The American Academy of Pediatrics Committee on Drugs recently published a statement on drugs in human milk (64). Of the nonprescription drugs included in the statement, aspirin and other salicylates are the only ones that were considered to have had significant effects on some nursing infants and that should be taken by nursing mothers with caution. Nonprescription drugs usually considered compatible with breast-feeding include acetaminophen, ibuprofen, pseudoephedrine, triprolidine, cascara, danthron, senna, vitamins, and fluorides. The amount of caffeine in caffeine-containing beverages is not harmful, but higher doses could cause irritability and poor sleep patterns in infants. There are a large number of nonprescription drugs for which data on their transfer into breast milk and their possible clinical effects are not available. (See discussion on breast-feeding in Chapter 18, *Infant Formula Products.*)

SUMMARY

Nonprescription drugs are an important component of the health care system. Properly used, these products can relieve minor physical complaints of patients and permit physicians to concentrate on more serious illnesses.

If used improperly, nonprescription drugs can create a multitude of problems. Many people diagnose their symptoms, select a nonprescription product, and monitor their therapeutic response. As pharmacists continue to expand their patient counseling services and people learn of these services, they will seek the assistance of pharmacists whenever they are in doubt about self-medication.

To be of greatest service to patients, pharmacists must continually update their therapeutic knowledge and improve their interpersonal communication skills. The result will be better-informed patients, who will not only use the professional services of pharmacists but also recognize the contributions of pharmacists to health care.

REFERENCES

1   M. Montagne and B. Bleidt, *U.S. Pharmacist*, *14*, 53 (1988).

2   *Drug Topics*, *133 (8)*, 32 (1989).

3   D. A. Knapp and R. S. Beardsley, *Am. Pharm.*, NS19, 37 (1979).

4   D. E. Knapp et al., *Med. Market. Media*, *10*, 28 (1975).

5   *J. NARD*, *10*, 22–23 (1980).

6   "The Schering Report I. Pharmacists and Consumers. A Fresh Look from Both Sides of the Counter," Schering Laboratories, Kenilworth, N.J., 1979.

7   H. A. Monsanto and H. L. Mason, *Drug Intell. Clin. Pharm.*, *23*, 218 (1989).

8   "The Schering Report VI. Agenda for the Future. A Look at Some Key Issues Confronting Pharmacists," Schering Laboratories, Kenilworth, N.J., 1984.

9   J. J. Wroblewski, *Drug Topics*, *126*, 45 (1982).

10   K. Gannon, *Drug Topics*, *133*, 28 (1989).

11   L. A. Morris and S. R. Moore, *Am. Pharm.*, NS23, 21 (1983).

12   D. R. Miller and T. P. Foster, *Drug Intell. Clin. Pharm.*, *19*, 140 (1985).

13   N. V. Carroll and J. P. Gagnon, *Drug Intell. Clin. Pharm.*, *17*, 648 (1983).

14   M. M. Werler et al., *Am. J. Epidemiol.*, *129*, 415 (1989).

15   T. R. Covington, oral presentation at the 120th Annual Meeting of the American Pharmaceutical Association, Academy of General Practice, Boston, Mass., July 23, 1973.

16   H. R. Manasse et al., *Am. Pharm.*, NS23, 24 (1983).

17   B. J. Andrew, *Am. J. Pharm. Ed.*, *37*, 290 (1973).

18   B. M. Korsch et al., *Pediatrics*, *42*, 855 (1968).

19   V. Francis et al., *N. Engl. J. Med.*, *280*, 535 (1969).

20   A. F. Shaughnessy, *Am. Pharm.*, NS28, 38 (1988).

21   P. W. Keys and M. J. Manolios, *Drug Intell. Clin. Pharm.*, *32*, 828 (1975).

22 P. L. Ranelli, *Soc. Sci. Med.*, *13A*, 733 (1979).

23 M. R. DiMatteo et al., *Med. Care*, *18*, 376 (1980).

24 G. Chermak and M. Jinks, *Drug Intell. Clin. Pharm.*, *15*, 377 (1981).

25 D. L. Smith, "Medication Guide for Patient Counseling," Lea and Febiger, Philadelphia, Pa., 1977, pp. 1–25.

26 D. Epstein, *Drug Topics*, *132*, 15 (1988).

27 R. E. Vestal, *Drugs*, *16*, 358 (1978).

28 D. P. Richey and A. D. Bender, *Ann. Rev. Pharmacol. Toxicol.*, *17*, 49 (1977).

29 P. P. Lamy and R. E. Vestal, *Hosp. Prac.*, *11*, 111 (1976).

30 P. O. Morselli, *Clin. Pharmacokinet.*, *1*, 81 (1976).

31 G. Udkow, *Am. J. Dis. Child.*, *132*, 1025 (1978).

32 A. Rane and J. T. Wilson, *Clin. Pharmacokinet.*, *1*, 2 (1976).

33 F. L. Willington, *Geriatrics*, *35*, 41 (1980).

34 M. E. Meyer and H. H. Schuna, *Drug Intell. Clin. Pharm.*, *23*, 171 (1989).

35 T. H. Shepard, *Curr. Prob. Ped.*, *10*, 5 (1979).

36 *Federal Register*, *44*, 37434 (1980).

37 *Federal Register*, *45*, 32550 (1980).

38 J. F. Tourville, *Hosp. Pharm.*, *12*, 386 (1977).

39 L. Millcovich and B. J. VanDenBerg, *Am. J. Obstet. Gynecol.*, *125*, 244 (1976).

40 D. P. Hays, *Drug Intell. Clin. Pharm.*, *15*, 542 (1981).

41 P. L. Doering and R. B. Stewart, *J. Am. Med. Assoc.*, *239*, 843 (1978).

42 W. A. Blyer et al., *J. Am. Med. Assoc.*, *213*, 2046 (1970).

43 P. C. Rubin et al., *Br. Med. J.*, *292*, 614 (1986).

44 D. G. Corby, *Pediatrics*, *62* (suppl.), 930 (1978).

45 R. B. Lewis and J. D. Schulman, *Lancet*, *2*, 1159 (1973).

46 E. Colins and G. Turner, *Lancet*, *2*, 335 (1975).

47 W. A. Bleyer and R. T. Breckenridge, *J. Am. Med. Assoc.*, *213*, 2049 (1970).

48 R. R. Haslman et al., *J. Ped.*, *84*, 556 (1974).

49 H. Niederhoff and H. P. Zahradnik, *Amer. J. Med.*, Symposium #5A, 117 (1983).

50 FDA Executive Director Regional Office Talk Paper, January 18, 1980.

51 J. E. Goyan, Health and Human Services news release, September 4, 1980.

52 *FDA Drug Bull.*, *11*, 19 (1980).

53 P. W. Weathersbee et al., *Postgrad. Med.*, *62*, 64 (1977).

54 S. Linn et al., *N. Engl. J. Med.*, *306*, 141 (1982).

55 V. A. Szucs-Myers and L. J. Mirva, *Drug. Intell. Clin. Pharm.*, *22*, 614 (1988).

56 H. Jick et al., *J. Am. Med. Assoc.*, *245*, 1329 (1981).

57 S. Shapiro et al., *J. Am. Med. Assoc.*, *247*, 2381, (1982).

58 J. L. Mills et al., *J. Am. Med. Assoc.*, *248*, 2148 (1982).

59 American Academy of Pediatrics Committee on Environmental Hazard, *Pediatrics*, *57*, 411 (1976).

60 J. E. Fielding, *N. Engl. J. Med.*, *298*, 337 (1978).

61 S. K. Clarren and D. W. Smith, *N. Engl. J. Med.*, *298*, 1063 (1978).

62 S. E. Shaywitz et al., *J. Ped.*, *96*, 978 (1980).

63 J. S. G. Biggs and J. A. Allan, *Drugs*, *21*, 69 (1981).

64 American Academy of Pediatrics Committee on Drugs, *Pediatrics*, *84*, 924 (1989).

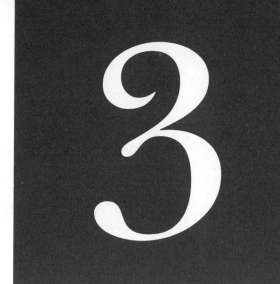

William E. Gilbertson

THE FDA'S OTC DRUG REVIEW

Over-the-counter (OTC) drugs play an increasingly vital role in America's health care system. Today, 6 out of every 10 medications bought by the consumer are OTC drugs. Consumers have developed a "take-charge" attitude toward their own health care. Aided by recently marketed OTC medical devices, they often diagnose the condition and then monitor the treatment progress. For example, home test kits that detect hidden blood in the stool can be useful in diagnosing colitis or colon cancer. Compounding this self-treatment trend is the expanding availability of OTC drugs that have been reclassified from prescription status; these drugs provide the consumer with even greater choices. (See Chapter 1, *The Self-Care Movement*.)

Historically, OTC drugs have been used to treat symptoms of minor discomfort, illness, or injury. Examples include taking an analgesic tablet for a headache, applying a first-aid preparation to a skinned knee, taking a cough suppressant to soothe a nagging cough accompanying a cold, and even using antiperspirants (which are considered drugs because they affect a body function) to prevent excessive underarm wetness. However, some OTC drugs contain prophylactic ingredients that are also capable of treating and curing certain minor conditions. For example, an antifungal agent is capable of curing the fungal infection of athlete's foot.

Obviously, self-medication should include only drugs proven safe and effective, but how can a consumer or pharmacist be sure that all OTC medications—especially those products that have been marketed for many years before the current laws requiring clinical proof of safety and effectiveness—will work as claimed in the labeling? In an effort to assure consumers that all OTC drugs are safe and effective, the Food and Drug Administration (FDA) has been conducting a massive review of the active ingredients in OTC drug

products to ensure that they contain safe and effective ingredients and bear fully informative labeling. This intensive review was initiated in 1972.

BACKGROUND AND STRUCTURE OF THE OTC DRUG REVIEW

Safety, effectiveness, and proper labeling have not always been characteristic of medications used in the United States. The first major federal legislation regulating drugs was the Pure Food and Drugs Act of 1906. "Unsafe" and "nonefficacious" drug products were not prohibited by the statute; drugs were required only to meet standards of strength and purity claimed by manufacturers. Drug safety was not required by law until the passage of the 1938 Federal Food, Drug, and

Editor's Note: The terms "over-the-counter drugs" and "nonprescription drugs" are virtually synonymous. APhA prefers the term "nonprescription" as more accurate and consistent (i.e., with the comparison term "prescription-legend"). However, the terms "over-the-counter" and "OTC" have been used routinely by the FDA in referring to its massive review of this class of drugs and are used in this chapter. In the remaining chapters of this edition of the *Handbook*, "over-the-counter" and "OTC" are used only when reference is made to the FDA's review project or its component elements.

With just a few exceptions (e.g., infant formulas, suntan products, diaper rash products), the terms "patient" and "consumer" are generally interchangeable in the discussion of nonprescription drug selection and use. Although APhA's preference is to use "patient"—to emphasize the health care thrust of the pharmacist's role in dispensing such products—the FDA's preference is to use "consumer"; hence, this latter term is used consistently in this chapter.

Cosmetic Act (the Act). Legislation for a new law had been under consideration since 1933, and one factor speeding final passage was the deaths of more than 100 individuals, many of them children, who used elixir of sulfanilamide containing ethylene glycol, a toxic solvent, as the vehicle. The 1938 law required that all new drugs be proven safe for human use before they could be marketed.

The 1962 Drug Amendments to the Act required that all drugs also be shown to be effective for their intended uses. This legislation required the FDA to review the effectiveness of the 4,500 new drug products, including 512 OTC drugs, that since 1938 had been approved for safety. In the mid-1960s, the FDA reviewed 4,000 prescription drugs through the National Academy of Sciences/National Research Council (NAS/NRC) review, followed by an FDA implementation procedure called the Drug Efficacy Study Implementation (DESI). As the DESI review was nearing completion, clearly it was time for the FDA to take a further look at the OTC drug marketplace.

More than 300,000 individual OTC drug products are marketed, but according to labeling claims, these products contain only about 700 active ingredients. The number of individual products may seem large because each manufacturer's or distributor's labeled product is considered a separately marketed drug product. In determining the logistics of the review, the FDA decided that a product-by-product review would not be feasible because of the sheer volume of OTC pharmaceuticals. Practicality dictated a review that focused on the ingredients used in these products, subdivided by therapeutic category (see Table 1). For example, instead of examining individual antacid products, of which there are estimated to be more than 8,000, the FDA evaluated only the active ingredients, such as aluminum hydroxide and magnesium carbonate. Because it is an ingredient process, the FDA's OTC drug review is vastly different from that applied to prescription drugs, which evaluates finished dosage forms.

The Advisory Panel Review

The OTC drug review is a three-phase rulemaking process (each phase requiring a *Federal Register* publication) culminating in the establishment of standards (monographs or nonmonographs) for each OTC therapeutic drug category (see Figure 1). The first phase was accomplished by advisory review panels, each of which included as voting members a pharmacist, a pharmacologist or toxicologist, physicians and other scientifically qualified individuals, and nonvoting technical liaison members representing consumer and industry

interests. The panels were charged with reviewing the ingredients in OTC drug products to determine whether these ingredients could be generally recognized as safe and effective for use in self-treatment. They were also charged with reviewing claims and recommending appropriate labeling, including therapeutic indications, dosage instructions, and warnings about side effects and potential misuse.

According to the terms of the review, the panels classified ingredients in three categories as follows:

- Category I—generally recognized as safe and effective for the claimed therapeutic indication;

- Category II—not generally recognized as safe and effective or unacceptable indications;

- Category III—insufficient data available to permit final classification.

The panel phase of the OTC drug review extended for almost 10 years, with more than 300 individuals participating in this unprecedented project. Between 1972 and 1981, an initial determination was made on the safety and effectiveness of more than 700 ingredients for therapeutic claims ranging from antiflatulent to antimicrobial and from hair restorer to pinworm remedy. These findings were based on a review of 14,000 volumes of data submitted largely by manufacturers but also by consumers, pharmacists, and other interested parties. The panels also based their judgments on their members' own clinical experience and expertise, on marketing experience of ingredients, and on controlled and uncontrolled clinical trials. The panels also relied heavily on the published literature. Isolated case reports, random experience, testimonials, and reports lacking sufficient details to permit scientific evaluation were not considered.

The FDA received 58 reports from the panels. These reports and proposed monographs, summarizing the panels' recommendations to the Commissioner of Food and Drugs, were published as advance notices of proposed rulemaking (ANPRs) in the *Federal Register*. Each publication invited public comment.

FDA's Review and Proposal

The second phase of the OTC drug review is the FDA's evaluation of the panels' findings, based on public comment and on new data that may have become available. The agency then publishes its tentative conclusions as a proposed rule (tentative final monograph). This document offers the first clear signal of the agency's ultimate intentions. After the publication of the tentative final monograph, a period of time is allotted

TABLE 1 Product categories by which FDA is reviewing OTC ingredients

Acne
Anorectal
Antacid
Anthelmintic
Anticaries
Antidiarrheal
Antiemetic
Antiflatulent
Antifungal
   Diaper rash[a]
Antimicrobials
   Alcohol (topical)
   Antibiotics (first aid)
   Antiseptics (topical)
   Diaper rash[a]
   Mercurials
Antiperspirant
Aphrodisiac
Benign prostatic hypertrophy
Boil ointments
Camphorated oil
Cholecystokinetic
Corn and callus remover
Cough/cold/allergy/bronchodilator/antiasthmatic
combinations
   Anticholinergic
   Antihistamine
   Antitussive
   Bronchodilator
   Expectorant
   Nasal decongestant
Dandruff/seborrhea/psoriasis
Daytime sedative
Deodorants (internal)
Digestive aids
Exocrine pancreatic insufficiency
External analgesic
   Astringents (wet dressings)[b]
   Diaper rash[a]
   Fever blister/cold sore (external)[b]
   Insect bites and stings
   Male genital desensitizers
   Poison (ivy/oak/sumac) treatment/prevention[b]

Fever blister/cold sore (internal)
Hair grower/loss
Hexachlorophene
Hormone (topical)
Hypo/hyperphosphatemia
Ingrown toenail relief
Insect repellents (internal)
Internal analgesic
   Leg muscle cramps
Laxative
Menstrual
Nailbiting/thumbsucking deterrent
Nighttime sleep aid
Ophthalmic
Oral health care
Oral mucosal injury
Overindulgence remedies
   Ingredients intended to minimize or
   prevent inebriation
Pediculicides
Poison treatment
   Antidotes—toxic ingestion
   Emetic
Relief of oral discomfort
Salicylanilides (TBS)
Skin bleaching
Skin protectant
   Astringents (wet dressings)[b]
   Diaper rash[a]
   Fever blister/cold sore (external)[b]
   Insect bites and stings[b]
   Poison (ivy/oak/sumac) treatment/prevention[b]
Smoking deterrent
Stimulant
Stomach acidifier
Sunscreen
Sweet spirits of nitre
Topical otic (earwax)
Topical otic (swimmer's ear)
Vaginal contraceptive
Vaginal drug
Vitamin/mineral
Wart remover
Weight control

[a] See also: Antimicrobials, external analgesics, and skin protectants
[b] See also: Skin protectants

for objections or for requests for a hearing before the Commissioner of Food and Drugs; new data may also be submitted during this period. This is a lengthy but necessary public process, involving both scientific and legal forces. After carefully considering objections and new data and after processing hearing requests, the agency

issues a final rule, usually in the form of a final monograph. Other final regulations, sometimes referred to as nonmonographs (where data are insufficient to establish any ingredients in a monograph), are also developed. These regulations describe ingredients and therapeutic claims that cannot lawfully be marketed.

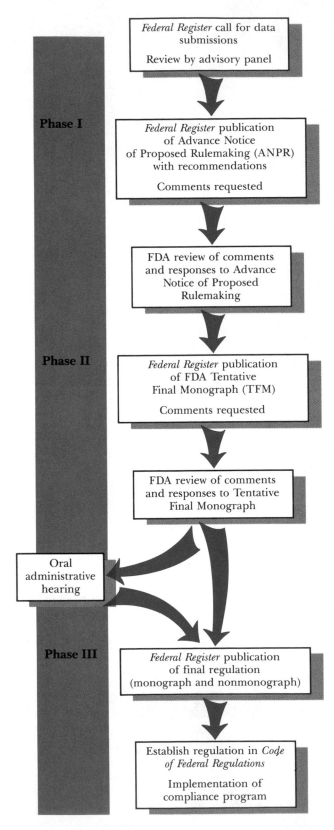

Phase I

Federal Register call for data submissions

Review by advisory panel

Federal Register publication of Advance Notice of Proposed Rulemaking (ANPR) with recommendations

Comments requested

FDA review of comments and responses to Advance Notice of Proposed Rulemaking

Phase II

Federal Register publication of FDA Tentative Final Monograph (TFM)

Comments requested

FDA review of comments and responses to Tentative Final Monograph

Oral administrative hearing

Phase III

Federal Register publication of final regulation (monograph and nonmonograph)

Establish regulation in *Code of Federal Regulations*

Implementation of compliance program

FIGURE 1 FDA's OTC drug review process.

Establishment of OTC Drug Monographs

The publication of final regulations is the third and last phase of the review process; many of the chapters of this handbook are based on information described in final monographs. Marketing preclearance of OTC drug products by the FDA is not required if these standards are met because the monographs represent the regulatory standards for the marketing of OTC drug products not covered by new drug applications (NDAs). Each final monograph will be included annually in the *Code of Federal Regulations* (CFR). Usually, monographs become effective 1 year after publication in the *Federal Register*; after that date, affected OTC drug products must meet the monograph specifications. The FDA's compliance program ensures that the applicable products conform with the regulation.

After the last OTC drug monograph is published in final form, new conditions that are not specified in the final regulations, including ingredients, combinations of ingredients, indications, and labeling, will still need to be reviewed. Manufacturers have two approaches to gain marketing clearance: submit supportive data in the form of a petition to amend a final monograph to include the new marketing conditions, or submit an NDA for OTC use.

Monographs contain the following components: reference to general provisions, active ingredients, and labeling. In some cases, procedures for testing the final dosage form may be included.

General Provisions

The general provision section specifies pertinent regulations detailing required conditions that are common to all OTC drug categories, such as manufacturing practices and drug registration. It also encompasses inactive ingredients, requiring suitable ingredients that are safe and do not interfere with the effectiveness of the formulation or with tests to be performed on the final product. Color additives may be used only in accordance with certain other provisions of the Act.

Although the Act requires only the labeling of the active ingredients in OTC drug products, the Nonprescription Drug Manufacturers Association has adopted a voluntary labeling program to identify the inactive ingredients used in medications. Although inactive ingredients have a history of safe use, a small percentage of people are sensitive to particular substances. This voluntary program enables consumers to identify the presence of substances to which they are allergic.

The general provision section contains labeling requirements such as all OTC drug labeling must contain the general warning: "Keep this and all drugs out of the reach of children."

Another general warning for pregnant and nursing mothers is required on all but a few exempted drugs. The warning is "As with any drug, if you are pregnant or nursing a baby, seek the advice of a health professional before using this product."

Active Ingredients

The monograph identifies the active ingredients that can be used in specific OTC drug products; it also identifies ingredients that may be combined with other active ingredients, not only from the same monograph (drug category) but also from other monographs. An example of the latter would be the combination of an antacid with an analgesic. In this case, combinations of specific antacid and analgesic ingredients judged to be safe and effective are identified under the pertinent subsections of each monograph. Stipulations are also set forth on the number of active ingredients that may be combined in one product.

Labeling

The labeling section contains the indications for the product; warnings against misuse, including drug interaction precautions; directions for use, including the time interval (frequency) and dosage for specific age groups; and any specialized labeling. A monograph may also contain professional labeling; that is, labeling provided to health professionals but not to the general public. For example, professional labeling indicates that aspirin may reduce the risk of myocardial infarct and that antacid may be used in ulcer therapy.

Testing Procedures

The monograph identifies any testing of a finished dosage form that is necessary before the product is marketed. For example, a battery of acid neutralization tests is now required for all antacid products because the agency has finalized the monograph for this class of drugs. Each antacid ingredient must be included in the product at a level that contributes at least 25% of the total acid-neutralizing capacity of the product, and the finished product must contain at least 5 mEq of acid-neutralizing capacity and result in a pH of 3.5 or greater at the end of the 10-minute test period.

Another example of required testing is the demonstration of the bioavailability of fluoride ions in fluoride dentifrices. Biological tests such as enamel solubility reduction, fluoride uptake by enamel, and animal caries reduction are conducted to ensure the anticaries effectiveness of such products. Manufacturers must ensure that their fluoride dentifrice formulations demonstrate the bioavailability of the fluoride in two of the three biological tests.

Establishment of Nonmonographs

Occasionally, the publication of the final regulation results in a nonmonograph rather than a monograph regulation. These nonmonographs also appear in the CFR. The nonmonograph regulation may occur when an ingredient or a particular product provides insignificant benefits when compared with the risk from use. For example, zirconium, once widely used in aerosol antiperspirants, was removed from aerosol drug and cosmetic products because of the potential for particulate zirconium to cause granuloma formation in the lungs. A lack of toxicologic data adequate to establish a safe level for use led the agency to conclude that because safer alternative aerosol antiperspirant ingredients are available, the adverse benefit-to-risk ratio precluded the use of zirconium in aerosolized products.

A nonmonograph regulation may also occur when OTC marketing of a particular ingredient or product is potentially hazardous. For example, camphorated oil, marketed primarily as a topical counterirritant or liniment, was often mistaken for castor oil, cod liver oil, mineral oil, olive oil, cough medicine, or other drug products. The OTC marketing of these drug products resulted in a large number of accidental ingestions of camphorated oil; toxicity often resulted from ingestion, primarily in infants and young children. Therefore, because of the potential hazard of poisoning, the benefit of using such products was judged insignificant when compared with the risk. The decision to remove camphorated oil from the OTC market was largely attributable to the efforts of a New Jersey pharmacist who for several years collected statistics on camphorated oil poisoning from poison control centers and pediatricians throughout the United States.

Atropine sulfate and all other active ingredients considered for use as anticholinergics in cough and cold products to relieve excessive secretions of the nose and eyes have been determined by the agency to be not effective for inclusion in an OTC drug monograph. The agency stated in the tentative final monograph that there was a lack of adequate studies available to support the continued use of these ingredients. In response to the tentative final monograph, no substantive data were received that would have allowed any anticholinergic ingredient to be upgraded to Category I. As a result of inadequate data, the nonmonograph was established.

The FDA has also determined that none of the ingredients marketed in OTC drug products to promote hair growth and prevent hair loss are generally recognized as safe and effective. Through all three stages of the rulemaking process, these ingredients remained in nonmonograph status. In spite of considerable public response, mostly as consumer complaints, the FDA concluded that the labeling claims are either false, misleading, or unsupported by scientific data.

Drugs Reclassified from Prescription to OTC Marketing Status

Perhaps the most significant unanticipated outcome of the OTC drug review has been the reclassification ("switching") of prescription drug products. Nearly 30 drugs (and many more drug products) have been reclassified as OTC since the review began (e.g., pyrantel pamoate and hydrocortisone). This reclassification of drugs to OTC status is seen by many as an effective means of providing consumers with more effective medications and curtailing the high cost of our health care system. Pharmacists should find many new opportunities with this expanding segment of the OTC marketplace. (See Chapter 1, *The Self-Care Movement*, and Chapter 2, *Patient Assessment and Consultation*.)

Criteria for Reclassification

Until 1951, federal laws did not contain a criterion for determining whether a drug should be limited to prescription use. This decision was left to the manufacturer; therefore, different manufacturers made different decisions about the same drug formulations, leading to confusion among manufacturers, regulators, and health professionals. There were questions about FDA's authority to limit drug prescribing to physicians. To end the confusion, Congress enacted an amendment (introduced by two pharmacists, Representative Durham and Senator Humphrey) to the basic law, which specified three classes of drugs that were required to be limited to prescription use:

- Certain habit-forming drugs listed by name in the Act;

- Drugs not safe for use except under the supervision of a licensed practitioner because of toxicity or other potentiality for harmful effect, the method of use, or the collateral measures necessary to use;

- Drugs limited to prescription under an NDA.

These statutory definitions are still the principal criteria for prescription/OTC classification. In considering reclassification, the second criterion is probably the most essential and worthy of close examination. The assessment of the overall margin of safety includes not only those considerations described in the statute (toxicity, potential for harmful effects, and collateral measures necessary to use) but also abuse and misuse potential and a favorable benefit-to-risk ratio.

Certain drugs that are needed to treat serious disease conditions may cause adverse side effects. These drugs must be carefully used to achieve the appropriate level of effectiveness without endangering the patient's safety; they are too toxic for OTC marketing and will continue to be classified as prescription drugs. On the other hand, almost any drug can be misused with some toxic result; the possibility that a drug can be misused is not a sufficient basis for a prescription classification. Because all drugs have both benefits and risks, some degree of risk must be tolerated to receive the benefits of the drug. For example, antihistamine drugs may cause drowsiness, but consumers can be informed of the risks through adequate labeling.

It is difficult to set exacting standards or reclassification criteria because many factors must be carefully considered, as illustrated in Figure 2. The classification must be judgmental, based on the various factors related to each drug's use. In contrast, some drugs have been limited to prescription use because of concerns of adverse effects with intentional misuse—not because the drug is believed to be inherently toxic—as with amyl nitrite, now a prescription drug.

The collateral measures necessary to use a drug can be many and varied; for example, the continued safe use of a drug may require routine medical examinations or laboratory work. One may believe that the prescription–OTC classification is dependent upon whether the condition being treated is self-diagnosable. Federal law does not require that a drug used for any condition that cannot be self-diagnosed must be placed on prescription status. Moreover, the FDA has not applied the law in this manner because numerous OTC drugs are currently marketed for conditions that are not susceptible to self-diagnosis by consumers. Insulin is the classic example because consumers cannot self-diagnose diabetes; the use of bronchodilators for the treatment of asthma is another example.

Mechanisms for Reclassification

The federal regulations provide three mechanisms for prescription exemptions: the switch regulation, supplemental NDA approval, and advisory panel recommendation.

The so-called "switch regulation" provides that drugs limited to prescription use under an NDA can be exempted from that limitation if the FDA determines that the prescription requirements are unnecessary for the protection of the public health. The regulation allows a proposal to exempt a drug from prescription status to be initiated by the FDA or by any interested person. Before the OTC drug review, which began in 1972, the FDA reclassified about 25 ingredients. The last reclassification under the regulation was in 1971 for tolnaftate.

A prescription drug that has an approved NDA can also be reclassified to OTC use through filing and approval of a supplemental NDA. Under this procedure, the FDA determines whether the drug previously limited under the terms of its NDA has now been shown to

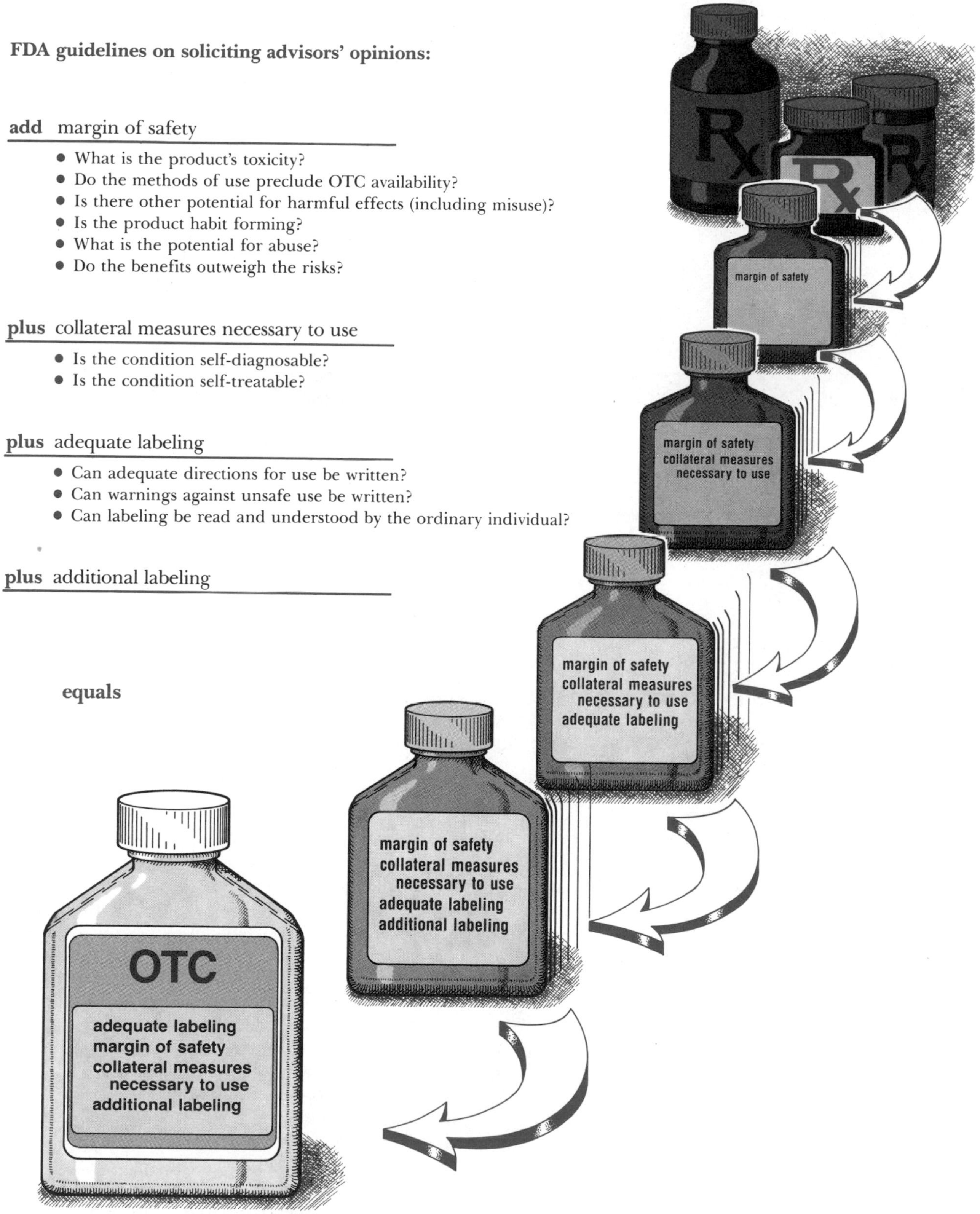
FDA guidelines on soliciting advisors' opinions:
add margin of safety
What is the product's toxicity?
Do the methods of use preclude OTC availability?
Is there other potential for harmful effects (including misuse)?
Is the product habit forming?
What is the potential for abuse?
Do the benefits outweigh the risks?
plus collateral measures necessary to use
Is the condition self-diagnosable?
Is the condition self-treatable?
plus adequate labeling
Can adequate directions for use be written?
Can warnings against unsafe use be written?
Can labeling be read and understood by the ordinary individual?
plus additional labeling
equals
Rx
margin of safety
margin of safety
collateral measures
necessary to use
margin of safety
collateral measures
necessary to use
adequate labeling
margin of safety
collateral measures
necessary to use
adequate labeling
additional labeling
OTC
adequate labeling
margin of safety
collateral measures
necessary to use
additional labeling

FIGURE 2 Reclassifying prescription drugs as OTC drugs.

| **TABLE 2**   Drug ingredients reclassified from prescription-to-OTC drug status |

Acidulated phosphate fluoride
Brompheniramine maleate
Chlorpheniramine maleate
Diphenhydramine hydrochloride
Diphenhydramine monocitrate
Doxylamine succinate
Dyclonine hydrochloride
Ephedrine sulfate
Epinephrine hydrochloride
Haloprogin
Hydrocortisone
Hydrocortisone acetate
Metaproterenol sulfate
Methoxyphenamine hydrochloride

Miconazole nitrate
Nystatin
Oxymetazoline hydrochloride
Phenylephrine hydrochloride
Phenyltoloxamine citrate
Promethazine hydrochloride
Pseudoephedrine hydrochloride
Pseudoephedrine sulfate
Pyrantel pamoate
Sodium fluoride
Stannous fluoride
Theophylline salts
Xylometazoline hydrochloride

be safe for OTC use.

Under either the switch regulation or the supplemental NDA approval, the reclassified drug product remains a "new drug" requiring premarket approval and periodic reports to the FDA.

Finally, under the OTC drug review system, the advisory panels were asked to make recommendations on any drugs that could be safely converted to OTC status. The OTC advisory panels recommended changing 27 ingredients from prescription use to OTC drug availability. The panels judged that the ingredients listed in Table 2 could be safely used by consumers in self-treatment without professional supervision.

Throughout the OTC drug review, the FDA encouraged manufacturers of drugs under consideration to reformulate and relabel their products to comply with panel recommendations before completion of the rulemaking proceeding. Therefore, the public receives the benefits of the review—the elimination of ingredients of questionable safety or effectiveness and the deletion of exaggerated labeling claims—before the issuance of final regulations, which often requires years of additional procedure to be completed. Such changes are permissible because the FDA has the discretion to withhold enforcement under the Act. Because these changes depend on enforcement policy, the FDA may issue a final monograph that requires manufacturers to abandon those changes and comply with different requirements. In 1975, the FDA issued an enforcement policy specifically directed to changes made in the marketing status of prescription drugs under consideration in the OTC drug review to include an opportunity for FDA review of such changes before they occurred. The status of these various active ingredients in the rulemaking process is shown in Tables 3 and 4.

Examples of Reclassification

Hydrocortisone   First included in the OTC external analgesic report of December 1979, hydrocortisone was recommended as a topical antipruritic at concentrations of 0.25–0.50%. With publication of the report, hydrocortisone was legally marketable as an OTC drug under the conditions of the proposed monograph. Even though the drug is currently dually marketable (i.e., prescription/OTC) at these strengths, the final monograph will provide a clear distinction—and ultimately a single channel of distribution for specific concentrations and indications.

Metaproterenol   In October 1982, the FDA proposed a monograph for OTC bronchodilator drug products. Included in this document was the agency's basic concurrence on the cough and cold panel's recommendations and the agency's own decision to classify the prescription drug metaproterenol sulfate in a metered-dose inhalation aerosol as a Category I drug. With that publication, immediate marketing was permitted. This was the first time that the FDA, on its own initiative, had recommended reclassifying the marketing status of a prescription drug in the context of the OTC drug review. Previous reclassifications had been recommended by advisory panels. After OTC marketing began in January 1983, the medical community voiced considerable criticism. By May, the FDA had received approximately 120 letters, some supporting the agency's actions, but many expressing concern about the drug's potential for misuse and inappropriate use by young children.

Before proposing the reclassification of metaproterenol, the agency carefully reviewed the safety and

TABLE 3 Prescription-to-OTC drug status appearing in FDA tentative final monographs

Tentative final monograph	Active ingredient(s)	Indication
Anorectal (published 8/15/88)	Epinephrine 0.005–0.01%	Vasoconstrictor
	Epinephrine hydrochloride 0.005–0.01%	Vasoconstrictor
	Phenylephrine hydrochloride 0.25%	Vasoconstrictor
	Ephedrine sulfate 0.1–1.25%	Vasoconstrictor
Anthelmintic (published 8/24/82)	Pyrantel pamoate (oral) 11 mg/kg	Anthelmintic (for pinworms)
Anticaries (published 9/30/85)	Sodium fluoride rinse 0.05%	Anticaries
	Stannous fluoride rinse 0.1%	Anticaries
	Stannous fluoride gel 0.4%	Anticaries
	Acidulated phosphate fluoride rinse 0.02% fluoride	Anticaries
Antiemetic (published 7/13/79)	Diphenhydramine hydrochloride (oral)[a] 25–50 mg	Antiemetic
Antihistamine (published 1/15/85)	Brompheniramine maleate (oral) 4 mg/4–6 hrs (adult) 2 mg/4–6 hrs (children 6 to under 12)	Antihistamine
	Chlorpheniramine maleate (oral) 4 mg/4–6 hrs (adult) 2 mg/4–6 hrs (children 6 to under 12)	Antihistamine
	Diphenhydramine hydrochloride (oral) 25–50 mg/4–6 hrs (adult) 12.5–25 mg/4–6 hrs (children 6 to under 12)	Antihistamine
	Dexbrompheniramine maleate (oral)[b,c] 2 mg/4–6 hrs (adult) 1 mg/4–6 hrs (children 6 to under 12)	Antihistamine
	Dexchlorpheniramine maleate (oral)[c,d] 2 mg/4–6 hrs (adult) 1 mg/4–6 hrs (children 6 to under 12)	Antihistamine
	Triprolidine hydrochloride (oral)[b,c] 2.5 mg/6–8 hrs (adult) 1.25 mg/6–8 hrs (children 6 to under 12)	Antihistamine
Antihistamine amendment (published 8/24/87)	Doxylamine succinate (oral) 7.5–12.5 mg/4–6 hrs (adult)	Antihistamine
Antitussive (published 10/19/83)	Benzonatate (oral)[e] 100 mg/4–6 hours	Antitussive
	Chlophedianol hydrochloride (oral)[f] 25 mg/6–8 hrs	Antitussive
Bronchodilator (published 10/26/82)	Metaproterenol sulfate inhalation[g] 1–2 inhalations, each containing 0.65 mg/3 hrs	Bronchodilator
Cold, cough, allergy, bronchodilator, and antiasthmatic combinations (published 8/12/88)	Promethazine hydrochloride (oral)[h] 6.25 mg/4–6 hrs (adult) 3.125 mg/4–6 hrs (children 6 to under 12)	Antihistamine combinations for relief of symptoms of common cold

(continued)

TABLE 3 *continued*

Tentative final monograph	Active ingredient(s)	Indication
Cholecystokinetic (proposed amendment of final monograph published 8/15/88)	Hydrogenated soybean oil[i]	Gallbladder diagnostic agent
External analgesic (published 2/8/83)	Hydrocortisone (topical) 0.25–0.5%	Antipruritic
	Hydrocortisone acetate (topical) 0.25–0.5%	Antipruritic
External analgesic amendment (published 7/30/86)	Hydrocortisone (topical) 0.25–0.5%	Antipruritic (add claims for seborrheic dermatitis and psoriasis)
	Hydrocortisone acetate (topical) 0.25–0.5%	Antipruritic (add claims for seborrheic dermatitis and psoriasis)
External analgesic amendment (published 8/25/88)	Hydrocortisone (topical) 0.25–0.5%	Antipruritic (for external anal itching; add warnings and directions)
	Hydrocortisone acetate (topical) 0.25–0.5%	Antipruritic (for external anal itching; add warnings and directions)
Nasal decongestant (published 1/15/85)	Oxymetazoline hydrochloride (topical) 0.05%	Nasal decongestant
	Pseudoephedrine hydrochloride (oral) 60 mg/4–6 hrs (adult) 30 mg/4–6 hrs (children 6 to under 12) 15 mg/4–6 hrs (children 2 to under 6)	Nasal decongestant
	Pseudoephedrine sulfate (oral) 60 mg/4–6 hrs (adult) 30 mg/4–6 hrs (children 6 to under 12) 15 mg/4–6 hrs (children 2 to under 6)	Nasal decongestant
	Xylometazoline hydrochloride (topical) 0.1% (adult) 0.05% (children 6 to under 12)	Nasal decongestant
Nighttime sleep aid (notice published on 4/23/82 after TFM published)	Diphenhydramine hydrochloride (50 mg) and diphenhydramine monocitrate (76 mg)	Nighttime sleep aid
Oral health care (published 1/27/88)	Dyclonine hydrochloride 0.05–0.10% solution or suspension, up to 4 times daily; 1–3 mg in a solid dosage form every 2 hours as needed	Anesthetic/analgesic

[a] Category III recommendation; OTC marketing permitted on 4/30/87.
[b] Previously marketed OTC under approved NDAs.
[c] Not considered by an OTC advisory review panel.
[d] OTC marketing not permitted until comments on proposal are evaluated.
[e] Comments evaluated; nonmonograph ingredient on 8/12/87; OTC marketing not permitted; may be marketed by prescription only.
[f] Comments evaluated; OTC marketing permitted on 8/12/87.
[g] The agency rescinded OTC marketing status on 6/3/83.
[h] OTC marketing proposed in combination only, but the agency rescinded OTC marketing status on 9/5/89.
[i] Comments evaluated; OTC marketing permitted on 2/28/89.

effectiveness record of the drug, which is a member of the same family of drugs as epinephrine. The agency pointed out that metaproterenol had a record of safe and effective use under an approved NDA for 9 years and that, based on a review of the adverse reaction reports for the drug while undergoing clinical studies and since being approved for marketing, the agency believed that the drug could be used OTC. To ensure the safe use of the drug, the agency proposed extensive labeling information.

By using the OTC rulemaking process, the agency provided an opportunity for public comment that is unavailable when approving an NDA or a supplemental NDA. However, because of the controversy that developed, in May 1983 a special meeting of the FDA's standing pulmonary–allergy drugs advisory committee was called in an effort to provide a public forum for discussion of this issue. Several individuals and professional organizations made formal presentations.

The complexity of the issue was apparent, and in voting to recommend that the FDA rescind its proposal to make metaproterenol an OTC drug, the committee did not reach a clear consensus but ultimately voted 4 to 3 in favor of recommending to the FDA that the drug be restricted to prescription status. The committee also believed that this issue merited further discussion. In the meantime, it has been concluded that products containing metaproterenol should be limited to prescription sales. Firms marketing these products have again limited them to prescription dispensing.

Ibuprofen Ibuprofen is a relatively recent new drug in the OTC analgesic armamentarium. It is available OTC via NDAs—not by monograph. The agency does not consider ibuprofen to be reclassified because the 200-mg strength currently available OTC was never marketed in the United States. Experience with ibuprofen marketed at prescription strengths (300, 400, 600, 800 mg) is pertinent but does not support the general recognition that the product can be used safely and effectively by the consumer alone.

Some have argued that there are enough public data to include ibuprofen in the monograph system. However, although the public availability of data is necessary to general recognition for purpose of the OTC review, it does not necessarily lead to general recognition among experts that a prescription drug is safe for OTC use. Published data relating primarily to the prescription strengths of ibuprofen were not regarded as sufficient to support general recognition. The FDA's arthritis advisory committee reviewed ibuprofen and recommended OTC status.

Even if it could be established that the 200-mg strength of ibuprofen had become generally recognized as safe and effective as a result of the investigations reported in the medical literature, the FDA has concluded that ibuprofen in that strength should be regarded as a new drug because it has not been used to a material extent and for a material time. A drug that has not been so used is not appropriately included in the monograph system.

TABLE 4 Prescription-to-OTC drug status appearing in FDA final rules

Final monograph	Active ingredient(s)	Indication
Anthelmintic (published 8/1/86)	Pyrantel pamoate (oral) 11 mg/kg	Anthelmintic (for pinworms)
Antiemetic (published 4/30/87)	Diphenhydramine hydrochloride (oral)[a] 25–50 mg	Antiemetic
Antitussive (published 8/12/87)	Chlophedianol hydrochloride (oral)[a] 25 mg/6–8 hrs (adult) 12.5 mg/6–8 hrs (children 6 to under 12)	Antitussive
	Benzonatate (oral)[b] 100 mg/4–6 hours	Antitussive
Cholecystokinetic amendment of final monograph (published 2/28/89)	Hydrogenated soybean oil[c]	Gallbladder diagnostic agent
Nighttime sleep aid (published 2/14/89)	Diphenhydramine hydrochloride (50 mg) and diphenhydramine citrate (76 mg)	Nighttime sleep aid

[a] OTC marketing permitted upon publication of final rule.
[b] Comments evaluated; OTC marketing not permitted; may be marketed by prescription only.
[c] Comments evaluated; OTC marketing permitted upon publication of final amendment of final monograph.

Promethazine The cough and cold panel classified promethazine hydrochloride in Category I as an OTC antihistamine. The agency dissented from the panel's classification in the preamble to the panel's 1976 report. The dissent was based in part on the degree of drowsiness produced by the ingredient and the possible adverse effects, such as extrapyramidal disturbances, that might occur, especially in children. In the 1985 antihistamine tentative final monograph, the agency stated that, based on additional data, concerns regarding the occurrence of extrapyramidal effects and the concern that children seem particularly liable to develop adverse central nervous system (CNS) reactions to promethazine had been adequately addressed. Therefore, at that time, the FDA did not believe that these possible adverse effects should preclude use of this ingredient at proposed OTC oral dosages. However, the agency placed single-ingredient products in Category III because of concerns that tardive dyskinesia, a rare but serious CNS reaction, might occur with prolonged use. The agency noted that the drug has not been used extensively on a long-term basis as a single ingredient for antihistamine, allergic rhinitis, or antiallergy use, and that consumers who use OTC antihistamines to treat such symptoms often use these products for a prolonged period. The agency also noted that use of promethazine as a prescription drug is primarily in combination products for short-term relief of acute cough and cold symptoms.

Subsequently, in a related 1988 tentative final monograph for OTC combination drug products, the agency proposed that cough–cold combination products containing promethazine hydrochloride be classified as Category I, used only for short-term (7 days) relief of symptoms of the common cold. By that action, OTC marketing for this limited use was permitted. Claims for use of these drug products in treating the symptoms of allergic rhinitis were specifically excluded from the labeling. However, based on new information, the agency received a citizen petition and letters from a number of physicians objecting to OTC drug status. The major concern expressed was the possibility that use in children under 2 years of age may be associated with the occurrence of sudden infant death syndrome (SIDS), and that OTC availability could dramatically increase overuse in children of this age. In response to these concerns, the FDA's pulmonary–allergy drugs advisory committee met to discuss these issues and evaluate the new information. By a vote of 7 to 1, the advisory committee recommended to the FDA that these drug products not be marketed OTC at this time. It should be noted that during this deliberation period the major drug manufacturer participated in the proceedings and responsibly did not market the product. Subsequent *Federal Register* notices announced that promethazine-containing combination drug products could not be marketed OTC at this time, but the FDA did reopen the record to allow additional information to be filed.

DRUG INFORMATION— LABELING AND ADVERTISING

Consumer Labeling

Obviously, the information in the labeling of a nonprescription product must be clearly presented. The OTC drug regulations require that labeling be stated in terms that are likely to be read and understood by the average consumer, including those of low comprehension, under customary conditions of purchase and use. In addition to evaluating the content of the labeling recommended by the panels, the agency also evaluates the language used to ensure that it is likely to be understandable to the consumer.

As a result of the OTC drug review, the labeling of every OTC drug product will be revised. A typical OTC drug product and the required labeling information are illustrated for a cough mixture in Figure 3.

Professional Labeling

Some monographs now contain professional labeling that provides to health professionals specific information not included in OTC drug labeling. The agency has proposed in the internal analgesic tentative final monograph, as part of professional labeling, the inclusion of the ingredient aspirin for "reducing the risk of recurrent transient ischemic attacks (TIAs) or stroke in men" and "to reduce the risk of death and/or nonfatal myocardial infarction in patients with a previous myocardial infarction or unstable angina pectoris." The agency's proposed changes, pending public response, will be implemented upon publication of the final monograph for these products. Obviously, consumers are aware of these uses from the news media, their physicians, and other sources. The agency considers it in the public interest to allow dissemination of this information before any final monograph.

What's on the label:

Product information for consumers, required or recommended by the U.S. Food and Drug Administration and OTC Advisory Review Panels for a typical nonprescription product

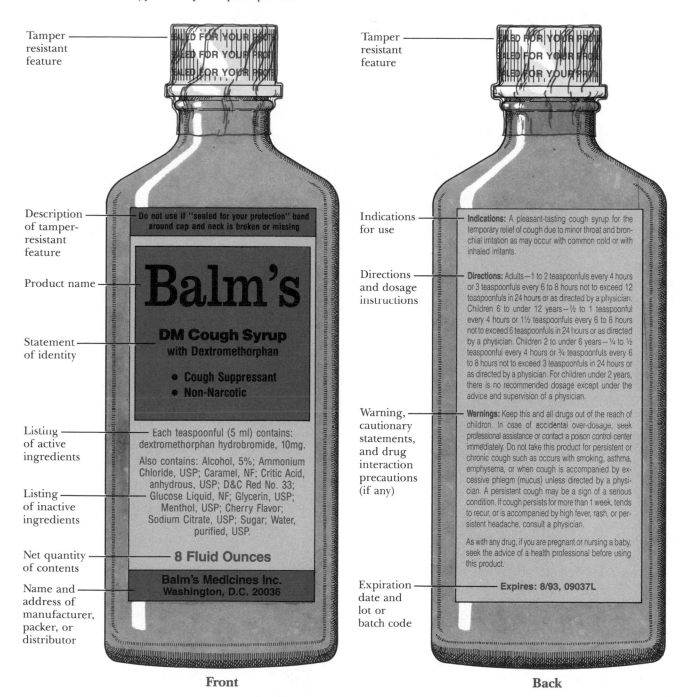

Tamper resistant feature

Description of tamper-resistant feature

Product name

Statement of identity

Listing of active ingredients

Listing of inactive ingredients

Net quantity of contents

Name and address of manufacturer, packer, or distributor

Do not use if "sealed for your protection" band around cap and neck is broken or missing

Balm's

DM Cough Syrup
with Dextromethorphan

- Cough Suppressant
- Non-Narcotic

Each teaspoonful (5 ml) contains: dextromethorphan hydrobromide, 10mg.

Also contains: Alcohol, 5%; Ammonium Chloride, USP; Caramel, NF; Critic Acid, anhydrous, USP; D&C Red No. 33; Glucose Liquid, NF; Glycerin, USP; Menthol, USP; Cherry Flavor; Sodium Citrate, USP; Sugar; Water, purified, USP.

8 Fluid Ounces

Balm's Medicines Inc.
Washington, D.C. 20036

Front

Tamper resistant feature

Indications for use

Directions and dosage instructions

Warning, cautionary statements, and drug interaction precautions (if any)

Expiration date and lot or batch code

Indications: A pleasant-tasting cough syrup for the temporary relief of cough due to minor throat and bronchial irritation as may occur with common cold or with inhaled irritants.

Directions: Adults—1 to 2 teaspoonfuls every 4 hours or 3 teaspoonfuls every 6 to 8 hours not to exceed 12 teaspoonfuls in 24 hours or as directed by a physician. Children 6 to under 12 years—½ to 1 teaspoonful every 4 hours or 1½ teaspoonfuls every 6 to 8 hours not to exceed 6 teaspoonfuls in 24 hours or as directed by a physician. Children 2 to under 6 years—¼ to ½ teaspoonful every 4 hours or ¾ teaspoonfuls every 6 to 8 hours not to exceed 3 teaspoonfuls in 24 hours or as directed by a physician. For children under 2 years, there is no recommended dosage except under the advice and supervision of a physician.

Warnings: Keep this and all drugs out of the reach of children. In case of accidental over-dosage, seek professional assistance or contact a poison control center immediately. Do not take this product for persistent or chronic cough such as occurs with smoking, asthma, emphysema, or when cough is accompanied by excessive phlegm (mucus) unless directed by a physician. A persistent cough may be a sign of a serious condition. If cough persists for more than 1 week, tends to recur, or is accompanied by high fever, rash, or persistent headache, consult a physician.

As with any drug, if you are pregnant or nursing a baby, seek the advice of a health professional before using this product.

Expires: 8/93, 09037L

Back

Whereas prescription drug labels for the patient carry minimal information, FDA requires that OTC labels be much more detailed so that consumers can properly use the products without the advice of a health professional.

FIGURE 3   Required labeling information on OTC drug products.

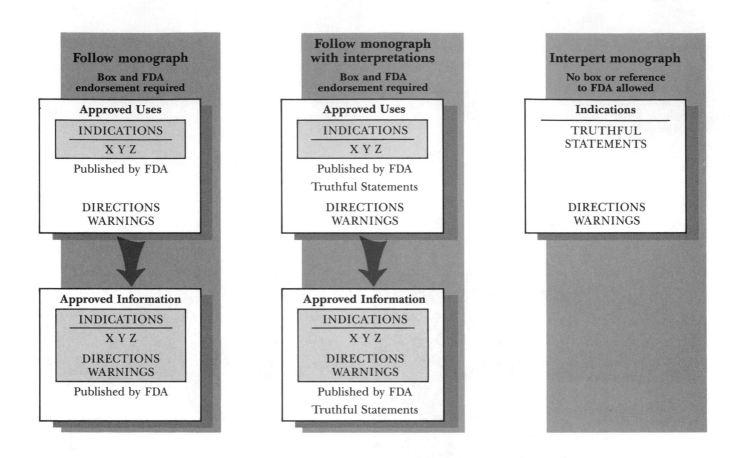

FIGURE 4   FDA's current policy as it relates to indications. Reprinted from *American Pharmacy, NS28 (11)*, 25 (1988).

Future Labeling

One heavily criticized policy of the OTC drug review was the agency's long-standing position that limited labeling terminology to the exact language developed and approved through the review process. This policy did not allow for synonymous terms or any variation in the labeling specified in the applicable drug monograph. The agency received many comments and objections on this "exclusivity policy," particularly regarding indications for use.

Because of the broad scope of this policy, the FDA conducted an open public forum at which interested parties presented their views. Manufacturers and trade associations contended that the exclusivity policy was unconstitutional because it unlawfully restrained free speech, was arbitrary and capricious, and was not authorized by the Act. Consumer groups urged the FDA to retain the policy to avoid confusion and deception and to facilitate comparisons among products. The

American Association of Retired Persons, a major consumer group, took the position that although it is important that limitations be placed on labeling to avoid confusion, alternative wording of labeling claims could also be advantageous.

Recognizing that, within limits, there are numerous ways of accurately stating the same concept, the agency concluded that by implementing new regulations, it could still meet its responsibilities of ensuring accurate and truthful labeling while providing greater flexibility for product use terminology. These regulations, which are now finalized, establish three ways of stating the indications for use in OTC drug labeling (see Figure 4).

The first style follows the monograph and requires that the labeling be contained in a prominent and conspicuous location, that it is easily read at time of purchase, and that it uses terminology describing the indications for use that have been established in the applicable final monograph. The terminology would be within a boxed area designated "**Approved Uses**" each time it appears in the labeling (e.g., on the outer carton, on the inner bottle label, and in any package insert). The manufacturer could also include other OTC labeling requirements within the boxed area. In such cases, the boxed area would be designated "**Approved Information**," rather than "**Approved Uses**." A statement that the information in the box was published by the FDA would appear within or close to the boxed area. In lieu of such a statement, manufacturers could modify the designation of the boxed area to read "**FDA Approved Uses**" or "**FDA Approved Information**," as appropriate, or "**Uses** (or "**Information**") **Approved by the Food and Drug Administration**," or use other similar wording.

The agency anticipates that consumers will look for the approved labeling when purchasing OTC drugs, thereby providing an incentive for manufacturers to use this alternative.

The second style follows the monograph but allows interpretations. In addition to the wording required in the boxed area (first style), the label and labeling could contain, outside the boxed area, alternative wording to describe indications for use established under an applicable monograph, as long as the additional wording is not false or misleading.

The third style interprets the monograph and permits manufacturers to state the indications for use in a prominent and conspicuous place in the labeling, using synonymous, truthful, and nonmisleading language. The interpretation describes those indications for use that have been developed in a relevant monograph, subject to the prohibition in the Act against false or misleading labeling. However, such alternative terminology could not be boxed and could not contain the "**Approved Uses**" or "**Approved Information**" designation or any statement asserting or implying that the indications statement appearing in the prominent and conspicuous area was published by the FDA. Any alternative language could not be inconsistent with that indication for use or imply or indicate a use that is not established under a relevant monograph. Alternative language representing or suggesting that use of the drug is safe and effective for indications other than those established in an appropriate final monograph would render the drug product a new drug for which an approved NDA would be required.

Advertising

The FDA does not regulate or have authority over OTC drug advertising. Authority rests with the Federal Trade Commission (FTC), which, until recently, proposed to allow in OTC drug advertising only those indications established in the FDA final monographs. The FTC, however, has rejected this approach to regulating OTC drug advertising. It will instead decide cases individually, considering the FDA's findings on the safety and effectiveness of OTC drugs in weighing advertising claims.

THE PHARMACIST AS A SOURCE OF HEALTH INFORMATION

The pharmacist has a vital role in disseminating the information from the FDA's OTC drug review; the pharmacist represents a direct communications link to the consumer and can be particularly helpful in providing information regarding new OTC reclassifications, reformulations, and revised labeling. The labeling is critical to a product's proper use and effectiveness, but not all consumers will read the labeling on OTC drug products. Therefore, the pharmacist can perform a valuable professional service at the time of an OTC drug purchase by calling the consumer's attention to labeling, particularly to important directions or warnings; this counseling is especially important for drugs recently reclassified from prescription to OTC marketing status. Pharmacists can also explain labeling when it is not understood by consumers and provide helpful supplementary information in the process. Likewise, the prescription-to-OTC trend offers tremendous opportunities for interactions between pharmacists and patients. Because of consumers' growing interest in their own health, availability of medical services, and cost containment, the prescription-to-OTC reclassification trend will surely extend into the next century, and the role of pharmacist as a health care counselor will greatly expand. (See Chapter 2, *Patient Assessment and Consultation*.)

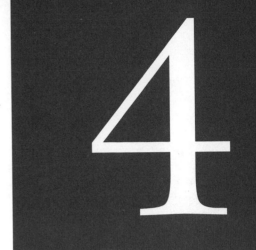

Susan Pawlak Meyer

IN-HOME DIAGNOSTIC PRODUCTS

*Q*uestions to ask in patient/consumer counseling

Blood Pressure Monitoring

Do you or anyone in your family have a history of high blood pressure?

Are you taking any medications to treat or control high blood pressure?

Do you know what blood pressure values are regarded as normal for you? Do you know what your blood pressure values have been?

Do you presently monitor your blood pressure? If so, when do you normally take your blood pressure readings (i.e., time of day, before or after what activity)? If not, do you wish to purchase a blood pressure monitor? Will you take your blood pressure readings by yourself, or will someone assist you?

Fecal Occult Blood Tests

How old are you?

Have you ever suffered from any disorder of the bowel?

Have you or anyone in your family had colorectal cancer?

Have any family members suffered from stomach or colon problems (e.g., ulcers, hemorrhoids)?

Are you currently taking any drug products, nonprescription or prescription?

Ovulation Prediction Tests

Are you currently taking any medications, nonprescription or prescription?

Do you have any chronic medical conditions?

Are you now consulting or have you previously consulted a doctor who specializes in fertility problems?

Have you ever used an ovulation prediction product? If so, how did you use it?

Pregnancy Tests

How late is your period?

Are you currently taking any medications, nonprescription or prescription?

Do you have any chronic medical conditions?

Have you ever used a pregnancy test before? If so, which one?

In-home test kits are becoming more important in health care because of increased emphasis on preventive medicine, increased public health awareness, increased awareness of technology, and the strong trend toward self-care. Sales of in-home tests are expected to exceed $1 billion by the early 1990s (1, 2). Recent advances in biotechnology have made it possible for more tests to be done at home (3) and have made test kits easier to use. A major technological development has been the use of an enzyme-linked immunoassay (ELISA) with monoclonal antibodies (organic molecules that uniquely bind to a target substance) to detect the presence of specific substances. Because of their specificity, the use of monoclonal antibodies has led to the development of highly sensitive, accurate, and reliable in-home tests.

Some test kits are designed to detect the signs of a condition (e.g., fecal occult blood in colorectal cancer), while others monitor a chronic condition and its treatment (e.g., blood glucose testing in diabetes).* In-home kits contribute to the patient's overall health care by encouraging early detection and treatment or careful maintenance of various conditions (4).

The in-home test kit market creates an important patient education role for pharmacists because these kits can provide useful information and be cost-effective only if they are used and interpreted correctly (5). Most manufacturers of in-home test kits claim accuracy of more than 95% if the user strictly adheres to the instructions and recommended procedure. For example, patients need to know the appropriate time to use a particular in-home test, how to use it properly, and how to interpret test results. Therefore, it is increasingly important for the pharmacist's knowledge to remain current as new test products are introduced and as existing tests, once done only by physicians, become available to the public in pharmacies.

HOME BLOOD PRESSURE MONITORING

Hypertension affects approximately 25% of the adult population in the United States. It is estimated that several million more persons suffer from the dis-ease, but remain undiagnosed. Left untreated, high blood pressure can result in stroke, heart disease, and kidney disease, all of which may be fatal. Through early diagnosis and compliance with a treatment regimen, hypertension can be controlled and the long-term complications avoided (6, 7).

Blood pressure measurements have two components: systolic and diastolic. Systolic pressure is the pressure exerted against the arterial wall during cardiac contraction (8). Diastolic pressure is resting pressure, or the pressure exerted against the arterial wall between cardiac contractions. Several factors may affect an individual's blood pressure, including recent exercise, body position at the time of pressure measurement, stress, emotional excitement, illness, and diet (9).

There are two types of indirect measurement of blood pressure: auscultatory and oscillometric. Mercury and aneroid meters involve auscultation, with the use of a stethoscope, of Korotkoff's sounds, which are produced by the motion of the arterial wall in response to changes in arterial pressure. As cuff pressure increases during the measurement procedure, blood flow is obstructed as the brachial artery is compressed. As cuff pressure is gradually released, blood flow is reestablished and Korotkoff's sounds are heard in different phases. Phase I corresponds to systolic pressure and can be identified when at least two consecutive "taps" are heard as pressure is decreased. The nature of the sounds changes over the next three phases. Diastolic pressure is identified as Phase V, the disappearance of sound (8).

Oscillometric cuffs measure blood pressure by detecting blood surges underneath the cuff as it is deflated. Blood pressure measurements are calculated from changes in the force of the surges.

Types of Blood Pressure Meters

Mercury

The mercury sphygmomanometer consists of a cuff attached to a column of mercury encased in a glass gauge, which rises and falls in relation to cuff pressure (Figure 1). Use of this type of meter requires a stethoscope. The mercury sphygmomanometer is the most accurate and reliable type of blood pressure meter available (10). It is factory calibrated and requires recalibration only if the mercury gauge does not read "0" when the cuff is deflated. However, the mercury sphygmomanometer is bulky and inconvenient to transport. Also, it contains breakable glass parts and carries the potential for toxic leaks of mercury. Proper use of the mercury meter and stethoscope requires good hearing ability and proper positioning of the gauge (i.e., the mercury column must be vertical) (11).

---

*Editor's Note: Urine glucose test kits, used in monitoring diabetes care and treatment, are discussed in Chapter 16, *Diabetes Care Products*. To avoid duplication, they are not covered in this chapter even though they are important in-home diagnostic products.

Aneroid

The aneroid blood pressure meter consists of a cuff and an attached circular dial that displays pressure readings (Figure 2). The needle on the dial moves clockwise as cuff pressure increases and counterclockwise as cuff pressure decreases. As does the mercury sphygmomanometer, the aneroid meter requires the use of a stethoscope. This type of meter is relatively compact and portable, and the gauge works in any orientation. Aneroid meters are relatively inexpensive, but require calibration by an expert at least once a year. Good eyesight and hearing are essential for obtaining accurate blood pressure measurements with an aneroid meter (11).

Automated

The third type of in-home blood pressure meter is the battery-operated electronic or digital meter (Figure 3). Because electronic auscultatory cuffs include a microphone to automatically detect blood sounds, a stethoscope and good hearing ability are not required. However, the cuff must be placed so that the microphone is directly over the artery for blood sounds to be detected.

Electronic oscillometric monitors are also available. Because these meters do not monitor blood

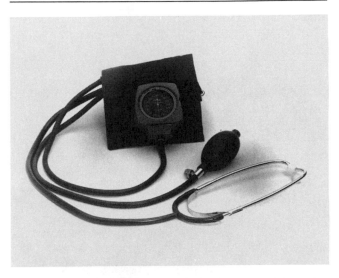

FIGURE 2   Aneroid sphygmomanometer. Reprinted from *Am. Pharm.*, *NS29*, 579 (1989).

sounds, correct placement of the cuff is not important in obtaining an accurate measurement. Cuffless oscillometric meters require the patient only to place a finger in the appropriate area of the monitor to obtain a blood pressure reading.

Automated blood pressure meters are convenient for patients to use and require less skill than those requiring auscultation of Korotkoff's sounds. However, these monitors are relatively expensive (12), require calibration at least yearly, and may be less accurate than mercury and aneroid devices (13).

Advantages of Ambulatory Blood Pressure Monitoring

General blood pressure monitoring in the community (e.g., stationary customer service monitors in pharmacies, health fair screenings) increases chances of detecting elevated blood pressure in persons who have not recently been evaluated (13). Ambulatory blood pressure monitoring also allows patients diagnosed with hypertension to actively participate in their own health care. By closely observing and measuring the effects of medications and lifestyle on blood pressure, the patient may become more motivated and compliant with therapy. Compliance and tight control of blood pressure can help the patient avoid the long-term health complications of hypertension. Better monitoring and reporting of blood pressure measured between clinic or office visits can help the physician evaluate therapy effectiveness and determine therapy changes.

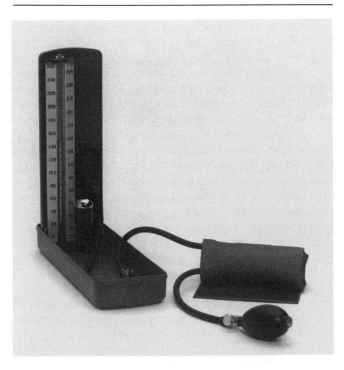

FIGURE 1   Mercury sphygmomanometer. Reprinted from *Am. Pharm.*, *NS29*, 578 (1989).

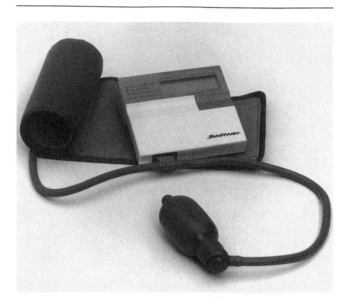

FIGURE 3   Electronic blood pressure meter. Reprinted from *Am. Pharm.*, *NS29*, 579 (1989).

Studies have shown that clinic and physician office measurements of blood pressure may result in the misdiagnosis of mild to moderate hypertension. This artificially elevated blood pressure, a response to the stress associated with a physician visit, is referred to as the "white coat" phenomenon. In-home self-monitoring of blood pressure over a 24-hour period provides much more valuable data in evaluating blood pressure status. These ambulatory measurements are also more predictive of end organ damage and cardiovascular complications associated with hypertension (14–17).

Patient Education

The pharmacist can provide many services for the hypertensive patient. Compliance with drug and nondrug therapies is often a problem for hypertensive patients. Monitoring of a patient's drug therapy regimen for timely prescription drug renewals is important. Additionally, the pharmacist can offer encouragement and stress the importance of lifestyle changes (e.g., sodium restriction, weight loss, exercise, smoking cessation), which are often an integral part of the overall control of hypertension (18).

The pharmacist can also provide important information to users of in-home blood pressure monitors. Proper technique and adherence to the manufacturer's instructions are crucial to obtaining accurate and reli-

able blood pressure measurements. A first-time user of a blood pressure monitor should be encouraged to compare initial readings with those of a health care professional to ensure that the monitor is calibrated and working properly. The pharmacist should educate the patient about activities and factors that may affect blood pressure readings. Patients should recognize that they may observe fluctuations of 20–30 mm Hg if multiple readings are taken each day (17, 19). The pharmacist should also caution the patient against adjusting medication dosages on the basis of in-home blood pressure readings. Patients should be encouraged to consult their physicians if a problem is encountered or pressure remains uncontrolled. All hypertensive patients should be encouraged to see their physicians for regular evaluation.

FECAL OCCULT BLOOD TEST KITS

Patients at Risk

Colorectal cancer is the second most common fatal cancer in the United States after lung cancer, for both males and females (20, 21). Colorectal cancer most often begins as a superficial lesion that, as it progresses, tends to invade the intestinal wall and metastasize to other organs. If detected early, however, colorectal cancer may be more successfully treated through surgery and/or other therapies. Therefore, early detection of cancerous lesions while localized can improve the prognosis and significantly increase survival rates (22). Certain subgroups of the population are at a higher risk for the development of cancers of the anus, colon, or rectum. Individuals with a personal history of inflammatory bowel disease, prior colorectal cancer, female genital cancer, or breast cancer are at increased risk. In addition, persons with a family history of polyposis, colorectal polyps, or colorectal cancer also have a higher than average risk (23). Persons at risk for the development of colorectal cancers also include those 40 years of age and older; this risk doubles with each decade after 50 years of age and appears to peak at 70 (20). The American Cancer Society has recommended that routine screening for colorectal cancer begin at 40 years of age with an annual digital rectal exam; persons 50 years of age and older should have an annual stool guaiac test and, after two initial negative sigmoidoscopies 1 year apart, should repeat a sigmoidoscopy every 3–5 years (24).

Biochemical Basis for Fecal Occult Blood Tests

One of the indicators of colorectal cancer is the presence of occult blood (i.e., concealed and in small quantities) in the feces. Blood found on the surface of the stool is most likely from a source in the lower gastrointestinal (GI) tract. (See Chapter 26, *Hemorrhoidal Products*.) Matrixed blood (i.e., blood found within the stool, not on the surface) is most likely from sources in the upper GI tract, such as bleeding peptic ulcer. Tests for in-home use are designed to detect fecal occult blood with a colorimetric assay for hemoglobin. Hemoglobin possesses peroxidase activity and oxidizes the test reagent to produce a noticeable color change. It is important to note that a positive result with this type of test does not indicate the presence of cancer, only the presence of blood within the GI tract, which may be indicative of any number of conditions. Also, because cancerous lesions may bleed intermittently and fail to be detected with a single test, testing is recommended for three consecutive bowel movements.

Product Information

The first generation of in-home fecal occult blood tests required the patient to obtain a stool specimen from the toilet bowl and place a smear onto a slide. Manufacturers have discontinued marketing of these tests, Hemoccult Home Test (Menley James) and Fleet DeteCAtest (Fleet), for in-home use because of problems with convenience and acceptance by the patient. However, slide tests are still used in physician offices and clinics as well as in mass screening programs. For the slide tests, the patient must apply a small sample of fecal matter to each of the two test areas on the cardboard slide for each of three consecutive bowel movements. The slides are then returned to the clinic or laboratory for application of a developing solution and interpretation of results. Appearance of a blue color indicates a positive result for the presence of blood. Both matrixed and stool surface blood can be detected with this method.

The second-generation fecal occult blood test, Early Detector (Warner-Lambert), requires an anal pat with the provided pad to obtain a fecal sample. The patient then wets the test area and the two activity indi-cator control spots on the bottom of the pad with a developer solution. If blood is present in the sample, the hemoglobin will oxidize the test reagent (guaiac), and a blue color will appear within 60 seconds. Any trace of blue color in the test area indicates the presence of blood in the sample. To verify that the test and solution are properly working, the positive activity indicator control spot turns blue when the developer solution is sprayed on it. The negative activity indicator control spot does not change color. The pad is biodegradable and can be flushed down the toilet after the results are recorded (25).

Each Early Detector kit contains three test pads to allow for testing on three consecutive bowel movements. Testing over a period of time is necessary because even if lesions are present, they may not continuously bleed. However, if a positive result is obtained on the first or second test, there is no need to perform the remaining tests. Patients should immediately contact their physicians after obtaining a positive result. With the anal pat method, the matrix of the stool is broken and occult blood within the stool from bleeding lesions higher in the GI tract may be detected.

The third-generation fecal occult blood tests do not require stool handling by the patient. The available nonprescription test kits, CS-T or ColoScreen Self-Test (Helena Laboratories) and EZ Detect (NMS Pharmaceuticals), contain materials for three tests. A new third-generation product, ColoCare (Helena Laboratories), is currently available for physician distribution, hospital use, and mass screening programs. Eventually ColoCare will be packaged for nonprescription distribution and will replace CS-T (26).

With the third-generation tests, a test pad is dropped, printed side up, into the toilet bowl following a bowel movement and observed for color change. If there is a clinically significant amount of blood on the surface of the stool, it disperses and floats on the surface of the toilet bowl water. The hemoglobin oxidizes the reagent in the test pad and causes a visible color change. Third-generation tests are more likely to detect blood from lesions lower in the GI tract because blood from these lesions is usually within the outer mucous surface of the stool.

The reagents used in these third-generation tests are susceptible to interference by toilet bowl cleaners, deodorants, and disinfectants. Therefore, the test user should remove any cleaner from the tank, flush twice before testing, and not throw toilet paper into the bowl until the test is complete.

The CS-T pad is floated in the toilet bowl, printed side up, immediately after a bowel movement. The pad is observed for 15–30 seconds for the appearance of a red-orange color in any of the four stool test areas on the pad. This color change, a result of oxidation of guaiacol derivatives, should be considered a positive result for the presence of hemoglobin. There are two pad check areas in the middle of the pad; one should turn red-orange and the other should not. If one pad check area does not react appropriately, the test results are considered invalid. The patient need not touch the pad at any time. It is biodegradable and should be flushed after the results are recorded (27).

The test reagents in the ColoCare pad are tetramethylbenzidine and cumene hydroperoxide. The test procedure is the same as described for CS-T. However, the appearance of a blue or green color in the test area indicates a positive result. ColoCare has two check areas at the bottom of the pad; the area on the left should always turn blue or green as a guide for color comparison, and the area on the right should not change color (28).

The EZ Detect kit contains five test pads and a positive control chemical package. Before using EZ Detect, the patient should use one test pad to check water quality. If any trace of blue appears in the cross area when the pad is floated in the toilet water without a specimen, another toilet bowl should be used for the tests. The EZ Detect test pad uses the same testing procedure as CS-T. Three consecutive bowel movements are tested. The reagent in the EZ Detect test pad is a reduced chromogen, tetramethylbenzidine, which produces a blue cross on the test pad when oxidized in the presence of hemoglobin. The reaction may take up to 2 minutes to develop. If no positive results are obtained for the three tests, a test pad quality check may be performed with the remaining pad. The patient should flush the toilet and empty the contents of the positive control chemical package into the bowl as it refills. The remaining test pad should be floated in the water, printed side up. A blue cross appearing within 2 minutes indicates that the test pads were working properly. If the blue cross does not appear, test results were invalid and the patient should call the assistance number provided with product (29).

Patient Counseling

The pharmacist can play an important role in personal health care by encouraging persons over 50 years of age to perform annual fecal occult blood tests, to participate in public screening programs, or to see their physicians for such tests. Colorectal lesions and polyps grow slowly and may remain asymptomatic for an extended period. However, if detected early, colorectal lesions can be treated. The pharmacist should also provide several instructions and warnings to users of in-home fecal occult blood test kits. To avoid inaccurate results, the patient must thoroughly read the manufac-

turer's instructions before testing and closely follow the recommended testing procedure. For at least 2 or 3 days before performing the first test and during the testing period, patients should avoid the ingestion of medications such as aspirin, potassium products, and iron-containing products. These agents may cause GI irritation and bleeding, which may cause false-positive results. Use of rectal ointments and medications should also be avoided for 2 days before and during testing. The reagents in CS-T and Early Detector, guaiac and guaiacol derivatives, are prone to interference from dietary sources of peroxidase or hemoglobin, such as red meats, broccoli, horseradish, turnips, and cauliflower. Therefore, the pharmacist should instruct users of those two products to avoid these types of foods for at least 2 days before and during the testing period. Also, ingestion of vitamin C may give false-negative results with those two products because it is a reducing substance. Literature accompanying the ColoCare product also instructs the user to avoid red meats and vitamin C before and during testing. An advantage of EZ Detect is that the patient does not have to restrict intake of foods with peroxidase activity that may cause false-positive results with tests containing guaiac or guaiacol derivatives. Furthermore, ingestion of vitamin C will not cause a false-negative result as it may with the other fecal occult blood tests.

Patients should be encouraged to increase roughage and fiber in their diets before using any fecal occult blood test kit. Roughage aids in the passage of the stool and facilitates detection of lesions that may bleed only intermittently. Examples of foods that should be eaten are popcorn, peanuts, bran cereal, whole grains, and vegetables (other than those which are high in peroxidase). (See Chapter 15, *Laxative Products*.)

Because interpretation of the results of these tests involves evaluation of a color change, color-blind or vision-impaired persons will require assistance when observing the test area on the pad.

The pharmacist should also stress that concurrent medical conditions, such as peptic duodenal ulcers and colitis, may cause false-positive results. However, an in-home fecal occult blood test kit may detect blood produced by these conditions and lead to their subsequent diagnosis and treatment. A test for fecal occult blood should not be performed if the patient is experiencing any of the following: menstrual bleeding, bleeding hemorrhoids, or constipation.

The pharmacist should stress to users of in-home fecal occult blood test kits that a positive result does not necessarily indicate that colorectal cancer is present. These tests are designed only to detect hidden blood in the stool, a symptom of multiple GI disorders. Patients obtaining a positive result with a fecal occult blood test should be immediately and tactfully referred to a physician for a complete evaluation. Only further testing by medical personnel can diagnose or rule out colorectal cancer.

OVULATION PREDICTION AND PREGNANCY KITS

The Female Reproductive Cycle

A brief discussion of the hormonal changes that occur throughout the female reproductive cycle and in early pregnancy will facilitate the understanding of the chemical basis for in-home ovulation prediction and pregnancy tests. (See Chapter 7, *Menstrual Products*.) Hormonal control of the female reproductive cycle, which is approximately 28 days long, involves negative feedback loops. At the beginning of the cycle (day 1 through approximately day 13), low levels of circulating estrogen and progesterone cause gonadotropin-releasing hormone (Gn-RH) to be secreted by the hypothalamus, which in turn stimulates the release of follicle-stimulating hormone (FSH) and low levels of luteinizing hormone (LH) from the anterior pituitary. This combination of hormones promotes the development of several follicles within an ovary during each cycle. However, at one point in the development, one follicle continues to mature while the others regress. At midcycle (day 14 or 15), circulating LH levels increase significantly and cause final maturation of the follicle. Ovulation, rupturing of the follicle and release of the ovum, occurs 20–48 hours after this LH surge. Cells in the ruptured follicle then luteinize and form the corpus luteum, which begins to secrete progesterone and estrogen. For 7 or 8 days following ovulation, the corpus luteum continues to develop and secrete estrogen and progesterone, which inhibit further secretion of FSH and LH. (See Chapter 7, *Menstrual Products*.) If fertilization occurs, the hormone human chorionic gonadotropin (hCG) is produced by trophoblastic cells. HCG causes the corpus luteum to continue to produce progesterone and estrogen, which forestall the onset of menses while the placenta develops and becomes functional. As early as the seventh day after conception, the placenta produces hCG, which continues to increase in concentration during early pregnancy. Some hCG is excreted in the urine; maximum levels of hCG are reached 6 weeks after conception. HCG levels decline over the following 4–6 weeks and then stabilize for the remainder of the pregnancy.

If fertilization does not occur during a cycle, the corpus luteum degenerates, circulating levels of progesterone and estrogen diminish, and menses occur (days 1–5). Resulting low levels of progesterone and estrogen cause release of Gn-RH from the hypothalamus, and the hormonal cycle begins again (30, 31).

Basal Thermometry

Before the introduction of in-home ovulation prediction test kits, basal body temperature (BBT) readings were the only self-testing procedure available to the public to help determine when ovulation occurred. The basal resting temperature is usually below normal during the first part of the female reproductive cycle. Following ovulation, this temperature rises to a level closer to 98.6° F (37° C). However, because the BBT increase is not detected until after ovulation has occurred, only a few hours (less than 24) of the woman's fertile period remain during which conception is most likely to occur. (See Chapter 25, *Contraceptive Methods and Products*.)

Because the only equipment necessary for BBT monitoring is a basal thermometer, this method is much less expensive than in-home ovulation prediction test kits. Basal temperatures can be measured orally, rectally, or vaginally each morning before arising; however, the chosen method must be used consistently because the temperature will vary depending on the measurement site. BBT may be a useful initial approach for a couple attempting to conceive. It is inexpensive and, if fertilization has not occurred within a few months, the woman has more accurate data regarding her cycle length to facilitate the selection of an in-home ovulation prediction kit.

Ovulation Prediction Kits

In-home test kits to determine when a woman is most fertile predict ovulation by detecting the surge in LH levels with monoclonal antibodies specific for LH in the urine. The LH surge precedes ovulation by 20–48 hours and can usually be detected in the urine 8–12 hours after it occurs in the serum. Therefore, depending on the in-home test kit used, ovulation should be expected to occur within 1 or 2 days after the surge is detected in the urine. Following ovulation, the ovum remains viable for 12–24 hours. Because sperm can survive for up to 72 hours after intercourse, the optimal days for fertilization include the 2 days preceding ovulation, the day ovulation occurs, and the day following ovulation. Therefore, detection of the LH surge indicates the beginning of the fertile period. However, the patient must understand that the ovulation prediction tests are not indicated for use in contraception because intercourse before ovulation may still result in pregnancy.

Product Information

In-home ovulation prediction tests were first marketed in the United States in 1985. These tests contain monoclonal antibodies specific for LH and use ELISA to elicit a color change proportional to the level of LH in the urine. A significant increase in the intensity of the color over baseline indicates the LH surge. Different ovulation prediction test kits contain supplies for five to ten tests. Theoretically, the earlier testing begins in a cycle and the more consecutive days tested, the greater the likelihood of predicting ovulation.

Before using an ovulation prediction kit, the woman must determine the period of time when ovulation is most likely to occur. To do so, she should calculate the average length of her last three menstrual cycles. Each product contains a chart based on the calculated average cycle length to assist the user in determining which day of her cycle to begin testing. For example, with the 9-day OvuQUICK Self-Test for Ovulation Prediction (Monoclonal Antibodies, Inc.), a woman whose cycle length is 29 days would begin testing on day 10 of her cycle (first day of menstrual bleeding is day 1) (32). With the First Response Ovulation Predictor Test (Tambrands, Inc.), which contains materials for 6 days of testing, a woman whose cycle is 29 days would begin testing on day 13 (33). Calculation of the time period in which ovulation is most likely to occur should be done carefully so that a baseline can be established and the LH surge detected. If the woman's cycle varies by more than 3 or 4 days each month, she should use the length of the shortest cycle to determine when to start testing. Six days of testing are adequate for detection of the LH surge and ovulation prediction in approximately 66% of ovulating women (33). By increasing the testing period to 10 consecutive days, the probability of detecting the LH surge is increased to 95% (34).

Because ovulation prediction kits for in-home testing use monoclonal antibodies, the possibility of interference from other substances is minimal. Commonly used nonprescription drug products, such as analgesics, decongestants, antihistamines, antitussives, and expectorants, should not interfere with the test results (32, 34, 35). However, medications used to promote ovulation (e.g., menotropins, danazol) may give a false-positive result because LH levels are artificially elevated. The true LH surge can be detected in patients receiving clomiphene if testing does not begin until 1 day after

therapy ends (33). Medical conditions associated with high levels of LH such as menopause and polycystic ovary syndrome may cause false-positive test results. A false-positive result may also be obtained if the user is already pregnant (36). If the patient has recently discontinued use of oral contraceptives, the start of ovulation may be delayed for one or two cycles. Use of in-home ovulation prediction test kits by such individuals is not appropriate until fertilization has been unsuccessfully attempted for several months following discontinuation of the oral contraceptives.

Patient Counseling

The pharmacist can provide users of in-home ovulation prediction test kits with important information to ensure proper use of the test and to increase the probability of accurate test results. The multiple steps involved in these tests increase the potential for procedural errors. The pharmacist should review the proper test procedure with the patient and emphasize the importance of strict adherence to the manufacturer's instructions. Timing of the component steps in the test procedure is crucial and requires a clock or timer. If the patient is unable to conduct the test immediately after the sample is collected, the urine may be refrigerated for up to 12 hours. Before conducting the test later in the day, the patient should allow the sample to reach room temperature by letting it stand for 20–30 minutes. Some sediment may accumulate on the bottom of the sample container while it is refrigerated. It is important that the patient not shake the sample or redisperse the sediment.

Some of the test kits require first morning urine, in which LH is the most concentrated. Others will work with a sample taken at any time during the day. Instructions for Answer (Carter Products), OvuKIT (Monoclonal Antibodies, Inc.), and OvuQUICK specifically state that first morning urine is not to be used (32, 35). For these tests, it is important for the user to obtain the sample at the same time each day of testing and to restrict fluid intake for 1 or 2 hours before obtaining the sample so that the urine will not be too dilute (37). Once the LH surge is detected, the patient can discontinue testing. Any remaining tests can be stored for use during the next cycle if fertilization does not occur (32, 34). If a woman obtains an intense color the first day of testing, she has started too late in the cycle and ovulation may have already occurred. She should stop testing for that cycle and, if pregnancy does not occur, begin testing a few days earlier in the next cycle.

The pharmacist should realize that the desire to conceive can be an emotional issue for couples using ovulation prediction kits and that empathy in communicating with these clients is important. Couples who are unable to conceive after two or three cycles, even when ovulation was detected, should be referred to a gynecologist or fertility specialist. Also, the pharmacist may inform the couple about Resolve, Inc., a national nonprofit organization that assists infertile couples through a free telephone counseling service, referral to medical services, support groups, public education, and publications. The toll free number for Resolve, Inc., is 800-662-1016 (except in Massachusetts). Infertile couples may also be advised to check telephone directories for local organizations.

Pregnancy Test Kits

In-home pregnancy tests are designed to detect the presence of hCG in the urine. In-home testing makes it possible to detect pregnancy early in the first trimester when crucial behavioral and lifestyle changes can prevent harm to the fetus (37). There are two types of in-home pregnancy tests: those based on a hemagglutination inhibition reaction and those that use monoclonal antibody technology.

Hemagglutination Inhibition Reaction Tests

The first-generation of in-home pregnancy test kits use the hemagglutination inhibition reaction. The e.p.t. Pregnancy Test Kit (Warner-Lambert), the first such test to be approved for in-home use, became available in 1977. Hemagglutination inhibition reaction test kits include a test tube containing red blood cells coated with an hCG-antigen and an hCG-antiserum. If hCG is present in the urine sample, it complexes with the antiserum and uncoats the red blood cells. These uncoated red blood cells fall to the bottom of the test tube and form a donut-shaped ring, which is considered a positive result for pregnancy. The original hemagglutination inhibition tests require rather high levels of hCG to be present to produce a positive result. These levels are usually achieved approximately 9 days after the missed onset of menses. Therefore, a false-negative result will be obtained if a hemagglutination inhibition test is used too early after conception or too late into the pregnancy when circulating hCG levels have decreased (i.e., after week 6 of pregnancy).

Answer 2 (Carter Products) is a hemagglutination inhibition test with monoclonal antibodies; it may be used as early as the day after a woman expected her period to begin. However, because hCG levels may not be adequate for detection, a second test is included in the package. If the first test result is negative, the user is instructed to wait until day 6 and test again.

The hemaglutination inhibition tests have some disadvantages. They take a relatively long time (30–60 minutes) to perform. Also, these tests are very sensitive to vibration; the slightest movement caused by a nearby appliance or telephone may yield erroneous results.

Monoclonal Antibody Tests

Early in the 1980s, a second generation of in-home pregnancy tests became available as a result of developments in monoclonal antibody technology. These second-generation pregnancy tests use ELISA to produce a color change indicating a positive result. If hCG is present in the urine sample, it is trapped by the hCG antibody. A second antibody attached to an enzyme complexes with the trapped hCG and the enzyme produces a color change on a plastic test stick or in a solution, depending on the product. The in-home pregnancy tests using monoclonal antibodies are very sensitive and can detect low levels of hCG. Monoclonal antibody pregnancy tests also require less time to complete (3–30 minutes, depending on the product) than do the hemagglutination inhibition tests. If correctly used, monoclonal antibody pregnancy tests for in-home use have a reported accuracy of more than 95% (38–40).

Sources of Interference

When a hemagglutination inhibition reaction test is used, cross-reactivity with elevated levels of LH may yield a false-positive result. Some medications that may cause increased LH secretion from the anterior pituitary include antiparkinsonian drugs, carbamazepine and other anticonvulsants, and phenothiazines. Oral contraceptives may cause a periodic elevation of LH and will also interfere with hemagglutination inhibition pregnancy tests. Medical conditions such as menopause, thyrotoxicosis, hematuria, and proteinuria can also cause false-positive results. A false-negative result may also be obtained if diluted urine is tested. Therefore, hemagglutination inhibition pregnancy tests require the sample to be first morning urine because it is the most concentrated.

Because of monoclonal antibody technology, the second-generation pregnancy tests are more sensitive for hCG and less susceptible to interference from other substances. However, urine collected in a waxed cup may cause erroneous results because extraneous wax particles can clog the test matrix. False-negative results may occur with monoclonal antibody pregnancy tests if the test is performed too early after conception or if the urine sample was refrigerated and not allowed to return to room temperature. Also, test sticks must be rinsed in cold water because warm or hot water could remove the monoclonal antibody during the procedure.

Patient Counseling

The pharmacist can provide users of in-home pregnancy tests with important information to ensure proper use of the test and increase the probability of an accurate test result. The pharmacist should review the proper test procedure with the patient and emphasize the importance of strict adherence to the manufacturer's instructions. With most in-home pregnancy tests, timing of the steps is crucial for accurate results. If the patient is unable to conduct the test immediately after the sample is collected, the urine may be stored in a refrigerator for up to 12 hours. Before conducting the test later in the day, the patient should allow the sample to return to room temperature by letting it stand for 20–30 minutes. Some sediment may accumulate in the bottom of the sample container while it is refrigerated. It is important that the patient not shake the sample or redisperse the sediment before testing. If the urine sample is cloudy or pink, or has a strong odor, it should not be used for an in-home pregnancy test because inaccurate results are likely to occur.

If the woman has selected a hemagglutination inhibition reaction test, the pharmacist should emphasize the susceptibility of the test to any source of vibration and advise her not to place the test tube near a telephone or appliances such as refrigerators or blenders.

If the test results are negative, the patient should review the procedure to make sure she performed the test properly. Then, she should wait the recommended number of days suggested by the manufacturer and repeat the test if menses have not yet begun. If the second test remains negative, the patient should contact her physician. Other underlying medical reasons for lack of menstruation may require diagnosis and treatment by trained medical personnel.

If the result of an in-home pregnancy test is positive, the patient should assume she is pregnant and arrange for an appointment with a physician. Behaviors known to be harmful to the fetus, such as alcohol ingestion, smoking, and illicit drug use, should be immediately discontinued. Prescription, as well as nonprescription, medication intake should be discussed with the physician. Pregnant diabetics should monitor blood glucose levels very carefully because normoglycemia decreases fetal morbidity and mortality.

When assisting in product selection, the pharmacist should consider specific product features and patient characteristics. For example, if a woman is testing early after possible conception, a two-test kit may be appropriate. Also, some monoclonal antibody tests require fewer steps, are less complicated to use, and can be performed quickly and discreetly.

THE FUTURE OF IN-HOME TEST KITS

As the products of biotechnology become more sophisticated, easier to use, and less costly, it is expected that more tests will become available on a nonprescription basis for in-home use. Manufacturers will continue to strive to make their products more accurate and reliable. Test kits to determine and monitor blood cholesterol levels; to detect the presence of sexually transmitted diseases, yeast infections, and streptococcal throat infections; and to use in therapeutic drug monitoring are expected to become available on a nonprescription basis in the near future (1, 41, 42). Self-monitoring of drug levels may play an important role in the overall health care and maintenance of patients with hypertension, arrhythmias, seizure disorders, asthma, and other chronic conditions. However, it is stressed to pharmacists and other health professionals that patients must know how to use and interpret the information provided by these tests and know their limitations. Interpretation of test results related to an individual patient and diagnosis of medical conditions remains in the domain of the physician. The role of the pharmacist as an educator on the use of in-home test and monitoring products should continue to grow as more tests become available. Because of the concern that patients may not correctly interpret test results or act appropriately after they obtain the test results, some manufacturers of diagnostics may allow dissemination of these products only through health professionals such as pharmacists. This will help ensure the intended outcome of the test.

REFERENCES

1 *Med. Advert. News, 7 (18)*, 6, 7 (1988).
2 M. C. Smith and D. D. Garner, *U.S. Pharmacist, 12 (6)*, 24–28 (1987).
3 M. Wilson, *Am. Drug., 193 (2)*, 107–113, 147 (1986).
4 M. Ratafia, *Med. Market. Media, 20 (8)*, 15–25 (1985).

5 R. Feierman and P. V. Shea, *Am. Drug.*, *199 (5)*, 62–68 (1989).

6 M. Moser, "High Blood Pressure and What You Can Do About It," Benjamin Company, Elmsford, N.Y., 1987, p. 3.

7 "Questions About Weight, Salt, and High Blood Pressure," National Institutes of Health, Department of Health and Human Services, Pub. No. 87-1459, Bethesda, Md., 1987.

8 M. N. Hill, *Am. J. Nurs.*, *80 (5)*, 942–946 (1980).

9 M. Moser, "High Blood Pressure and What You Can Do About It," Benjamin Company, Elmsford, N.Y., 1987, p. 7.

10 G. R. Schmidt and J. H. Wenig, *Am. Pharm.*, *NS29 (9)*, 25–30 (1989).

11 R. Y. Miller, *U.S. Pharmacist*, *11 (8)*, 60–64 (1986).

12 J. Bagley, *Am. Drug.*, *194 (6)*, 102–107 (1986).

13 C. M. Grim, *Calif. Pharm.*, *37 (3)*, 31–35 (1989).

14 M. A. Weber, *Am. Heart J.*, *116 (4)*, 1118–1123 (1988).

15 T. G. Pickering, *Hypertension*, *11 (no. 3, pt. 2)*, II96–100 (1988).

16 G. Mancia and G. Parati, *Am. Heart. J.*, *116 (4)*, 1134–1140 (1988).

17 C. J. Lavie et al., *Am. Heart J.*, *116 (4)*, 1146–1151 (1988).

18 D. O. Fedder, *U.S. Pharmacist*, *11 (7)*, 66–72 (1986).

19 T. G. Pickering, *Am. Heart J.*, *116 (4)*, 1141–1145 (1988).

20 G. V. Stajich and J. Rakos, Jr., in "Clinical Pharmacy and Therapeutics," 4th ed., E. T. Herfindal et al., Eds., Williams and Wilkins, Baltimore, Md., 1988, p. 920.

21 S. J. Winawer et al., *CA*, *32 (2)*, 100–112 (1982).

22 T. T. Nostrant and J. A. P. Wilson, *Postgrad. Med.*, *73 (6)*, 131–139 (1986).

23 G. V. Stajich and J. Rakos, Jr., in "Clinical Pharmacy and Therapeutics," 4th ed., E. T. Herfindal et al., Eds., Williams and Wilkins, Baltimore, Md., 1988, p. 921.

24 American Cancer Society, *CA*, *30 (4)*, 208–215 (1980).

25 Early Detector product information, Warner-Lambert Company, Inc., Morris Plains, N.J., 1987.

26 Sharon Matthews, Helena Laboratories, Beaumont, Tex., personal communication, 1989.

27 CS-T product information, Helena Laboratories, Beaumont, Tex., 1987.

28 ColoCare product information, Helena Laboratories, Beaumont, Tex., 1988.

29 EZ-Detect product information, NMS Pharmaceuticals, Inc., Newport Beach, Calif., 1987.

30 T. P. Reiders et al., "Methods of Birth Control: Assessment Skills for Pharmacists," Syntex Laboratories, Palo Alto, Calif., 1985, pp. 2–5.

31 J. K. Inglis, "A Textbook of Human Biology," 3rd ed., Pergamon Press, New York, N.Y., 1986, pp. 252–253.

32 OvuQUICK Self-Test for Ovulation Prediction product information, Monoclonal Antibodies, Inc., Mountain View, Calif., 1988.

33 First Response Ovulation Prediction Test product information, Tambrands, Inc., Palmer, Mass., 1988.

34 QTest for Ovulation Prediction product information, Becton-Dickinson and Company, Franklin Lakes, N.J., 1986.

35 OvuKIT Self-Test for Ovulation Prediction product information, Monoclonal Antibodies, Inc., Mountain View, Calif., 1988.

36 Use of the OvuSTICK Self-Test, Monoclonal Antibodies, Inc., Mountain View, Calif., 1984.

37 *Pharm. Times*, *55 (3)*, 107–108 (1989).

38 Clearblue Easy product information, Whitehall Laboratories, New York, N.Y.

39 Answer Quick and Simple product information, Carter Products, Cranbury, N.J., 1989.

40 e.p.t. Stick product information, Parke-Davis Consumer Products, Morris Plains, N.J., 1990.

41 J. Chi, *Drug Topics*, *130 (15)*, 28–34 (1986).

42 B. Robinson, *Drug Topics*, *132 (5)*, 42 (1988).

ELECTRONIC OSCILLOMETRIC BLOOD PRESSURE MONITOR PRODUCT TABLE

Product (Manufacturer)	Description
Model BP-3 060014 (Healthcheck)	microphoneless pulsonic comfort cuff helps assure correct placement blood pressure and pulse displayed on a large screen in less than 45 seconds manual inflate, automatic deflate easy to read instruction booklet vinyl storage case
Model CX-5 060020 (Healthcheck)	cuffless available with standard and large finger rings automatic inflate and deflate memory for most recent reading digital display of blood pressure and pulse multi-lingual instructions
Model CX-10 10025 (Healthcheck)	cuffless available with standard and large finger rings automatic inflate and deflate 14-reading memory adaptor for optional printer digital display of blood pressure and pulse calendar and clock feature graphic display of data multi-lingual instructions
Digital Electronic Blood Pressure Monitor with Pulse Meter and Mikeless Cuff Model 1060 (Lumiscope)	no stethoscope required digital display of blood pressure and pulse uses 4 AA batteries "D"-bar self-adjusting cuff, auto deflate, error codes, auto "off"
Digital Finger Automatic Oscillometric Blood Pressure Monitor Model 1082 (Lumiscope)	takes accurate blood pressure and pulse readings from finger no arm cuff or stethoscope required finger adjuster for correct fit LCD read-out
Deluxe Digital Automatic Oscillometric Blood Pressure Monitor Model 1081 (Lumiscope)	large digital display automatic inflate and deflate preset inflate pressures uses 4 AA batteries
Deluxe Digital Automatic Oscillometric Blood Pressure Monitor Model 1091 (Lumiscope)	large digital display clock feature built-in printer for hard copy of blood pressure, pulse, time and date automatic inflate and deflate preset inflate pressures uses 4 AA batteries
Deluxe Digital Automatic Oscillometric Blood Pressure Monitor Model 1095 (Lumiscope)	large digital display clock feature built-in printer for hard copy of blood pressure, pulse, time and date capable of producing bar graph of all readings in memory automatic inflate and deflate 7-reading memory preset inflate pressures uses 4 C batteries

FECAL OCCULT BLOOD TEST KITS TABLE

Product (Manufacturer or Supplier)	Sizes Available or Description	Comments
ColoScreen Self-Test (CS-T) (Helena Laboratories)	3 specimen pads	use for three consecutive bowel movements. Flush toilet twice before each bowel movement. Pad is floated in toilet bowl with specimen. Observe 15 to 30 seconds. One pad check area will turn red-orange, the other will not. Positive result is appearance of red-orange color in stool test area.
ColoCare (Helena Laboratories) (will eventually replace CS-T)	package size not yet determined	use for three consecutive bowel movements. Flush toilet twice before each bowel movement. Pad is floated in toilet bowl with specimen. Observe 30 seconds. Pad check area on left will turn blue and/or green, the other will not. Positive result is appearance of blue and/or green color in test area.
EZ-Detect (Biomerica)	3 specimen pads	use for three consecutive bowel movements. Flush toilet twice before each bowel movement. Pad is floated in toilet bowl with specimen. Observe for up to 2 minutes. Positive result is appearance of a blue cross on the test pad.
Early Detector (Parke-Davis Consumer Products)	3 specimen pads spray developer	use for three consecutive bowel movements. Patient must obtain sample with anal wipe. Reagent tablet added to liquid in spray bottle. Developer sprayed on pad, observed for appearance of blue color. Result obtained in one minute.

OVULATION PREDICTION TEST KITS TABLE

Product (Manufacturer or Supplier)	Sizes Available	Time for Procedure	Indication of Positive Result	Comments
Answer (Carter Products)	6-day kit	30 minutes	color of lower Color Bead is significantly darker green or green-blue than the previous day.	do not use first morning urine. Collect urine at the same time each day. Do not shake stored sample. Positive result indicates ovulation should occur within 24-36 hours.
Clearplan Easy (Whitehall)	5-day kit	5 minutes	positive result when color of line in large window is similar or darker than line in small window	test same time each day. Morning urine not required. Positive result indicates ovulation should occur in next 24-36 hours. Blue line in small window shows that test is complete.
First Response Ovulation Predictor (Hygeia)	5-day kit 3-day refill	10 minutes	positive result when color in test well is darker than reference color.	use first morning urine. Do not shake stored urine. Positive result indicates ovulation should occur within 12-24 hours.
Fortel (Biomerica)	9-day kit	30 minutes	positive result when color of liquid is significantly darker blue than the previous day.	use first morning urine.
OvuQUICK (Monoclonal Antibodies, Inc.)	6-day kit 9-day kit	4 minutes	positive result when color of test result area on test pad matches or is darker than the reference spot.	use urine collected between 10 am and 8 pm. Do not use first morning urine. Collect at the same time each day over the testing period. Positive result indicates ovulation should occur within 24-40 hours.
OvuKIT (Monoclonal Antibodies, Inc.)	6-day kit 9-day kit	1 hour	positive result when blue color on test stick is darker than the Surge Guide test.	use urine collected between 10 am and 8 pm. Do not use first morning urine. Collect at the same time each day over the testing period. Positive result indicates ovulation should occur within 24-40 hours.
QTest for Ovulation (Becton-Dickinson)	5-day kit	35 minutes	positive result is markedly darker blue on test pad area as compared to previous day. "Error control" pad should remain white or pale blue.	collect urine at any time, but at same time each day over the testing period. Do not shake stored urine. Positive result indicates ovulation should occur within 20-44 hours.

PREGNANCY TEST KITS TABLE MONOCLONAL ANTIBODIES

Product (Manufacturer or Supplier)	Sizes Available	Time for Procedure	Indication of Positive Result	Comments
Advance (Advanced Care Products)	1 test per kit	30 minutes	color change from white to blue on tip of test stick is positive result.	day 1 test. Collect first morning urine. Do not shake stored urine.
Answer Plus (Carter Products)	1 test per kit	30 minutes	color change from yellow to bluish green on the lower Color Bead is a positive result.	can test day after period was expected to begin. Collect first morning urine.
Answer Plus 2 (Carter Products)	2 tests per kit	30 minutes	color change from yellow to bluish-green on the lower Color Bead is a positive result.	can test day after period was expected to begin. Collect first morning urine.
Answer Quick & Simple (Carter Products)	1 test per kit	3 minutes	color key has three test areas. Top area is control and should turn pink-purple. The middle comparison test area should remain white. If lower result test area changes from white to pink-purple, the test is positive.	can test day after period was expected to begin. Does not require first morning urine.
Clearblue (Whitehall)	2 tests per kit	30 minutes	color change to blue on test stick tip is a positive result.	can test day after period was expected to begin.
Clearblue Easy (Whitehall)	1 test per kit 2 tests per kit	3 minutes	blue line in large window is positive result.	can test day period is due. Is a one-step test. Test stick is held in stream of first morning urine to wet tip. Must hold stick upright during testing. Blue line in small window indicates test is complete.
e.p.t. Stick (Parke-Davis Consumer Products)	1 test per kit 2 tests per kit	30 minutes	color change from white to pink on tip of test stick is positive result.	day 1 test. Collect first morning urine. Urine collection container is shallow. Do not shake stored urine.
Fact Plus (Advanced Care Products)	1 test per kit	5-8 minutes	appearance of "+" on plus cube is positive for pregnancy. Negative result is indicated by appearance of a dark "-" on plus cube.	can test on first day of missed period.
First Response 5-minute Test for Pregnancy (Hygeia Sciences)	1 test per kit	5 minutes	appearance of pink color in test well is positive result.	can test day 1 of missed period. Collect urine sample at any time during day.
QTest for Pregnancy (Becton-Dickinson)	1 test per kit 2 tests per kit	9 minute positive, 16 minute negative	appearance of blue color on test pad area of test strip which is darker than 'error control' pad. Error control pad should remain white or pale blue.	can test day of missed period. Collect first morning urine. Do not shake stored urine.

PREGNANCY TEST KITS TABLE
HEMAGGLUTINATION INHIBITION WITH MONOCLONAL ANTIBODIES

Product (Manufacturer or Supplier)	Sizes Available	Time for Procedure	Indication of Positive Result	Comments
Answer (Carter Products)	1 test per kit	60 minutes	formation of red ring or button at the bottom of the test tube.	can test 3 days after period was expected to begin. Collect first morning urine. Test is sensitive to vibration.
Answer 2 (Carter Products)	2 tests per kit	60 minutes	formation of red ring or button at the bottom of the test tube.	can test day after period was expected to begin. Collect first morning urine. Test is very sensitive to vibration. If first test is negative, wait 5 days and test again.

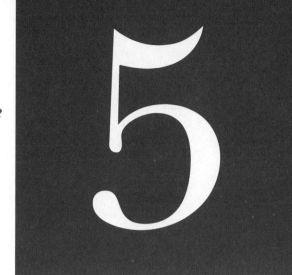

W. Kent Van Tyle

INTERNAL ANALGESIC PRODUCTS

Questions to ask in patient/consumer counseling

Where is the pain? Is it in one place or does it spread to other parts of the body?

What type of pain do you have? Is it sharp, dull, aching, knifelike, etc.?

Does the pain occur at any particular time of the day? Does anything make it worse or better?

Do you have any other symptoms that you feel might be associated with the pain you have or any idea as to the reason for the pain (physical injury)?

What pain reliever has worked for you before?

What have you already taken? How much and for how long?

Does aspirin upset your stomach?

Have you ever had an allergic reaction to aspirin?

Do you now have or have you ever had asthma, allergies, or ulcers?

Are you now taking medication for gout, arthritis, or diabetes?

Are you now taking medication that thins your blood?

Have you ever had any problem with your blood being slow to clot?

(If appropriate) How high is your fever, and how long have you had a fever?

Internal analgesics are used to relieve pain. Certain compounds in this group also possess pharmacologic activities that make them valuable for reducing elevated body temperature and for ameliorating various inflammatory conditions.

Even though pain is a common experience, it is not a simple condition to define. Pain is a sensation, but it is also an interpretation of that sensation that can be influenced by many factors. Fatigue, anxiety, fear, and the anticipation of more pain all affect the perception of and reaction to pain. Studies show that various personality types may experience pain differently; the introverted personality has a lower pain threshold than the extrovert (1). In addition, the perception of pain may be modified significantly by suggestion. Studies indicate that approximately 35% of patients suffering pain from a variety of causes report their pain as being "satisfactorily relieved" by placebo (2).

ETIOLOGY

Pain is usually a protective mechanism, occurring when tissue is damaged or when cells are altered by pain stimuli that threaten to damage tissue. Pain resulting from a functional disturbance or pathology is called "organic" pain. In contrast, "psychogenic" pain is a symptom of an underlying emotional disturbance and is not a consequence of organic pathology.

57

Origin and Perception of Pain

Pain is categorized, according to its origin, as either somatic or visceral. Somatic pain arises from the musculoskeletal system or skin; visceral pain originates from the organs or viscera of the thorax and abdomen.

Free nerve endings serve as pain receptors* to initiate nerve impulses that travel through specialized pain fibers (nociceptive afferent fibers) through the spinal cord and/or brain stem to specific receiving areas of the brain. These receptors are found throughout the superficial skin layers and in certain deeper tissues such as membranous bone covering, arterial walls, muscles, tendons, joint surfaces, and membranes lining the skull. Pain-evoking stimuli have in common the ability to injure cells and to release proteolytic enzymes and polypeptides that stimulate nerve endings and initiate the pain impulse (3). Prostaglandins sensitize nerve endings to polypeptide-induced stimulation (4).

Pain fibers enter the dorsal roots of the spinal cord and interconnect with other nerve cells that cross to the opposite side of the cord and ascend to the brain. Nociceptive neural pathways project to the thalamus and cerebral cortex where recognition and interpretation of the nature and location of the pain impulse occur.

Pain initiation, transmission, and perception are essentially the same for both visceral and somatic pain. One important distinction, however, is that highly localized visceral damage rarely causes severe pain. Diffuse stimulation of nerve endings throughout an organ is required to produce significant visceral pain. Conditions producing visceral pain include ischemia of organ tissue, chemical destruction of visceral tissue, spasm of visceral smooth muscle, and physical distention of an organ or stretching of its associated mesentery (3).

In evaluating the etiology and therapy of pain, it is important to recognize the potential for referred pain. Referred pain is perceived as coming from a part of the body other than that part actually initiating the pain signal. Unlike somatic pain, visceral pain cannot be localized by the brain as coming from a specific organ. Instead, most visceral pain is interpreted by the brain as coming from various skin or muscle segments (it is "referred" to various body surface areas) (Table 1). When a pharmacist is advising the patient as to the need for or potential benefit of nonprescription analgesic products, an appreciation for the sites of referred visceral pain is invaluable. Failure to recognize the possibility of

---

Editor's Note: The technical term "nociceptor" is currently used in the scientific research literature as a more definitive term to connote "a receptor that is stimulated by injury; a receptor for pain." However, in the interest of consistency, the more familiar term "pain receptor" will continue to be used throughout this edition of the *Handbook*.

TABLE 1	Body surface areas associated with referred visceral pain
Origin of visceral pain	**Localization of pain on body surface**
Appendix	Around umbilicus localizing in right lower quadrant of abdomen
Bladder	Lower abdomen directly over bladder
Esophagus	Pharynx, lower neck, arms, midline chest region
Gallbladder	Upper central portion of abdomen; lower right shoulder
Heart	Base of neck, shoulders, and upper chest; down arms (left side involvement more frequent than right)
Kidney and ureters	Regions of lower back over site of affected organ; anterior abdominal wall below and to the side of umbilicus
Stomach	Anterior surface of chest or upper abdomen
Uterus	Lower abdomen

Adapted from A. C. Guyton, "Textbook of Medical Physiology," 6th ed., W. B. Saunders, Philadelphia, Pa., 1981, pp. 618–620, and L. Zetzel, in "Textbook of Medicine," Vol. 1, 13th ed., P. B. Beeson and W. McDermott, Eds., W. B. Saunders, Philadelphia, Pa., 1971, p. 1327.

referred visceral pain could mean that a serious visceral pathology might go undiagnosed and untreated while ineffective self-medication with nonprescription analgesics is attempted. Consequently, effective medical treatment may be dangerously delayed.

Pain Responsive to Nonprescription Analgesics

The analgesic products available for self-medication are more effective in treating musculoskeletal (somatic) pain than visceral pain (5). Nonprescription analgesic therapy is used most frequently for headache or for pain associated with peripheral nerves (neuralgia), muscles (myalgia), or joints (arthralgia).

Headache

The most common form of pain is headache. An estimated 15% of the population experiences headache pain each week (6). Headache may be classified as either intracranial or extracranial, depending on the area of the initiation of the pain (7).

Intracranial headache results from inflammation or traction of sensitive, primarily vascular, intracranial structures. Its etiology includes tumor, abscess, hematoma, or infection. Intracranial headache is uncommon, but because of the potential seriousness of its underlying causes, this type of headache requires immediate medical attention.

Because headache may be a symptom of a serious underlying pathology, the pharmacist should evaluate the potential for intracranial headache and should be prepared to recommend medical attention when appropriate. Intracranial headache produced by tumor or meningeal traction is "deep, aching, steady, dull, and seldom rhythmic or throbbing" (8). The pain may be continuous, is generally more intense in the morning, and may be associated with nausea and vomiting. Pain location cannot be used to differentiate headache of intracranial origin. Concomitant disturbances in sensory function such as blurred vision, dizziness, or hearing loss or changes in personality, behavior, speech patterns, or memory are signals to seek immediate medical attention.

The more common headache forms are extracranial and of diverse etiology. Migraine headache is characterized by intense throbbing, hemicranial pain lasting from several hours to 2 days. The pain may be preceded by visual disturbances; numbness and tingling in the lips, face, or hands; and dizziness and confusion. As the pain increases in intensity, it is often accompanied by nausea, vomiting, and photophobia (3, 8, 9). A hereditary association is seen in 60–80% of patients with migraine; there is a 3:1 female predominance; and stress, hormonal changes, dietary chemicals, and other environmental factors can trigger an attack (10–12). Abnormalities in platelet aggregation resulting in increased plasma serotonin levels are seen in patients with migraine. Increased platelet aggregation occurs during the preheadache phase and parallels increased plasma serotonin levels (13–15). Preheadache vasoconstriction occurs in a migraine, possibly in response to the increased plasma serotonin levels, and is followed by both intracranial and extracranial vasodilation (16). Because of the resulting vascular tone loss, the arteries begin to pulsate with the rising and falling intravascular pressure, and intense pain results from the distention and traction of the affected arteries (12, 16). Drugs, such as aspirin, that inhibit platelet aggregation and the associated serotonin release may be of prophylactic value in reducing the frequency of migraine attacks (17, 18).

The tension (or muscle contraction) headache is the result of spasms of the somatic musculature of the neck and scalp. Symptoms include a feeling of tightness or pressure at the base of the head or in the muscles of the back of the neck. Pain with a tension headache is often located in the forehead or at the base of the skull and is usually bilateral.

The sinus headache may be distinguished from headache of other etiology because its location is restricted to the frontal area of the head and behind or around the eyes. Sinus headaches often recur and subside at the same time each day, and the pain often is intensified by bending over. Sinus pain may be present upon awakening and may subside after a few hours with facilitated sinus drainage. Accompanying symptoms include rhinorrhea, nasal congestion, and a feeling of sinus pressure. The underlying cause is irritation and edema of the nasal and sinus mucous membranes with resultant pressure placed on sinus walls. Infection or allergy is the usual cause, and short-term decongestant therapy often is helpful in facilitating sinus drainage and reducing intrasinus pressure. (See Chapter 8, *Cold and Allergy Products.*)

In addition to being a symptom of sinus headache, pain around or behind the eyes may be caused by uncorrected visual problems associated with difficulty in focusing on near or far objects. An attempt to gain clear vision by tonic ciliary muscle contractions may result in extraocular muscle spasm and referred retro-orbital pain. If retro-orbital headache recurs persistently, referral for ophthalmologic examination is indicated. Recurrent facial or mandibular pain may indicate the need for professional dental examination and treatment.

Neuralgia

Pain generated along the course of a sensory nerve is called neuralgia. The trigeminal nerve frequently is affected, and trigeminal neuralgia is characterized by sharp, stabbing pain in the face or jaw region occurring in brief, agonizing episodes. The cause of trigeminal neuralgia is unknown, but apparently it is not the result of organic damage to the nerve (19, 20). Because of the intense pain of trigeminal neuralgia, therapy with drugs more potent than those available in nonprescription medications may be required.

Dull, aching facial pain localized in the trigeminal nerve area may occur in association with or during recovery from an upper respiratory tract infection. Although the pain often is described as "neuralgia," the exact etiology usually is unknown. Nevertheless, nonprescription analgesics frequently are helpful in alleviating this type of facial pain.

Myalgia

Pain from skeletal muscle (myalgia) is common. The most frequent cause is strenuous exertion of an unconditioned body. However, prolonged tonic contraction produced by tension or by maintaining a certain body position for extended periods also may produce muscle pain (7). Myalgia usually responds well to nonprescription analgesics and adjunctive treatment with rubefacients, counterirritants, and heat. (See Chapter 32, *External Analgesic Products.*)

Arthralgia

The most frequent cause of joint pain is inflammation of the synovial membrane (synovitis) or the associated bursae (bursitis). Joints that require free movement between two bones are constructed to maintain the articulating ends of the bones bathed in a lubricating synovial fluid. The two opposing bone ends are held in position by tough, fibrous tissue that forms an enclosure around the bone ends. The inner lining of this fibrous enclosure is the synovial membrane, which produces the lubricating synovial fluid (21). Bursae are saclike structures that contain fluid formed at sites of joint friction (where a tendon passes over a bone).

Rheumatoid arthritis is a chronic inflammation of synovial membranes, often occurring at multiple sites and having a predilection for smaller joints such as those of the hands, fingers, wrists, feet, and toes. Symptoms include joint stiffness, especially after arising in the morning, pain with joint motion, and swelling and tenderness of affected joints. Studies indicate that approximately 2.5–3% of the adult population has this condition, the highest incidence occurring in people over 40 (22). Although the cause of rheumatoid arthritis is obscure, hereditary factors have been demonstrated, and an immunologic mechanism has also been proposed.

Because of the slow, subtle nature of the onset of rheumatoid arthritis, many people attempt self-medication in the initial stages on the premise that advancing age inevitably brings aches and pains. As the disease progresses, it is a common practice to increase the dosage of nonprescription analgesics voluntarily to maintain relief from arthritic pain. The pharmacist should caution the patient about the potential for chronic toxicity, drug interactions, or other adverse effects and should watch for symptoms that indicate overmedication or progression of the disease. Also, because rheumatoid arthritis is a progressive, degenerative disease, medical attention must be encouraged to institute physical therapy and exercise so that the maximum mobility of affected joints is maintained.

Bursitis

This condition may be caused by trauma, gout, infection, or rheumatoid arthritis. Although the shoulder is the most common site of bursa inflammation, the knee (housemaid's knee) and the elbow (tennis elbow) also may be affected. Common symptoms include pain and limited motion of the affected joint. Depending on the severity, the pain usually will respond to nonprescription analgesic therapy. Limiting motion of the affected joint often hastens recovery (23, 24).

TREATMENT

On the basis of careful patient history evaluation, the pharmacist should decide whether the pain or fever can be self-medicated or if physician referral is necessary. If the condition is amenable to self-medication with a nonprescription analgesic/antipyretic, the pharmacist should recommend an appropriate product.

Salicylates

Because of their historical significance, extent of use, and spectrum of pharmacologic activity, the salicylates represent the prototype of nonnarcotic analgesics. They produce their pharmacologic effects primarily through the production of salicylate ion in the body. Several forms of salicylate are available.

The salicylates have analgesic, antipyretic, and anti-inflammatory activity and are most effective in treating mild to moderate pain of the dull, aching type that originates in somatic structures. Salicylates produce analgesia peripherally by inhibiting impulse production in pain receptors (5, 25–27). Prostaglandins sensitize peripheral pain receptors, making them more sensitive to chemical or mechanical initiation of pain impulses (4, 27). Salicylates inhibit prostaglandin synthesis and desensitize pain receptors to the initiation of pain impulses by decreasing prostaglandin production at inflammation and trauma sites (28).

Salicylate therapy for fever reduction is initiated most frequently in children because of their propensity for fever-induced convulsions. Salicylates effectively reduce elevated body temperature by causing the hypothalamic thermoregulatory center to reestablish a normal set point. Heat production is not inhibited, but rather heat loss is augmented by increased cutaneous blood flow and sweating induced by the reset thermoregulatory center. Salicylates exert their antipyretic effect by inhibiting prostaglandin production in the hypothalamus (5, 29, 30).

TABLE 2 Recommended pediatric single dosage schedule for aspirin and acetaminophen

Age of child (years)	Number of 80-mg pediatric dosage units to be taken every 4 hours[a]	Dose (mg) every 4 hours	Maximum total 24-hour dosage (mg)
Under 2[b]			
2 to under 4	2	160	800
4 to under 6	3	240	1,200
6 to under 9	4	320	1,600
9 to under 11	5	400	2,000
11 to under 12	6	480	2,400

[a] Not to exceed five single doses in 24 hours. No child should be given a nonprescription analgesic for more than 5 days or a nonprescription antipyretic for more than 3 days except under the advice and supervision of a physician.

[b] There is no recommended dosage except under the advice and supervision of a physician.

Adapted from the Report of the Advisory Review Panel on OTC Internal Analgesic and Antirheumatic Drug Products, *Federal Register*, *42(131)*, 35368 and 35445-50 (1977).

The adult oral aspirin dosage considered to be safe for self-medication by the FDA advisory review panel on over-the-counter (OTC) internal analgesic and antirheumatic drug products is 325–650 mg every 4 hours while symptoms persist, not to exceed 4 g in 24 hours. On the basis of pharmacokinetic considerations, the panel recommends that the maximum single dose be 975 mg (31). This is to be administered only once as a single dose or as the initial (loading) dose in a multiple-dose regimen. Single analgesic–antipyretic doses of salicylate usually yield plasma salicylate concentrations below 6 mg/100 ml (5). These dosage recommendations apply to aspirin used either as an analgesic or as an antipyretic. The panel's recommendations for pediatric aspirin dosage are summarized in Table 2.

Although the efficacy of salicylates in treating inflammatory conditions such as rheumatic fever and rheumatoid arthritis is well established, the mechanism by which these beneficial effects are produced is not. Studies show that the anti-inflammatory effect of salicylates is the result of their inhibition of prostaglandin synthesis (28, 32). E-type prostaglandins are formed at inflammation sites where they produce vasodilation and potentiate plasma exudate formation produced by other mediators such as histamine and bradykinin (33, 34). Research in animals shows a correlation between potentiation of plasma exudate formation and the vasodilator activity of prostaglandins and suggests that prostaglandins probably do not increase vascular permeability and plasma exudate formation directly in inflammation (35). Therefore, at least part of the anti-inflammatory effect of salicylates is attributable to decreased prostaglandin synthesis at inflammation sites, with a resultant decrease in vasodilation and plasma exudate formation.

Aspirin dosages of 4–6 g per day are effective in relieving symptomatic pain associated with rheumatoid arthritis and produce plasma salicylate concentrations of 15–30 mg/100 ml (5). Nonprescription labeling regulations for aspirin direct the patient not to exceed 4 g in 24 hours. Consequently, self-medication with aspirin for arthritis may be inadequate therapy because the aspirin dose required for efficacy is often greater than that deemed safe for self-medication (36). Furthermore, some patients may require higher aspirin doses to attain adequate salicylate serum levels for optimal anti-inflammatory effects.

Contraindications to Salicylate Use

Impaired Platelet Aggregation and Hypoprothrombinemia Aspirin, but not other salicylates, may compromise hemostasis by irreversibly inhibiting platelet aggregation; all salicylates can decrease plasma prothrombin levels. In a normal individual, a single 650-mg dose of aspirin approximately doubles the mean bleeding time for 4–7 days (5, 37). This increase in bleeding time is due primarily to inhibited platelet aggregation and not to hypoprothrombinemia. Decreased platelet aggregation is the result of an irreversible aspirin-induced inhibition of prostaglandin synthesis in the platelet (38–40). Salicylate doses of more than 6 g per day are required to reduce plasma prothrombin levels, and the minimal prolongation of prothrombin time that occurs with these doses is rarely clinically significant (5, 37). Salicylates reduce plasma prothrombin levels by interfering with the use of vitamin K for prothrombin synthesis (41).

Platelet aggregation is an important hemostatic mechanism, especially in capillaries and other small blood vessels. When small vessel damage occurs, platelets adhere to exposed collagen fibers and aggregate to form a plug. A fibrin network forms, and a clot develops to stop bleeding from the damaged vessel. Platelet aggregation is an extremely important mechanism for controlling the oozing type of capillary bleeding. Aspirin may potentiate capillary bleeding from the gastrointestinal (GI) tract, post-tonsillectomy tonsillar bed, and tooth sockets following dental extractions (42–44). Consequently, aspirin therapy should be discontinued at least 1 week before surgery, and aspirin should be used to relieve the pain of tonsillectomy or dental extraction only under the advice and supervision of a physician or dentist. Additionally, the FDA advisory review panel on OTC internal analgesic and antirheumatic drug products recommends the following warning on all oral aspirin products to be chewed (chewable tablets or gums): "Do not take this product for at least 7 days after tonsillectomy or oral surgery except under the advice and supervision of a physician" (45).

Many patients are under the false impression that for "tooth" or "throat" pain, local placement of aspirin is more beneficial. Pharmacists should be aware of the potential dangers of gum ulceration with this practice and advise their patients appropriately.

Aspirin use should be avoided by individuals with hypoprothrombinemia, vitamin K deficiency, hemophilia, or history of other clotting disorders, and by those with a history of peptic ulcer or GI bleeding. In contrast to aspirin, acetaminophen does not affect platelet aggregation or bleeding time (37, 42). In both normal patients and hemophiliacs, a 6-week course of acetaminophen (1,950 mg per day) has no clinically meaningful effect on bleeding time or platelet aggregation (46). Therefore, acetaminophen is a useful analgesic for patients in whom concern about hemostasis contraindicates aspirin use.

Impaired Uric Acid Elimination Salicylates affect uric acid secretion and reabsorption by the renal tubules. The result is dependent on the dosage of salicylate administered. In low dosages of 1–2 g per day, salicylates inhibit tubular uric acid secretion without affecting reabsorption. Consequently, low salicylate dosages of 1–2 g per day reduce urate excretion by the kidney, elevate plasma urate levels, and may precipitate an acute gout attack. Moderate dosages (2–3 g per day) usually have no effect on uric acid secretion, and high dosages (>5 g per day) may increase uric acid excretion, resulting in decreased plasma urate levels. However, effective uricosuric dosages of salicylates are poorly tolerated, making aspirin a poor choice as a uricosuric agent (5). For this reason, self-medication with salicylates by individuals with a history of gout should be discouraged.

GI Irritation and Bleeding Dyspepsia with heartburn, epigastric distress, and nausea or vomiting occurs in approximately 5% of patients taking aspirin (47). More common than dyspepsia is mild GI bleeding following aspirin ingestion in 40–70% of patients. The GI blood loss usually is in the range of 2–6 ml per day, but as much as 10 ml per day has been reported with normal analgesic dosages (48, 49). GI blood loss usually is not clinically significant, but prolonged aspirin use may result in continued blood loss and a persistent iron-deficient anemia (50, 51). Gastroscopic examination in salicylate-treated patients often reveals ulcerative and hemorrhagic lesions of the gastric mucosa, although lesions are not always visible in those experiencing blood loss (5, 6, 52). Occult blood tests of stool are frequently false-positive in patients taking aspirin. Aspirin use should be discontinued 3 days before such tests.

Massive GI bleeding characterized by the vomiting of blood (hematemesis) or the presence of large amounts of digested blood in the stools (melena) has been linked to aspirin ingestion. Approximately 30–40% of hospital admissions for hematemesis and/or melena are attributable to prior salicylate use (53–55). Individuals who take aspirin at least 4 days a week during a 12-week period have a significantly greater likelihood of suffering major GI bleeding than the less frequent user or nonuser of aspirin. The incidence rate of hospital admissions for major upper GI bleeding attributable to regular aspirin use is estimated to be about 15 cases per 100,000 admissions per year (56). Aspirin is contraindicated in individuals having a history of peptic ulcer disease or GI bleeding because it may activate latent ulcers or aggravate existing ones. In addition, ingesting alcohol with aspirin appears to increase the incidence of GI bleeding, and patients taking aspirin daily should be advised of the potential hazards of alcohol ingestion (57, 58).

Aspirin Hypersensitivity In predisposed individuals, aspirin may produce a hypersensitivity reaction characterized by any of the following symptoms: shortness of breath, skin rash and edema, hives (urticaria), severe asthma attack, anaphylaxis with laryngeal edema, bronchoconstriction, and shock. Aspirin hypersensitivity occurs most frequently in persons having a history of asthma or chronic urticaria. Up to 20% of such persons may exhibit aspirin hypersensitivity (59–62). In contrast, the incidence of aspirin hypersensitivity in the general population is estimated to be 0.3% (63).

The two major types of aspirin hypersensitivity differ in mechanism and type of response (64). Asthma patients usually exhibit shortness of breath or bronchospastic symptoms in response to aspirin. Evidence suggests that asthma-like symptoms are related to prostaglandin synthesis inhibition by aspirin, and cross-sensitivity has been demonstrated with other prostaglandin synthesis inhibitors including flufenamic acid, ibuprofen, indomethacin, mefenamic acid, and phenylbutazone (65–67). It should be noted that ibuprofen has a high incidence (>90%) of cross-reactivity in aspirin-sensitive patients (68). Acetaminophen rarely shows cross-sensitivity in this group (65).

The second aspirin-hypersensitive group, those with chronic urticaria, most frequently exhibits skin reactions such as rash or hives. The mechanism for this reaction is uncertain; however, an imbalance of plasma prostaglandins has been reported in this group (69, 70). This group may be more susceptible to cross-sensitivity with acetaminophen but the frequency is still low (71). Acetaminophen sensitivity has been estimated at 5–6% in persons intolerant to aspirin (72).

A history of asthma, chronic urticaria, or aspirin hypersensitivity contraindicates aspirin use for self-medication. In addition, a history of asthma-like reactions to the prostaglandin synthesis inhibitors also contraindicates self-medication with aspirin. Limited studies on cross-sensitivity suggest that acetaminophen may be an acceptable analgesic/antipyretic drug. Finally, persons with known aspirin hypersensitivity should be cautioned about using other nonprescription medications that may contain aspirin, salicylates, or ibuprofen. (See Chapter 9, *Asthma Products*.)

Drug Interactions Uricosuric agents such as probenecid and sulfinpyrazone are effective in treating gout because they block the tubular reabsorption of uric acid. Salicylates inhibit the uricosuric effects of both drugs by blocking this inhibitory effect on uric acid reabsorption (73, 74). Consequently, the concurrent administration of salicylates with either probenecid or sulfinpyrazone should be avoided because of the possibility of precipitating acute gouty attacks, hyperuricemia, or urate stone formation. Occasionally, salicylate doses of 650 mg or less, which do not produce serum salicylate levels above 5 mg/100 ml, do not appear to significantly affect probenecid uricosuria (75).

Because salicylates are highly protein bound and affect hemostasis and GI mucosa, hemorrhaging can occur if salicylates are administered with oral anticoagulants. The effect of oral anticoagulants on bleeding time may be enhanced by the salicylates, and the severity of salicylate-induced GI bleeding may be augmented as a result of hemostasis impairment by anticoagulant drugs (76). It is advised that the concurrent administration of salicylates and oral anticoagulants be avoided. For analgesic/antipyretic activity, acetaminophen is recommended for self-medication in patients receiving oral anticoagulant therapy (76).

Lowering of blood glucose levels by the sulfonylurea oral hypoglycemics may be enhanced when a salicylate is administered concurrently. Salicylates displace tolbutamide and chlorpropamide from plasma protein binding sites and have intrinsic hypoglycemic activity when taken by diabetics (5, 77). Controlled clinical studies documenting the significance of this interaction are lacking. However, in view of existing evidence, it is advisable to closely monitor diabetics who are receiving both salicylates and a sulfonylurea hypoglycemic agent,

especially when the drug is started or doses are changed. In recommending a nonprescription analgesic for concurrent administration, the pharmacist should take into consideration that acetaminophen seems to have less potential for interaction than the salicylates. (See Chapter 16, *Diabetes Care Products*.)

All anti-inflammatory drugs, both steroidal and nonsteroidal, used to treat arthritis and other inflammatory diseases are potentially ulcerogenic. Because of possible enhanced GI erosion when these agents are used in combination with a salicylate, it is recommended that persons taking prescription anti-inflammatory drugs should not self-medicate concurrently with salicylates (78). There is no clinical evidence to suggest additive or synergistic anti-inflammatory activity with the concurrent administration of nonsteroidal anti-inflammatory drugs (NSAIDs) and salicylates. In this regard, the ulcerogenic potential with salicylates would make acetaminophen a more appropriate choice of therapy (79).

Alcohol is known to potentiate the erosive effects of aspirin on the GI tract and to increase fecal blood loss (80, 81). However, it was recently reported that alcohol potentiates the prolongation of bleeding time produced by aspirin and ibuprofen (82). Both the magnitude and the duration of the bleeding time response are increased by the ingestion of alcohol up to 36 hours after the ingestion of aspirin. The magnitude and duration of the increased bleeding time are highly variable, and have been suggested to be sufficient to produce spontaneous bleeding (83). Although the clinical significance of this interaction seems minimal based on the widespread use of both drugs without deleterious results, it is prudent to caution the patient with a history of GI bleeding about the concurrent use of aspirin and alcohol. It has also been suggested that patients receiving aspirin for its antiplatelet effect should be cautioned about the potential hazard of concurrent alcohol use (81).

Aspirin has been reported to decrease the antihypertensive effect of captopril in sodium-restricted patients receiving the drug for hypertension. It is postulated that the long-term antihypertensive effects of captopril may result from the release of vasodilating prostaglandins, and aspirin interferes with their release. Patients receiving captopril for the control of blood pressure should be cautioned about self-medication with aspirin or other inhibitors of prostaglandin synthesis (84).

Salicylate Toxicity Mild salicylate toxicity may occur in adults or children after repeated administration of large doses. Symptoms may include dizziness, ringing in the ears (tinnitus), difficulty in hearing, nausea, vomiting, diarrhea, mental confusion, and lassitude (5). Skin eruptions may appear if salicylates are continued for a week or longer, and more pronounced symptoms of the central nervous system (CNS) may develop, such as incoherent speech, delirium, or hallucinations.

The mean lethal aspirin dose in adults is between 20 and 30 g, and the toxic dose for children is 150 mg/kg (85–87). Symptoms of salicylate poisoning include those cited for mild toxicity and hyperventilation, dimness of vision, mental confusion, delirium, hallucinations, convulsions, and coma. Acid-base disturbances are prominent and range from respiratory alkalosis to metabolic acidosis. Initially, salicylate effects on the respiratory center in the medulla produce hyperventilation and respiratory alkalosis. In severely intoxicated adults and in most children under 5, respiratory alkalosis rapidly changes to metabolic acidosis (5, 86, 87).

Salicylate poisoning affects other physiologic functions. The metabolic rate is increased, resulting in increased heat production and fever. Children are more prone than adults to develop high fever in salicylate poisoning (86, 87). Hypoglycemia results from increased tissue glucose use and may be especially serious in children (5). Bleeding may occur from the GI tract because of erosion of the mucosal lining, or hemorrhaging from other sites may occur as a consequence of salicylate inhibition of platelet aggregation (85, 87).

Emergency management of aspirin poisoning is designed to remove it from the stomach. Because of the rapid absorption of salicylates from the GI tract, emptying the stomach at home or en route to an emergency medical facility is advised. Vomiting should be induced even if the patient has vomited spontaneously. Adults should be given 30 ml of syrup of ipecac followed by 8 oz of water, clear liquids, or carbonated beverages and ambulated to stimulate emesis (88). If emesis does not occur in 20–30 minutes, the process should be repeated with the same ipecac dose. Children 1–12 years of age should be given 15 ml of syrup of ipecac followed by a smaller volume of liquid; children under 1 year of age should have emesis induced only under medical supervision. Administering liquids or ipecac to a person who is convulsing or to one who is not completely conscious is absolutely contraindicated (85, 87). It should also be noted that any patient suspected of taking a CNS depressant agent should not be given an emetic. Because it takes several minutes for the emetic to act, aspiration pneumonia may occur if the patient becomes obtunded before emesis.

An activated charcoal slurry, prepared by diluting each 10 g of charcoal with at least 80 ml of diluent, may be given orally and is very effective in delaying salicylate absorption from the stomach. For adults the dose is 30–100 g of activated charcoal diluted according to instructions; for children the dose is 15–30 g of activated charcoal diluted according to instructions. (See Chapter 12, *Emetic and Antiemetic Products.*)

Biopharmaceutics of Aspirin-Containing Products

The rate-limiting step for achieving therapeutic blood levels with solid dosage forms of aspirin is dissolution in the GI fluids rather than absorption from the gut (89). Factors affecting the dissolution rate include the degree of GI motility, the gastric fluid pH, gastric fluid volume, and the diffusion layer pH (the region of high salicylate concentration surrounding the dissolving aspirin particles). Aspirin's dissolution rate is increased by raising the volume and pH of the surrounding medium (90). Including alkaline buffering agents in the table formulation produces an elevated pH in the diffusion layer, increasing the aspirin dissolution rate. If formulated properly, buffered aspirin has significantly greater dissolution and absorption rates than nonbuffered aspirin (43, 91–93). However, there is no evidence from controlled clinical studies that buffered aspirin provides a more rapid onset or greater degree of pain relief than nonbuffered aspirin (91, 93).

The degree of salicylate-induced gastric irritation and erosion is a function of the salicylate concentration and the duration of exposure at the gastric mucosal surface. Although aspirin solutions also may produce GI erosion, undissolved aspirin particles are thought to be primarily responsible for gastric mucosal damage because they produce high salicylate concentrations at mucosal surfaces in the region of their diffusion layer (94). Buffered aspirin tablets produce less GI bleeding than nonbuffered tablets, presumably because they dissolve more rapidly, reducing the exposure time of the gastric mucosa to the offending aspirin particles (91, 95). Aspirin dissolution is favored when tablets are taken with a full glass (8 oz) of fluid.

Aspirin is absorbed more rapidly in solution than from either buffered or nonbuffered tablets because the dissolution factor is eliminated (92). Highly buffered aspirin solutions having a neutralizing capacity of at least 20 mEq of hydrochloric acid significantly decrease the amount of gastric bleeding (96, 97). However, the effervescent-type buffered aspirin solutions achieve their buffering action at the expense of a high sodium content. For this reason their use should be avoided by patients whose sodium intake is restricted. In addition, there is no valid evidence that highly buffered aspirin solutions produce more rapid or effective analgesia than either plain or buffered aspirin tablets (91).

Enteric-coated aspirin is specially formulated to prevent tablet dissolution until it reaches the more alkaline pH of the small intestine, preventing the gastric distress associated with dissolution in the stomach. However, aspirin absorption from enteric-coated tablets may be highly erratic. Tablets sometimes dissolve prematurely in the stomach and sometimes they do not dissolve at all (98). The variable aspirin absorption from enteric-coated tablets also is caused by differences in the tablets' gastric retention time (99, 100). However, enteric coating may reduce the likelihood of gastric and duodenal mucosal injury (101, 102). Studies indicate that current formulations of enteric-coated aspirin produce serum salicylate levels not significantly different from regular aspirin (103).

Timed-release aspirin is a formulation using encapsulation techniques attempting to prolong the product's duration of action. Such products are not useful for rapid pain relief because their absorption is delayed. However, the prolonged absorption may make timed-release aspirin useful as a bedtime medication. One study showed that 6–8 hours after ingestion of a single 1,300-mg aspirin dose the total serum salicylate concentration is significantly higher with the timed-release product tested than with regular tableted aspirin (104). Timed-release aspirin has been implicated in hemorrhagic gastritis and an increased incidence of deafness, but definitive clinical studies are not available (105–107).

Other Aspirin and Salicylate Dosage Forms

Choline salicylate is the only liquid salicylate preparation available. It is absorbed from the stomach more rapidly than aspirin in tablet form, but this property has little clinical significance (108). Evidence suggests that choline salicylate is less potent than aspirin as an analgesic/antipyretic; however, it may produce less GI bleeding and distress (25, 108, 109). A dose of 435 mg of choline salicylate is equivalent to 325 mg of sodium salicylate. The recommended adult dosage is 435–870 mg every 4 hours, not to exceed 5,220 mg in 24 hours (108). The liquid form is often useful for arthritic patients who have difficulty swallowing tablets.

Magnesium salicylate is equivalent to sodium salicylate in analgesic/antipyretic potency. Claims remain to be proven that it might be indicated when aspirin cannot be tolerated (108). In addition, the possibility of systemic magnesium toxicity exists in persons with renal insufficiency who take maximum daily doses of magnesium salicylate. The recommended adult dosage is 325–650 mg every 4 hours, not to exceed 4 g in 24 hours (108). The FDA, however, is considering revision of the recommended adult dosage for magnesium salicylate. Magnesium salicylate is available as the tetrahydrate; as a consequence, the salicylate content of approximately 375 mg of magnesium salicylate tetrahydrate is equivalent to 325 mg of sodium salicylate.

Sodium salicylate produces blood salicylate levels as high as equimolar doses of aspirin; however, it is probably less effective than aspirin as an analgesic/antipyretic (110). The sodium content of the maximum daily sodium salicylate dose (25 mEq) is sufficient to contraindicate its use in persons on sodium-restricted diets. The recommended adult dosage of sodium salicylate is 325–650 mg every 4 hours, not to exceed 4 g in 24 hours (108).

Salsalate (salicylsalicylic acid) is the salicylate ester of salicylic acid. It is absorbed principally from the small intestine and is hydrolyzed to salicylate during absorption and in the liver and other tissues. However, up to 15% of an oral dose is not hydrolyzed to salicylate, but rather is conjugated with glucuronic acid and is excreted in urine. Therefore, the amount of salicylate derived from salsalate is up to 15% less than the amount derived from aspirin when the drugs are given in doses that would theoretically provide equivalent amounts of salicylate (111). There are few comparative efficacy studies of salsalate and aspirin, but the analgesic effects of salsalate are considered to be comparable to those of aspirin. Salsalate reportedly does not affect platelet aggregation and produces less GI bleeding than aspirin (111, 112). The recommended dosage is 500–1,000 mg every 4 hours not to exceed 6,000 mg in 24 hours (112).

Aspirin and Pregnancy

Evidence from studies in laboratory animals and from retrospective studies in humans suggests that aspirin use during the latter months of pregnancy has adverse effects on both the mother and the fetus. The administration of 200 mg/kg per day of aspirin to rats during the last 6 days of pregnancy produced a prolongation of labor, a prolongation of parturition time, and increased in utero fetal death (113).

A 20-year retrospective study of 103 women who took more than 3,250 mg of aspirin a day during the last 6 months of pregnancy suggests that aspirin has detrimental effects during pregnancy. In comparison with control groups of women, those using aspirin had significantly longer gestation periods, longer labor periods, and greater blood loss at delivery. These effects on pregnancy may be related to the inhibition of prostaglandin synthesis, platelet aggregation, and prothrombin synthesis by aspirin (114).

Studies of 144 women who used nonprescription analgesic preparations containing aspirin during pregnancy reached similar conclusions (115, 116). The major effects reported for regular aspirin use during pregnancy included an increased frequency of anemia during pregnancy, a prolonged gestation period, an increased incidence of complicated deliveries, a high incidence of antepartum and postpartum hemorrhage, increased perinatal mortality, and decreased neonate birth weight.

Interpretation of these results is complicated, however, by a higher incidence of smoking in the aspirin-using group and by the fact that the nonprescription analgesic products used by these women were combinations of either aspirin, salicylamide, and caffeine or aspirin, phenacetin, and caffeine. Smoking in itself has been established to have numerous detrimental effects on pregnancy including lower birth weight of the neonate, increased perinatal mortality, and increased spontaneous abortion (117). Another study of 1,515 mother–child pairs exposed to aspirin for at least 8 days a month during at least 6 months of the pregnancy found "no evidence that aspirin as used by pregnant women in the United States is related to perinatal mortality or low birth weight" (118). It is possible therefore that the differences in perinatal mortality and birth weight reported in Australian studies are due to confounding factors such as smoking rather than totally to aspirin use (115, 116).

In attempting to reconcile the Australian (115, 116) and Boston Collaborative Drug Surveillance Program reports, the amount and frequency of aspirin use also must be considered (118). In the Australian study the group of women showing the greatest incidence of detrimental aspirin effect on pregnancy admitted taking nonprescription analgesic preparations every day during the pregnancy. This dosage represented a higher frequency of aspirin use than that evaluated in the Boston study.

Aspirin readily crosses the placenta and may be found in higher concentration in the blood of the neonate than in that of the mother (116, 119, 120). Salicylate elimination is slow in the neonate because of the reduced capacity to form glycine and glucuronic acid conjugates in the liver as well as the reduced urinary excretion resulting from low glomerular filtration rates in the newborn (119, 121). Consequently, analgesic aspirin taken by the mother before delivery may decrease platelet aggregation in the neonate and may affect hemostasis in both the mother and neonate (122, 123). In a group of 10 maternal–neonatal pairs in which aspirin (5–10 g) had been ingested by the mother within 5 days before delivery, a marked increase in the incidence of hemostatic abnormalities was reported in both mothers and offspring. Six of 10 mothers had an abnormal fall in hemoglobin levels postpartum and four of these six had direct evidence of abnormal blood loss including labial hematoma, intraoperative bleeding during cesarean and postpartum hemorrhage. Nine out of 10 of the infants born to these mothers had mucosal or superficial bleeding characterized by profuse petechiae, subconjunctival hemorrhage, hematuria, and bleeding from a circumcision site (124). It has been suggested that neonates are more sensitive to the platelet effects of aspirin than are adults because platelet adhesiveness and aggregation are impaired in the neonate (125, 126).

Neonatal intracranial hemorrhage has been reported to occur with higher frequency in infants born to mothers who took aspirin during the week before delivery. Of 108 premature infants who were evaluated for intracranial hemorrhage by computed tomographic scanning between days 3 and 7 postpartum, 53 (49%) developed intracranial hemorrhage. The incidence was significantly greater in infants born to mothers who had taken aspirin during the week before delivery than in infants born to mothers who had used acetaminophen or no aspirin during the same period (127). Consequently, it is recommended that aspirin not be taken during the last 3 months of pregnancy unless under the supervision of a physician and that acetaminophen is the preferred drug for self-medication during the last trimester.

Aspirin and Reye's Syndrome

Reye's syndrome is an acute, potentially fatal illness in children and young adults. It is characterized by vomiting, progressive CNS damage, signs of hepatic injury, and hypoglycemia (128). Influenza or chickenpox usually precedes the acute onset of vomiting or neurologic symptoms, and the peak incidence is during the winter months, correlating with the peak incidence of influenza. From 1977 to 1984, between 198 and 548 cases were reported each year, with a mortality rate of 22–42% (129).

Typically the child with Reye's syndrome will be recovering from either influenza or chickenpox and will abruptly develop intractable vomiting. Subsequently, the child presents neurologic symptoms such as listlessness, lethargy, disorientation, hostility, combativeness, inability to recognize family members, incessant moaning or screaming, twitching, and jerking. From this stage the child can rapidly progress to coma and death within 3–5 days (130).

Three case-controlled retrospective studies reported between 1980 and 1982 by the state health departments of Arizona (131), Michigan (132), and Ohio (133) have suggested an association between the development of Reye's syndrome and the ingestion of aspirin during the antecedent viral illness. These reports led the Committee on Infectious Disease of the American Academy of Pediatrics to conclude that "there is high probability that the administration of aspirin contributes to the causation of Reye's syndrome" and to recommend that "aspirin not be prescribed under usual circumstances for children with varicella (chickenpox) or those suspected of having influenza" (134). Although these studies have been criticized on methodological grounds (130, 135, 136), a review of the existing data by the Centers for Disease Control prompted a reiteration of the above position.

As a result of the uncertainty raised by these reports, it was suggested that the Public Health Service (PHS) coordinate a new, well-controlled study to clarify the role of aspirin in the development of Reye's syndrome. A task force comprised of members of the National Institutes of Health, the FDA, and the Centers for Disease Control designed and implemented a new epidemiologic study to evaluate the association between medication use and Reye's syndrome. Final results of the PHS study, reported in 1987, showed "a strong statistical association with the ingestion of salicylates during the antecedent illness and prior to the onset of Reye's syndrome" (137). In 1989, a case-controlled study attempting to eliminate possible bias in the PHS study also demonstrated a significant association between the use of aspirin during an antecedent viral illness and the development of Reye's syndrome (138). Therefore, based on the best available epidemiologic information, pharmacists should continue to advise parents that there is an increased risk of Reye's syndrome associated with the use of salicylates in children and young adults who have an influenza-like illness or chickenpox.

Aspirin and Antiplatelet Therapy

The use of aspirin under medical supervision for the prophylaxis or therapy of platelet-mediated thromboembolic or atherosclerotic disease has aroused considerable interest. When blood vessel damage occurs, platelets aggregate and adhere to collagen and other components of the damaged vessel wall, release granular contents including adenosine diphosphate (ADP), aggregate, and release thromboxane A_2, a prostaglandin produced from arachidonic acid. Its release promotes further platelet aggregation, and it is a potent vasoconstrictor. The vessel wall also produces a prostaglandin called prostacyclin, a powerful vasodilator that inhibits both platelet adherence to the vessel wall and platelet aggregation. Prostacyclin seems to control homeostasis by limiting thrombus formation at sites of vessel wall damage. Its antiaggregatory effect counters the proaggregatory effect of platelet thromboxane A_2 (139, 140).

Aspirin irreversibly inhibits prostaglandin-dependent platelet aggregation and thromboxane A_2 synthesis by acetylating and inhibiting the cyclo-oxygenase enzyme in platelets (141, 142). Aspirin destroys the ability of circulating platelets to synthesize prostaglandins and thromboxane A_2 for the life of the platelet (approximately 10 days), decreasing its ability to aggregate. Aspirin also acetylates vascular cyclo-oxygenase and inhibits the synthesis of prostacyclin in blood vessels, thereby allowing platelets to aggregate, a potential prothrombotic event. Earlier studies suggested that low dosages of aspirin (20–40 mg per day) possibly inhibit synthesis of thromboxane A_2 while only minimally affecting the synthesis of prostacylclin; however, more recent evidence is contradictory and does not support this theory (143, 144). Of the nonprescription salicylates, only as-

pirin irreversibly inhibits platelet aggregation; other salicylates have only a transient effect on platelet prostaglandin synthesis and aggregation (145, 146).

Several clinical studies suggest that antiplatelet therapy is effective in preventing transient ischemic attack (TIA) and stroke. A TIA is a sudden interruption of the blood flow to a portion of the brain or retina, resulting in symptoms of neurologic deficit lasting from a few seconds to 24 hours. Emboli consisting of platelet-fibrin masses or debris from atherosclerotic lesions are the most common cause (147). The risk of stroke in a patient who has had a TIA is approximately 5–6% a year with the greatest risk in the 3 months following the first attack (147).

The Canadian Cooperative Stroke Study found that a dose of 1,300 mg of aspirin per day produced a 48% decrease in the incidence of stroke and death in men who had had a TIA within 3 months of entering the study. However, no significant benefit of aspirin was found in women (148). A similar study in the United States also employing 1,300 mg of aspirin per day demonstrated a reduction in TIAs during the first 6 months following entry into the study, but no difference between the responses of men and women was demonstrated (149). More recently, a United Kingdom TIA study group conducted a study on aspirin and TIA by randomly selecting 2,435 male and female TIA patients and placing them in three treatment groups: members of one group received 300 mg of aspirin a day, members of a second group received 1,200 mg of aspirin a day, and members of the control group received placebos. At the end of the 4-year mean treatment interval, the odds of suffering a nonfatal myocardial infarct, nonfatal stroke, or vascular death were 18% less in the two groups receiving aspirin. No significant difference in response was noted between these two groups except that the group receiving the lower dosage experienced less GI toxicity (150).

A recent analysis of 13 antiplatelet drug trials in patients with a history of cerebrovascular disease demonstrated a 22% (standard deviation ±5%) reduction in first myocardial infarct, stroke, or vascular death with antiplatelet drug therapy. The trials included four antiplatelet treatments: low dosages of aspirin (300–325 mg a day), high dosages of aspirin, sulfinpyrazone only, or high dosages of aspirin with dipyridamole (151). Comparison of the effects of the four treatments showed no significant differences.

Numerous observations suggest a link between platelet-induced thromboembolism and myocardial infarct. In animal models of myocardial ischemia, aggregated platelets have been found in the coronary vessels, which may produce occlusion and myocardial injury (152). Patients dying suddenly with coronary atherosclerosis but no infarct often show platelet aggregates in the myocardial microcirculation (153). Several clinical studies have shown that patients with coronary artery disease have increased platelet aggregation and decreased platelet survival (154). The rationale for the use of antiplatelet drugs in patients with ischemic heart disease is to prevent the formation of a platelet-fibrin thrombus and its subsequent embolization in the coronary microcirculation (155).

Recently, the results of 10 antiplatelet drug trials in patients with a history of myocardial infarct were pooled to evaluate clinical efficacy of antiplatelet treatments in this risk group. Of the ten trials, eight used aspirin (alone or with dipyridamole) and two used sulfinpyrazone. The pooled analysis demonstrated a 25% (standard deviation ±4%) reduction in vascular events defined as myocardial infarct, stroke, or vascular death. No significant difference was found between the various antiplatelet therapies (151). It is estimated that without aspirin therapy, 78 out of 100 patients will survive 1 year following a myocardial infarct, and that if given aspirin 83 out of 100 will survive (156). It should also be noted that in three of the myocardial reinfarct trials cited above, stroke incidence was reduced by 20%.

Aspirin has been shown to be protective against myocardial infarct and death in patients with unstable angina. Males diagnosed with unstable angina and documented coronary artery disease were given 342 mg of aspirin daily in a buffered aqueous solution. At the end of 12 weeks, there was a 51% reduction in nonfatal myocardial infarct and mortality in the aspirin-treated group as compared to the placebo-treated group (157). Recently the International Study of Infarct Survival Collaborative Group conducted a large randomized trial in which low dosages of aspirin (160 mg a day) were administered to patients who had suffered myocardial infarct. After 5 weeks, highly significant reductions were noted in stroke (45%), reinfarct (49%), and vascular death (22%) (158).

In 1988 and 1989, the results of the first two, large-scale, prospective trials evaluating aspirin in the primary prevention of cardiovascular events and death were reported. Participants enrolled in these studies had no previous history of cardiovascular disease. The Physicians' Health Study randomly assigned 22,071 male doctors to three treatment groups: members of one group received 325 mg of aspirin every other day, members of a second group received beta carotene, and members of the control group received placebos. The effect of low dosages of aspirin on cardiovascular events was evaluated within an average follow-up time of 60 months. The aspirin-treated group showed a 44% reduction in the risk of myocardial infarct as well as a statistically nonsignificant trend of increased risk of stroke. The data on the effect of low dosages of aspirin on stroke and cardiovascular death were inconclusive because of the inadequate numbers of participants with these end points. Analysis of trial data showed that al-

though reduction in the risk of myocardial infarct was apparent only among participants 50 years of age and older, this benefit was present at all levels of cholesterol (159, 160).

A similar study in Great Britain randomly assigned 5,139 healthy male physicians to either an aspirin-treated group (500 mg a day) or a group with instructions to avoid all aspirin-containing products. At the end of 6 years, the study's data did not show aspirin having any effect on reducing stroke, myocardial infarct, or total mortality. However, differences in study size and design have been used to explain the discrepancy in results of the two studies (161, 162).

In response to widespread publicity about the results of the Physicians' Health Study, patients will inevitably seek information from their pharmacist about possible self-medication with aspirin for the prophylaxis of future cardiovascular events. When responding to such inquiries, the pharmacist should emphasize the demonstrated benefits of lowering plasma cholesterol, controlling blood pressure, stopping smoking, increasing exercise, and normalizing body weight in reducing cardiovascular risk. In the study, the use of even 325 mg of aspirin every other day was associated with increased risk of peptic ulceration and bleeding; therefore, patients with a history of peptic ulceration or other bleeding disorder should not self-medicate with aspirin. Because low-dose aspirin prophylaxis may also increase the risk of stroke, patients at increased risk of stroke from uncontrolled hypertension should not self-medicate with aspirin prophylaxis. Finally, the reduction in risk of myocardial infarct associated with aspirin prophylaxis has been shown only in males over 50 years of age. This risk reduction cannot be extrapolated to other segments of the population.

Salicylamide

Although it is structurally similar to salicylates, salicylamide is not hydrolyzed to salicylic acid in the body, and its pharmacologic activity resides in the salicylamide molecule itself (163). Salicylamide's unusual pharmacokinetic character complicates interpretation of its efficacy and formulation factors. Oral salicylamide doses below 600 mg are almost completely metabolized to inactive metabolites during transit through the GI mucosa and hepatic circulation before reaching the systemic circulation. Consequently, "breakthrough doses" greater than 600 mg are required to saturate the intestinal and hepatic enzyme systems and to achieve effective systemic concentrations (164, 165).

Salicylamide has been shown to have greater analgesic effects than aspirin in animals (166, 167); however, studies in humans with pathologic pain have shown that salicylamide is not superior to aspirin in doses below 600 mg and is indistinguishable from placebo (25, 166). Salicylamide has proven consistently inferior to aspirin as an antipyretic in both animal and human studies and is estimated to be about half as potent as aspirin as an antipyretic (31, 168). Persons allergic to aspirin usually have no cross-sensitivity to salicylamide, and salicylamide does not increase prothrombin time (164, 169). The FDA advisory review panel on OTC internal analgesic and antirheumatic drug products concluded that salicylamide is probably ineffective in the recommended adult dosages of 300–600 mg every 4 hours when used as a single analgesic or antipyretic agent. The panel also concluded that there is insufficient evidence of efficacy when salicylamide is used as an adjuvant in combination with other analgesic–antipyretic ingredients. Higher doses (1,000 mg per 4 hours, not to exceed 6,000 mg in 24 hours) may be effective; however, there is insufficient evidence supporting the safety of salicylamide. There is no recommended dosage for children under 12 years of age except under the advice and supervision of a physician (164).

Ibuprofen

Ibuprofen has been available in the United States as a prescription anti-inflammatory/analgesic since 1974. In 1984, the FDA approved ibuprofen for sale without a prescription with a lower recommended daily dosage than when dispensed as a prescription drug. Ibuprofen is a peripherally acting analgesic, producing a reversible inhibition of cyclo-oxygenase and the subsequent inhibition of prostaglandin synthesis in tissues. It also has clinically useful anti-inflammatory properties that result from its inhibition of prostaglandin synthesis and other effects on the immune system (170, 171). Ibuprofen has no effect on the pituitary–adrenocortical axis. Like the salicylates, the analgesic effect is seen with lower dosages than is the anti-inflammatory effect (172). Whereas the anti-inflammatory dose is 300–600 mg every 4–6 hours with not more than 2,400 mg in 24 hours, the analgesic dose is 200–400 mg every 4–6 hours with not more than 1,200 mg in 24 hours (173).

Numerous studies have documented the analgesic efficacy of ibuprofen. In postsurgical dental pain, 400 mg of ibuprofen was more effective than aspirin (650 mg), codeine (60 mg), and *d*-propoxyphene HCl (65 mg). A dose-effect relationship has been demonstrated for ibuprofen analgesia in the range of 100–400 mg; however, with doses greater than 400 mg there is no demonstrable enhancement of analgesic efficacy either

in peak effect or duration (174). Comparative studies demonstrate that on a milligram-to-milligram basis, ibuprofen is approximately 3.5 times more potent than aspirin as an analgesic and that the analgesic effect lasts at least 6 hours (175). By comparison, aspirin and codeine usually provide only 4 hours or less of analgesia.

Ibuprofen has been shown in numerous clinical trials to be effective in relieving the symptoms of primary dysmenorrhea. Primary dysmenorrhea is estimated to occur in up to 50% of women during their reproductive years and is characterized by uterine cramps, backache, vomiting, diarrhea, headache, mild fever, and malaise. The symptoms occur shortly before and during the onset of menses and result from increased endometrial production of prostaglandins during this period (176, 177). With the exception of aspirin, all NSAIDs tested are effective in relieving the symptoms of primary dysmenorrhea. Ibuprofen is equal to indomethacin, but clearly superior to salicylate, aspirin, acetaminophen, and propoxyphene for symptomatic relief of primary dysmenorrhea (176). A review of the inhibition of prostaglandin synthesis for the symptomatic treatment of dysmenorrhea covered 11 trials in which 308 women were given ibuprofen for menstrual pain. An average of 66% of the women reported excellent or complete relief of pain, and an average of 22% reported slight or no pain relief (the remainder included a placebo response) (178). Symptomatic relief results from the reversible inhibition of cyclo-oxygenase and the subsequent inhibition of prostaglandin production in the uterus. The recommended dosage of ibuprofen for primary dysmenorrhea is 400–800 mg initially followed by 400 mg 4 times a day for the 2 or 3 days that symptoms persist (177). (See Chapter 7, *Menstrual Products*.)

The most common side effects of ibuprofen are gastrointestinal, including indigestion, nausea, epigastric pain, and diarrhea. NSAIDs produce dose-dependent GI mucosal injury with ulceration and bleeding. Ibuprofen produces less GI irritation and injury than aspirin, and dosages of 1,200 mg per day or less produce little ulceration or bleeding (170, 179, 180).

In dosages of 600–1,800 mg per day, ibuprofen increases bleeding time as a result of inhibition of platelet aggregation. However, in contrast to aspirin, ibuprofen's effect on platelet aggregation is reversible within 24 hours after discontinuation of the drug (179, 181). Ibuprofen has been shown safe to use in patients with hemophilia, but caution is advised (181). Ibuprofen does not affect whole blood clotting time or prothrombin time (179).

Because of ibuprofen's effect on bleeding time, concern has been expressed about its possible interaction with oral anticoagulant therapy. In addition, ibuprofen is more than 99% bound to plasma albumin, creating the potential for enhanced anticoagulant effects resulting from protein binding displacement of the oral anticoagulant by ibuprofen. In dosages of 1,200–2,400 mg per day, ibuprofen does not appear to affect the hypothrombinemia produced by warfarin (182). However, because binding displacement can occur (183), it is recommended that coagulation studies be carefully monitored at the beginning of ibuprofen therapy in patients being maintained on warfarin (184). In addition, because alcohol ingestion has been shown to potentiate 3.5-fold the bleeding time prolongation produced by ibuprofen, patients taking ibuprofen and warfarin should be advised not to consume alcohol (82).

Ibuprofen may decrease renal function and cause sodium and water retention. This effect is the result of inhibition of renal prostaglandin synthesis and may worsen or precipitate congestive heart failure (1, 185). Renal blood flow and glomerular filtration rate decreased in patients with mild impairment of renal function who took 1,200 mg per day of ibuprofen for 1 week (186). Advanced age, hypertension, use of diuretics, diabetes, or atherosclerotic cardiovascular disease appear to increase the risk of renal toxicity with ibuprofen (187). Consequently, patients with a history of congestive heart failure or impaired renal function should self-medicate with ibuprofen with caution, if at all. In addition, 7 days of therapy with ibuprofen (1,600 mg) in congestive heart failure patients stabilized on digoxin produced a 60% increase in serum digoxin concentrations (188). Consequently, patients with congestive heart failure stabilized on digoxin should be counseled to avoid self-medication with ibuprofen. Also, ibuprofen dosages of 2,400 mg per day for 3 weeks has produced a 5.8 mm Hg increase in mean arterial pressure in patients receiving antihypertensive medication. It has been hypothesized that ibuprofen attenuates the effectiveness of antihypertensive therapy by interfering with the production of certain vasodilator and natriuretic prostaglandins (189). In contrast, 1 g of acetaminophen every 8 hours did not adversely affect control of blood pressure. Consequently, patients taking antihypertensive medication should be counseled not to self-medicate with ibuprofen for an extended period of time; however, acetaminophen can be safely recommended for these patients.

Caution must be exercised with the use of ibuprofen in patients with a history of asthma, urticaria, or aspirin sensitivity. Prostaglandin synthesis inhibitors can produce bronchospasm in patients with asthma, and a dose of 50 mg of ibuprofen is reported to decrease expiratory flow in aspirin-sensitive patients (190). The abrupt onset of rash and hives has also been reported in an aspirin-sensitive patient who took a single 400-mg dose of ibuprofen (191). Allergic reactions to ibuprofen, including high fever, rash, and elevated liver function tests, also have been documented in patients with systemic lupus erythematosus or juvenile

rheumatoid arthritis (192, 193).

Although there is no evidence of fetal malformation or adverse fetal effect resulting from in utero ibuprofen exposure (194), it is recommended that all NSAIDs, including ibuprofen, be avoided during pregnancy, especially during the third trimester. In lactating women taking up to 2,400 mg per day of ibuprofen, there is no measurable excretion of ibuprofen into breast milk (195, 196).

Data from postmarketing surveillance in this country (194) and in England (197) suggest that ibuprofen produces minimal toxicity when taken in overdose. In the 9 years following its introduction into the United States, 67 ibuprofen overdose cases were reported. Of these, 36% were in children under 3 years of age. Of the 67 reported cases, three had a fatal outcome. The three fatalities were all adults and were complicated by the ingestion of other drugs or trauma. Of the 116 overdose cases reported by the National Poisons Information Service in London, only one resulted in death. This was a 67-year-old woman with a history of arthritis, angina, and depression who took an unknown quantity of ibuprofen together with aspirin. She died shortly after hospital admission from hypotension and cardiac arrest. Commonly reported symptoms of ibuprofen overdose include drowsiness, sweating, abdominal pain, nausea, vomiting, nystagmus, headache, tinnitus, coma, and hypotension. Based on alleged doses ingested, it appears that doses greater than 10 g have the potential for producing moderate to severe symptoms. Unless contraindicated by convulsions or unconsciousness, appropriate first aid for ibuprofen overdose includes the induction of vomiting with syrup of ipecac.

Acetaminophen

Acetaminophen is an analgesic–antipyretic and is effective in treating mild to moderate pain such as headache, neuralgia, and musculoskeletal pain (198). Although the mechanism and site of action of acetaminophen have not been definitely established (5), it appears they involve central prostaglandin inhibition (198–200). Studies document the analgesic efficacy of acetaminophen in dosage of 325–650 mg (201–203). The recommended adult dosage of acetaminophen is 325–650 mg every 4 hours, not to exceed a total of 4 g in 24 hours. Table 2 gives the recommended pediatric dosage for acetaminophen. Although comparative analgesic effectiveness is difficult to establish because of the nature of existing clinical testing procedures, acetaminophen is similar in potency to aspirin as an analgesic and antipyretic. However, a single 1,000-mg dose of acetaminophen is less effective than 600 mg of aspirin in relieving pain associated with rheumatoid arthritis when it is given as an analgesic supplement to regular anti-inflammatory drug therapy (204).

Although there are reports of minimal anti-inflammatory activity with acetaminophen, the *p*-aminophenols have no therapeutic use as anti-inflammatory drugs (5, 198).

Toxicity of Acetaminophen

Because it lacks many undesirable effects produced by aspirin, acetaminophen has gained favor in the United States as the "common household analgesic" (5, 205–209). However, there is also growing concern that increasing household availability and the public's lack of recognition of acetaminophen toxicity will produce a new health hazard (210–213). Acute acetaminophen poisoning may produce fatal hepatic necrosis (214–216). Chronic excessive use of acetaminophen (>5 g per day) for several weeks can produce hepatotoxicity, which is potentiated by chronic alcohol consumption (217–219).

In adults, symptoms of acute toxicity may occur following the ingestion of 10–15 g of acetaminophen (5, 220, 221). A single oral ingestion of 15–25 g is seriously hepatotoxic and potentially fatal (222–224). However, estimates of the ingested acetaminophen dose are not reliable predictors of potential hepatotoxicity. Plasma acetaminophen levels should be determined following ingestion of a potentially toxic amount; nomograms have been established to relate plasma acetaminophen levels to the likelihood of hepatotoxicity (225, 226). The plasma acetaminophen half-life is prolonged in cases of hepatotoxicity and is a valuable predictor of hepatic necrosis. If the plasma acetaminophen half-life exceeds 4 hours, hepatic necrosis is likely to occur (227).

The progression of symptoms with acute acetaminophen poisoning includes vomiting within a few hours; anorexia, nausea, and stomach pain within 24 hours; evidence of hepatotoxicity in 2–4 days with jaundice; and death in 2–7 days (5, 220). In addition, kidney damage, disturbances in clotting mechanisms, metabolic acidosis, hypoglycemia, and myocardial necrosis may occur (5, 211, 212). A latent period with no visible symptoms follows the initial symptoms. This can be deceptive to both the patient and physician. In nonfatal cases, the hepatic damage is usually reversible (228). Emergency first aid for acetaminophen poisoning should include emesis with syrup of ipecac (228). Activated charcoal will reduce acetaminophen absorption significantly but is most effective if given immediately after emesis within 30 minutes of acetaminophen ingestion (229). The benefit of activated charcoal must be evaluated if oral administration of acetylcysteine is anticipated because the charcoal may prevent adequate absorption of the antidote (230, 231). If given to the patient, activated charcoal can be removed by gastric lavage before administering acetylcysteine. The dosages and contraindications for syrup of ipecac and activated charcoal previously discussed for salicylate poisoning also apply to acetaminophen overdose. (See Chapter 12, *Emetic and Antiemetic Products*.)

The oral administration of a solution of acetylcysteine (Mucomyst) is effective without significant toxicity in preventing the hepatic necrosis of acetaminophen poisoning (232, 233). Although acetylcysteine is most effective in preventing hepatic necrosis when given within 10 hours of an acetaminophen overdose, it is still effective when given up to 24 hours after the overdose (234). The dosage of acetylcysteine recommended for acetaminophen poisoning includes a loading dose of 140 mg/kg, followed in 4 hours with a maintenance dosage regimen of 70 mg/kg every 4 hours for a total of 18 doses. Acetylcysteine should be diluted with a soft drink or unsweetened grapefruit juice to 5% (235). Evidence suggests that intravenous (IV) administration of acetylcysteine is safe and effective; in the United States, the IV product is available only as an Investigational New Drug (IND) (236).

Analgesic Renal Toxicity

Reports linking chronic analgesic use to renal papillary necrosis and interstitial nephritis first appeared in the 1950s (237–240). The syndrome is characterized by a symptomatic sloughing of renal papillary tissue, sometimes with the elimination of "brown lumps" of necrotic tissue in the urine. Tissue necrosis may be accompanied by oliguria, nausea and vomiting, massive diuresis, or hematuria. Anemia may be present as the syndrome progresses, and final stages include renal insufficiency, hypertension, and death (241).

Analgesic nephropathy has been linked most consistently to the use of phenacetin-containing analgesic combination products. Current opinion suggests that aspirin alone is not an initiator of nephropathy but that it may worsen or perpetuate the progression of papillary necrosis and renal dysfunction (242–248). Aspirin-induced inhibition of prostaglandin synthesis has been suggested to contribute to the nephrotoxicity of aspirin–phenacetin combinations by causing ischemic changes in Henle's loop, which predisposes the tissue to phenacetin-induced necrosis (249, 250).

In the United States, phenacetin-containing products have been involved in almost all reported cases of analgesic-induced kidney disease (249). Numerous epidemiologic studies suggest temporal and dose relationships between phenacetin ingestion and renal dysfunction, and follow-up studies in countries that completely removed phenacetin from nonprescription use support the causality assumption (251–257). As a result, phenacetin has been removed from all nonprescription analgesic products by order of the FDA. Recently, the regular use of acetaminophen has been associated with an increased risk for chronic renal disease (258), but the magnitude of this finding is yet to be determined.

PRODUCT SELECTION GUIDELINES

In evaluating the relative merits of nonprescription internal analgesic products, the choices are aspirin, acetaminophen, or ibuprofen and the various formulations of these substances.

Aspirin is the most frequently used nonprescription analgesic. It is specifically contraindicated because of its effects on hemostasis or GI erosion or in cases of hypersensitivity, third trimester pregnancy, or drug interaction. Buffered aspirin and choline salicylate have the advantage of producing less GI distress. Highly buffered aspirin solutions produce less GI erosion but contain large amounts of sodium and should not be used by individuals on low-sodium diets. Enteric-coated aspirin products may reduce the likelihood of GI erosion but have a longer onset of action because of their delayed and possibly incomplete absorption. The delayed onset of such products precludes their use in acute pain when prompt relief is desired.

In many cases, acetaminophen is the drug of choice. It is less likely to trigger asthma-like symptoms in asthmatics, but hypersensitivity reactions to the drug have been reported (259). Because acetaminophen does not cause gastric mucosal erosion and does not affect platelet function, it may be recommended for individuals with a history of peptic ulcer disease (260). Although acetaminophen in doses of 650 mg 4 times a day for 2 weeks significantly increased prothrombin time, two 650-mg doses 4 hours apart did not (261, 262). In addition, a 6-week course of acetaminophen (1,950 mg a day) did not affect bleeding time or platelet aggregation (46). Consequently, the intermittent use of acetaminophen by individuals receiving oral anticoagulant therapy should present no serious interaction. Because of its lack of anti-inflammatory activity, acetaminophen is not an acceptable substitute for aspirin in treating rheumatoid arthritis and similar inflammatory conditions. Acetaminophen is usually not as effective as aspirin if the pain has an inflammatory component, such as with a sprain. Acetaminophen is the nonprescription analgesic of choice for patients taking uricosuric drugs because it does not antagonize the uricosuric effect (259). In addition, acetaminophen's stability in

solution provides a convenient and palatable pediatric dosage form.

Ibuprofen is equal to or more potent than aspirin for the relief of mild to moderate pain and is especially useful in postsurgical dental pain and pain associated with inflammation. Although ibuprofen produces less GI injury than aspirin (263), acetaminophen is still preferable to ibuprofen in patients with a history of GI bleeding. Ibuprofen is more effective than either aspirin or acetaminophen for the relief of primary dysmenorrhea pain and should be recommended as the nonprescription drug of choice for this purpose. Ibuprofen should be avoided in patients with a history of renal failure or congestive heart failure, especially if the patient is stabilized on digoxin. Although ibuprofen does not affect the hypoprothrombinemia produced by warfarin or other oral anticoagulants, it should be used with caution in patients taking oral anticoagulants. In such patients, it is preferable to recommend acetaminophen because it does not affect platelet aggregation and does not influence the protein binding of drugs such as warfarin. Nonprescription doses of ibuprofen do not affect blood glucose in type 2 (adult onset) diabetic patients; consequently, ibuprofen can be used by diabetics who are controlled with insulin or oral hypoglycemic drugs (264). Similarly, because ibuprofen does not affect uric acid excretion by the kidney, it can be used in patients with a history of gout or who are taking uricosuric drugs. Because ibuprofen may alter the binding of aspirin to the cyclo-oxygenase enzyme and its subsequent irreversible acetylation, it is recommended that ibuprofen not be taken by patients who are using low-dose aspirin for antiplatelet therapy (265). Acetaminophen should be recommended to such patients because it does not affect aspirin-induced inhibition of platelet aggregation (266). Ibuprofen should be avoided in patients with a history of aspirin sensitivity or systemic lupus erythematosus because severe reactions to ibuprofen have been reported in such patients. Self-medication with ibuprofen should be avoided in patients taking prescription NSAIDs because of possible enhanced toxicity when two NSAIDs are given together.

Historically, many nonprescription analgesic products have been combinations of ingredients, often containing varying proportions of drugs such as aspirin, phenacetin, acetaminophen, salicylamide, or caffeine. The intent of such combinations has been to produce greater analgesic efficacy while minimizing side effects by reducing the total amount of analgesic present. Few well-controlled studies support the enhanced efficacy of such combinations. Two studies suggest that the venerable aspirin–phenacetin–caffeine combination (APC) is more effective than either the aspirin or phenacetin component alone (267, 268). However, other studies do not support this conclusion (269), and it might seem

TABLE 3   Factors influencing the choice of analgesic agents

Patient	Drug
CONDITION BEING TREATED	EFFICACY OF DRUG
Type of pain	Analgesic potency
Accompanying symptoms	Antipyretic potency
Frequency of dose and duration of treatment	Anti-inflammatory potency
	Onset and duration of effect formulation factors
PATIENT PROFILE	UNTOWARD EFFECTS OF DRUG
Age of patient	General acute and chronic toxicity
Drug allergy or idiosyncrasies	Allergenic potential and cross-sensitivity with other drugs
Pathologic conditions or susceptibility to untoward effects	Relative tendency to produce untoward effects
Concomitant use of other drugs, therapeutic diets, or diagnostic procedures	Potential to modify pharmacologic activities of other drugs or endogenous compounds

only of historical interest because many combination products have removed the phenacetin component because of its implication in analgesic renal toxicity. A well-designed study in cancer patients was unable to show that the combination of aspirin and acetaminophen was more effective in relieving cancer pain than either component alone (270). However, the APC combination was more effective than either aspirin or acetaminophen or the combination of the two (271). In studies of pain occurring after dental extractions and episiotomies, the addition of 65 mg of caffeine to 500 mg of acetaminophen appeared to enhance the analgesic effect of acetaminophen (272).

SUMMARY

The appropriate choice of an analgesic/antipyretic agent involves a consideration of both patient and drug factors (Table 3). In determining the drug of choice for

recommendation, the pharmacist must consider the condition being treated; the nature and origin of the pain or fever; accompanying symptoms; a history of asthma, urticaria or other allergic disease, hypersensitivity reactions, peptic ulcer, or clotting disorders; and the concomitant use of other medication. In addition, product selection must include evaluation of the product's proven efficacy for the condition being treated, formulation factors that may give the patient more prompt relief or fewer side effects, and the potential for adverse effects from the product ingredients.

REFERENCES

1   D. R. Haslam, *Br. J. Psychol., 58,* 139 (1967).

2   H. K. Beecher, in "Nonspecific Factors in Drug Therapy," K. Rickels, Ed., Charles C. Thomas, Springfield, Ill., 1968, p. 27.

3   A. C. Guyton, "Textbook of Medical Physiology," 7th ed., W. B. Saunders, Philadelphia, Pa., 1986, pp. 572–605.

4   S. H. Ferriera et al., *Prostaglandins, 16,* 31 (1978).

5   "The Pharmacological Basis of Therapeutics," 7th ed., A. G. Gilman, L. S. Goodman, T. W. Rall, and F. Murad, Eds., New York, N.Y., 1985, pp. 674–715.

6   M. L. Tainter and A. J. Ferris, "Aspirin in Modern Therapy," Sterling Drug, New York, N.Y., 1969, p. 43.

7   H. G. Wolff, "Headache and Other Head Pain," 2nd ed., Oxford University Press, New York, N.Y., 1963.

8   "Textbook of Medicine," 15th ed., P. B. Beeson, W. McDermott, and J. B. Wyngaarden, Eds., W. B. Saunders, Philadelphia, Pa., 1979, pp. 728–733.

9   "Harrison's Principles of Internal Medicine," 10th ed., R. G. Petersdorf et al., Eds., McGraw-Hill, New York, N.Y., 1983, pp. 18–20.

10   J. R. Saper, *J. Am. Med. Assoc., 239,* 2380, 2480 (1978).

11   V. S. Caviness, Jr. and P. O'Brien, *N. Eng. J. Med., 302,* 446 (1980).

12   R. J. Scheite and J. R. Hills, *Am. J. Hosp. Pharm., 37,* 365 (1980).

13   S. V. Deshmukh and J. S. Meyer, *Stroke, 7,* 11 (1976).

14   J. R. Couch, *Neurology, 26,* 348 (1976).

15   S. V. Deshmukh and J. S. Meyer, *Headache, 17,* 101 (1977).

16   J. Edmeads, *Headache, 17,* 148 (1977).

17   D. J. Dalessio, *J. Am. Med. Assoc., 239,* 52 (1978).

18   B. P. O'Neill and J. D. Mann, *Lancet, 2,* 1179 (1978).

19   "Textbook of Medicine," 15th ed., P. B. Beeson et al., Eds., W. B. Saunders, Philadelphia, Pa., 1979, p. 727.

20 "The Merck Manual," 15th ed., Merck, Rahway, N.J., 1987, p. 1107.

21 W. S. Gilmer, Jr., in "Concepts of Disease," J. B. Brunson and E. A. Gall, Eds., Macmillan, New York, N.Y., 1971, p. 746.

22 "Textbook of Medicine," 15th ed., P. B. Beeson et al., Eds., W. B. Saunders, Philadelphia, Pa., 1979, p. 186.

23 "The Merck Manual," 15th ed., Merck, Rahway, N.J., 1987, p. 979.

24 "Textbook of Medicine," 15th ed., P. B. Beeson et al., Eds., W. B. Saunders, Philadelphia, Pa., 1979, p. 205.

25 R. K. Lim et al., *Arch. Int. Pharmacodyn. Ther., 152,* 25 (1964).

26 R. J. Capetola et al., *J. Clin. Pharmacol., 23,* 545 (1983).

27 S. H. Ferreira, *Nature New Biol., 240,* 200 (1972).

28 J. R. Vane, *Nature New Biol., 231,* 232 (1971).

29 R. J. Flower, *Am. Heart J., 86,* 844 (1973).

30 M. Perlow et al., *J. Infect. Dis., 132,* 157 (1975).

31 *Federal Register, 42,* 35360–3 (1977).

32 S. H. Ferreira and J. R. Vane, *Annu. Rev. Pharmacol., 14,* 57 (1974).

33 A. Willis, *J. Pharm. Pharmacol., 21,* 126 (1969).

34 T. J. Williams and M. J. Peck, *Nature, 270,* 530 (1977).

35 T. J. Williams, *Br. J. Pharmacol., 56,* 341P (1976).

36 *Federal Register, 42,* 35453–61 (1977).

37 J. H. Weiss, in "Aspirin, Platelets and Stroke," W. S. Fields and W. K. Hass, Eds., W. H. Green, St. Louis, Mo., 1971, p. 51.

38 H. J. Weiss and L. M. Aledort, *Lancet, 2,* 495 (1967).

39 J. B. Smith and A. L. Willis, *Nature, 231,* 235 (1971).

40 H. J. Weiss, *Am. Heart J., 92,* 86 (1976).

41 K. P. Link et al., *J. Biol. Chem., 147,* 463 (1943).

42 C. Pochedly and G. Ente, *Pediatr. Clin. N. Am., 19,* 1104 (1972).

43 S. H. Reuter and W. W. Montgomery, *Arch. Otolaryngol., 80,* 214 (1964).

44 *Federal Register, 42,* 35385 (1977).

45 *Federal Register, 42,* 35412 (1977).

46 C. H. Mielke, D. Heiden et al., *J. Am. Med. Assoc., 235,* 613 (1976).

47 A. Muir, in "Salicylates—An International Symposium," A. St. J. Dixon et al., Eds., J. & A. Churchill, London, England, 1963, p. 230.

48 L. T. Stubbe, *Br. Med. J., 2,* 1062 (1958).

49 M. I. Grossman et al., *Gastroenterology, 40,* 383 (1961).

50 W. H. J. Summerskill and A. S. Alvarez, *Lancet, 2,* 925 (1958).

51 H. Heggarty, *Br. Med. J., 1,* 491 (1974).

52 H. E. Paulus and M. W. Whitehouse, *Annu. Rev. Pharmacol., 13,* 107 (1973).

53 A. Muir and I. A. Cossar, *Br. Med. J., 2,* 7 (1955).

54 H. F. Lange, *Gastroenterology, 33,* 778 (1957).

55 A. S. Alverez and W. H. J. Summerskill, *Lancet, 2,* 920 (1958).

56 M. Levy, *N. Eng. J. Med., 290,* 1158 (1974).

57 K. Goulston and A. R. Cooke, *Br. Med. J., 4,* 664 (1968).

58 C. D. Needham et al., *Gut, 12,* 819 (1971).

59 G. A. Settipane and F. H. Chafee, *J. Allergy Clin. Immunol., 53,* 200 (1974).

60 B. Giraldo et al., *Ann. Intern. Med., 71,* 479 (1969).

61 B. T. Fein, *J. Allergy, 29,* 598 (1971).

62 M. Moore-Robinson and R. P. Warin, *Br. Med. J., 4,* 262 (1967).

63 R. A. Settipane et al., *Allergy, 35,* 149 (1980).

64 *Federal Register, 42,* 35397–99 (1977).

65 A. Szczeklik et al., *Br. Med. J., 1,* 67 (1975).

66 A. Szczeklik and G. Czerniawska-Mysik, *Lancet, 1,* 488 (1976).

67 A. Szczeklik et al., *J. Allergy Clin. Immunol., 58,* 10 (1976).

68 G. A. Settipane, *Arch. Int. Med., 141,* 328 (1981).

69 S. I. Asad et al., *Clin. Allergy, 13,* 459 (1983).

70 S. I. Asad et al., *Brit. Med. J., 288,* 745 (1984).

71 J. A. M. Phills et al., *J. Allergy Clin. Immunol., 49,* 97 (1972).

72 G. A. Settipane, *Arch. Intern. Med., 111,* 328 (1981).

73 T. F. Yu et al., *J. Clin. Invest., 42,* 1330 (1963).

74 "Evaluations of Drug Interactions," 3rd ed., C. V. Mosby, St. Louis, Mo., pp. 58–59.

75 P. D. Hansten, "Drug Interactions," 4th ed., Lea and Febiger, Philadelphia, Pa., 1979, p. 255.

76 "Evaluations of Drug Interactions," 3rd ed., C. V. Mosby, St. Louis, Mo., pp. 156–157.

77 H. Wishinsky et al., *Diabetes, 11,* (suppl.) 18 (1962).

78 *Federal Register, 42,* 35453 (1971).

79 D. R. Millet, *Drug. Intell. Clin. Pharm., 7,* 1513 (1981).

80 K. Goulston and A. R. Cooke, *Br. Med. J., 4,* 664 (1968).

81 "Evaluations of Drug Interactions." A. F. Shinn and R. P. Shrewsbury, Eds., C. V. Mosby, St. Louis, Mo., 1985, pp. 34–35.

82 D. Deykin et al., *New Eng. J. Med., 306,* 852 (1982).

83 W. V. Kageler et al., *Am. J. Ophthalmol., 82,* 631 (1976).

84 "Evaluations of Drug Interactions," A. F. Shinn and R. P. Shrewsbury, Eds., C. V. Mosby, St. Louis, Mo., 1985, p. 308.

85 R. E. Gosselin et al., "Clinical Toxicology of Commercial Products," 5th ed., Williams and Wilkins, Baltimore, Md., 1984, pp. 368–375.

86 A. R. Temple, *Pediatrics, 62* (suppl.), 873 (1978).

87 H. B. Andrews, *Am. Fam. Physician, 8,* 102 (1973).

88 D. L. Uden et al., *Ann. Emerg. Med., 10,* 79 (1981).

89 G. Levy and J. R. Leonards, in "The Salicylates—A Critical Bibliographic Review," M. J. H. Smith and P. K. Smith, Eds., Interscience, New York, N.Y., 1966, pp. 5–47.

90 G. Levy, in "Salicylates—An International Symposium," A. St. J. Dixon et al., Eds., J. & A. Churchill, London, England, 1963, pp. 9–16.

91 *Med. Lett. Drugs Ther., 16,* 57 (1974).

92 J. R. Leonards, *Clin. Pharmacol. Ther., 4,* 476 (1963).

93 *Federal Register, 42,* 35378 (1977).

94 K. W. Anderson, in "Salicylates—An International Symposium," A. St. J. Dixon et al., Eds., J. & A. Churchill, London, England, 1963, pp. 217–223.

95 J. R. Leonards and G. Levy, *Arch. Intern. Med., 129,* 457 (1972).

96 J. R. Leonards and G. Levy, *Clin. Pharmacol. Ther., 10,* 571 (1969).

97 P. H. Wood et al., *Br. Med, J., 1,* 669 (1962).

98 L. Stubbe et al., *Br. Med. J., 1,* 675 (1962).

99 E. Nelson, *Clin. Pharmacol. Ther., 4,* 283 (1963).

100 J. R. Leonards and G. Levy, *J. Am. Med. Assoc., 193,* 99 (1965).

101 F. L. Lanza et al., *N. Eng. J. Med., 303,* 136 (1980).

102 G. R. Silvoso et al., *Ann. Intern. Med., 91,* 517 (1979).

103 J. J. Oroczo-Alcala and J. Baum, *Arthritis Rheum., 22,* 1034 (1979).

104 L. E. Hollister, *Clin. Pharmacol. Ther., 13,* 1 (1972).

105 J. R. Hoon, *J. Am. Med. Assoc., 229,* 841 (1974).

106 R. R. Miller, *J. Clin. Pharmacol., 18,* 468 (1978).

107 R. John, *J. Am. Med. Assoc., 230,* 823 (1974).

108 *Federal Register, 42,* 35417–21 (1977).

109 "Drugs of Choice—1980/1981," W. Modell, Ed., C. V. Mosby, St. Louis, Mo., 1980, p. 205.

110 "AMA Drug Evaluations," 5th ed., Publishing Science Group, Littleton, Mass., 1983, p. 92.

111 "Drug Information 84," G. K. McEvoy and G. M. McQuarrie, Eds., American Society of Hospital Pharmacists, Bethesda, Md., 1984, pp. 96–597.

112 *Federal Register, 42,* 35442 (1977).

113 H. Tuchmann-Duplessis et al., *Toxicology, 3,* 207 (1975).

114 R. B. Lewis and J. D. Schulman, *Lancet, 2,* 1159 (1973).

115 E. Collins and G. Turner, *Lancet, 2,* 335 (1975).

116 G. Turner and E. Collins, *Lancet, 2,* 338 (1975).

117 J. E. Fielding, *N. Eng. J. Med., 298,* 337 (1978).

118 S. Shapiro et al., *Lancet, 1,* 1375 (1976).

119 G. Levy and L. K. Garrettson, *Pediatrics, 53,* 201 (1974).

120 P. A. Palmisano and G. Cassady, *J. Am. Med. Assoc., 209,* 556 (1969).

121 G. Levy, *Pediatrics, 62* (suppl.), 867 (1978).

122 W. A. Bleyer and R. T. Breckenridge, *J. Am. Med. Assoc., 213,* 2049 (1970).

123 R. R. Haslam et al., *J. Pediatr., 84,* 556 (1974).

124 M. J. Stuart et al., *N. Eng. J. Med., 307,* 909 (1982).

125 M. M. Mull and W. E. Hathaway, *Pediatr. Res., 4,* 229 (1970).

126 D. G. Corby and I. Schulman, *J. Pediatr., 79,* 13 (1971).

127 C. M. Rumack et al., *Obstet. Gynecol., 58,* 52S (1981).

128 "Harrison's Principles of Internal Medicine," 10th ed., R. G. Petersdorf et al., Eds., McGraw-Hill, New York, N.Y., 1983, pp. 1819–1820.

129 *J. Am. Med. Assoc., 253,* 751 (1985).

130 J. P. Orlowski, *Postgrad. Med., 75,* 47 (1984).

131 K. M. Starko et al., *Pediatrics, 66,* 859 (1980).

132 R. J. Waldman et al., *J. Am. Med. Assoc., 247,* 3089 (1982).

133 J. T. Halpin et al., *J. Am. Med. Assoc., 248,* 687 (1982).

134 V. A. Fulginiti et al., *Pediatrics, 69,* 810 (1982).

135 J. T. Wilson and R. D. Brown, *Pediatrics, 69,* 822 (1982).

136 D. H. Murphy, *Amer. Pharm., NS24,* 41 (1984).

137 E. S. Hurwitz et al., *J. Am. Med. Assoc., 257,* 1905 (1987).

138 B. W. Forsyth et al., *J. Am. Med. Assoc., 261,* 2517 (1989).

139 S. Moncada and J. R. Vane, *Pharmacol. Rev., 30,* 293 (1979).

140 J. F. Mustard et al., *Annu. Rev. Med., 31,* 89 (1980).

141 G. J. Roth et al., *Proc. Nat. Acad. Sci., 72,* 3073 (1975).

142 J. B. Smith and A. L. Willis, *Nature New Biol., 231,* 235 (1971).

143 J. Hirsh, *Chest, 95* (suppl.), 12S (1989).

144 P. A. Kyrle et al., *Circulation 75,* 1025 (1987).

145 J. J. Kocsis et al., *Prostaglandins, 3,* 141 (1973).

146 G. DeGaetano et al., *Lancet, 2,* 974 (1982).

147 H. J. M. Barnett, *Med. Clin. N. Am., 63,* 649 (1979).

148 Canadian Cooperative Study Group, *N. Eng. J. Med., 299,* 53 (1978).

149 W. S. Fields et al., *Stroke, 8,* 301 (1977).

150 UK-TIA Study Group, *Br. Med. J., 296,* 316 (1988).

151 Antiplatelet Trialist's Collaboration, *Br. Med. J., 296,* 320 (1988).

152 H. Vik-Mo, *Scand. J. Haematol., 19,* 68 (1977).

153 J. W. Haerem, *Artheroscelrosis, 15,* 199 (1972).

154 P. P. Steele et al., *Circulation, 48,* 1194 (1972).

155 J. Mehta, *J. Am. Med. Assoc., 249,* 2818 (1983).

156 P. C. Elwood, *Drugs, 28,* 1 (1984).

157 H. D. Lewis, Jr. et al., *N. Eng. J. Med., 309,* 396 (1983).

158 ISIS 2 (International Study of Infarct Survival) Collaborative Group, *Lancet, 2,* 349 (1988).

159 The Steering Committee of the Physician's Health Study Research Group. Preliminary Report, *N. Eng. J. Med., 318,* 262 (1988).

160 The Steering Committee of the Physician's Health Study Research Group, *N. Eng. J. Med., 321,* 129 (1989).

161 R. Peto et al., *Br. Med. J., 296,* 313 (1988).

162 V. Fuster et al., *N. Eng. J. Med., 321,* 183 (1989).

163 D. C. Brodie and I. J. Szekely, *J. Am. Pharm. Assoc. Sci. Ed., 40,* 414 (1951).

164 *Federal Register, 42,* 35439–35442 (1977).

165 L. Fleckenstein et al., *Clin. Pharmacol. Ther., 17,* 233 (1975).

166 E. R. Hart, *J. Pharmacol. Exp. Ther., 89,* 205 (1947).

167 E. M. Bavin et al., *J. Pharm. Pharmacol., 4,* 872 (1952).

168 A. J. Vignec and M. Gasparik, *J. Am. Med. Assoc., 167,* 1821 (1958).

169 A. J. Quick, *J. Pharmacol. Exp. Ther., 128,* 95 (1960).

170 T. G. Kantor, *Ann. Int. Med., 91,* 877 (1979).

171 P. Amadio, *Am. J. Med., 77,* 17 (1984).

172 L. S. Simon and J. A. Mills, *N. Eng. J. Med., 302,* 1237 (1980).

173 *Med. Lett., 26,* 63 (1984).

174 S. A. Cooper, *Ann. Rev. Pharmacol. Toxicol., 23,* 617 (1983).

175 R. R. Miller, *Pharmacotherapy, 1,* 21 (1981).

176 W. Y. Chan, *Ann. Rev. Pharmacol. Toxicol., 23,* 131 (1983).

177 M. Y. Dawood, *Am. J. Med., 77*(1A), 87 (1984).

178 P. R. Owen, *Am. J. Obstet. Gynecology, 148,* 96 (1984).

179 G. L. Royer et al., *Am. J. Med., 77*(1A), 25 (1984).

180 F. L. Lanza, *Am. J. Med., 77*(1A), 19 (1984).

181 B. A. McIntyre et al., *Clin. Pharmacol. Ther., 24,* 616 (1978).

182 J. A. Penner and P. H. Albrecht, *Curr. Ther. Res., 18,* 862 (1975).

183 J. T. Slattery and G. Levy, *J. Pharm. Sci., 66,* 1060 (1977).

184 "Evaluations of Drug Interactions," 3rd ed., A. F. Shinn and R. P. Shrewsbury, Eds., C. V. Mosby, St. Louis, Mo., 1985, p. 174.

185 R. T. Schooley et al., *J. Am. Med. Assoc., 237,* 1716 (1977).

186 G. Ciabattoni et al., *N. Eng. J. Med., 310,* 279 (1984).

187 J. L. Blackshear et al., *Arch. Int. Med., 143,* 1130 (1983).

188 F. P. Quattrochi et al., *Drug, Intel. Clin. Pharm., 17,* 286 (1983).

189 K. L. Radack and C. C. Deck, *Ann. Int. Med., 107,* 628–635 (1987).

190 D. E. Furst, *Am. J. Med., 77,* 51 (1984).

191 G. J. Merrit and R. I. Seele, *Am. J. Hosp. Pharm., 35,* 1245 (1978).

192 B. Mandell et al., *Ann. Int. Med., 85,* 209 (1976).

193 D. A. Stempel and J. J. Miller, *J. Pediatr., 90,* 657 (1977).

194 W. S. Barry et al., *Am. J. Med., 77,* 35 (1984).

195 R. J. Townsend and T. J. Benedetti, *Am. J. Obstet. Gynecol., 149,* 184 (1984).

196 R. T. Weibert, *Clin. Pharm., 1,* 457 (1981).

197 H. Court and G. N. Volans, *Adv. Drug React. Ac. Pois. Rev., 3,* 1 (1984).

198 L. O. Randall, in "Physiological Pharmacology," Vol. 1, W. S. Root and F. G. Hofmann, Eds., Academic, New York, N.Y., 1963, pp. 356–369.

199 B. B. Brodie and J. Axelrod, *J. Pharmacol. Exp. Ther., 97,* 58 (1949).

200 A. H. Conney et al., *J. Pharmacol. Exp. Ther., 151,* 133 (1966).

201 F. B. Flinn and B. B. Brodie, *J. Pharmcol. Exp. Ther., 94,* 76 (1948).

202 S. L. Wallenstein and R. W. Houde, *Fed. Proc., 13,* 414 (1954).

203   D. R. L. Newton and J. M. Tanner, *Br. Med. J.*, *2*, 1096 (1956).

204   E. C. Huskisson, *Br. Med. J.*, *4*, 196 (1974).

205   M. Swanson, *Drug. Intell. Clin. Pharm.*, *7*, 6 (1973).

206   P. A. Parks and J. Banks, *Ann. N.Y. Acad. Sci.*, *123*, 198 (1965).

207   L. O. Boreus and F. Sandberg, *Acta Physiol. Scand.*, *28*, 261 (1953).

208   E. Manor et al., *J. Am. Med. Assoc.*, *236*, 2777 (1976).

209   E. E. Czapek, *J. Am. Med. Assoc.*, *235*, 636 (1976).

210   J. R. DiPalma, *Am. Fam. Physician*, *13*, 142 (1976).

211   E. Sutton and L. F. Soyka, *Clin. Pediatr. (Philadelphia)*, *12*, 692 (1973).

212   H. Matthew, *Clin. Toxicol.*, *6*, 9 (1973).

213   R. Goulding, *Pediatrics*, *52*, 883 (1973).

214   D. G. Davidson and W. N. Eastham, *Br. Med. J.*, *2*, 497 (1966).

215   P. G. Rose, *Br. Med. J.*, *1*, 381 (1969).

216   R. Clark et al., *Lancet*, *1*, 66 (1973).

217   J. D. Barker et al., *Ann. Intern. Med.*, *87*, 299 (1977).

218   L. Harvey et al., *Ann. Intern. Med.*, *92*, 511 (1980).

219   C. J. McClain et al., *J. Am. Med. Assoc.*, *244*, 251 (1980).

220   A. T. Proud and W. N. Wright, *Br. Med. J.*, *3*, 557 (1970).

221   M. Black, *Gastroenterology*, *78*, 382 (1980).

222   J. Koch-Weser, *N. Eng. J. Med.*, *295*, 1297 (1976).

223   J. Ambre and M. Alexander, *J. Am. Med. Assoc.*, *238*, 500 (1977).

224   B. McJunkin et al., *J. Am. Med. Assoc.*, *236*, 1874 (1976).

225   B. Rumack and H. Matthew, *Pediatrics*, *55*, 871 (1975).

226   L. F. Prescott et al., *Lancet*, *2*, 109 (1976).

227   L. F. Prescott et al., *Lancet*, *1*, 519 (1971).

228   E. P. Krenzelok et al., *Am. J. Hosp. Pharm.*, *34*, 391 (1977).

229   G. Levy and J. B. Houston, *Pediatrics*, *58*, 432 (1976).

230   B. H. Rumack and R. S. Peterson, *Pediatrics*, *62* (suppl.), 898–903 (1978).

231   A. S. Manoguerra, *Clin. Toxicol.*, *14*, 151–155 (1979).

232   R. G. Peterson and B. H. Rumack, *J. Am. Med. Assoc.*, *237*, 2406 (1977).

233   B. H. Rumack and R. G. Peterson, *Pediatrics*, *62* (suppl.), 898 (1978).

234   M. J. Smilkstein et al., *N. Eng. J. Med.*, *319*, 1557–1562 (1988).

235   R. D. Scalley and C. S. Conner, *Am. J. Hosp. Pharm.*, *35*, 964 (1978).

236   L. F. Prescott, *Arch. Intern. Med.*, *141*, 386 (1981).

237   O. Spuhler and H. N. Zollinger, *Z. Klin. Med.*, *151*, 1 (1953).

238   L. F. Prescott, *J. Pharm. Pharmacol.*, *18*, 331 (1966).

239   J. H. Shelley, *Clin. Pharmacol. Ther.*, *8*, 427 (1967).

240   M. H. Gault et al., *Ann. Intern. Med.*, *68*, 906 (1968).

241   B. Koch et al., *Can. Med. Assoc. J.*, *98*, 9 (1968).

242   L. F. Prescott, *Scott. Med. J.*, *14*, 82 (1969).

243   P. Kincaid-Smith et al., *Med. J. Aust.*, *1*, 203 (1968).

244   M. A. McIver and J. B. Hobbs, *Med. J. Aust.*, *1*, 197 (1975).

245   U. C. Dubach et al., *Lancet*, *1*, 539 (1975).

246   R. D. Emkey and J. Mills, *J. Rheumatol.*, *1*, 126 (1974).

247   A. F. Macklon et al., *Br. Med. J.*, *1*, 597 (1974).

248   R. J. Bulger et al., *Ann. Rheum. Dis.*, *27*, 339 (1968).

249   *Federal Register*, *42*, 35424–30 (1977).

250   R. S. Hanra and P. Kincaid-Smith, *Br. Med. J.*, *3*, 559 (1970).

251   K. Grimlund, *Acta Med. Scand.*, *174*, 3 (1963).

252   A. F. Burry et al., *Med. J. Aust.*, *1*, 873 (1966).

253   N. R. Eade and L. Lasanga, *J. Pharmacol. Exp. Ther.*, *155*, 301 (1967).

254   V. Bengtsson, *Acta Med. Scand.*, *388*, 5 (1962).

255   H. H. Pearson, *Med. J. Aust.*, *2*, 308 (1967).

256   D. Bell et al., *Br. Med. J.*, *3*, 378 (1969),

257   D. R. Wilson, *Can. Med. Assoc. J.*, *107*, 752 (1972).

258   D. P. Sandler et al., *N. Eng. J. Med.*, *320*, 1238–1243 (1989).

259   *Med. Lett. Drugs Ther.*, *13*, 74 (1971).

260   C. H. Mielke, Jr., and A. F. Britten, *N. Eng. J. Med.*, *282*, 1270 (1970).

261   A. M. Antlitz et al., *Curr. Ther. Res.*, *10*, 501 (1968).

262   A. M. Antlitz and L. F. Awalt, *Curr. Ther. Res.*, *11*, 360 (1969).

263   G. Pasero, *Minerva Med.*, *64*, 2497 (1973).

264   N. L. Mork and R. P. Robertson, *West. J. Med.*, *139*, 46 (1983).

265   G. H. Rao et al., *Arteriosclerosis*, *3*, 383 (1983).

266   G. H. Rao et al., *Prostaglandins Leukotrienes Med.*, *9*, 109 (1982).

267   T. J. DeKornfeld et al., *J. Am. Med. Assoc.*, *182*, 1315 (1962).

268   R. O. Bauer et al., *J. Med.*, *5*, 317 (1974).

269   W. T. Beaver, *Am. J. Med.*, *77*, 38 (1984).

270   W. L. Wallenstein, in "Proceedings of the Aspirin Symposium," Aspirin Foundation, London, Eng., pp. 5–10, 1975.

271   E. M. Laska et al., *J. Am. Med. Assoc.*, *251*, 1711 (1984).

272   E. M. Laska et al., *Clin. Pharmacol. Ther.*, *33*, 498 (1983).

INTERNAL ANALGESIC PRODUCT TABLE

Product[a] (Manufacturer)	Aspirin	Salicyl- amide	Acetami- nophen	Ibuprofen	Caffeine	Sodium	Other Ingredients
Acephen Suppositories (G & W Labs)			120 mg 325 mg 650 mg			NS[b]	hydrogenated vegetable oil, polysorbate 80
Aceta (Century)			325 mg 500 mg 32 mg/ml (elixir)				alcohol, 7% (elixir)
Acetaminophen (Various manufacturers)			325 mg 500 mg 650 mg				
Acetaminophen Capsules (Various manufacturers)			500 mg				
Acetaminophen Chewable Tablets (Various manufacturers)			80 mg				
Acetaminophen Drops (Various manufacturers)			100 mg/ml				
Acetaminophen Elixir (Various manufacturers)			24 mg/ml 26 mg/ml 32 mg/ml				
Acetaminophen Liquid[c] (UDL Labs)			32 mg/ml				
Acetaminophen Suppositories (Various manufacturers)			120 mg 300 mg 325 mg 650 mg				
Acetaminophen Uniserts (Upsher-Smith)			120 mg 325 mg 650 mg				
Actamin (Buffington)			325 mg 500 mg		NS[b]	free	
Actamin Super (Buffington)			500 mg		65 mg	free	
Addaprin (Dover)				200 mg		free	
Adult Analgesic Pain Reliever (DeWitt)	400 mg				32 mg		
Adult Strength Headache Relief Formula (DeWitt)			325 mg				phenyltoloxamine citrate, 30 mg
Advil (Whitehall)				200 mg		0.004 mEq	

INTERNAL ANALGESIC PRODUCT TABLE, continued

Product[a] (Manufacturer)	Aspirin	Salicyl-amide	Acetami-nophen	Ibuprofen	Caffeine	Sodium	Other Ingredients
Alka-Seltzer (Miles)	324 mg					567 mg	sodium bicarbonate, 1.9 g citric acid, 1 g
Alka-Seltzer Extra Strength (Miles)	500 mg						sodium bicarbonate, 1.9 g citric acid, 1 g
Alka-Seltzer, Flavored (Miles)	324 mg					506 mg	sodium bicarbonate, 1.7 g citric acid, 1.2 g saccharin flavor
Allerest Headache Strength (Fisons)			325 mg			NS[b]	chlorpheniramine maleate, 2 mg phenylpropanolamine hydrochloride, 18.7 mg
Allerest, No Drowsiness (Fisons)			325 mg			NS[b]	pseudoephedrine hydrochloride, 30 mg
Allerest, Sinus Pain Formula (Fisons)			500 mg			NS[b]	phenylpropanolamine hydrochloride, 18.7 mg chlorpheniramine maleate, 2 mg
Aminofen (Dover)			325 mg 500 mg		free	free	
Anacin Caplets and Tablets (Whitehall)	400 mg				32 mg	0.001 mEq	
Anacin, Maximum Strength (Whitehall)	500 mg				32 mg	0.002 mEq	
Anacin-3, Regular Strength (Whitehall)			325 mg			0.03 mEq	
Anacin-3, Children's (Whitehall)			80 mg/chewable tablet 30 mg/ml (liquid[c])			NS[b]	flavor
Anacin-3 Infants' Drops[c] (Whitehall)			100 mg/ml				saccharin sorbitol flavor
Anacin-3, Maximum Strength (Whitehall)			500 mg			< 0.5 mEq	
Analval (Vale)	227 mg		162 mg		32 mg		
Anodynos (Buffington)	420 mg	35 mg			NS[b]	free	
Apacet Chewable Tablets (Parmed)			80 mg				

INTERNAL ANALGESIC PRODUCT TABLE, continued

Product[a] (Manufacturer)	Aspirin	Salicyl- amide	Acetami- nophen	Ibuprofen	Caffeine	Sodium	Other Ingredients
Arthritis Pain Formula (Whitehall)	500 mg (micronized)					0.01 mEq	aluminum hydrox- ide, 27 mg magnesium hydrox- ide, 100 mg
Arthritis Pain Formula, Aspirin Free (Whitehall)			500 mg			0.006 mEq	
Arthropan Liquid (Purdue Frederick)						NS[b]	choline salicylate, 174 mg/ml (equi- valent to 130 mg of aspirin)
A.S.A. Enseals (Lilly)	325 mg 650 mg				NS[b]	NS[b]	
A.S.A. Suppositories (Lilly)	325 mg 650 mg						
Ascriptin (Rorer)	325 mg					NS[b]	magnesium hydrox- ide, 50 mg aluminum hydrox- ide gel, dried, 50 mg calcium carbonate
Ascriptin A/D (Rorer)	325 mg					NS[b]	magnesium hydrox- ide, 75 mg aluminum hydrox- ide gel, dried, 75 mg calcium carbonate
Ascriptin, Extra Strength (Rorer)	500 mg						magnesium hydrox- ide, 80 mg aluminum hydrox- ide gel, dried, 80 mg calcium carbonate
Aspercin (Otis Clapp)	325 mg 500 mg					free	
Aspergum (Schering- Plough)	228 mg					0.003 mEq	
Aspermin (Buffington)	325 mg 500 mg					free	
Aspirin (Various manufacturers)	325 mg 500 mg 650 mg						
Aspirin, Buffered (Various manufacturers)	325 mg						buffers
Aspirin, Childrens (Various manufacturers)	65 mg 75 mg 81 mg						
Aspirin Free Pain Relief (Hudson)			325 mg 500 mg				

INTERNAL ANALGESIC PRODUCT TABLE, continued

Product[a] (Manufacturer)	Aspirin	Salicyl- amide	Acetami- nophen	Ibuprofen	Caffeine	Sodium	Other Ingredients
Aspirin Suppositories (Various manufacturers)	60 mg 120 mg 125 mg 130 mg 195 mg 200 mg 300 mg 325 mg 600 mg 650 mg 1.2 g					NS[b]	
Aspirtab (Dover)	325 mg 500 mg					free	
Banesin (Forest)			500 mg			free	
Bayer Aspirin (Glenbrook)	325 mg					< 0.01 mEq	
Bayer Aspirin, Maximum (Glenbrook)	500 mg					< 0.01 mEq	
Bayer Chil- dren's Aspirin (Glenbrook)	81 mg					< 0.01 mEq	saccharin flavor
Bayer 8-Hour Timed-Release (Glenbrook)	650 mg					< 0.01 mEq	
BC Tablet and Powder	325 mg/ tablet 650 mg (powder)	95 mg/tablet 195 mg (powder)			16 mg/ tablet 32 mg (powder)	free	
BC Arthritis Strength Powder (Block)	742 mg	222 mg			36 mg	free	
Bromo-Seltzer (Warner- Lambert)			325 mg/ capful			33 mEq/ capful	sodium bicarbo- nate, 2.78 g/ capful citric acid, 2.22 g/ capful
Buffaprin (Buffington)	325 mg 500 mg					free	magnesium oxide
Buffasal (Dover)	325 mg 500 mg					free	magnesium oxide
Bufferin, Arthritis Strength Tri- Buffered Caplets (Bristol-Myers Products)	500 mg					< 0.04 mEq	calcium carbonate, 222.3 mg magnesium oxide, 88.9 mg magnesium carbo- nate, 55.6 mg
Bufferin, Extra Strength Tri- Buffered (Bristol-Myers Products)	500 mg					< 0.04 mEq	calcium carbonate, 222.3 mg magnesium oxide, 88.9 mg magnesium carbo- nate, 55.6 mg

INTERNAL ANALGESIC PRODUCT TABLE, continued

Product[a] (Manufacturer)	Aspirin	Salicyl-amide	Acetami-nophen	Ibuprofen	Caffeine	Sodium	Other Ingredients
Bufferin, Tri-Buffered (Bristol-Myers)	325 mg					0.03 mEq	calcium carbonate, 158 mg magnesium oxide, 63 mg magnesium carbonate, 34 mg
Buffets II (JMI)	226.8 mg		162 mg		32.4 mg		aluminum hydroxide, 50 mg
Buffex (Hauck)	325 mg						dihydroxyaluminum aminoacetate
Buffinol (Otis Clapp)	325 mg 500 mg				NS[b]	free	magnesium oxide sugar lactose
Cama Arthritis Pain Reliever (Dorsey)	500 mg					NS[b]	magnesium hydroxide, 150 mg aluminum hydroxide gel, dried, 150 mg
Congespirin For Children Chewable (Bristol-Myers Products)			81 mg			NS[b]	phenylephrine hydrochloride, 1.25 mg
Cope (Mentholatum)	421 mg				32 mg		magnesium hydroxide, 50 mg aluminum hydroxide, 25 mg
Dapa (Ferndale)			325 mg				
Dapa Extra Strength Capsules (Ferndale)			500 mg				
Dasin (Beecham Labs)	130 mg				8 mg		atropine sulfate, 0.13 mg ipecac, 3 mg camphor, 15 mg
Datril Extra Strength Caplets and Tablets (Bristol-Myers Products)			500 mg			NS[b]	
DeWitt Pills (DeWitt)		108.2 mg			6.5 mg	NS[b]	potassium nitrate, 56.4 mg uva ursi extract, 32.4 mg buchu leaves, 7.8 mg
Doan's Original (Ciba)							magnesium salicylate, 325 mg magnesium stearate microcrystalline cellulose polyethylene glycol stearic acid

INTERNAL ANALGESIC PRODUCT TABLE, continued

Product[a] (Manufacturer)	Aspirin	Salicyl-amide	Acetami-nophen	Ibuprofen	Caffeine	Sodium	Other Ingredients
Doan's Extra Strength (Ciba)							magnesium salicy-late, 500 mg hydroxypropyl methylcellulose magnesium stearate microcrystalline cellulose polyethylene glycol polysorbate 80 propylene glycol stearic acid titanium dioxide
Dolanex[d] (Lannett)			65 mg/ml				alcohol, 23%
Dolcin (Dolcin Corp.)	240.5 mg					NS[b]	calcium succinate monohydrate, 182 mg
Dorcol Children's Non-Aspirin Fever & Pain Reducer (Sandoz Consumer)			32 mg/ml				
Duradyne (Forest)	230 mg		180 mg		15 mg	NS[b]	
Dyspel (Dover)			325 mg		free	free	atropine sulfate, 0.06 mg ephedrine sulfate, 8 mg
Ecotrin Regular Strength (SmithKline Beecham)	325 mg					0.001 mEq	
Ecotrin Maximum Strength (SmithKline Beecham)	500 mg					0.001 mEq	
Emagrin (Otis Clapp)	357 mg	32.5 mg			NS[b]	free	
Empirin (Burroughs Wellcome)	325 mg					free	
Excedrin Extra Strength Caplets and Tablets (Bristol-Myers Products)	250 mg		250 mg		65 mg	NS[b]	
Excedrin P.M. Tablets and Caplets (Bristol-Myers Products)			500 mg			NS[b]	diphenhydramine citrate, 38 mg

INTERNAL ANALGESIC PRODUCT TABLE, continued

Product[a] (Manufacturer)	Aspirin	Salicyl- amide	Acetami- nophen	Ibuprofen	Caffeine	Sodium	Other Ingredients
Excedrin, Sinus Caplets and Tablets (Bristol-Myers Products)			500 mg				pseudoephedrine hydrochloride, 30 mg
Feverall, Children's Suppositories (Upsher-Smith)			120 mg				
Feverall, Junior Strength Suppositories (Upsher-Smith)			325 mg				
Gemnisyn (Kremers-Urban)	325 mg		325 mg				
Genapap, Children's Chewable (Goldline)			80 mg				
Genapap, Children's Elixir[c] (Goldline)			32 mg/ml				flavor
Genapap, Extra Strength (Goldline)			500 mg				
Genapap, Infants' Drops[c] (Goldline)			100 mg/ml				flavor
Genebs (Goldline)			325 mg				
Genebs Extra Strength (Goldline)			500 mg				
Genpril (Goldline)				200 mg			
Gensan (Goldline)	400 mg				32 mg		
Goody's Extra Strength (Goody's)	260 mg		130 mg		16.25 mg	NS[b]	
Goody's Headache Powder (Goody's)	520 mg		260 mg		32.5 mg	< 0.001 mEq	lactose potassium chloride
Halenol (Halsey)			325 mg				
Halenol Children's Liquid[c] (Halsey)			32 mg/ml				
Halenol Extra Strength (Halsey)			500 mg				
Haltran (Upjohn)				200 mg			

INTERNAL ANALGESIC PRODUCT TABLE, continued

Product[a] (Manufacturer)	Aspirin	Salicyl-amide	Acetami-nophen	Ibuprofen	Caffeine	Sodium	Other Ingredients
Legatrin (Night Leg Cramp Relief) (O'Conner)							quinine sulfate, 162.5 mg
Liquiprin Children's Elixir (SmithKline Beecham)			32 mg/ml				dextrose fructose sucrose flavor
Liquiprin Solution (SmithKline Beecham)			48 mg/ml			< 0.03 mEq/ml	
Lurline PMS (Fielding)			500 mg				pamabrom, 25 mg pyridoxine, 50 mg
Magnaprin (Rugby)	325 mg						magnesium hydroxide, 75 mg aluminum hydroxide, 75 mg
Magnaprin Arthritis Strength (Rugby)	325 mg						magnesium hydroxide, 150 mg aluminum hydroxide, 150 mg
Measurin Timed-Release (Winthrop)	650 mg					NS[b]	
Meda Cap (Circle)			500 mg				
Meda Tab (Circle)			325 mg				
Medipren Caplets and Tablets (McNeil)				200 mg			
Menoplex (Fiske)			325 mg				phenyltoloxamine citrate, 30 mg
Menstra-Eze (Reese)			325 mg				pyrilamine maleate, 20 mg
Midol Caplets, Original Formula (Glenbrook)	454 mg				32.4 mg		cinnamedrine hydrochloride, 32.4 mg
Midol for Cramps Caplets, Maximum Strength (Glenbrook)	500 mg				32.4 mg		cinnamedrine hydrochloride, 14.9 mg
Midol PMS Capsules (Glenbrook)			500 mg				pamabrom, 25 mg pyrilamine maleate, 15 mg
Mobigesic (B.F. Ascher)						NS[b]	phenyltoloxamine citrate, 30 mg magnesium salicylate, 325 mg

INTERNAL ANALGESIC PRODUCT TABLE, continued

Product[a] (Manufacturer)	Aspirin	Salicyl-amide	Acetami-nophen	Ibuprofen	Caffeine	Sodium	Other Ingredients
Momentum (Whitehall)	500 mg					0.009 mEq	phenyltoloxamine citrate, 15 mg
Motrin-IB (Upjohn)				200 mg			
Myapap Drops[c,d] (Gen-King)			100 mg/ml				
Neogesic (Rev.) (Vale)	194.4 mg		129.6 mg		32 mg		
Neopap Suppositories (Alcon)			125 mg				
Norwich Aspirin (Vicks Health Care)	325 mg						
Norwich Extra Strength (Vicks Health Care)	500 mg						
Nuprin Caplets and Tablets (Bristol-Myers Products)				200 mg			
Oraphen-PD (Great Southern)			24 mg/ml				alcohol, 5% flavor
Pabalate (A.H. Robins)						88.4 mg	sodium salicylate, 0.3 g sodium aminoben-zoate, 0.3 g
PAC (Upjohn)	400 mg				32 mg	< 0.01 mg	
Pain-Eze + (Reese)			650 mg				
Pain Reliever Tablets (Rugby)	250 mg		250 mg		65 mg		
Pamprin (Chattem)			400 mg				pamabrom, 25 mg pyrilamine maleate, 15 mg
Pamprin Maxi-mum Cramp Relief Caplets and Capsules (Chattem)			500 mg				pamabrom, 25 mg pyrilamine maleate, 15 mg
Panadol (Glenbrook)			500 mg				
Panadol, Chil-dren's Chewable[d] (Glenbrook)			80 mg				flavor

INTERNAL ANALGESIC PRODUCT TABLE, continued

Product[a] (Manufacturer)	Aspirin	Salicylamide	Acetaminophen	Ibuprofen	Caffeine	Sodium	Other Ingredients
Panadol, Children's Liquid[c,d] (Glenbrook)			32 mg/ml				saccharin sorbitol flavor
Panadol, Infants' Drops[c,d] (Glenbrook)			100 mg/ml				saccharin flavor
Panex (Hauck)			325 mg				
Panex 500 (Hauck)			500 mg				
Panodynes Analgesic (Keystone)	260 mg	64.8 mg	64.8 mg		16.2 mg	free	
Phenaphen Caplets (Robins)			325 mg				
Prēmsyn PMS Caplets and Capsules (Chattem)			500 mg				pamabrom, 25 mg pyrilamine maleate, 15 mg
Presalin (Hauck)	260 mg	120 mg	120 mg				aluminum hydroxide, 100 mg
Rid-A-Pain (Pfeiffer)		97.2 mg	226.8 mg		32.4 mg	NS[b]	
S-A-C (Lannett)		230 mg	150 mg		30 mg		
Salabuff (Ferndale)	324 mg				16.2 mg		aluminum hydroxide-mangesium carbonate, co-dried gel
Salatin Capsules (Ferndale)	259.2 mg		129.6 mg		16.2 mg		
Saleto (Hauck)	210 mg	65 mg	115 mg		16 mg		
Salocol (Hauck)	210 mg	65 mg	115 mg		16 mg		
Sinarest (Fisons)			325 mg 500 mg			NS[b]	phenylpropanolamine hydrochloride, 18.7 mg chlorpheniramine maleate, 2 mg
Sinarest, No Drowsiness (Fisons)			500 mg			NS[b]	pseudoephedrine hydrochloride, 30 mg
Sine-Aid Maximum Strength (McNeil)			500 mg				pseudoephedrine hydrochloride, 30 mg
Snaplets-FR Granules (Baker-Cummins)			80 mg				

INTERNAL ANALGESIC PRODUCT TABLE, continued

Product[a] (Manufacturer)	Aspirin	Salicyl- amide	Acetami- nophen	Ibuprofen	Caffeine	Sodium	Other Ingredients
Sodium Salicylate (Various manufacturers)							sodium salicylate, 325 mg 650 mg
Stanback Powder and Max Powder (Stanback)	650 mg 850 mg					NS[b]	
St. Joseph Aspirin (Schering-Plough)	325 mg					free	
St. Joseph Low Dose Adult Aspirin (Schering-Plough)	81 mg (chewable)					free	
St. Joseph Aspirin-Free Infant Drops[c,d] (Schering-Plough)			80 mg/0.8 ml			NS[b]	
St. Joseph Aspirin-Free Liquid for Children[c,d] (Schering-Plough)			80 mg/2.5 ml			NS[b]	
St. Joseph Aspirin-Free Tablets for Children (Schering-Plough)			80 mg			NS[b]	flavor
Supac (Mission)	230 mg		160 mg		33 mg		calcium gluconate, 60 mg
Suppap-120 Suppositories (Raway)			120 mg				
Suppap-325 Suppositories (Raway)			325 mg				
Suppap-650 Suppositories (Raway)			650 mg				
Synabrom (Ferndale)			325 mg				pamabrom, 25 mg cinnamedrine hydrochloride, 14.9 mg
Tapanol Extra Strength (Republic)			500 mg				
Tempra Chewable Tablets (Mead Johnson)			80 mg 160 mg				

INTERNAL ANALGESIC PRODUCT TABLE, continued

Product[a] (Manufacturer)	Aspirin	Salicyl- amide	Acetami- nophen	Ibuprofen	Caffeine	Sodium	Other Ingredients
Tempra Drops[c] **and Syrup**[c] (Mead Johnson)			100 mg/ml (drops) 32 mg/ml (syrup)			0.08 mEq/ ml (drops) 0.03 mEq/ ml (syrup)	
Tenol (Vortech)			325 mg			NS[b]	
Tenol-Plus (Vortech)	250 mg		250 mg		65 mg		
Trigesic (Squibb)	230 mg		125 mg		30 mg	free	
Tri-Pain Caplets (Ferndale)	162 mg	162 mg	162 mg		16.2 mg		
Tylenol Chil- dren's Chew- able Tablets, Drops[c]**, Elixir**[c] (McNeil)			80 mg/chew- able tablet 100 mg/ml (drops) 32 mg/ml (elixir)			0.04 mEq/ chewa- ble tablet 0.04 mEq/ ml (drops) 0.02 mEq/ ml (elixir)	saccharin (drops) sorbitol (elixir) sucrose (elixir)
Tylenol Extra Strength Caplets, Gel- caps, Tablets, Liquid (McNeil)			500 mg/ caplet, gel- cap, tablet 33.3 mg/ml (liquid)			< 0.04 mEq/ tablet 0.02 mEq/ ml (liquid)	alcohol, 8.5% (liquid)
Tylenol Junior Strength (McNeil)			160 mg			0.04 mEq	
Tylenol Regu- lar Strength Caplets and Tablets (McNeil)			325 mg/ caplet, tablet				
Uracel 5 (Vortech)						NS[b]	sodium salicylate, 324 mg
Ultraprin (Otis Clapp)				200 mg		free	
Valadol (Squibb)			325 mg				
Valesin (Vale)	150 mg	150 mg	150 mg				
Valorin (Otis Clapp)			325 mg 500 mg			free	
Valorin Super (Otis Clapp)			500 mg		NS[b]	free	
Valprin (Buffington)				200 mg		free	

INTERNAL ANALGESIC PRODUCT TABLE, continued

Product[a] (Manufacturer)	Aspirin	Salicyl- amide	Acetami- nophen	Ibuprofen	Caffeine	Sodium	Other Ingredients
Vanquish Caplet (Glenbrook)	227 mg		194 mg		33 mg	free	magnesium hydrox-ide, 50 mg aluminum hydrox-ide gel, dried, 25 mg
Verin (Hauck)	650 mg						
Wesprin Buffered (Wesley)	325 mg						aluminum hydroxide magnesium hydroxide

[a] Tablet unless specified otherwise.
[b] Quantity not specified.
[c] Alcohol free.
[d] Sugar free.

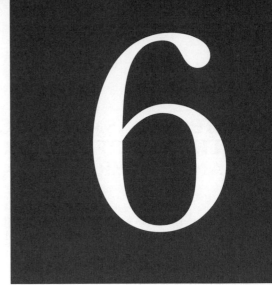

Thomas E. Lackner

ANTIPYRETIC DRUG PRODUCTS

*Q*uestions to ask in patient/consumer counseling

How long have you been ill?

What is your temperature? How did you measure the temperature (i.e., by the oral, axillary, rectal, tympanic, or palpation method)?

How long have you had this fever?

What activities preceded this fever?

Do you have any other symptoms?

What medication or other treatment have you used to treat the fever?

Have you ever had chickenpox?

What prescription medications are you taking?

What nonprescription medications are you taking?

Have you ever had a convulsion, seizure, or brain disorder?

Have you ever had an ulcer or stomach problem?

Do you take any anticoagulants or medications that interfere with blood clotting?

Do you have any type of bleeding problem or blood clotting disease?

Do you have gout?

Have you ever had asthma, nasal polyps, or a breathing problem?

Have you ever had hives or a recurrent skin rash?

What allergies or reactions have you ever had to drugs, foods, dyes, or food additives?

Almost everyone will experience a fever sometime in life; fever is one of the most common abnormalities experienced by children. Serious complications of fever are uncommon and are usually the result of inappropriate treatment, rather than a consequence of the fever itself (1). Pharmacists and other health professionals can reduce the risk of complications by helping consumers to better understand fever and its appropriate management.

Fever is a sign of an upward displacement of the body's thermoregulatory "set-point" and is manifested as an abnormally elevated body temperature. A fever is generally recognized as an oral temperature above 100°F (37.8°C), a rectal temperature exceeding 101°F (38.3°C), or an axillary (armpit) temperature greater than 98.6°F (37.0°C) (2–5). Fever can occur with or without serious underlying pathophysiology. Normal rectal temperatures in healthy children may approach 101°F (38.3°C) in the late afternoon or after physical activity (4–9).

MECHANISMS OF NORMAL THERMOREGULATION AND FEVER

Body heat is primarily the product of basal metabolic processes and muscle activity (10, 11). At rest, the liver is the principal source of body heat; during exercise, muscles elicit a substantial amount of heat. Metabolic activity is largely influenced by adrenal medullary and thyroid hormones. Heat loss is primarily achieved by conduction, evaporation, and radiation from the skin. The rate of heat loss is directly proportional to the cutaneous blood flow rate, which in turn is under the control of the hypothalamic regulatory center.

Body temperature is regulated by a thermoregulatory center located in the anterior hypothalamus (10–12). Temperature-sensitive neurons in both the hypothalamus and the skin continuously transmit information about body temperature to the hypothalamic thermostat. Physiologic and behavioral mechanisms can then be invoked to maintain the body temperature. Examples of behavioral adaptations to temperature changes or extremes include putting on extra clothing, adjusting the air conditioning, rubbing the hands together for warmth, or seeking out the shade of a tree for relief from the hot sun. Compensatory physiologic mechanisms involve heat dissipation (sweating, vasodilation, hyperventilation) in response to heat or heat production and/or conservation (shivering, vasoconstriction) in response to cold. Compensatory effects are mediated by alterations in the secretory rates of thyroid-stimulating hormone and catecholamines. Normal thermoregulation prevents wide fluctuations in body temperature so that the average body temperature is usually maintained at 97.7–99.5°F (36.5–37.5°C).

Numerous fever-producing substances, called pyrogens, can increase the thermoregulatory set-point (2, 13, 14). Pyrogens can be categorized as exogenous or endogenous, depending on their place of origin. Exogenous pyrogens are those substances that are foreign to the body. Most febrile episodes can be attributed to infection by various microorganisms (exogenous pyrogens), including viruses, bacteria, fungi, yeasts, and protozoa. Despite some evidence that elevated temperatures associated with bacterial infection are generally higher than those with viral infections, there is no absolute temperature at which these infections can be differentiated (15–17). Furthermore, there is no reason to believe that viral and bacterial infections can be distinguished by the magnitude of temperature reduction with antipyretic drug therapy (18).

Clinical data suggest that the febrile response to exogenous pyrogens, such as infection, is often diminished in elderly patients. The reason for this effect is unknown (19). Consequently, the presence of infection may not be easily recognized in the elderly.

Other causes of fever include malignancies, certain drugs, tissue damage (e.g., myocardial infarct, surgery), metabolic disorders, antigen–antibody interactions, and dehydration. Each of these factors can cause the production and release of small molecular weight proteins, known as endogenous pyrogens, from liver and spleen cells, monocytes, eosinophils, and neutrophils. All exogenous pyrogens exert their effect through the actions of endogenous pyrogen. Fever caused by the release of endogenous pyrogens from the malignant cells of acute leukemia, histiocytic lymphoma, and Hodgkin's disease is difficult to distinguish from an infectious etiology in such patients. However, evidence indicates that naproxen or indomethacin ameliorates neoplastic fever but not fever associated with infection (20).

Experimental evidence in animals strongly suggests that prostaglandins of the E series are produced in response to circulating endogenous pyrogens and that the E prostaglandins act on the anterior hypothalamus to elevate the set-point, thereby producing fever (14, 21–28). Endogenous pyrogens increase the concentration of E prostaglandins in cerebrospinal fluid, and drugs that inhibit the synthesis of E prostaglandins in response to endogenous pyrogens possess antipyretic activity. In response to E prostaglandins and changes in monoamine concentration, the hypothalamus directs the reestablishment of body temperature to correspond to the new elevated set-point (2, 8, 14). Within hours, the body temperature reaches this new set-point, and fever results. During the period of upward temperature readjustment, symptoms of chills and shivering are experienced as peripheral heat conservation and production mechanisms, such as peripheral vasoconstriction and increased skeletal muscle tone, are activated. The new set-point is regulated by a negative feedback system so that temperatures rarely exceed 106°F (41°C) (29–32).

HYPERTHERMIA

Temperature elevation can also occur in a condition referred to as hyperthermia (8, 33, 34). However, in contrast to fever, a normal thermoregulatory set-point is maintained in hyperthermia. Body temperature rises when the compensatory thermoregulatory response to heat production or retention is inadequate (i.e., heat production and retention predominate over heat dissipation). For example, excessive physical activity on a hot, humid day can greatly increase body temperature and overcome compensatory vasodilation and sweating, resulting in heat stroke (33, 34). The loss of large amounts of fluid by sweating may further increase the morbidity and mortality of hyperthermia by causing dehydration (35). Heat dissipation by evaporation of sweat may be suppressed by high humidity while heat production is accelerated during exercise. Sweating diminishes with increasing age so that elderly individuals may be particularly sensitive to hyperthermia. Body temperatures associated with heat stroke generally exceed 107.6°F (42°C) and can result in delirium, coma, anhidrosis (suppression of perspiration with hot, dry skin), and death (36, 37). Without aggressive management, the mortality of hyperthermia can approach 80%, and those who survive may be afflicted with permanent neurologic deficits, such as ataxia (muscular incoordination) and severe dysarthria (difficulty in speaking clearly and fluently).

Because of the potentially fatal complications of heat stroke, treatment should always be referred to a physician. Most clothing should be removed and the coolest and most ventilated location made available. Ice-water sponging and manual skin massage can be initiated to facilitate heat loss while awaiting additional medical aid. The cornerstone of treatment of heat stroke is immersion of the hospitalized patient in an ice-water bath to ensure heat dissipation. Antipyretic agents are of no benefit in the treatment of hyperthermia because the thermoregulatory set-point is not elevated in this condition (36, 37).

Hyperthermia may also accompany endocrine disorders, such as thyrotoxicosis and pheochromocytoma, which increase the basal metabolic rate (38).

DRUG FEVER

Many drugs are reported to cause fever. Table 1 lists the drugs most frequently implicated in this condition (39). The actual incidence of drug fever is unknown but it probably accounts for more than 3% of adverse drug reactions (39). Drug-induced fever probably is not related to atopy, gender, age, or systemic lupus erythematosus as was previously believed (39). Recognition of drug-induced fever is important because failure to discontinue use of the offending agent can result in death. However, drug-induced fever is often unrecognized due to lack of consistent signs and symptoms.

The majority of drug-related fevers occur as hypersensitivity reactions or are idiosyncratic in nature (40–42). However, drugs may also elicit fever by interfering with peripheral heat dissipation, increasing the basal metabolic rate, invoking a cellular immune response, structurally mimicking endogenous pyrogens, and inflicting direct tissue damage.

Sometimes it is the method of administration, rather than the drug itself, that results in fever (42).

TABLE 1 Agents responsible for episodes of drug fever[a]

Cardiovascular (38)
Alpha methyldopa (16)
Quinidine (13)
Procainamide (6)
Hydralazine
Nifedipine
Oxprenelol

Antimicrobial (46)
Penicillin G (9)
Ampicillin (2)
Methicillin (6)
Cloxacillin (2)
Cephalothin (7)
Cephapirin
Cephamandole
Tetracycline (2)
Lincomycin
Sulfonamide (2)
Sulfa-trimethoprim
Streptomycin[b]
Vancomycin
Colistin
Isoniazid (5)
Para-aminosalicylic acid
Nitrofurantoin (2)
Mebendazole

Antineoplastic (12)
Bleomycin (3)
Daunorubicin
Procarbazine
Cytarabine
Streptozocin (2)
6-mercaptopurine
L-asparaginase
Chlorambucil
Hydroxyurea

Central nervous system (30)
Diphenylhydantoin (11)
Carbamazepine (3)
Chlorpromazine
Nomifensine (2)
Haloperidol
Triamterene
Benztropine[b]
Thioridazine (2)
Trifluoperazine[b]
Amphetamine (2)
Lysergic acid (5)[b]

Anti-inflammatory (3)
Ibuprofen
Tolmetin
Aspirin

Other (19)
Iodide (6)
Cimetidine (2)
Levamisole
Metoclopramide
Clofibrate
Allopurinol
Folate
Prostaglandin E_2 (2)
Ritodrine
Interferon (2)
Propylthiouracil

[a] Numbers in parentheses show number of episodes induced by drugs responsible for several episodes.
[b] Fever seen during drug overdose.
Reprinted with permission from P. A. Mackowiak and C. F. LeMaistre, *Ann. Intern. Med., 106*, 729 (1987).

Examples of such reactionary fevers are thrombophlebitis and septicemia from intravenous catheterization, phlebitis from the careless administration of potentially caustic agents (e.g., rapid infusion of vancomycin), and the release of endogenous pyrogens from sterile abscesses formed after multiple intramuscular injections.

Some drugs can elevate body temperature by altering normal thermoregulatory mechanisms. Large doses of phenothiazines or anticholinergic agents can decrease sweating (reduced heat dissipation), and thyroid hormones can increase the metabolic rate (increased heat generation) (31, 40). Other drugs can modify behavioral response to the climatic temperature. For example, obtundation (decreased level of consciousness) from sedatives may impair the usual behavioral withdrawal response from a high environmental temperature, resulting in hyperthermia.

Occasionally, fever may be a direct result of the pharmacologic effect of a drug. The release of endotoxin from spirochetes following the initiation of antibiotic therapy (e.g., penicillin for syphilis) can result in high fever, chills, hypotension, myalgias, and leukocytosis (40, 42). This phenomenon, known as the Jarisch–Herxheimer reaction, may occur within hours after the initiation of parenteral antispirochetal therapy. Fever may also result from the release of endogenous pyrogen associated with cellular necrosis following cancer chemotherapy (41). Similarly, administration of drugs that possess oxidizing activity to individuals having a glucose-6-phosphate dehydrogenase (G6PD) deficiency may cause fever secondary to the release of endogenous pyrogen from damaged erythrocytes (40, 42).

Drugs, or drug metabolites, and certain biological preparations can behave as antigens and cause hypersensitivity. Although drug fever usually develops after 7–10 days of treatment, fever and other symptoms may occur shortly after drug administration when previous exposure and sensitization has occurred (40, 41). Drug fever caused by antineoplastic agents often begins within 7 days; fever caused by cardiac drugs may not occur for more than 10 days (39).

Drug fever is distinguished by fever during or shortly after treatment with a drug previously reported to cause fever or other allergic symptoms, fever accompanied by other manifestations of allergy, and temperature elevation despite patient improvement (43). One recent study of drug-induced fevers identified skin rash in only 18% of patients, and less than half of these individuals experienced urticaria (39). Furthermore, a generally mild eosinophilia was present in only 22% of the patients. The presence of a high fever and shaking chills occurred in some patients with drug fever, which prevents reliably distinguishing drug fever from infection. Relative bradycardia is uncommon with drug fever (39). Although diurnal temperature variation accompanying a drug fever is often minimal, this fever pattern is not a reliable diagnostic sign of a drug fever.

The management of drug-induced fever involves the discontinuation of the suspected agent whenever possible, and if feasible, all drugs should be temporarily discontinued. If the fever has been caused by a drug, the patient's temperature will generally decrease within 24–48 hours after the drug is withdrawn (41). After considering the patient's safety and the need for a de-

finitive identification of the offending drug, each drug can be reinstituted one at a time with observation for fever recurrence. If an implicated drug cannot be discontinued, corticosteroids may be given to suppress fever and to minimize other allergic symptoms (41). A fever associated with drug administration can be prevented by giving careful attention to proper catheter placement and care, avoiding frequent intramuscular injections, and adhering to recommended infusion rates (42). Dosage reduction of phenothiazines, anticholinergic agents, and thyroid hormone can decrease elevated temperatures and should be considered if these drugs are suspected of causing fever, particularly in elderly individuals.

Fever may therefore result from a variety of factors, ranging from a relatively harmless, transient viral infection to a condition associated with malignancy. Attention to related signs and symptoms will help distinguish between such disorders. When appropriate, treatment of fever should be directed against the underlying cause. The foremost reason for treating fever is to alleviate patient discomfort. The perception of fever among individuals is highly variable. Although some individuals quite accurately detect an elevation in their body temperature, others (for example, those with tuberculosis) may be unaware of temperatures as high as 103°F (39.4°C) (44). Furthermore, fever may be ignored because of other, more unpleasant concomitant symptoms. The symptoms associated with fever may include headache, sweating, generalized malaise, tachycardia, arthralgias without arthritis, back pain, irritability, and anorexia (4, 45). Very high temperatures may cause dulled intellectual functioning, disorientation, and delirium, especially in individuals with preexisting dementia, cerebral arteriosclerosis, or alcoholism. Decreasing a high temperature may alleviate central nervous system (CNS) symptoms in some individuals, depending on the underlying cause and preexistent disease.

In contrast to drug-induced hyperthermia, certain drugs can cause hypothermia. Phenothiazines can cause either hyperthermia or hypothermia by interfering with thermoregulation in the CNS (17). Consequently, body temperature is affected by ambient air temperature (e.g., body temperature will fall with exposure to cold). Corticosteroids can also depress body temperature, even in febrile patients (17). However, corticosteroids are ineffective in treating heat stroke (17).

TEMPERATURE MEASUREMENT

The normal body temperature varies according to the age of the individual, physical and emotional stress, environmental temperature, the time of day, and the anatomical site at which the temperature is measured (2, 4, 9, 29, 30, 46, 47). Body temperature may be measured at axillary, oral, rectal, or tympanic (ear canal) sites. The rectal temperature is usually regarded to be the most accurate estimate of actual body temperature. However, results from a study of hospitalized children found no significant difference between temperature measurement at rectal and axillary sites (48). The risks associated with taking a rectal temperature include injuries resulting from broken glass, retention of the thermometer, rectal perforation, and peritonitis (49). An oral temperature should not be taken when the individual is mouth-breathing or hyperventilating, has recently had oral surgery, is not fully alert, is uncooperative or confused, or is a child under 3 years of age (maintaining a tight seal around the thermometer is difficult for young children) (50–52). Most individuals, particularly children, prefer the axillary or oral sites for temperature measurement (48). During the course of an illness, the same thermometer should be used because the accuracy of different brands of thermometers may vary (53, 54).

Mercury-in-glass and electronic thermometers are commonly used for temperature measurement. Both are accurate when used appropriately (54–56). Mercury-in-glass thermometers can break, rendering them useless and potentially dangerous. Although the elemental mercury used in modern day thermometers is nonabsorbable through the gastrointestinal (GI) tract and is nontoxic, many patients still fear mercury poisoning from a broken thermometer. The real danger from a broken thermometer is glass fragments; therefore, patients should be instructed to discard chipped thermometers. In addition, mercury-in-glass thermometers register slowly and must be disinfected before each use. Mercury-in-glass thermometers should be stored in a cool location and out of direct sunlight because they may be damaged by excessive heat (54). Advantages of mercury-in-glass thermometers over electronic thermometers are patient familiarity, low cost, light weight, and compact size. Electronic thermometers register quickly (about 30 seconds for equilibration) and are not subject to glass breakage and the risk of cuts. The use of disposable covers with the electronic thermometer eliminates the need for disinfection following their use. In addition, the electronic digital temperature display is easier to read than the traditional glass thermometer.

Thermometers intended for oral use have a long thin bulb to reach well under the tongue. In contrast, the bulb of the rectal thermometer is short and thick, permitting insertion in the rectum with little risk of breakage. Although a rectal thermometer can be used for oral temperature measurement, an oral thermometer should never be inserted into the rectum because of the risk of breakage and injury to rectal tissue. The use of the security-type rectal thermometer should be restricted to either rectal or oral routes because effective sterilization is difficult and cross-infection is a greater risk. To ensure a reliable measurement, the individual should not engage in vigorous physical activity or artificially heat or cool the oral cavity by smoking or by drinking hot or cold beverages for at least 5 minutes (preferably 20 minutes) before the temperature is measured (51).

Before measuring oral temperature using a mercury-in-glass thermometer, an inspection should be made for cracks or imperfections. Next the thermometer is disinfected by drawing it through a swab moistened with an antiseptic (e.g., alcohol or Betadine) and then rinsed with cool water (hot water should never be used because this may break the thermometer). After disinfection, the thermometer is calibrated by rotating it at eye level or slightly below eye level to confirm that the displayed temperature is below 96°F (35.5°C). If the reading exceeds this value, the thermometer is shaken in a rapid downward motion until the height of the mercury column falls below this level. The pharmacist, when counseling about mercury-in-glass thermometers, should demonstrate the correct shaking motion. The user should also be advised to shake the thermometer over a bed or other soft surface to reduce the likelihood of breakage. The thermometer is then placed under the tongue, positioned slightly to one side of the mouth, and left in place for 2–4 minutes. Although most literature reports recommend insertion for 6–10 minutes, many people consider 3 minutes an adequate time. There is evidence that 3 minutes is sufficient, however, further study is needed to resolve this controversy (57). Alternatively, the temperature measurement can be repeated for 1-minute periods after an initial 3-minute reading until a similar temperature is recorded. The patient's lips should be sealed to hold the thermometer in place and to prevent air from flowing over it (50, 52). Saliva should be removed from the thermometer by wiping from the stem toward the bulb. After the recorded temperature is noted, the mercury is shaken down to less than the 96°F (35.5°C) level and disinfected as described previously.

To measure an oral temperature with an electronic thermometer, the probe is removed from the thermometer base in which it is stored. The temperature setpoint is verified as specified by the manufacturer. The thermometer probe is then inserted into a probe sheath following the same instructions for placement in the mouth as those for the glass thermometer. After the electronic thermometer indicates that the temperature measurement has been completed, the probe is removed, the sheath is discarded, and the temperature display is read. Finally, the probe is returned to the base to reset the thermometer. Electronic thermometers can be used in children as young as 3 years of age because they are not breakable if bitten and therefore pose no risk of cuts. Children under 3 years of age are frequently unable to maintain a tight seal around the thermometer and so require rectal or axillary temperature measurement.

The average oral temperature in adults is 98.6°F (37°C), with a normal range of 97.7–99.5°F (36.5–37.5°C) (4–9).

To measure a rectal temperature using a mercury-in-glass thermometer, a rectal (security bulb) thermometer should be disinfected and calibrated in the same manner as described for oral temperature measurement. Then, the thermometer bulb is lubricated with a water-soluble lubricant to allow easy passage through the anal sphincter and to reduce the risk of trauma. Adults should lie on their side with their legs flexed to about a 45° angle from their abdomen. In adults, the bulb should be inserted about 1½ to 2 inches into the rectum using finger placement on the thermometer stem as a guide. To facilitate passage of the thermometer through the anal sphincter, the patient should be told to take a deep breath which helps to divert the individual's attention to another activity. Insertion of a thermometer into the rectum of an individual with hemorrhoidal tissue should be particularly gentle because forceful insertion can cause pain and injury. Rectal measurement in infants and children is best accomplished by placing the child face down over the parent's lap, separating the buttocks with the thumb and forefinger of one hand, and inserting a rectal thermometer in a direction pointing toward the child's umbilicus with the other hand (58). In infants, the thermometer should be inserted into the rectum to the length of the bulb; in children, the thermometer should be inserted about 1 inch into the rectum (58). The thermometer should be held in place for 3 minutes. The thermometer should be withdrawn from the rectum in a straight line along its angle of insertion. The thermometer should be cleaned of feces by wiping from the stem toward the bulb. The temperature should be read at eye level or slightly below eye level. Finally, the thermometer should be disinfected as previously described for the oral method using a mercury-in-glass thermometer, and any remaining lubricant should be wiped away from the anus.

The patient should never be left unattended while the thermometer remains in place because a positional change may cause the thermometer to be expelled or broken. Rectal temperature measurement is contraindicated in people who have had recent rectal surgery or injury, or who have rectal pathology (e.g., obstructive hemorrhoids), or in newborn infants (newborns are very susceptible to mucosal perforation) (59). The average normal rectal temperature is about 99.5°F (37.5°C) (4–9). The average rectal temperature at 18 months of age is 100°F (37.8°C), although 50% of infants may have normal rectal temperatures exceeding 100°F (9). Many parents cannot take a rectal temperature correctly or read the thermometer accurately (60). Confusion often results from the difference between the centigrade and Fahrenheit scales and normal variations in temperature among rectal, oral, and axillary sites of measurement. These differences should be emphasized when instructing individuals on the use of the thermometer.

An axillary temperature measurement is recommended in adults who are not candidates for oral or rectal temperature measurement (e.g., a somnolent individual recovering from rectal surgery) and may be preferred in children under 5 years of age because intrusive procedures can be very frightening to preschool children. Axillary temperature measurement is accomplished by placing a thermometer under the arm (in the armpit) and holding the arm pressed against the body for 10 minutes. The average normal axillary temperature is about 97.5°F (36.5°C) (4–9).

Experience with skin thermometers, adhesive temperature strips that are applied to the skin and change color over a particular temperature range, indicates that they are not accurate (61). In fact, in one study they failed to detect 66% of fevers of 100°F (37.8°C) or higher (62).*

Thorough hand washing should precede and follow all temperature measurements, regardless of the method or site that is used.

An individual's normal body temperature varies consistently throughout the day (i.e., circadian rhythm) (17). This circadian rhythm is absent in neonates and infants under 2 years of age and is greater in children than adults. The temperature can vary by as much as 1.5°F (0.9°C) in adults and 2.5°F (1.5°C) in children. Circadian variation is manifest even during febrile illness (17).

An individual's body temperature peaks daily between 5 and 7 p.m., and reaches its lowest point between 3 and 5 a.m. (2). This normal diurnal, or daily, variation occurs regardless of age, sleep state, or work pattern. For this reason, many individuals with a febrile illness can have a relatively normal temperature in the early morning. Furthermore, a moderately high evening temperature associated with circadian variation should not be misinterpreted as a fever.

An individual with a fever should restrict physical activity. Strenuous exercise (e.g., long-distance running) can cause a temporary rise in body temperature to

---

Note Added in Proof: Body temperature can also be determined by tympanic measurement: a probe placed at the ear canal measures body temperatures by sensing infrared radiation [M. Benzinger, *J. Am. Med. Assoc.*, *209*, 1207 (1969), and T. Shinozaki et al., *Crit. Care Med.*, *16*, 148 (1988).] Tympanic temperature measurement is accurate, easy to perform, and completed within two seconds. Unfortunately, the measurement apparatus is very expensive relative to the glass-in-mercury and electronic thermometers; consequently, its use is presently limited to instances where a large number of measurements must be made.

more than 104°F (40°C), particularly on hot days or if excessive clothing is worn (28, 36, 37, 47). Therefore, it is important to remember that the temperature associated with an illness can be erroneously elevated if measured too soon (within about 10 minutes) after exercise.

Subjective assessment by parents typically involves palpating a part of the body, such as the forehead. However, it has been found that fever was unrecognized by the palpation method in 26% of children with documented fever, and 6% of afebrile children were thought to have a fever (60).

TREATMENT

The decision to treat fever is based on several considerations. Arguments against treatment include the generally benign and self-limited course of fever, the possible elimination of a diagnostic or prognostic sign, the attenuation of enhanced host defenses, the possible therapeutic effect of fever, and the untoward effects of antipyretic drugs (63–66).

Because fever is not a specific sign, the diagnostic or prognostic value of fever alone does not generally warrant withholding antipyretic therapy. In addition, there is no correlation between the magnitude nor pattern (i.e., persistent, intermittent, recurrent, prolonged) of temperature elevation and the underlying etiology or severity of the disease (31, 32, 67, 68). Furthermore, when associated with an infectious disease, effective antibiotic therapy is generally guided by microbiologic cultures (69). In the febrile neutropenic patient with negative cultures, antipyretic therapy should be periodically interrupted to determine the need for continued antibiotic therapy (70, 71). An agent lacking anti-inflammatory activity, such as acetaminophen, should be used when anti-inflammatory effects may mask the clinical signs of the disease (e.g., rheumatic fever) (72).

The issue of the physiologic benefits of fever with respect to disease is quite controversial (63, 64, 73–77). If fever is considered to be an adaptive response, one can argue that some therapeutic benefit might result from the presence of an elevated temperature (63). Although the growth of some pathogenic microorganisms in man is impaired by higher than normal temperatures, the benefits of fever appear to be restricted to regional infections (e.g., cutaneous infection) (77). Despite the possibility that a low-grade fever might enhance certain host defense mechanisms (e.g., increase leukocyte motility), there is no conclusive evidence that fever favorably alters the course of infectious diseases (64, 73). Acetaminophen does *not* alleviate symptoms of chickenpox in children and may even prolong illness

(i.e., delay scabbing) (78). Data from animal studies suggest that abolition of fever may actually enhance and prolong viral shedding (79). In addition, aspirin has been associated with increased shedding of rhinovirus in adults (80).

Serious complications of fever are rare. Harmful effects (dehydration, delirium, seizures, coma, and irreversible neurologic or muscular damage) are most likely to occur at temperatures in excess of 106°F (41°C) (29–32). However, the body temperature rarely exceeds 106°F in otherwise healthy individuals. A greater risk for higher temperatures exists in patients with brain tumors or hemorrhage, CNS infections, or preexisting neurologic damage, or in those who are less able to dissipate heat (32, 81). Even lower body temperatures may be life threatening in patients with heart disease because of an increased demand for oxygen in conjunction with increased cardiac output and heart rate (10, 45).

Febrile seizures occur in about 2–4% of all children between 6 months and 6 years of age (82–86). Febrile seizures are those associated with fever and occurring in the absence of another cause (e.g., acute metabolic disorder or CNS inflammation). Simple febrile seizures last no more than 15 minutes, have no features characteristic of a focal origin, and do not recur during a single febrile episode (87). Although somewhat controversial, significant neurologic sequelae (e.g., impaired intellectual development) are believed to be unlikely following a single pediatric febrile seizure that is not complicated by status epilepticus (82, 88, 89). However, the prevalence of epilepsy (2–3%) may be higher following a febrile seizure, particularly after a complex seizure or when severe electroencephalogram abnormalities exist (83, 85, 89). Unlike simple febrile seizures, complex febrile seizures are repetitive during the course of a single febrile episode, are longer than 15 minutes' duration, and exhibit signs characteristic of a focal origin; complex seizures are believed to be precipitated by fever in individuals with epilepsy or such a predilection (84, 85). Although both the magnitude and the rate of the temperature increase appear to be critical determinants in precipitating febrile seizures, the temperature at which a particular child will experience a seizure is unpredictable (90). The majority of initial febrile seizures occur in children under 3 years of age (86, 91). Seizures occurring after the age of 3 are usually unrelated to fever. The risk of a febrile seizure is increased in children who have experienced a previous febrile seizure (especially before 1 year of age or a complex febrile seizure) or who have a documented seizure or other CNS disorder, or when there is a family history of febrile seizures (86, 89, 92).

It is generally recommended that chronic prophylaxis against febrile seizures with antiepileptic drugs be reserved for individuals at high risk of subsequent epilepsy. For such continuous administration, phenobarbital or sodium valproate have been the prophylactic drugs of choice (93, 94).* Recent information indicates that short-term rectal administration (i.e., treatment with onset of fever) of diazepam is also effective in reducing febrile seizure recurrence (89). The low average number of doses of diazepam administered (five) in this study minimized the risks of an altered lifestyle, long-term adverse effects, and the cost of therapy associated with the chronic use of phenobarbital and sodium valproate (93, 94). Compliance with the rectal administration of diazepam is good when thorough instructions are given and the treatment is acceptable to the parents (89). Rectal absorption of the drug from suspensions and suppositories is slower, and peak serum concentrations are lower than absorption from solutions (95). Therefore, a rectal solution may be preferred when a more rapid onset is needed. Serious adverse effects, such as respiratory depression, are rare with rectally administered diazepam (89). Despite claims that short-term prophylaxis is ineffective because the fever often cannot be detected in time to initiate treatment to prevent a seizure, only about 4% of children experienced a seizure that was attributed to unrecognized fever in the study of this method of treatment (89).

Status epilepticus, which is characterized by recurrent or repetitive seizures without intervening periods of normal consciousness, occurs in only about 1–2% of children who experience a febrile seizure (82, 96, 97). Unlike simple febrile seizures, status epilepticus can result in permanent brain damage, renal failure, cardiorespiratory arrest, and death if not controlled (92, 98).

In general, treatment of fever with oral antipyretic agents is recommended only if the oral temperature exceeds 102°F (39°C) and/or if the individual is uncomfortable (29). When a lower temperature is present, nonpharmacologic intervention is usually sufficient, but antipyretic treatment should be initiated and the physician contacted at the first evidence of fever in a child predisposed to seizures. In such individuals, antipyretic medication should be given every 4 hours with one dose given during the night; therapy should be continued for at least 24 hours. The need for additional therapy, such as anticonvulsant medication, should be determined by the physician.

If a seizure occurs, sponging with tepid water should be initiated and the physician notified immediately. Nonpharmacologic treatment should consist of

parental reassurance in the case of the febrile child, an adequate fluid intake to replenish imperceptible losses, light clothing, removal of blankets, and maintenance of the room temperature at 78°F (26°C).

When the body temperature exceeds 104°F (40°C), body sponging with tepid (lukewarm) water can be instituted to facilitate heat dissipation. Ideally, sponging should follow oral antipyretic therapy by 1 hour to permit the reduction of the hypothalamic set-point, thereby permitting a more sustained temperature lowering response (6, 76, 99). Unlike acetaminophen and salicylates, topical sponging does not reduce the hypothalamic set-point. Sponging with lukewarm or tepid water is sufficient because only a small temperature gradient between the body and the sponging medium is necessary to achieve an effective antipyretic response (99). Ice-water baths or sponging with hydroalcoholic solutions (e.g., isopropyl or ethyl alcohol) are uncomfortable and unnecessary. In addition, serious alcohol poisoning, including coma, can result from the cutaneous absorption or inhalation of topically applied alcohol solutions (99–102). In a case of extreme hyperthermia where the temperature exceeds 106°F (41°C), sponging or immersion in ice water is appropriate (36, 37).

NONSTEROIDAL ANTI-INFLAMMATORY DRUGS

The selection of an antipyretic agent should be based on its clinical effectiveness, the incidence and severity of adverse effects associated with its use, its contraindications, the convenience of its administration, and the cost of therapy. Acetaminophen and aspirin are the most popular and effective antipyretic agents available today. Under most circumstances, both are equally effective and have similar times to onset of effect, times-to-peak antipyretic activity, and duration of action (103–107). Both salicylates and acetaminophen exert antipyretic activity by lowering an elevated temperature set-point, which is accomplished through the inhibition of prostaglandin synthesis and release at the thermoregulatory center. When concurrent anti-inflammatory effects are desired, salicylates should be used because acetaminophen lacks significant anti-inflammatory activity.

The onset of antipyretic activity after an oral dose of either agent occurs within about 30 minutes to 1 hour. Maximum temperature reduction is evident between 2 and 3 hours after the dose, and antipyretic effects are sustained for about 4–6 hours (103–107).

Note Added in Proof: However, emerging evidence raises doubt about the benefit of continuous prophylaxis with phenobarbital; two reports failed to find a decrease in the seizure recurrence rate, and cognitive performance may be impaired even after the drug is discontinued [R. W. Newton, *Arch. Dis. Child.*, *63*, 1189 (1988), and J. R. Farwell et al., *N. Engl. J. Med.*, *322*, 364 (1990).]

Because the average maximum reduction in temperature is usually only 2–3°F (0.5°–1.5°C) "normalization" of temperature will probably not occur. However, because the most important objective of fever management is to relieve patient discomfort, temperature normalization may be unnecessary.

Because acetaminophen and aspirin have similar antipyretic activities, product selection should be based on the side effects of each agent, concurrent diseases that may preclude the use of either drug, the convenience of administration, and the cost of therapy.

Although studies of the antipyretic effect of several nonsteroidal anti-inflammatory drugs (NSAIDs) are in progress, ibuprofen is currently the only such agent approved for treatment of fever (108–110). Ibuprofen is available without a prescription in a strength of 200 mg. Ibuprofen is not yet approved for use in children under 12 years of age, nor is it currently available in the United States in a liquid dosage form for children. Approval for the use of ibuprofen in children may be forthcoming because doses of 6–10 mg/kg have been shown to be equally safe and effective as aspirin (10 mg/kg) and acetaminophen (12.5 mg/kg) (108, 109). In addition, ibuprofen appears to have a longer duration of action than aspirin or acetaminophen (108, 109, 111, 112). Adverse effects with the short-term administration of ibuprofen for treating self-limiting fever are minimal and include stomach upset, mild heartburn, or pain (108). GI side effects can be minimized by administration with food or milk.

There is currently no evidence that NSAIDs other than salicylates cause Reye's syndrome (113–115). However, the possibility of such an association cannot be entirely refuted because other NSAIDs have just recently been approved for treatment of febrile illness.

The recommended antipyretic dosage of ibuprofen in adults is 1 or 2 tablets or caplets every 4–6 hours as needed, with a maximum daily dosage of 6 tablets or caplets. Ibuprofen should not be used with salicylates or other products containing ibuprofen because of an increased risk of GI injury and bleeding (116). Ibuprofen should not be used during the last 3 months of pregnancy.

The antipyretic utility of other anti-inflammatory drugs such as naproxen will be established by ongoing clinical trials.

UNTOWARD EFFECTS

Although serious gastroduodenal injury from aspirin may occur, GI symptoms may be minimal or absent (117, 118). Occult blood loss or acute GI hemorrhage can occur with salicylate administration (66). It is believed that occult blood loss results from local erosion of the gastric mucosa. In the absence of underlying pathology, the ingestion of aspirin tablets causes an average 4- to 12-fold increase in blood loss over the normal daily loss of 0.5 ml (119–123). In most patients this represents a median loss of about 1 teaspoon per day. However, rare cases have been reported of individuals losing nearly 4 fluid ounces of blood each day (124). Chronic aspirin ingestion, particularly in large or frequent doses, may cause the loss of enough blood to precipitate iron deficiency anemia (125, 126). Although such extended use is uncommon in the treatment of an isolated fever, awareness of this potential is important in the long-term treatment necessary for the febrile, septic neutropenic patient. Salicylates can greatly potentiate blood loss in patients who are actively bleeding from the GI tract and can actually precipitate acute GI hemorrhage, particularly in patients with a history of peptic ulcer disease or other underlying bleeding risks (117, 118, 127–130). However, short-term administration (single or repeated doses within a 24-hour period) of aspirin has rarely been implicated in cases of duodenal ulceration.

The aggregation of platelets following damage to small blood vessels is an important hemostatic mechanism. Therapeutic antipyretic doses of aspirin impair this response by inhibiting platelet aggregation for the life of the platelet. The platelet-inhibiting effect of aspirin is of particular concern in individuals with underlying hematologic disorders, such as hemophilia or a clotting factor deficiency, and in those undergoing surgical procedures, such as a tonsillectomy or dental extraction (131–138). Prolongation of the bleeding time by 2- to 10-fold by aspirin may increase the risk of serious bleeding in these individuals during treatment and for 4–10 days following its discontinuation (134, 139). Platelet aggregation is not inhibited by other salicylates.

Aspirin and some other nonsteroidal anti-inflammatory agents can evoke acute airway obstruction in sensitive patients within minutes to hours after their ingestion. Severe attacks are associated with cyanosis and coma and are occasionally fatal (140–152). Salicylate intolerance may also precipitate abdominal cramps, angioedema, urticaria, rhinitis, and purpura, and may involve nearly 28% of children and 16% of adults with asthma as identified by a deterioration in pulmonary function test performance (142–147). Such intolerance is usually manifested as an exacerbation of urticaria in individuals with chronic urticaria, and as bronchospasm in persons having asthma or nasal polyps. Cross-sensitivity does not appear to occur with sodium salicylate, salicylamide, or choline salicylate in aspirin-intolerant individuals (150).

Reye's syndrome is an acute neurologic disorder characterized by encephalopathy along with fatty degeneration of the liver (153–156). A nonspecific viral prodrome is followed by persistent vomiting, and later, altered consciousness (delirium rapidly progressing to stupor and finally coma and possible seizures) and possible death (153, 155–157). Hepatic dysfunction occurs with elevations of serum ammonia, aspartate transaminase (AST), prolongation of the prothrombin time, and decreased serum glucose (153–157). Substantial evidence implicates aspirin (salicylates) as a provocative factor in the pathogenesis of Reye's syndrome, particularly in conjunction with viral illnesses such as chickenpox or influenza (158–160). The risk of Reye's syndrome appears to be greatest in children and teenagers but may occur in adults as well. A continuing downward trend in the reported cases of Reye's syndrome has been noted since the risk of salicylate use and Reye's syndrome became widely publicized (161).

The Food and Drug Administration (FDA) has categorized the teratogenic potential of drugs and requires product labels to bear pregnancy warnings. Infrequent, low doses of salicylates [aspirin (Category D) and salsalate or magnesium salicylate (Category C)] probably pose no significant risk to mother or child during the pregnancy (162). However, aspirin should be avoided during the latter portion of the last trimester because increased blood loss during delivery, prolongation of labor, and possible prepartal bleeding may occur (131, 163–166). In addition, excessive salicylate dosage can prolong gestation, reduce neonatal birth weight, and block the ductus arteriosis, resulting in fetal pulmonary hypertension (167). Salicylates enter breast milk in low concentrations, and antiplatelet effects can occur in the infant (168–173).

In combination with phenacetin and caffeine, a possible association between aspirin and renal toxicity has been reported (174, 175). Subsequent studies indicated that the combined phenacetin and salicylate constituents were the most probable nephrotoxins, rather than the aspirin alone (176). In the United States, antipyretic compounds no longer contain phenacetin. Serious renal toxicity is unlikely from the short-term administration of antipyretic doses of aspirin alone (176).

Individuals with a deficiency of G6PD are frequently susceptible to hemolytic anemia following exposure to drugs that have oxidant properties. At very high salicylate concentrations (exceeding about 500 mg/dl) oxidant activity can be expected. However, oxidant activity and red blood cell hemolysis is highly unlikely with doses of salicylates used in treating fever (177).

Low doses of less than 2 g per day of aspirin can impair urate excretion and should be used only under the supervision of a physician in patients who have gout (116).

Aspirin may rarely cause hepatitis, particularly in individuals with systemic lupus erythematosus, juvenile rheumatoid arthritis, rheumatic fever, adult rheumatoid arthritis, or other collagen disease (178, 179).

Acetaminophen is devoid of many of the adverse effects that accompany the use of salicylates (116, 150–152, 164–166, 180–186). Although bronchospasm may occur rarely in asthmatics given acetaminophen, this appears to be much less likely than with salicylates (150–152). Cross-sensitivity to acetaminophen in aspirin-sensitive patients has been reported but is uncommon (152).

The greatest concern with acetaminophen is the potentially fatal hepatotoxicity that is associated with acute overdoses of greater than about 200 mg/kg (187). Hepatic necrosis results from the covalent binding of a toxic intermediate metabolite of acetaminophen to hepatocytes. The signs and symptoms of toxicity during the first 12 to 24 hours after ingestion are nausea, vomiting, loss of appetite, and sweating. This may be followed by apparent symptomatic improvement lasting up to 4 days. However, despite apparent clinical improvement, the patient may exhibit rising liver enzymes, hypoprothrombinemia, and the development of right upper quadrant pain. Three to 5 days after ingestion, abdominal pain, hepatic tenderness, jaundice, and hepatic failure can occur (187). The risk of toxicity following an acute overdose appears to be greater in adults than in children. It is not known why children are spared the most severe toxicities, but it is thought to result from more severe and earlier vomiting and differences in drug metabolism (188–191).

The general management of an acute overdose of acetaminophen should include the induction of emesis with syrup of ipecac and clear liquids or gastric lavage. The presence of seizures, loss of the gag reflex, coma, a decreasing level of consciousness, or the concomitant ingestion of caustic or volatile substances will require the use of gastric lavage. Plasma acetaminophen concentrations over 200 mcg/ml and 50 mcg/ml at 4 and 12 hours after ingestion, respectively, are associated with severe liver damage. Toxicity is unlikely with concentrations under 150 mcg/ml and 30 mcg/ml at 4 and 12 hours, respectively. The elimination half-life of acetaminophen is not a reliable predictor of impending hepatotoxicity. Early administration of acetylcysteine (within 10 to 16 hours of the ingestion) can reduce the risks of hepatic damage. Whenever the use of acetylcysteine is contemplated, activated charcoal should not be given because it may interfere with the absorption of acetylcysteine. Acetylcysteine should be administered in an initial oral dose of 140 mg/kg (diluted 1 to 3 in a soft drink, grapefruit juice, or plain water) followed by 70 mg/kg every 4 hours for a total of 17 doses. If vomiting occurs within 1 hour after a dose is given, the dose of acetylcysteine should be repeated.

It is not known with certainty whether the long-term administration of acetaminophen results in liver damage. Although a few anecdotal reports suggest the possibility of toxic hepatitis or chronic active hepatitis after chronic acetaminophen ingestion, the excessive dosages and/or additional contributing factors cited in these reports suggest that such toxicity occurs rarely, if at all (192–200). In addition, the short-term use of acetaminophen in therapeutic dosages in patients with preexisting liver disease is not associated with an increased risk of hepatotoxicity (200–203).

Excretion of acetaminophen into breast milk is minimal and is apparently harmless to the infant in the setting of infrequent antipyretic doses (168–173).

Acetaminophen has been implicated in causing kidney damage. It is believed that renal tissue damage is incurred through the oxidizing activity that results in the inhibition of G6PD that normally protects tissues against damage from oxidizing substances (204, 205). The risk of renal damage does not appear to be increased by occasional use of acetaminophen (206).

Hemolysis of red blood cells is not increased by the consumption of acetaminophen in individuals who have a deficiency of G6PD. Therefore, acetaminophen can be used without concern of developing a hemolytic anemia (207).

DRUG INTERACTIONS

Serious drug interactions with the short-term use of antipyretic dosages of acetaminophen or salicylates are possible—particularly with aspirin (116). In addition to the GI irritant effect and antiplatelet activity of aspirin, concomitant administration with oral anticoagulants such as warfarin can displace the anticoagulant from plasma proteins and increase anticoagulant activity and the risk of bleeding (116). Acetaminophen has been associated with a slight increase in the prothrombin time (about 4.5 seconds) in patients receiving oral anticoagulants, but it is regarded as safer than aspirin in this situation because it is devoid of antiplatelet activity and does not cause GI bleeding (116). The infrequent and short-term use of acetaminophen in treating the fever of a self-limited illness is unlikely to cause a significant increase in the risk of bleeding. Daily administration of moderate to high doses of salicylates can diminish the uricosuric effect of probenecid and sulfinpyrazone (116). Salicylates are reported to significantly increase the bone marrow depression and hepatotoxicity associated with the use of methotrexate by possibly inhibiting renal excretion and/or plasma protein displacement (116). Therefore, a smaller dose of methotrexate or a larger dose of leucovorin may be required.

Methotrexate plasma levels should also be monitored. Salicylates may potentiate the hypoglycemic effect of sulfonylureas; hence, this effect may require a corresponding reduction in the sulfonylurea dose (116). Lithium serum levels, pharmacologic effect, and potential for toxicity may be increased with concurrent administration of ibuprofen, naproxen, indomethacin, and piroxicam (116). The concurrent use of ibuprofen and other NSAIDs with oral anticoagulants may increase the risk of bleeding (116). Other drug interactions have been reported, but these either are not well documented or are not likely to produce significant clinical consequences.

DOSAGE CONSIDERATIONS

Acetaminophen is frequently underdosed, especially in younger, lighter patients (208). The underdosing of acetaminophen often results from parents' reuse of the 0.8 ml dropper provided with infant drops (80 mg/0.8 ml) to measure a dose of an equivalent volume of acetaminophen elixir (160 mg/5 ml) when incorrectly assuming the same strength. In addition, rapidly growing infants quickly outgrow previous dose requirements. Therefore, recalculation of the dose according to present body weight and the 15 mg/kg measure is recommended at the time of each treatment course (208).

The recommended oral antipyretic dose of aspirin and acetaminophen for children 2–11 years of age is 10–15 mg/kg of total body weight every 4–6 hours as needed up to a maximum daily dose of 65 mg/kg for up to 5 days. The dosing of either agent in infants under 2 years of age should be directed by a physician (Tables 2 and 3) (107, 131, 209). One manufacturer recommends that an acetaminophen dose of 40 mg be taken by mouth every 4 hours by infants under 4 months of age, 80 mg for those 4–11 months and 120 mg for those 1 to 2 years of age, although this regimen has not been approved by the FDA. (The data are on file with McNeil Consumer Products Co., Fort Washington, Pa.) The recommended adult dose of either agent is 650 mg every 4–6 hours as needed for up to 10 days (131). Although a dose calculated according to body weight is most accurate, age-related dose instructions are a more practical guide for the lay public (Table 2) (131). The palatability of aspirin can be improved by dissolving the tablet in a small amount of water in a spoon and mixing this with jelly or by using a commercial flavored aspirin product. The use of rectal suppositories of aspirin and acetaminophen should be avoided because rectal ab-

TABLE 2   Recommended antipyretic doses

Body weight	Age[a]	Single dose (mg)[b]
ACETAMINOPHEN		
10–15 mg/kg	less than 4 mo.[c]	40
total body	4–11 mo.[c]	80
weight	12–23 mo.[c]	120
	2–3 yr	160
	4–5 yr	240
	6–8 yr	320
	9–10 yr	400
	11–12 yr	480
	more than 12 yr (adult)	650
ACETYLSALICYLIC ACID		
10–15 mg/kg	less than 2 yr	physician directed
total body	2–3 yr	162
weight	4–5 yr	243
	6–8 yr	324
	9–10 yr	405
	11–12 yr	486
	more than 12 yr (adult)	650

[a] Use of antipyretic agents in children under 2 years of age should be supervised by a physician.
[b] Individual doses may be repeated every 4 to 6 hours as needed up to 4 to 5 daily doses.
[c] Adapted with permission from A. R. Temple, *Pediatr. Pharmacol.*, *3*, 321 (1983).

sorption is slower, incomplete, and unreliable (17). However, when aspirin or acetaminophen cannot be given orally (e.g., if the patient is vomiting), rectal suppositories at a dosage of 25–50% greater than the usual oral dosage has been recommended (17). Excessive aspirin dosage should be avoided because the manifestations of early salicylate toxicity such as nausea, vomiting, restlessness, irritability, ringing in the ears (tinnitus), hyperthermia, and rapid breathing (hyperpnea) may mimic the signs and symptoms of the disease being treated (187).

The FDA advisory review panel on over-the-counter (OTC) analgesics and antipyretics recommends that repeated dosing (i.e., for more than 5 days) of acetaminophen or salicylates be avoided, whenever possible, in infants and children under 12 years of age. This recommendation is based on a lack of pharmacokinetic and pharmacodynamic data in this patient population and limited information indicating that the clearance of these drugs from the body is reduced (131, 210). Repeated doses of salicylates or acetaminophen should be avoided in neonates because drug clearance may be reduced with liver and renal immaturity; the appropri-

ate frequency of dosing in neonates is therefore uncertain. A cooling blanket may be used in lieu of antipyretic agents for neonates (211–215).

Neither the dose nor the frequency of administration of salicylates or acetaminophen require alteration in elderly patients (216–220).

The dosing interval of acetaminophen should be extended to 8 hours in patients with renal dysfunction (when the rate of glomerular filtration falls below 10 ml/min) because of the danger of accumulation of active drug metabolites. Patients with lesser degrees of renal impairment require no dose adjustment (221). A supplemental dose of acetaminophen is recommended after hemodialysis but is unnecessary after peritoneal dialysis (221). Patients having a glomerular filtration rate of less than 10 ml/min should not be given salicylates because these drugs may further reduce renal function when renal blood flow is dependent on prostaglandin activity (221). A supplemental dose of salicylate

TABLE 3   Available dosage forms

Form	Content (mg per ml or solid form)
ACETAMINOPHEN	
Elixir/syrup	24, 32[a], 33, 65[a]
Drops	48, 100[a]
Chewable tablet	80[a]
Tablet	325
Capsule	325, 500, 650
Caplet	325
Suppositories	120, 325, 650
Effervescent granules	325/capful measure
Wafer	120
ACETYLSALICYLIC ACID	
Tablet	65, 81, 325, 500, 650
Chewable tablet	81[a]
Gum	228[a]
Capsule	325, 488
EC[b] tablet	325, 488, 500, 650, 975
EC[b] encapsulated granules	325, 500
Time-released tablet	650
Suppository	130, 195, 300, 325, 600, 650
Buffered tablet	324, 325, 486, 488, 500
Capsule	325, 500
Effervescent tablet	324
IBUPROFEN	
Tablet	200
Caplet	200

[a] Flavored preparations
[b] EC = Enteric-coated

is recommended following either peritoneal dialysis or hemodialysis (221).

PRODUCT SELECTION GUIDELINES

In general, acetaminophen is the preferred antipyretic agent. Adults may be given aspirin in the absence of a specific contraindication (e.g., previous episode of intolerance to a nonsteroidal anti-inflammatory agent or allergy to tartrazine dye) and when concomitant anti-inflammatory activity is desired. The use of salicylates is not recommended in individuals, especially children and teenagers, who have a viral illness (114, 161). Acetaminophen is also recommended for individuals with blood coagulation defects, a predisposition to bleeding (e.g., platelet defects or ongoing treatment with anticoagulant drugs), active bleeding, steroid-dependent asthma, chronic urticaria, nasal polyps, peptic ulcer disease, alcoholism, or gout. Acetaminophen is also recommended for patients who have cancer or are undergoing cancer chemotherapy (especially with methotrexate) and for patients in the last 3 months of pregnancy. Oral antipyretic agents are ineffective in the treatment of hyperthermia and drug fever; non-pharmacologic therapy should be instituted under the direction of a physician in the case of temperatures exceeding 104°F (40°C).

The amount of antacid contained in commercial "buffered" aspirin preparations is insufficient to protect the gastroduodenal mucosa from erosive damage (180, 222, 223), although a small amount of antacid may relieve the mild GI discomfort that is sometimes associated with the use of plain uncoated aspirin. The use of enteric-coated aspirin preparations significantly reduces gastroduodenal erosion (224). In contrast to the enteric-coated products first developed, the absorption and pharmacologic effects of the newer enteric-coated products have been shown to be equivalent to plain aspirin (223, 225, 226). Aspirin should be taken with food or milk to minimize GI upset, even though this does not prevent GI bleeding. Oral administration of either aspirin or acetaminophen is preferred over rectal administration because of the inferior and unreliable bioavailability of the latter (227, 228).

The combined use of salicylates and acetaminophen or the use of both drugs in an alternating schedule is not recommended. The concurrent administration of acetaminophen and aspirin has resulted in a greater temperature reduction than that achieved with either agent alone, and the antipyretic effect after combined therapy is sustained beyond that of either agent when used alone (128, 229). However, further study is needed to evaluate the possible benefits and risks that might accompany such administration. The potential benefit of prolonged antipyresis during sleep by bedtime administration of such a combination product has been suggested (2). There is concern, however, that the hepatotoxic potential of acetaminophen and the untoward effects of salicylate may be increased by combined treatment (71). A regimen of alternating the administration of salicylates and acetaminophen has not been proven to be clinically superior to use of either agent alone in the course of a fever. In addition, an alternating schedule is likely to be confusing and more likely to result in medication error.

PATIENT INFORMATION

Pharmacists and other health professionals should educate consumers about the proper assessment and treatment of fever. Medication errors can be reduced through consumer education efforts (230). Patients should also be instructed on the proper use of thermometers by demonstrating the method that is planned for use at home. Furthermore, parents should be reminded that rectal termperatures are 1 degree higher than oral temperatures. Acetaminophen is the preferred antipyretic agent for infants, children, and young adults; salicylates should *not* be given to treat fever that is associated with chickenpox, viral upper respiratory infections, or influenza-like illness in these individuals.

Patients and parents should be assured that fever is usually a benign, self-limited disorder and that the purpose of treatment is to alleviate the patient's discomfort. Oral antipyretic agents can usually be withheld until the temperature exceeds 102°F (39°C) or the patient becomes uncomfortable (see Table 4 for centigrade-Fahrenheit conversion formula and selected equivalents). Lower temperatures may be managed by nonpharmacologic measures. Sponging with tepid water should be reserved for temperatures exceeding 104°F (40°C) that follow a seizure or that have not responded to treatment with oral antipyretic agents. With the exception of an individual predisposed to seizures, sleep should not be interrupted to administer an antipyretic agent or to measure the temperature because a restful sleep is also presumed to be important.

Unnecessary antipyretic medication in adults can be avoided by measuring the temperature before giving each dose. Because frequent temperature measurements may not be acceptable to the child nor adhered to by the parents, the child's behavior and complaints

TABLE 4 Temperature equivalents

Centigrade = $\frac{5}{9}$ (°F − 32)

Fahrenheit = ($\frac{9}{5}$ × °C) + 32

Example conversions:

Centigrade	Fahrenheit
36°	96.8°
37°	98.6°
38°	100.4°
39°	102.2°
40°	104.0°
41°	105.8°
42°	107.6°

should serve as guides to the need for giving repeated, scheduled doses to the child. If the presence of fever is uncertain or discomfort persists despite treatment, the temperature should be remeasured. Patients should be alerted to the fact that aspirin and acetaminophen may be components in many other nonprescription products, and that the use of more than one agent may result in inadvertent overdosage of acetaminophen or aspirin.

A physician should be notified and antipyretic therapy should be instituted routinely in a febrile child who has experienced a previous febrile seizure or who has a documented history of seizures or another CNS disorder, or when there is a family history of seizures. If a seizure occurs, topical sponging should be initiated and the physician should be notified immediately.

Other conditions that warrant physician consultation are persistent vomiting and mental status changes such as increasing lethargy, irritability, and delirium in children being treated with salicylates. The appearance of tinnitus, difficulty in breathing (or rapid breathing), nausea, vomiting, restlessness, spontaneous or uncontrolled bleeding, the appearance of "dot and blot" hemorrhages (petechiae), or dysuria during salicylate therapy warrants immediate referral to a physician. A physician should also be contacted in the case of a whimpering infant, pain, sore throat, or a temperature exceeding 104°F (40°C) despite the administration of antipyretic agents. An isolated fever of more than 24 hours' duration, fever relapse, fever associated with any illness of more than 72 hours' duration, or unresponsiveness to treatment are additional conditions that require physician consultation. The possibility of subtle manifestations of life-threatening infections in infants supports the recommendation of physician consultation when a fever occurs in a child under 6 months of age (29).

Antiplatelet effects of salicylates in the nursing infant are unlikely to be clinically significant, but acetaminophen can be substituted if this is a concern (169–173).

Parents should be instructed to keep antipyretic agents, as well as all other medications, out of the reach of children and in a cool, dry location. A poison control center or physician should be contacted immediately if an overdose of either acetaminophen or a salicylate is suspected. (See the appendix in Chapter 12, *Emetic and Antiemetic Products*, for a listing of major poison control centers.)

SUMMARY

Fever is generally a benign, self-limited disorder. The primary purpose of treatment is to alleviate discomfort, and therefore a conservative approach to antipyretic treatment is recommended. Selection of an antipyretic drug should be based on the desirable pharmacologic properties of the drug and the medical history of the patient. In general, acetaminophen is the antipyretic agent of choice, but caution must be exercised in its use to achieve maximum antipyretic effects and to avoid inadvertent overdose.

REFERENCES

1 B. D. Schmitt, *Pediatrics, 74* (suppl.), 929 (1984).

2 C. A. Dinarello and S. M. Wolff, *N. Engl. J. Med., 298,* 607 (1978).

3 J. T. Stitt, *Fed. Proc., 40,* 2835 (1981).

4 A. Iliff et al., *Child Develop., 23,* 238 (1952).

5 E. Atkins and P. Bodel, *Fed. Proc., 38,* 57 (1979).

6 F. H. Lovejoy, Jr., *Pediatrics, 62* (suppl.), 904 (1978).

7 J. J. Drago et al., *J. Foot Surgery, 21,* 269 (1982).

8 H. A. Bernheim et al., *Ann. Intern. Med., 91,* 261 (1979).

9 R. A. Hoekelman, in "A Guide to Physical Examination," 3rd ed., B. Bates, Ed., Lippincott, Philadelphia, Pa., 1986, pp. 41–42, 457.

10 M. Cabanac, *Annu. Rev. Physiol., 37,* 415 (1975).

11 I. S. Edelman, *N. Engl. J. Med., 290,* 1303 (1974).

12 T. H. Benzinger, *J. Am. Med. Assoc., 209,* 1200 (1969).

13 E. Atkins, *Physiol. Rev., 40,* 580 (1960).

14 A. S. Milton, *J. Pharm. Pharmacol., 28,* 393 (1976).

15 W. B. Caspe et al., *Pediatr. Infect. Dis., 2,* 131 (1983).

16 M. E. Weisse et al., *Pediatr. Infect. Dis., 6,* 1091 (1987).

17 M. I. Lorin, in "The Febrile Child: Clinical Management of Fever and Other Types of Pyrexia," John Wiley & Sons, New York, N. Y., 1982, pp. 227–228.

18 M. Wasserman et al., *J. Amer Ger. Soc., 37,* 537 (1989).

19 P. C. Jones et al., *Gerontol., 30,* 182 (1984).

20 J. C. Chang, *Postgrad. Med., 84,* 71 (1988).

21 G. H. Willies et al., *Neuropharmacology, 15,* 9 (1976).

22 W. Feldberg and K. P. Gupta, *J. Physiol., 228,* 41 (1973).

23 W. Feldberg et al., *J. Physiol., 234,* 279 (1973).

24 W. Feldberg and P. N. Saxena, *J. Physiol., 217,* 547 (1971).

25 W. Feldberg and P. N. Saxena, *J. Physiol., 219,* 739 (1971).

26 C. A. Harvey and A. S. Milton, *J. Physiol., 250,* 18P (1975).

27 C. A. Harvey et al., *J. Physiol., 248,* 26P (1975).

28 A. S. Milton and Wendlandt, *J. Physiol., 207,* 76P (1970).

29 B. D. Schmitt, *Am. J. Dis. Child., 134,* 176 (1980).

30 E. F. DuBois, *Am. J. Med. Sci., 217,* 361 (1949).

31 W. A. Tomlinson, *J. Am. Med. Assoc., 129,* 693 (1975).

32 P. L. McCarthy and T. F. Dolan, *Am. J. Dis. Child., 130,* 849 (1976).

33 X. J. Musacchia, *Fed. Proc., 38,* 27 (1979).

34 J. Z. Sullivan-Bolyai et al., *Public Health Rep., 94,* 466 (1979).

35 L. O. Lamke et al., *Acta Chir. Scand., 146,* 81 (1980).

36 E. B. Ferris, Jr. et al., *J. Clin. Invest., 17,* 249 (1938).

37 J. P. Knochel, *Arch. Intern. Med., 133,* 841 (1974).

38 J. T. Stitt, *Fed. Proc., 38,* 39 (1979).

39 P. A. Mackowiak and C. F. LeMaistre, *Ann. Intern. Med., 106,* 728 (1987).

40 R. Patterson and J. Anderson, *J. Am. Med. Assoc., 248,* 2637 (1982).

41 J. D. Hasday, *Drug Ther., 78,* December (1980).

42 D. W. Martin et al., *West. J. Med., 129,* 321 (1978).

43 H. W. Murray and J. J. Mann, *Ann. Intern. Med., 83,* 84 (1975).

44 R. R. MacGregor, *Am. J. Med., 58,* 221 (1975).

45 S. M. Wolff, in "Cecil Textbook of Medicine," 17th ed., J. B. Wyngaarden and L. H. Smith, Eds., W. B. Saunders, Philadelphia, Pa., 1985, pp. 1470–1473.

46 R. W. Steale, in "Pediatric Therapy," 5th ed., H. C. Shirkey, Ed., C. V. Mosby, St. Louis, Mo., 1975, p. 331.

47 L. H. Newburgh, "Physiology of Heat Regulation," W. B. Saunders, Philadelphia, Pa., 1949, pp. 109–192.

48 M. J. Eoff and B. Joyce, *Am. J. Nurs., 81,* 1010 (1981).

49 J. Lau and G. Ong, *Nurses Drug Alert, 6,* 31 (1982).

50 D. Tandberg, *N. Engl. J. Med., 308,* 945 (1983).

51 *Health Devices, 2,* 3 (1972).

52 R. Erickson, *Int. J. Nurs. Stud., 13,* 199 (1976).

53 *Consumer Rep., 31,* 388 (1966).

54 R. Erickson, *Nurs. Res., 29,* 157 (1980).

55 N. J. Shanks et al., *Br. Med. J., 287,* 1263 (1983).

56 H. A. Knapp, *Am. J. Surg., 112,* 139 (1966).

57 N. C. Baker et al., *Nurs. Res., 33,* 109 (1984).

58 R. A. Hoekelman, in "A Guide to Physical Examination," 3rd ed., B. Bates, Ed., Lippincott, Philadelphia, Pa., 1986, pp. 41–42, 456.

59 E. I. Greenbaum et al., *Pediatrics, 44,* 539 (1969).

60 M. E. Siebenaler, *Amer. J. Maternal Child Nursing, 10,* 71 (1985).

61 K. S. Reisinger, *Pediatrics, 64,* 4 (1979).

62 E. M. Lewit et al., *J. Am. Med. Assoc., 247,* 321 (1982).

63 J. F. Donaldson, *Hosp. Pract., 16* (1981).

64 N. J. Roberts, Jr., *Microbiol. Rev., 43,* 241 (1979).

65 G. D. Benson, *Am. J. Med., 75* (5A), 85 (1983).

66 K. J. Ivey, *Am. J. Med., 75* (5A), 53 (1983).

67 D. M. Musher et al., *Arch. Intern. Med., 139,* 1225 (1979).

68 P. A. Pizzo et al., *Pediatrics, 55,* 468 (1975).

69 J. P. Phair, *Arch. Intern. Med., 139,* 1219 (1979).

70 P. A. Pizzo et al., *Am. J. Med., 67,* 194 (1979).

71 A. K. Done, *Am. J. Med., 74* (6A), 27 (1983).

72 A. K. Done, *Pediatrics, 23,* 774 (1959).

73 J. Klastersky and E. H. Kass, *J. Infect. Dis., 128,* 81 (1970).

74 J. F. Enders and M. F. Shaffer, *J. Exp. Med., 64,* 7 (1936).

75 D. L. Walker and W. D. Boring, *J. Immunol., 80,* 39 (1958).

76 R. C. Stern, *Pediatrics, 59,* 92 (1977).

77 D. Robard, *N. Engl. J. Med., 305,* 808 (1981).

78 T. F. Doran et al., *J. Pediatr., 114,* 1045 (1989).

79 P. A. Brunell, *Pediatr. Infect. Dis., 1,* 304 (1982).

80 E. Stanley et al., *J. Am. Med. Assoc., 231,* 1248 (1975).

81 Y. Akerren, *Acta Pediatr., 31,* 1 (1943).

82 J. G. Millichap, *J. Pediatr., 56,* 364 (1960).

83 K. B. Nelson and J. H. Ellenberg, *N. Engl. J. Med., 295,* 1029 (1976).

84 E. M. Ouellette, *Pediatr. Clin. North Am., 21,* 467 (1974).

85 M. A. Fishman, *J. Pediatr., 94,* 177 (1979).

86 C. M. Verity et al., *Br. Med. J., 290,* 1307 (1985).

87 J. H. Ellenberg and K. B. Nelson, *Arch. Neurol., 35,* 17 (1978).

88 E. M. Ouellette, *Drug Ther., 2,* 37 (1977).

89 C. M. Verity et al., *Br. Med. J., 290,* 1311 (1985).

90 F. U. Knudsen, *Pediatrics, 106,* 487 (1985).

91 J. G. Millichap, *Pediatrics, 23,* 76 (1959).

92 W. G. Lennox, *Pediatrics, 11,* 341 (1953).

93 B. Meldrum, *Neuropeadiatrie, 9,* 203 (1978).

94 E. Ngwane and B. Bower, *Br. Med. J., 280,* 353 (1980).

95 N. M. Graves and R. L. Kriel, *Pediatr. Neurol., 3,* 321 (1987).

96 S. M. Wolff et al., *Pediatrics, 59,* 378 (1977).

97 J. Aicardi and J. J. Chevrie, *Epilepsia, 11,* 187 (1970).

98 J. M. Oxbury and C. W. M. Whitty, *Brain, 94,* 733 (1971).

99 R. W. Steele et al., *J. Pediatr., 77,* 824 (1970).

100 S. W. McFadden and J. E. Haddow, *Pediatrics, 43,* 622 (1969).

101 R. F. Garrison, *J. Am. Med. Assoc., 152,* 317 (1958).

102 E. H. Senz and D. L. Goldfarb, *J. Pediatr., 53,* 322 (1958).

103 M. T. Colgan and A. A. Mintz, *J. Pediatr., 50,* 552 (1957).

104 A. W. Eden and A. Kaufman, *Am. J. Dis. Child., 114,* 284 (1967).

105 J. Hunter, *Arch. Dis. Child., 48,* 313 (1973).

106 L. Tarlin and P. Landrigan, *Am. J. Dis. Child., 124,* 880 (1972).

107 S. Similia et al., *Eur. J. Pediatr., 121,* 15 (1975).

108 P. D. Walson et al., *Clin. Pharmacol. Ther., 46,* 9 (1989).

109 M. E. Mortensen and R. M. Rennebohm, in "The Pediatric Clinics of North America," vol. 36, J. L. Blumer and M. D. Reed, Eds., 1989, p. 1113.

110 J. T. Wilson, *Ther. Drug. Monitor., 7,* 2 (1985).

111 U. K. Sheth et al., *J. Clin. Pharmacol.*, 20, 672–675 (1980).

112 B. B. Gaitonde et al., *J. Assoc. Physicians India.*, 21, 599 (1973).

113 S. M. Hall et al., *Arch. Dis. Child.*, 63, 857 (1988).

114 E. S. Hurwitz et al., *J. Am. Med. Assoc.*, 257, 1905 (1987).

115 D. Wells, Centers for Disease Control, Atlanta, Ga., personal communication, 1989.

116 "Drug Interaction Factors," J. B. Lippincott, St. Louis, Mo., 1989.

117 J. W. Hoftiezer et al., *Gastroenterology*, 78, 1183 (1980).

118 J. W. Hoftiezer et al., *Gut*, 23, 692 (1982).

119 J. A. Beirne et al., *Clin. Pharmacol. Ther.*, 16, 821 (1974).

120 J. R. Leonards and G. Levy, *Arch. Intern. Med.*, 129, 457 (1972).

121 J. R. Leonards and G. Levy, *Clin. Pharmacol. Ther.*, 14, 62 (1973).

122 J. R. Leonards et al., *N. Engl. J. Med.*, 289, 1020 (1973).

123 F. E. Silverstein et al., *Arch. Intern. Med.*, 141, 322 (1981).

124 R. N. Pierson et al., *Am. J. Med.*, 31, 259 (1961).

125 G. E. Bergman and J. L. Naiman, *J. Pediatr.*, 88, 501 (1976).

126 H. Heggarty, *Br. Med. J.*, 1, 491 (1974).

127 H. Jick, *Arch. Intern. Med.*, 141, 316 (1981).

128 D. Coggon et al., *Gut*, 23, 340 (1982).

129 G. E. Shambaugh, Jr., *J. Am. Med. Assoc.*, 218, 1573 (1971).

130 M. I. Grossman et al., *Gastroenterology*, 40, 383 (1961).

131 *Federal Register*, 42, 35366 (1977).

132 C. H. Mielke, Jr., *Arch. Intern. Med.*, 141, 305 (1981).

133 G. Masotti et al., *Lancet*, 2, 1213 (1979).

134 M. M. Kaneshiro et al., *N. Engl. J. Med.*, 281, 1039 (1969).

135 A. J. Quick, *Am. J. Med. Sci.*, 252, 265 (1966).

136 A. J. Quick, *Am. J. Med. Sci.*, 254, 392 (1967).

137 R. A. Binder et al., *Am. J. Dis. Child.*, 127, 371 (1974).

138 S. H. Reuter and W. W. Montgomery, *Arch. Otolaryngol.*, 80, 214 (1964).

139 D. Treacher et al., *Lancet*, 2, 1378 (1978).

140 M. Weinberger, *Pediatrics*, 62 (suppl), 910 (1978).

141 D. A. Mathison et al., *J. Allergy Clin. Immunol.*, 69, 135 (1982).

142 *J. Allergy Clin. Immunol.*, 58, 10 (1976).

143 C. H. A. Walton et al., *Can. Med. Assoc. J.*, 76, 1016 (1957).

144 M. Moore-Robinson and R. P. Warin, *Br. Med. J.*, 4, 262 (1967).

145 R. W. Lamson and R. Thomas, *J. Am. Med. Assoc.*, 99, 107 (1932).

146 B. R. Dysart, *J. Am. Med. Assoc.*, 101, 446 (1933).

147 N. Francis et al., *J. Allergy*, 6, 504 (1935).

148 J. R. McDonald et al., *J. Allergy Clin. Immunol.*, 50, 198 (1972).

149 G. S. Rachelefsky et al., *Pediatrics*, 56, 443 (1975).

150 M. Samter and R. F. Beers, *Ann. Intern. Med.*, 68, 975 (1968).

151 A. Szczeklik et al., *J. Allergy Clin. Immunol.*, 58, 10 (1976).

152 A. Szczeklik et al., *Br. Med. J.*, 1, 67 (1975).

153 R. D. K. Reye et al., *Lancet*, 2, 749 (1963).

154 J. C. Partin et al., *N. Engl. J. Med.*, 285, 1339 (1971).

155 B. A. Shaywitz et al., *Pediatrics*, 66, 198 (1980).

156 K. E. Bove et al., *Gastroenterology*, 69, 685 (1975).

157 L. Corey et al., *Pediatrics*, 60, 702 (1977).

158 K. M. Starko et al., *Pediatrics*, 66, 859 (1980).

159 *U.S. Morbidity and Mortality Weekly Reports*, 34, 13 (1985).

160 *U.S. Morbidity and Mortality Weekly Reports*, 31, 289 (1982).

161 *FDA Drug Bulletin*, 18(2), (1988).

162 S. Shapiro et al., *Lancet*, 1, 1375 (1976).

163 R. B. Lewis and J. D. Schulman, *Lancet*, 2, 1159 (1973).

164 L. K. Garrettson et al., *Clin. Pharmacol. Ther.*, 17, 98 (1975).

165 W. A. Bleyer and R. T. Breckenridge, *J. Am. Med. Assoc.*, 213, 2049 (1970).

166 D. G. Corby and I. Schulman, *J. Pediatr.*, 79, 307 (1971).

167 M. Niederhoff and H. P. Zahradnik, *Am. J. Med.*, 75 (5A), 117 (1983).

168 C. M. Berlin et al., *Pediatr. Pharmacol.*, 1, 135 (1980).

169 J. W. A. Findlay et al., *Clin. Pharmacol. Ther.*, 29, 625 (1981).

170 P. O. Anderson, *Drug Intell. Clin. Pharm.*, 11, 208 (1977).

171 C. M. Berlin, Jr., et al., *Clin. Pharmacol. Ther.*, 27, 245 (1980).

172 S. H. Erickson and G. L. Oppenheim, *J. Fam. Pract.*, 8, 189 (1979).

173 G. Levy, *J. Pediatr.*, 62 (suppl.), 867 (1978).

174 M. H. Gault et al., *Ann. Intern. Med.*, 68, 906 (1968).

175 T. Murray and M. Goldberg, *Annu. Rev. Med.*, 26, 537 (1976).

176 R. D. Emkey and J. A. Mills, *J. Am. Med. Assoc.*, 247, 55 (1982).

177 B. E. Glader, *J. Pediatr.*, 89, 1027 (1976).

178 H. J. Zimmerman, *Arch. Intern. Med.*, 141, 333 (1981).

179 R. R. Rich and J. Johnson, *Arthritis Rheum.*, 16 (1973).

180 A. M. Rudolph, *Arch. Intern. Med.*, 141, 358 (1981).

181 P. C. Johnson and T. Driscoll, *Curr. Ther. Res.*, 30, 79 (1981).

182 K. Goulston and A. Skyring, *Gut*, 5, 463 (1964).

183 D. H. Loebl et al., *J. Am. Med. Assoc.*, 237, 976 (1977).

184 C. H. Jackson et al., *Can. Med. Assoc. J.*, 131, 25 (1984).

185 C. K. Kasper and S. I. Rapaport, *Ann. Intern. Med.*, 77, 189 (1972).

186 C. H. Mielke, Jr., and A. F. H. Britten, *N. Engl. J. Med.*, 282, 1270 (1970).

187 "Poisindex," Micromedex, Englewood, Colo., 1985.

188 S. A. Kanada et al., *Am. J. Hosp. Pharm.*, 35, 330 (1978).

189 R. C. Peterson and B. H. Rumack, *Arch. Intern. Med.*, 141, 390 (1981).

190 R. P. Miller et al., *Clin. Pharmacol. Ther.*, 19, 284 (1976).

191 B. H. Lauterberg et al., *J. Pharmacol. Exp. Ther.*, 213, 54 (1980).

192 S. N. Alam et al., *J. Pediatr.*, 90, 130 (1977).

193 R. E. Mancini et al., *Res. Commun. Chem. Pathol. Pharmacol.*, 27, 603 (1980).

194 J. D. Barker, Jr., et al., *Ann. Intern. Med.*, 87, 299–301 (1977).

195 A. J. Ware et al., *Ann. Intern. Med.*, 88, 267–268 (1978).

196 G. K. Johnson and K. G. Tolman, *Ann. Intern. Med.*, 87, 302–304 (1977).

197 H. L. Bonkowsky et al., *Lancet*, 1, 1016–18 (1978).

198 T. J. Meredith and R. Goulding, *Postgrad. Med. J.*, 56, 459–473 (1980).

199 J. Neuberger et al., *J. R. Soc. Med.*, 73, 701–707 (1980).

200 "Aspirin or Paracetamol?" *Lancet*, 2, 287 (1981).

201 J. A. H. Forrest et al., *Eur. J. Clin. Pharmacol.*, 15, 427–431 (1979).

202 P. B. Andreasen and L. Hutters, *Acta Med. Scand.*, 624 (suppl.), 99–105 (1979).

203 G. D. Benson, *Clin. Pharmacol. Ther.*, 33, 95–101 (1983).

204 G. Duggin and G. Mudge, *J. Pharmacol. Exp. Ther.*, 199, 10 (1976).

205 G. Duggin and G. Mudge, *J. Pharmacol. Exp. Ther.*, 199, 1 (1976).

206 D. P. Sandler et al., *N. Engl. J. Med.*, 320, 1238 (1989).

207 L. M. Fraser, *Ann. N.Y. Acad. Sci., 151,* 777 (1968).

208 B. Gribetz and S. A. Cronley, *Pediatrics, 80,* 630 (1987).

209 J. T. Wilson, et al., *Ther. Drug Monit., 4,* 147 (1982).

210 M. C. Nahata et al., *Eur. J. Clin. Pharmacol., 27,* 57 (1984).

211 G. Levy and L. K. Garrettson, *Pediatrics, 53,* 201 (1974).

212 G. Levy et al., *Pediatrics, 55,* 818 (1975).

213 E. Nelson and T. Morioka, *J. Pharm. Sci., 52,* 864 (1963).

214 A. J. Cummings et al., *Br. J. Pharmacol., 29,* 150 (1976).

215 L. F. Prescott et al., *Clin. Pharmacol. Ther., 9,* 605 (1968).

216 E. J. Triggs et al., *Eur. J. Clin. Pharmacol., 8,* 55 (1975).

217 R. H. Briant et al., *J. Am. Geriatr. Soc., 24,* 359 (1980).

218 S. A. M. Salem and I. H. Stevenson, *Br. J. Clin. Pharmacol., 4,* 397 P (1977).

219 G. Cuny et al., *Gerontology, 25,* 49 (1979).

220 C. M. Castledon et al., *Age and Aging, 6,* 138 (1977).

221 W. M. Bennett et al., *Am. J. Kidney Dis., 3,* 155 (1983).

222 O. O. Lockard et al., *Gastrointest. Endosc., 26,* 5 (1980).

223 F. L. Lanza et al., *N. Engl. J. Med., 303,* 136 (1980).

224 J. W. Hoftiezer et al., *Lancet, 2,* 609 (1980).

225 W. T. Beaver, *Am. J. Med. Sci., 250,* 577 (1965).

226 A. T. Canada and A. H. Little, *Curr. Ther. Res., 18,* 727 (1975).

227 S. N. Pagay et al., *J. Pharm. Sci., 60,* 600 (1971).

228 M. M. Nowak et al., *Pediatrics, 54,* 23 (1974).

229 R. W. Steele et al., *Am. J. Dis. Child., 123,* 204 (1972).

230 R. Casey et al., *Pediatrics, 73,* 600 (1984).

ANTIPYRETIC PRODUCT TABLE

Product[a] (Manufacturer)	Aspirin	Salicyl-amide	Aceta-minophen	Ibu-profen	Caffeine	Sodium	Other Ingredients
Acephen Suppositories (G&W Laboratories)			120 mg 325 mg 650 mg			NS[b]	hydrogenated vegetable oil polysorbate 80
Aceta Elixir & Tablets (Century Pharm)			160 mg/5 ml (elixir) 325 mg/ tablet 500 mg/ tablet				alcohol, 7% (elixir)
Acetaminophen (Various manufacturers)			325 mg 500 mg 650 mg				
Acetamino-phen Capsules (Various manufacturers)			500 mg				
Acetamino-phen Chewable Tablets (Various manufacturers)			80 mg				
Acetamino-phen Drops (Various manufacturers)			100 mg/ml				
Acetamino-phen Elixir (Various manufacturers)			120 mg/5 ml 130 mg/5 ml 160 mg/5 ml				
Acetamino-phen Liquid[c] (UDL Labs)			160 mg/5 ml				
Acetamino-phen Suppositories (Various manufacturers)			120 mg 300 mg 325 mg 650 mg				
Acetamino-phen Uniserts (Upsher-Smith)			120 mg 325 mg 650 mg			NS[b]	
Actamin (Buffington)			325 mg 500 mg		65 mg	free	
Advil (Whitehall)				200 mg		0.004 mEq	
Alka-Seltzer (Miles Labs)	324 mg					567 mg	sodium bicarbo-nate, 1.9 g citric acid, 1 g
Alka-Seltzer Flavored (Miles Labs)	324 mg					506 mg	sodium bicarbo-nate, 1.7 g citric acid, 1.2 g saccharin flavor

ANTIPYRETIC PRODUCT TABLE, continued

Product[a] (Manufacturer)	Aspirin	Salicyl- amide	Aceta- minophen	Ibu- profen	Caffeine	Sodium	Other Ingredients
Alka-Seltzer Extra Strength (Miles Labs)	500 mg						sodium bicarbo- nate, 1.9 g citric acid, 1 g
Anacin (Whitehall)	400 mg 500 mg				32 mg 32 mg	0.001 mEq 0.002 mEq	
Anacin-3 (Whitehall)			325 mg 500 mg			0.03 mEq < 0.5 mEq	
Anacin-3[c] Chil- dren's[c] & Infants'[c] Aspirin Free (Whitehall)			80 mg/chew- able tablet 160 mg/5 ml (liquid) 80 mg/0.8 ml (drops)				saccharin (drops) sorbitol (drops) cherry flavor (chew- able tablet, liquid) fruit flavor (drops)
Anodynos (Buffington)	NS[b]	NS[b]			NS[b]	free	
Apacet Chewa- ble Tablets (Parmed)			80 mg				
Arthritis Pain Formula (Whitehall)	500 mg (micronized)					0.01 mEq	aluminum hydrox- ide, 27 mg magnesium hydrox- ide, 100 mg
Arthritis Pain Formula Aspirin Free (Whitehall)			500 mg				
Arthropan Liquid (Purdue Frederick)						NS[b]	choline salicylate, 174 mg/ml (equi- valent to 130 mg of aspirin)
A.S.A. (Lilly)	325 mg 650 mg						
A.S.A. Enseals (Lilly)	325 mg 650 mg				NS[b]	NS[b]	
A.S.A. Pulvules (Lilly)	325 mg						
Ascriptin Caplets (Rorer)	325 mg					NS[b]	magnesium hydrox- ide, 50 mg aluminum hydrox- ide, 50 mg calcium carbonate
Ascriptin A/D Caplets (Rorer)	325 mg					NS[b]	magnesium hydrox- ide, 75 mg aluminum hydrox- ide, 75 mg calcium carbonate
Ascriptin Extra Strength Caplets (Rorer)	500 mg						magnesium hydrox- ide, 80 mg aluminum hydrox- ide, 80 mg calcium carbonate

ANTIPYRETIC PRODUCT TABLE, continued

Product[a] (Manufacturer)	Aspirin	Salicyl-amide	Aceta-minophen	Ibu-profen	Caffeine	Sodium	Other Ingredients
Aspercin (Otis Clapp)	325 mg 500 mg					free	
Aspergum Chewing Gum (Schering-Plough)	228 mg					0.003 mEq	cherry or orange flavor
Aspirin (Various manufacturers)	325 mg 500 mg 650 mg						
Aspirin, Buffered (Various manufacturers)	325 mg						buffers
Aspirin, Children's (Various manufacturers)	65 mg 75 mg 81 mg						
Aspirin Free Pain Relief (Hudson)			325 mg 500 mg				
Aspirin Suppositories (Various manufacturers)	60 mg 120 mg 125 mg 130 mg 195 mg 200 mg 300 mg 325 mg 600 mg 650 mg 1.2 g					NS[b]	
Banesin (Forest)			500 mg			free	
Bayer Aspirin (Glenbrook)	325 mg					< 0.01 mEq	
Bayer, Maxi-mum Aspirin Tablets and Caplets (Glenbrook)	500 mg						
Bayer Child-ren's Chewable Aspirin (Glenbrook)	81 mg					0.004 mEq	saccharin orange flavor
Bayer 8-hour Timed-Release Aspirin (Glenbrook)	650 mg					< 0.01 mEq	
BC (Block)	325 mg	95 mg			16 mg		
BC Powder (Block)	650 mg	195 mg			32 mg		
BC Powder Arthritis Strength (Block)	742 mg	222 mg			36 mg		

ANTIPYRETIC PRODUCT TABLE, continued

Product[a] (Manufacturer)	Aspirin	Salicyl-amide	Aceta-minophen	Ibu-profen	Caffeine	Sodium	Other Ingredients
Bromo-Seltzer (Warner-Lambert)			325 mg/ capful			33 mEq/ capful	sodium bicarbonate, 2.78 g/capful citric acid, 2.22 g/ capful
Buffaprin[d] (Buffington)	325 mg 500 mg					free	magnesium oxide
Buffasal (Dover)	325 mg 500 mg					free	magnesium oxide
Bufferin (Bristol-Myers Products)	324 mg						magnesium carbonate aluminum glycinate
Bufferin, Arthritis Strength (Bristol-Myers Products)	500 mg						magnesium carbonate aluminum glycinate
Bufferin, Extra Strength (Bristol-Myers Products)	500 mg						magnesium carbonate aluminum glycinate
Bufferin, Tri-Buffered (Bristol-Myers Products)	325 mg					NS[b]	magnesium carbonate, 34 mg magnesium oxide, 63 mg calcium carbonate, 158 mg
Bufferin, Tri-Buffered Arthritis Strength Caplets (Bristol-Myers Products)	500 mg					NS[b]	calcium carbonate, 222.3 mg magnesium oxide, 88.9 mg magnesium carbonate, 55.6 mg
Bufferin, Tri-Buffered Extra Strength (Bristol-Myers Products)	500 mg						calcium carbonate, 222.3 mg magnesium oxide, 88.9 mg magnesium carbonate, 55.6 mg
Buffets II (JMI)	226.8 mg		162 mg		32.4 mg		aluminum hydroxide, 50 mg
Buffex (Hauck)	325 mg						dihydroxyaluminum aminoacetate
Buffinol[d] (Otis Clapp)	325 mg 500 mg					free	magnesium oxide
Cama Arthritis Pain Reliever (Sandoz Consumer)	500 mg						magnesium oxide, 150 mg aluminum hydroxide, 150 mg
Cama In-Lay Tablets (Sandoz Consumer)	600 mg					NS[b]	magnesium hydroxide, 150 mg aluminum hydroxide gel, dried, 150 mg

ANTIPYRETIC PRODUCT TABLE, continued

Product[a] (Manufacturer)	Aspirin	Salicyl-amide	Aceta-minophen	Ibu-profen	Caffeine	Sodium	Other Ingredients
CoAdvil (Whitehall)				200 mg			pseudoephedrine hydrochloride, 30 mg
Conacetol (CMC)			325 mg				
Congespirin For Children Chewable (Bristol-Myers Products)			81 mg			NS[b]	phenylephrine hydrochloride, 1.25 mg
Cope (Mentholatum)	421 mg				32 mg		magnesium hydrox-ide, 50 mg aluminum hydrox-ide, 25 mg
Dapa (Ferndale)			324 mg				
Dapa, Extra Strength Capsules (Ferndale)			500 mg				
Dasin Capsules (Beecham)	130 mg				8 mg		atropine sulfate, 0.13 mg ipecac, 3 mg camphor, 15 mg
Datril Extra Strength Caplets and Tablets (Bristol-Myers Products)			500 mg			NS[b]	
Doan's, Original (Ciba Consumer)							magnesium salicy-late, 325 mg
Doan's, Extra Strength (Ciba Consumer)							magnesium salicy-late, 500 mg
Dolanex Elixir[d] (Lannett)			325 mg/5 ml				alcohol, 23%
Dolcin (Dolcin)		240.5 mg				NS[b]	calcium succinate monohydrate, 182 mg
Dorcol Chil-dren's Fever and Pain Reducer Liquid (Sandoz Consumer)			160 mg/5 ml				sucrose
Duradyne (Forest)	230 mg		180 mg		15 mg		
Ecotrin & Eco-trin Maximum (SmithKline Beecham)	325 mg 500 mg					0.001 mEq	

ANTIPYRETIC PRODUCT TABLE, continued

Product[a] (Manufacturer)	Aspirin	Salicyl- amide	Aceta- minophen	Ibu- profen	Caffeine	Sodium	Other Ingredients
Empirin (Burroughs Wellcome)	325 mg					free	
Excedrin Caplets and Tablets (Bristol-Myers Products)	250 mg		250 mg		65 mg		
Excedrin PM (Bristol-Myers Products)			500 mg			NS[b]	diphenhydramine citrate, 38 mg
Feverall, Children's Suppositories (Upsher-Smith)			120 mg				
Feverall, Junior Strength Suppositories (Upsher-Smith)			325 mg				
Gemnisyn (Kremers-Urban)	325 mg		325 mg				
Genapap, Children's Chewable (Goldline)			80 mg				
Genapap, Children's Elixir[c] (Goldline)			160 mg/5 ml				cherry flavor
Genapap, Extra Strength (Goldline)			500 mg				
Genapap, Infants' Drops[c] (Goldline)			100 mg/ml				fruit flavor
Genebs (Goldline)			325 mg				
Genebs Extra Strength (Goldline)			500 mg				
Genpril (Goldline)				200 mg			
Genprin (Goldline)	325 mg						
Gensan (Goldline)	400 mg				32 mg		
Halenol and Halenol Extra Strength (Halsey)			325 mg 500 mg				
Halenol Children's Liquid[c] (Halsey)			160 mg/5 ml				cherry flavor

ANTIPYRETIC PRODUCT TABLE, continued

Product[a] (Manufacturer)	Aspirin	Salicyl- amide	Aceta- minophen	Ibu- profen	Caffeine	Sodium	Other Ingredients
Liquiprin Children's Elixir[c] (SmithKline Beecham)			160 mg/5 ml				dextrose fructose sucrose cherry flavor
Liquiprin Infants' Drops[c] (SmithKline Beecham)			48 mg/ml			< 0.03 mEq/ml	fruit flavor
Magnaprin (Rugby)	325 mg						magnesium hydrox- ide, 75 mg aluminum hydrox- ide, 75 mg
Magnaprin, Arthritis Strength (Rugby)	325 mg						magnesium hydrox- ide, 150 mg aluminum hydrox- ide, 150 mg
Measurin (Winthrop Pharm)	650 mg (timed release)				NS[b]		
Meda Cap (Circle)			500 mg				
Meda Tab (Circle)			325 mg				
Menoplex (Fiske)			325 mg				phenyltoloxamine citrate, 30 mg
Midol Caplets, Original Formula (Glenbrook)	454 mg				32.4 mg		cinnamedrine hydrochloride, 14.9 mg
Midol for Cramps Caplets, Maxi- mum Strength (Glenbrook)	500 mg				32.4 mg		cinnamedrine hydrochloride, 14.9 mg
Midol PMS Capsules (Glenbrook)			500 mg				pamabrom, 25 mg pyrilamine maleate, 15 mg
Mobigesic (B.F. Ascher)						NS[b]	phenyltoloxamine citrate, 30 mg magnesium salicy- late, 325 mg
Myapap Drops[c,d] (Gen-King)			100 mg/ml				
Neogesic (Rev.) (Vale)	184.4 mg		129.6 mg		32.4 mg		dihydroxyaluminum acetate
Neopap Suppositories (Alcon)			125 mg				
Norwich Aspirin and Extra Strength (Vicks Health Care)	325 mg 500 mg						

ANTIPYRETIC PRODUCT TABLE, continued

Product[a] (Manufacturer)	Aspirin	Salicyl- amide	Aceta- minophen	Ibu- profen	Caffeine	Sodium	Other Ingredients
Nuprin (Bristol-Myers Products)				200 mg			
Oraphen-PD Elixir (Great Southern)			120 mg/5 ml				alcohol, 5% cherry flavor
Pabalate (A.H. Robins)						88.4 mg	sodium salicylate, 0.3 g sodium aminoben- zoate, 0.3 g
P-A-C (Upjohn)	400 mg				32 mg		tartrazine
Pain-Eze + (Reese)			650 mg				
Pain Reliever Tablets (Rugby)	250 mg		250 mg		65 mg		
Pamprin (Chattem)			400 mg				pamabrom, 25 mg pyrilamine maleate, 15 mg
Pamprin Maxi- mum Cramp Relief Caplets and Capsules (Chattem)			500 mg				pamabrom, 25 mg pyrilamine maleate, 15 mg
Panadol Caplets and Tablets (Glenbrook)			500 mg				
Panadol, Child- rens[c,d] **and Infants'**[c,d] (Glenbrook)			80 mg/chew- able tablet 160 mg/5 ml (liquid) 80 mg/0.8 ml (drops)				saccharin (liquid, drops) sorbitol (liquid) fruit flavor (chewa- ble tablet, liquid, drops)
Panex (Hauck)			325 mg				
Panex 500 (Hauck)			500 mg				
Phenaphen (A.H. Robins)			325 mg				
Prēmsyn PMS Caplets and Capsules (Chattem)			500 mg				pamabrom, 25 mg pyrilamine maleate, 15 mg
Presalin (Hauck)	260 mg	120 mg	120 mg				aluminum hydrox- ide, 100 mg
Rid a Pain (Pfeiffer)		97.2 mg	226.8 mg		32.4 mg		
S-A-C (Lannett)		230 mg	150 mg		30 mg		

ANTIPYRETIC PRODUCT TABLE, continued

Product[a] (Manufacturer)	Aspirin	Salicyl-amide	Aceta-minophen	Ibu-profen	Caffeine	Sodium	Other Ingredients
Salabuff (Ferndale)	324 mg				16.2 mg		aluminum hydroxide magnesium carbonate co-dried gel
Salatin Capsules (Ferndale)	259.2 mg		129.6 mg		16.2 mg		
Saleto (Hauck)	210 mg	65 mg	115 mg		16 mg		
Salocol (Hauck)	210 mg	65 mg	115 mg		16 mg		
Snaplets-FR Granules (Baker Cummins)			80 mg				
Sodium Salicylate (Various manufacturers)							sodium salicylate, 325 mg, 650 mg
St. Joseph Aspirin (Schering-Plough)	325 mg					free	
St. Joseph Low Dose Adult Aspirin (Schering-Plough)	81 mg (chewable)					free	
St. Joseph Aspirin-Free for Children and Infants[c,d] (Schering-Plough)			80 mg/chewable tablet 80 mg/0.8 ml (drops)			NS[b]	saccharin (drops) fruit flavor (chewable tablet, drops)
St. Joseph Aspirin-Free Fever Reducer for Children[c,d] (Schering-Plough)		160 mg/5 ml (liquid)					saccharin sorbitol
Supac (Mission)	230 mg		160 mg		33 mg		calcium gluconate, 60 mg
Suppap-120 Suppositories (Raway)			120 mg				
Suppap-325 Suppositories (Raway)			325 mg				
Suppap-650 Suppositories (Raway)			650 mg				
Tapanol Extra Strength (Republic)			500 mg				

ANTIPYRETIC PRODUCT TABLE, continued

Product[a] (Manufacturer)	Aspirin	Salicyl- amide	Aceta- minophen	Ibu- profen	Caffeine	Sodium	Other Ingredients
Tempra (Mead Johnson)			160 mg				
Tempra Chewa- ble Tablets (Mead Johnson)			80 mg				
Tempra Syrup[c] and Drops[c] (Mead Johnson)			160 mg/5 ml (syrup) 80 mg/0.8 ml (drops)			0.03 mEq/ml (syrup) 0.08 mEq/ml (drops)	cherry flavor (syrup) grape flavor (drops)
Tenol (Vortech)			325 mg			NS[b]	
Tenol-Plus (Vortech)	250 mg		250 mg		65 mg		
Trigesic (Squibb)	230 mg		125 mg		30 mg		
Tri-Pain Caplets (Ferndale)	162 mg	162 mg	162 mg		16.2 mg		
Tylenol, Child- ren's[c] and Infants'[c] (McNeil)			80 mg/chew- able tablet 100 mg/ml (drops) 32 mg/ml (elixir)			< 0.04 mEq/ chewa- ble tablet < 0.04 mEq/ml (drops) 0.02 mEq/ml (elixir)	sorbitol (elixir) sucrose (elixir) saccharin (drops) fruit or grape flavor (chewable tablet) cherry or grape fla- vor (elixir) fruit flavor (drops)
Tylenol Extra Strength (McNeil)			500 mg (tablet, gel- cap, caplet) 33.3 mg/ml (liquid)			< 0.04 mEq (tablet, gelcap, caplet) 0.02 mEq/ml (liquid)	alcohol, 9% (liquid) sorbitol (liquid) sucrose (liquid) mint flavor (liquid)
Tylenol Junior Strength Swallowable (McNeil)			160 mg				
Tylenol Regu- lar Strength (McNeil)			325 mg (tablet, caplet)			< 0.04 mEq/ tablet	
Uracel 5 (Vortech)						NS[b]	sodium salicylate, 324 mg
Valadol (Squibb)			325 mg				
Valesin (Vale)	150 mg	150 mg	150 mg				
Valorin (Otis Clapp)			325 mg 500 mg			free	

ANTIPYRETIC PRODUCT TABLE, continued

Product[a] (Manufacturer)	Aspirin	Salicyl-amide	Aceta-minophen	Ibu-profen	Caffeine	Sodium	Other Ingredients
Vanquish Caplets (Glenbrook)	227 mg		194 mg		33 mg		magnesium hydroxide, 50 mg aluminum hydroxide, 25 mg
Verin (Hauck)	650 mg (timed release)						
Wesprin Buffered (Wesley)	325 mg						aluminum hydroxide magnesium hydroxide

[a] Tablet unless specified otherwise.
[b] Quantity not specified.
[c] Alcohol free.
[d] Sugar free.

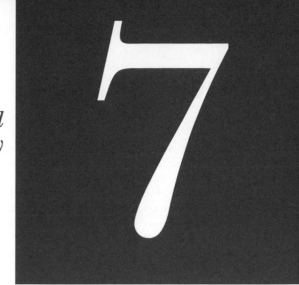

Catherine Angell Sohn and
Barbara H. Korberly

MENSTRUAL PRODUCTS

Questions to ask in patient/consumer counseling

When was your last menstrual period? Was it late or early?

Do you use any contraceptive measures?

When does your pain occur in relation to the onset of your menstrual period?

How do your present symptoms vary from those of your normal cycle (flow, duration, and intensity)?

Are you under the care of a physician?

Do you have any vaginal discharge accompanied by pain, itching, pus, blood, or foul odor?

What have you already done to treat this problem?

Do you have any known drug allergies (aspirin)?

Are you taking any medication for another condition?

Do you use tampons or sanitary napkins?

Menstruation (menses) is a regular physiologic condition in women during their childbearing years. In addition to blood loss, many women experience unpleasant symptoms during various phases of the menstrual cycle, such as headaches, fluid retention, breast tenderness, irritability, anxiety, backache, abdominal pain and cramping, and depression.

The presence and intensity of these symptoms vary widely from one woman to another. The pharmacist should be able to interview a woman and assess her symptoms to determine their severity and whether physician referral is warranted. In addition, the pharmacist should be able to evaluate the many nonprescription preparations so that effective therapy and adjunctive measures can be recommended to alleviate the patient's premenstrual or menstrual discomfort.

Recognition of the illness identified as "toxic shock syndrome" has focused attention on tampons, the risk associated with their use, and recommendations for their correct use.

MENSTRUAL CYCLE

The female's reproductive years are characterized by monthly rhythmic changes in rates of secretion of female hormones necessary for reproduction. This rhythmic pattern is called the female sexual cycle or menstrual cycle. Two functions of the menstrual cycle are to release a mature ovum (egg) from an ovary and to prepare the uterine endometrium for implantation of the embryo should the ovum be fertilized during its course through the fallopian or uterine tube. In the absence of fertilization, the degenerated ovum is discarded along with the endometrial lining in the menstrual flow that passes through the cervix, down the vaginal canal, and out of the body (Figure 1A) (1). (See Chapter 25, *Contraceptive Methods and Products.*)

Menstruation is this periodic, physiologic discharge of blood, mucus, and cellular debris from the uterine mucosa, which occurs at more or less regular intervals from puberty to menopause, except during pregnancy and lactation. The normal menstrual cycle is coordinated with the ovarian cycle and depends on the integrated functions of the endocrine and nervous system. Menarche, the occurrence of the first menstrual period, is a function of the maturation process of the young female. It is preceded by the development of required organ systems, a growth spurt, and early signs and appearance of secondary sexual characteristics. It usually occurs at the end of the pubertal process.

The average age at which menstruation begins is between 12 and 13 years, but its onset may be as early as 10 and as late as 16 years of age. The onset of menstruation depends on such variables as race, genetic factors, environmental temperature conditions, and nutritional status. Menopause is the cessation of menstrual function. It occurs on the average at 51 years of age, but ranges between 45 and 55 years of age (2).

The average duration of the normal female menstrual cycle is 28 days. The first day of menstrual flow is considered to be day 1 of each cycle. Each cycle may be as short as 20 days or as long as 45 days in normal, healthy women. There is great variation among women and within the cycle of any individual woman. Variations in the menstrual cycle occur in relation to the woman's age, physical and emotional well-being, extent and intensity of exercise, and environmental factors.

The duration of menstrual flow is also variable. The usual duration is 3–7 days, but it can be as short as 2 days or as long as 8 days. For any individual woman, the menstrual flow is fairly constant. The average amount of blood and tissue debris lost in menstruation is about 70 ml, but many women lose considerably more (3). Women under 35 years of age tend to lose more blood than those over 35. Although it is difficult to quantitate the amount of blood lost, studies indicate that a slight lowering of hemoglobin may occur even in healthy women with adequate diets. The blood loss during menstruation may range from 40 to 100 ml (4).

The menstrual discharge has a characteristic dark reddish color because of the blood and mucosal breakdown products. The offensive odor of the menstrual flow is attributable to decomposed blood elements and the vulvar sebaceous gland secretions. In addition to the blood elements, the flow contains cervical mucus, vaginal mucosa, numerous bacteria, and degenerated endometrial particles. The odor and secretions of menstruation must be differentiated from the foul-sweet odor of trichomoniasis and gardnerella infections and the heavy, creamy secretions of vaginal yeast infections.

(See Chapter 27, *Personal Care Products.*) These conditions usually warrant referral to a physician for diagnosis and treatment.

PHYSIOLOGY

Hormone release is regulated by complex neuroendocrine feedback systems that are not yet fully understood.

The hypothalamus releases luteinizing hormone-releasing hormone (LH-RH). Under the influence of LH-RH, the anterior pituitary gland releases luteinizing hormone (LH) and follicle stimulating hormone (FSH). LH and FSH are also called gonadotropic hormones. Under the influence of LH and FSH, the ovaries secrete estrogens and progesterone.

As previously stated, the primary results of the female sexual cycle are maturation of an ovum and development of the uterine endometrium to provide a life support system for a fertilized ovum (embryo). Maturation of the ovum is the function of the ovarian cycle, and preparation of the uterus is the function of the endometrial cycle.

The ovarian cycle is regulated by cyclical increases and decreases in the concentrations of the gonadotropic hormones LH and FSH (Figure 2). At the beginning of each month of the female sexual cycle, at about the onset of menstruation, the concentration of FSH starts to increase. This hormonal increase causes follicles to develop within the ovary (follicular phase) (Figure 3), stimulating the maturation of an ovum as well as the release of estrogen from the ovary. The higher concentrations of estrogen trigger the release of LH from the anterior pituitary. LH causes final maturation of the follicle and release of the mature ovum (ovulation) around day 14. The high concentrations of LH also cause the empty follicle to develop into the corpus luteum (luteal phase), which over the next 11–12 days secretes increasing concentrations of progesterone and estrogen (Figure 3). As the corpus luteum regresses on about the 26th day of the female cycle, the anterior pituitary gland increases secretion of FSH again (Figure 2), initiating new growth of a follicle and maturation of an ovum.

The endometrium, under the influence of the two ovarian hormones, estrogen and progesterone, exhibits characteristic cyclic changes that can be divided into the menstrual phase, proliferative phase (estrogenic or follicular phase), and secretory phase (progestational or luteal phase).

During menstruation (days 1–5) much of the endometrium is sloughed, leaving a thin endometrial lining.

A

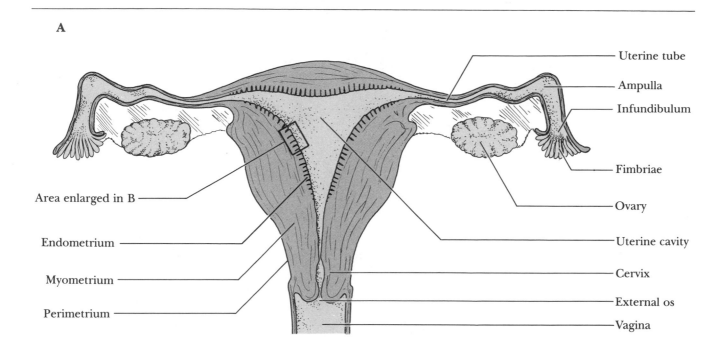

Uterine tube

Ampulla

Infundibulum

Fimbriae

Ovary

Uterine cavity

Cervix

External os

Vagina

Area enlarged in B

Endometrium

Myometrium

Perimetrium

B

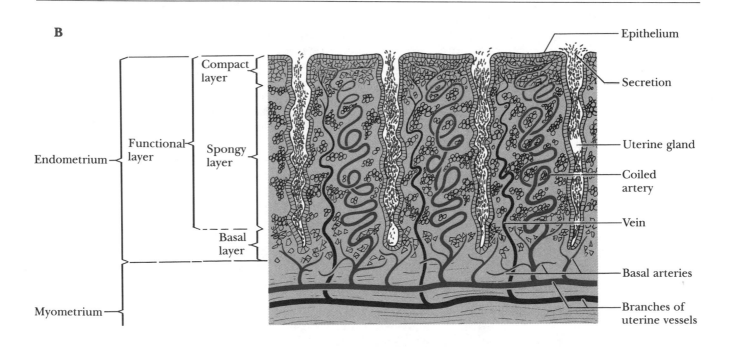

Epithelium

Secretion

Uterine gland

Coiled artery

Vein

Basal arteries

Branches of uterine vessels

Endometrium

Functional layer

Compact layer

Spongy layer

Basal layer

Myometrium

FIGURE 1A and B A, diagrammatic frontal section of the uterus and uterine tubes. The ovaries and vagina are also indicated. B, enlargement of the area outlined in A. Modified with permission from K. L. Moore, "The Developing Human," 2nd ed., W. B. Saunders, Philadelphia, Pa., 1977.

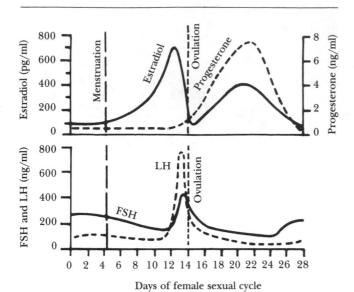

FIGURE 2   Plasma concentrations of the gonadotropins and ovarian hormones during the normal female sexual cycle. Reprinted with permission from A. C. Guyton, "Textbook of Medical Physiology," 6th ed. W. B. Saunders, Philadelphia, Pa., 1981, p. 1006.

Under the influence of estrogens secreted by the ovaries, the stromal cells, epithelial gland cells, and blood vessels of the endometrium proliferate rapidly (Figure 1B). By the time ovulation takes place on day 14, the endometrium is 2–3 mm thick (1). The proliferative phase of the endometrial cycle takes place from about day 5 to day 14 of the typical 28-day cycle (Figure 3).

During the secretory phase (days 15–27), progesterone from the newly formed corpus luteum of the ovary causes marked swelling and secretory development of the endometrium. The glandular cells begin to secrete small amounts of epithelial fluid, lipid and glycogen stores increase significantly in the stromal cells, and the blood supply increases in proportion to the secretory activity. The thickness of the endometrium approximately doubles during the secretory phase so that toward the end of the monthly cycle the endometrium has a thickness of 4–6 mm (1).

On approximately day 27, estrogen and progesterone concentrations decrease sharply because of the regression of the corpus luteum. Tissue fluid and secretions decrease, as does the thickness of the endometrium. During the 24 hours preceding menstruation (day 28), the blood vessels leading to the mucosal layers of the endometrium become vasospastic, causing the endometrial tissues to become ischemic. It is thought that prostaglandins, primarily the PGF alpha group, cause the intense arterial spasm and smooth muscle contraction that occur just before menstruation (1).

Necrosis and small vessel hemorrhage begin to develop, causing the outer layers of the endometrium to separate from the uterus. The sloughed tissue and blood in the uterine cavity initiate further uterine contractions that expel the uterine contents, starting the menstrual flow (day 1 of the new cycle) (1).

MENSTRUAL ABNORMALITIES

Dysmenorrhea

Dysmenorrhea is painful menstruation, one of the most common gynecologic disorders in nulliparous women. Typically, dysmenorrhea diminishes as a woman ages, has sexual intercourse, or gives birth (5). About 50% of women are affected by mild cramplike symptoms that occur at the onset of menses, restrict normal activities, and disappear within 1–3 days. About 10% of women experience severe cramping pain over the lower abdomen, which is often accompanied by systemic symptoms including nausea, vomiting, diarrhea, headache, and dizziness. These symptoms may be incapacitating and occur most often just prior to or during the first few days of menses.

When dysmenorrhea occurs in the absence of any pelvic disease it is referred to as primary dysmenorrhea. When dysmenorrhea occurs because of an underlying condition, such as endometriosis, fibroids, or pelvic inflammatory disease (PID), it is termed secondary dysmenorrhea.

Although psychogenic factors may affect the assessment of pain, there has been no evidence that these factors are important in the etiology of dysmenorrhea. Clinical data support the theory that endogenous prostaglandins play a role in primary dysmenorrhea (6). The intrauterine production of prostaglandins at menstruation may be regulated by ovarian steroid hormones, such as progesterone, which are at high concentrations after ovulation and before the development of menstruation. Evidence of increased concentrations of prostaglandins and prostaglandin metabolites has been found in the menstrual fluid, endometrium, and peripheral circulation of women with primary dysmenorrhea. Because endogenous prostaglandins may play a role in primary dysmenorrhea, any drug that inhibits their synthesis may be effective in reducing pain and other systemic symptoms.

Intrauterine devices (IUDs) used for contraception may cause severe uterine bleeding or pain. This is generally because the IUD causes endometrial compression and myometrial distention. It has been postulated that endometrial trauma induced by the presence of the IUD may enhance the biosynthesis of prostaglandins, which would be the etiology for secondary dysmenorrhea. These problems often necessitate removal of the device.

Amenorrhea

Amenorrhea is the lack of menstruation. Amenorrhea is classified as primary if the female has never menstruated and secondary if there is a cessation of menses for longer than 3 months. Primary amenorrhea usually refers to the failure of menses to occur before the 18th birthday and is usually associated with chromosomal, pituitary, or ovarian dysfunction (4).

The most common causes of secondary amenorrhea are pregnancy, lactation, and menopause. Menstruation does not occur in pregnancy because of the secretion of progesterone and estrogen from the corpus luteum and, later, because of the formation of the placenta, which secretes tremendous amounts of progesterone to maintain the endometrium during pregnancy. Menstruation stops at menopause because the ovaries fail to respond to gonadotropins.

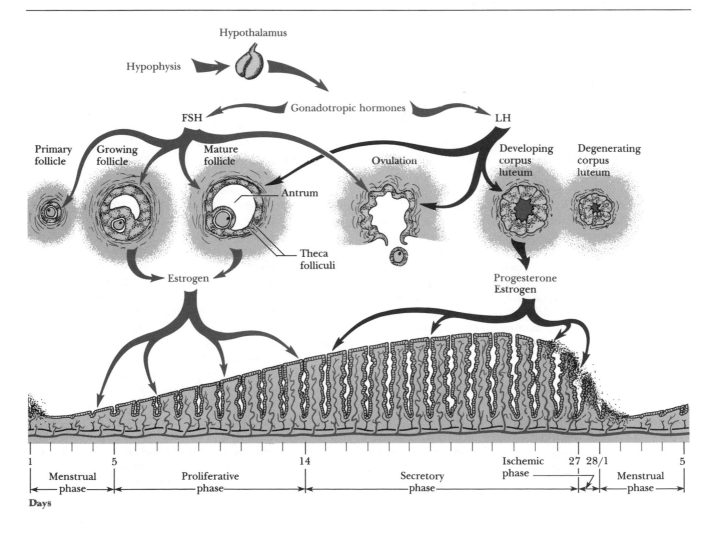

FIGURE 3   Schematic drawing illustrating the interrelations of the hypothalamus, hypophysis (pituitary gland), ovaries, and endometrium. One complete menstrual cycle and the beginning of another are shown. Changes in the ovaries, called the ovarian cycle, are promoted by the gonadotropic hormones (FSH and LH). Hormones from the ovaries (estrogens and progesterone) then promote changes in the structure and function of the endometrium. Thus, the cyclical activity of the ovary is intimately linked with changes in the uterus. From K. L. Moore, "The Developing Human," 2nd ed., W. B. Saunders, Philadelphia, Pa., 1977.

Breast-feeding will inhibit ovulation and menstruation in about 50% of nursing mothers. It is hypothesized that the nervous signals from the breasts to the hypothalamus that cause prolactin secretion during suckling simultaneously inhibit LH-RH by the hypothalamus, thus inhibiting release of the gonadotropic hormones, LH and FSH (1). Although breast-feeding without supplementation of formula provides some protection against pregnancy, it cannot be relied on as a contraceptive measure (7).

When evaluating amenorrhea in a patient who is not pregnant, lactating, or postmenopausal, ovarian function should be determined. Causes of amenorrhea in women of childbearing age include prolonged strenuous exercise and the cessation of oral contraceptive therapy. Such cases usually require physician supervision but rarely reflect any serious problem.

Intermenstrual Pain and Bleeding

Intermenstrual pain (termed "mittelschmerz") usually occurs at midcycle and may last from a few hours to a few days. The pain may be accompanied by various amounts of bleeding.

There appears to be a relationship among intermenstrual pain, bleeding, and ovulation. The etiology of the pain is unknown but may be inflammation of the ovulatory site itself or peritoneal irritation from follicular fluid released at ovulation (4). The bleeding may be caused by a temporary decrease in estrogen concentrations and, if slight, no treatment is necessary. If bleeding is severe, diagnostic measures should be used to rule out other etiologies such as intrauterine lesions.

Premenstrual Syndrome

Many women suffer from a recurrent complex of symptoms known as premenstrual syndrome (PMS). Although symptoms usually begin 1–7 (and up to 14) days before the onset of menses, they may also occur toward the end of menses (8). The onset of symptoms varies among women but is usually constant in the cycle of any individual woman.

PMS encompasses a variety of symptoms with severity ranging from mild to incapacitating. Questionnaire data indicate that 70–90% of women experience recurrent PMS, with 20–40% reporting some degree of temporary mental or physical incapacitation (7). However, most women have only mild to moderate symptoms that do not interfere with their daily activities. In about 5–8% of women, symptoms are severe enough to cause functional impairment. Symptoms of PMS include the following:

- Psychologic—irritability, lethargy, depression, anxiety, sleep disorders, crying spells, hostility;

- Neurologic—headache (migraines usually occur the week preceding menstruation), dizziness, fainting, seizures (occur rarely in epileptic patients);

- Breasts—tenderness, swelling;

- Gastrointestinal—constipation, abdominal bloating, abdominal cramping, craving for sweets;

- Extremities—edema;

- Urinary—less frequent urination;

- Skin—acne.

The most common psychologic symptom of PMS is tension. The onset of premenstrual tension is often heralded by sudden mood swings and is characterized by depression, irritability, and lethargy. An increased thirst or appetite accompanied by a craving for sweets and salty foods is common.

One of the most common physical symptoms experienced by women is premenstrual edema or bloating, especially apparent as enlarged or tender breasts, abdominal swelling, swollen feet or ankles, and a puffy face. If the edema is severe, weight gain of up to 9 lb may result. However, the majority of women gain no more than 5 lb. Once menstruation has begun, there is noticeable polyuria and rapid disappearance of edema.

The pathogenesis of PMS remains speculative; however, evidence suggests that it is associated with the cyclic nature of the hypothalamic–pituitary–ovarian axis (9). It has been suggested that PMS results from the precipitous drop in progesterone concentrations that occurs at the time of menstruation or from elevated estrogen concentrations. Others suggest that high levels of prolactin, deficiencies in vitamin B_6 or vitamin A, or hypoglycemia may produce the symptoms. Many have suggested an underlying psychogenic disorder. Another hypothesis suggests that because water retention is so common, premenstrual edema may be a manifestation of an underlying neuroendocrine disorder involving estrogen, aldosterone, vasopressin, prolactin, and/or dopamine (9). However, it appears that symptoms result from changing concentrations of prostaglandins and neurotransmitters that ultimately affect mood. Increased prostaglandin serum may be responsible for many symptoms seen in PMS, such as joint pains, breast tenderness, headaches, and nausea (10). One hypothesis concerning PMS suggests that the intermediate lobe of the pituitary gland may be involved through effects of melanocyte-stimulating hormone and endorphins (9). No one hypothesis has yet explained the full spectrum of PMS symptoms.

PATIENT ASSESSMENT

Most women who purchase nonprescription menstrual products are otherwise healthy but are experiencing midcycle or premenstrual fluid retention, headache, or abdominal cramping characteristic of PMS. Before recommending any product for a patient, the pharmacist should establish whether the symptoms are related to normal functional menstrual discomforts, if they are similar to symptoms of previous cycles, or if they are unusually severe for her typical menstrual pattern.

All women should be aware of warning symptoms that could signal serious disease. Pharmacists should refer a patient to her physician for any of the following: abnormal bleeding, failure to menstruate, abnormal vaginal discharge, excessive pain preceding and during menstruation, painful intercourse, lumps in the breast, and/or abnormal nipple discharge.

If evaluation indicates that the discomfort is related to the woman's normal menstrual cycle, the pharmacist should inquire about products previously taken for relief of symptoms so as to avoid recommending any product that has failed to give relief. It is important to determine whether the patient has taken a full therapeutic dose of an agent because some nonprescription products promoted for menstrual and premenstrual symptoms contain doses of ingredients that would be subtherapeutic if given alone. The presence or absence of salicylate allergy (aspirin allergy) should always be verified. Recommendations for any nonprescription product should be accompanied by appropriate patient counseling regarding proper use and dosing and any other adjunctive measures.

Dysmenorrhea

Before recommending any product for a patient, the pharmacist should establish the onset of pain in relation to menses. Primary dysmenorrhea produces pain that occurs before or during the first 2 days of menses. Pain associated with dysmenorrhea generally tapers over 1 or 2 days. Pain that occurs during the first few days of menses and increases in severity throughout menses may suggest underlying pathology; these patients with secondary dysmenorrhea should be referred to a physician for evaluation.

Amenorrhea

Any patient developing primary or secondary amenorrhea must be evaluated by a physician. The most common causes of secondary amenorrhea are pregnancy, lactation, prolonged or strenuous physical exercise (such as jogging), menopause, and withdrawal of oral contraceptives. Other etiologies that must be considered are disorders of the hypothalamus, pituitary gland, adrenal gland, ovaries, and uterus.

Intermenstrual Pain and Bleeding

Women may experience pain and bleeding for brief periods between menses. This discomfort is generally associated with ovulation. Therapeutic doses of nonprescription analgesics may be recommended, but if pain is severe, or if bleeding continues for more than 2 days, the patient should be referred to a physician (11).

Premenstrual Syndrome

PMS is a recognized clinical entity affecting a large portion of the female population (9). Because no single etiology has been established, many treatment alternatives have been proposed based on anecdotal reports. However, many women may not require medication. Initial therapy should include education, moderate, regular exercise, and identification and reduction of stress factors. The efficacy of various vitamin therapies remains unsubstantiated by double-blind trials and are regarded as placebo therapy. Additional trials using agents such as bromocriptine, agonists of gonadotropin-releasing hormone, diuretics, and psychoactive drugs have demonstrated some improvement in the patients treated (12–14). However, additional large-scale studies that are well-controlled and double-blind are needed to document the safety and efficacy of any single treatment in the management of PMS.

Pharmacologic Treatment

The Food and Drug Administration (FDA), in its tentative final monograph for orally administered over-the-counter (OTC) menstrual drug products, reviews the agents considered safe and effective for relieving symptoms related to the menstrual period (15).

Several nonprescription drug products are available for the treatment of dysmenorrhea and premenstrual syndrome.

Analgesics

In the treatment of primary dysmenorrhea, the first objective is to rule out secondary dysmenorrhea. Selection of a drug for primary dysmenorrhea should begin with the nonprescription analgesics. Clinical trials have shown that nonsteroidal prostaglandin inhibitors provide significant relief from primary dysmenorrhea. Ibuprofen, up to 1,200 mg a day, has been approved as a nonprescription product. Ibuprofen (400 mg) provides significantly greater relief than aspirin (650 mg) in the treatment of menstrual pain (16, 17). The approved analgesic dosage for nonprescription ibuprofen is 200 mg every 4–6 hours while symptoms persist; if pain does not respond to 200 mg, 400 mg may be taken, not to exceed 1,200 mg a day. Many nonprescription menstrual products contain either aspirin or acetaminophen as the analgesic. Aspirin is an inhibitor of prostaglandin synthesis. The exact effect of acetaminophen on prostaglandin synthesis is unclear. However, both acetaminophen and aspirin are safe and effective for menstrual pain when taken according to label directions in dosages of 325–650 mg every 4 hours, 325–500 mg every 3 hours, or 650–1,000 mg every 6 hours, not to exceed 4,000 mg a day (18). (See Chapter 5, *Internal Analgesic Products*.)

Before recommending aspirin, the pharmacist should question the patient regarding aspirin allergy; disease states that may preclude the use of salicylates, such as bleeding disorders, ulcers, and asthma; and any current medications, such as anticoagulants, probenecid, phenytoin, and oral hypoglycemic agents, that may interact with these compounds.

Because primary dysmenorrhea occurs in ovulatory cycles, oral contraceptives that suppress ovulation and lower the prostaglandin concentration have been used. Prescription nonsteroidal anti-inflammatory agents and oral contraceptives require the recommendation and supervision of a physician.

Diuretics

The FDA's tentative final monograph on OTC menstrual drug products reviews diuretics for use in elimination of water accumulation during the premenstrual and menstrual periods, thereby relieving symptoms of water retention and weight gain, bloating, swelling, and a full feeling (15). Ammonium chloride, caffeine, and pamabrom have been classified as safe and effective as diuretics in nonprescription menstrual products.

Ammonium Chloride Ammonium chloride is an acid-forming salt with limited value (4–5 days' duration) in promoting diuresis. There are no large-scale studies of the use of this diuretic alone in PMS. However, one double-blind crossover clinical trial compared the effectiveness of ammonium chloride (325 mg) and caffeine (100 mg) with placebo for the relief of symptoms associated with premenstrual weight gain in 22 women. The combination of ammonium chloride and caffeine induced a statistically significant greater reduction in weight compared with placebo [mean weight change of ≤ 1.5 lb (0.7 kg)]. Subjective evaluation indicated an improved mental state in subjects given ammonium chloride and caffeine compared with those given placebo (19).

Ammonium chloride is safe for use as a diuretic in the treatment of water accumulation symptoms of the premenstrual and menstrual periods in an oral dose of up to 3 g a day administered in divided doses 3 times daily for periods of up to 6 days.

Large doses of ammonium chloride (4–12 g a day) are associated with gastrointestinal and central nervous system symptoms. The drug is contraindicated in patients with impaired renal and liver function because metabolic acidosis may result.

Caffeine As a member of the xanthine family, caffeine promotes diuresis by inhibition of renal tubular reabsorption of sodium and chloride. Caffeine is safe and effective for use as a diuretic for relief of water accumulation symptoms (bloating, swelling, and a full feeling) of the premenstrual and menstrual periods in dosages of 100–200 mg every 3 or 4 hours. Doses over 100 mg may provoke gastric irritation by augmenting gastric secretions. Patients should also be advised that products containing caffeine may cause sleeplessness if taken within 4 hours of bedtime. Coffee, cola, or tea drinkers should be cautioned against an additive effect when taking caffeine-containing products.

Pamabrom Pamabrom is marketed in combination with analgesics and antihistamines for the relief of PMS. As a derivative of theophylline, pamabrom has weak diuretic properties. Pamabrom has been recognized as safe and effective in relieving water accumulation symptoms of the premenstrual and menstrual periods when used in dosages of 50 mg up to 4 times daily (not to exceed 200 mg daily).

Miscellaneous Ingredients

Several smooth muscle relaxants, antihistamines, and sympathomimetic amines have been evaluated for their use in relieving cramps associated with primary dysmenorrhea and PMS. None of the agents are considered Category I. Some preparations contain extracts of botanical and vegetable herbs. None of these agents have been classified Category I.

Alternative Therapy

A rational, professional approach to treating PMS consists of dietary modification to prevent edema formation through salt restriction before menstruation. However, for a patient significantly troubled with premenstrual edema, the pharmacist may refer the patient to her physician who may prescribe a mild diuretic.

RELATED MENSTRUAL PRODUCTS

Feminine Cleansing Products

The pharmacist should be familiar with the available feminine hygiene products and should know what, if anything, to recommend under a given set of circumstances. (See Chapter 27, *Personal Care Products*.)

Feminine Napkins and Tampons

Feminine napkins are pads that are used to absorb menstrual or other vaginal discharges. They are made of absorbent cotton, synthetic, or cellulose (derived from wood pulp) material covered with a lightweight paper gauze to reduce irritation. A layer of cellulose or thin plastic is incorporated into the side of the pad worn away from the perineum to minimize leakage and soiling of undergarments.

Feminine napkins are available in a wide variety of sizes and absorbencies. Some require a belt to hold them in place on the perineum so they can effectively absorb the menstrual flow, but most newer styles are held in place with adhesive strips on the underside of the pad, which affixes to the undergarment.

Because most women experience their heaviest menstrual flow on day 2 of the menstrual cycle, "super" napkins or "maxi" pads may be used at this time. The napkins should be frequently changed to minimize the development of unpleasant odors arising from the breakdown of blood products and vaginal secretions.

During days of heaviest flow, napkins may need to be changed every 2–4 hours; changing every 4–6 hours may be adequate for days of lesser menstrual flow. Frequent changing of sanitary pads also helps to minimize the degree of irritation or chafing of the upper inner thigh associated with napkin use. Dusting this area with a talcum powder may also alleviate chafing. The goal is to allow maximum absorption of discharged fluid and to minimize odor and risk of irritation and infection.

"Mini" or "light" pads and "junior" or "teen" napkins are designed to accommodate the smaller anatomy and lighter flow of the adolescent female. The narrower width of the pads may reduce chafing and irritation. Many women prefer the new, less cumbersome light pads for the first and last days of their cycles. These light pads or the new, thin shields also may be used to protect undergarments from being stained by vaginal cream, suppository leakage, or normal vaginal secretions.

Tampons are intravaginal inserts, made of cellulose or synthetic materials, designed to absorb menstrual or other vaginal discharge. They have the advantage over feminine napkins of being worn internally, which lessens chafing, odor, bulkiness, and irritation. Until reports associated tampon use with toxic shock syndrome, marketing data estimated that 70–80% of menstruating women in the United States used tampons (20). Some women use both a tampon and napkin on days of heavy menstrual flow or on days when they know their schedule will not permit frequent changing. However, this prolonged wearing should be discouraged because evidence associates this practice with a higher risk of microvaginal ulceration and infection (21).

Tampons which are labeled "deodorant" have been renamed by the FDA as "scented" because none of the available products contain an effective antimicrobial agent (22). Some fragrance materials may cause local irritation and allergic reactions, such as allergic contact dermatitis, because mucosal surfaces readily absorb these materials.

Before 1977, all tampons were made of rayon or rayon and cotton materials. Since then, 44% of tampon products (65% of the estimated market) have contained newer, more absorbent synthetic materials. Both absorbency types have been documented to cause vaginal mucosal drying, epithelial changes, and microulcerations; however, the incidence is much higher in women using the superabsorbent tampons. Most microulcerations are asymptomatic and resolve spontaneously, but some were still present in preovulatory phase in up to 31% of women examined. Tampon use over a period of several months to years has also been associated with cervicovaginal ulcerations. The immediate and long-term clinical significance of these findings has yet to be demonstrated.

The FDA's advisory review panel in the division of obstetrics and gynecology evaluated feminine napkins and tampons and classified unscented menstrual pads into performance Class I. This classification indicates that the device meets only the general controls applicable to all devices. The FDA advisory review panel has classified scented menstrual pads and both unscented and scented menstrual tampons into performance Class II, which requires the future development of standards to ensure the safety and efficacy of the products (22).

TOXIC SHOCK SYNDROME

Toxic shock syndrome (TSS) is an illness that can develop in young, otherwise healthy, women in association with tampon use during menstruation. Most cases occur in women under 30 years of age, with the highest incidence occurring in the 15–19-year-old group (20, 23, 24). The disease complex is characterized by the sudden onset of:

- High fever (102° F or 38.9° C or greater);
- Diffuse erythematous, macular, sunburn-like rash that subsequently desquamates, most notably on the palms and soles;
- Dizziness caused by a sudden drop in blood pressure; low systolic blood pressure of < 90 mm Hg in an adult (shock or hypotension).

In addition, the patient with TSS may present with at least four of the following symptoms:

- Nausea, vomiting, or diarrhea;
- Severe myalgias;
- Sore throat;
- Renal failure (decrease in urinary output);
- Low platelet counts, bruising, and/or bleeding;
- Hepatic failure (rise in enzyme levels and bilirubin);
- Irritability, disorientation, and/or coma;
- Hypotension, shock, arrhythmias, and/or adult respiratory distress syndrome.

Steps should be taken to rule out meningococcemia, Rocky Mountain spotted fever, or bacterial sepsis. Ninety-five percent of TSS cases occur in women during or within 48 hours of ending their menstrual period (especially days 2–4). Blood and throat cultures are negative for bacteria; however, vaginal cultures are frequently positive.

More than 408 cases of TSS have been reported to the Centers for Disease Control (CDC), with a mortality of 10%. The estimates of a woman's risk for development of TSS range from 3 to 6.2 cases per 100,000 women of menstruating age (12–49 years) per year. Risk was determined to be highest in women using tampons continually throughout menstruation (20). The etiologic agent is suspected to be a select type of *Staphylococcus aureus*, colonizing the skin or vagina, which produces an enterotoxin that subsequently is absorbed and is responsible for the systemic complex of symptoms. A large number of cases of TSS occurred in women using the superabsorbent synthetic cellulose tampons, marketed under the brand name Rely (Procter and Gamble); however, TSS has been documented with all brands in a study reported to the CDC including (in decreasing order of frequency) Rely (used by 71% of patients), Playtex (19%), Tampax (5%), Kotex (2%), and o.b. (2%) (25). The Rely brand tampons were removed from the market by the manufacturer under a consent agreement with the FDA, although it had not been documented that the increased rate of occurrence was directly related to the Rely product. It has been proposed that the different frequency of occurrence could be due to greater use of the Rely product in the population at risk. However, the risk factors for TSS remain controversial because subsequent studies by the CDC failed to demonstrate a significant difference in occurrence in patients who developed TSS versus control subjects who did not, based on brand of tampon, degree of absorbency, inclusion of a deodorant (fragrance) ingredient, or frequency of tampon changing (23). Several confirmed cases of TSS have been associated with the use of the vaginal contraceptive sponge. In addition, TSS has been linked to diaphram use when removal was delayed beyond 24 hours.

The relatively high mortality in young, otherwise healthy women, initially reported to be between 3% and 10%, has most frequently been associated with severe hypotensive shock. Successful treatment may necessitate administration of large volumes of intravenous fluids to maintain circulation and cardiac output. Occasionally, dialysis has been necessary for management of transient uremia and renal failure. The use of beta-lactamase-resistant antibiotics such as nafcillin or a cephalosporin has not affected the outcome of severity of individual cases of TSS, but has reduced the rate of reoccurrence (24).

Current recommendations to patients regarding TSS include:

- Women who use tampons and who have not had TSS are at a very low risk of TSS and need not change their pattern of tampon use; however, they may decrease an already small risk by avoiding the use of tampons entirely.

- Tampons should be changed 4–6 times a day.

- Women may consider intermittent use of tampons and sanitary napkins (using tampons for only a portion of the menstrual cycle or using sanitary napkins at night if tampons are worn during the day).

- Patients developing sudden onset of high fever, sunburn-like rash, hypotension, vomiting, and diarrhea should immediately remove tampons and seek emergency medical treatment (fluids may be required for shock and possible beta-lactamase-resistant antibiotics for vaginal *Staphylococcus aureus*).

- Women who have had TSS are at a much higher risk (up to 45% in one study) of developing recurrences, and should not use tampons for several menstrual cycles after their illness unless eradication of *Staphylococcus aureus* from vaginal secretions has been documented.

The pharmacist is in a unique setting to evaluate the data on TSS and educate patients on current recommendations. The FDA advisory review committee has evaluated product labeling and consumer information inserts on tampon use and TSS. The warning statement required on packages of menstrual tampons is as follows (25):

> **WARNING** Tampons have been associated with toxic shock syndrome, a rare disease that can be fatal. You can almost entirely avoid the risk of getting this disease by not using tampons. You can reduce the risk by using tampons on and off during your period. If you have a fever of 102° or more and vomit or get diarrhea during your period, remove the tampon at once and see a doctor right away.

SUMMARY

Premenstrual and menstrual pain is a frequent problem in the majority of women. In most cases, nonprescription analgesics such as ibuprofen, aspirin, or acetaminophen are efficacious. In some women, diuretics for premenstrual edema may be required. The pharmacist should remember that menstruation is a normal physiologic process, even though the premenstrual syndrome has now been well described. The majority of women function normally and require minimal pharmacologic intervention.

Specific problems identified in this chapter, such as dysmenorrhea, amenorrhea, and significant premenstrual edema, require careful evaluation and physician referral in most instances.

REFERENCES

1 A. C. Guyton, "Textbook of Medical Physiology," 6th ed., W. B. Saunders, Philadelphia, Pa., 1981, pp. 1005–1016.
2 C. B. Hammond and W. S. Maxson, *Clin. Obstet. Gynecol.*, *29*, 407 (1986).
3 R. C. Benson, "Handbook of Obstetrics and Gynecology," Lange Medical, Los Altos, Calif., 1980, pp. 28–37.
4 "Harrison's Principles of Internal Medicine," 11th ed., E. Braunwald et al., Eds., McGraw-Hill, New York, N.Y., 1988, pp. 214–215.
5 N. J. Wenzlott, *Drug. Intell. Clin. Pharm.*, *18*, 22 (1984).
6 M. Y. Dawood, "Dysmenorrhea," *Clin. Obstet. Gynecol.*, *26*, 719 (1983).
7 "Current Obstetric and Gynecologic Diagnosis and Treatment," R. C. Benson, 3rd ed., Lange Medical, Los Altos, Calif., 1980, pp. 112–119.
8 M. A. Smith and E. Q. Young Kin, *Clin. Pharm.*, *5*, 788–796 (1986).
9 R. L. Reid and S. S. Yen, *Am. J. Obstet. Gynecol.*, *135*, 85 (1981).
10 P. W. Budoff, "No More Menstrual Cramps and Other Good News," Putnam and Sons, New York, N.Y., 1980, pp. 53–75.
11 E. R. Novak, G. S. Jones, and H. W. Jones, "Novak's Textbook of Gynecology," 9th ed., Williams and Wilkins, Baltimore, Md., 1976, pp. 58–96.
12 Z. H. Chakmakjian, *J. Reprod. Med.*, *28*, 532 (1983).
13 K. N. Muse, *N. Engl. J. Med.*, *311*, 1345 (1984).
14 K. E. Lyon, *J. Reprod. Med.*, *29*, 705 (1984).
15 *Federal Register*, *53*, 46194–202 (1988).
16 S. Shapiro and K. Diem, *Cur. Ther. Res.*, *30*, 327–334 (1981).
17 M. Y. Dawood, *Am. J. Med.*, *77*, 87–94 (1984).
18 *Federal Register*, *53*, 46257 (1988).
19 J. J. Hoffman, *Curr. Ther. Res.*, *26*, 575 (1979).
20 J. P. Davis et al., *N. Engl. J. Med.*, *303*, 1429 (1980).
21 E. G. Friedrich and K. A. Siegesmund, *Obstet. Gynecol.*, *55*, 149 (1980).
22 *Federal Register*, *45*, 12713 (1980).
23 K. N. Shands et al., *N. Engl. J. Med.*, *303*, 1436 (1980).
24 *Morbid. Mortal. Weekly Rep.*, *30*, 25 (1981).
25 *Federal Register*, *45*, 69840 (1980).

MENSTRUAL PRODUCT TABLE

Product[a] (Manufacturer)	Analgesic	Diuretic	Antihistamine	Caffeine	Other Ingredients
Advil (Whitehall)	ibuprofen, 200 mg				
A-Nuric (Alvin Last)		buchu powdered extract, 65 mg couch grass powdered extract, 65 mg hydrangea powdered extract, 32.5 mg corn silk powdered extract, 32.5 mg			
Aqua-Ban (Thompson Medical)		ammonium chloride, 325 mg		100 mg	
Aqua-Ban Plus (Thompson Medical)		ammonium chloride, 650 mg		200 mg	iron, 6 mg (as ferrous sulfate)
Diurex (Alva Amco)	potassium salicylate salicylamide	uva ursi buchu		NS[b]	juniper berries methylene blue magnesium trisilicate
Diurex Long Acting (Alva Amco)	potassium salicylate	uva ursi buchu		NS[b]	riboflavin
Diurex-2 (Alva Amco)	potassium salicylate salicylamide	uva ursi buchu		NS[b]	iron juniper berries methylene blue magnesium trisilicate
Femcaps (Buffington)	acetaminophen, 325 mg			32.5 mg	ephedrine sulfate, 8 mg atropine sulfate, 0.03 mg
Fluidex (O'Connor)		buchu powdered extract, 65 mg couch grass powdered extract, 65 mg corn silk powdered extract, 32.5 mg hydrangea powdered extract, 32.5 mg			
Fluidex with Pamabrom (O'Connor)		pamabrom, 50 mg			
Haltran (Upjohn)	ibuprofen, 200 mg				
Humphrey's No. 11 (Humphrey's Pharmacal)					cimicifuga, 3X pulsatilla, 3X sepia, 3X

MENSTRUAL PRODUCT TABLE, continued

Product[a] (Manufacturer)	Analgesic	Diuretic	Antihistamine	Caffeine	Other Ingredients
Lydia E. Pinkham Tablets (CooperVision)					extract of Jamaica dogwood pleurisy root licorice dried ferrous sulfate, 75 mg
Lydia E. Pinkham Vegetable Compound Liquid (CooperVision)					extract of Jamaica dogwood pleurisy root licorice alcohol, 13.5%
Menoplex Tablets (Fiske)	acetaminophen, 325 mg		phenyltoloxamine citrate, 30 mg		
Menstra-Eze (Reese)	acetaminophen, 325 mg		pyrilamine maleate, 20 mg		
Midol, Maximum Strength (Glenbrook)	acetaminophen, 500 mg		pyrilamine maleate, 15 mg		
Midol PMS (Glenbrook)	acetaminophen, 500 mg	pamabrom, 25 mg	pyrilamine maleate, 15 mg		
Midol, Regular Strength (Glenbrook)	acetaminophen, 325 mg		pyrilamine maleate, 12.5 mg		
Midol 200 (Glenbrook)	ibuprofen, 200 mg				
Multi Symptom Menstrual Discomfort Relief Formula (DeWitt)	acetaminophen, 325 mg	pamabrom, 25 mg	pyrilamine maleate, 12.5 mg		
Nuprin (Bristol-Myers Products)	ibuprofen, 200 mg				
Odrinil (Fox)		pamabrom, 25 mg			
Pamprin (Chattem)	acetaminophen, 325 mg	pamabrom, 25 mg	pyrilamine maleate, 12.5 mg		
Pamprin Extra Strength Multi-Symptom Relief Formula (Chattem)	acetaminophen, 400 mg	pamabrom, 25 mg	pyrilamine maleate, 15 mg		
Pamprin-IB (Chattem)	ibuprofen, 200 mg				
Pamprin Maximum Cramp Relief Caplets and Capsules (Chattem)	acetaminophen, 500 mg	pamabrom, 25 mg	pyrilamine maleate, 15 mg		

MENSTRUAL PRODUCT TABLE, continued

Product[a] (Manufacturer)	Analgesic	Diuretic	Antihistamine	Caffeine	Other Ingredients
Panadol Caplets and Tablets (Glenbrook)	acetaminophen, 500 mg				
Panadol Jr.[b,c] (Glenbrook)	acetaminophen, 160 mg				
Premsyn PMS Caplets and Capsules (Chattem)	acetaminophen, 500 mg	pamabrom, 25 mg	pyrilamine maleate, 15 mg		
Sunril (Schering)	acetaminophen, 300 mg	pamabrom, 50 mg	pyrilamine maleate, 25 mg		
Trendar (Whitehall)	ibuprofen, 200 mg				
Tri-Aqua (Pfeiffer)		buchu triticum uva ursi zea		100 mg	

[a] Tablet unless specified otherwise.
[b] Quantity not specified.
[c] Sugar free.
[d] Alcohol free.

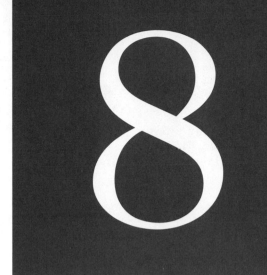

Bobby G. Bryant and Thomas P. Lombardi

COLD AND ALLERGY PRODUCTS

*Q*uestions to ask in patient/consumer counseling

What symptoms do you have? Do you have a runny or stuffy nose, sore throat, cough, fever, or earache? Do you have red, itchy eyes, sneezing, postnasal drip, or muscle aches?

―――――

How long have you had these symptoms?

―――――

Do members of your family have a history of allergies, asthma, or atopic dermatitis?

―――――

Do you have any respiratory disease (breathing problems) such as asthma or bronchitis?

―――――

Do you have atopic dermatitis or any other chronic skin disorder?

―――――

Do you have diabetes, glaucoma, heart disease, thyroid problems, or high blood pressure? Are you under a physician's care for this? Are these conditions controlled? If so, how are they controlled?

―――――

What medications are you taking? How long have you been taking them?

―――――

Which products have you used for your cold and allergy symptoms? Were they effective? Have you had any problems taking them?

―――――

Does your job require you to remain alert to prevent an accident?

―――――

Although the common cold and allergic rhinitis are etiologically different, they present similar symptoms and respond to similar management approaches. This chapter provides the pharmacist with the information necessary to identify and distinguish between the common cold and allergic rhinitis, as well as other disorders that may mimic them, and to advise the patient on the proper use of cold and allergy products.

TYPES OF DISORDERS

The common cold is a mixture of symptoms affecting the upper respiratory tract (Figure 1). It is also called a "cold," acute rhinitis, infectious rhinitis, coryza, or catarrh. The symptoms, which are usually acute and self-limiting, may be caused by one of many viruses. The main anatomical sites of infection may vary; therefore, a cold may present symptoms, individually or in combination, of the nose (rhinitis), throat (pharyngitis), larynx (laryngitis), or bronchi (bronchitis). The intensity of symptoms may vary from hour to hour. A reasonable approach is to treat the patient symptomatically, with individual drugs (1).

Allergic rhinitis is the antibody-mediated reaction of the nasal mucosa to one or more inhaled antigens. It may be perennial because of the year-round presence of antigenic substances, or it may be seasonal and correspond with the periodic appearance of offending antigens. The most common type of allergic rhinitis, "hay fever" or pollenosis, is seasonal.

Upper Respiratory Tract

The nose is a respiratory organ. As a passageway for airflow into and out of the lungs, it humidifies and warms inspired air and filters inhaled particles. Several anatomical features aid the performance of these functions. The nasal cavity is divided by a central septum and finger-like projections (turbinates) that extend into the cavity, increasing the nasal surface area (Figure 2).

The nasal passageway surface is coated with a thin layer of mucus, a moderately viscous, mucoproteinaceous liquid secreted continuously by the mucous glands. Under normal conditions, foreign bodies such as dust, bacteria, powder, and oil droplets are trapped in the film and carried out of the nose into the nasopharynx. The turbinates facilitate this action by causing many eddies in the flowing air, forcing it to rebound in different directions before finally completing its passage through the nose. This rapid change in airflow enables air-suspended particles to precipitate against the nasal surfaces. High vascularity and resultant high-blood flow within the nasal mucosa help warm and humidify the inspired air.

Nerve control of the nasopharyngeal vascular bed is derived from both sympathetic and parasympathetic divisions of the autonomic nervous system. Stimulation of the sympathetic fibers causes decreased activity of the mucous glands and vasoconstriction that reduces the size of the turbinates, thus widening the nasal passageway. Parasympathetic stimulation increases mucus production and narrows the airways by vasodilation and vascular engorgement of the mucosal tissue. Treatment may be directed toward eliciting a sympathetic re-

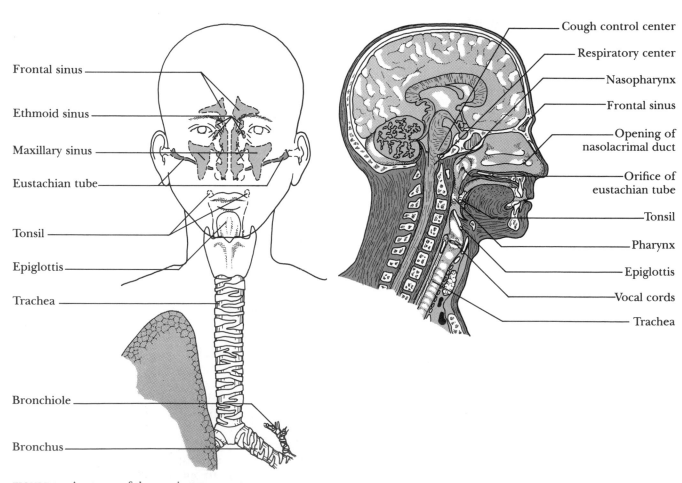

FIGURE 1   Anatomy of the respiratory passages,

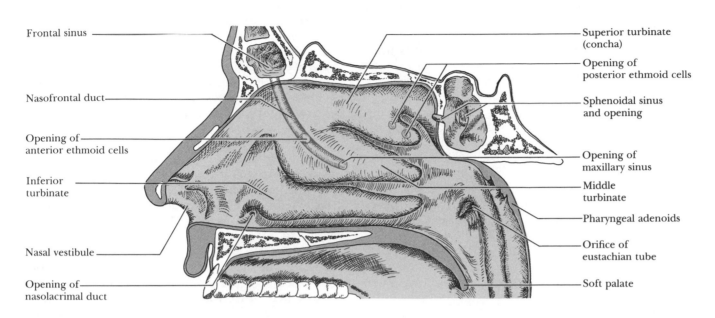

Frontal sinus

Nasofrontal duct

Opening of
anterior ethmoid cells

Inferior
turbinate

Nasal vestibule

Opening of
nasolacrimal duct

Superior turbinate
(concha)

Opening of
posterior ethmoid cells

Sphenoidal sinus
and opening

Opening of
maxillary sinus

Middle
turbinate

Pharyngeal adenoids

Orifice of
eustachian tube

Soft palate

FIGURE 2   The nose and paranasal sinus. Reprinted with permission from "Medical Notes on the Common Cold," Burroughs Wellcome Co., Publication No. PI99-2, Research Triangle Park, N.C., 1972.

sponse, blocking a parasympathetic response, or both.

The epithelium of the nasal passageways is ciliated. The constant beating of the cilia causes the mucus film to be moved continually toward the nasopharynx, carrying with it trapped particles to be expectorated or swallowed (2). Because this ciliary movement is one of the body's main defense mechanisms, care should be taken to avoid agents that impair this movement. Oils, especially mineral oil, and the overuse of topically applied decongestants may interfere with normal ciliary movement. Dust, fumes, smoke, and lack of humidity may also impair ciliary movement (3).

The mucus is rich in lysozymes and contains glycoproteins and immunoglobulins (4). Lysozymes are an important defense against bacteria because they readily digest the lipid and carbohydrate cell walls of some bacteria and are responsible for the digestion of the cell walls of pollens and the subsequent release of antigenic substances. Mucous glycoproteins may temporarily inhibit some viruses by combining with the virus protein coat. The union of inhibitor (mucous glycoprotein) and virus is reversible; therefore, these inhibitors probably do no more than delay host cell invasion by the virus particles. Immunoglobulins of low molecular weight, mainly IgA and IgG, also are contained in the mucus secretion. Although present in low concentrations, they may decrease the infectivity of certain viruses.

Viruses that attach to and invade respiratory tract host cells stimulate the infected cell to produce inter-

feron. Interferon protects neighboring, noninfected cells by inducing them to produce an antiviral protein that inhibits viral replication, thus preventing subsequent viral infection. Interferon is active not only against the virus that caused its production but also against other unrelated viruses (5). Research is directed toward a better understanding of this substance as well as stimulating its endogenous development.

The cough reflex is an essential body defense mechanism by which the respiratory airways leading to the lungs are kept free of foreign matter. The cough reflex functions in a perfectly healthy person as well as in a diseased person; however, its manifestation is frequently a symptom of some pathologic condition. All areas of the respiratory tract (the trachea, larynx, bronchi, and terminal bronchioles) are sensitive to foreign matter and other causes of irritation such as irritant gases and infection. A cough may be caused by the stimulation of receptors (mechanoreceptors and chemoreceptors) located in the mucosa of the airways and lungs. Afferent impulses pass along nerve pathways to the cough center in the medulla, which coordinates efferent impulses to the diaphragm and intercostal and abdominal muscles. An automatic sequence of events leads to the cough response, the rapid expulsion of air from the lungs, which carries the foreign bodies that initiated the reflex. Localized bronchoconstriction also may play an important role in the stimulation of the cough reflex.

The sneeze reflex is similar to the cough reflex, except that it clears the nasal passages instead of the lower respiratory tract. Irritation in the nasal passages initiates the sneeze reflex. The afferent impulses from the nose travel to the medulla, where the reflex is triggered. A series of reactions similar to those for the cough reflex take place. In addition, the uvula is depressed, so that large amounts of air pass rapidly through the nose, as well as through the mouth, helping to clear the nasal passages of foreign matter (2).

The passageways of the trachea and lungs are lined with a ciliated, mucus-coated epithelium that aids in removing foreign matter. As in the nasal passageways, the cilia in the trachea and lungs beat toward the pharynx, carrying mucus and trapped particles out of the respiratory tract to be expectorated or swallowed.

The Common Cold

The common cold has been described as the single most expensive illness in the United States. In fact, the common cold causes more time lost from work and school than all other diseases combined. The common cold accounts for 161 million days of restricted activity, 26 million days of school absence, and 23 million days of work absence, according to the National Interview Health Survey of 1985 (6, 7).

The common cold resulted in approximately 27 million physician visits in 1985. A 1980 survey reports that drugs were recommended in 94% of visits for upper respiratory tract infections, pharyngitis, and tracheitis. An average of two drugs was prescribed per patient (8).

Most colds do not result in medical attention and are self-treated. More than 800 nonprescription cough and cold preparations are on the market with annual sales exceeding $2 billion in the United States (9). With approximately 50% of cough and cold preparations purchased in pharmacies, pharmacists should interact and assist the self-medicating patient with the proper selection and administration of cough and cold preparations.

The common cold can be spread directly from person to person with no intermediate source such as food, water, or animals. The only means by which spreading may be prevented is by isolating the infected individual. However, by the time a cold has been detected, the virus undoubtedly has already been transmitted to others through respiratory droplets (5).

There is an apparent relationship between the season of the year and the common cold. The exact etiologic relationship is not known, but it is usual to observe three peak seasons of common colds per year. One of these occurs in the autumn, a few weeks after schools open; another occurs in midwinter; and a third occurs in the spring. These separate epidemics are associated with different viruses, each of which may have its own seasonal epidemiology. The U.S. Public Health Service studies show that during the winter quarter, approximately 50% of the population experience a common cold; during the summer quarter, only about 20% are stricken with a cold (10).

The patient's age is related to the incidence of the common cold and to its complications. Children 1–5 years of age are most susceptible, and each child averages 6–12 respiratory illnesses per year, most of which are common colds. Some practitioners believe that infants under 6 months of age are somewhat resistant to cold viruses, but this finding may be attributed to the infants' relatively infrequent exposure to different environments. This may also be partially explained by residual immunologic prevention from placental crossover while in utero or from acquisition of antibody in breast milk. Individuals 25–30 years old average about six respiratory illnesses per year; older adults average two or three. Women, primarily 20–30 years of age, appear to be afflicted by colds more frequently than males of the same age or older patients. This could be attributed to exposure to children with colds (6). Young children are more prone to complications of the common cold, such as middle ear inflammation (otitis media) and pneumonia; adults also suffer from these complications (4, 10).

Poor nutritional state, fatigue, and emotional disturbances are associated with greater susceptibility to infection as well as increased severity of infection and greater likelihood of complications (10). Body chills or wet feet in themselves do not induce the common cold. However, if the virus is a recent invader, exposure probably is a contributory factor because it is associated with a vasomotor effect that decreases the nasal mucosal temperature by several degrees. As a result of this temperature change, many people experience symptoms of nasal irritation, such as sneezing and serous discharge. Changes in the nasal mucosa and a subsequent change in the character of the mucus may then facilitate viral invasion (10).

Allergic disorders involving the nasopharynx, such as hay fever, also seem to facilitate infection. The probable mechanism is the inflammatory changes occurring in the mucosa as a result of the antigen–antibody reaction, which may facilitate subsequent viral invasion.

Etiology

Viruses cause the common cold. More than 120 different viral strains that produce common cold symptoms in humans have been isolated (10). Known causative organisms include rhinoviruses (approximately 60 serologic types), adenoviruses, coxsackieviruses, influenza viruses, parainfluenza viruses, and respiratory syncytial viruses. Of these, the rhinoviruses comprise the largest etiologic group, probably accounting for more than half of all common colds in adults (10). A significant number, 5–10%, of common colds are associated with more than one virus, and evidence of simultaneous infection with two viruses is not rare (4, 10).

Viruses differ from bacteria by their existence within the host cell, their chemical composition, their mode of replication, and their responsiveness to drug therapy (5). The process of a viral infection is divided into three states: entry into the host cell and nucleic acid release, genome replication and viral protein synthesis, and assembly of new virus particles and their release from the cell to infect additional host cells (11). There probably are several mechanisms by which the virus penetrates the host cell, but none is well defined. Once inside the host cell, the virus is attacked by host cell enzymes and possibly other substances, releasing the viral nucleic acid. In the second state of infection, the virus uses metabolic pathways of the host cell itself to duplicate the viral genome and synthesize viral proteins. Finally, these components are assembled into new, mature virus particles and are released by the host cell. The release may be rapid and may be accompanied by lysis and death of the host cell, although cell death may not always result. The new virus particles then infect adjacent cells by the same cycle.

When host cell injury or death occurs, the body's inflammatory defense mechanism is activated, causing pathologic changes and subsequent symptoms. These clinical manifestations of infection are not evident, however, until after extensive viral replication and inflammation have occurred.

Specific immunity against illness from reinfection with the same strain of virus was demonstrated in volunteers; this clinical immunity is apparent for about 2 years after infection. Reinfection, however, is not entirely prevented and usually results in a modified illness. The specificity of the antibody and its concentration at the infection site appear to be critical in the likelihood and extent of reinfection (4). These characteristics also underscore the difficulty of developing comprehensive vaccines to prevent the common cold.

Pathophysiology and Symptoms

Symptoms associated with the common cold are a manifestation of the pathologic changes (inflammation) that occur in the respiratory epithelium, secondary to viral invasion. The pathologic changes that make up the inflammatory response to one or more viruses are excess blood flow in the area (hyperemia), abnormal fluid accumulation in the intercellular spaces (edema), and profuse watery discharge from the nasal mucous membrane (rhinorrhea) (10).

The severity of the cellular damage (and hence the degree of inflammation and symptoms) is related to the type and virulence of the infecting virus and the extent of the infection. Various strains of influenza virus may cause more damage to the respiratory epithelium than other viruses that cause the common cold. Therefore, "flu" symptoms are usually more severe than cold symptoms, and the predisposition to secondary bacterial complications is greater.

Although colds commonly involve the nasal structure, other sites along the respiratory tract may be affected. This condition is due to the predilection of certain viruses for pharyngeal, laryngeal, or bronchial cells and to the extension of the infectious process from the original invasion site (5).

Because the incubation period for these viral infections is relatively short (1–4 days), patients often report a rapid onset and progression of symptoms. Virus shedding usually begins 1–2 days before the onset of symptoms and is associated with epithelial sloughing and regeneration. A few days later, during the symptomatic phase, peak viral replication and host cell injury occur. With the intervention of host defenses such as production and release of interferon, virus excretion declines after several days and symptoms decrease (4).

The clear, watery fluid that initially flows from the irritated nasal epithelium (nasal discharge or rhinorrhea) is the hallmark of the common cold. Although it is initially clear, it is followed shortly by a much thicker and tenacious mucoid and purulent secretion, largely composed of dead epithelial cells and white blood cells. The quantity of epithelial cells shed may be so high at times as to give the appearance of purulence. It is commonly assumed that these mucopurulent secretions are the result of secondary bacterial infection; however, this is not always the case. Viruses may cause inflammatory reactions of their own, and secretions occur even when there has been no change in the nasal bacterial flora (12).

Nasal congestion (engorgement of the nasal vasculature and thus swelling of the nasal turbinates) encroaches on the nasal lumen, which is also burdened with increased secretions. Nasal discharge and congestion are the most commonly described discomforts associated with the common cold.

The combination of nasal irritation, discharge, and congestion (which cause further irritation) gives rise to sneezing. Sneezing is not as discomforting as the discharge and congestion, and subsides when the infection and secretions clear.

Pharyngitis also may occur during a cold (4). This throat symptom is usually described as a "dryness" or "soreness" rather than actual pain such as that associated with bacterial pharyngitis or acute tonsillitis. Nonbacterial pharyngitis is attributed to edema of the pharyngeal mucosa, which activates sensory nerve fibers as the viral infection spreads to deeper tissue.

Environmental factors also may lead to pharyngitis. Overuse of tobacco products and ingestion of large amounts of concentrated, alcohol-containing beverages or other irritating substances are associated with pharyngeal irritation and sore throat. Rarely, inhalation of an irritant gas is an etiologic factor for nonbacterial pharyngitis.

Diseases in which pharyngitis may be a symptom include not only the common cold but also streptococcal infection of the throat, scarlet fever, tonsillitis, influenza, measles, and smallpox. It is important that the etiology be uncovered so that appropriate measures may be taken. An acute sore throat with a nonbacterial infection usually has a much slower onset than bacterial pharyngitis. Nonbacterial pharyngitis is characterized by milder constitutional symptoms, normal or slightly elevated temperature, and a dry, raspy, or tickling sensation in the throat when swallowing.

This irritation of the pharynx ("tickling") also may cause a nonproductive cough. In addition, the cough may result from irritation of tracheal or bronchial mucous membranes caused by the direct extension of the inflammation or from infectious material dripping from the nasopharynx (postnasal drip). At its onset the cough is usually dry and nonproductive. Later stages of the common cold are characterized by heavy bronchial congestion resulting from the cellular debris of local phagocytic activity added to the respiratory tract fluids in the bronchial and nasal passage secretions and draining into the lower respiratory tract. Ciliary activity may not be sufficient to remove these fluids, and coughing is necessary to clear the lower tract of accumulated secretions.

Another possible manifestation of the common cold is laryngitis, which is associated with hoarseness or loss of voice. It may be caused by the spread of infection, or it may be an irritation secondary to drainage from the nasopharynx.

A hot or warm sensation ("feverishness") is another fairly common complaint. In general, little or no fever is actually present. Finally, headache, which usually occurs in the early stages of the cold, may be caused by the infection and inflammation of the nasal passages and paranasal sinuses.

Complications

In an otherwise healthy individual the common cold is self-limiting; the course of symptoms is 5–7 days. It is not uncommon (but not inevitable) for complications to develop during or immediately following a common cold. The pharmacist should be familiar with possible complications, their causes, and how they are treated. Viral infection induces swelling and some exudation, but it causes no significant change in the bacterial flora of the nasopharynx. If the inflammatory changes are of sufficient magnitude, passages connecting the paranasal sinuses and middle ear become obstructed; under these conditions, infection may occur from secondary bacterial growth. In addition, it has been reported that viral infections trigger a substantial proportion of wheezing attacks in young asthmatic children, chronic bronchitics, and patients with emphysema (13, 14).

The most common bacterial complications to colds are purulent sinusitis (approximately 0.5% adults), otitis media (approximately 2% adults), bacterial pneumonia, and tonsillitis (13, 14).

Young children are especially prone to pneumonia and otitis media. Five percent or more of children develop secondary otitis media following a cold (14). This occurs because a child's eustachian tubes are short, relatively horizontal, and rather narrow. This configuration facilitates fluid accumulation in the middle ear as well as rapid blockage in response to only a slight degree of inflammation. A young child's bronchiolar passages also are smaller in diameter than those of older children and adults and become blocked more easily. The smaller passages and the child's lack of conscious effort to cough up accumulated fluids in the lower tract lead to stasis of the fluids, inflammation, and secondary bacterial infection.

These complications usually manifest themselves by worsening of local symptoms (earache, headache, or cough), development of a fever, and failure of the cold to improve in the expected time. Such manifestations in a person with a recent cold probably are caused by secondary bacterial invaders for which culture and sensitivity tests and appropriately prescribed antibiotic therapy are indicated.

Conditions Mimicking the Common Cold

Other infectious diseases present initial manifestations identical to those of the common cold (15). The pharmacist should be aware of these disorders because some of them have potentially serious implications for which a physician should be consulted. Using strictly palliative therapy in situations that may not be self-limiting has little or no effect on the underlying problem and may delay necessary and more appropriate treatment. A patient's "sore throat," alone or in conjunction with other symptoms, may be caused by bacteria, a virus, or another irritative process. For example, a sore throat in a child may be a bacterial pharyngitis caused by beta-hemolytic species of *Streptococcus*, or "strep throat." If symptomatic therapy alone is recommended and the child is suffering from beta-hemolytic streptococcal pharyngitis, the possible sequela of rheumatic fever or glomerulonephritis may develop. Appropriate antibiotic therapy may help prevent these dangerous sequelae.

Sore throat in children is usually bacterial; it should be evaluated by a physician as soon as possible; symptomatic therapy should be employed to provide relief until a physician can be seen. Sore throat in adults may be due to a variety of causes, some of which may be amenable to self-medication. However, if bacterial pharyngitis is suspected, the patient should be referred to a physician (Table 1).

Influenza A viral respiratory tract infection that may mimic a cold is called influenza, or the "flu." Flu is usually distinguishable from the common cold by its epidemic or pandemic occurrence and by fever, dry cough, generalized joint and muscle ache, and more significant malaise. Although generally symptomatic, treatment of flu is usually more vigorous than treatment of a common cold. Complications, especially secondary bacterial infections, are more likely to develop (12), especially in elderly and debilitated patients, who should be referred to a physician when influenza is suspected. Influenza vaccines are readily available and generally recommended for annual prophylaxis in these patient populations.

Measles Measles (rubeola) is a highly contagious disease caused by a deoxyribonucleic acid (DNA) virus. The incidence of measles has been drastically reduced by active immunization practices. When it does occur, measles is associated with a prodrome that includes fever, rhinitis, dry cough, and conjunctivitis. Initially, it is difficult to distinguish from the common cold. However, in about 3 days, a red rash develops over the face, trunk, and extremities. The appearance of Koplik's spots is characteristic of measles. These spots usually appear 1 to 2 days before the rash. They are white or gray marks often described as "table salt crystals" and appear most frequently on the mucous membranes of the cheek. The patient should be isolated and, although treatment is symptomatic, a physician should be notified because secondary bacterial infection and postmeasles encephalitis or subacute sclerosing panencephalitis (SSPE) may develop. These complications rarely occur in the United States. Infection with rubeola provides long-lasting immunity to the disease (16).

Pharmacists should be aware of local public health regulations that require the reporting of measles.

German Measles Another viral disease in which arthralgia, fever, malaise, lymphadenopathy, and rhinitis coincide with eruption of a fine red rash is German measles (rubella). It is recommended that this disorder be brought to a physician's attention because of possible complications. An important concern is the devastating effect that rubella infection may have on a fetus.

TABLE 1 Distinguishing bacterial from nonbacterial sore throats

	Bacterial sore throat	Nonbacterial sore throat
Onset	Rapid	Slower
Soreness	Marked	Seldom marked
Constitutional symptoms	Marked	Mild
Upper and lower respiratory symptoms	Present in 50% of cases	Usual
Lymph nodes	Large, tender	Slight enlargement, not tender

Adapted from V. Bulteau, *Med. J. Aust.*, 2, 1053 (1966).

Maternal infection has been associated with miscarriage, spontaneous abortion, and fetal abnormalities. If a pregnant woman is exposed to a case of rubella (proven or suspected), she must be referred to a physician to determine her degree of immunity to the virus. Vaccination to rubella has significantly decreased the incidence of German measles in the United States. Immunization is encouraged for all children by the age of 18 months (16).

Allergy A history of allergy and a review of symptoms help differentiate allergic rhinitis from the common cold. Hay fever may be suspected in young children who suffer from repeated coldlike symptoms in a seasonal pattern. Persistent symptoms of a cold are often the first clue to allergic rhinitis. Because a cold usually lasts only several days, a patient who has a stuffy nose for several weeks may have allergic rhinitis or some other form of noninfectious rhinitis.

Treatment of the Common Cold

Self-medication of the common cold is intended to palliate symptoms. There are no curative remedies, only drugs that bring temporary relief while the cold runs its course and the normal body defenses attempt to remove the viral invaders and repair the damage. In general, additional bed rest and prevention of chilling add to the patient's comfort. Adequate fluid intake is necessary to prevent dehydration, and humidification of room air may contribute to loosening of respiratory secretions. A well-balanced diet should be maintained.

Single agent therapy offers the ability to design a regimen directed at each symptom; however, many agents contain multiple medications. These combination products may be effective and provide a convenient dosage form when the patient has multiple symptoms. However, combination products are usually more expensive, are limited by fixed doses in the preparation, and may have additive adverse effects (17).

Nasal Congestion and Discharge Treatment of nasal congestion not only relieves the discomfort but also prevents excessive nose blowing, which may further irritate mucous membranes and the nostrils. Excessive nose blowing also may force infected fluids into nasal sinuses and the eustachian tubes, extending the infection and discomfort. Decongestants (sympathomimetic amines) applied as drops or spray to the nasal mucosa or administered systemically are effective vasoconstrictors that help decrease edema and swelling of the nasal mucosa, therefore enlarging the nasal airways. The watery nasal discharge experienced in the early stages of the common cold may be minimized by decongestant use.

Cough The first step in attempting to control a cough is to provide the respiratory tract with adequate fluids by increasing oral fluid intake, humidifying the inspired air, or both. If the cough is productive and frequency is tolerable, ensuring adequate fluid intake may be all that is needed. If the cough is dry, hyperactive, and annoying, a cough suppressant (antitussive) is indicated. If the cough is productive or congested, an expectorant may be useful because it theoretically will enhance the removal of sputum from the upper respiratory tract (18). Antitussives and expectorants are frequently combined in nonprescription products. Regardless of the character of the cough, if it is bothersome and not related to asthma, a cough suppressant may be beneficial. This is particularly true if the cough interferes with sleep. Any increase in cough by persons with any chronic obstructive lung disease (asthma, emphysema) should be referred to a physician. (See Chapter 9, *Asthma Products*.) The tickling sensation in the pharynx that causes a cough may be treated initially with a demulcent, such as hard candy or cough drops, but if the cough becomes more intense, a cough suppressant may be recommended (1).

Dry or Sore Throat A sore throat in a child is difficult to evaluate and should not be self-medicated. The child should be seen by a physician.

Lozenges and gargles containing antiseptics and topical anesthetics are heavily promoted for treating sore throat. However, aside from a demulcent effect, the use of an antibacterial lozenge or gargle is irrational because the antibacterial ingredients are not effective against viruses.

If the throat is dry or raspy, hard candy may be used to stimulate saliva flow, which acts as a demulcent. A frequently overlooked measure in soothing an inflamed throat is the regular use of a warm, normal saline gargle (2 tsp of salt per qt of water). If these measures do not provide adequate relief, lozenges or sprays containing a local anesthetic (phenol, hexylresorcinol, or benzocaine) may be used every 3–4 hours for temporary symptomatic relief.

Laryngitis Acute laryngitis presents a therapeutic problem—the only direct way to reach the inflamed laryngeal tissue is by inspired air. Lozenges and gargles do nothing to relieve hoarseness; their ingredients or the saliva that they stimulate does not reach this area. Water vapor inhalation (steam or cool mist) several times a day may be beneficial in acute laryngitis. The value of adding any medications to steam has not been established. Active or passive inhalation of irritants such as cigarette smoke should be avoided. The voice should be rested as much as possible.

Feverishness and Headache Vague complaints of feverishness and headache, although not necessarily occurring together, may be treated with the same remedies. In conjunction with fluid and rest, proper dosages of aspirin, acetaminophen, or ibuprofen are usually effective because of their analgesic/antipyretic properties. Fever (oral temperature higher than 98.9–99.6° F or 37.2–37.6° C or rectal temperature higher than 99.9–100.6° F or 37.7–38.1° C) is seldom associated with the common cold, and the benefit of the antipyretic property of aspirin, acetaminophen, or ibuprofen is doubtful. When a fever is present and persists for more than 24 hours in spite of treatment, a physician should be consulted. In the interim, an antipyretic will provide temporary relief of fever symptoms. If fever persists in spite of those medical measures, the patient should be sponged or bathed in cool or tepid, not cold, water. The use of cold water will promote shivering, which may in turn increase the core body temperature. The use of diluted isopropyl alcohol (50:50 in water) also has been recommended as adjunctive antipyretic therapy. In spite of this sponging solution's proven effectiveness, its use has been associated with several drawbacks (19). First, significantly more discomfort has been identified with its use when compared to tepid water. Second, coma caused by acute alcohol poisoning has been associated in patients when isopropyl alcohol has been used (19, 20). Finally, alcohol will denature the proteins in the skin and cause drying. Therefore, the alcohol solution should not be used; the most rational approach to fever reduction in adults and children is use of an antipyretic, such as aspirin, acetaminophen, or ibuprofen, and/or tepid water sponging (21). (See Chapter 6, *Antipyretic Drug Products*.)

Evidence suggests a relationship between aspirin use for fever associated with viral infection and the increased incidence of Reye's syndrome. Therefore, aspirin should be used with extreme caution in children and adolescents with fever associated with viral infection (22, 23). See Chapter 6, *Antipyretic Drug Products* for further discussion of Reye's syndrome.

Physician-directed treatment is usually unnecessary unless there is concern that the patient has a disease other than a cold, the symptoms are severe, or secondary complications are present or suspected. Severely debilitated patients, however, should consult their physician, as should patients with other chronic disorders (such as emphysema and cystic fibrosis) for whom respiratory infection may pose serious problems or the usual nonprescription remedies are contraindicated.

Allergic Rhinitis

Etiology

Allergic rhinitis may begin at almost any age, although the incidence of first onset is greatest in children and young adults and decreases with age. Heredity seems to play a role. Allergic rhinitis itself is not genetically transmitted; however, the heightened predisposition to become sensitized after exposure to adequate concentrations of an allergen is transferred (24).

Pollens from plants that depend on wind for crosspollination and mold spores are the main agents responsible for seasonal allergic rhinitis. Ragweed pollen accounts for about 75% of seasonal rhinitis in the United States; grass pollens, 40%; and tree pollens, about 9%. Approximately 25% of individuals with seasonal rhinitis suffer from both grass and ragweed allergic rhinitis and about 5% suffer from all three allergies (25).

The seasonal appearance of symptoms reflects the pollen or spores in the air. Of the airborne mold spores, species of *Alternaria* and *Hormodendrum* are the most common (26). These spores are most prevalent from mid-March to late November. Tree pollination begins in late March and extends to early June. Grasses generally pollinate from mid-May to mid-July. Ragweed pollen has a long season, extending from early August to early October or to the first killing frost. The pollinating season for a particular plant in a given locale is relatively constant from year to year. Weather conditions such as temperature and rainfall influence the amount of pollen produced but not the actual onset or termination of a specific season (24). The appearance of seasonal allergic rhinitis symptoms is influenced by the patient's geographic location and specific hypersensitivities.

Perennial allergic rhinitis symptoms are usually caused by house dust, animal dander, and feathers. Occupational causes may include wheat flour, various grains, cotton and flax seeds, enzymes used in detergents, paint fumes, topical sprays, and industrial solvents. Foods and medications may also contain allergens such as sulfites and bisulfites. The continued presence of the allergens results in symptoms that persist more or less year-round. Some patients may also exhibit perennial allergic rhinitis symptoms with seasonal exacerbations. Nonspecific irritants such as tobacco smoke, chalk dust, road dust, and heavily polluted air may also contribute to symptoms in an allergic patient (27).

Vasomotor rhinitis is a nonallergic, noninfectious rhinitis characterized by watery, profuse nasal discharge and congestion. Often the symptoms are provoked by changes in environmental temperature or posture and by exposure to volatile irritants. This form of rhinitis can be differentiated by the lack of eosinophils in the nasal secretions; no evidence of sensitization to specific antigens can be demonstrated.

Pathophysiology

Allergic rhinitis symptoms may be due to many different etiologic allergens. These allergens, which are primarily protein in nature, may, when deposited on the nasal mucosa, initiate an inflammatory response by the body and produce symptoms characteristic of allergic rhinitis.

The pathologic inflammatory process of seasonal allergic rhinitis develops within minutes after an allergen is deposited on the nasal mucous membrane of an allergy-prone individual. Pollen itself is not believed to be directly antigenic. However, the body reacts to the pollen, as it does to any foreign substance, and the lysozyme component of nasal mucus degrades the pollen cell wall to allow for the release of the proteinaceous contents. This released protein may be an antigen. The antigen stimulates lymphoid tissue in the respiratory tract to produce a specific type of immunoglobulin, IgE (reagin). These reaginic antibodies have a special affinity for circulating basophils and tissue mast cells. The cells pick up many IgE molecules on their surfaces and thus become sensitized. Subsequent exposure to the same antigen, by its deposition on nasal mucosa, causes an antigen–antibody reaction, which causes the sensitized host cells to release vasoactive chemical mediators. These mediators of inflammation include histamine, eosinophilic and neutrophilic chemotactic factors, and mast cell proteases. Prostaglandin D_2, leukotrienes, and platelet-activating factor are also released (28).

The nasal mucosa is particularly vulnerable to this immediate type of allergic reaction because the allergen is deposited directly where it may act locally and because the mediators are very active vasodilators that are released in a highly vascularized area. The immediate effects are vasodilation, increased vascular permeability, and increased mucus secretion, all of which are responsible for the symptoms.

The longer the symptoms persist, from whatever cause, the more the patient will note chronic and irreversible changes such as thickening of the mucosal epithelium, connective tissue proliferation, loss of epithelial cilia, and development of polyps of the nose or sinuses.

Symptoms

Major symptoms of allergic rhinitis are edema and symptoms resulting from the engorgement of the nasal mucosa; sneezing, rhinorrhea, nasal pruritus, and nasal congestion are the most common. Sudden sneezing attacks may consist of 10–20 sneezes in rapid succession (Table 2).

Rhinorrhea is typically a clear, watery discharge that may be quite profuse and continuous. Purulent discharge does not occur in uncomplicated allergic rhinitis; its presence indicates a secondary infection.

The nasal congestion of allergic rhinitis is due to swollen turbinates. If the nasal obstruction is severe, it may cause headaches or earaches. With continuous, severe nasal congestion, loss of smell and taste may occur. Itching of the nose, particularly in children, may cause frequent nose rubbing.

Conjunctival symptoms commonly associated with allergic rhinitis include itching and lacrimation. These symptoms are caused by the trapping of pollen grains in the conjunctival sac and subsequent antigen–antibody reaction as well as possible lacrimal duct congestion caused indirectly by the nasal congestion. Patients with severe eye symptoms often complain of photophobia and sore, tired eyes. Dark circles or greater than normal discolorations beneath the eyes are called "allergic shiners." This discoloration is more common in perennial rhinitis than in the seasonal variant.

A characteristic of seasonal allergic rhinitis is the periodicity of its appearance. A careful patient history indicates when the symptoms began and the intervals at which they were exacerbated. With seasonal rhinitis, the allergic reaction often begins with sneezing and progresses to rhinorrhea, then possibly to severe nasal obstruction, at which time sneezing may be absent and rhinorrhea minimal. Perennial rhinitis is more likely to begin with nasal obstruction and postnasal discharge than with sneezing and rhinorrhea (29).

The symptoms of allergic rhinitis may exhibit periodicity even within the season. Most patients tend to exhibit more intense symptoms in the morning and on windy days because of increased pollen in the air. Symptoms may diminish when it rains and the pollen is cleared from the air.

TABLE 2 Characteristics of the various types of rhinitis

| Rhinitis | Allergic | | Infectious | Nonallergic (vasomotor) |
	Seasonal	Perennial		
Etiology	IgE-mediated immunologic reaction	IgE-mediated immunologic reaction	Respiratory infection	Autonomic nervous system disorder
Seasonal pattern	Yes	Present year-round	Often worse in winter	Worse in changing seasons
Recurrences	Mild symptoms between attacks	Mild symptoms between attacks	Clears completely	Frequently continuous
Family history of allergy	Common	Common	Occasional	Occasional
Systemic symptoms	Rare	Rare	Common	Rare
Other allergic symptoms (asthma, eczema)	Common	Common	Occasional	Occasional
Pruritus	Yes	Yes	No	Mild or absent
Fever	No	No	Occasional	No
Conjunctivitis	Yes	Yes	No	No
Discharge	Water-like	Water-like	Mucopurulent	Water-like
Paroxysmal sneezing	Yes	Yes	No	Yes

It is more difficult to associate perennial rhinitis than seasonal rhinitis with the environment; the patient history may be helpful in these cases. The most common perennial allergens are house dust and household pet dander with which the patient may be in contact during all seasons. Many patients with perennial allergic rhinitis have continuous symptoms because of the presence of dander or dust in their environment. However, other patients who have overlapping allergies can be symptomatic each season for different reasons. The patient with allergies to mold, grass, ragweed, and house dust may be symptomatic year-round.

Generally, allergic rhinitis tends to show increasingly severe symptoms for 2 or 3 years until a somewhat stable condition is reached. With seasonal allergic rhinitis, symptoms then tend to be exacerbated annually. There is no effective means of predicting whether symptoms will increase or decrease in severity. In fact, for reasons not well understood, hypersensitivity may disappear after several years.

The pharmacist may differentiate seasonal allergic rhinitis from perennial allergic rhinitis by questioning the patient about the appearance and disappearance of symptoms. The presence of acute exacerbations is important in differentiating seasonal allergic rhinitis from perennial allergic rhinitis. Patients with seasonal allergic rhinitis generally have a marked increase in symptoms corresponding to an increase in the amount of allergen in the air. The treatment is similar with both of these conditions.

Complications

Patients with allergic rhinitis may develop complications of chronic nasal inflammation including recurrent otitis media with hearing loss, sinusitis, and loss of epithelial cilia. Hyposmia (decreased sense of smell acuity), nasal polyps, and vocal changes may be caused by chronic mucosal inflammation, which would explain why these complications are more often seen in patients with the perennial form (30). Complications of allergic rhinitis seem to be more prominent in children. Often a child develops a characteristic manner of rubbing the nose upward with the palm of the hand to relieve itching and spread the nasal wall, producing better nasal ventilation. This persistent rubbing is called the "allergic salute" and may lead to the development of a fold on the bridge of the nose called an "allergic crease." Nasal allergy in children may also lead to bony structural changes in the palate and a depression of cheek bone prominence. The resultant crowding of the incisor teeth is called the Gothic arch. Other related facial growth patterns have been identified in children with allergic rhinitis (31, 32). Children with chronic, recurrent rhinitis may develop a hearing impairment due to the involvement of the eustachian tube and middle ear.

Approximately 20% of patients with allergic rhinitis have middle ear abnormalities (33).

Allergic rhinitis and asthmatic attacks often may be precipitated by the same agents. If allergic rhinitis symptoms are prolonged, a persistent cough and a feeling of constriction in the chest or asthmatic wheezing may follow. These are dangerous signals—a warning of possible asthma onset. Because one-third or more of all patients with allergic rhinitis may develop asthma, these signs should be the basis for directing the patient to a physician for diagnosis and treatment (34). (See Chapter 9, *Asthma Products*.)

Perennial allergic rhinitis is associated with chronic symptoms that may lead to anatomical changes within the nasal and sinus cavities. The resulting complications include loss of epithelial cilia and development of nasal polyps. Because the symptoms are chronic and complications may develop, all perennial allergic rhinitis sufferers should be under a physician's care.

Conditions Mimicking Allergic Rhinitis

It is important for pharmacists to recognize common disease entities that may mimic signs or symptoms of allergic rhinitis. The main clinical entity in differential diagnosis of seasonal allergic rhinitis is infectious rhinitis. A mucopurulent discharge, the possibility of fever and other systemic symptoms, and the lack of pruritus often distinguish infectious rhinitis (Table 2). Chronic sinusitis, recurrent infectious rhinitis, abnormalities of nasal structures such as septal deviations, and nonseasonal, nonallergic, noninfectious rhinitis of unknown etiology (vasomotor rhinitis) may be confused with perennial allergic rhinitis (15). A physician should be consulted to differentiate among these conditions.

Other conditions that may mimic allergic rhinitis symptoms are rhinitis medicamentosa, reserpine rhinitis, foreign bodies in the nose, and cerebrospinal rhinorrhea. Rhinitis medicamentosa is a condition resulting from the overuse of topically applied vasoconstrictors. The pharmacist may identify this condition by questioning the patient about past use of nose drops or sprays for nasal congestion.

Preparations containing reserpine or other antiadrenergic antihypertensives may cause marked nasal congestion. Often, this side effect is transient and subsides with continued antihypertensive administration. However, if it persists and is bothersome, topical decongestant treatment may be tried.

In rare instances the presence of a foreign body in the nose may be mistaken for chronic allergic rhinitis. Examination by a physician is necessary. Cerebrospinal rhinorrhea may follow a head injury; it is characterized by the discharge of a clear, watery fluid, usually from one nostril.

Treatment of Allergic Rhinitis

Allergic rhinitis treatment involves:

- Avoidance of allergens when possible to prevent the immunologic response;

- Injection of allergen extracts to alter the immunologic response to the allergens (immunotherapy);

- Pharmacologic treatment to minimize or counteract the consequences of the immunologic response once it has occurred.

In most cases of allergic rhinitis, total avoidance of the allergen is difficult because airborne allergens are so widely distributed and, in most cases, patients are sensitive to more than one allergen. However, avoidance of certain situations (burning leaves, sleeping with the bedroom windows open, and driving in the countryside when pollen counts are especially high) decreases exposure to environments or situations conducive to encountering potential allergens. The mechanical filters in most air conditioners help reduce the number of allergens if they are changed regularly (monthly), if doors and windows are kept closed, and if the air is recirculated. An electrostatic precipitator or other high-efficiency mechanical filter used in conjunction with a central heating and air conditioning unit is even more effective in reducing house dust and other potential allergens. An effective environmental control for allergy to house dust is covering the bed mattress (where the dust mite lives) with a plastic cover and sealing the pillow in a plastic casing.

When brief exposure to an allergen is unavoidable, a proper face mask effectively filters the inhaled air. Such masks are sold by industrial or scientific supply firms as well as pharmacies for protection against noxious dust. The commonly used gauze masks are ineffective. The pharmacist should explain to the patient specific measures that decrease the likelihood of exposure to the offending allergen.

Immunotherapy (hyposensitization) attempts to raise a person's threshold for symptoms following exposure to the allergen. Although the mechanisms of immunotherapy are not understood completely, it is believed that blocking antibodies are produced when the patient is given a continuing series of allergen injections in specified incremental doses. A successful treatment regimen enables the patient to develop increased allergen tolerance. The indications for immunotherapy, a relatively long-term treatment, are relative rather than absolute. For example, if a patient's symptoms are mild and last only a few weeks, the patient may be well managed by symptomatic therapy alone. For those whose reaction to the allergens is much more severe or who cannot tolerate symptomatic treatment, immunotherapy may be considered.

Immunotherapy begins with the proper identification of the offending allergen, most commonly by skin tests measuring the patient's response to test allergens introduced intracutaneously. After the offending allergen is identified, an extract is injected in small amounts at frequent intervals. Studies indicate that in pollen allergy, 70–80% of the patients treated with immunotherapy experience beneficial results (24, 34, 35). However, most of the studies on the efficacy of immunotherapy relate to successes with ragweed and grass.

Immunotherapy does not cure the disease but reduces the number of symptoms, making it easier to control the allergy by symptomatic medication. Patients who experience allergic rhinitis symptoms throughout the year, whose allergic reactions tend to be severe, and who do not demonstrate a beneficial response from self-medication may be candidates for immunotherapy and should be advised by the pharmacist to seek the aid of a physician.

PHARMACOLOGIC AGENTS

The primary pharmacologic agents used in treating these disorders are antihistamines (H_1-blockers) and adrenergic agonists (decongestants). Antihistamines are valuable because they competitively inhibit the effects of any histamine released as a result of the antigen–antibody reaction. The alpha-adrenergic agonists, on the other hand, reverse the effects of histamine or viral inflammation by constricting dilated blood vessels, thereby diminishing nasal congestion.

Antihistamines

Histamine is a potent common biogenic amine found in every body tissue; most, however, is found in the mast cells and basophils. Mast cells are primarily located in the skin, respiratory tract, and gastrointestinal (GI) tract. In these cells, histamine is localized and stored in granules; it generally becomes active only when the cells are lysed. It may be released as a result of an antigen–antibody reaction (allergy) or physical damage (trauma or infection). Histamine has its most significant effects on the cardiovascular system, exocrine glands, and smooth muscles. Its major effects in allergic rhinitis are profound vasodilation, increased capillary permeability, and edema. These effects are more pronounced in highly vascularized areas such as the nose.

Histamine is released primarily in allergic reactions. It may be released in colds, but this remains controversial (36). The symptomatology varies according to the amount of histamine released. In allergy the antigen–antibody reaction leads to cellular damage of specific sensitized cells (mast cells) and consequent release of histamine that initiates the local inflammatory response. In colds, the local inflammatory response results from widespread cellular injury caused by virus particle invasion. Therefore, the vasodilation and resultant edema associated with a cold may be attributed not only to histamine release but also (and perhaps predominantly) to the body's inflammatory defense and the release of other inflammatory mediators.

Antihistamines are chemical agents that exert their effect in the body primarily by competitively blocking the actions of histamine at receptor sites (37). They are classified as "pharmacologic antagonists" of histamine with a mechanism of action analogous to other pharmacologic antagonists such as antiadrenergics and anticholinergics. They do not prevent histamine release, but act by competitive inhibition; therefore, if the histamine concentration at the receptor site exceeds the drug concentration, histamine effects predominate. It has been observed that most antihistamines can be classified as either H_1-receptor blockers, which block the smooth muscle response, or H_2-receptor blockers, whose primary effect is blocking histaminic stimulation of gastric acid secretion (38). Those antihistamines that block the H_1 receptor are potentially useful in treating allergic rhinitis and, to a lesser extent, colds.

Although antihistaminic activity is the dominant effect of these agents, antihistamines are structurally similar to other pharmacologic classes of drugs (anticholinergic, local anesthetic, and ganglionic-blocking and adrenergic-blocking agents) and exert various combinations and degrees of side effects. In some cases, the side effects have been used to achieve a therapeutic goal, such as central nervous system (CNS) depression for insomnia and local anesthetic effects for pruritus. However, these side effects, especially drowsiness, may be bothersome and potentially dangerous.

The most commonly used nonprescription antihistamines and their usual dosages are shown in Table 3. Brompheniramine maleate, chlorpheniramine maleate, doxylamine succinate, phenindamine tartrate, pheniramine maleate, promethazine maleate, pyrilamine maleate, and thonzylamine hydrochloride are recognized by the Food and Drug Administration (FDA) over-the-counter (OTC) advisory review panel on cold, cough, allergy, bronchodilator, and antiasthmatic drug products as being safe for nonprescription use and effective in suppressing the symptoms of allergic rhinitis when taken in the dosage specified. Conclusive evidence is still lacking as to the safety and effectiveness of phenyltoloxamine citrate (1).

Antihistamines are most effective in controlling allergic rhinitis (1), and are rarely effective in vasomotor rhinitis.

Some regular antihistamine users may find that they do not obtain the same degree of relief after several weeks or months. One reason for this decreased effectiveness is that some antihistamines are capable of hepatic enzyme induction, resulting in increased metabolism in the liver. Enzyme induction by antihistamines is a possible cause of diminished effectiveness of other drugs; however, the clinical significance of such interactions is undetermined. The various antihistamine classes differ in their capacity to induce hepatic enzymes. Some practitioners have found that if tolerance develops, some patients may benefit by switching to another antihistamine. Further studies are needed to evaluate the effectiveness of this technique.

Although antihistamines have no ability to prevent or abort the common cold, they are found in many cold remedies. The rationale for their inclusion in these products probably stems from their anticholinergic action, which decreases the amount of mucus secretion, relieving the rhinorrhea. Although some people experience a drying effect, the anticholinergic activity of the antihistamines is actually very weak, and this action may be insignificant at the dosage levels of the various nonprescription preparations.

In general, antihistamines possess a high therapeutic index (toxic dose/therapeutic dose), and serious toxicities are seldom noted in adults. At recommended labeled doses, most nonprescription antihistamines also are safe for use in children. As with most drugs, however, accidental overdose in children may lead to profound symptoms, such as excitement, ataxia, incoordination, muscular twitching, generalized convulsions with pupillary dilation, and skin flushing. Treatment is symptomatic and usually requires supportive therapy with artificial respiration.

The major contraindication to antihistamine use, which is the agent's sedative property, is relative. Degrees of drowsiness associated with antihistamines vary. The ethanolamines, such as diphenhydramine hydrochloride, have a pronounced tendency to induce sedation. The alkylamines (chlorpheniramine maleate) possess weak sedative properties, and the ethylenediamines (pyrilamine maleate) have intermediate sedative properties (39). Although most individuals acquire a tolerance to this effect, the alkylamines probably are the most suitable agents for daytime use (39). In one study, persistent drowsiness was reported to be uncommon when therapy was initiated with a low dose of drug at bedtime, and the dose increased progressively over a 10-day period as tolerated (40). If a person's job or other activities require a high degree of mental alertness, any antihistamine must be used cautiously until its effect is determined by the individual. The effects of

TABLE 3 Antihistamine dosage

Drug (by chemical class)	Dosage (maximum/24 hours)		
	Adults	**Children 6 to <12 years**	**Children 2 to <6 years**
ETHANOLAMINES			
Diphenhydramine hydrochloride	25–50 mg every 4–6 hours (300 mg)	12.5–25 mg every 4–6 hours (150 mg)	6.25 mg every 4–6 hours (37.5 mg)
Doxylamine succinate	7.5–12.5 mg every 4–6 hours (75 mg)	3.75–6.25 mg every 4–6 hours (37.5 mg)	Professional labeling only: 1.9–3.125 mg every 4–6 hours (18.75 mg)
Phenyltoloxamine citrate	50 mg every 4–6 hours (300 mg)	Information inadequate to establish dosage	Information inadequate to establish dosage
ETHYLENEDIAMINES			
Pyrilamine maleate	25–50 mg every 6–8 hours (200 mg)	12.5–25 mg every 6–8 hours (100 mg)	6.25–12.5 mg every 6–8 hours (50 mg)
Thonzylamine hydrochloride	50–100 mg every 4–6 hours (600 mg)	25–50 mg every 4–6 hours (300 mg)	12.5–25 mg every 4–6 hours (150 mg)
ALKYLAMINES			
Pheniramine maleate	12.5–25 mg every 4–6 hours (150 mg)	6.25–12.5 mg every 4–6 hours (75 mg)	3.125–6.25 mg every 4–6 hours (37.5 mg)
Brompheniramine maleate	4 mg every 4–6 hours (24 mg)	2 mg every 4–6 hours (12 mg)	1 mg every 4–6 hours (6 mg)
Chlorpheniramine maleate	4 mg every 4–6 hours (24 mg)	2 mg every 4–6 hours (12 mg)	1 mg every 4–6 hours (6 mg)
MISCELLANEOUS			
Phenindamine tartrate	25 mg every 4–6 hours (150 mg)	12.5 mg every 4–6 hours (75 mg)	6.25 mg every 4–6 hours (37.5 mg)

The FDA advisory review panel on OTC cold, cough, allergy, bronchodilator, and antiasthmatic products has recommended all of these ingredients as safe and effective (Category I) except phenyltoloxamine citrate, for which there is insufficient evidence (Category III). At the time of this writing, the final status of several other antihistamine agents had not been fully resolved by the FDA; these include dexbrompheniramine, dexchlorpheniramine, and triprolidine.

alcohol and other CNS depressants, including hypnotics, sedatives, analgesics, and antianxiety agents, may be enhanced by the antihistamines. If concurrent administration is necessary, caution must be exercised because of the increased possibility of drowsiness (39, 41, 42). Patients should be warned of "hidden" sources of alcohol contained in some nonprescription medications.

Recently, a number of antihistamines have been introduced that offer the advantage of less or no sedation. These newer agents are characterized by lack of anticholinergic effects, longer duration, and less ability to "cross over" the blood brain barrier into the CNS. It is believed that this latter effect makes these agents less soporific (43). Although these newer agents are restricted to prescription use in the United States, manufacturers are attempting to have them reclassified for nonprescription marketing as they are in several foreign countries (44).

Many commercial products contain both an antihistamine and a decongestant. These products may have less tendency to cause sedation because of the decongestant component, and may offset the sedative effect of the antihistamine (45).

A paradoxical effect frequently seen in children is CNS stimulation rather than depression, causing insomnia, nervousness, and irritability (phenindamine).

For this reason, antihistamines must be used cautiously in children with convulsive disorders or hyperkinesis (1, 35). The anticholinergic properties of an antihistamine may predominate in some individuals. Antihistamines may cause dry mouth, blurred vision, urinary retention (in older males suffering from an enlarged prostate), and constipation as a result of their anticholinergic effects; these effects, however, are usually associated with high doses. In the past, some practitioners believed that antihistamines should not be given to asthmatics because of the potential drying effect on the respiratory tract. However, these products have proven very useful in patients whose asthma has an allergic component and are now routinely used (46, 47). The physician may elect a trial course of antihistamine therapy in patients not adequately controlled with the usual antiasthmatic regimen (4).

The cholinergic-blocking effect of antihistamines has a quantitatively unpredictable additive effect with anticholinergic drugs. Although excessive blocking effects are usually of minor clinical significance, effects such as urinary retention, constipation, and dry mouth may be bothersome in certain populations (1).

The cholinergic-blocking properties of the antihistamines may pose a problem for patients taking an anticholinesterase to control narrow-angle glaucoma. Such an effect is unpredictable; because of the potential consequences, such patients probably should take antihistamines only under a physician's supervision. Ninety-five percent of all patients with glaucoma have the wide-angle type, and antihistamines are not contraindicated in these patients.

Hypersensitivity reactions may develop with the antihistamines, but this effect is more common with topical application than with systemic use (38). Antihistamine overdose may cause dermatitis, psychosis, convulsions, and facial dyskinesias (47–50).

Topical Decongestants

Various sympathomimetic amines have been used to provide relief from the nasal stuffiness of colds and allergic rhinitis. These drugs, which differ primarily in their duration of action, are contained in many nonprescription products promoted for hay fever and colds. Nasal decongestants stimulate the alpha-adrenergic receptors of the vascular smooth muscle, constricting the dilated arteriolar network within the nasal mucosa and reducing blood flow in the engorged edematous nasal area. This constriction results in shrinkage of the engorged mucous membranes, which promotes drainage, improves nasal ventilation, and relieves the feeling of stuffiness.

The ideal topical decongestant agent should have a prompt and prolonged effect. It should not produce systemic side effects, irritation to the mucosa with resultant harmful interference on the action of the cilia of the respiratory tract, or rebound congestion. An ideal topical sympathomimetic amine has not yet been found (51).

Intranasal application of commercially available decongestants provides prompt and dramatic decrease of nasal congestion. Shrinking of the mucous membrane not only makes breathing easier but also permits the sinus cavities to drain.

It is important that the patient follows the decongestant's label directions regarding the frequency and duration of use. Topical application of these drugs is often followed by a rebound phenomenon (rhinitis medicamentosa) in which the nasal mucous membranes become even more congested and edematous as the drug's vasoconstrictor effect subsides. This secondary congestion is believed to result from ischemia caused by the drug's intensive local vasoconstriction and local irritation of the topically applied agent itself. If the use of a topical nasal decongestant is restricted to 3 or 4 days or less, rebound congestion is minimal; with chronic use or overuse of these agents, rebound nasal stuffiness may become quite pronounced. This phenomenon may begin a vicious cycle because it leads to more frequent use of the agent that causes it. To determine the possible existence of this condition, the pharmacist should question a patient about prior use of nasal sprays, drops, or inhalants. If the pharmacist suspects that the patient is experiencing this rebound phenomenon, the patient should be referred to a physician. Attempts to treat the iatrogenic symptoms with additional topical sympathomimetic drugs create a cycle that is extremely difficult to break. Topical decongestant therapy should be discontinued, and systemic decongestants and/or isotonic saline drops or spray may be used.

The patient should be instructed on the proper administration of topical decongestants to obtain maximum relief without encountering side effects from the drug's systemic absorption. These products are available as drops or sprays. Nasal decongestant sprays are packaged in flexible plastic containers that produce a fine mist when squeezed. The patient should administer nasal sprays in the upright position, squeezing once into each nostril. The nose should be blown to remove mucus 3–5 minutes after spraying. If still congested, the patient should administer another dose, which should reach farther into the nasal cavities and to the surfaces of the turbinates.

Some persons prefer to administer the decongestant solution with a nasal atomizer. Most commercial spray containers are designed to deliver the approximate dose with one squeeze; the atomizer, however, is not so calibrated. Also, using an atomizer may increase the possibility of contaminating the solution. If the patient prefers to use a nasal atomizer, instructions should be provided on the proper use of the particular atomizer, including the liquid level and proper placement within the nostril and the hazards of misuse. The patient should be instructed to remove the solution and rinse the atomizer after use to guard against solution contamination. Naphazoline solutions should not be used in atomizers containing aluminum parts because drug degradation will result.

Nasal drops usually do not cover the entire nasal mucosa and may pass to the pharynx, where they may be swallowed. Although systemic absorption through the nasal mucosa is minimal because of the local vasoconstriction induced by the drug, if an excess amount drains through the nasal passage and is swallowed, absorption and systemic effects are then possible. Proper administration minimizes the amount of medication swallowed.

To administer nasal drops, the patient should recline on a bed with the head tilted back over the edge or should recline on the side with the head held lower than the shoulders. The drops should be placed in the lower nostril; the dropper should not touch the nasal surface. After the drops have been instilled into each nostril, the patient should breathe through the mouth and remain in the reclining position for about 5 minutes. To ensure more uniform absorption of the medication, the head should be turned from side to side while the patient is reclining.

A topical decongestant in spray form is probably more convenient for adults and older children. Sprays also may afford better decongestion by reaching greater areas of the mucous membranes. Drops are the most effective means of administering a topical decongestant to children under 6 years of age because of their smaller nostril openings.

Several agents are commonly used as topical nasal decongestants. The primary difference lies in their intensity and duration of action (Table 4).

Ephedrine

Ephedrine is the prototype of the topical sympathomimetic decongestant. Various ephedrine salts provide rapid nasal decongestion applied topically in 0.5–1.0% concentrations. Ephedrine's peak effects are achieved 1 hour after administration. The aqueous solution of topical ephedrine as drops or sprays is the only vehicle recommended by the FDA advisory review panel on OTC cold, cough, allergy, bronchodilator, and antiasthmatic drug products because oily solutions may lead to lipoid pneumonia (1). Products containing ephedrine should be shielded from direct light, because decomposition will be hastened by such exposure. Discolored ephedrine solutions should not be used. Ephedrine in a concentration of 0.5% should be administered as 2 or 3 drops or sprays for adults or as 1 or 2 drops or sprays for children 6–12 years of age, not more frequently than every 4 hours. Ephedrine is not recommended for children under 6 years of age except under the advice and supervision of a physician (52).

Phenylephrine

Phenylephrine hydrochloride is an effective nonprescription nasal decongestant. It is commonly applied as 2 or 3 drops or sprays of a 0.25–1.0% solution every 4 hours. The use of stronger solutions is hazardous, except under a physician's direction. This agent may produce a marked irritation of the nasal mucosa in some individuals, in addition to the irritation already present from the pathologic condition of the allergic disorder or cold. If this reaction occurs, phenylephrine use should be stopped immediately.

Phenylephrine hydrochloride is also available as an aqueous jelly. A small amount of jelly is placed in each nostril and snuffed well back into the nasal passage. This dosage form is not convenient and is not widely used, and its effectiveness has not been established. Theoretically, a more prolonged decongestant effect may be achieved with nasal jellies, which may have an emollient and protective action on the nasal mucosa, but these effects also have not been proven (53). Nasal decongestant jellies are used most commonly by otorhinolaryngologists for office examination or treatment.

Naphazoline

Naphazoline hydrochloride is a more potent vasoconstrictor than phenylephrine hydrochloride. It produces CNS depression, rather than stimulation when it is absorbed systemically. Because of its systemic effects, this agent is not recommended for use in children under 6 years of age except under the advice and supervision of a physician (1). Naphazoline hydrochloride is commonly administered as 1 or 2 drops or sprays of a 0.05% solution every 6 hours. It may be irritating to the mucosa and may sting when administered; use should be discontinued if this effect persists or worsens.

Oxymetazoline and Xylometazoline

Longer acting topical nasal decongestants, such as oxymetazoline hydrochloride and xylometazoline hydrochloride, have a decongestant effect that may last 5 or 6 hours, with a gradual decline thereafter (1, 54–56). Because of these agents' long duration of action, they are used only twice a day; therefore, they are easier to use, and rhinitis medicamentosa or rebound congestion may be less likely to occur. Overuse or prolonged use of

TABLE 4 Topical nasal decongestant dosage

Drug	Concentration	Dosage		
		Adults, drops or sprays	Children 6 to <12 years drops or sprays	Children 2 to <6 years*
Ephedrine (various salts)	0.5%	2–3 (≥4 hours)	1–2 (≥4 hours)	—
Naphazoline hydrochloride	0.05%	1–2 (≥6 hours)	Not recommended (refer to 0.025%)	—
	0.025%	—	1–2 (≥6 hours)	—
Oxymetazoline hydrochloride	0.05%	2–3 (morning and evening)	Same as for adults	Not recommended (refer to 0.025%)
	0.025%	—	—	2–3 (morning and evening)
Phenylephrine hydrochloride	1%	2–3 (≥4 hours)	Not recommended (refer to 0.25%)	Not recommended (refer to 0.125%)
	0.25%	Same as 1%	2–3 (≥4 hours)	Not recommended (refer to 0.125%)
	0.125%	—	—	2–3 drops (≥4 hours)
Xylometazoline hydrochloride	0.1%	2–3 (8–10 hours)	Not recommended (refer to 0.05%)	Not recommended (refer to 0.05%)
	0.05%	—	2–3 (8–10 hours)	2–3 (8–10 hours)

The FDA advisory review panel on cold, cough, allergy, bronchodilator, and antiasthmatic products has recommended these ingredients as safe and effective (Category I) at the dosages specified. Only drops should be used in children 2 to <6 years because the spray is difficult to use in small nostrils. These products should not be used in patients with chronic rhinitis because of the risk of rhinitis medicamentosa.

* For children under 6 there is no recommended dosage of ephedrine, naphazoline, or oxymetazoline except under the advice and supervision of a physician.

these agents is associated with chronic rhinitis, nasal congestion, and nasal irritability (34). Oxymetazoline may be administered as 2 or 3 drops or sprays in the morning and evening; xylometazoline may be administered in the same amount every 8–10 hours (1).

Levodesoxyephedrine and Propylhexedrine

Levodesoxyephedrine and propylhexedrine are sympathomimetic amines that are volatile and commonly used in inhalants. Both of these aromatic amines are classified as Category I when used as two inhalations in each nostril not more frequently than every 2 hours. Although children 6 years of age and over may use the adult dose of propylhexedrine, the dose of levodesoxyephedrine should be halved to 1 inhalation not more frequently than every 2 hours. Neither product is promoted for use in children under 6 years of age.

The use of nasal inhalers is associated with potential problems, such as the loss of the active agent when the cap is not properly replaced. Also, there may not be sufficient nasal airflow to distribute the agent throughout the nasal cavity. These agents have been implicated as being irritating to the nasal mucosa and as interfering with ciliary action, as have all effective topical nasal decongestants. As with other topical amines, overuse produces side effects of local irritation and rebound congestion.

Oral Decongestants

Oral administration of sympathomimetic amines distributes the drug through the systemic circulation to the vascular bed of the nasal mucosa. The oral decongestant agents have the advantage of a longer duration of action than certain topically applied decongestants. However, they cause less intense vasoconstriction than the topically applied sprays or drops. Oral agents have not been associated with rebound congestion or rhinitis medicamentosa because of their lesser degree of vasoconstriction and the lack of local drug irritation (39).

These agents do not exert their action exclusively on the vasculature of the nasal mucosa; in doses large enough to bring about nasal decongestion, they also affect other vascular beds (39). Although the vasoconstriction produced by oral decongestants usually does not increase blood pressure, individuals predisposed to hypertension may experience a change in blood pressure. These decongestants may cause cardiac stimulation and the development of arrhythmias in predisposed individuals. Sympathomimetic agents may be a problem in patients with glucose intolerance or insulin-dependent diabetes mellitus (IDDM or type I), because these drugs increase blood glucose levels. However, hyperglycemia is a beta$_2$-adrenergic effect and most oral decongestants (except ephedrine) contain primarily alpha-adrenergic stimulating properties. Labeling instructions on products containing sympathomimetics should indicate that patients with hypertension, hyperthyroidism, diabetes mellitus, or ischemic heart disease should use these products only on the advice of a physician. (See Chapter 16, *Diabetes Care Products*.)

Sympathomimetic amines are contraindicated in patients receiving monoamine oxidase (MAO) inhibitor therapy for depression because a hypertensive crisis may result. They should be used cautiously in hypertensive patients stabilized with guanethidine (57). These warnings apply largely to the oral agents and are not likely to occur with topically applied drugs.

Ephedrine, phenylpropanolamine hydrochloride, phenylephrine hydrochloride, and pseudoephedrine are oral sympathomimetic amines commonly incorporated into cold and allergy products (Table 5). According to classification by the FDA advisory review panel, only phenylpropanolamine, phenylephrine, and pseudoephedrine have been shown to be effective as oral decongestants (1).

Ephedrine

According to the FDA advisory review panel on cold, cough, allergy, bronchodilator, and antiasthmatic drug products, ephedrine is effective as a bronchodilator for asthma but has not been proven effective as a nasal decongestant (58). Taken orally, in doses of 12.5–25 mg every 4 hours for adults and children 12 years of age and over, ephedrine is effective as a bronchodilator for use in treating symptoms of asthma. The bronchodilator effects usually appear within 30 min-

utes to 1 hour after oral administration. Ephedrine has CNS stimulatory effects.

Phenylpropanolamine

Phenylpropanolamine hydrochloride resembles ephedrine in its action, but it is somewhat more active as a vasoconstrictor and less active as a CNS stimulant and bronchodilator. The peak effect occurs approximately 3 hours after administration.

Phenylephrine

Phenylephrine hydrochloride is rapidly metabolized in the GI tract, and the amount delivered to the bloodstream through oral administration is hard to predict, but effectiveness as an oral decongestant has been demonstrated (1). Phenylephrine is a common ingredient of cold preparations; however, it may be present in inadequate dosage levels. Because of the unique properties of phenylephrine and its GI absorption, it is important to select products that contain the full and appropriate FDA recommended dosage.

Pseudoephedrine

Pseudoephedrine is another effective vasoconstrictor. It has less vasopressor action than ephedrine and causes little CNS stimulation. The dosages given in Table 5 reflect a recent relabeling requirement following an FDA decision that data on safety and effectiveness do not support the advisory review panel's original recommendation for a 360-mg adult daily dosage of pseudoephedrine. The FDA's latest labeling requirement sets the adult daily dosage at 240 mg. The daily dosage for children 6–12 years of age has been changed from 180 mg to 120 mg and for children 2–6 years of age, from 90 mg to 60 mg. The peak effect of a 60-mg dose occurs approximately 4 hours after administration. Because pseudoephedrine has a short duration of effect, several companies have marketed slow-release formulations to maintain more constant relief from nasal airway obstruction. Patients who have nasal stuffiness interfering with nighttime sleep may benefit from a slow-release pseudoephedrine formulation.

Antitussives and Expectorants

The cough associated with the common cold may be either productive or nonproductive (dry cough). The productive cough is useful if it helps to remove accumulated secretions and debris (phlegm) from the lower tract. Although a patient with "chest congestion" is

TABLE 5 Oral nasal decongestant dosage

Drug	Dosage (maximum/24 hours)		
	Adults	Children 6 to <12 years	Children 2 to <6 years*
Phenylephrine	10 mg every 4 hours (60 mg)	5 mg every 4 hours (30 mg)	2.5 mg every 4 hours (15 mg)
Phenylpropanolamine	25 mg every 4 hours (150 mg)	12.5 mg every 4 hours (75 mg)	6.25 mg every 4 hours (37.5 mg)
Pseudoephedrine	60 mg every 6 hours (240 mg)	30 mg every 6 hours (120 mg)	15 mg every 6 hours (60 mg)

The FDA advisory review panel on nonprescription cold, cough, allergy, bronchodilator, and antiasthmatic products has recommended these ingredients as safe and effective (Category I) at the dosages specified.

*There is no recommended dosage for children under 2 years of age except under the advice and supervision of a physician.

expected to expectorate phlegm ("productive" cough) during coughing, this does not always occur. It would be inappropriate, however, to describe the cough as "nonproductive" because this description usually is related to dry, noncongested coughing. For the sake of distinction in this section as well as rationale for product selection later, a cough will be classified in one of the following categories:

- Congested/productive—cough associated with chest congestion and the expectoration of phlegm;

- Congested/nonproductive—cough associated with chest congestion and scant expectoration of phlegm;

- Dry/nonproductive—cough not associated with chest congestion.

By referring to these categories the pharmacist will be able to determine when and which type of an agent should be used. Coughs in the first two categories could be undiagnosed symptoms of asthma because intermittent asthmatics may only develop symptoms during a viral respiratory infection.

Excessive coughing, particularly if it is dry and nonproductive, not only is discomforting but also tends to be self-perpetuating because the rapid air expulsion further irritates the tracheal and pharyngeal mucosa. The general classes of pharmacologic agents available for self-medication are expectorants and cough suppressants. Table 6 indicates the sites at which the cough reflex may be blocked as well as the mechanism of the agents.

Expectorants

Use of expectorants in clinical practice is a controversial issue revolving around doubts of therapeutic efficacy. The controversy stems from lack of strong, supportive, objective data showing that an expectorant decreases sputum viscosity or eases expectoration more than does a placebo. One study evaluating guaifenesin concludes that "from a scientific point of view this drug probably has no rational use in clinical medicine as an expectorant" (59). Other literature also questions the efficacy of expectorants, stating that "the use of expectorants is based primarily on tradition and the widespread subjective clinical impression that they are effective" (39). The apparent difficulty in accumulating objective evidence stems from two factors: insufficient evidence as to which physiochemical property of respiratory secretions correlates best with ease of expectoration, and a lack of appropriate techniques and instrumentation to measure the effect on respiratory secretions (1). One study failed to objectively show that guaifenesin had any effect on sputum consistency in patients with chronic bronchitis (60). However, several studies suggest that guaifenesin is effective by subjectively decreasing cough frequency, chest discomfort, and thickness and quantity of sputum and facilitates the raising of sputum (61, 62). The FDA advisory review on allergy, bronchodilator, and antiasthmatic drug products has reclassified guaifenesin as the only expectorant in Category I (generally recognized as safe and effective) (18). All other expectorants remain classified as Category III (available data are insufficient to classify as safe and effective, and further testing is required) (18).

Increasing fluid intake and maintaining adequate humidity of the inspired air are important to respiratory tract fluid mucus production and therefore are essential in cold therapy. These measures may be accomplished by increasing fluid intake to 6–8 glasses a day in patients who do not have fluid restrictions and by using a cool mist or hot steam vaporizer (see section on adjunctive therapy).

TABLE 6	Blockade of cough reflex	
Site	**Mechanism**	**Blocking agents**
Sensory nerves	Reduction of primary irritation; inhibition of broncho-constriction; inhibition of afferent impulses	Demulcents/expectorants; bronchodilators; local anesthetics
Cough center (medulla)	Depression	Opiate and nonopiate suppressants
Motor nerves	Inhibition of efferent impulses	Local anesthetics

Adapted from H. Salem and D. M. Aviado, *Drug Inform. J.*, *8*, 111 (1974).

Subjective findings constitute the basis for continued expectorant use. Table 7 lists the usual dose and dosage range of the most commonly used expectorants.

There are no apparent absolute contraindications to the use of orally administered expectorants. The toxicity associated with expectorant drugs varies among agents. Most expectorants are considered to be safe yet lack effectiveness data. In general, the most common adverse effect to anticipate is gastric upset.

Ammonium Chloride Ammonium chloride is believed to increase the amount of respiratory tract fluid by reflex stimulation of bronchial mucous glands resulting from irritation of the gastric mucosa. In the presence of renal, hepatic, or chronic heart disease, doses of 5 g have caused severe poisoning (63). A relative contraindication exists when ammonium chloride is used in patients with hepatic, renal, or pulmonary insufficiency; doses larger than those recommended may predispose to metabolic acidosis. Because ammonium chloride acidifies the urine, it may affect the excretion of other drugs (57). This effect probably is not significant because the usual daily dosage range as a systemic acidifier is 4–12 g, which is greatly in excess of the safe range for nonprescription use (64).

Guaifenesin (Glyceryl Guaiacolate) Guaifenesin, in the doses recommended for nonprescription use, also is thought to act by reflex gastric stimulation. In spite of its mechanism of action, its use at these doses is seldom associated with gastric upset and nausea. However, one controlled study has shown that guaifenesin neither increases the volume of sputum production nor decreases viscosity (60). Other studies have shown that guaifenesin is subjectively more effective than placebo for expectorant activity (62, 63). The FDA advisory review panel on OTC cold, cough, allergy, bronchodilator, and antiasthmatic drug products has reclassified guaifenesin as the only Category I expectorant.

Ipecac Syrup Administration of 0.5–1.0 ml of ipecac syrup (see Table 7 for concentration) 3 or 4 times a day is believed to increase respiratory secretion flow by gastric irritation. Although no longer commercially available, special care should be used not to use the fluidextract of ipecac. Although little is known regarding the toxicity associated with ipecac at dosages used for expectoration, the chief alkaloids, emetine and cephaeline, are very toxic. The primary toxicity of concern is cardiac and neuromuscular; several cases have resulted in death (65, 66). Fatalities have occurred from the administration of ipecac in emesis-producing dosages over prolonged periods of time and from the administration of the more potent fluidextract of ipecac. For this reason, the FDA review panel recommended a 1-week time limit when OTC ipecac preparations are used for self-medication. Ipecac is not recommended for this use in children under 6 years of age.

Terpin Hydrate Terpin hydrate, a volatile oil derivative, is believed to act by direct stimulation of lower respiratory tract secretory glands in the dosage recommended for nonprescription use. Because of the elixir's high alcohol content, the potential for alcohol abuse should be recognized; however, because of its added codeine content, misuse is associated far more frequently with terpin hydrate and codeine elixir. Terpin hydrate elixir is not recommended for use in children under 12 years of age (1). Some GI distress, such as nausea and vomiting, has been noted with the recommended dosage.

Beechwood Creosote and Potassium Guaiacolsulfonate The apparent usefulness of beechwood creosote and potassium guaiacolsulfonate as expectorants is due to the local irritating effects of guaiacol, the major constitutent of the former and the active moiety of the latter. Guaiacol, like guaifenesin, apparently increases respiratory tract fluid by a gastric reflex action. It is believed that potassium guaiacolsulfonate is metabolized in vivo to liberate guaiacol, but this has not been clearly established.

Although a dosage for beechwood creosote has been proposed, the FDA panel was unable to establish a dosage for potassium guaiacolsulfonate (1, 64).

Other ingredients of unproven effectiveness that are added to cold products for their claimed expectorant properties include:

TABLE 7 Expectorant dosage, where specified, considered safe

Drug	Dosage (maximum/24 hours)		
	Adults	Children 6 to <12 years	Children 2 to <6 years*
Ammonium chloride	300 mg every 2–4 hours	150 mg every 2–4 hours	75 mg every 2–4 hours
Beechwood creosote	250 mg every 4–6 hours (1,500 mg)	125 mg every 4–6 hours (750 mg)	62.5 mg every 4–6 hours (375 mg)
Guaifenesin	200–400 mg every 4 hours (2,400 mg)	100–200 mg every 4 hours (1,200 mg)	50–100 mg every 4 hours (600 mg)
Potassium guaiacolsulfonate	Not established	Not established	Not established
Ipecac syrup	0.5–1.0 ml (of syrup containing not less than 123 mg and not more than 157 mg of total ether-soluble alkaloids of ipecac/100 ml) 3 or 4 times a day	0.25–0.5 ml (of syrup containing not less than 123 mg and not more than 157 mg of total ether-soluble alkaloids of ipecac/100 ml) 3 or 4 times a day	Not recommended
Terpin hydrate	200 mg every 4 hours (1,200 mg)	100 mg (of terpin hydrate alone or in a nonalcoholic mixture, not the elixir for children under 12) every 4 hours (600 mg)	50 mg (of terpin hydrate alone or in a nonalcoholic mixture, not the elixir for children under 12) every 4 hours (300 mg)

The FDA advisory review panel on OTC cold, cough, allergy, bronchodilator, and antiasthmatic drug products has concluded that available data are sufficient to classify guaifenesin as Category I. All other expectorants lack data to permit reclassification in Category I and remain in Category III.

*There is no recommended dosage for children under 2 years of age except under the advice and supervision of a physician.

- Benzoin preparations;
- Camphor;
- Eucalyptus oil;
- Menthol;
- Peppermint oil;
- Pine tar;
- Sodium citrate;
- Tolu;
- Turpentine oil.

Antitussives

Antitussives (cough suppressants) are indicated when there is a need to reduce the frequency of a cough, especially when it is dry and nonproductive (39). Antitussives are also frequently used by patients with productive or congested coughs. Theoretically antitus-sives may be counterproductive because of the suppressant effects on the mechanism of secretion removal; however, use of these agents may be warranted if the productive cough is particularly bothersome, for example, if the patient is unable to sleep. Otherwise antitussives should not be used in patients with productive or congested coughs. The mechanism by which the narcotic and non-narcotic agents affect a cough's intensity and frequency depends on the principal site of action: CNS depression of the cough center in the medulla, or suppression of the nerve receptors within the respiratory tract (1).

Codeine Codeine is the standard antitussive against which all other antitussives are measured (33). The FDA advisory review panel on cold, cough, allergy, bronchodilator, and antiasthmatic drug products has concluded that under usual conditions of therapeutic use, codeine has low-dependency liability (67). The average adult antitussive dose is 15 mg (with a range of

TABLE 8 Antitussive dosage

Drug	Dosage (maximum/24 hours)		
	Adults	Children 6 to <12 years	Children 2 to <6 years[a]
Codeine[b]	10–20 mg every 4–6 hours (120 mg)	5–10 mg every 4–6 hours (60 mg)	2.5–5 mg every 4–6 hours (30 mg)
Dextromethorphan	10–20 mg every 4 hours or 30 mg every 6–8 hours (120 mg)	5–10 mg every 4 hours or 15 mg every 6–8 hours (60 mg)	2.5–5 mg every 4 hours or 7.5 mg every 6–8 hours (30 mg)
Diphenhydramine hydrochloride	25 mg every 4 hours (150 mg)	12.5 mg every 4 hours (75 mg)	6.25 mg every 4 hours (37.5 mg)
Noscapine hydrochloride[c]	15–30 mg every 4–6 hours (180 mg)	7.5–15 mg every 4–6 hours (90 mg)	3.75–7.5 mg every 4–6 hours (45 mg)

The FDA advisory review panel on OTC cold, cough, allergy, bronchodilator, and antiasthmatic products has recommended all of these ingredients as safe and effective (Category I) except noscapine hydrochloride, for which there is insufficient evidence (Category III).
[a] There is no recommended dosage for children under 2 years of age except under the advice and supervision of a physician.
[b] The FDA recommends that the labels on OTC agents containing codeine not give dosage information for children under 6 years of age.
[c] Category III, additional evidence of safety and effectiveness required.

10–20 mg). At this dosage, codeine provides effective cough relief (see Table 8 for children's dosage). Stringent controls have been placed on codeine-containing nonprescription products as a result of their misuse. There is no danger of psychologic physical dependence when codeine is used in recommended amounts for short periods; however, dependence may develop after prolonged use (68). On a weight basis, the respiratory depressant effect of codeine is about one-fourth that of morphine. Even when the dose is increased, commensurate increase in respiratory depression does not necessarily occur. In dosages commonly used in nonprescription cough products, in otherwise healthy persons, the effects on respiration are not apparent. Codeine is thought by some investigators to have a drying effect on the respiratory mucosa; this property would be detrimental in asthma and emphysema patients because of the increased viscosity of respiratory fluids and decreased cough reflex. The FDA advisory review panel on OTC cold, cough, allergy, bronchodilator, and antiasthmatic drug products has suggested that label dosage recommendations for products containing codeine be limited to patients over 6 years of age. Physician consultation is suggested for children under 6 years of age because of a slightly greater chance of respiratory depression caused by the codeine (69).

In clinical practice the adverse effects most commonly encountered with codeine include nausea, drowsiness, lightheadedness, and constipation, especially when recommended dosage levels are exceeded. Allergic reactions and pruritus also may occur but are not as common. These reactions may be more common in patients who are atopic or in those prone to allergic reactions; however, antitussive codeine doses generally are well tolerated (70). Codeine's CNS effects are additive to that of other CNS depressants; therefore, such agents should be used cautiously when given concurrently.

The FDA has recommended that all products containing codeine be dispensed with a measuring device when the product is to be used for children between 2 and 6 years of age (69).

Codeine use is contraindicated in individuals with chronic pulmonary disease, where mucosal drying and slight respiratory depression, in addition to impairment of the clearing of the airway of secretions, may be additionally detrimental (1). Codeine should be avoided by patients who have experienced codeine-induced allergic manifestations (pruritus or rash). Codeine is safe and effective when used as directed for cough.

Dextromethorphan Dextromethorphan is a methylated dextro-isomer of levorphanol, but, unlike its analgesic counterpart, it has no significant analgesic properties and does not depress respiration or predispose to addiction (38). Some investigators believe that dextromethorphan and codeine are equipotent, some give a slight edge to codeine, and others support dextromethorphan as the superior antitussive (71). Therefore, because of the probable equal effectiveness, dextromethorphan may be indicated in patients for whom adverse effects of codeine may be particularly bothersome. Unlike codeine, increasing the dose of dextromethorphan to 30 mg does not increase its antitussive effects.

Adverse effects produced by dextromethorphan hydrobromide at recommended nonprescription dosages are mild and infrequent. Drowsiness and GI upset are the most common complaints. Accidental poisonings in children have resulted in symptoms of stupor and gait disturbances, with rapid recovery after emesis and activated charcoal (72). Larger dosages in the abuse range have produced intoxication with bizarre behavior but no dependence (70).

Dextromethorphan hydrobromide at nonprescription dosages (Table 8) is a safe and effective antitussive for which there are no apparent contraindications except hypersensitivity to this agent (1).

Diphenhydramine Diphenhydramine hydrochloride is a safe and effective antihistamine and antitussive.

Objective results of clinical studies indicate that diphenhydramine, in 25- and 50-mg doses, significantly reduced coughing in chronic cough patients. Diphenhydramine's antitussive effect is due to a central mechanism involving the medullary cough center. A peripheral action may also contribute to its effectiveness, but further studies will be necessary to establish this point. (See Table 8 for dosage recommendations.)

The adverse effects associated with diphenhydramine hydrochloride are typical of other antihistamines. The most commonly encountered adverse effects are sedation and anticholinergic (atropine-like) effects. Because of these properties, diphenhydramine hydrochloride should not be taken by individuals in whom anticholinergics are contraindicated (those with narrow-angle glaucoma or prostatic hypertrophy) or in situations where mental alertness is required, such as driving a car. There has been one case of dependence attributed to a product containing diphenhydramine (73).

Because of its additive CNS depressant effect, diphenhydramine should be used cautiously in individuals taking tranquilizers, sedatives, or hypnotics. Likewise, ingesting alcohol will have additive depressant effects, and caution must be exercised in taking diphenhydramine hydrochloride. Because of additive anticholinergic effects, diphenhydramine hydrochloride should be used cautiously in patients taking other anticholinergic drugs (74). Caution should also be used when combining this agent with other antitussives such as codeine. Diphenhydramine hydrochloride, like codeine and dextromethorphan hydrobromide, is a safe and effective antitussive but has a high likelihood of producing side effects, which must be kept in mind when recommending it.

Camphor-Containing Ointments Camphor-containing ointments have been reclassified as Category I agents (generally recognized as safe and effective) by the FDA advisory review panel on OTC cold, cough, allergy, bronchodilator, and antiasthmatic drug products. The proposed mechanism of action is believed to occur because inhalation of the aromatic vapors causes a local anesthetic action, which produces an antitussive effect. Camphor has been shown to be safe and effective for reducing cough when externally applied to the chest and throat of young children. The FDA advisory review panel on OTC topical analgesic, antirheumatic, otic, burn, and sunburn prevention and treatment drug products has concluded that topical agents containing as much as 11% of camphor are safe for external use. Products used for the antitussive effect contain approximately 5% camphor (69).

Toxicity may occur if the camphor is ingested. The primary toxic effect reported is seizures. Patients should be counseled to avoid use near the mouth and nose to prevent accidental internal ingestion.

Noscapine Noscapine is an opium alkaloid related to papaverine. It is used in only a few nonprescription preparations. It has been reported to reduce the frequency and severity of allergic cough (64). Nevertheless, the FDA advisory review panel has suggested additional testing to establish its effectiveness (1). Noscapine's antitussive effectiveness is dose related, and although some investigators believe that it is equipotent on a weight basis to codeine, safe nonprescription adult dosages range from 15 to 30 mg every 4–6 hours, not to exceed 180 mg a day (Table 8).

In therapeutic doses, noscapine shows little or no effect on the CNS or respiratory system and has neither analgesic properties nor addictive liabilities. Constipation and other GI reactions have not been encountered to a significant degree. Noscapine is apparently safe at currently available nonprescription dosages, but effectiveness has yet to be proven.

The following ingredients may have antitussive properties but need to be tested for effectiveness:

- Beechwood creosote;
- Benzonatate;
- Camphor (lozenges);
- Caramiphen edisylate (ethanedisulfonate);
- Carbetapentane citrate;

- Cod liver oil;

- Elm bark;

- Ethylmorphine hydrochloride;

- Eucalyptol/eucalyptus oil (topical/inhalant);

- Horehound (horehound fluidextract);

- Menthol/peppermint oil (topical/inhalant);

- Thymol (topical/inhalant);

- Turpentine oil (spirits of turpentine or rectified turpentine oil) (topical/inhalant).

Oral Antibacterials and Anesthetics

A sore throat may indicate a more serious disease that demands medical attention (for example, streptococcal pharyngitis), and self-treatment may mask the symptoms. When the sore throat symptom is not related to environmental factors, to allergic rhinitis, or to a cold, a physician should be consulted. Failure to consult a physician may result in a worsening of the condition and development of complications. For self-medication of sore throat symptoms, many products promote relief, but only those containing local anesthetics have any basis for effectiveness. Because most of these products are lozenges, sprays and mouthwashes, gargles, and throatwashes, effectiveness is limited to the mucous membranes of the oral tract that can be reached by the dosage form. Local anesthetics have no beneficial effect for the treatment of laryngitis because of the inability for drug delivery to the site of disease.

Antibacterial Agents

The primary purpose of a mouthwash is to cleanse and soothe. Most mouthwashes are promoted for bad breath with the suggestion that these products kill germs. The American Dental Association Council on Dental Therapeutics does not recognize substantial contributions to oral health from medicated mouthwashes (75). Much of the controversy surrounding the use of these products stems from the problems associated with substantiating germicidal or germistatic claims. There is no method that effectively compares the germicidal activity in the test tube with that in the oral cavity. There is also no adequate evidence that individuals benefit from a nonspecific change in the oral cavity flora; it is possible that alteration of the normal oral cavity flora actually may allow invasion by pathogenic organisms. In addition, most infectious sore throats are viral in origin, and using a lozenge or gargle promoted as an "antibacterial" does not influence the viral pharyngitis.

The antimicrobial substances in most commercial mouthwashes are phenols, alcohol, quaternary ammonium compounds, volatile oils, oxygenating agents, and iodine-containing preparations. However, these agents are believed to be of little value in treating sore throat symptoms.

Anesthetic Agents

A possible benefit of oral mouthwashes and gargles is derived from the anesthetic compounds they contain. These agents temporarily desensitize the sensory nerves in the pharyngeal mucosa, affording transient relief. The danger remains, however, in masking a symptom of a condition that may be harmful. Many commercially available lozenges also are promoted to treat sore throat symptoms. They usually contain an antibacterial agent in combination with a local anesthetic. The beneficial effect of these combinations is probably caused by the anesthetic agent.

Much controversy surrounds the effectiveness of the different anesthetic ingredients in lozenges and mouthwashes promoted for sore throats. The value and effectiveness of a local anesthetic agent usually are established by testing on human skin, oral mucosa, or tongue, not by pharyngeal tests. Consequently, patient satisfaction is probably the best indicator of these products' effectiveness until they meet the regulations being proposed by the FDA advisory review panel on OTC dentifrice and dental care drug products.

Benzocaine Benzocaine will produce local anesthesia in concentrations of 5–20%. Concentrations of less than 5% are not considered beneficial. There are currently no nonprescription sore throat preparations containing an effective benzocaine concentration.

Phenol and Phenol-Containing Salts Phenol and phenol-containing salts are included in several nonprescription liquids and lozenges. They are generally effective antibacterial agents in concentrations of 0.5–1.5% (76).

Benzyl Alcohol Benzyl alcohol is an effective oral anesthetic agent used in concentrations up to 10%.

The pharmacist should recommend a product that contains an effective dose of a local anesthetic and a minimum of extraneous compounds, because their effectiveness or value is doubtful. Moreover, extraneous compounds may increase the risk of a hypersensitivity reaction. The pharmacist also should try to follow up on patient response to recommended agents to suggest alternative nonprescription therapy for pharyngeal soreness.

Anticholinergics

Anticholinergics, such as atropine, theoretically can dry excessive nasal secretions associated with the common cold. They have been shown to have no effect on sneezing or congestion caused by the common cold (77, 78). High dosages are necessary for the therapeutic effect (79). The dosages of anticholinergics that were commonly found in nonprescription cold medications (0.06–0.2 mg total alkaloids) were ineffective in accomplishing the intended objective. To make up for this therapeutic shortcoming, these agents are usually found in products that also contain an antihistamine. The additive anticholinergic effect obtained from such a combination theoretically may help reduce secretions resulting from the common cold, but this claim remains to be proven for specific combinations. Such a combination exposes the patient to the antihistamine's unwanted sedative effects. It seems irrational to combine the therapeutic effect of one drug (in subtherapeutic amounts) with an unpredictable side effect of another in an attempt to achieve the effects obtainable with a larger (therapeutic) dose of the former.

Drug interactions involving anticholinergics are unlikely at the dosages used in cold or allergy remedies that do not contain other ingredients with anticholinergic effects. However, hypersensitivity to these relatively small amounts does occur. If a hypersensitive individual also suffers from narrow-angle glaucoma or enlarged prostate, a physician should be contacted before a preparation containing an anticholinergic is taken. These products should also be used with caution in nonhypersensitive patients with cardiovascular disease and glaucoma.

Pending further definitive dosage data, the anticholinergics available in nonprescription products should not be considered significant contributors to the relief of cold or allergy symptoms (1). The FDA review panel on drugs for OTC use had found that no anticholinergic agent is safe and effective for the treatment of the common cold. Any nonprescription product containing any anticholinergic intended for the treatment of the cold is considered misbranded (79).

Antipyretics/Analgesics

Patients with the common cold seldom have an actual clinical fever. More often they have a feeling of warmth but little or no temperature elevation. The usefulness of aspirin or acetaminophen lies in relieving the discomforts of generalized aches and pains or malaise associated with the viral infection. (See Chapter 5, *Internal Analgesic Products*.)

Ascorbic Acid (Vitamin C)

The claim that ascorbic acid is effective in preventing and treating the common cold is controversial. Linus Pauling, who popularized the use of ascorbic acid for the cold, recommends 1–5 g of ascorbic acid per day as a prophylactic measure and as much as 15 g per day to treat a cold (80). Many studies have been conducted, and although some have shown trends in favor of ascorbic acid's effectiveness, these studies have not shown the vitamin to be unequivocally effective in any dosage in either preventing colds or reducing their severity or duration (81, 82).

The potential for adverse effects associated with these large dosages is also debated. The most frequently noted adverse effect is diarrhea. Precipitation of urate, oxalate, or cystine stones in the urinary tract has been seen, although the potential for this problem increases with higher dosages of 1 g or above. The effects on the urinary excretion of other drugs also must be investigated because of ascorbic acid's ability to acidify the urine (83).

Urinary acidification increases the possibility of aminosalicylic acid crystalluria in patients receiving aminosalicylic acid in the free acid form. It also increases the excretion of drugs that are weak bases (e.g., amphetamines), reducing their effect, and increases renal tubular salicylate reabsorption, increasing serum salicylate concentrations. Ascorbic acid in dosages large enough to acidify the urine (4–12 g a day) should not be given with aminosalicylic acid and should be used cautiously when salicylates are taken in large dosages (3–5 g a day).

Ascorbic acid has been implicated in an interaction with warfarin in which the anticoagulant's hypoprothrombinemic effect was diminished (41, 57). Only isolated incidents were reported, however, and it is believed that the interaction either was dose dependent or occurred only in certain patients. Until further clarification is provided, practitioners should be aware of the possible interaction and inquire about ascorbic acid intake from single or multiple vitamin preparations by patients who respond erratically to an anticoagulant. The possibility of an exaggerated hypoprothrombinemic response also must be kept in mind when these patients stop taking the vitamin. The use of high-dose ascorbic acid has been demonstrated to raise ethinyl estradiol plasma levels in women taking estradiol-containing oral contraceptives (84). The clinical importance of this interaction is not known, but it potentially could be serious.

Diabetic patients who are taking ascorbic acid and monitoring their condition by testing their urine using glucose oxidase test kits may encounter false negative results; the copper reduction method may produce false positive results (57).

Zinc Gluconate

Zinc gluconate has been shown to inhibit rhinovirus growth in vitro and may be useful for the treatment and prophylaxis of the common cold (85). The exact antiviral mechanism is unknown (86). Studies have shown that zinc gluconate lozenges are well tolerated and decrease the signs and symptoms of the rhinovirus cold (86).

The only adverse effect of the lozenges reported by volunteers was altered taste of some foods and was considered minimal (86).

Despite the positive in vitro support, the efficacy of zinc gluconate for the treatment and prophylaxis of the cold remains controversial.

Adjunctive Therapy

Inhaling water vapor is an adjunctive therapeutic measure that provides a demulcent action on the respiratory mucosa and adds to and dilutes respiratory tract fluid, decreasing its viscosity (12). Humidifying inspired air may aid in the relief of cough and hoarseness accompanying laryngitis and associated colds. Inhalation of humidified, warm air has also been shown to reduce symptoms of allergic rhinitis and increase nasal patency without adverse effects (87). Humidification may be a prophylactic measure against upper respiratory infections when people are exposed to low relative humidities. This is usually the case during the winter months, when doors and windows are closed and the heat is on. The mucus viscosity increases with inspiration of dry air, and irritation of the respiratory mucosa may develop, creating a predisposition to viral or bacterial invasion. The relative humidity may be as low as 10% in the home on a cold day; 40–50% is necessary for comfort, and 60–80% is better for persons with respiratory problems. However, at this level, condensation on windows and walls is a limiting factor.

The oldest method of humidifying the air involves generating steam from a pot of boiling water or, more commonly, from an electric steam vaporizer. Newer methods involve formation of a cool mist by pumping water through a fine screen or by ultrasonically dispersing the water. Both methods disperse fine droplets of water. Therapeutically, the steam vaporizer does not seem to offer an advantage over the cool mist type. The cool mist vaporizers are safe in that they do not generate heat or hot water; however, they are noisier and humidify somewhat more slowly than the steam vaporizers, they become quickly contaminated, and they may lower room temperature because the water particles absorb heat from the surrounding air, chilling the air and causing air saturation at a lower temperature. In one study, 24 hospitalized patients contracted systemic infections with *Acinetobacter calcoaceticus* during a 4-month period; cold-air humidifiers at patients' bedsides were implicated as the source of infection in six. The outbreak was terminated with the removal of the humidifiers (88). It is important to follow the manufacturer's directions for cleaning the unit to avoid bacterial overgrowth. Steam vaporizers do not incur the hazards of contamination and do not lower room temperature.

If humidification is supplemented with a volatile substance (menthol or compound benzoin tincture), a steam vaporizer must be used. It has not been established whether these volatile substances are of therapeutic value, and therefore they may have no advantage over inhaling plain water vapor. In some cases they may even cause irritation of the respiratory tract and could be potentially dangerous if they reached high concentrations in a small enclosed room.

As an adjunctive measure, humidifying the inspired air is important. Either a steam-generated unit or a cool mist vaporizer may be used as prophylaxis and should be used at the cold's onset. It is also important to increase oral fluid intake (6–8 glasses of fluid a day) to prevent dehydration during a cold.

Devices have been introduced that force dry, hot air into the nose and mouth in an attempt to destroy the virus and therefore treat and "cure" the common cold. There is no evidence to support any claims that these devices either relieve the symptoms or cure the common cold (89).

PRODUCT SELECTION GUIDELINES

The effectiveness of many products available for self-medication of colds may be questionable, but they are generally safe when used as directed. Allergic rhinitis treatment provides comfort until the acute symptoms subside. Experience may influence selection. Nevertheless, the pharmacist must be prepared to distinguish between the common cold and allergic rhinitis on the basis of symptoms, recognize complications that may arise or have arisen, and recommend the proper approaches for control of the symptoms (self-medication or consulting a physician), including drugs, adjunctive measures, and duration of treatment.

Patient Considerations

When symptoms usually associated with the common cold are present, recognizing the underlying disorder is not difficult. However, recognition of the allergic rhinitis condition is often more involved. In both conditions the pharmacist should conduct a brief but careful history of the present illness. This history should provide information useful in distinguishing one disorder from another and in identifying those disorders that should or should not be self-medicated. The following specific points should be investigated:

- Abruptness of onset;
- Symptomatology;
- Intensity;
- Duration;
- Recurrence;
- Other medications being used;
- Family history of atopy.

Common cold onset generally is associated with a prodrome ("running nose" or dry throat); in fact, it is very common for people to predict that they are "coming down with a cold."

Early in a cold's development the symptoms are not very intense. As the infection runs its course, the symptoms may get worse, subject to patient variability and depending on the infecting organism. The intensity of symptoms in allergic rhinitis is based on the amount of allergen encountered and the degree of individual hypersensitivity. Generally, the symptoms are most intense following allergen exposure and subside over time unless additional exposures are encountered.

Duration of cold symptoms is a very important detail in deciding which course of action should be taken. Typically, the common cold lasts 4–7 days. If the problem persists beyond this time with no apparent improvement or if the cold symptoms tend to be recurrent, a physician should be consulted for an evaluation. Duration of allergic rhinitis symptoms is extremely variable, partially because of individual sensitivity to the allergen. If the patient has received no relief in 10 days of self-treatment, physician evaluation and proper management are indicated.

The recurrent nature of seasonal allergic rhinitis is a hallmark in differentiating this condition from other nonallergic respiratory conditions. The recurrence of symptoms often follows high pollen counts or patient activities that result in increased allergen exposure. If the symptomatology is present throughout the year or if it persists after the first killing frost, the condition may be perennial allergic rhinitis. Referral to a physician is desirable with perennial allergic rhinitis because of the prolonged duration of symptoms and the potential for developing complications.

Information on medications that have already been tried will aid the pharmacist not only in assessing the patient's current status but also in selecting a product. If, in the pharmacist's judgment, the measures were appropriate and were not effective, the patient should be encouraged to see a physician. If no medication was tried or if inadequate or inappropriate measures were taken, the pharmacist should recommend a more appropriate course of therapy. When a patient seeks the pharmacist's assistance in selecting a cold or allergy remedy, the pharmacist should question the individual about the presence of other acute or chronic illnesses. This process may identify patients for whom certain preparations should be used cautiously, if at all.

Orally administered preparations containing sympathomimetics should be given only on the advice of a physician to patients with hyperthyroidism (the patient is already predisposed to tachycardia and arrhythmias), hypertension (especially moderate to severe, where additional peripheral vasoconstriction may cause significant blood pressure elevation), diabetes mellitus (especially in insulin-dependent diabetics and in cases where glycogenolysis may cause the diabetes to go out of control), and ischemic heart disease or angina (where an increase in heart rate may precipitate an acute angina attack and possibly a subsequent myocardial infarct). These concerns center primarily on the oral administration of sympathomimetic decongestants, where systemic effects are predictable. Judiciously administered decongestant drops, sprays, or inhalations provide a local intranasal action without significant concern of systemic absorption.

Theoretically, all of these effects may occur when the sympathomimetics reach the systemic circulation. In practice, however, the effect on diabetic patients has not been a particular problem, except in extremely unstable (brittle) diabetics. The question often arises: "Should a diabetic patient take a liquid cough or cold preparation containing sugar?" The syrup vehicle may contain as much as 85% (weight per volume) sucrose, and each gram of sucrose has about 4 cal (17 kcal/tsp). If 4 tsp (about 70 kcal) are taken in 1 day, the additional (nondietary) calories may be clinically significant in a brittle diabetic. Consequently, a sugar-free preparation is preferable. In a stable diabetic, however, these additional calories probably would be of little concern. (See Chapter 16, *Diabetes Care Products*.)

Another factor that pharmacists should consider when counseling a diabetic patient is the alcohol content of the product to be used. Alcohol, like sucrose, will provide calories, more calories, in fact, than an equal weight of sucrose. Because most liquid cough remedies contain alcohol (1–25%, each gram providing about 7 kcal), it is clear that a brittle diabetic taking a recommended dose might experience some difficulty with diabetes control.

Persons taking disulfiram also must be cautious of alcohol in cough syrups. However, the minimum amount necessary to trigger an adverse reaction has not been established.

Products containing alcohol should also be used with caution in children. Adverse effects may be associated with excessive use.

The anticholinergic properties of antihistamines are usually not prominent in nonprescription preparations. However, the anticholinergic effects of atropine and other belladonna alkaloids in some allergy and cold remedies pose a potential problem. In cases of glaucoma or urinary retention secondary to prostatic hypertrophy, preparations containing anticholinergic agents and antihistamines, especially in combination, should be used only on a physician's advice.

The pharmacist should have a medication history to avoid possible drug interactions and to identify and avoid drug allergies or idiosyncrasies. In addition, a history of chronic use of topical nasal decongestants may help identify rhinitis medicamentosa.

Product Considerations

Because of the number of cold and allergy products (single-entity and combinations), it is important that the pharmacist become familiar with a few preparations, especially those found safe and effective by FDA advisory review panels and those found empirically useful, and recommend these products preferentially. The pharmacist who recommends a nonprescription product must know what effect is sought, which drug entity will produce this effect, how much of the drug is necessary to produce this effect, and which nonprescription product satisfactorily meets these needs. The dosage of each ingredient should be compared to the FDA recommended dosage for the appropriate age of the ultimate user.

If only one effect is sought (e.g., nasal decongestion), a preparation with a single agent in a full therapeutic dose should be used. When more than one effect is desired, selection becomes more complex. Several single-entity products may be used, but a combination product will usually be preferable to the patient. The pharmacist should be selective in recommending a combination because many of these preparations are extreme examples of "shotgun therapy."

Combinations recommended by the FDA advisory review panels provide a reasonable basis for selection when directions for use are followed carefully.

The pharmacist should select a combination product containing the desired agents in full therapeutic doses, with as few additional ingredients as possible. This goal, however, seldom is achievable. The pharmacist must decide which effect is most important and select the combination on the basis of the agent that will

produce this effect. For example, antihistamine efficacy in common cold treatment is doubtful, and this drawback is magnified by the subtherapeutic doses contained in some nonprescription remedies. Therefore, an antihistamine–decongestant product should be selected on the basis of the decongestant, with only secondary consideration being given to the antihistamine. Alternatively, the antihistamine is the important ingredient when selecting a product for allergic rhinitis.

There is no evidence that incorporating other ancillary agents or other ingredients of the same pharmacologic class in a subtherapeutic dose provides more relief or even as much relief as one agent in its full therapeutic dose. There is also no evidence that supports an increased efficacy when two or more antihistamines are combined within a product (90). The addition of a decongestant in sufficient dosage to the antihistamine in the allergic rhinitis product is rational and may provide additional relief of symptoms as well as theoretically counteracting drowsiness caused by antihistamines.

Combination products containing analgesic and antipyretic agents generally should not be recommended. Their routine use carries the risk of masking a fever that may indicate a bacterial infection. Also, if an adverse effect should occur, confusion would exist as to which agent was the culprit. Such agents should be administered separately and only when needed.

Similarly, preparations that do not disclose the amounts of ingredients on the package should not be recommended. It would be difficult for a pharmacist to justify recommending a product to ameliorate a symptom when there is no indication as to how much of the active ingredients the product contains.

In general, the use of timed-release preparations allows better patient compliance and increased patient convenience. However, some practitioners feel that these advantages may be outweighed by the fact that drug bioavailability in this dosage form may be neither uniform nor reliable. The pharmacist's recommendation of a timed-release preparation should be based on the presence of indicated agents in therapeutic doses and on the pharmacist's experience and the product's success record.

Much controversy surrounds the advantages of oral nasal decongestants over the topical agents. Proponents of oral decongestants state that these agents can affect all respiratory membranes, that they are unaffected by the character of mucus, that they do not induce pathologic changes in the nasal mucosa, and that they relieve nasal obstruction without the additional irritation of locally applied medication.

There is also evidence to support the value of topically applied vasoconstrictors (91). Although nasal sprays and drops do not represent the ideal dosage form, they do provide rapid relief. Because the relief is so dramatic, the patient tends to overuse topical agents, risking drug-induced irritation of the nasal mucosa, alteration of the mucosal ciliary movement, and possibly rhinitis medicamentosa.

Combining topical therapy with oral decongestant therapy is also a controversial procedure. However, judicious use of an oral decongestant proven safe and effective along with a fast-acting topical agent presents a definite advantage. With this combination, the patient experiences rapid relief from the topically applied decongestant and possibly a greater degree of relief through the systemic circulation from the oral agent if given in an adequate dosage. Depending on the topical agent being used, a longer lasting effect also is possible with this combined therapy.

Patient Consultation

In almost all cases of self-medication, the pharmacist is the first and only knowledgeable professional contacted. If the pharmacist takes the time to identify the patient's problem and ensure proper product selection, advice regarding proper use also must be considered essential to fulfilling professional responsibility.

Patients cannot always be depended on to read, understand, and follow the package instructions. There is a tendency to believe in the philosophy that "if one is good, two are better." Because of the movement toward formulating nonprescription drug products in accordance with the FDA recommended dosages, this is not the case. Pharmacists should caution patients against increasing the dosage or frequency of administration of any medication.

Even when antihistamines are taken in recommended amounts, they may cause transient drowsiness. Patients should be advised of this effect, especially if they are taking a prescription medication that also depresses the CNS. Patients should be advised of the possible effects and should determine what effect the antihistamine has on them before engaging in activities requiring mental alertness, such as driving an automobile or operating heavy machinery. The patient should also be specifically warned of the additive sedation that will occur if the antihistamine is combined with alcohol.

Nasal solutions may become contaminated. The pharmacist should recommend that the tip of the dropper or the spray applicator be rinsed in hot water after use, that only one person use the spray or drop applicator, and that the bottle or spray be discarded when the medication is no longer needed. Contamination of the nasal dropper also may be minimized by not touching the nose or the nasal surface with the dropper itself.

In patients with allergic rhinitis, the presence of coughing, wheezing, tightness in chest (asthma), pain above the teeth, on the sides of the nose, or around the eyes (sinusitis), and earache are all indications for medical advice. In addition, if nonprescription drugs are not markedly effective or if side effects are persistent even at reduced dosages, the patient should consult a physician.

Nondrug measures (humidification, increased fluid intake, and local heat) may be recommended, and although these suggestions may not seem acceptable to the patient who desires a medication, they may be quite beneficial. The pharmacist's recommendation that the patient use humidification and increase fluid intake is in the patient's best interest. Using saline gargles several times a day helps relieve an inflamed throat. Patients using saline gargles should be warned against swallowing the solution. These solutions should also be used with caution by patients with cardiac disease, hypertension, or renal failure or by patients who are on salt-restricted diets. Tepid (not cold) water sponge baths, with or without an antipyretic, usually cause an elevated temperature to fall.

A cold usually lasts 7 days. The duration of therapy depends on which day in the course of the cold the medication is begun. If symptoms persist beyond the arbitrary, yet fairly reliable, 7-day limit in spite of adequate therapy, a physician should be consulted. If after 2 or 3 days of therapy the symptoms do not improve or become more intense, or if a fever, a very painful sore throat, or a cough productive of a mucopurulent sputum develops, the patient should seek a physician's diagnosis of the condition.

It is important that the patient realizes that a cold will usually resolve itself in spite of the medication and other measures recommended, that the medication is intended only to relieve discomfort, and that relief should occur in a week or less. The concern for duration of self-medication stems not only from the potential adverse effects of some medications but also from the minority of cold sufferers who may develop complications, such as secondary bacterial infections. If the pharmacist does not stipulate a time limit for therapy, patients may unknowingly continue self-medicating with little effect, prolonging their discomfort and delaying the time for a physician's diagnosis and appropriate treatment.

Product selection must be based not only on the presence of an effective agent in a therapeutic amount but also on underlying disorders that may be influenced adversely by the recommended therapy. Having chosen the product, the pharmacist must then ensure that the patient knows how to take the medication and what to expect from it with regard to symptomatic relief as well as adverse effects. The patient must be told for how long the medication should be taken. Realizing that questions may arise later, the pharmacist should encourage the patient to return or call back.

SUMMARY

By evaluating the presenting symptoms the pharmacist usually can distinguish the common cold from disorders such as influenza or allergic rhinitis and offer proper suggestions for treatment. The pharmacist also can offer the allergic rhinitis sufferer medications to provide symptomatic relief. By conducting a careful history and recognizing the pertinent symptoms, a partial diminution of the symptoms may be achieved through advice and medication.

Recommendations for the common cold should be directed at relieving symptoms; those for allergic rhinitis should be directed at preventing symptoms. The pharmacist's endorsement of a shotgun remedy is irrational because the intensity of symptoms will vary from hour to hour. Recommending a particular product is also irresponsible if the product contains agents in less than therapeutic amounts.

Common cold treatment objectives include reducing nasal secretions, opening congested nasal passages, reducing frequency of a cough, soothing a sore throat, overcoming the hoarseness of laryngitis, and relieving feverishness and headache. For allergic rhinitis the treatment is directed at blocking or competing with the effect of released histamine, relieving nasal congestion, and palliating secondary symptoms such as pharyngitis and headache. Effective treatments for nasal congestion include topically applied phenylephrine hydrochloride (0.25–1.0%) used every 4 hours, if needed, or oxymetazoline hydrochloride (0.05%) used twice a day, if needed. To augment the effects of the topical decongestant, an oral nasal decongestant also may be recommended. Pseudoephedrine, 60 mg every 4 hours, or phenylpropanolamine, as much as 50 mg 3 times a day, is usually effective.

The very few oral nasal decongestants available as single-entity products should be recommended. Topically applied products should contain only the decongestant. For example, antihistamines add no beneficial effect to a topical decongestant preparation and may increase the likelihood of a hypersensitivity reaction. Oral antihistamines in combination with nasal decongestants may be indicated in allergic rhinitis, but should be avoided in the treatment of cold because of the lack of evidence to support the beneficial effect of their use in the treatment of the cold.

The frequency of cough resulting from colds can usually be controlled by humidification of the inspired air (with hot or cold vaporizer) and/or use of medication. A demulcent to the mucosa (hard candy or cough drop), an expectorant (guaifenesin), a cough suppressant (codeine or dextromethorphan), and/or the antihistamine diphenhydramine, used as an antitussive, are included in the armamentarium for the treatment of a cough associated with a cold. Humidification should be started early in the course of a cold and continued throughout. Products that contain a cough suppressant in combination with an expectorant should not be recommended. In the case of a dry cough, the dosage of the cough suppressant is the criterion by which a product is selected. Productive coughs should not be treated with cough suppressants. Administration of 15 mg of codeine or dextromethorphan usually decreases the cough's frequency and intensity.

The dry, sore throat present in colds and, to a lesser extent, in allergic rhinitis may be relieved by dissolving a piece of hard candy in the mouth to stimulate saliva flow. Frequent warm normal saline gargles may relieve symptoms. Topical antibacterials for a viral infection or allergic rhinitis are unwarranted. Significant relief may be obtained from a lozenge or throat spray containing an anesthetic such as hexylresorcinol or phenol in sufficient concentration. A sore throat that is markedly sore and accompanied by swollen lymph nodes, fever, and constitutional symptoms may be caused by bacterial rather than viral infection. The patient should be directed to seek medical care for appropriate diagnostic tests and antimicrobial therapy. For nonbacterial pharyngitis, a sore throat product may be used for as long as the symptom persists.

Laryngitis may be managed by water vapor inhalation, voice rest, and avoidance of inhaled irritants such as tobacco smoke. Dissolving lozenges in the mouth, gargling, and use of a throat spray do little to soothe the inflamed laryngeal tissues. Steam vapors, by virtue of reaching the more distal laryngeal tissue, may be more useful.

Relief from feverishness and headache may be provided by using an analgesic/antipyretic, such as aspirin, acetaminophen, or ibuprofen. Products containing these agents in combination with other ingredients are not recommended. Taking an antipyretic agent regularly during the common cold or acute allergic rhinitis masks the possible development of fever, which could indicate a secondary bacterial infection. An antipyretic agent should be used to bring acute relief only as needed. Products containing aspirin or other salicylates should be avoided in children and adolescents because of the associated risk of Reye's syndrome.

Antihistamines are effective at abating symptoms of allergic rhinitis; however, their role in the treatment of symptoms associated with the common cold is controversial and, at best, only adjunctive because of mild anticholinergic drying effects. Chlorpheniramine maleate, administered orally in doses of as much as 4 mg, is effective in the treatment of allergic rhinitis and only slightly sedative. There is marked individual variability among the different antihistamines. The pharmacist should be aware of this variability and should be prepared to suggest an alternative if relief is not obtained with the original agent. Most antihistamines in commercial products are found in combination with other ingredients. A combination of these agents may be best used to treat allergic disorders. The only rational combination for allergic rhinitis treatment is an oral antihistamine with an oral nasal decongestant. Other ingredients found in nonprescription products are of dubious efficacy.

The duration of therapy depends on when during the course of a cold the patient decides to start treatment. In any case, the patient should be able to stop treatment on the sixth or seventh day of the cold. Slight symptoms, such as cough, may persist for another day or so and should be treated, if necessary.

The duration of treatment of allergic rhinitis should be limited to 3 days when topical nasal decongestants are used, in order to minimize the chances of rhinitis medicamentosa. Generally, oral decongestant therapy should be limited to 10 days. The patient's need of the oral agents for longer than 10 days may indicate the development of complications, and the patient should be referred to a physician. An antihistamine product may be used prophylactically for acute allergic rhinitis during seasons when exposure to allergens is increased.

Patients who have a common cold or allergic rhinitis offer the pharmacist many opportunities to be involved. Although pharmacists often cannot counsel every cold or hay fever sufferer, they should be available on request and volunteer as other professional responsibilities permit.

REFERENCES

1 *Federal Register, 41,* 38312 (1976).

2 A. C. Guyton, "Textbook of Medical Physiology," 6th ed., W. B. Saunders, Philadelphia, Pa., 1981, p. 487.

3 "Mechanisms in Respiratory Toxicology," Vol. I, H. Witchi and P. Nettesheim, Eds., CRC Press, Boca Raton, Fla., pp. 262–263.

4 "Cecil Textbook of Medicine," 18th ed., J. B. Wyngarden and L. H. Smith, Jr., Eds., W. B. Saunders, Philadelphia, Pa., 1988, pp. 1750–1757.

5 A. G. Christie, "Infectious Disease—Epidemiology and Clinical Practice," 4th ed., Churchill Livingston, New York, N.Y., 1987, pp. 416–17, 442, 444–5, 459.

6 S. J. Sperber and F. G. Hayden, *Antimicrob. Agents Chemother., 32,* 409 (1988).

7 "Current Estimates from the National Health Interview Survey, United States, 1985," Vital and Health Statistics Series 10, No. 160, National Center for Health Statistics, Public Health Service, Washington, D.C., 1986.

8 B. K. Cypress, in "The National Ambulatory Medical Care Survey, United States, 1980," National Center for Health Statistics, Vital and Health Statistics Series 13, No. 71, Public Health Service, Washington, D.C., 1983, pp. 1–47.

9 S. R. Lowenstein and T. A. Parrino, *Adv. Intern. Med., 32,* 207 (1987).

10 "Medical Notes on the Common Cold," Burroughs Wellcome, Research Triangle Park, N.C., 1972.

11 W. B. Pratt, "Chemotherapy of Infection," Oxford University Press, New York, N.Y., 1977, pp. 413–415.

12 B. Lachman, *Am. Pharm., NS27,* 51 (1987).

13 J. Price, *Br. Med. J., 288,* 1666 (1984).

14 I. Gregg, *Eur. J. Resp. Dis., 64,* 369 (1983).

15 "Current Medical Diagnosis and Treatment, 1987," M. A. Krupp et al., Eds., Appleton and Lange, Norwalk, Ct., 1987, p. 119.

16 V. A. Serrano Murphy and G. Bubica, "Applied Therapeutics—The Clinical Use of Drugs," 4th ed., L. Y. Young and M. A. Koda-Kimble, Eds., Applied Therapeutics, Inc., Vancouver, Wash., 1988, pp. 1817–1860.

17 P. Refinetti et al., *Curr. Ther. Res., 30,* 33 (1981).

18 *Federal Register, 54,* 8495 (1989).

19 R. W. Steele et al., *J. Pediatr., 77,* 824 (1970).

20 S. W. McFadden and J. E. Haddow, *Pediatrics, 43,* 622 (1969).

21 *Federal Register, 42,* 35346 (1977).

22 *Morbid. Mortal. Week. Rep., 31,* 289 (1982).

23 M. F. Rogers et al., *Pediatrics, 75,* 260 (1985).

24 A. J. Ricketti, "Allergic Diseases—Diagnosis and Management," R. Patterson, Ed., Lippincott, Philadelphia, Pa., 1985, pp. 207–231.

25 W. B. Sherman, "Hypersensitivity Mechanisms and Management," W. B. Saunders, Philadelphia, Pa., 1968.

26 J. M. O'Loughlin, *Drug Ther., 4,* 47 (1974).

27 L. Tuft, "Allergy Management in Clinical Practice," C. V. Mosby, St. Louis, Mo., 1973, pp. 185–238.

28 W. E. Serafin and K. F. Austen, *N. Engl. J. Med., 317,* 30 (1987).

29 P. M. Seebohm, *Postgrad. Med., 53,* 52 (1973).

30 J. A. Church, *Clin. Pediatr., 19,* 657 (1980).

31 G. M. Trask et al., *Am. J. Orthod. Dentofacial Orthop., 92,* 286 (1987).

32 G. G. Shapiro, *J. Allerg. Clin. Immunol., 82,* 935 (1988).

33 J. M. Bernstein et al., *Otolaryngol. Head Neck Surg., 89,* 874 (1981).

34 F. E. R. Simons, *Ped. Clin. N. Am., 35,* 1053 (1988).

35 R. K. Bush, *Hosp. Form., 23,* 245 (1988).

36 R. M. Naclerio et al., *Pediatr. Infect. Dis. J., 7,* 218 (1988).

37 "International Encyclopedia in Medicine," 2nd ed., J. R. DiPalma, Ed., McGraw-Hill, New York, N.Y., 1982, pp. 335–345.

38 "Goodman and Gilman's The Pharmacological Basis of Therapeutics," 7th ed., A. G. Gilman et al., Eds., Macmillan, New York, N.Y., 1985, pp. 607–610, 621.

39 "Drug Evaluations," 6th ed., American Medical Association, Chicago, Ill., 1986, pp. 371, 374, 1042.

40 L. Schaaf et al., *J. Allerg. Clin. Immunol., 63,* 129 (1979).

41 "Evaluations of Drug Interactions," A. F. Shinn, Ed., C. V. Mosby, Princeton, N.J., 1987, pp. 4/25, 15/5.

42 *Med. Lett. Drug. Ther., 753,* 105 (1987).

43 *Am. J. Hosp. Pharm., 46,* 1512 (1989).

44 H. M. Druce and M. A. Kaliner, *J. Am. Med. Assoc., 259,* 260 (1988).

45 F. E. R. Simons, "The Child With Asthma. Report of the Sixth Canadian Ross Conference in Pediatrics," F. E. R. Simons, Ed., Ross Laboratories, Montreal, Canada, 1986, pp. 140–145.

46 D. E. Maddox and C. E. Reed, *Ann. Allerg., 59,* 43 (1987).

47 B. J. Thack et al., *N. Engl. J. Med., 293,* 486 (1975).

48 V. J. Cirillo and K. F. Tempero, *Am. J. Hosp. Pharm., 33,* 1200 (1976).

49 C. Hale and T. Heins, *Med. J. Austr., 1,* 112 (1978).

50 D. S. Pearlman, *Drugs, 12,* 258 (1976).

51 "Drill's Pharmacology in Medicine," J. R. DiPalma, Ed., McGraw-Hill, New York, N.Y., 1971, pp. 655.

52 *Federal Register, 41,* 38397 (1976).

53 E. W. Martin, "Techniques of Medication," Lippincott, Philadelphia, Pa., 1979, p. 91.

54 J. T. Connell, *Ann. Allergy, 27,* 541 (1969).

55 G. Aschan and B. Drettner, *Eye Ear Nose Throat Mon., 43,* 66 (1964).

56 *Federal Register, 41,* 38398 (1976).

57 P. D. Hasten and J. R. Horn, "Drug Interactions," 6th ed., Lea and Febiger, Philadelphia, Pa., 1989.

58 *Federal Register, 41,* 38370 (1976).

59 S. R. Hirsch, *Drug Ther., 5,* 179 (1976).

60 S. R. Hirsch et al., *Chest, 63,* 9 (1973).

61 J. J. Kuhn et al., *Chest, 82,* 713 (1982).

62 R. E. Robinson et al., *Curr. Ther. Res., 22,* 284 (1977).

63 C. J. Polson and R. N. Tattersall, "Clinical Toxicology," Lippincott, Philadelphia, Pa., 1973, p. 92.

64 "The United States Dispensatory," 27th ed., A. Osol and R. Pratt, Eds., Lippincott, Philadelphia, Pa., 1973, pp. 354, 571, 794, 947.

65 J. McLeod, *N. Engl. J. Med., 268,* 146 (1963).

66 B. R. Manno and J. E. Manno, *Clin. Toxicol., 10,* 221 (1977).

67 *Federal Register, 41,* 38339 (1976).

68 M. Borde and S. H. Nizamie, *Lancet, 1,* 760 (1988).

69 *Federal Register, 52,* 30049 (1987).

70 Committee on Drugs, American Academy of Pediatrics, *Pediatrics, 62,* 118 (1978).

71 H. Matthys et al., *J. Intern. Med., 11,* 92 (1983).

72 B. Katona and S. Wason, *N. Engl. J. Med., 314,* 993 (1986).

73 S. MacRury et al., *Postgrad. Med., 63,* 587 (1987).

74 Product information, Parke, Davis and Company, Morris Plains, N.J.

75 "Accepted Dental Therapeutics," 38th ed., American Dental Association, Chicago, Ill., 1979.

76 J. C. Valle-Jones, *Practitioner, 227,* 1037 (1983).

77 M. J. Gaffery et al., *Am. Rev. Respir. Dis., 135,* 241 (1987).

78 P. Borum, *Postgrad. Med., 63,* 61 (1987).

79 *Federal Register, 50,* 46582 (1985).

80 L. Pauling, "Vitamin C and the Common Cold," Freeman, San Francisco, Calif., 1970.

81 *Med. Lett. Drug Ther., 16,* 85 (1974).

82 J. L. Coulehan, *Postgrad. Med., 66,* 153 (1979).

83 *Med. Lett. Drug Ther., 12,* 105 (1970).

84 D. J. Black et al., *Br. Med. J., 282,* 1516 (1981).

85 J. C. Godfrey, *Antimicrob. Agents Chemother., 32,* 605 (1988).

86 W. Al-Nakib et al., *J. Antimicrob. Chemother., 20,* 893 (1987).

87 D. Ophir et al., *Ann. Allerg., 60,* 239 (1988).

88 P. W. Smith and R. M. Massanari, *J. Am. Med. Assoc., 237,* 795 (1977).

89 *Med. Lett. Drug Ther., 31,* 8 (1989).

90 L. Hendeles et al., *Am. J. Hosp. Pharm., 37,* 1496 (1980).

91 *Ann. Otol. Laryngol. Rhinol., 86,* 310 (1977).

COLD, ALLERGY, COUGH PRODUCT TABLE

Product (Manufacturer)	Dose Form	Decongestant	Antihistamine
Aceta-Gesic Relief of Pain (Rugby)	tablet		phenyltoloxamine citrate, 30 mg
Actagen (Goldline)	syrup	pseudoephedrine hydrochloride, 30 mg/5 ml	triprolidine hydrochloride, 1.25 mg/5 ml
	tablet	pseudoephedrine hydrochloride, 60 mg	triprolidine hydrochloride, 2.5 mg
Actidil (Burroughs Wellcome)	syrup		triprolidine hydrochloride, 1.25 mg/5 ml
	tablet		triprolidine hydrochloride, 2.5 mg
Actifed (Burroughs Wellcome)	capsule tablet	pseudoephedrine hydrochloride, 60 mg	triprolidine hydrochloride, 2.5 mg
	syrup	pseudoephedrine hydrochloride, 30 mg/5 ml	triprolidine hydrochloride, 1.25 mg/5 ml
Actifed Plus (Burroughs Wellcome)	capsule tablet	pseudoephedrine hydrochloride, 30 mg	triprolidine hydrochloride, 1.25 mg
Actifed 12-Hour (Burroughs Wellcome)	capsule	pseudoephedrine hydrochloride, 120 mg	triprolidine hydrochloride, 5 mg
Actifed with Codeine (Burroughs Wellcome)	syrup	pseudoephedrine hydrochloride, 30 mg/5 ml	triprolidine hydrochloride, 1.25 mg/5 ml
Alamine[b] (Vortech)	liquid	phenylephrine hydrochloride, 5 mg/5 ml	chlorpheniramine maleate, 2 mg/5 ml
Alamine-C (Vortech)	liquid	pseudoephedrine hydrochloride, 30 mg/5 ml	chlorpheniramine maleate, 2 mg/5 ml
Alamine Expectorant (Vortech)	liquid	pseudoephedrine hydrochloride, 30 mg/5 ml	
Alamine Expectorant Modified Formula (Vortech)	liquid	pseudoephedrine hydrochloride, 30 mg/5 ml	
Alka-Seltzer Plus Cold (Miles)	tablet	phenylpropanolamine bitartrate, 24 mg	chlorpheniramine maleate, 2 mg
Alka-Seltzer Plus Night-Time Cold (Miles)	tablet	phenylpropanolamine bitartrate, 24 mg	diphenhydramine citrate, 38 mg
Alleract Decongestant (Burroughs Wellcome)	caplet tablet	pseudoephedrine hydrochloride, 60 mg	triprolidine hydrochloride, 2.5 mg
Aller-Chlor (Rugby)	tablet		chlorpheniramine maleate, 4 mg
	syrup		chlorpheniramine maleate, 2 mg/5 ml
Allerest (Fisons)	tablet	phenylpropanolamine hydrochloride, 18.7 mg	chlorpheniramine maleate, 2 mg
Allerest Children's (Fisons)	tablet	phenylpropanolamine hydrochloride, 9.4 mg	chlorpheniramine maleate, 1 mg
Allerest Headache Strength (Fisons)	tablet	phenylpropanolamine hydrochloride, 18.7 mg	chlorpheniramine maleate, 2 mg
Allerest No Drowsiness (Fisons)	tablet	pseudoephedrine hydrochloride, 30 mg	
Allerest Sinus Pain Formula (Fisons)	tablet	phenylpropanolamine hydrochloride, 18.7 mg	chlorpheniramine maleate, 2 mg
Allerest, 12 Hour (Fisons)	caplet	phenylpropanolamine hydrochloride, 75 mg	chlorpheniramine maleate, 12 mg

Analgesic	Expectorant	Cough Suppressant	Other Ingredients
acetaminophen, 325 mg			
			alcohol, 4% sorbitol
			sorbitol (syrup)
acetaminophen, 500 mg			
		codeine phosphate, [a] 10 mg/5 ml	alcohol, 4.3% sorbitol
			alcohol, 5%
		codeine phosphate,[a] 10 mg/5 ml	alcohol, 5%
	guaifenesin, 100 mg/5 ml	codeine phosphate,[a] 10 mg/5 ml	alcohol, 7.5%
	guaifenesin, 100 mg/5 ml	codeine phosphate,[a] 10 mg/5 ml	alcohol, 20%
aspirin, 325 mg			
aspirin, 325 mg			sodium, 506 mg lemon flavor
			saccharin sorbitol
acetaminophen, 325 mg			
acetaminophen, 325 mg			
acetaminophen, 500 mg			

COLD, ALLERGY, COUGH PRODUCT TABLE, continued

Product (Manufacturer)	Dose Form	Decongestant	Antihistamine
Allerfrin OTC (Rugby)	syrup	pseudoephedrine hydrochloride, 30 mg/5 ml	triprolidine hydrochloride, 1.25 mg/5 ml
	tablet	pseudoephedrine hydrochloride, 60 mg	triprolidine hydrochloride, 2.5 mg
Allergy Relief Medicine (Various manufacturers)	tablet	phenylpropanolamine hydrochloride, 25 mg	chlorpheniramine maleate, 4 mg
AllerMax (Pfeiffer)	caplet		diphenhydramine hydrochloride, 25 mg
			diphenhydramine hydrochloride, 50 mg
All-Nite Cold Formula (Major)	liquid	pseudoephedrine hydrochloride, 10 mg/5 ml	doxylamine succinate, 1.25 mg/5 ml
Ambenyl-D Decongestant Cough Formula (Forest)	liquid	pseudoephedrine hydrochloride, 30 mg/5 ml	
Amonidrin (Forest)	tablet		
Anodynos Forte (Buffington)	tablet	phenylephrine hydrochloride, 5 mg	chlorpheniramine maleate, 2 mg
Anti-Tuss (Century)	syrup		
Aprodine (Major)	tablet	pseudoephedrine hydrochloride, 60 mg	triprolidine hydrochloride, 2.5 mg
A.R.M. (SmithKline)	caplet	phenylpropanolamine hydrochloride, 25 mg	chlorpheniramine maleate, 4 mg
Banophen (Major)	capsule tablet		diphenhydramine hydrochloride, 25 mg
Bayer Children's Cold (Glenbrook)	tablet	phenylpropanolamine hydrochloride, 3.125 mg	
Bayer Cough Syrup for Children (Glenbrook)	syrup	phenylpropanolamine hydrochloride, 9 mg/5 ml	
Benadryl Decongestant Kapseals (Parke-Davis)	capsule	pseudoephedrine hydrochloride, 60 mg	diphenhydramine hydrochloride, 25 mg
Benadryl Plus (Parke-Davis)	tablet	pseudoephedrine hydrochloride, 30 mg	diphenhydramine hydrochloride, 12.5 mg
Benadryl Plus Nighttime (Parke-Davis)	liquid	pseudoephedrine hydrochloride, 30 mg/5 ml	diphenhydramine hydrochloride, 25 mg/5 ml
Benadryl 25 (Parke-Davis)	capsule tablet		diphenhydramine hydrochloride, 25 mg
Benylin (Parke-Davis)	liquid		diphenhydramine hydrochloride, 12.5 mg/5 ml
Benylin D (Parke-Davis)	elixir	pseudoephedrine hydrochloride, 30 mg/5 ml	diphenhydramine hydrochloride, 12.5 mg/5 ml

Analgesic	Expectorant	Cough Suppressant	Other Ingredients
acetaminophen, 167 mg/5 ml		dextromethorphan hydro-bromide, 5 mg/5 ml	alcohol, 25%
	guaifenesin, 100 mg/5 ml	dextromethorphan hydro-bromide, 15 mg/5 ml	alcohol, 9.5% menthol saccharin sorbitol sucrose
	guaifenesin, 200 mg		
salicylamide, 32.5 mg acetaminophen, 357 mg			caffeine
	guaifenesin, 100 mg/5 ml		alcohol, 3.5%
aspirin, 81 mg			
		dextromethorphan hydro-bromide, 7.5 mg/5 ml	alcohol, 5% saccharin sorbitol cherry flavor
acetaminophen, 500 mg			
acetaminophen, 500 mg/5 ml			alcohol, 10% saccharin honey-lemon flavor
	ammonium chloride, 125 mg/5 ml sodium citrate, 50 mg/5 ml		alcohol, 5%
			alcohol, 5% saccharin sucrose menthol

COLD, ALLERGY, COUGH PRODUCT TABLE, continued

Product (Manufacturer)	Dose Form	Decongestant	Antihistamine
Benylin DM Cough Syrup (Parke-Davis)	liquid		
Benylin Expectorant (Parke-Davis)	liquid		
BQ Cold (Bristol-Myers)	tablet	phenylpropanolamine hydrochloride, 12.5 mg	chlorpheniramine maleate, 2 mg
Breonesin[b] (Winthrop)	capsule		
Bromatap[b] (Goldline)	elixir	phenylpropanolamine hydrochloride, 12.5 mg/5 ml	brompheniramine maleate, 2 mg/5 ml
Bydramine Cough (Major)	syrup		diphenhydramine hydrochloride, 12.5 mg/5ml
Cenafed (Century)	syrup	pseudoephedrine hydrochloride, 30 mg/5 ml	
	tablet	pseudoephedrine hydrochloride, 30 mg or 60 mg	
Cenafed Plus (Century)	tablet	pseudoephedrine hydrochloride, 60 mg	triprolidine hydrochloride, 2.5 mg
Cerose-DM[b] (Wyeth-Ayerst)	liquid	phenylephrine hydrochloride, 10 mg/5 ml	chlorpheniramine maleate, 4 mg/5 ml
Cheracol (Upjohn)	syrup		
Cheracol D (Upjohn)	syrup		
Cheracol Plus (Upjohn)	liquid	phenylpropanolamine hydrochloride, 25 mg/15 ml	chlorpheniramine maleate, 4 mg/15 ml
Cheralin Expectorant (Lannett)	liquid		
Chexit (Sandoz)	tablet	phenylpropanolamine hydrochloride, 25 mg	pheniramine maleate, 12.5 mg pyrilamine maleate, 12.5 mg
Chlor-Rest (Rugby)	tablet	phenylpropanolamine hydrochloride, 18.7 mg	chlorpheniramine maleate, 2 mg
Chlor-Trimeton (Schering)	syrup		chlorpheniramine maleate, 2 mg/5 ml
	tablet		chlorpheniramine maleate, 4 mg
Chlor-Trimeton Decongestant (Schering)	tablet	pseudoephedrine sulfate, 60 mg	chlorpheniramine maleate, 4 mg
Chlor-Trimeton Long-Acting Decongestant Repetabs (Schering)	tablet	pseudoephedrine sulfate, 120 mg	chlorpheniramine maleate, 8 mg
Chlor-Trimeton Long-Acting Repetabs (Schering)	tablet, timed release		chlorpheniramine maleate, 8 mg
Chlor-Trimeton Maximum Strength (Schering)	tablet		chlorpheniramine maleate, 12 mg

Analgesic	Expectorant	Cough Suppressant	Other Ingredients
	ammonium chloride, 125 mg/5 ml sodium citrate, 50 mg/5 ml	dextromethorphan hydrobromide, 10 mg/5 ml	alcohol, 5%
	guaifenesin, 100 mg/5 ml	dextromethorphan hydrobromide, 5 mg/5 ml	alcohol, 5%
acetaminophen, 325 mg			sucrose
	guaifenesin, 200 mg		
			alcohol, 2.3% saccharin sorbitol grape flavor
			alcohol, 5%
		dextromethorphan hydrobromide, 15 mg/5 ml	alcohol, 2.4% saccharin
	guaifenesin, 100 mg/5 ml	codeine phosphate[a], 10 mg/5 ml	alcohol, 4.75%
	guaifenesin, 100 mg/5 ml	dextromethorphan hydrobromide, 10 mg/5 ml	alcohol, 4.75%
		dextromethorphan hydrobromide, 20 mg/15 ml	alcohol, 8%
	potassium guaiacolsulfonate, 88 mg/5 ml ammonium chloride, 88 mg/5 ml antimony potassium tartrate, 1 mg/5 ml		alcohol, 3%
acetaminophen, 325 mg	terpin hydrate, 180 mg	dextromethorphan hydrobromide, 30 mg	

COLD, ALLERGY, COUGH PRODUCT TABLE, continued

Product (Manufacturer)	Dose Form	Decongestant	Antihistamine
Chlor-Trimeton Sinus (Schering)	caplet	phenylpropanolamine hydro-chloride, 12.5 mg	chlorpheniramine maleate, 2 mg
CoAdvil (Whitehall)	caplet	pseudoephedrine hydrochloride, 30 mg	
Co-Apap (Various manufacturers)	tablet	pseudoephedrine hydrochloride, 30 mg	chlorpheniramine maleate, 2 mg
Codimal (Central)	capsule tablet	pseudoephedrine hydrochloride, 30 mg	chlorpheniramine maleate, 2 mg
Codimal DM[b] (Central)	syrup	phenylephrine hydrochloride, 5 mg/5 ml	pyrilamine maleate, 8.3 mg/5 ml
Codimal Expectorant (Central)	liquid	phenylpropanolamine hydro-chloride, 25 mg/5 ml	
Codimal PH (Central)	syrup	phenylephrine hydrochloride, 5 mg/5 ml	pyrilamine maleate, 8.3 mg/5 ml
Codistan No. 1 (Vortech)	syrup		
Coldonyl (Dover)	tablet	phenylephrine hydrochloride, 5 mg	
Colrex Expectorant (Reid-Rowell)	liquid		
Comtrex (Bristol-Myers)	caplet tablet	pseudoephedrine hydrochloride, 30 mg	chlorpheniramine maleate, 2 mg
	liquid	pseudoephedrine hydrochloride, 10 mg/5 ml	chlorpheniramine maleate, 0.65 mg/5 ml
	liqui-gel	phenylpropanolamine hydro-chloride, 12.5 mg	chlorpheniramine maleate, 2 mg
Comtrex, Allergy-Sinus (Bristol-Myers)	caplet tablet	pseudoephedrine hydrochloride, 30 mg	chlorpheniramine maleate, 2 mg
Comtrex Cough Formula (Bristol-Myers Products)	liquid	pseudoephedrine hydrochloride, 15 mg/5 ml	
Conar (Beecham Labs)	syrup	phenylephrine hydrochloride, 10 mg/5 ml	
Conar-A (Beecham Labs)	tablet	phenylephrine hydrochloride, 10 mg	
Conar Expectorant (Beecham Labs)	liquid	phenylephrine hydrochloride, 10 mg/5 ml	
Conex (Forest)	liquid	phenylpropanolamine hydro-chloride, 12.5 mg/5 ml	
Conex D.A. (Forest)	tablet	phenylpropanolamine hydro-chloride, 37.5 mg	chlorpheniramine maleate, 4 mg
Conex Plus (Forest)	tablet	phenylpropanolamine hydro-chloride, 25 mg	chlorpheniramine maleate, 4 mg
Conex with Codeine (Forest)	syrup	phenylpropanolamine hydro-chloride, 12.5 mg/5 ml	

Analgesic	Expectorant	Cough Suppressant	Other Ingredients
acetaminophen, 500 mg			
ibuprofen, 200 mg			
acetaminophen, 325 mg		dextromethorphan hydro-bromide, 15 mg	
acetaminophen, 325 mg			
	sodium citrate, 216 mg/5 ml citric acid, 50 mg/5 ml	dextromethorphan hydro-bromide, 10 mg/5 ml	alcohol, 4%
	guaifenesin, 100 mg/5 ml sodium citrate, 1.5 mg/5 ml		
	sodium citrate, 216 mg/5 ml citric acid, 50 mg/5 ml	codeine phosphate[a], 10 mg/5 ml	
	guaifenesin, 100 mg/5 ml	dextromethorphan hydro-bromide, 15 mg/5 ml	alcohol, 1.4%
acetaminophen, 325 mg			
	guaifenesin, 100 mg/5 ml		alcohol, 4.7% mint flavor
acetaminophen, 325 mg		dextromethorphan hydro-bromide, 10 mg	alcohol, 20% (liquid) sucrose (liquid)
acetaminophen, 108.5 mg/ 5 ml		dextromethorphan hydro-bromide, 3.35 mg/5 ml	sorbitol (liqui-gel)
acetaminophen, 325 mg		dextromethorphan hydro-bromide, 10 mg	
acetaminophen, 500 mg			
acetaminophen, 125 mg/ 5 ml	guaifenesin, 50 mg/5 ml	dextromethorphan hydro-bromide, 7.5 mg/5 ml	alcohol, 20% menthol saccharin sucrose
		dextromethorphan hydro-bromide, 15 mg/5 ml	tangerine flavor
acetaminophen, 300 mg	guaifenesin, 100 mg	dextromethorphan hydro-bromide, 15 mg	
	guaifenesin, 100 mg/5 ml	dextromethorphan hydro-bromide, 15 mg/5 ml	peach/apricot flavor
	guaifenesin, 100 mg/5 ml		methylparaben, 0.13% propylparaben, 0.03%
			sucrose, 20 mg
acetaminophen, 325 mg			
	guaifenesin, 100 mg/5 ml	codeine phosphate[a], 10 mg/5 ml	methylparaben, 0.13% propylparaben, 0.03%

COLD, ALLERGY, COUGH PRODUCT TABLE, continued

Product (Manufacturer)	Dose Form	Decongestant	Antihistamine
Congespirin for Children, Aspirin Free (Bristol-Myers)	chewable tablet cough syrup	phenylpropanolamine hydrochloride, 1.25 mg/tablet	
Congestac (SmithKline)	caplet	pseudoephedrine hydrochloride, 60 mg	
Contac (SmithKline)	capsule, timed release	phenylpropanolamine hydrochloride, 75 mg	chlorpheniramine maleate, 8 mg
Contac Jr.[b,c] (SmithKline)	liquid	pseudoephedrine hydrochloride, 15 mg/5 ml	
Contac Maximum Strength Cold Formula (SmithKline)	caplet	phenylpropanolamine hydrochloride, 75 mg	chlorpheniramine maleate, 12 mg
Contac Nighttime Cold Medicine (SmithKline)	liquid	pseudoephedrine hydrochloride, 10 mg/5 ml	doxylamine succinate, 1.25 mg/ 5 ml
Contac Severe Cold Formula (SmithKline)	caplet	phenylpropanolamine hydrochloride, 12.5 mg	chlorpheniramine maleate, 2 mg
Co-Pyronil 2 Pulvules (Dista)	capsule	pseudoephedrine hydrochloride, 60 mg	chlorpheniramine maleate, 4 mg
Coricidin (Schering)	tablet		chlorpheniramine maleate, 2 mg
Coricidin D (Schering)	tablet	phenylpropanolamine hydrochloride, 12.5 mg	chlorpheniramine maleate, 2 mg
Coricidin Demilets (Schering)	chewable tablet	phenylpropanolamine hydrochloride, 6.25 mg	chlorpheniramine maleate, 1 mg
Coricidin Maximum Strength Sinus Headache (Schering)	tablet	phenylpropanolamine hydrochloride, 12.5 mg	chlorpheniramine maleate, 2 mg
Coryban-D (Leeming)	tablet	pseudoephedrine hydrochloride, 60 mg	triprolidine hydrochloride, 2.5 mg
Cough Formula (PBI)	liquid		doxylamine succinate, 3.75 mg/ 5 ml
Cough Formula with Expectorant (PBI)	liquid	pseudoephedrine hydrochloride, 20 mg/5 ml	
Covangesic (Wallace)	tablet	phenylpropanolamine hydrochloride, 12.5 mg phenylephrine hydrochloride, 7.5 mg	chlorpheniramine maleate, 2 mg pyrilamine maleate, 12.5 mg
Cremacoat 1 (Richardson-Vicks)	syrup		
Cremacoat 2 (Richardson-Vicks)	syrup		
Dallergy-D (Laser)	capsule	pseudoephedrine hydrochloride, 120 mg	chlorpheniramine maleate, 12 mg
	syrup[c]	phenylephrine hydrochloride, 5 mg/5 ml	chlorpheniramine maleate, 2 mg/5 ml

Analgesic	Expectorant	Cough Suppressant	Other Ingredients
acetaminophen, 81 mg/ tablet		dextromethorphan hydro- bromide, 5 mg/5 ml (syrup)	fruit flavor (tablet) saccharin (tablet) sucrose (tablet and syrup) sorbitol (syrup) orange flavor (syrup)
	guaifenesin, 400 mg		
acetaminophen, 160 mg/ 5 ml		dextromethorphan hydro- bromide, 5 mg/5 ml	saccharin sorbitol berry flavor
acetaminophen, 167 mg/ 5 ml		dextromethorphan hydro- bromide, 5 mg/5 ml	alcohol, 25% saccharin sorbitol sugar
acetaminophen, 500 mg		dextromethorphan hydro- bromide, 15 mg	
acetaminophen, 325 mg			
acetaminophen, 325 mg			
acetaminophen, 80 mg			saccharin
acctaminophen, 500 mg			
		dextromethorphan hydro- bromide, 15 mg/5 ml	alcohol, 10%
	guaifenesin, 67 mg/5 ml	dextromethorphan hydro- bromide, 10 mg/5 ml	alcohol, 10%
acetaminophen, 275 mg			
		dextromethorphan hydro- bromide, 10 mg/5 ml	alcohol, 10%
	guaifenesin, 67 mg/5 ml		alcohol, 10% sorbitol
			syrup: raspberry/vanilla flavor sugar

COLD, ALLERGY, COUGH PRODUCT TABLE, continued

Product (Manufacturer)	Dose Form	Decongestant	Antihistamine
Daycare (Richardson-Vicks)	caplet	pseudoephedrine hydrochloride, 30 mg	
	liquid	pseudoephedrine hydrochloride, 10 mg./5 ml	
Dehist (Forest)	capsule	phenylpropanolamine hydrochloride, 75 mg	chlorpheniramine maleate, 8 mg
Delsym[c] (McNeil)	suspension		
Demazin (Schering)	syrup	phenylpropanolamine hydrochloride, 12.5 mg/5 ml	chlorpheniramine maleate, 2 mg/5 ml
Demazin Repetabs (Schering)	tablet	phenylpropanolamine hydrochloride, 25 mg	chlorpheniramine maleate, 4 mg
Dexophed (Various manufacturers)	tablet	pseudoephedrine sulfate, 120 mg	dexbrompheniramine maleate, 6 mg
Dihistine (Various manufacturers)	elixir	phenylephrine hydrochloride, 5 mg/5 ml	chlorpheniramine maleate, 2 mg/5 ml
Dilone (Richardson-Vicks)	tablet		phenyltoloxamine citrate, 30 mg
Dimacol (Robins)	caplet	pseudoephedrine hydrochloride, 30 mg	
Dimetane (Robins)	elixir		brompheniramine maleate, 2 mg/5 ml
	tablet, timed release		brompheniramine maleate, 4 mg brompheniramine maleate, 8 mg, 12 mg
Dimetane Decongestant (Robins)	elixir	phenylephrine hydrochloride, 5 mg/5 ml	brompheniramine maleate, 2 mg/5 ml
	tablet	phenylephrine hydrochloride, 10 mg	brompheniramine maleate, 4 mg
Dimetapp (Robins)	elixir	phenylpropanolamine hydrochloride, 12.5 mg/5 ml	brompheniramine maleate, 2 mg/5 ml
	extentab	phenylpropanolamine hydrochloride, 75 mg	brompheniramine maleate, 12 mg
	tablet	phenylpropanolamine hydrochloride, 25 mg	brompheniramine maleate, 4 mg
Diphen Cough (PBI)	syrup		diphenhydramine hydrochloride, 12.5 mg/5 ml
Disophrol (Schering)	tablet	pseudoephrine sulfate, 60 mg	dexbrompheniramine maleate, 2 mg
Disophrol Chronotabs (Schering)	tablet, timed release	pseudoephedrine sulfate, 120 mg	dexbrompheniramine maleate, 6 mg
DM Cough (PBI)	syrup		
Dondril Anticough (Whitehall)	tablet	phenylephrine hydrochloride, 5 mg	chlorpheniramine maleate, 1 mg
Dorcol Children's (Sandoz)	syrup	pseudoephedrine hydrochloride, 15 mg/5 ml	
Dorcol Children's Decongestant (Sandoz)	liquid	pseudoephedrine hydrochloride, 15 mg/5 ml	
Dorcol Children's Formula (Sandoz)	liquid	pseudoephedrine hydrochloride, 15 mg/5 ml	chlorpheniramine maleate, 1 mg/5 ml

Analgesic	Expectorant	Cough Suppressant	Other Ingredients

acetaminophen, 325 mg
acetaminophen, 108 mg/5 ml
	guaifenesin, 100 mg
	guaifenesin, 33.3 mg/5 ml
		dextromethorphan hydrobromide, 10 mg
		dextromethorphan hydrobromide, 3.3 mg/5 ml
			liquid:
			  alcohol, 10%
			  saccharin

		dextromethorphan polistirex (equivalent to 30 mg/5 ml dextromethorphan hydrobromide)	orange flavor
			alcohol, 7.5%
acetaminophen, 325 mg			caffeine, 30 mg pineapple flavor
	guaifenesin, 100 mg	dextromethorphan hydrobromide, 10 mg	saccharin

			elixir:
			  alcohol, 3%
			  saccharin

			elixir:
			  alcohol, 2.3%
			  sorbitol
			  grape flavor

			elixir:
			  alcohol, 2.3%
			  saccharin
			  sorbitol
			  grape flavor

		dextromethorphan hydrobromide, 10 mg/5 ml	alcohol, 5%
		dextromethorphan hydrobromide, 10 mg	
	guaifenesin, 50 mg/5 ml	dextromethorphan hydrobromide, 5 mg/5 ml	
			sorbitol
			sorbitol sucrose

COLD, ALLERGY, COUGH PRODUCT TABLE, continued

Product (Manufacturer)	Dose Form	Decongestant	Antihistamine
Drinophen (Lannett)	capsule	phenylpropanolamine hydrochloride, 15 mg	
Dristan, Advanced Formula (Whitehall)	caplet tablet	phenylephrine hydrochloride, 5 mg	chlorpheniramine maleate, 2 mg
Dristan AF (Aspirin-Free) (Whitehall)	tablet	phenylephrine hydrochloride, 5 mg	chlorpheniramine maleate, 2 mg
Dristan Maximum Strength (Whitehall)	caplet	pseudoephedrine hydrochloride, 30 mg	
Dristan Room Vaporizer (Whitehall)	aerosol spray		
Drixoral (Schering)	tablet, extended release	pseudoephedrine sulfate, 120 mg	dexbrompheniramine maleate, 6 mg
	syrup	pseudoephedrine sulfate, 30 mg/5 ml	dexbrompheniramine maleate, 2 mg/5 ml
Drixoral Non-Drowsy Formula (Schering)	tablet, extended release	pseudoephedrine sulfate, 120 mg	
Drixoral Plus (Schering)	tablet, extended release	pseudoephedrine sulfate, 60 mg	dexbrompheniramine maleate, 3 mg
Duadacin (Hoechst-Roussel)	capsule	phenylpropanolamine hydrochloride, 12.5 mg	chlorpheniramine maleate, 2 mg
Efricon Expectorant (Lannett)	liquid	phenylephrine hydrochloride, 5 mg/5 ml	chlorpheniramine maleate, 2 mg/5 ml
Emagrin Forte (Otis Clapp)	tablet	phenylephrine hydrochloride, 5 mg	
Excedrin Sinus (Bristol-Myers)	caplet tablet	pseudoephedrine hydrochloride, 30 mg	
Extreme Cold Formula (Major)	caplet	phenylpropanolamine hydrochloride, 12.5 mg	chlorpheniramine maleate, 2 mg
Fedahist (Schwarz Pharma)	tablet	pseudoephedrine hydrochloride, 60 mg	chlorpheniramine maleate, 4 mg
Fedahist Decongestant (Schwarz Pharma)	syrup	pseudoephedrine hydrochloride, 30 mg/5 ml	chlorpheniramine maleate, 2 mg/5 ml
Fedahist Expectorant (Schwarz Pharma)	liquid	pseudoephedrine hydrochloride, 30 mg/5 ml	
Fedahist Expectorant Pediatric (Schwarz Pharma)	drops	pseudoephedrine hydrochloride, 7.5 mg/ml	
Fendol (Buffington)	tablet	phenylephrine hydrochloride, 5 mg	
Fiogesic (Sandoz)	tablet	pseudoephedrine hydrochloride, 30 mg	
Formula 44 Cough Mixture (Richardson-Vicks)	liquid		chlorpheniramine maleate, 2 mg/5 ml

Analgesic	Expectorant	Cough Suppressant	Other Ingredients
acetaminophen, 200 mg aspirin, 230 mg			caffeine, 15 mg
acetaminophen, 325 mg			caffeine, 16.2 mg
acetaminophen, 325 mg			
acetaminophen, 500 mg			
			camphor, 0.7% thymol, 0.1% eucalyptol, 0.4% menthol, 1.2% alcohol, 16.6%
acetaminophen, 500 mg			
acetaminophen, 325 mg			
	ammonium chloride, 90 mg/ 5 ml potassium guaiacolsulfonate, 90 mg/5 ml sodium citrate, 60 mg/5 ml	codeine phosphate[a], 10.96 mg/5 ml	
acetaminophen, 260 mg	guaifenesin, 100 mg		caffeine
acetaminophen, 500 mg			
acetaminophen, 500 mg			
			saccharin sorbitol sucrose grape flavor
	guaifenesin, 200 mg/5 ml		saccharin sorbitol
	guaifenesin, 40 mg/ml		saccharin sorbitol
salicylamide, 65 mg acetaminophen, 355 mg	guaifenesin, 100 mg		caffeine
aspirin, 325 mg			
		dextromethorphan hydro- bromide, 15 mg/5 ml	alcohol, 10% sugar

COLD, ALLERGY, COUGH PRODUCT TABLE, continued

Product (Manufacturer)	Dose Form	Decongestant	Antihistamine
Formula 44D Decongestant Cough Mixture (Richardson-Vicks)	liquid	pseudoephedrine hydrochloride, 20 mg/5 ml	
Formula 44M (Richardson-Vicks)	liquid	pseudoephedrine hydrochloride, 15 mg/5 ml	
4-Way Cold (Bristol-Myers)	tablet	phenylpropanolamine hydrochloride, 12.5 mg	chlorpheniramine maleate, 2 mg
Genac (Goldline)	tablet	pseudoephedrine hydrochloride, 60 mg	triprolidine hydrochloride, 2.5 mg
Genahist (Goldline)	elixir		diphenhydramine hydrochloride, 12.5 mg/5 ml
Genaminc (Goldline)	syrup	phenylpropanolamine hydrochloride, 12.5 mg/5 ml	chlorpheniramine maleate, 2 mg/5 ml
Genaphed (Goldline)	tablet	pseudoephedrine hydrochloride, 30 mg	
Genatap (Goldline)	elixir	phenylpropanolamine hydrochloride, 12.5 mg/5 ml	brompheniramine maleate, 2 mg/5 ml
Genatuss (Goldline)	syrup		
Genatuss DM (Goldline)	syrup		
Gencold (Goldline)	capsule	phenylpropanolamine hydrochloride, 75 mg	chlorpheniramine maleate, 8 mg
Gen-D-Phen (Goldline)	syrup		diphenhydramine, 12.5 mg/5 ml
Genex (Goldline)	capsule	phenylpropanolamine hydrochloride, 18 mg	
Genite (Goldline)	liquid	pseudoephedrine hydrochloride, 10 mg/5 ml	doxylamine succinate, 1.25 mg/5 ml
GG-Cen (Central)	capsule syrup		
Glyate (Geneva Generics)	syrup		
Guaituss-DM (Various manufacturers)	liquid		
Halls Mentho-Lyptus Decongestant (Warner-Lambert)	liquid	phenylpropanolamine hydrochloride, 18.75 mg/5 ml	
Halotussin-DM (Various manufacturers)	syrup		
Hista-Compound No. 5 (Vortech)	tablet		chlorpheniramine maleate, 2 mg

Analgesic	Expectorant	Cough Suppressant	Other Ingredients
	guaifenesin, 67 mg/5 ml	dextromethorphan hydrobromide, 10 mg/5 ml	alcohol, 10% saccharin
acetaminophen, 125 mg/5 ml	guaifenesin, 50 mg/5 ml	dextromethorphan hydrobromide, 7.5 mg/5 ml	alcohol, 20% saccharin
acetaminophen, 325 mg			
			alcohol, 14%
			alcohol, 2.3% saccharin sorbitol grape flavor
	guaifenesin, 100 mg/5 ml		alcohol, 3.5%
	guaifenesin, 100 mg/5 ml	dextromethorphan hydrobromide, 15 mg/5 ml	alcohol, 1.4% sucrose saccharin glucose
			alcohol, 5%
acetaminophen, 325 mg			
acetaminophen, 167 mg/5 ml		dextromethorphan hydrobromide, 5 mg/5 ml	alcohol, 25% tartrazine

	guaifenesin, 200 mg
	guaifenesin, 100 mg/5 ml
			syrup:
			  alcohol, 10%
			  saccharin
			  sorbitol
			  grape flavor

	guaifenesin, 100 mg/5 ml		alcohol, 3.5%
	guaifenesin, 100 mg/5 ml	dextromethorphan hydrobromide, 15 mg/5 ml	alcohol, 1.4%
		dextromethorphan hydrobromide, 7.5 mg/5 ml	alcohol, 22% menthol sorbitol eucalyptus oil sucrose cherry flavor
	guaifenesin, 100 mg/5 ml	dextromethorphan hydrobromide, 15 mg/5 ml	alcohol, 1.4%
acetaminophen, 150 mg salicylamide, 175 mg			

COLD, ALLERGY, COUGH PRODUCT TABLE, continued

Product (Manufacturer)	Dose Form	Decongestant	Antihistamine
Histadyl E.C. (Lilly)	syrup	pseudoephedrine hydrochloride, 60 mg/5 ml	chlorpheniramine maleate, 4 mg/5 ml
Histatab Plus (Century)	tablet	phenylephrine hydrochloride, 5 mg	chlorpheniramine maleate, 2 mg
Hydramine Cough (Goldline)	syrup		diphenhydramine hydrochloride, 12.5 mg/5 ml
Hydriodic Acid (Lilly)	syrup		
Isoclor (Fisons)	liquid	pseudoephedrine hydrochloride, 30 mg/5 ml	chlorpheniramine maleate, 2 mg/5 ml
	tablet	pseudoephedrine hydrochloride, 60 mg	chlorpheniramine maleate, 4 mg
Isoclor Timesules (Fisons)	capsule, timed release	pseudoephedrine hydrochloride, 120 mg	chlorpheniramine maleate, 8 mg
Kolephrin (Pfeiffer)	caplet	pseudoephedrine hydrochloride, 30 mg	chlorpheniramine maleate, 2 mg
Kolephrin/DM (Pfeiffer)	caplet	pseudoephedrine hydrochloride, 30 mg	chlorpheniramine maleate, 2 mg
Kolephrin GG/DM Expectorant[c] (Pfeiffer)	liquid		
Kophane Cough and Cold Formula[c] (Pfeiffer)	syrup	phenylpropanolamine hydrochloride, 5 mg/5 ml	chlorpheniramine maleate, 0.5 mg/5 ml
Lanatuss Expectorant[b,c] (Lannett)	liquid	phenylpropanolamine hydrochloride, 5 mg/5 ml	chlorpheniramine maleate, 2 mg/5 ml
Mediquell (Warner-Lambert)	chewy squares		
Myfedrine (PBI)	liquid	pseudoephedrine hydrochloride, 30 mg/5 ml	
Myfedrine Plus (PBI)	liquid	pseudoephedrine hydrochloride, 30 mg/5 ml	chlorpheniramine maleate, 2 mg/5 ml
Myminic (PBI)	syrup	phenylpropanolamine hydrochloride, 12.5 mg/5 ml	chlorpheniramine maleate, 2 mg/5 ml
Myminic Expectorant (PBI)	liquid	phenylpropanolamine hydrochloride, 12.5 mg/5 ml	
Myminicol[c] (PBI)	liquid	phenylpropanolamine hydrochloride, 12.5 mg/5 ml	chlorpheniramine maleate, 2 mg/5 ml
Myphetapp (PBI)	elixir	phenylpropanolamine hydrochloride, 12.5 mg/5 ml	brompheniramine maleate, 2 mg/5 ml
Mytussin (PBI)	syrup		
Mytussin DM (PBI)	syrup		
Naldecon DX Adult[b,c] (Bristol Labs)	liquid	phenylpropanolamine hydrochloride, 18 mg/5 ml	
Naldecon DX Children's[b,c] (Bristol Labs)	syrup	phenylpropanolamine hydrochloride, 6.25 mg/5 ml	

Analgesic	Expectorant	Cough Suppressant	Other Ingredients
		codeine phosphate[a], 10 mg/ 5 ml	alcohol, 5% saccharin sucrose
			alcohol, 5%
	hydrogen iodide, 70 mg/5 ml		
			liquid: sorbitol grape flavor
acetaminophen, 325 mg			
acetaminophen, 325 mg		dextromethorphan hydro-bromide, 10 mg	
	guaifenesin, 150 mg/5 ml	dextromethorphan hydro-bromide, 15 mg/5 ml	sucrose, 1130 mg/5 ml
	ammonium chloride, 90 mg/5 ml sodium citrate	dextromethorphan hydro-bromide, 10 mg/5 ml	cherry flavor
	guaifenesin, 100 mg/5 ml sodium citrate, 197 mg/5 ml citric acid, 60 mg/5 ml		
		dextromethorphan hydro-bromide, 15 mg	
	guaifenesin, 100 mg/5 ml		alcohol, 5%
		dextromethorphan hydro-bromide, 10 mg/5 ml	
			alcohol, 2.3% grape flavor
	guaifenesin, 100 mg/5 ml		alcohol, 3.5%
	guaifenesin, 100 mg/5 ml	dextromethorphan hydro-bromide, 15 mg/5 ml	alcohol, 1.4%
	guaifenesin, 200 mg/5 ml	dextromethorphan hydro-bromide, 15 mg/5 ml	saccharin sorbitol
	guaifenesin, 100 mg/5 ml	dextromethorphan hydro-bromide, 5 mg/5 ml	alcohol, 5% sucrose

COLD, ALLERGY, COUGH PRODUCT TABLE, continued

Product (Manufacturer)	Dose Form	Decongestant	Antihistamine
Naldecon DX Pediatric[b] (Bristol Labs)	drops	phenylpropanolamine hydrochloride, 6.24 mg/ml	
Naldecon EX Pediatric (Bristol Labs)	drops	phenylpropanolamine hydrochloride, 6.25 mg/ml	
Naldecon Senior DX[b,c] (Bristol Labs)	liquid		
Naldecon Senior EX[b,c] (Bristol Labs)	liquid		
Naldegesic (Bristol Labs)	tablet	pseudoephedrine hydrochloride, 15 mg	
Napril (Randob)	tablet	pseudoephedrine hydrochloride, 60 mg	chlorpheniramine maleate, 4 mg
Nidryl (Geneva Generics)	elixir		diphenhydramine hydrochloride, 12.5 mg/5 ml
Nolahist (Carnrick)	tablet		phenindamine tartrate, 25 mg
Noraminic (Vortech)	syrup	phenylpropanolamine hydrochloride, 12.5 mg/5 ml	chlorpheniramine maleate, 2 mg/5 ml
Noratuss II Expectorant[b,c] (Vortech)	liquid	pseudoephedrine hydrochloride, 15 mg/5 ml	
Nordryl Cough (Vortech)	syrup		diphenhydramine hydrochloride, 12.5 mg/5 ml
Nortussin (Vortech)	syrup		
Novahistine[b] (Lakeside)	elixir	phenylephrine hydrochloride, 5 mg/5 ml	chlorpheniramine maleate, 2 mg/5 ml
Novahistine DH (Lakeside)	liquid	pseudoephedrine hydrochloride, 30 mg/5 ml	chlorpheniramine maleate, 2 mg/5 ml
Novahistine DMX (Lakeside)	syrup	pseudoephedrine hydrochloride, 30 mg/5 ml	
Novahistine Expectorant (Lakeside)	liquid	pseudoephedrine hydrochloride, 30 mg/5 ml	
Nycoff[b] (Dover)	tablet		
Nycold Medicine (Rugby)	liquid	pseudoephedrine hydrochloride, 10 mg/5 ml	doxylamine succinate, 1.25 mg/5 ml
NyQuil Nighttime Cold Medicine (Richardson-Vicks)	liquid	pseudoephedrine hydrochloride, 10 mg/5 ml	doxylamine succinate, 1.25 mg/5 ml
Oranyl[b] (Otis Clapp)	tablet	pseudoephedrine hydrochloride, 30 mg	
Oranyl Plus[b] (Otis Clapp)	tablet	pseudoephedrine hydrochloride, 30 mg	
Ornex (SmithKline)	caplet	pseudoephedrine hydrochloride, 30 mg	

Analgesic	Expectorant	Cough Suppressant	Other Ingredients
	guaifenesin, 30 mg/ml	dextromethorphan hydrobromide, 5 mg/ml	alcohol, 0.6% saccharin sorbitol
	guaifenesin, 30 mg/ml		alcohol, 0.6% sucrose
	guaifenesin, 200 mg/5 ml	dextromethorphan hydrobromide, 15 mg/5 ml	saccharin sorbitol
	guaifenesin, 200 mg/5 ml		
acetaminophen, 325 mg			
			alcohol, 14%
	guaifenesin, 50 mg/5 ml	dextromethorphan hydrobromide, 3.75 mg/5 ml	
			alcohol, 5%
	guaifenesin, 100 mg/5 ml		alcohol, 3.5% cherry flavor
			alcohol, 5% sorbitol
		codeine phosphate[a], 10 mg/5 ml	alcohol, 5% sugar saccharin sorbitol
	guaifenesin, 100 mg/5 ml	dextromethorphan hydrobromide, 10 mg/5 ml	alcohol, 10% saccharin sorbitol
	guaifenesin, 100 mg/5 ml	codeine phosphate[a], 10 mg/5 ml	alcohol, 7.5% saccharin sorbitol invert sugar
		dextromethorphan hydrobromide	
acetaminophen, 167 mg/5 ml		dextromethorphan hydrobromide, 5 mg/5 ml	alcohol, 25% mint flavor
acetaminophen, 167 mg/5 ml		dextromethorphan hydrobromide, 5 mg/5 ml	alcohol, 25% saccharin tartrazine
acetaminophen, 500 mg			
acetaminophen, 325 mg			

COLD, ALLERGY, COUGH PRODUCT TABLE, continued

Product (Manufacturer)	Dose Form	Decongestant	Antihistamine
Orthoxicol (Upjohn)	syrup	phenylpropanolamine hydrochloride, 8.3 mg/5 ml	chlorpheniramine maleate, 1.3 mg/5 ml
Pedia Care Cold Formula (McNeil)	liquid	pseudoephedrine hydrochloride, 15 mg/5 ml	chlorpheniramine maleate, 1 mg/5 ml
Pedia Care Cough-Cold Formula (McNeil)	liquid	pseudoephedrine hydrochloride, 15 mg/5 ml	chlorpheniramine maleate, 1 mg/5 ml
Pedia Care Cough-Cold Formula, Chewable (McNeil)	tablet	pseudoephedrine hydrochloride, 7.5 mg	chlorpheniramine maleate, 0.5 mg
Percogesic (Richardson-Vicks)	tablet		phenyltoloxamine citrate, 30 mg
Pertussin CS (Pertussin Labs)	liquid		
Pertussin ES (Pertussin Labs)	liquid		
Pertussin PM (Pertussin Labs)	liquid	pseudoephedrine hydrochloride, 10 mg/5 ml	doxylamine succinate, 1.25 mg/5 ml
Pfeiffer's Allergy (Pfeiffer)	tablet		chlorpheniramine maleate, 4 mg
Phanadex (Pharmakon)	syrup	phenylpropanolamine hydrochloride, 25 mg/5 ml	pyrilamine maleate, 40 mg/5 ml
Phanatuss Cough[b] (Pharmakon)	syrup		
PhenAPAP No. 2 (Rugby)	tablet	pseudoephedrine hydrochloride, 30 mg	
PhenAPAP Sinus Headache & Congestion (Rugby)	tablet	pseudoephedrine hydrochloride, 30 mg	chlorpheniramine maleate, 2 mg
Phendry (LuChem)	elixir		diphenhydramine hydrochloride, 12.5 mg/5 ml
Phenetron Compound (Lannett)	tablet		chlorpheniramine maleate, 2 mg
Phenhist[b] (Rugby)	elixir	phenylephrine hydrochloride, 5 mg/5 ml	chlorpheniramine maleate, 2 mg/5 ml
Phenylgesic (Goldline)	tablet		phenyltoloxamine citrate, 30 mg
Pinex (Alvin Last)	syrup		
Pinex Concentrate (Alvin Last)	syrup		

Analgesic	Expectorant	Cough Suppressant	Other Ingredients
		dextromethorphan hydrobromide, 6.7 mg/5 ml	alcohol, 8%
			sorbitol
		dextromethorphan hydrobromide, 5 mg/5 ml	
		dextromethorphan hydrobromide, 2.5 mg	
acetaminophen, 325 mg			
	guaifenesin, 25 mg/5 ml	dextromethorphan hydrobromide, 3.5 mg/5 ml	alcohol, 8.5% sorbitol sugar
		dextromethorphan hydrobromide, 15 mg/5 ml	alcohol, 9.5% sorbitol sugar
acetaminophen, 167 mg/ 5 ml		dextromethorphan hydrobromide, 5 mg/5 ml	alcohol, 2.5% saccharin sucrose
	glyceryl guaiacolate, 100 mg/ 5 ml potassium citrate, 75 mg/5 ml citric acid, 35 mg/5 ml	dextromethorphan hydrobromide, 15 mg/5 ml	grape flavor sugar
	guaifenesin, 85 mg/5 ml potassium citrate, 75 mg/5 ml citric acid, 35 mg/5 ml	dextromethorphan hydrobromide, 10 mg/5 ml	menthol saccharin sorbitol solution, 70%
acetaminophen, 500 mg			
acetaminophen, 325 mg			
			alcohol, 14%
aspirin, 390 mg			caffeine, 32 mg
acetaminophen, 325 mg			
		dextromethorphan hydrobromide, 7.5 mg/5 ml	sugar honey alcohol, 3%
		dextromethorphan hydrobromide, 7.5 mg/5 ml (when diluted to 16 fl. oz.)	sugar honey alcohol, 16% (3% when diluted)

COLD, ALLERGY, COUGH PRODUCT TABLE, continued

Product (Manufacturer)	Dose Form	Decongestant	Antihistamine
Poly-Histine Expectorant (Bock)	syrup	phenylpropanolamine hydrochloride, 12.5 mg/5 ml	
Primatuss Cough Mixture 4 (Rugby)	liquid		doxylamine succinate, 3.75 mg/5 ml
Primatuss Cough Mixture 4D (Rugby)	liquid	phenylpropanolamine hydrochloride, 12.5 mg/5 ml	
Propagest (Carnrick)	tablet	phenylpropanolamine hydrochloride, 25 mg	
Pruni-codeine[b] (Lilly)	liquid		
Pseudoephedrine Hydrochloride (Various manufacturers)	tablet	pseudoephedrine hydrochloride, 30 mg or 60 mg	
Pseudogest (Major)	tablet	pseudoephedrine hydrochloride, 30 mg or 60 mg	
Pseudo-gest Plus (Major)	tablet	pseudoephedrine hydrochloride, 60 mg	chlorpheniramine maleate, 4 mg
Pyrroxate (Upjohn)	capsule	phenylpropanolamine hydrochloride, 25 mg	chlorpheniramine maleate, 4 mg
Quelidrine Cough (Abbott)	syrup	phenylephrine hydrochloride 5 mg/5 ml ephedrine hydrochloride, 5 mg/5 ml	chlorpheniramine maleate, 2 mg/5 ml
Queltuss (Forest)	tablet		
Quiet Night (PBI)	liquid	pseudoephedrine hydrochloride, 10 mg/5 ml	doxylamine succinate, 1.25 mg/5 ml
REM (Alvin Last)	liquid		
Robitussin (Robins)	syrup		
Robitussin-CF (Robins)	syrup	phenylpropanolamine hydrochloride, 12.5 mg/5 ml	
Robitussin-DM (Robins)	syrup		
Robitussin Night Relief Colds Formula (Robins)	liquid	phenylephrine hydrochloride, 1.67 mg/5 ml	pyrilamine maleate, 8.3 mg/5 ml
Robitussin-PE (Robins)	syrup	pseudoephedrine hydrochloride, 30 mg/5 ml	
Ru-Tuss (Boots-Flint)	liquid	phenylephrine hydrochloride, 5 mg/5 ml	chlorpheniramine maleate, 2 mg/5 ml
Ru-Tuss Expectorant (Boots-Flint)	liquid	pseudoephedrine hydrochloride, 30 mg/5 ml	
Ryna[b,c] (Wallace)	liquid	pseudoephedrine hydrochloride, 30 mg/5 ml	chlorpheniramine maleate, 2 mg/5 ml

Analgesic	Expectorant	Cough Suppressant	Other Ingredients
	guaifenesin, 100 mg/5 ml		saccharin sucrose cherry/strawberry flavor
		dextromethorphan hydro- bromide, 7.5 mg/5 ml	alcohol, 10%
	guaifenesin, 100 mg/5 ml	dextromethorphan hydro- bromide, 10 mg/5 ml	alcohol, 10% cherry flavor
	terpin hydrate, 29 mg/5 ml	codeine sulfate[a], 10 mg/5 ml	alcohol, 25% saccharin pinus strobus, 175 mg/5 ml prunus serotina, 263 mg/5 ml sanguinaria, 44 mg/5 ml
acetaminophen, 500 mg			
	ammonium chloride, 40 mg/ 5 ml ipecac fluid extract, 0.005 ml/ 5 ml	dextromethorphan hydro- bromide, 10 mg/5 ml	alcohol, 2% sucrose
	guaifenesin, 100 mg/5 ml	dextromethorphan hydro- bromide, 15 mg/5 ml	alcohol, 1.4%
		dextromethorphan hydro- bromide, 5 mg/5 ml	tartrazine mint/cherry flavor
	citric acid sodium citrate	dextromethorphan hydro- bromide, 5 mg/5 ml	sugar
	guaifenesin, 100 mg/5 ml		alcohol, 3.5%
	guaifenesin, 100 mg/5 ml	dextromethorphan hydro- bromide, 10 mg/5 ml	alcohol, 4.75% saccharin sorbitol
	guaifenesin, 100 mg/5 ml	dextromethorphan hydro- bromide, 15 mg/5 ml	alcohol, 1.4% saccharin
acetaminophen, 167 mg/ 5 ml		dextromethorphan hydro- bromide, 5 mg/5 ml	alcohol, 25% saccharin sorbitol
	guaifenesin, 100 mg/5 ml		alcohol, 1.4% saccharin
			alcohol, 5%
	guaifenesin, 100 mg/5 ml	dextromethorphan hydro- bromide, 10 mg/5 ml	alcohol, 10%
			sorbitol

COLD, ALLERGY, COUGH PRODUCT TABLE, continued

Product (Manufacturer)	Dose Form	Decongestant	Antihistamine
Ryna-C[b] (Wallace)	liquid	pseudoephedrine hydrochloride, 30 mg/5 ml	chlorpheniramine maleate, 2 mg/5 ml
Ryna-CX[b,c] (Wallace)	liquid	pseudoephedrine hydrochloride, 30 mg/5 ml	
Silexin[b,c] (Otis Clapp)	syrup tablet		
Sinapils (Pfeiffer)	tablet	phenylpropanolamine hydrochloride, 12.5 mg	chlorpheniramine maleate, 1 mg
Sinarest (Fisons)	tablet	phenylpropanolamine hydrochloride, 18.7 mg	chlorpheniramine maleate, 2 mg
Sinarest Extra Strength (Fisons)	tablet	phenylpropanolamine hydrochloride, 18.7 mg	chlorpheniramine maleate, 2 mg
Sinarest No-Drowsiness (Fisons)	tablet	pseudoephedrine hydrochloride, 30 mg	
Sine-Aid Maximum (McNeil)	caplet	pseudoephedrine hydrochloride, 30 mg	
Sine-Aid Sinus Headache (McNeil)	tablet	pseudoephedrine hydrochloride, 30 mg	
Sine-Off Maximum Strength Allergy/Sinus (SmithKline)	caplet	pseudoephedrine hydrochloride, 30 mg	chlorpheniramine maleate, 2 mg
Sine-Off Maximum Strength No Drowsiness Formula (SmithKline)	caplet	pseudoephedrine hydrochloride, 30 mg	
Sine-Off Sinus Medicine (SmithKline)	tablet	phenylpropanolamine hydrochloride, 12.5 mg	chlorpheniramine maleate, 2 mg
Singlet (Lakeside)	tablet	pseudoephedrine hydrochloride, 60 mg	chlorpheniramine maleate, 4 mg
Sinulin (Carnrick)	tablet	phenylpropanolamine hydrochloride, 25 mg	chlorpheniramine maleate, 4 mg
Sinutab Allergy Formula Sustained Action (Parke-Davis)	tablet	pseudoephedrine sulfate, 120 mg	dexbrompheniramine maleate, 6 mg
Sinutab Maximum Strength (Parke-Davis)	caplet tablet	pseudoephedrine hydrochloride, 30 mg	chlorpheniramine maleate, 2 mg
Sinutab Maximum Strength Without Drowsiness (Parke-Davis)	tablet	pseudoephedrine hydrochloride, 30 mg	
Snaplets-D (Baker Cummins)	granules	phenylpropanolamine hydrochloride, 6.25 mg/pack	chlorpheniramine maleate, 1 mg/pack
Snaplets-DM (Baker Cummins)	granules	phenylpropanolamine hydrochloride, 6.25 mg/pack	
Snaplets-Multi (Baker Cummins)	granules	phenylpropanolamine hydrochloride, 6.25 mg/pack	chlorpheniramine maleate, 1 mg/pack
Sorbutuss (Dalin)	liquid		

Analgesic	Expectorant	Cough Suppressant	Other Ingredients
		codeine phosphate[a], 10 mg/ 5 ml	saccharin sorbitol
	guaifenesin, 100 mg/5 ml	codeine phosphate[a], 10 mg/ 5 ml	saccharin sorbitol
	guaifenesin (syrup)	dextromethorphan hydrobromide	benzocaine (tablet)
acetaminophen, 327 mg			caffeine, 32.5 mg
acetaminophen, 325 mg			
acetaminophen, 500 mg			
acetaminophen, 500 mg			
acetaminophen, 500 mg			
acetaminophen, 325 mg			
acetaminophen, 500 mg			
acetaminophen, 500 mg			
aspirin, 325 mg			
acetaminophen, 650 mg			
acetaminophen, 650 mg			
acetaminophen, 500 mg			
acetaminophen, 500 mg			
		dextromethorphan hydro- bromide, 5 mg/pack	
		dextromethorphan hydro- bromide, 5 mg/pack	
	potassium citrate, 85 mg/5 ml citric acid, 35 mg/5 ml guaifenesin, 100 mg/5 ml ipecac fluid extract, 0.05 min/ 5 ml	dextromethorphan hydro- bromide, 10 mg/5 ml	

COLD, ALLERGY, COUGH PRODUCT TABLE, continued

Product (Manufacturer)	Dose Form	Decongestant	Antihistamine
St. Joseph Cold Tablets for Children (Schering-Plough)	chewable tablet	phenylpropanolamine hydrochloride, 3.125 mg	
St. Joseph Cough Suppressant for Children (Schering-Plough)	syrup		
Sudafed (Burroughs Wellcome)	tablet	pseudoephedrine hydrochloride, 30 mg or 60 mg	
Sudafed, Children's (Burroughs Wellcome)	liquid	pseudoephedrine hydrochloride, 30 mg/5 ml	
Sudafed Cough (Burroughs Wellcome)	syrup	pseudoephedrine hydrochloride, 15 mg/5 ml	
Sudafed Plus (Burroughs Wellcome)	syrup	pseudoephedrine hydrochloride, 30 mg/5 ml	chlorpheniramine maleate, 2 mg/5 ml
	tablet	pseudoephedrine hydrochloride, 60 mg	chlorpheniramine maleate, 4 mg
Sudafed Sinus (Burroughs Wellcome)	caplet	pseudoephedrine hydrochloride, 30 mg	
Sudafed 12 Hour (Burroughs Wellcome)	capsule, timed release	pseudoephedrine hydrochloride, 120 mg	
Sudanyl[b] (Dover)	tablet	pseudoephedrine hydrochloride, 30 mg	
Super Anahist (Warner-Lambert)	tablet	pseudoephedrine hydrochloride, 30 mg	
Teldrin (SmithKline)	capsule, timed release		chlorpheniramine maleate, 12 mg
Terpin Hydrate w/Dextromethorphan Hydrobromide (Various manufacturers)	elixir		
TheraFlu Flu and Cold Medicine (Sandoz)	packet	pseudoephedrine hydrochloride, 60 mg	chlorpheniramine maleate, 4 mg
TheraFlu Flu, Cold and Cough Medicine (Sandoz)	packet	pseudoephedrine hydrochloride, 60 mg	chlorpheniramine maleate, 4 mg
Threamine DM[c] (Various manufacturers)	liquid	phenylpropanolamine hydrochloride, 12.5 mg/5 ml	chlorpheniramine maleate, 2 mg/5 ml
Tolu-Sed[b] (Scherer)	syrup		
Tolu-Sed DM[b] (Scherer)	liquid		
Triaminic Allergy (Sandoz)	tablet	phenylpropanolamine hydrochloride, 25 mg	chlorpheniramine maleate, 4 mg
Triaminic Chewable (Sandoz)	tablet	phenylpropanolamine hydrochloride, 6.25 mg	chlorpheniramine maleate, 0.5 mg
Triaminic Cold[c] (Sandoz)	syrup	phenylpropanolamine hydrochloride, 12.5 mg/5 ml	chlorpheniramine maleate, 2 mg/5 ml
	tablet	phenylpropanolamine hydrochloride, 12.5 mg	chlorpheniramine maleate, 2 mg
Triaminic-DM[c] (Sandoz)	liquid, timed release	phenylpropanolamine hydrochloride, 12.5 mg/5 ml	

Analgesic	Expectorant	Cough Suppressant	Other Ingredients
acetaminophen, 80 mg			sucrose, 96.2 mg
	sodium citrate	dextromethorphan hydrobromide, 7.5 mg/5 ml	
	guaifenesin, 100 mg/5 ml	dextromethorphan hydrobromide, 5 mg/5 ml	alcohol, 2.4%
			sucrose (syrup)
acetaminophen, 500 mg			
acetaminophen, 325 mg			
	terpin hydrate, 85 mg/5 ml	dextromethorphan hydrobromide, 10 mg/5 ml	
acetaminophen, 500 mg			lemon flavor sucrose
acetaminophen, 500 mg		dextromethorphan hydrobromide, 20 mg	lemon flavor sucrose
		dextromethorphan hydrobromide, 10 mg/5 ml	saccharin sorbitol
	guaifenesin, 100 mg/5 ml	codeine phosphate[a], 10 mg/5 ml	alcohol, 10%
	guaifenesin, 100 mg/5 ml	dextromethorphan hydrobromide, 10 mg/5 ml	alcohol, 10%
			saccharin sucrose, 52.5 mg
			sorbitol (syrup) sucrose (syrup) saccharin (tablet)
		dextromethorphan hydrobromide, 10 mg/5 ml	sorbitol sucrose

COLD, ALLERGY, COUGH PRODUCT TABLE, continued

Product (Manufacturer)	Dose Form	Decongestant	Antihistamine
Triaminic Expectorant (Sandoz)	liquid	phenylpropanolamine hydrochloride, 12.5 mg/5 ml	
Triaminic Expectorant with Codeine (Sandoz)		phenylpropanolamine hydrochloride, 12.5 mg/5 ml	
Triaminic Nite Light[c] (Sandoz)	liquid	pseudoephedrine hydrochloride, 15 mg/5 ml	chlorpheniramine maleate, 1 mg/5 ml
Triaminic-12 (Sandoz)	tablet, timed release	phenylpropanolamine hydrochloride, 75 mg	chlorpheniramine maleate, 12 mg
Triaminicin (Sandoz)	tablet	phenylpropanolamine hydrochloride, 25 mg	chlorpheniramine maleate, 4 mg
Triaminicol Multi-Symptom Cold (Sandoz)	syrup[c]	phenylpropanolamine hydrochloride, 12.5 mg/5 ml	chlorpheniramine maleate, 2 mg/5 ml
	tablet	phenylpropanolamine hydrochloride, 12.5 mg	chlorpheniramine maleate, 2 mg
Tricodene[b] (Pfeiffer)	liquid		chlorpheniramine maleate, 0.5 mg/5 ml
Tricodene Forte (Pfeiffer)	liquid	phenylpropanolamine hydrochloride, 12.5 mg/5 ml	chlorpheniramine maleate, 2 mg/5 ml
Tricodene NN Cough and Cold Medication (Pfeiffer)	syrup	phenylpropanolamine hydrochloride, 5 mg/5 ml	chlorpheniramine maleate, 0.5 mg/5 ml
Tricodene No. 1 (Pfeiffer)	liquid		pyrilamine maleate, 4.15 mg/5 ml
Tricodene Pediatric (Pfeiffer)	liquid	phenylpropanolamine hydrochloride, 12.5 mg/5 ml	
Tricodene Sugar Free[b] (Pfeiffer)	liquid		chlorpheniramine maleate, 0.5 mg/5 ml
Trind[b] (Mead Johnson)	liquid	phenylpropanolamine hydrochloride, 12.5 mg/5 ml	chlorpheniramine maleate, 2 mg/5 ml
Trind-DM[b] (Mead Johnson)	liquid	phenylpropanolamine hydrochloride, 12.5 mg/5 ml	chlorpheniramine maleate, 2 mg/5 ml
Tri-Nefrin Extra Strength (Pfeiffer)	tablet	phenylpropanolamine hydrochloride, 25 mg	chlorpheniramine maleate, 4 mg
Triofed (Various manufacturers)	syrup	pseudoephedrine hydrochloride, 30 mg/5 ml	triprolidine hydrochloride, 1.25 mg/5 ml
Triphenyl[c] (Rugby)	syrup	phenylpropanolamine hydrochloride, 12.5 mg/5 ml	chlorpheniramine maleate, 2 mg/5 ml
Triphenyl Expectorant (Rugby)	liquid	phenylpropanolamine hydrochloride, 12.5 mg/5 ml	
Tripodrine (Danbury)	tablet	pseudoephedrine hydrochloride, 60 mg	triprolidine hydrochloride, 2.5 mg
Tussagesic (Sandoz)	tablet	phenylpropanolamine hydrochloride, 25 mg	pheniramine maleate, 12.5 mg pyrilamine maleate, 12.5 mg

Analgesic	Expectorant	Cough Suppressant	Other Ingredients
	guaifenesin, 100 mg/5 ml		alcohol, 5% saccharin sorbitol sucrose
	guaifenesin, 100 mg/5 ml	codeine phosphate[a], 10 mg/5 ml	alcohol, 5% saccharin sorbitol
		dextromethorphan hydro-bromide, 7.5 mg/5 ml	sorbitol sucrose grape flavor
acetaminophen, 650 mg			

		dextromethorphan hydro-bromide, 10 mg/5 ml
		dextromethorphan hydro-bromide, 10 mg
			syrup:
			  saccharin
			  sorbitol
			  sucrose

	ammonium chloride, 90 mg/5 ml sodium citrate	dextromethorphan hydro-bromide, 10 mg/5 ml	sorbitol mannitol saccharin
		dextromethorphan hydro-bromide, 10 mg/5 ml	sucrose, 3000 mg/5 ml
	ammonium chloride, 90 mg/5 ml sodium citrate	dextromethorphan hydro-bromide, 10 mg/5 ml	
		codeine phosphate[a], 8 mg/5 ml	sucrose, 1665 mg/5 ml
		dextromethorphan hydro-bromide, 10 mg/5 ml	sucrose, 3000 mg/5 ml
	ammonium chloride, 90 mg/5 ml sodium citrate	dextromethorphan hydro-bromide, 10 mg/5 ml	sorbitol mannitol saccharin
			alcohol, 5% sorbitol orange flavor
		dextromethorphan hydro-bromide, 7.5 mg/5 ml	alcohol, 5% sorbitol fruit flavor
	guaifenesin, 100 mg/5 ml		alcohol, 5%
acetaminophen, 325 mg	terpin hydrate, 180 mg	dextromethorphan hydro-bromide, 30 mg	

COLD, ALLERGY, COUGH PRODUCT TABLE, continued

Product (Manufacturer)	Dose Form	Decongestant	Antihistamine
Tussar DM[c] (Rorer)	syrup	pseudoephedrine hydrochloride, 30 mg/5 ml	chlorpheniramine maleate, 2 mg/5 ml
Tussar-2 (Rorer)	syrup		chlorpheniramine maleate, 2 mg/5 ml
Tussciden Expectorant (Cenci)	liquid		
Tussex Cough (Various manufacturers)	syrup	phenylephrine hydrochloride, 5 mg/5 ml	
Ty-Cold (Major)	tablet	pseudoephedrine hydrochloride, 30 mg	chlorpheniramine maleate, 2 mg
Tylenol Allergy Sinus (McNeil)	caplet	pseudoephedrine hydrochloride, 30 mg	chlorpheniramine maleate, 2 mg
Tylenol Cold Medication (McNeil)	liquid	pseudoephedrine hydrochloride, 10 mg/5 ml	chlorpheniramine maleate, 0.67 mg/5 ml
Tylenol Cold No Drowsiness (McNeil)	caplet	pseudoephedrine hydrochloride, 30 mg	
Tylenol Multi-Symptom Cold (McNeil)	caplet tablet	pseudoephedrine hydrochloride, 30 mg	chlorpheniramine maleate, 2 mg
Tylenol Sinus Maximum Strength (McNeil)	caplet tablet	pseudoephedrine hydrochloride, 30 mg	
Ursinus Inlay-Tabs (Sandoz)	tablet	pseudoephedrine hydrochloride, 30 mg	
Valihist (Otis Clapp)	tablet	phenylephrine hydrochloride, 5 mg	chlorpheniramine maleate, 2 mg
Vicks Children's Cough[c] (Richardson-Vicks)	syrup		
Viro-Med (Whitehall)	tablet	pseudoephedrine hydrochloride, 30 mg	chlorpheniramine maleate, 2 mg

[a] Schedule V drug; nonprescription sale forbidden in some states.
[b] Sugar free.
[c] Alcohol free.

Analgesic	Expectorant	Cough Suppressant	Other Ingredients
		dextromethorphan hydrobromide, 15 mg/5 ml	sucrose
	guaifenesin, 105 mg/5 ml	codeine phosphate[a], 10 mg/5 ml	alcohol, 6% saccharin sucrose
	guaifenesin, 100 mg/5 ml		
	guaifenesin, 100 mg/5 ml	dextromethorphan hydrobromide, 10 mg/5 ml	
acetaminophen, 325 mg		dextromethorphan hydrobromide, 15 mg	
acetaminophen, 500 mg			
acetaminophen, 108.3 mg/ 5 ml		dextromethorphan hydrobromide, 5 mg/5 ml	alcohol, 7%
acetaminophen, 325 mg		dextromethorphan hydrobromide, 15 mg	
acetaminophen, 325 mg		dextromethorphan hydrobromide, 15 mg	
acetaminophen, 500 mg			
aspirin, 325 mg			
acetaminophen, 325 mg			caffeine
	guaifenesin, 50 mg/5 ml	dextromethorphan hydrobromide, 3.5 mg/5 ml	saccharin sucrose cherry flavor
acetaminophen, 500 mg		dextromethorphan hydrobromide, 15 mg	

TOPICAL DECONGESTANT PRODUCT TABLE

Product (Manufacturer)	Application Form	Sympathomimetic Agent	Preservative	Other Ingredients
Adrenalin Chloride (Parke-Davis)	nasal drops	epinephrine hydrochloride, 0.1%	chlorobutanol sodium bisulfite	
Afrin 12-Hour (Schering)	nasal drops nasal spray (metered pump)	oxymetazoline hydrochloride, 0.05%	benzalkonium chloride, 0.2 mg/ml phenylmercuric acetate, 0.02 mg/ml	sorbitol, 57 mg/ml glycine, 3.8 mg/ml sodium hydroxide
Afrin 12-Hour Cherry (Schering)	nasal spray	oxymetazoline hydrochloride, 0.05%	benzalkonium chloride phenylmercuric acetate	glycine sorbitol aromatics
Afrin 12-Hour Menthol (Schering)	nasal spray	oxymetazoline hydrochloride, 0.05%	benzalkonium chloride phenylmercuric acetate	camphor eucalyptol glycine menthol sorbitol
Afrin 12-Hour Pediatric (Schering)	nasal drops	oxymetazoline hydrochloride, 0.025%	benzalkonium chloride, 0.2 mg/ml phenylmercuric acetate, 0.02 mg/ml	glycine, 3.8 mg/ml sorbitol, 57.1 mg/ml
Alconefrin 12 (Webcon)	nasal drops	phenylephrine hydrochloride, 0.16%		
Alconefrin 25 (Webcon)	nasal drops nasal spray	phenylephrine hydrochloride, 0.25%		
Alconefrin 50 (Webcon)	nasal drops	phenylephrine hydrochloride, 0.5%		
Allerest (Fisons)	nasal spray	oxymetazoline hydrochloride, 0.05%	sodium bisulfite benzalkonium chloride EDTA	saline phosphate buffer
Benzedrex (SmithKline)	inhaler	propylhexedrine, 250 mg		aromatics menthol
Chlorphed-LA (Hauck)	nasal spray	oxymetazoline hydrochloride, 0.05%	phenylmercuric acetate	
Coricidin (Schering)	nasal mist	oxymetazoline hydrochloride, 0.05%	benzalkonium chloride phenylmercuric acetate, 0.02 mg/ml	glycine sorbitol
Doktors (Scherer)	nasal drops nasal spray	phenylephrine hydrochloride, 0.25%	chlorobutanol sodium bisulfite benzalkonium chloride	
Dristan (Whitehall)	inhaler nasal spray (metered-dose pump)	propylhexedrine (inhaler) phenylephrine hydrochloride, 0.5% (spray)	benzalkonium chloride, 0.02% (spray) thimerosal, 0.002% (spray)	pheniramine maleate, 0.2% (spray) menthol eucalyptol
Dristan Long-Lasting (Whitehall)	nasal spray (metered-dose pump)	oxymetazoline hydrochloride, 0.05%	benzalkonium chloride, 0.02% thimerosal, 0.002%	
Dristan Long-Lasting Menthol (Whitehall)	nasal spray	oxymetazoline hydrochloride, 0.05%	benzalkonium chloride, 0.02% thimerosal, 0.002%	menthol camphor eucalyptol
Dristan Menthol (Whitehall)	nasal spray	phenylephrine hydrochloride, 0.5%	benzalkonium chloride, 0.02% thimerosal, 0.002%	pheniramine maleate, 0.2% camphor eucalyptol menthol methyl salicylate

TOPICAL DECONGESTANT PRODUCT TABLE, continued

Product (Manufacturer)	Application Form	Sympathomimetic Agent	Preservative	Other Ingredients
Duramist Plus (Pfeiffer)	nasal spray	oxymetazoline, 0.05%	thimerosal, 0.002%	
Duration (Schering-Plough)	nasal spray	oxymetazoline hydrochloride, 0.05%	phenylmercuric acetate, 0.002%	
Duration Mentholated Vapor Spray (Schering-Plough)	nasal spray	oxymetazoline hydrochloride, 0.05%	phenylmercuric acetate, 0.002%	menthol camphor eucalyptol
Efedron (Hyrex)	nasal jelly	ephedrine hydrochloride, 0.6%	chlorobutanol	aromatics
4-Way Fast Acting Menthol and Regular (Bristol-Myers)	nasal spray	phenylephrine hydrochloride, 0.5% naphazoline hydrochloride, 0.05%	thimerosal, 0.005%	pyrilamine maleate, 0.2%
4-Way Long Lasting (Bristol-Myers)	nasal spray	oxymetazoline hydrochloride, 0.05%	phenylmercuric acetate, 0.002%	
Genasal (Goldline)	nasal solution	oxymetazoline hydrochloride, 0.05%	phenylmercuric acetate	
Myci-Spray (Misemer)	nasal spray	phenylephrine hydrochloride, 0.25%		pyrilamine maleate, 0.15%
Neo-Synephrine Extra (Winthrop)	nasal drops nasal spray	phenylephrine hydrochloride, 1%	benzalkonium chloride thimerosal, 0.001%	
Neo-Synephrine Maximum-12 Hour (Winthrop)	nasal pump nasal spray	oxymetazoline hydrochloride, 0.05%	benzalkonium chloride thimerosal, 0.001%	
Neo-Synephrine Mild (Winthrop)	nasal drops nasal spray	phenylephrine hydrochloride, 0.25%	benzalkonium chloride thimerosal, 0.001%	
Neo-Synephrine Pediatric (Winthrop)	nasal drops	phenylephrine hydrochloride, 0.125%	benzalkonium chloride thimerosal, 0.001%	
Neo-Synephrine Regular (Winthrop)	nasal drops nasal jelly nasal pump nasal spray	phenylephrine hydrochloride, 0.5%	benzalkonium chloride thimerosal, 0.001% phenylmercuric acetate, 0.002% (jelly)	
Nichols Nasal Douche Powder (Alvin Last)	powder (for isotonic reconstitution)			sodium bicarbonate sodium chloride sodium borate menthol eucalyptol
Nostril 1/4% Mild (Boehringer-Ingelheim)	nasal spray	phenylephrine hydrochloride, 0.25%	benzalkonium chloride, 0.004%	boric acid sodium borate
Nostril 1/2% Regular (Boehringer-Ingelheim)	nasal spray	phenylephrine hydrochloride, 0.5%	benzalkonium chloride, 0.004%	boric acid sodium borate
Nostrilla, Long Acting 12-Hour (Boehringer-Ingelheim)	nasal spray	oxymetazoline hydrochloride, 0.05%	benzalkonium chloride, 0.02%	glycine sorbitol solution
NTZ Long Lasting (Winthrop)	nasal drops nasal spray	oxymetazoline hydrochloride, 0.05%	benzalkonium chloride phenylmercuric acetate, 0.002%	

TOPICAL DECONGESTANT PRODUCT TABLE, continued

Product (Manufacturer)	Application Form	Sympathomimetic Agent	Preservative	Other Ingredients
Otrivin (Ciba)	nasal drops nasal spray	xylometazoline hydrochloride, 0.1%	benzalkonium chloride, 1:5000	potassium chloride potassium phosphate monobasic sodium chloride sodium phosphate dibasic
Otrivin Pediatric (Ciba)	nasal drops	xylometazoline hydrochloride, 0.05%	benzalkonium chloride, 1:5000	potassium chloride potassium phosphate monobasic sodium chloride sodium phosphate dibasic
Oxymetazoline Hydrochloride (Various manufacturers)	nasal spray	oxymetazoline hydrochloride, 0.05%		
Phenylephrine Hydrochloride (Various manufacturers)	nasal solution	phenylephrine hydrochloride, 0.25%, 1%		
Privine (Ciba)	nasal drops nasal spray	naphazoline hydrochloride, 0.05%	benzalkonium chloride, 1:5000 EDTA	hydrochloric acid sodium chloride
Rhinall (Scherer)	nasal drops nasal spray	phenylephrine hydrochloride, 0.25%	chlorobutanol sodium bisulfite benzalkonium chloride	
Rhinall-10 (Scherer)	nasal drops	phenylephrine hydrochloride, 0.2%	chlorobutanol sodium bisulfite benzalkonium chloride	
Sinarest (Fisons)	nasal spray	oxymetazoline hydrochloride, 0.05%	sodium bisulfite benzalkonium chloride EDTA	saline phosphate buffer
Sinex (Richardson-Vicks)	nasal spray	phenylephrine hydrochloride, 0.5%	thimerosal, 0.001%	menthol eucalyptol camphor
Sinex-L.A. (Richardson-Vicks)	nasal spray	oxymetazoline hydrochloride, 0.05%	thimerosal, 0.001%	
St. Joseph (Schering-Plough)	nasal spray (metered dose)	phenylephrine hydrochloride, 0.125%	cetylpyridinium chloride phenylmercuric acetate, 0.002%	
Twice-A-Day (Major)	nasal solution	oxymetazoline hydrochloride, 0.05%		
Va-Tro-Nol (Richardson-Vicks)	nasal drops	ephedrine sulfate, 0.5%	thimerosal, 0.001%	menthol eucalyptol camphor
Vicks Inhaler (Richardson-Vicks)	inhaler	levodesoxyephedrine, 50 mg		menthol camphor bornyl acetate
Xylometazoline Hydrochloride (Various manufacturers)	nasal spray	xylometazoline hydrochloride, 0.1%		

TOPICAL DECONGESTANT PRODUCT TABLE, continued

MISCELLANEOUS NASAL PRODUCTS

Product (Manufacturer)	Application Form	Preservative	Other Ingredients
Ayr (B.F. Ascher)	nasal drops nasal spray	benzalkonium chloride thimerosal	sodium chloride, 0.65%
HuMIST Saline (Scherer)	nasal spray	chlorobutanol	sodium chloride, 0.65%
NãSal Saline Nasal Moisturizer (Winthrop)	nasal drops nasal spray	benzalkonium chloride thimerosal, 0.001%	sodium chloride, 0.65%
Ocean Mist (Fleming)	nasal spray		benzyl alcohol sodium chloride, 0.65%
Pretz (Parnell)	nasal solution	EDTA benzalkonium chloride	sodium chloride, 0.6%
Salinex (Muro)	nasal drops nasal spray	EDTA benzalkonium chloride	sodium chloride, 0.4%

LOZENGE PRODUCT TABLE

Product (Manufacturer)	Anesthetic	Antibacterial Agent	Cough Suppressant	Expectorant	Other Ingredients
Cēpacol (Lakeside)	benzyl alcohol, 3%	cetylpyridinium chloride, 1:1500			sucrose, 1 g
Cēpacol Troches (Lakeside)	benzocaine, 10 mg	cetylpyridinium chloride, 1:1500			sucrose, 1 g
Cēpastat[a] (Lakeside)		phenol[b], 1.45%			menthol, 0.12% eucalyptus oil, 0.04% sorbitol
Cēpastat Cherry[a] (Lakeside)		phenol[b], 0.73%			menthol, 0.12% sorbitol mannitol
Children's Chloraseptic (Richardson-Vicks)	benzocaine, 5 mg				
Children's Hold 4-Hour Cough Suppressant (SmithKline Beecham)			dextromethor-phan, 3.75 mg		phenylpropanolamine, 6.25 mg
Chloraseptic Cherry and Menthol (Richardson-Vicks)		phenol[b], 32.5 mg			flavor sucrose
Chloraseptic Cool Mint (Richardson-Vicks)	benzocaine, 6 mg				menthol, 10 mg flavor sucrose
Conex (Forest)	benzocaine, 5 mg	cetylpyridinium chloride, 0.5 mg			methylparaben, 2 mg propylparaben, 0.5 mg sucrose, 738 mg
Hall's Mentho-Lyptus (Warner-Lambert)					menthol eucalyptus oil flavor
Hold 4-Hour Cough Suppressant (SmithKline Beecham)			dextromethor-phan hydro-bromide, 5 mg		
Isodettes Sore Throat Lozenges (Goody's)		phenol[b], 32.5 mg			
Lanazets Improved (Lannett)	benzocaine, 5 mg	cetylpyridinium chloride, 1 mg			
Larynex[a] (Dover)	benzocaine				
Listerine Antiseptic (Warner-Lambert)		hexylresorcinol, 2.4%			flavor

LOZENGE PRODUCT TABLE, continued

Product (Manufacturer)	Anesthetic	Antibacterial Agent	Cough Suppressant	Expectorant	Other Ingredients
Listerine Maximum Strength Throat (Warner-Lambert)		hexylresorcinol, 4 mg			
Medikets (Halsey)	benzocaine, 10 mg	cetylpyridinium chloride, 2.5 mg			
Mycinettes[a] (Pfeiffer)	benzocaine, 15 mg	cetylpyridinium chloride, 2.5 mg			
N'Ice Cough Lozenges[a] (SmithKline Beecham)					menthol, 3-6 mg (depending on flavor) sorbitol
Oracin[a] (Richardson-Vicks)	benzocaine, 6.25 mg				menthol, 0.08%
Oradex-C (Commerce)	benzocaine, 10 mg	cetylpyridinium chloride, 2.5 mg			
Protac (Republic)	benzocaine, 10 mg	cetylpyridinium chloride, 2.5 mg			
Robitussin-DM Cough Calmers (Robins)			dextromethorphan hydrobromide, 7.5 mg	guaifenesin, 50 mg	sucrose, 3.63 g
Sepo (Otis Clapp)	benzocaine, 14 mg				
Silexin (Otis Clapp)	benzocaine, 7.9 mg		dextromethorphan hydrobromide, 5 mg		
Soretts (Lannett)	benzocaine, 32 mg				licorice extract, 8 mg menthol, 0.5 mg
Spec-T (Squibb)	benzocaine, 10 mg				
Spec-T Sore Throat/Cough Suppressant Lozenges (Squibb)	benzocaine, 10 mg		dextromethorphan hydrobromide, 10 mg		tartrazine
Spec-T Sore Throat/Decongestant Lozenges (Squibb)	benzocaine, 10 mg				phenylephrine hydrochloride, 5 mg phenylpropanolamine hydrochloride, 10.5 mg tartrazine
Sucrets (SmithKline Beecham)		hexylresorcinol, 2.4 mg			
Sucrets Children's Cherry Flavored Sore Throat Lozenges (SmithKline Beecham)	dyclonine hydrochloride, 1.2 mg				citric acid corn syrup silicon dioxide sucrose flavor

LOZENGE PRODUCT TABLE, continued

Product (Manufacturer)	Anesthetic	Antibacterial Agent	Cough Suppressant	Expectorant	Other Ingredients
Sucrets Cold Decongestant Formula (SmithKline Beecham)					phenylpropanolamine hydrochloride, 25 mg
Sucrets Cough Control Formula (SmithKline Beecham)			dextromethorphan hydrobromide, 7.5 mg		
Sucrets Maximum Strength Sore Throat Lozenges (SmithKline Beecham)	dyclonine hydrochloride, 3 mg				citric acid corn syrup silicon dioxide sucrose flavor
Synthaloids (Buffington)	benzocaine, 12 mg				calcium-iodine complex
T-Caine (Schein)	benzocaine, 5 mg				
Thorets[a] (Buffington)	benzocaine, 18 mg				
Throat Discs (Marion)					capsicum peppermint oil anise oil cubeb glycyrrhiza extract linseed anethole oleoresin mineral oil sucrose starch acacia gum tragacanth
Trocaine (Vortech)	benzocaine, 10 mg	cetylpyridinium chloride, 2.5 mg		terpin hydrate, 15 mg	
Tymatro (Jones Medical)	benzocaine, 5 mg	cetylpyridinium chloride, 1.5 mg			flavor
Tyrobenz (Hauck)	benzocaine, 10 mg				cherry custard flavor
Vicks Cough Silencers (Richardson-Vicks)	benzocaine, 1 mg		dextromethorphan hydrobromide, 2.5 mg		tartrazine menthol anethole peppermint oil
Vicks Formula 44 Cough Control Discs (Richardson-Vicks)	benzocaine, 1.25 mg		dextromethorphan hydrobromide, 5 mg		menthol, 4.3 mg
Vicks Throat Lozenges (Richardson-Vicks)	benzocaine, 5 mg				menthol camphor eucalyptus oil

LOZENGE PRODUCT TABLE, continued

Product (Manufacturer)	Anesthetic	Antibacterial Agent	Cough Suppressant	Expectorant	Other Ingredients
Victors Regular Flavor (Richardson-Vicks)					menthol, 3.69 mg (square) 3.44 mg (football)
Victors Cherry Flavor (Richardson-Vicks)					menthol, 2.97 mg (square) 2.61 mg (football)

[a] Sugar free.
[b] Phenol is also an anesthetic.

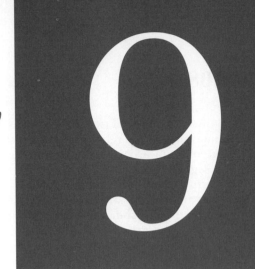

H. William Kelly and Celeste Lindley

ASTHMA PRODUCTS

Q*uestions to ask in patient/consumer counseling*

Has a physician diagnosed your condition as asthma?

Are you under the care of a physician?

Do you have any other medical problems such as heart disease, seizures, high blood pressure, hyperthyroidism, or diabetes?

What prescription or nonprescription medications are you taking?

Which asthma products have you used before? Were they effective?

Did they cause any problems (side effects)? If so, what were they?

The respiratory system is a series of airways, starting with the nose and mouth and leading ultimately to the terminal air sacs or alveoli. The mouth and nasal passages lead to the pharynx, which branches into the esophagus and the trachea. The trachea divides into the two large mainstem bronchi that supply air to the lungs. Each bronchus progressively divides into smaller airways (bronchioles), leading through the alveolar ducts to the alveoli (1). Layers of smooth muscle are wrapped around the airways in diminishing amounts as the airways progress toward the alveoli.

As an airway branches, the walls become progressively thinner. At the level of the alveoli, all that remains is a thin layer of cells surrounded by pulmonary capillaries. Respiration, which is the exchange of gases, occurs in the alveoli. Oxygen passes across the alveolar walls into the capillaries, and carbon dioxide diffuses in the opposite direction.

The lungs are essentially elastic air sacs suspended in the airtight thoracic cavity. The movable walls of this cavity are formed by the sternum, ribs, and diaphragm. As the thoracic cavity expands, the pressure within the cavity becomes less than the atmospheric pressure, air enters, and the lungs expand. This process is accomplished by means of two simultaneous mechanisms. The diaphragm, when relaxed, is a dome-shaped muscle that extends upward into the thoracic cavity. As the diaphragm contracts, it becomes flattened and moves downward into the abdomen, causing an increase in the longitudinal size of the thoracic cavity. The ribs are attached to the spinal vertebrae and join together at the sternum (breastbone). Contraction of the external intercostal muscles raises the ribs, causing an elevation and forward movement of the sternum and an increase in the diameter of the chest cavity. During inspiration, the diaphragm and the ribs move simultaneously, expanding the thoracic cavity, and the lungs fill with air. Expiration results from relaxation of the ventilatory muscles and the elastic recoil force of the alveoli and airways.

During normal inspiration, inhaled air is cleaned and humidified before it is delivered to the alveoli. The nasal cavities are lined with highly vascular mucous membranes and ciliated epithelial cells. As air passes over these areas, it is warmed, humidified, and filtered. Dust particles, bacteria, and other foreign matter are trapped in the mucus and propelled toward the pharynx by the movement of the nasal cilia. Humidification and filtration continue as air passes through the trachea, bronchi, and bronchioles. The airway's mucous membrane consists of ciliated epithelial cells interspersed with mucous-producing goblet cells. Trapped particles are moved upward with the mucus by the wavelike movement of the cilia and are deposited in the oral cavity where they are either expelled or swallowed.

Bronchial smooth muscle tone and mucus secretion are under neural and humoral control (Figure 1). Afferent nerves leading from irritant receptors in the mucosal epithelium produce reflex bronchoconstriction, increased mucus production, and cough through cholinergic innervation of bronchial smooth muscle and goblet cells from the vagus nerve. Smooth muscle of the airway is only sparsely innervated by the adrenergic system through the first six generations of airways; however, smooth muscle throughout the entire airway contains beta-adrenergic receptors. Alpha-adrenergic stimulation produces smooth muscle contraction (primary vascular), and beta$_2$-adrenergic stimulation produces smooth muscle relaxation. The nonadrenergic, noncholinergic (NANC) nervous system is the principal inhibitory system of the airways, counteracting the cholinergic excitatory system. Stimulation of this system through the vagus nerve primarily produces bronchodilation but can also produce bronchoconstriction. Neurotransmission through the NANC is mediated by neuropeptides, which have not been conclusively identified. It appears that vasoactive intestinal peptide (VIP) acts as an inhibitory transmitter and substance P as an excitatory transmitter. Under normal circumstances these systems maintain normal bronchomotor tone.

Epidemiology and Etiology of Asthma

The American Thoracic Society has defined bronchial asthma as "a disease characterized by an increased responsiveness of the trachea and bronchi to various stimuli and manifested by a widespread narrowing of the airways that changes in severity either spontaneously or as a result of therapy" (3).

The 1979 National Institute of Allergy and Infectious Diseases (NIAID) Task Force on Asthma estimated that more than 9 million persons suffer from asthma (about 4% of our population) (4). As many as 7% of all Americans have had asthma during their lifetime. The estimated cost of asthma in the United States in 1979 was $2.4 billion (5). The estimated number of deaths caused by asthma was 1,872, with an additional 4,401 deaths in which asthma was a significant contributing factor (5). Of major concern are recent studies showing an increase in the death rates for asthma in the United States and other countries (6–8). In 1977, the death rate in the United States reached a nadir of 0.6/100,000 population but by 1984 it almost doubled, to 1.1/100,000 population (7, 8). Although the most dramatic increase in death rates was in the elderly, all age ranges have been affected. The cause is unclear. It is important to note that the most precipitous increases occurred in urban areas and for black and Hispanic patients. In retrospective studies, fatalities have been linked to failure to institute therapy with high-dose corticosteroid early in the course of acute exacerbation. Asthma is the most common cause of school absenteeism and hospital admissions in children. Annually, asthma was responsible for almost 7 million physician office visits and for more than 2 million days in the hospital (5).

Symptomatic asthma is more prevalent in children (8–10%) than adults; the age of onset for 50% of all subjects was under 10 years of age (9). The prevalence rate for asthma is slightly higher in males than in females (9). Long-term follow-up studies of asthmatic children indicate that 50–70% go into permanent or temporary symptom-free remission by adulthood. In many of the patients, symptoms significantly decrease in severity. Therefore, children who develop asthma have a good overall prognosis. However, 30% of children with asthma will have chronic symptoms into adulthood, and there is increasing evidence that chronic asthma may result in irreversible chronic obstruction.

In the past patients were characterized as having either extrinsic (allergenic) or intrinsic (nonallergenic) asthma. A personal or family history of allergy, seasonal variation in symptoms, positive skin tests, and elevated circulating immunoglobulin E (IgE) levels were considered characteristics of extrinsic asthma. Recent find-

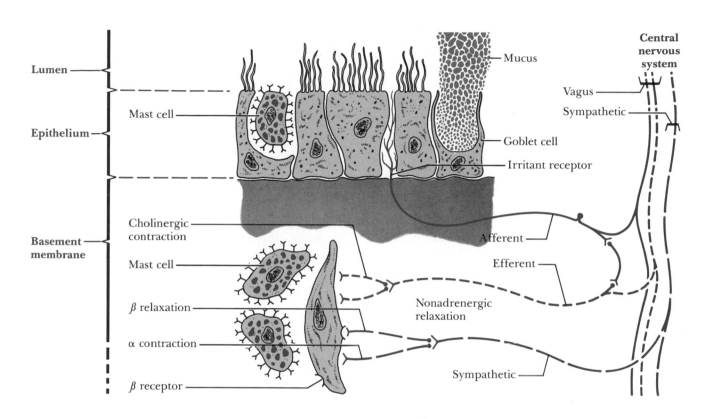

FIGURE 1 Innervation of the airways by the sympathetic, cholinergic, and nonadrenergic inhibitory systems. Mast cell concentration increases from the epithelial lumen to the submucosa. Adapted with permission from "Pharmacotherapy: A Pathophysiologic Approach," J. Dipiro et al., Eds., Elsevier Science Publishing, New York, N.Y., 1989, p. 350.

ings suggest that all asthmatics have elevated serum IgE levels, and that there are no differences between intrinsic and extrinsic asthma. However, the exact etiology of asthma is still unknown. Asthma may be a heterogeneous group of diseases with a similar final common expression, or it may require a specific set of coincidental conditions such as genetic predisposition and environmental exposures. Regardless, it is now clear that asthma is a lung disorder and not an emotional, allergic, or infectious disease. Despite our improved understanding of the pathophysiology of asthma, the lack of a specific etiology frequently results in classifying asthma according to its predominant environmental trigger.

Asthma exacerbations are generally precipitated by respiratory tract infection, particularly viral infection; inhaled allergens such as pollen, dust, or mold; inhaled air pollutants; exercise; or occupational and industrial irritants or drugs (11). Many triggers may induce an exacerbation in a patient's symptoms. An identifiable allergen is the major precipitating factor in about 35–55% of the asthmatic population, and respiratory infections are a major factor in about 40%. About 2–10% of asthmatics develop acute asthma following ingestion of aspirin and other nonsteroidal anti-inflammatory drugs (12).

Pathophysiology of Asthma

The mechanism by which asthma attacks occur continues to be a major area of research, and has recently been reviewed (13). The common finding in all patients with asthma is hyperreactivity of the tracheobronchial tree. The hyperreactivity is characterized by airway smooth muscle contraction, mucosal inflammation and edema, and mucus hypersecretion (Figure 2). When patients with allergies and asthma are exposed to an antigen, sensitized mast cells become activated and release chemical mediators of immediate hypersensitivity (histamine, leukotrienes, eosinophil chemotactic factor, prostaglandins, and others). These chemical mediators are capable of constricting bronchiolar smooth muscle, increasing vascular permeability, aggregating platelets, and stimulating an inflammatory reaction. However, the allergic reaction is not the only etiology of the patient's hyperreactivity. These patients also produce bronchospasm upon exposure to nonspecific stimuli such as exercise, irritants, and cold air hyperventilation. Moreover, a large number of patients with allergies or hay fever do not have asthma (12).

An imbalance in neuronal control may be involved. Neural control of the lungs is channeled through the parasympathetic and NANC fibers in the vagus nerve and the sympathetic fibers that arise from ganglia in the thorax. Normal tone of the bronchiolar smooth muscle is maintained by the vagus. Direct stimulation of the vagus causes constriction of the trachea, bronchi, and large bronchioles as well as increased goblet cell secretion and dilated pulmonary vessels, resulting in bronchospasm and excess mucus production. Activation of the irritant receptors produces stimulation of cholinergic pathways, resulting in a cough reflex and bronchospasm. Bronchospasm is the constriction of smooth muscles that line the tracheobronchial tree, resulting in a decrease in airway caliber and air flow. The NANC nervous system normally modulates the effect of the cholinergic nervous system (2). The recent discovery that the inhibitory neuropeptide VIP is absent in the lungs of asthmatics and is present in nonasthmatics may explain the bronchial hyperreactivity (14). There is minimal sympathetic innervation of the lungs; however, the airway smooth muscles contain numerous $beta_2$-receptors.

The activities of the mast cell and bronchiolar smooth muscle appear to be modulated by the intracellular concentration of the cyclic nucleotides 3':5' guanosine monophosphate (cyclic GMP) and 3':5' adenosine monophosphate (cyclic AMP). Cyclic GMP enhances the release of the chemical mediators from mast cells and promotes bronchoconstriction. Cholinergic activity stimulates the production of cyclic GMP. Cyclic AMP, on the other hand, promotes smooth muscle relaxation and inhibits mast cell mediator release. Beta$_2$-adrenergic stimulation increases cyclic AMP.

A relative decrease in beta$_2$-adrenergic activity has been proposed as a mechanism for bronchoconstriction (13). In asthmatics, administration of a beta$_2$-blocking agent may precipitate an attack. In contrast, nonasth-

matic patients whose beta-receptors have been completely blocked by drugs such as propranolol do not experience bronchospasm. It has been shown that chronic treatment with beta$_2$-agonists can produce a down regulation of beta$_2$-receptors; however, recent studies have failed to detect a significant beta blockade in asthma.

It has become increasingly evident that asthma is an inflammatory disease of the lungs, and that the severity of a patient's asthma and the degree of bronchial hyperreactivity correlate with the degree of inflammation (13). The bronchial smooth muscle of asthmatics does not respond to contracting substances such as histamine, serotonin, or acetylcholine with greater contraction than the bronchial smooth muscle of nonasthmatics. The chronic inflammation of the asthmatic's airways, however, produces smooth muscle hyperplasia, basement membrane hypertrophy, and increased mucus production, mucosal edema, and epithelial sloughing. These pathophysiologic changes (Figure 2) narrow the airway lumen of asthmatics so that contraction of the smooth muscle can result in complete closure of the airway (15). Therefore, inflammation of the airways, coupled with the possible lack or decrease of normal neuronal inhibitory control, results in the bronchial hyperreactivity that is characteristic of asthma.

The degree of the airway's hyperreactivity can be measured by having an asthmatic inhale increasing concentrations of pollens, or chemicals such as histamine, cold air, sulfur dioxide, or methacholine until the patient's tests of pulmonary function, usually forced expiratory volume in one second (FEV_1) or forced vital capacity (FVC), drop significantly (at least by 20%). The dose required to produce the drop is called the provocative dose or concentration (PD_{20} or PC_{20}) (16), which is the measure of the patient's hyperreactivity. This measure correlates with the severity of the patient's symptoms, need for medications, and reactivity to exercise and noxious environmental stimuli (16). An atopic patient's reactivity increases (PD_{20} to histamine or methacholine decreases) during a specific pollen season.

Symptoms

By definition, asthma is episodic in nature. Periods of airway obstruction may last from a few minutes to several days. The severity of obstruction is highly variable, producing mild symptoms or rapidly progressing to respiratory failure. Patients with more severe disease may have continuous symptoms that require chronic medication for control, while others may have normal pulmonary function between episodes and require only periodic medication.

The classic symptom of asthma is wheezing (a fine whistling sound) on expiration. In more severe obstruction, wheezing may occur on inspiration and expiration.

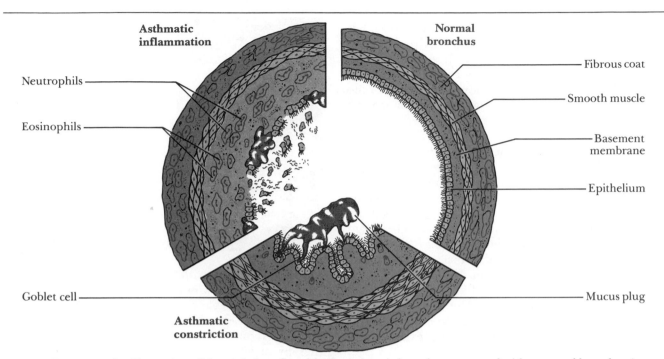

FIGURE 2 Representative illustration of the pathology found in the asthmatic bronchus compared with a normal bronchus (upper right section). Each section demonstrates how the lumen is narrowed. Edema of the basement membrane, mucus plugging, smooth muscle hypertrophy, and constriction contribute (lower section). Inflammatory cells producing epithelial desquammation fill the airway lumen with cellular debris and expose the airway smooth muscle to other mediators (upper left section). Adapted with permission from "Pharmacotherapy: A Pathophysiologic Approach," J. Dipiro et al., Eds., Elsevier Science Publishing, New York, N.Y., 1989, p. 349.

Coughing as a result of stimulation of the irritant receptors occurs commonly. Chronic cough may be the only presenting symptom in some patients with asthma. Patients may have normal spirometric pulmonary function tests between episodes, but many asthmatics have an increased bronchomotor tone, which is readily reversed with a bronchodilator drug. During attacks, asthmatics demonstrate a marked decrease in all measures of expiratory flow rate and patients often complain of a tightness in their chest and dyspnea (difficult breathing). Because outflow of air is obstructed to a greater degree than inflow, the lungs actually become overinflated and the patient has to breathe at higher lung volumes, making it more difficult to breathe.

PATIENT ASSESSMENT

In most cases, the patients themselves make the diagnosis of asthma after several episodes of intermittent shortness of breath and wheezing (11). Tightness in the chest and cough are frequently present and usually come and go with each attack. In some cases, however, chronic cough and shortness of breath may occur. Many patients have mild asthma that does not progress; in others, the condition may worsen and be accompanied by the following symptoms:

- Dyspnea and wheezing;
- Cough;
- Tachycardia;
- Retraction of the sternocleidomastoid muscle;
- Apprehension;
- Chest distention;
- Tenacious sputum;
- Flaring nostrils.

Sinus tachycardia with a pulse rate up to 120 contractions per minute is a very common finding (11). Sternocleidomastoid muscle retraction is a consistent finding in patients with severely impaired pulmonary function (11).

The question as to whether the pharmacist should evaluate patients' symptoms and recommend a nonprescription agent for the treatment of asthma is difficult to answer, but the following should be considered. If the symptoms are new and the patient has not been diagnosed by a physician as having asthma, physician referral for evaluation is essential. Nonprescription medication for asthma relief should never be used unless a diagnosis of asthma has been established by a physician. Diagnosis is important to rule out other causes of pulmonary symptoms such as physical obstruction from a tumor, congestive heart failure, and chronic bronchitis. It is also important to establish a baseline for disease severity, explore the etiology of the patient's asthma so that the triggering factor may be removed, and avoid nonprescription medication that may worsen other conditions.

For instance, if a patient with new pulmonary symptoms describes a history of hypertension or heart disease, physician referral is essential because patients with congestive heart failure may awaken in the middle of the night with dyspnea and cough resulting from pulmonary edema. Shortness of breath and chest pain in women taking oral contraceptives may be signs of pulmonary emboli rather than asthma, and the patient should be referred to a physician.

People with chronic bronchitis and emphysema have symptoms similar to asthma. However, these symptoms are usually continuous, not episodic, and should not be treated with nonprescription drugs except under a physician's care.

If a diagnosis of asthma has been established previously, it is important to determine how severe the symptoms are and which self-treatment approaches have already been tried. Patients need immediate medical help if they are unable to complete a full sentence without stopping for shortness of breath, if discomfort persists while at rest after bronchodilator administration, or if the bronchodilator does not completely relieve the symptoms. If a bronchodilator (aerosol, oral, or both) is being used, but the dyspnea becomes worse, a severe attack may be imminent, and patients should see a physician immediately. Patients with progressive dyspnea and wheezing, who are dependent on nonprescription products, may be in danger of severe pulmonary obstruction, which may require hospitalization.

It is important to note that the leading cause of death from asthma is underassessment of severity of an attack, which results in failure to seek medical care. In patients with intermittent asthma, or in those whose symptoms are relieved with therapy, evaluation of symptoms becomes more difficult. Significant airway obstruction may be present even when symptoms are absent. In this situation, spirometric measurements will most accurately reflect the status of airway function (11). In one group of patients who were symptomatic, the patients were more accurate in characterizing the severity of their airway obstruction than were experienced physicians on the basis of a physical examination (17). However, in another group of asthmatics, 15% of patients were unable to sense significant airway obstruction (18).

Although it is clear that symptoms of patients with mild, seasonal asthma or exercise-induced asthma are often relieved without medication, the difficulty is in

TABLE 1   Antiasthmatic medications

Drug class	Availability
ANTI-INFLAMMATORIES	
Cromolyn sodium	Rx
Nedocromil	Rx
Corticosteroids	Rx
BRONCHODILATORS	
Sympathomimetics	Rx & OTC
Methylxanthines	Rx & OTC
Anticholinergics	Rx

distinguishing these patients from those with significant airway obstruction who may go on to develop a severe attack. The available evidence suggests that this judgment can best be made by the objective measurement of pulmonary function. It therefore seems prudent that therapy of all patients with asthma should be determined on the basis of periodic pulmonary function tests.

TREATMENT

It is now clear from our understanding of the pathophysiology of asthma that treatment should be aimed at reversing or preventing inflammation and bronchospasm produced by smooth muscle contraction. Table 1 lists the currently available drugs used to treat asthma. Because the only drugs available for non-prescription therapy of asthma are bronchodilators, nonprescription therapy is expected only to provide symptomatic relief of acute bronchospasm and decrease exercise-induced asthma. This form of therapy does not decrease the underlying inflammation and bronchial hyperreactivity in asthmatics (13).

Drugs available without a prescription for the treatment of asthma are limited to epinephrine in aerosol dosage form; ephedrine alone and in combination dosage forms, such as with theophylline; and ephedrine, phenobarbital, and theophylline in combination dosage forms. Prescription bronchodilator drugs available for the treatment of asthma include aerosol isoproterenol, metaproterenol, terbutaline, pirbuterol, bitolterol, and isoetherine. Oral bronchodilator dosage forms include terbutaline, albuterol, metaproterenol, and single-entity theophylline. In addition to these agents, aerosolized atropine and ipratropium have been used to reduce bronchoconstriction while using oral and aerosolized corticosteroids, cromolyn and the cromolyn-like agent nedocromil to abate inflammation (Table 2).

General Pharmacology

Beta$_2$-adrenergic bronchodilators (albuterol and terbutaline) stimulate the enzyme adenylate cyclase, producing an increased intracellular cyclic AMP concentration. Anticholinergic bronchodilators (atropine) inhibit the formation of cyclic GMP (19). Similarly, drugs with the opposite effects, such as beta-blockers and cholinergics, can be expected to cause bronchospasm in patients with asthma (12). Other drugs that can induce bronchospasm are aspirin and other prostaglandin synthetase inhibitors, sulfites, and phenylephrine in some patients.

For clinical purposes, it is more important to understand the pharmacologic effects of stimulating the different autonomic receptors (Table 3). The effect of a nonselective drug such as ephedrine and epinephrine depends on the predominant receptor type in the tissue or organ. Thus epinephrine produces relaxation in the bronchi and constriction in the vasculature. The ideal drug for the treatment of asthma would induce bronchodilation and stimulate mucociliary clearance. The only desirable property of alpha-adrenergic stimulation is the decongestant effect, which has little utility in asthma. The concomitant effects of bronchoconstriction, vasoconstriction, urinary retention, and mydriasis

TABLE 2 Characteristics of bronchodilator drugs

Drug	Route of administration	Availability	Pharmacologic activity				Duration of action (hr)
			SYMPATHOMIMETIC			ANTICHOLINERGIC	
			Alpha	Beta$_1$	Beta$_2$		
Albuterol	Inhalation	Rx		+[a]	+++		4–6
	PO: tablets	Rx		+	+++		4–8
Bitolterol	Inhalation	Rx		+[a]	+++		4–6
Epinephrine	Inhalation	OTC	+++[a]	+++[a]	+++		0.5–1
	SC	Rx	+++	+++	+++		1
	SC suspension						4–6
Ephedrine	PO: syrup, capsules, combination tablets	OTC	+++	++	++		3–5
	IV, IM, SC	Rx					2–4
Isoproterenol	Inhalation	Rx		+++[a]	+++		1–2
	IV, SL	Rx		+++	+++		IV = <1 SL = 1–2
Isoetharine	Inhalation	Rx		++[a]	+++		1–2
Metaproterenol	Inhalation	Rx		+++[a]	+++		3–4
	PO: tablets, syrup	Rx		+++	+++		4
Pirbuterol	Inhalation	Rx		+[a]	+++		4–6
Terbutaline	Inhalation	Rx		+[a]	+++		4–6
	Tablet	Rx		+	+++		4–8
	SC	Rx					1.5–4
Theophylline (various salts)	PO: combination liquids & tablets	OTC	+	++[b]	++[b]		4–12
	PO: single entity liquids & tablets sustained release	Rx	+	++[b]	++[b]		4–8 8–24
	IV	Rx					4–12
Atropine	IV, inhalation	Rx				+++	4
Ipratropium bromide	Inhalation	Rx				+++	4–6

+ Relative intensity of effect.
[a]Inhalation confers more bronchial activity than systemic administration.
[b]Although theophylline is not a sympathomimetic drug, it causes the release of endogenous catecholamines.

are clearly undesirable and are reflective of the clinical adverse effects of systemically administered epinephrine or ephedrine (Table 2). In some patients with bronchospasm and rhinorrhea (hay fever), decongestant effects may be desirable. However, patients with bronchospasm and rhinorrhea who need a nasal decongestant may be treated more effectively with an alpha-adrenergic nasal spray and a bronchodilator that does not produce undesirable systemic alpha-adrenergic effects.

Beta$_1$-adrenergic stimulation (cardiac stimulation) is not a desirable effect, whereas beta$_2$-adrenergic stimulation most closely approaches the ideal drug characteristics in the treatment of asthma. Isoproterenol and metaproterenol have about the same beta$_1$ and beta$_2$ effects as opposed to the newer, relatively selective beta$_2$ drugs, including bitolterol, terbutaline, pirbuterol, and albuterol. Terbutaline, for example, induces bronchodilation and stimulates mucociliary clearance. However, up to 33% of patients on oral terbutaline may experience skeletal muscle tremor, which can be severe (20). The ultimate clinical benefit from using a systemic beta$_2$-agonist is unclear. Peripheral vasodilation from systemic beta$_2$-adrenergic stimulation decreases blood pressure, producing a compensatory increase in heart rate to maintain cardiac output (21). It is also known that 30–50% of cardiac beta-receptors are beta$_2$-receptors, and that beta$_2$-agonists can produce tachycardia by direct stimulation of these receptors. An early study comparing the relative effects of graded intravenous doses of isoproterenol (beta$_1$, beta$_2$) with albuterol (beta$_2$) found that albuterol produced less tachycardia at the same degree of bronchodilation. Isoproterenol produced a similar increase in both tachycardia and bronchodilation as the dose was increased (22). A study in patients with chronic obstructive pulmonary disease and preexisting premature ventricular contractions found that terbutaline (beta$_2$) produced a greater increase in heart rate and tended to produce a greater increase in premature ventricular contractions than theophylline or ephedrine at similar levels of bronchodilation (23). Hence, the newer beta$_2$-adrenergic stimulants should be regarded as "relatively selective" at best. An aerosol dosage form optimizes the bronchoselective action of the beta-agonists.

Anticholinergic drugs such as atropine are potent bronchodilators. However, when used systemically, the undesirable attendant pharmacologic effects (tachycardia, urinary retention, decreased mucociliary clearance, and mydriasis) limit the drugs' clinical utility. Aerosol administration greatly enhances atropine's bronchoselectivity. The lack of bronchoselectivity is caused by atropine's excellent systemic absorption. The quaternary ammonia derivative ipratropium bromide is poorly absorbed systemically and therefore provides greater bronchoselectivity and fewer side effects due to residual concentration in the lung.

Route of administration has a profound effect on the pulmonary selectivity of sympathomimetic and anticholinergic bronchodilators. At the same degree of bronchodilation, oral or intravenous terbutaline produces more tremor, hypotension, and tachycardia than does inhalation (21). The same is true for metaproterenol and epinephrine (24). When these drugs are inhaled, much less drug reaches the systemic circulation because the dose is smaller and the portion of the dose that is deposited in the mouth and swallowed (80% from a metered dose inhaler) is metabolized in the gut and liver. Local administration does not usually result in systemic effects at normal doses. It seems that the pattern of bronchodilation (large central bronchi versus small peripheral bronchioles) is similar by inhalation or systemic administration (24). Two significant advantages of the newer relatively selective beta$_2$-adrenergic stimulants are that they can be administered by mouth and their duration of action is longer.

Historically, there has been concern about patients becoming tachyphylactic or resistant to the bronchodilator effects of sympathomimetic bronchodilators. For an individual asthma patient who worsens, it would be difficult to determine if the drug has become ineffective because of tachyphylaxis or simply because the disease has worsened due to external or unidentified internal causes. The evidence indicates that there is both a down regulation (decreased number) and a decreased affinity which develops at the beta$_2$-receptor during chronic beta$_2$-agonist use (25). However, it reaches a plateau within a few weeks with no further deterioration. It appears to affect duration of action more than it does intensity of effect; corticosteroid therapy can prevent and reverse the tolerance. The clinical consequence of beta$_2$-agonist tolerance appears inconsequential.

Ingredients in Nonprescription Products

Epinephrine

Epinephrine is useful for the treatment of periodic and acute severe bronchospasm and also in prophylaxis against exercise-induced bronchospasm. For periodic asthma, epinephrine is administered by inhalation (metered aerosol or nebulized solution). Acute, severe asthma can be treated by subcutaneous injection or inhalation. Although the various epinephrine products differ slightly in the drug dose delivered, there is no difference between prescription or nonprescription inhalation epinephrine products.

TABLE 3 Clinical drug-induced effects on the various organs and tissues

Organ	Sympathomimetic			Anticholinergic
	Alpha	Beta$_1$	Beta$_2$	
Bronchopulmonary	Bronchoconstriction Decongestion		Bronchodilation Stimulation of mucociliary clearance	Bronchodilation Inhibition of mucociliary clearance
Heart		Increased heart rate, contractility, and automaticity	Increased heart rate	Increased heart rate
Peripheral blood vessels	Constriction		Dilation	
Urinary bladder	Difficulty in micturition			Difficulty in micturition
Eye	Mydriasis			Mydriasis Failure of accommodation
Skeletal muscle			Tremor	

Epinephrine has roughly equipotent alpha-, beta$_1$-, and beta$_2$-agonist effects, which are dose dependent. The effects of epinephrine are terminated as the drug is taken up by sympathetic nerve endings and by surrounding tissues (26). Epinephrine is metabolized in the nerve ending by monoamine oxidase, and in the tissues by catechol-*o*-methyltransferase. Epinephrine and isoproterenol are ineffective when taken by mouth because there is nearly complete metabolism by catechol-*o*-methyltransferase and sulfatase in the gastrointestinal tract and the liver. Adverse effects of epinephrine (tachycardia, cardiac arrhythmia, hypertension, tremor, and anxiety) are almost always associated with the parenteral route of administration. These effects would not be expected by the inhalation route except in an extreme overdose.

The peak effect of both epinephrine and isoproterenol aerosol occurs within 5–10 minutes. The peak effect of newer selective beta$_2$-agonists occurs between 15 and 30 minutes after administration. The duration of bronchodilation from epinephrine and isoproterenol is about 1–2 hours. The newer beta$_2$-agonists have a duration of bronchodilation of 4–6 hours; however the duration of protection from a significant asthmogenic stimulus (e.g., exercise, allergen challenge) is significantly shorter, only 2–3 hours (25). Thus, aerosol beta-agonists are not useful for chronic prophylaxis of asthma.

Probably the most significant problem associated with nonprescription epinephrine aerosols is that most patients do not administer the drug correctly. One study of hospitalized patients found that 47% did not use their aerosol correctly (27). The most commonly observed error was that the patient actuated the aerosol after the inspiration was complete. Even after the patients who used the aerosol incorrectly were taught the correct procedure, upon retesting at a later date approximately two-thirds had reverted to the incorrect techniques. These were patients who had serious diseases and would be expected to be under a physician's care.

Numerous studies investigating the optimal delivery of beta-adrenergic aerosols have been performed and recently reviewed (28, 29). The most commonly used delivery systems for the beta-adrenergic agonists are the chlorofluorocarbon-propelled, metered-dose canisters and the jet nebulizers with or without intermittent positive pressure breathing (IPPB). Numerous trials comparing the metered-dose canisters to nebulization and/or IPPB have failed to demonstrate a significant advantage for any of the methods. The metered-dose canisters are the most convenient form for administering aerosol beta-adrenergic agonists as well as the most cost effective.

Following actuation of a Freon-propelled canister, only approximately 10% of the dose is actually deposited in the lungs and 80% is deposited in the oropharynx and later swallowed. The remainder of the delivered dose is recovered from the canister and expired air. It has become increasingly recognized that inhalation technique and particle size are major determinants of the dose delivered to the lungs. A number of investigators have advocated various techniques to increase delivery, such as holding the canister away from an open mouth and timing the actuation late in inspiration. A series of recent studies have convincingly shown that the two most important variables are speed of inhalation and duration of breath holding. With a slow, deep inhalation and 10 seconds of breath holding, the time of canister actuation during inspiration was not a factor (29). This is an important finding because actuation of the canister after inspiration is complete is the most common error patients make. When accurate synchronization cannot be achieved, the patient may use a tube-spacer device, which acts as a holding chamber in which the medication is sprayed before inhalation, to improve deposition of aerosol into the lungs.

When a nonprescription epinephrine aerosol is purchased in a pharmacy, the pharmacist must instruct the patient on the correct administration technique. The correct procedure is to have the patient shake the canister thoroughly and then place the mouthpiece between the lips making sure the teeth and tongue are out of the way. An alternative method is for the patient to hold the mouthpiece an inch in front of the open mouth at level of the lips. The patient breathes out slowly and then activates the canister while taking a *slow,* deep breath. The inspiration continues to completion and the patient holds his breath at full inspiration for at least 10 seconds. A second dose may be administered at least 1 minute later. Waiting a few minutes between inhalations may allow the second dose to reach deeper into the small bronchioles and also allows the actuator to repressurize to ensure delivery of the correct dose. The pharmacist should watch the patient use the device to ensure that the instructions have been understood. If an aerosol is not administered correctly, it may be worthless in relieving bronchospasm. Also, all patients using inhalation devices should be periodically checked to ensure proper technique because studies have confirmed that even when initially instructed, many patients later develop poor technique.

In the 1960s in Great Britain, there were reports of a rapidly increasing mortality in asthmatic patients, particularly in children 10–14 years of age (30–32). It appeared that patients may have been overdosing themselves with nonprescription isoproterenol preparations that delivered a larger dose than was available in the United States. It was hypothesized that excessive exposure to the beta-agonist combined with the Freon propellant produced cardiac arrhythmias leading to sudden death. The epidemiologic data have been reevaluated, and autopsy data indicate that most deaths were caused by severe asthma attacks (33). Therefore, a more plausible explanation is that because of overdependence on aerosols, which were purchased without

medical supervision, the patients failed to recognize the severity of the problem and delayed seeking appropriate medical help.

Here lies the dilemma associated with the use of nonprescription drugs to treat bronchospasm from seasonal allergy, asthma, or chronic bronchitis. If the condition is self-limiting and does not become progressively worse, nonprescription bronchodilators may be effective, much like aspirin for relieving a simple headache. However, if the patient's condition worsens, competent medical care must be sought immediately. To tread this fine line can be dangerous, and the patient and the patient's family should know when to abandon self-treatment and immediately seek medical care. It should be remembered that in most cases of death from asthma, the severity of the obstruction had been underestimated by the physician or patient. Patients, with or without competent medical advice, continued inhaler treatment without relief.

The final monograph for over-the-counter (OTC) bronchodilator drug products was published by the Food and Drug Administration (FDA) in October 1986 (34). It addressed the issue of overuse of inhalers during acute attacks by requiring the following warning in bold face type: "Do not continue to use this product, but seek medical assistance immediately if symptoms are not relieved within 20 minutes or become worse." The final monograph placed epinephrine, epinephrine bitartrate, and epinephrine hydrochloride (racemic) in pressurized, metered-dose aerosol dosage forms and in aqueous solutions equivalent to 1% epinephrine for use with hand-held rubber bulb nebulizers in Category I. FDA further specified that when epinephrine is used in a pressurized metered-dose aerosol container, each inhalation should contain the equivalent of 0.16–0.25 mg of epinephrine base. Dosage recommendations adopted for metered-dose delivery systems for adults and children 4 years of age and older are as follows: Start with one inhalation, then wait at least 1 minute. If not relieved, use once more. Do not use again for at least 3 hours. When an aqueous solution at a concentration equivalent to 1% epinephrine base is used with a hand-held rubber bulb nebulizer, the inhalation dosage for adults and children 4 years of age or older are: 1 to 3 inhalations not more often than every 3 hours. For children under 4 years of age there is no recommended dosage except under the advice and supervision of a physician. The statement includes the directions that the use of these products by children should be supervised by an adult.

These products also require statements warning against exceeding the recommended dosages unless directed by a physician. Patients should be warned that excessive use of epinephrine-containing products may cause nervousness and rapid heart beat. Patients with heart disease, high blood pressure, thyroid disease, diabetes, or difficulty in urination due to enlargement of the prostate should avoid self-medication with these products except under the advice and supervision of a physician. In addition, patients taking a prescription antihypertensive or antidepressant drug are directed to consult their physician before using these products.

The products available when used in the manner described may be expected to provide temporary relief of shortness of breath, tightness in the chest, and wheezing caused by bronchial asthma. In the recommended dosage, it is unlikely that epinephrine will complicate cardiac disease or hypertension, or produce drug interactions. However, it must be recognized that some patients may have a tendency to overuse these products, particularly when relief of symptoms does not occur. If epinephrine is going to relieve bronchospasm, the effect should occur within 5–10 minutes after the last inhalation when the inhalor is used correctly. Pharmacists should advise patients to *seek medical attention if prompt relief does not occur* with recommended use of epinephrine-containing products.

Ephedrine

As a bronchodilator, ephedrine is useful only for treating mild to moderate seasonal or chronic asthma. Parenteral ephedrine is not recommended as a bronchodilator. Although ephedrine sulfate is available on a nonprescription basis for use as a single entity in a 25-mg capsule and a syrup, by far the most abundantly available preparations are combination tablets, elixirs, and suspensions. Drugs combined with ephedrine in these dosage forms include theophylline, phenobarbital, guaifenesin, and pyrilamine, as discussed below.

Ephedrine has roughly equivalent alpha, beta$_1$, and beta$_2$ activity. The pharmacologic actions of ephedrine are produced by an indirect effect whereby ephedrine induces the release of norepinephrine from sympathetic nerve endings. Because ephedrine causes the release of norepinephrine, the administration of ephedrine to a patient who has been receiving a monoamine oxidase inhibitor, which decreases the degradation and increases the storage of norepinephrine, could result in severe hypertension. Although this is a potentially fatal interaction, there is little clinical information available. Tricyclic antidepressants may partially block the action of ephedrine.

The major route of ephedrine elimination is as the unchanged drug in urine (35, 36). Although the average elimination half-life is 6 hours, the half-life will be decreased by urinary acidification and increased by alkalinization. Metabolic routes of elimination include nitrogen demethylation and oxidative deamination.

The peak bronchodilation effect occurs in 1 hour and lasts about 5 hours (37, 38). There is far more discussion of ephedrine tachyphylaxis or tolerance as a significant problem than is evidenced in the literature (37, 39).

The principal adverse effects of ephedrine are central nervous system (CNS) stimulation, nausea, tremors, tachycardia, and urinary retention. Other than urinary retention, this similar pattern of adverse effects is produced by theophylline. Of all the bronchodilators, CNS stimulation is produced only by ephedrine and theophylline. Reports indicate that chronic ephedrine overdosage may result in either severe cardiac toxicity or psychosis (40, 41). One report indicated that ephedrine may be a potential drug of abuse, producing symptoms of schizophrenia similar to those found in amphetamine psychosis. Ephedrine, like amphetamines, produces the release of catecholamines in the CNS. Ephedrine, caffeine, and phenylpropanolamine are frequent ingredients of drugs manufactured to physically resemble amphetamine dosage forms (42).

With the development of new orally active, selective, beta$_2$-agonists over the past decade, ephedrine has fallen into disfavor by many clinicians in the treatment of serious chronic or intermittent bronchospasm. Ephedrine is less potent and potentially more toxic, particularly in the CNS, than the newer orally active selective beta$_2$-agonists (terbutaline and albuterol) (43, 44). Ephedrine is considerably more hazardous to hypertensive patients. There appears to be little reason to recommend its use.

Ephedrine is available as a base, as hydrochloride and sulfate salts, and as racemic ephedrine hydrochloride. It is usually combined with other bronchodilator drugs. The tentative final monograph for OTC bronchodilator drug products placed products containing ephedrine in Category I—safe and effective. The dosage recommendation for adults and children over 12 years of age is 12.5–25 mg every 4 hours, not to exceed 150 mg in 24 hours. These dosage recommendations do not account for differences in salt forms of ephedrine. The FDA advisory review panel on OTC cough, cold, allergy, bronchodilator, and antiasthmatic drug products strongly recommended that ephedrine be available as scored tablets containing 12.5 mg and 25 mg of ephedrine to permit flexibility in dosage (45). These are now available from a number of manufacturers. Additionally, the panel recommended and the agency approved dosage recommendations for ephedrine-containing products in children between 2 and 12 years of age. These products are available to health professionals but not to the lay public. Based on these recommendations, it is likely that the panel and agency feel that ephedrine would be unsafe but not ineffective for unsupervised use in children 2–12 years of age.

Labeling requirements for ephedrine-containing products include a warning statement against exceeding the recommended dosage unless directed by a physician. If symptoms are not relieved within 1 hour or become worse, the product should be discontinued and a physician consulted immediately. Adverse effects include nervousness, tremor, sleeplessness, nausea, and loss of appetite.

The FDA advisory review panel on OTC cough, cold, allergy, bronchodilator, and antiasthmatic drug products recommended that ephedrine not be taken by patients with heart disease, high blood pressure, thyroid disease, diabetes, or difficulty in urination due to enlargement of the prostate gland. Ephedrine should not be taken concurrently with antihypertensive or antidepressant drugs. These warnings are reasonable and should be emphasized by the pharmacist when advising a patient who is purchasing ephedrine, particularly for the first time. The panel's maximum dosage recommendation (150 mg a day) is approximately one-half of the current maximum ephedrine hydrochloride dosage, which is allowable with current Tedral labeling (288 mg a day). This ephedrine dosage, contained in some commercial products, is likely to produce adverse effects in many patients and could be dangerous. Usually nonprescription ephedrine will not be purchased as a single-entity drug. The dosage form will usually contain theophylline and other drugs. The ephedrine dosage in these combinations is not different from that of single-entity ephedrine dosage forms. The above warnings deserve even more emphasis for combination dosage forms because both ephedrine and theophylline cause nervousness, tremor, sleeplessness, and nausea and can be dangerous in selected patients with seizure disorders or cardiac arrhythmias. The panel did not address the relative safety of single-entity versus combination ephedrine dosage forms.

Theophylline

Theophylline is effective in treating periodic, chronic, and acute, severe bronchospasm and in prophylaxis against exercise-induced bronchospasm. Several studies indicate that 5–20 mg/l is the therapeutic theophylline plasma concentration range (46–51). A plasma theophylline concentration above 20 mg/l can cause nausea, vomiting, cardiac tachyarrhythmias, and seizures. Critical reviews of theophylline clinical pharmacology are available (52, 53). Although there is little information directly comparing the relative efficacy and adverse effects of theophylline and beta$_2$-adrenergic stimulants, cardiac adverse effects, including tachycardia and arrhythmia, are uncommon within the therapeutic range (47, 50, 51). In a direct comparison of theophylline and terbutaline in patients with bronchoconstriction and premature ventricular contractions, at the same level of bronchodilation, theophylline produced both less tachycardia and fewer premature ventricular contractions (23). Theophylline is the only bronchodilator that increases gastric acidity (54).

In addition, theophylline decreases the lower esophageal sphincter pressure. Patients with peptic ulcers, heartburn, gastroesophageal reflux, or a hiatal hernia should be warned of this effect. Theophylline and ephedrine, the only oral nonprescription bronchodilators, are also the only bronchodilators that cause CNS stimulation.

Nonprescription theophylline dosage forms are available only in combination with ephedrine and other drugs. Prescription theophylline, or theophylline salts or complexes, are available in the following dosage forms: aqueous solution, elixir, uncoated tablet, enteric-coated tablet, sustained-release tablet and capsule, suppository, retention enema, and in intravenous (IV) and intramuscular (IM) injections. Aminophylline should not be given through intramuscular injection because it is painful and offers no advantage over other dosage forms. Nonprescription theophylline products contain anhydrous and hydrous theophylline and theophylline calcium salicylate. Prescription products contain these ingredients in addition to other salts (Table 4). None of these salts or complexes offer any therapeutic advantage over anhydrous theophylline.

The principal determinants of the theophylline plasma concentration for a given dosage regimen are the rate and extent of drug absorption (bioavailability) and drug clearance. Theophylline is rapidly and completely absorbed from uncoated tablets and oral solutions, and absorption may be complete with some sustained-release dosage forms (55–57). Food may decrease the rate of absorption of theophylline products and may interfere with extent of absorption of some sustained-release products (58). Theophylline absorption may be incomplete or erratic from enteric-coated tablets, suppositories, and some sustained-release products (59–60). Suppositories, which take about 6 hours to be completely absorbed, are frequently expelled too soon. For most purposes, the only dosage forms that are necessary are uncoated tablets, oral solutions, sustained-release tablets or capsules, and IV injections. Oral solutions are useful for patients who cannot swallow tablets. However, sprinkling the contents of bead-filled, sustained-release capsules on a small amount of food (1 tbsp) is more convenient and palatable. Sustained-release preparations may decrease the required dosing frequency (from every 6 hours to every 8 or 12 hours), and will make the theophylline plasma concentration less variable. Patients with a high theophylline clearance and short elimination half-life will have a large difference between the maximal (peak) and minimal (trough) theophylline plasma concentration. For example, theophylline plasma levels may vary from over 20 mg/l to under 5 mg/l at steady-state. Because both therapeutic and toxic effects of theophylline are correlated to the plasma drug concentration, it may be more desirable to decrease fluctuations in serum concentra-

TABLE 4 Theophylline content of various products

	Theophylline (%)
Theophylline anhydrous	100
Theophylline hydrous	91
Aminophylline	80
Oxtriphylline	65
Theophylline calcium salicylate	48
Theophylline sodium glycinate	50
Theophylline monoethanolamine	75

tion while maintaining an acceptable dosing interval by using a sustained-release preparation.

Theophylline clearance is primarily determined by hepatic metabolism with less than 10% eliminated unchanged in the urine. Theophylline clearance is increased by tobacco and marijuana smoking, charcoal-broiled beef, a high protein diet, phenytoin, rifampin, carbamazepine, and phenobarbital (60). Theophylline clearance is decreased by hepatic failure, severe congestive heart failure, viral respiratory infections, vaccines, severe pulmonary obstruction, propranolol (should not be used in patients with bronchospasm), erythromycin, troleandomycin, ciprofloxacin, enoxacin, norfloxacin, and cimetidine (60, 61). Compared with adults, children have a high theophylline clearance and premature infants have a low theophylline clearance (62, 63). There is no conclusive evidence that elderly patients have altered clearance. Studies have found altered disposition of theophylline in elderly patients with diseases that are known to decrease theophylline clearance. Theophylline clearance tends to be dynamic as changes occur in the severity of disease, as interacting drugs are added or discontinued, as smoking status changes, as diet changes, and as the patient ages (64). There is an indication that theophylline clearance is dose dependent (65). However, for most patients the assumption of first-order (linear) pharmacokinetics is sufficient for clinical dosage adjustments.

Dosing theophylline can be complex if the effects of the various factors that alter theophylline clearance are considered. Because these factors may alter theophylline clearance 2- to 3-fold, and the factors are variable, a fixed theophylline dosage for all patients (as is the case with nonprescription dosage recommendations) may not be safe or effective. Furthermore, the safest method of chronic theophylline dosing will use

theophylline plasma concentration determinations. Although it is unlikely that many patients taking a nonprescription theophylline product will have severe cardiac, hepatic, or pulmonary failure, it is likely that some patients may smoke, experience a viral respiratory infection, alter their diet, or use erythromycin, troleandomycin, or cimetidine.

The recommended dosage of theophylline should not be exceeded except under the advice and supervision of a physician, and it should not be taken if nausea, vomiting, or restlessness occurs. If asthmatic symptoms are not relieved within 1 hour or become worse, a physician should be contacted immediately. The drug is contraindicated in patients already taking a drug or suppository containing any form of theophylline, except under the supervision of a physician.

As with ephedrine, the FDA panel seemed to recognize that unsupervised use of theophylline in children may be unsafe. The dosage recommendations for Tedral (130 mg theophylline, 24 mg ephedrine hydrochloride, 8 mg phenobarbital) are adults, 1 or 2 tablets every 4 hours; children over 25 kg, one-half the adult dose. At the maximum recommended dosage of Tedral, an adult could receive 1,560 mg theophylline a day. If it is assumed that theophylline is completely absorbed and theophylline clearance is 40.9 ml/hr/kg for a 70-kg adult who is a nonsmoker, is not seriously ill, and has no other factor affecting theophylline clearance, the mean expected theophylline plasma concentration would be 22.7 mg/l (95% confidence interval 10–51 mg/l) (60). Using a similar projection for a 25-kg child who takes one Tedral tablet every 4 hours using a mean clearance of 87 ml/hr/kg (60), the expected mean theophylline plasma concentration would be 13.7 mg/l (range 5.4–38.4 mg/l).

The panel's recommendations are reasonable and certainly safer than the current labeling of nonprescription theophylline products. The fact that theophylline toxicity has not been commonly reported from nonprescription products is probably due to patients taking less than the maximum dosage recommendations and the possibility that patients who do become sick from an overdose recognize this and either discontinue the drug or decrease the dosage. The risk of severe toxicities is compounded if a patient who is already taking a prescription theophylline product adds to it a nonprescription theophylline-containing product.

Combination Products

The major ingredients in bronchodilator combination products are theophylline and ephedrine. Both drugs have been demonstrated individually to be effective bronchodilators. However, for the theophylline–ephedrine combination to offer an advantage over a single drug, it seems reasonable that the combination product should either achieve a greater degree of bronchodilation or produce fewer adverse effects at the same degree of bronchodilation.

To determine the maximal degree of bronchodilation from two single drugs and the combination, a study would need to increase the dose of each bronchodilator alone to the dose above which bronchodilation does not increase. Then, either the alternate drug could be added to determine if further bronchodilation could be achieved or a dose–response curve could be constructed with a fixed combination to maximal bronchodilation. Based on the studies reviewed, these criteria have not been met (24, 66–69). Most investigators have studied the bronchodilating effects of a single dose or multiple dosage regimen for theophylline, ephedrine, and the combination of theophylline and ephedrine in the same doses as when administered alone. In general, investigators find that the combination produces more bronchodilation than either single drug. But this does not exclude the possibility that the same degree of bronchodilation achieved with the combination could also be achieved by increasing the dose of either single drug. The doses chosen for theophylline in these studies often do not achieve theophylline plasma concentrations in the generally recommended therapeutic range.

Similarly, there is no evidence to indicate that at the same degree of bronchodilation, the combination of theophylline and ephedrine is less toxic than either single drug. To the contrary, the incidence of adverse effects seems to be higher (24, 60). This is not surprising because the adverse effect patterns are similar (e.g., nausea, agitation, and tachycardia) for theophylline and ephedrine. It would seem more rational to combine theophylline with an oral beta₂-agonist for which the adverse effect patterns are somewhat different (70). Even more advantageous might be the combination of theophylline with a beta₂-agonist aerosol.

Hence, the fixed combination of theophylline and ephedrine may offer no advantage over either single drug and may be more toxic.

Phenobarbital was originally added to the theophylline–ephedrine combination to offset the CNS stimulant properties of the bronchodilators. One study supported by the manufacturer of Tedral found that this proposed effect of phenobarbital could not be detected. If used in the maximum dosage, Tedral would supply an adult with 96 mg of phenobarbital a day. Theoretically, because phenobarbital is completely absorbed, a 70-kg adult with an average clearance of 3.0 ml/hr/kg would be estimated to have a steady-state phenobarbital plasma level of 19 mg/l (range 15–27 mg/l with an anticonvulsant therapeutic range of 10–30 mg/l) (71, 72). Because phenobarbital apparently offers no therapeutic advantage and may induce the metabolism of other drugs, it may unnecessarily complicate therapy.

Other Agents

Antihistamines Some combination asthma products contain antihistamines to antagonize histamine effects. However, they have no effect on other inflammatory mediators in asthma, and thus are usually ineffective as therapeutic agents for asthma. When hay fever or conjunctivitis accompany asthmatic symptoms, antihistamines may have some beneficial effects. It has been stated without supporting scientific evidence that because antihistamines have anticholinergic activity, bronchial secretions may be reduced, resulting in formation of thicker mucus that is more difficult to expectorate. It is unlikely that this would be a significant problem in ambulatory patients taking recommended antihistamine doses. In fact, most short-term trials of antihistamines in chronic asthma have demonstrated an improvement in symptoms and pulmonary functions. Therefore, asthma should not be considered a contraindication for antihistamines.

Expectorants Many asthma products contain expectorants, especially guaifenesin and potassium iodide. These agents are probably no more effective as expectorants than adequate hydration of the patient. Therefore their use in asthma is questionable. Because of the concern for iodide toxicity, the FDA advisory review panel on cough and cold drug products recommended that iodide-containing products (expectorants) be restricted to prescription status.

Antitussives Antitussives, such as codeine and dextromethorphan hydrobromide, are occasionally used in asthma products. Coughing is the major mechanism for removing bronchial secretions and mucus plugs. Therefore antitussives generally should not be used for asthma because the cough usually has a useful effect. The reflex cough induced by bronchospasm is relieved by bronchodilators, not antitussives.

PRODUCT SELECTION GUIDELINES

Before recommending a nonprescription product for asthma it is important that the pharmacist have a good understanding of the patient's general health and asthmatic condition. A complete patient profile alerts the pharmacist to conditions such as heart disease, diabetes, hypertension, aspirin sensitivity, and prescription medications being taken that can duplicate or interact with nonprescription products. It also may indicate the patient's compliance with drug regimens. Regular dosing with oral agents to maintain therapeutic drug blood levels is necessary to prevent asthma symptoms. Patients who consistently forget to take oral medications may do better by treating symptoms as they occur with an aerosolized product. Patients with chronic symptoms should be under the care of a physician; therapy should be aimed at reducing the patient's airway reactivity.

It must also be remembered that the patient is usually the best judge of whether a particular agent is effective. After recommending an agent, the pharmacist should alert the patient to discontinue the product and seek medical assistance if symptoms are not relieved within 1 hour or become worse. Nothing is gained by continuing ineffective therapy. When nonprescription medications do not provide sufficient relief, physician referral is the necessary next step.

Education in use of asthma medication is as important as drug choice. Improper use of aerosol agents may decrease effectiveness and increase side effects. If headache, nervousness, or palpitations occur, the medication should be discontinued. The mouthpiece should be washed daily with warm water to prevent clogging, and it should always be kept free of particles. Gargling after each use prevents dry mouth and throat irritation.

Patients with aspirin sensitivity should be cautioned that some asthma combination drug preparations contain aspirin. However, the FDA panel has recommended that no aspirin be included in products used for asthma (73). If nausea, vomiting, or restlessness occurs after taking nonprescription xanthine preparations, the dosage should be reduced. If an adverse effect occurs while taking theophylline, the drug should be stopped and medical attention sought to establish a safe and effective dosage. Excessive use of coffee, medications, or foods containing methylxanthines (caffeine, theobromine, or theophylline) should be avoided because they apparently increase the risk of theophylline toxicity. When stressful situations, such as exercise, are unavoidable, prophylactic use of an aerosol before exposure may prevent an asthmatic attack.

Mild seasonal or intermittent bronchospasm is usually self-limiting and may produce only discomfort. A patient who experiences seasonal asthma may feel comfortable with self-treatment, but unfortunately it is difficult to distinguish those patients who will worsen from those who will remain stable or improve. Although nonprescription epinephrine aerosol seems safe, there is no evidence that oral ephedrine or theophylline–ephedrine combination products are safer than prescription-only bronchodilators. Theophylline–ephedrine combinations at their current labeled dosages are probably not as safe as prescription aerosol bronchodilators or cromolyn. Combination products are currently being reevaluated for nonprescription availability.

The FDA advisory review panel on OTC cough, cold, allergy, bronchodilator, and antiasthmatic drug products recommended that bronchodilators are generally safe and effective for nonprescription use at recommended dosages in relieving the shortness of breath caused by bronchospasm. However, the panel emphasized that these preparations should not be used unless a diagnosis of asthma and a dosage schedule of nonprescription medicine has been established by a physician. In addition, patients with asthma may also require prescription drugs that may have serious dangers and side effects, requiring continued medical supervision (74).

Availability of nonprescription bronchodilators outside of pharmacies should also be a matter of concern. Who instructs patients purchasing an epinephrine aerosol in a grocery or department store on the correct manner of drug administration? Who warns patients in these environments about adverse effects and dosing, or checks on other drugs the patient is taking? Weight-reducing preparations sold in health food stores commonly contain ephedrine, caffeine, and phenylpropanolamine. These drugs are also purchased for their stimulant properties by drug abusers. In these situations, the nonprescription availability of these drugs may not be beneficial to the public health. There are inconsistencies in the availability of these nonprescription drugs, the labeled doses, and the current standards for appropriate asthma therapy.

SUMMARY

It seems that the most commonly available oral nonprescription bronchodilator preparation, which contains a fixed dose of theophylline, ephedrine, and phenobarbital, is less rational and, perhaps, less safe than many prescription bronchodilators.

There is no evidence to indicate that expectorant (guaifenesin) or antihistamine drugs contained in oral nonprescription bronchodilator combinations are beneficial (11, 72).

REFERENCES

1   J. B. West, "Respiratory Physiology—The Essentials," 3rd ed., Williams & Wilkins, Baltimore, Md., 1985.

2   M. A. Kaliner and P. J. Barnes, "The Airways—Neural Control in Health and Disease," Marcel Dekker, New York, N.Y., 1988.

3 American Thoracic Society, *Am. Rev. Resp. Dis., 85*, 762 (1962).

4 NIAID Task Force Report: Asthma and other Allergic Diseases, DHEW (National Institutes of Health) Publication No. 79–387, May 1979.

5 Tenth Report of the Director, National Heart, Lung and Blood Institute. *3*, Lung Disease. US Department of Health and Human Services. NIH Publication No. 84–2358, 1984.

6 S. R. Benatar, *N. Engl. J. Med., 314*, 423 (1986).

7 R. Evans et al., *Chest, 91* (suppl.), 65 (1987).

8 E. D. Robin, *Chest, 93*, 614 (1988).

9 D. B. Coultas and J. M. Samet, in "Childhood Asthma: Pathophysiology and Treatment," D. G. Tinkelman et al., Eds., Marcel Dekker, New York, N.Y., 1987, pp. 132–157.

10 B. Burrows et al., *N. Engl. J. Med., 320*, 271 (1989).

11 H. W. Kelly and R. L. Davis, in "Pharmacotherapy: A Pathophysiologic Approach," J. T. DiPiro et al., Eds., Elsevier, New York, N.Y., 1989, pp. 347–367.

12 H. W. Kelly, in "Pharmacotherapy: A Pathophysiologic Approach," J. T. DiPiro et al., Eds., Elsevier, New York, N.Y., 1989, pp. 397–407.

13 P. J. Barnes, *J. Allergy Clin. Immunol., 83*, 1013 (1989).

14 S. Ollerenshaw et al., *N. Engl. J. Med., 320*, 1244 (1989).

15 A. L. James et al., *Am. Rev. Respir. Dis., 139*, 242 (1989).

16 F. E. Hargreave et al., *J. Allergy Clin. Immunol., 68*, 347 (1981).

17 C. S. Shim and M. H. Williams, *Am. J. Med., 68*, 11 (1980).

18 A. R. Rubinfeld and M. C. F. Pain, *Lancet, 1*, 882 (1976).

19 N. Svedmyr and B. G. Simonson, *Pharmac. Ther. B., 3*, 397 (1978).

20 H. Formgren, *Scand. J. Resp. Dis., 56*, 321 (1975).

21 J. W. Paterson et al., *Br. J. Dis. Chest, 65*, 21 (1971).

22 G. Thiringer and N. Svedmyr, *Scand. J. Resp. Dis., 101*, (95) (1977).

23 A. S. Banner et al., *Arch. Intern. Med., 139*, 434 (1979).

24 C. Shim and M. H. Williams, Jr., *Ann. Intern. Med., 93*, 428 (1980).

25 H. W. Kelly, *Clin. Pharm., 4*, 393 (1985).

26 L. L. Iversen, *Br. J. Pharmacol., 41*, 571 (1971).

27 C. Shim and M. H. Williams, Jr., *Am. J. Med., 69*, 891 (1980).

28 S. P. Newman et al., *Eur. J. Respir. Dis., 62*, 3 (1981).

29 S. P. Newman et al., *Eur. J. Respir. Dis., 63* (Suppl. 119), 57 (1982).

30 J. M. Smith, *Lancet, 1*, 1042 (1966).

31 M. J. Greenberg and A. Pines, *Br. Med. J., 1*, 563 (1967).

32 P. D. Stolley, *Am. Rev. Resp. Dis., 105*, 883 (1972).

33 J. M. Esdaile et al., *Arch. Intern. Med., 147*, 543 (1987).

34 *Federal Register, 51*, 35326 (1986).

35 G. R. Wilkinson and A. H. Beckett, *J. Pharmacol. Exp. Ther., 162*, 139 (1968).

36 P. S. Sever et al., *Eur. J. Clin. Pharmacol., 9*, 193 (1975).

37 D. G. Tinkelman and S. E. Avner, *J. Am. Med. Assoc., 237*, 553 (1977).

38 T. D. James and H. A. Lyons, *J. Am. Med. Assoc., 241*, 704 (1979).

39 C. S. May et al., *Br. J. Clin. Pharmacol., 2*, 533 (1975).

40 W. V. Mieghem et al., *Br. Med. J., 1*, 816 (1978).

41 M. G. Roxanas and J. Spaulding, *Med. J. Aust., 2*, 639 (1977).

42 U.S. Drug Enforcement Administration, *Microgram, 13*, 143 (1980).

43 D. P. Taskin et al., *Chest, 68*, 155 (1975).

44 M. M. Weinberger and E. A. Bronsky, *J. Pediatr., 84*, 421 (1974).

45 *Federal Register, 41*, 38370 (1976).

46 R. Maselli et al., *J. Pediatr., 76*, 777 (1970).

47 J. W. Jenne et al., *J. Clin. Pharmacol. Ther., 13*, 349 (1972).

48 P. A. Mitenko and R. I. Ogilvie, *N. Engl. J. Med., 289*, 600 (1973).

49 J. Pollack et al., *Pediatrics, 60*, 840 (1977).

50 L. Hendeles et al., *Drug Intell. Clin. Pharm., 11*, 12 (1977).

51 M. H. Jacobs et al., *J. Am. Med. Assoc., 235*, 1983 (1976).

52 M. Bukowsky et al., *Ann. Intern. Med., 101*, 63 (1984).

53 J. R. Powell and J. E. Jackson, in "Applied Pharmacokinetics," W. E. Evans et al., Eds., Applied Therapeutics, San Francisco, Calif., 1981, pp. 139–166.

54 L. J. Foster et al., *J. Am. Med. Assoc., 241*, 2613 (1979).

55 R. A. Upton et al., *J. Pharmacokinet. Biopharm., 8*, 229 (1980).

56 R. A. Upton et al., *J. Pharmacokinet. Biopharm., 8*, 131 (1980).

57 M. Fixley et al., *Am. Rev. Resp. Dis., 115*, 955 (1977).

58 P. G. Welling et al., *J. Clin. Pharmacol. Ther., 17*, 475 (1975).

59 R. A. Upton et al., *J. Pharmacokinet. Biopharm., 8*, 151 (1980).

60 L. Hendeles et al., in "Applied Pharmacokinetics," W. E. Evans et al., Eds., Applied Therapeutics, Spokane, Wash., 1986, pp. 1105–1188.

61 D. J. Edwards et al., *Clin. Pharmacokinet., 15*, 194 (1988).

62 E. F. Ellis, *Pediatrics, 58*, 542 (1976).

63 J. V. Aranda et al., *N. Engl. J. Med., 295*, 413 (1976).

64 S. Vozeh et al., *J. Am. Med. Assoc., 240*, 1882 (1978).

65 L. J. Lesko, *Clin. Pharmacokinet., 4*, 449 (1979).

66 B. G. Simonsson and N. Svedmyr, *Pharmac. Ther. B., 3*, 239 (1977).

67 M. M. Weinberger et al., *J. Clin. Pharmacol. Ther., 17*, 585 (1975).

68 J. A. Sims et al., *J. Allergy Clin. Immunol., 62*, 15 (1978).

69 W. F. Taylor et al., *Ann. Allergy, 26*, 523 (1968).

70 H. W. Kelly, *Clin. Pharm., 3*, 386 (1984).

71 E. A. Nelson et al., *J. Clin. Pharmacol. Ther., 29*, 273 (1981).

72 J. D. Leopold et al., *Br. J. Clin. Pharmacol., 8*, 249 (1979).

73 *Federal Register, 41*, 38326 (1976).

74 *Federal Register, 41*, 38370 (1976).

ASTHMA AEROSOL PRODUCT TABLE

Product (Manufacturer)	Dosage Form	Epinephrine	Other Ingredients
Adrenalin Chloride (Parke-Davis)	solution for nebulization	1:100 epinephrine hydrochloride	benzethonium chloride sodium bisulfite
AsthmaHaler (SmithKline Beecham)	inhaler 350 doses/15 ml	0.16 mg base/spray (0.3 mg epinephrine bitartrate/spray)	
AsthmaNefrin (SmithKline Beecham)	solution for nebulization	2.25% base (as racemic epinephrine hydrochloride)	chlorobutanol, 0.5%
Breatheasy (Pascal)	inhaler	2.2% (as epinephrine hydrochloride)	benzyl alcohol, 1% isotonic salts, 0.5%
Bronitin Mist (Whitehall)	inhaler 466 doses/20 ml	0.16 mg base/spray (0.3 mg epinephrine bitartrate/spray)	freon propellant
Bronkaid Mist (Winthrop)	inhaler	0.27 mg base/spray	alcohol, 33%
Bronkaid Mist Suspension (Winthrop)	inhaler	0.16 mg base/spray (0.3 mg epinephrine bitartrate/spray)	
Dey-Dose Epinephrine (Dey Labs)	solution for nebulization	2.25% base (as racemic epinephrine hydrochloride)	
Epinephrine (Various manufacturers)	inhaler	0.2 mg epinephrine/spray	
Medihaler-Epi (Riker)	inhaler 300 doses/15 ml	0.16 mg base/spray (0.3 mg epinephrine bitartrate/spray)	
microNEFRIN (Bird)	solution for nebulization	2.25% base (as racemic epinephrine hydrochloride)	chlorobutanol, 0.5 g
Primatene Mist Solution (Whitehall)	inhaler 415 doses/15 ml	0.2 mg epinephrine/spray	alcohol, 34% freon propellant
Primatene Mist Suspension (Whitehall)	inhaler 233 doses/10 ml	0.16 mg base/spray (0.3 mg epinephrine bitartrate/spray)	
S-2 Inhalant Solution (Nephron)	solution for nebulization	2.25% base (as racemic epinephrine hydrochloride)	
Vaponefrin (Fisons)	solution for nebulization	2.25% base (as racemic epinephrine hydrochloride)	chlorobutanol, 0.5%

ASTHMA ORAL COMBINATION PRODUCT TABLE

Product (Manufacturer)	Dosage Form	Ephedrine	Theophylline	Other Ingredients
Amesec (Glaxo)	capsule	25 mg (as hydrochloride)	130 mg (as aminophylline)	
Asthmalixir (Reese)	elixir	2.4 mg/ml (as sulfate)	3 mg/ml	guaifenesin, 10 mg/ml phenobarbital[a], 0.8 mg/ml alcohol, 19% cherry flavor
Azma Aid (Various manufacturers)	tablet	24 mg (as hydrochloride)	118 mg	phenobarbital[a], 8 mg
Bronitin (Whitehall)	tablet	24.3 mg (as hydrochloride)	130 mg (hydrous)	guaifenesin, 100 mg pyrilamine maleate, 16.6 mg
Bronkaid (Winthrop)	tablet	24 mg (as sulfate)	100 mg (anhydrous)	guaifenesin, 100 mg
Bronkolixir (Winthrop)	elixir	2.4 mg/ml (as sulfate)	3 mg/ml	guaifenesin, 10 mg/ml phenobarbital[a], 0.8 mg/ml alcohol, 19%
Bronkotabs (Winthrop)	tablet	24 mg (as sulfate)	100 mg	guaifenesin, 100 mg phenobarbital[a], 8 mg
Guaiphed (Various manufacturers)	elixir	2.4 mg/ml (as sulfate)	3 mg/ml	guaifenesin, 10 mg/ml phenobarbital[a], 0.8 mg/ml
Phedral C.T. (Vortech)	tablet	24 mg (as hydrochloride)	130 mg	phenobarbital[a], 8 mg
Primatene (Whitehall)	tablet	24 mg (as hydrochloride)	130 mg (anhydrous)	
Primatene M (Whitehall)	tablet	24 mg (as hydrochloride)	130 mg (hydrous)	pyrilamine maleate, 16.6 mg
Primatene NS (Whitehall)	tablet	24 mg (as hydrochloride)	130 mg (anhydrous)	
Primatene P (Whitehall)	tablet	24 mg (as hydrochloride)	130 mg (hydrous)	phenobarbital[a], 8 mg
Tedral (Parke-Davis)	elixir suspension tablet	1.2 mg/ml (elixir) 2.4 mg/ml (suspension) 24 mg/tablet (all as hydrochloride)	6.5 mg/ml (elixir) 13 mg/ml (suspension) 130 mg/tablet	phenobarbital[a], 0.4 mg/ml (elixir) 0.8 mg/ml (suspension) 8 mg/tablet cherry flavor (elixir) licorice flavor (suspension)
Tedrigen (Goldline)	tablet	25 mg (as hydrochloride)	125 mg	phenobarbital[a], 8 mg
T.E.P. (Geneva Generics)	tablet	24 mg (as hydrochloride)	130 mg	phenobarbital[a], 8 mg
Theodrine (Rugby)	tablet	24 mg (as hydrochloride)	130 mg	phenobarbital[a], 8 mg
Theophenyllin (H.L. Moore)	tablet	24 mg (as hydrochloride)	130 mg	phenobarbital[a], 8 mg

[a] Limited availability according to state laws.

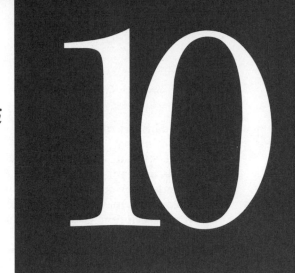

James P. Caro and Susan R. Dombrowski

SLEEP AID AND STIMULANT PRODUCTS

Q*uestions to ask in patient/consumer counseling*

Sleep Aid and Sedative Products

How long have you had a sleep problem? Do you have difficulty sleeping every night or only occasionally?

Is the problem related to falling asleep, staying asleep, or awakening too early?

Do you awaken during the night? If so, how often?

Do you feel excessively tired during the day?

Can you relate the sleep problem to a cause such as a change in work shifts, anxiety, or pain?

Are you taking any medication? If so, what are you taking and how often do you take it? At what time of day do you take it?

Do you drink alcohol or caffeine-containing beverages such as coffee, tea, and cola? How much do you drink daily? At what time of day do you drink these beverages?

Do you have any chronic diseases?

Are you under a physician's care?

Have you used sleep aid products previously? Which products did you use? Were they effective?

Stimulant Products

Have you ever used a stimulant product before? Did you experience any adverse effects?

Why do you want to use this product?

How long do you intend to use this product?

Do you regularly consume coffee, tea, cola, or other caffeinated beverages? Have you experienced adverse effects from drinking them?

What other medications, prescription and nonprescription, do you take?

Are you under a physician's care?

Are you pregnant or breast-feeding?

Do you smoke cigarettes?

Do you have anxiety, irritability, or any other nervous condition?

Insomnia is a remarkably common symptom that varies greatly in character, severity, and duration. For most people, it is a transient response to the stresses and disruptions that are part of everyday life. However, severe or protracted insomnia may be an important symptom of more serious disease—either physiologic or emotional. Moreover, many drugs play a role in causing insomnia.

Obviously, a critical first step in evaluating a patient complaining of insomnia is a careful review of the nature and history of the problem as well as a thorough medication history.

At the opposite end of the spectrum are individuals who need stimulants to stay awake. Boredom, fatigue, and extended periods of monotonous activity, such as highway driving, may induce sleepiness.

Nonprescription drugs are available to combat both of these problems. Pharmacists should counsel patients on the correct use of sedatives and stimulants and be prepared to suggest adjunct, nondrug solutions to the problem. Usually a restful sleep pattern can be established without drugs; for example, a leisurely walk before bedtime may relax the body enough to facilitate falling asleep. Excessive intake of caffeine either in beverages or stimulant products is unwise under any circumstances. Caffeine may have untoward effects, such as nervousness and irritability, and may contribute to insomnia.

SLEEP AID PRODUCTS

The Food and Drug Administration (FDA) advisory review panel on over-the-counter (OTC) sedative, tranquilizer, and sleep aid drug products has thoroughly reviewed and evaluated the active ingredients of sleep aid preparations. The panel's final report, issued in early 1989, calls for elimination of all nonprescription sedative agents except diphenhydramine and doxylamine succinate (1).

Physiology of Sleep

The sites and mechanisms of action of sleep-inducing drugs are largely unknown. Neurophysiologic investigations have yielded many theories concerning the influence of brain structures on consciousness and have provided some insight into the complex feedback systems that control consciousness. It is known that the brain stem coordinates the activity of these systems.

The brain stem contains the reticular activating system (RAS), which monitors and selectively limits all sensory input to the brain. Although this system responds to stimuli by arousing the brain, the cerebral cortex discriminates among stimuli even during sleep. For this reason, only selected stimuli produce arousal from sleep (2, 3). Recent evidence also suggests that modulators of immune response may play a role in the regulation of sleep (4).

Sleep is classified into two phases: rapid eye movement (REM), also known as paradoxical sleep, and nonrapid eye movement (non-REM) (Figure 1). During REM sleep, the body is physiologically more active than it is in non-REM stages. In young adults, REM sleep constitutes about 25% of a night's sleep. Non-REM sleep is subdivided into stages I–IV, according to increasing depth of sleep. In young adults, an initial awake period (sleep latency) is followed by a rapid progression through non-REM stages I–IV. This sequence is then reversed and followed by the first REM period of the night. This initial sequence of non-REM sleep before the first REM period (REM latency) lasts about 70 minutes. The first REM period is very short and is followed by another cycle. In each successive cycle, less time is spent in stage IV and more time is spent in the other stages, including REM. In the elderly, both sleep latency and REM latency increase, stage IV may decrease or be absent, and awakenings are more frequent (5).

In spite of detailed monitoring of these patterns and extensive investigations on the effects of sleep deprivation, the physiologic and psychologic functions of sleep are still unclear.

Etiology of Insomnia

The occasional inability to attain restful sleep is a common problem. About one-third of the population probably experiences insomnia at some time; insomnia occurs more frequently in women and the elderly (6). Although insomnia is usually transient and self-limiting, it may be of sufficient duration or severity to interfere with an individual's functioning during the waking hours. Severe or chronic insomnia may be a symptom of serious psychologic or physiologic illness. Careful review of the exact nature and history of the sleep problem will provide important information on its possible causes.

Situational Stress and Anxiety

Stress and anxiety may cause difficulty in falling asleep and are probably the most frequent causes of insomnia in young people. Usually acute and transient, stress and anxiety may include anything that causes worry or excitement.

Difficulty in falling asleep will be resolved when the precipitating cause is eliminated. When insomnia is a short-term (less than 1 week) problem that can be attributed to a specific situation, nondrug measures and

Young Adults

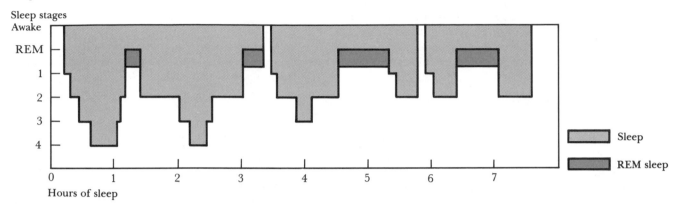

The Elderly

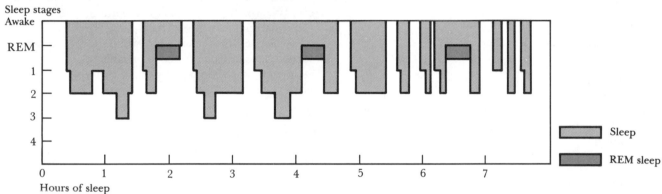

Insomniacs

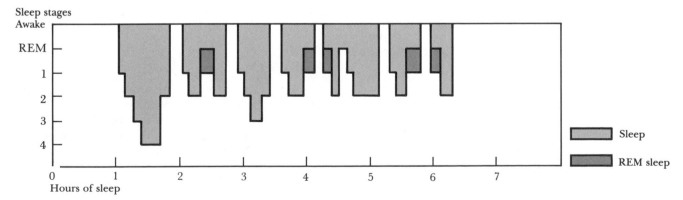

FIGURE 1   Hours of sleep and sleep stages in young adults, the elderly, and insomniacs. Adapted with permission from A. Kales, *Ann. Intern. Med., 68,* 1078–1104 (1968).

nonprescription preparations may provide sufficient relief. However, pharmacists should be aware that chronic insomnia is often a symptom of depression or other psychiatric disorder. Any patient complaining of insomnia along with loss of energy, weight loss or gain, severe anxiety, or decreased sex drive should be referred to a physician for a thorough evaluation.

Pain or Physical Discomfort

Pain of any type will disturb sleep. Obviously, the underlying cause of pain must be identified and treated. Several disorders including angina, vascular headache, and duodenal ulcer pain may be exacerbated during sleep because of increased autonomic activity during REM periods. Patients complaining of insomnia because of pain or discomfort should be questioned closely to determine whether self-treatment or referral to a physician is indicated. (See Chapter 5, *Internal Analgesic Products*.)

Change in Daily Rhythm

A change in work shift or the "jet lag" that frequently follows air travel across several time zones are typical occurrences that may precipitate insomnia. These changes, however, are self-limiting and generally respond to nondrug measures or nonprescription medication.

Age

Elderly individuals are prone to early or frequent awakening because sleep cycles change with age. These changes in sleep patterns are not harmful, and unless they are causing problems, such patients may simply need reassurance that these changes are part of the normal aging process. Sensitivity to caffeine increases with age so that individuals who previously consumed coffee or colas with impunity may find that these beverages are disturbing sleep (3).

Psychiatric Disorders

Some types of depression are associated with awakenings during the night or early morning. If anxiety occurs with depression, the patient may complain of difficulty in falling and remaining asleep. Referral to a physician is appropriate.

Conditions with Nocturnal Exacerbation

Autonomic nervous system bursts during REM sleep precipitate angina attacks, vascular headaches, and duodenal ulcer distress that disturb sleep. Asthma,

epilepsy, and lumbosacral and cervical disc disease also have been implicated in sleep disturbances.

Endocrine Abnormalities

Hypothyroidism and hyperthyroidism as well as other endocrine disorders disturb sleep patterns, but the mechanism is unknown.

Sleep Apnea

Sleep apnea, a sleep disturbance that is most common in men over 40 years of age, is manifested by loud, irregular snoring. In this syndrome, respiration actually stops for periods of 20–90 seconds many times during the night, resulting in partial awakening and sleep disruption. The patient is often unaware of irregular respiration and may complain only of feeling tired during the day. Researchers believe that sleep apnea is caused by a defect in central nervous system (CNS) respiratory control, which in some cases is complicated by an anatomical upper airway obstruction (7). Alcohol and other CNS depressants may exacerbate sleep apnea and should be avoided if apnea is a suspected diagnosis. It is estimated that sleep apnea is the cause of 1–5% of reported insomnias (7).

Nocturnal Myoclonus

The nocturnal myoclonus syndrome consists of recurrent, rhythmic movement of one or both legs. Although the patient may not actually awaken, sleep is disrupted; the patient may complain of sleeping poorly or feeling tired during the day. The patient may be unaware of the nocturnal movement, but complaints from a spouse may help identify a person with this syndrome. It is most prevalent in older patients and accounts for 10–15% of patients with chronic insomnia (7).

Drug Use

Many drugs may cause disruptions in sleep patterns. Paradoxically, these drugs include many of those commonly used to treat sleep disturbances. Certain anorexigenic preparations (prescription and nonprescription) containing CNS stimulants, caffeine, and aminophylline may cause nervousness and prevent sleep. Alcohol, amphetamines, barbiturates, diphenhydramine, ethchlorvynol, glutethimide, methyprylon, monoamine oxidase inhibitors, narcotics, scopolamine, and tricyclic antidepressants are drugs that cause sleep disturbances by suppressing REM sleep (7). Other drugs that disrupt sleep patterns include benzodiazepines, chloral hydrate, methyldopa, nicotine, phenytoin, reserpine, steroids, and thyroid preparations.

Ironically, the widely used benzodiazepine and barbiturate hypnotics disrupt sleep patterns by suppressing REM sleep. In addition, tolerance to the hypnotic effects of these agents develops quickly. As a result of these properties, patients get caught in a cycle of taking more medication to induce sleep, which in turn causes further disruption of sleep. When patients try to discontinue the medication after chronic use, the body responds with a compensatory rebound in REM that is accompanied by additional sleep disturbances and nightmares. The patient seeks relief by resuming drug use, and the cycle continues until professional intervention is sought.

Individuals who seek advice regarding treatment of insomnia should be carefully interviewed to obtain a complete medication history, including alcohol and caffeine use. Patients with a history of chronic drug use for insomnia should be referred to a physician for a thorough evaluation of possible causes and treatment.

Ingredients in Nonprescription Products

The FDA advisory review panel on OTC sedative, tranquilizer, and sleep aid drug products conducted a comprehensive review of all ingredients in these products, and the FDA's final ruling on the panel's recommendations became effective in February 1990 (1). After 15 years of extensive deliberations, diphenhydramine hydrochloride and citrate were the only active ingredients found to be safe and effective for nonprescription use; these products will continue to be marketed. In addition, nonprescription products containing doxylamine succinate are being marketed under approved New Drug Applications (NDAs).

Still unresolved is the issue of combination products containing analgesic and sleep aid ingredients. The FDA is currently reviewing additional data on these combinations and plans to issue a separate final ruling on them. In the meantime, these combinations will continue to be marketed.

The ingredients that have been eliminated from nonprescription sleep aids because of concerns about safety or effectiveness are methapyrilene fumarate and hydrochloride, phenyltoloxamine dihydrogen citrate, pyrilamine maleate, ammonium, potassium, and sodium bromide, scopolamine aminoxide hydrobromide, salicylamide, thiamine hydrochloride, and passionflower extract.

Ethanolamines

Diphenhydramine and doxylamine belong to the ethanolamine class of antihistamines, also known as aminoalkyl ethers. Other members of this class include carbinoxamine, clemastine, dimenhydrinate, diphenylpyraline, and phenyltoloxamine (8). Characteristically, the ethanolamines produce significant anticholinergic and sedative effects and a low incidence of adverse gastrointestinal (GI) effects; in fact, diphenhydramine has been used in the treatment of nausea caused by motion sickness (8). These properties make the ethanolamines well suited as sleep aids.

Diphenhydramine and doxylamine have similar profiles. Both are well absorbed following oral administration. Characteristics of these drugs upon oral administration are listed in Table 1.

Although exactly how antihistamines exert their CNS effects remains unclear, reports show a relationship between their CNS activity and their affinity for cerebral H_1 histamine receptors (9). Recent studies have shown that the drowsiness and mental impairment produced by diphenhydramine are well correlated with changes in plasma levels of the drug (10–12).

Antihistamines can induce symptoms of both CNS stimulation and depression. Drowsiness is the most common effect of therapeutic doses; excitation may be a symptom of intoxication. However, some people exhibit paradoxical excitation with therapeutic doses. Children, the elderly, and patients with CNS dysfunction are more prone to exhibit this effect (8). The CNS depressant action of antihistamines also is unpredictable because individuals vary in sensitivity to this effect and tolerance develops with continued use. Patients who use antihistamines should be warned not to drive an automobile or operate hazardous machinery until their response to the drug is known. Alcohol and other CNS depressants may add to the depressant effect and should be avoided.

Other side effects of antihistamines include dizziness, tinnitus, blurred vision, GI disturbances, and dry-

TABLE 1	Characteristics of diphenhydramine and doxylamine	
	Diphenhydramine	**Doxylamine**
Sedative dose	50 mg	25 mg
Time-to-peak level	1–4 hr	2–3 hr
Half-life	2.4–9.3 hr	10 hr

From "AHFS Drug Information 89," G. K. McEvoy, Ed., American Society of Hospital Pharmacists, Bethesda, Md., 1989, pp. 2–5, 16–19.

ness of the mouth and throat. Geriatric patients may be particularly susceptible to dizziness, sedation, and hypotension. Antihistamines may also cause CNS stimulation, resulting in nervousness and insomnia. However, this effect is uncommon and occurs primarily in children (8).

Although antihistamines have a wide margin of safety, potential poisoning should not be discounted if an acute overdose is taken, especially in combination with alcohol or other CNS depressants. Poisonings are most common in children, and symptoms are most severe in this group. The symptoms observed with intoxication result from the CNS effects and are characteristic of anticholinergic overdose (pupils become fixed and dilated, fever may be present, sweating may be decreased or absent, and excitement, hallucinations, and convulsions occur). In severe cases, these symptoms are followed by coma and cardiorespiratory collapse. Treatment consists of preventing the drug's absorption by inducing emesis and providing supportive measures such as ensuring hydration, assisting ventilation, and controlling convulsions (13, 14).

Because antihistamines have produced teratogenic effects in animals, they should be avoided by pregnant women. High doses may precipitate convulsions and should be used with caution in persons with epilepsy (8).

L-Tryptophan

This amino acid has been used to treat insomnia, depression, and migraine. For treating insomnia, doses of 1–3 g administered 20 minutes before bedtime have been effective in inducing sleep and decreasing sleep latency. However, the response is highly variable and additional studies are needed to determine the clinical usefulness of this agent, particularly in severe insomnia (15). L-Tryptophan has never been marketed as a sleep aid in the United States but has been available as a nutritional supplement. However, in late 1989, the FDA requested that manufacturers recall all products in which L-tryptophan was the sole or major component. This action was prompted by a strong link between the use of such products and subsequent development of eosinophilia-myalgia syndrome. Several hundred cases (including several deaths) of this rare blood disorder were reported. The symptoms include severe muscle and joint pain, swelling of the arms and legs, skin rash, and fever. These symptoms are accompanied by severe eosinophilia. At the time of this voluntary recall, it was unclear whether this syndrome is caused by L-tryptophan itself or by some contaminant resulting from the manufacturing process. Until these issues are clarified, pharmacists should strongly caution patients to avoid all use of concentrated L-tryptophan products.

Adjunctive Measures

Before recommending use of nonprescription sleep aid preparations, the pharmacist should encourage the following nondrug measures, as appropriate, to relieve insomnia (6):

- Drink a hot milk beverage at bedtime.

- Participate in stimulating daytime activities.

- Arise at a specific early hour each morning, regardless of the previous night's sleep. (After a few nights of poor sleep, improvement may occur, and sleep may become more regular.)

- Try not to worry if unable to sleep because anxiety can contribute to or cause insomnia.

- Abstain from or decrease consumption of beverages containing caffeine or alcohol, particularly in the evening.

- Avoid heavy meals several hours before bedtime.

- Avoid naps during the day.

- Perform light exercise such as taking a leisurely walk before bedtime.

- Avoid strenuous exercise before bedtime.

- Designate a specific time for sleep.

- Relax by engaging in activities such as reading in bed, watching television, or listening to relaxing music.

- Minimize external stimuli that might disturb sleep (use dark shades over the windows to keep out light; wear ear plugs to keep out noise).

Moreover, persons who request nonprescription sleep aid products should be advised that these products are only for occasional use for no more than 1 week. Pharmacists should caution all patients using these products that their coordination and alertness will be impaired, making driving or hazardous activities inadvisable and that concurrent use with alcohol or other CNS depressants will intensify these effects.

STIMULANT PRODUCTS

Caffeine is the only stimulant active ingredient recognized by the FDA as safe and effective for nonprescription use (16). It is used as an aid in staying awake and to restore alertness during fatigue or drowsiness. Nonprescription medications containing caffeine are commonly used by people studying for exams or driving long distances, particularly at night.

Caffeine is also used in combination with analgesics to treat headache (including migraine headache) and other types of pain (17). (See Chapter 5, *Internal Analgesic Products*.)

Caffeine (1,3,7-trimethylxanthine) and two structurally similar drugs, theophylline and theobromine, are known as methylxanthines (Figure 2). They share various pharmacologic properties but differ in potency. Caffeine has the most potent CNS stimulant action and the weakest cardiovascular and diuretic activity (18). Caffeine is the only methylxanthine that is used therapeutically as a stimulant.

Caffeine is a common component of the diet; the caffeine content of some foods and beverages is listed in Table 2. The caffeine content of coffee and tea is highly variable, depending on the method of preparation. Generally, automatic drip coffee has a higher caffeine content than percolated coffee, and the longer tea is allowed to steep, the greater its caffeine content (19).

The average American drinks two or three cups of coffee a day (20, 21). Overall, men drink more coffee and consume more caffeine than women (21). The average adult daily caffeine intake from all sources (coffee, tea, cola, etc.) is 210 mg (20). Even children's caffeine consumption can be substantial (20), averaging approximately 37–43 mg a day (20, 22).

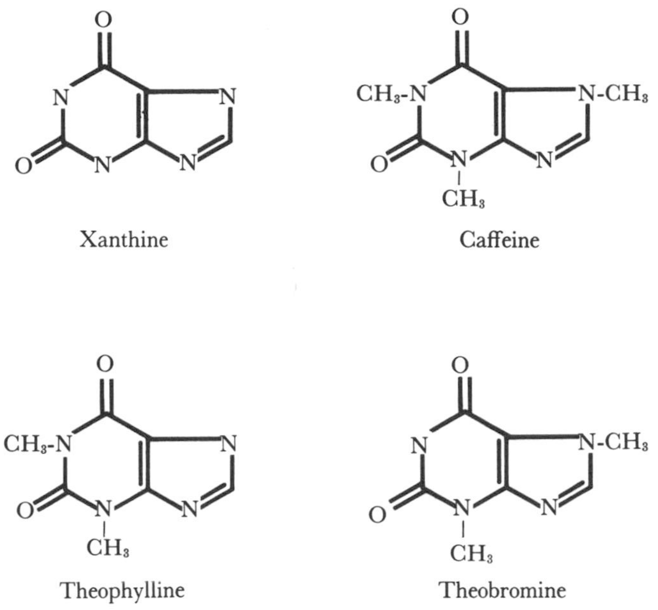

Caffeine's Mechanism of Action

The action of caffeine is complex. One proposed mechanism is an increase in the concentration of adenosine 3',5'-cyclic monophosphate (cyclic AMP) by inhibition of phosphodiesterase, the enzyme that causes cyclic AMP degradation. Cyclic AMP, in turn, produces an influx of calcium ions into the intracellular space, resulting in muscle contraction (23).

The calcium channel blocker nifedipine reverses the caffeine-induced increase in blood pressure and decrease in heart rate, thus demonstrating that caffeine's effect is mediated at least in part by the calcium channels (24).

Other research suggests that caffeine increases the intracellular concentration of calcium either by stimulating rapid release of calcium from the sarcoplasmic reticulum (intracellular calcium storage units) or by inhibiting the reuptake of calcium by the sarcoplasmic reticulum, rather than by affecting calcium influx through calcium channels (23, 25).

FIGURE 2   Structures of methylxanthines.

Some investigators have questioned the role of phosphodiesterase inhibition because the plasma concentrations of caffeine that affect blood pressure are below what is required to inhibit phosphodiesterase (26).

Another possible mechanism of caffeine's action is antagonism of adenosine receptors. Adenosine is used therapeutically to induce hypotension. It increases heart rate and cardiac output and decreases mean arterial blood pressure by decreasing peripheral vascular resistance (27). A single injection of caffeine counteracted the decrease in mean arterial pressure produced by adenosine infusion in rats, but caffeine alone did not increase mean arterial pressure (28).

Some investigators suggested that patients with hypertension may have altered adenosine receptors or circulating adenosine levels (29).

An increase in the sensitivity of myocardial contractile proteins to caffeine may be responsible for its inotropic effects, although this mechanism is more likely to occur at high caffeine concentrations (23).

A direct effect of caffeine on the adrenal medulla, resulting in epinephrine and norepinephrine release, has been proposed (30). However, inconsistencies in research results suggest that the effects of caffeine probably are not mediated largely by the sympathoadrenal or renin-angiotensin system (26, 29, 31).

TABLE 2 Approximate caffeine content of common foods and beverages

Food or beverage	Caffeine (mg)
5 oz brewed automatic drip coffee	60-180[a]
5 oz brewed percolator coffee	40-170[a]
5 oz instant coffee	30-120[a]
6 oz brewed Sanka decaffeinated coffee	3-5[b]
6 oz instant Sanka decaffeinated coffee	3-5[b]
5 oz brewed American tea	20-90[a]
5 oz brewed imported tea	25-110[a]
5 oz instant tea	28[c]
12 oz canned iced tea	22-36[d]
12 oz Jolt Cola	90[c]
12 oz Dr. Pepper	39.6[a]
12 oz Coca-Cola	45.6[a]
12 oz Pepsi-Cola	38.4[a]
12 oz Diet Coke	45.6[a]
12 oz Diet Pepsi	36.0[a]
12 oz Pepsi-Free	0[d]
12 oz 7-Up	0[d]
12 oz Sunkist Orange	0[d]
12 oz ginger ale	0[d]
5 oz cocoa beverage	4[a]
8 oz chocolate milk	5[a]
1 oz milk chocolate	6[a]
1 oz semisweet dark chocolate	20[a]
1 oz baking chocolate	26[a]
2/3 cup chocolate ice cream	4.5[e]
1/2 cup instant chocolate pudding	5.5[e]

[a]C. Lecos, *FDA Consumer, 18,* 14 (1984).

[b]*Med. Lett. Drugs Ther., 19,* 65 (1977).

[c]A. K. Henry and J. Feldhausen, "Drugs, Vitamins, and Minerals in Pregnancy," Fisher Books, Tucson, Ariz., 1989, p. 381.

[d]M. A. Raebel and J. Black, *Hosp. Pharm., 19,* 257 (1984).

[e]*J. Am. Med. Assoc., 252,* 803 (1984).

Central Nervous System Effects of Caffeine

Caffeine stimulates the cerebral cortex at low (threshold) doses and the medullary respiratory, vasomotor, and vagal centers at larger doses (Figure 3). Toxic amounts stimulate all areas of the brain and spinal cord, resulting in convulsions (32).

Caffeine improves alertness and mood and decreases fatigue. It postpones the development of boredom, fatigue, inattentiveness, and sleepiness (33). Experimental subjects reported feeling more alert, energetic, quick-witted, and attentive and less tired after receiving single oral caffeine doses of 250 and 500 mg than after receiving placebos (34).

A dose-related increase in subjective mood (self-rating on alertness and physical activity) occurred after single 150- and 300-mg oral doses of caffeine. However, these doses had no effect on objective performance of tasks requiring alertness and psychomotor coordination (35). Physical endurance and capacity and work output also are increased by caffeine. An effect on intelligence has not been demonstrated, although caffeine increases the capacity for sustained intellectual effort (33).

Caffeine increases sleep latency (time to fall asleep) and decreases sleep quality (36).

Caffeine has been used to counteract the effects of alcohol, although it does not increase alcohol metabolism (37). Caffeine partially counteracts the impairment in motor performance caused by alcohol (33). However, in a study designed to measure the effects of alcohol and caffeine on performance during stress, caffeine did not antagonize the alcohol-induced impairment in performance (38). Caffeine adds synergistically to the increase in reaction time caused by alcohol; it does not antagonize the effect of alcohol on reaction time (39). Caffeine also impairs hand steadiness (33). Coffee is commonly drunk to counteract the effects of alcohol before driving an automobile. The effectiveness of this practice may be due to the metabolism of alcohol that takes place during the time devoted to coffee drinking rather than to antagonism by caffeine (38).

The CNS effects associated with excessive caffeine intake include irritability, tremulousness, apprehension, restlessness, dizziness, lightheadedness, and insomnia (40).

Cardiovascular Effects of Caffeine

In a research setting, single doses of caffeine cause small increases in diastolic and systolic blood pressure (due to increases in vascular resistance rather than increases in cardiac output) and decreases in heart rate (probably as a result of a baroreceptor-mediated vagal reflex) (41). Caffeine-induced blood pressure increases are more pronounced for older subjects than for younger ones and for caffeine nonusers than for users, regardless of age (31).

However, chronic caffeine consumption is not thought to cause hypertension because tolerance develops to the acute effects on blood pressure. Patients with and without borderline hypertension experienced increases in blood pressure after single doses of caffeine, but significant increases did not persist beyond the first few days of a 7-day regimen (29, 42).

Caffeine may have different cardiovascular effects in the resting state and during stress (43, 44). It apparently acts primarily on the vasculature rather than on the heart during resting conditions (44). Caffeine increases vascular resistance in the resting state but not during stress (43). It has no effect on cardiac output and produces a slight decrease or no effect on heart rate at rest, but it adds to stress-induced increases in heart rate, cardiac output, and systolic blood pressure (43).

The arrhythmogenic potential of caffeine has been a subject of concern, particularly for patients with cardiovascular disease (45). In normal subjects, high doses of caffeine produced no significant changes in heart rate or rhythm (46). Moreover, in a study of patients receiving a single 300-mg dose of caffeine during the recovery phase after acute myocardial infarct, no relationship between caffeine and the occurrence or severity of ventricular arrhythmias was observed (47).

The effect of caffeine on patients with stable angina controlled by medication was studied at rest and during treadmill exercise. Caffeine did not affect treadmill exercise duration, time to onset of exercise-induced angina, myocardial function, or intensity of ischemia. No increase in the frequency or severity of atrial or ventricular arrhythmias occurred at rest or during exercise (48). Evidence linking caffeine to adverse effects on cardiac rhythm is inconclusive. Therefore, moderation in caffeine intake rather than complete abstinence is advisable for patients with cardiac rhythm disturbances, unless caffeine is known to aggravate the patient's condition (49).

Coffee consumption has been linked to elevations in serum total cholesterol and triglycerides (50–53). Significant reductions in serum total cholesterol were achieved in hypercholesterolemic men who abstained from coffee (52). However, caffeine may not be the component of coffee responsible for the observed relationship because cola and tea consumption were not associated with elevations in serum lipids (53).

A dose–response relationship between coffee consumption and coronary heart disease was found in prospective and case-control studies, although diet was not assessed (54, 55). Heavy coffee drinkers (five or more cups a day) were reported to have a twofold to threefold increased risk of coronary heart disease (sudden cardiac death, acute myocardial infarction, and angina pectoris) (54). One study found that in men the percentage of calories obtained from total and saturated fats and cholesterol is positively related to coffee consumption (53). Thus, the alleged link between coffee intake and coronary heart disease may be due to an atherogenic diet rather than to coffee. Other investigators failed to find an association between caffeine consumption and coronary heart disease (56, 57). Although moderation in caffeine use is advisable for patients at risk for heart disease, abstinence is probably unnecessary in the absence of more conclusive evidence implicating caffeine.

Caffeine constricts cerebral arteries and decreases cerebral blood flow (58). Caffeine's effectiveness in migraine and vascular headaches is attributed to its cerebral vasoconstriction. Caffeine could potentially decrease the delivery of drugs to the brain, an effect that would be most important for drugs whose site of action is the CNS. Caffeine also decreases hepatic blood flow (59). It may decrease the clearance (and potentially enhance the effect) of hepatically eliminated drugs (drugs with a high intrinsic hepatic clearance).

Other Caffeine Effects

Caffeine has the weakest diuretic activity of the methylxanthines (18). It increases renal blood flow and glomerular filtration rate (GFR) and blocks tubular reabsorption of sodium in the kidney, resulting in increased urinary excretion of sodium (36). Low-grade tolerance develops to this diuresis (18).

Weight-control benefits may be associated with caffeine use because of its thermogenic effect. A single 100-mg dose produced a 3–4% increase in resting metabolic rate over a 2.5-hour period, and a series of six 100-mg doses at 2-hour intervals resulted in an 8–11% increase in energy expenditure in both lean persons and those with a tendency to gain weight (60).

Caffeine also decreases serum potassium concentrations (61). Although it is not known whether tolerance develops to this effect, persons at risk for hypokalemia should be warned to limit their intake of caffeine.

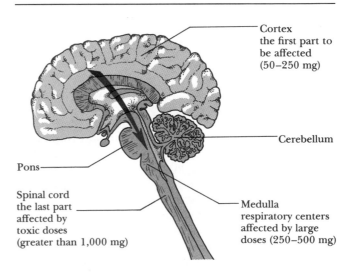

FIGURE 3   Sites of action of caffeine in the central nervous system.

Caffeine (and the other methylxanthines) dilates the bronchioles. Caffeine is as effective as theophylline in producing bronchodilation in asthmatic children (62). In an epidemiologic study of more than 70,000 adults, coffee drinkers were less likely to have asthma than were nondrinkers. An inverse dose–response relationship between coffee consumption and prevalence of asthma was reported (63).

Caffeine stimulates gastric acid secretion but to a significantly lesser extent than coffee that contains equivalent amounts of caffeine. Further, decaffeinated coffee stimulates gastric acid secretion to the same extent as regular coffee, suggesting that some other component of coffee is responsible for the observed acid secretion (64). Moreover, caffeine-free soft drinks produce the same gastric acid output as similar caffeine-containing beverages (65). The effect of coffee temperature on gastric acid secretion also was studied; comparable marked increases in gastric acid secretion were observed after drinking hot, warm, and cold coffee (66). Therefore, avoidance of caffeine (in beverages or stimulant products) by patients with peptic ulcer disease is not indicated unless caffeine aggravates their condition.

The effects of caffeine and regular and decaffeinated coffee on lower esophageal sphincter pressure were studied. Similar significant increases in pressure were produced by both regular and decaffeinated coffee, but no substantial changes were produced by caffeine. These findings negate the hypothesis that heartburn associated with drinking coffee is mediated by a caffeine-induced decrease in lower esophageal sphincter pressure (64).

Tolerance, Physical Dependence, and Withdrawal

Chronic use of caffeine is associated with tolerance, physical dependence, and a withdrawal syndrome. The mechanisms by which these conditions develop are unclear. Chronic caffeine intake is thought to produce an increase in density or sensitivity of adenosine receptors (28). This change could explain the headache associated with caffeine withdrawal because adenosine dilates cerebral blood vessels.

Induction of the hepatic microsomal enzymes responsible for caffeine's metabolism, resulting in decreased plasma caffeine concentrations, has been proposed as a possible mechanism for tolerance (67).

Tolerance develops to the sleep-disturbing (68), cardiovascular (29, 42), diuretic (18), and other effects of caffeine. A significantly higher number of coffee nondrinkers than coffee drinkers required more time than usual to fall asleep after 150 mg of caffeine at bedtime (68).

Development of tolerance to the effects of caffeine on blood pressure and heart rate occurs quickly (over 1–4 days) (42) and at relatively low levels of consumption (300 mg per day) (31). Tolerance also diminishes rapidly. In a laboratory setting, caffeine produced elevations in blood pressure in caffeine users after only 12 hours of abstinence, demonstrating that either tolerance diminishes within 12 hours or some caffeine consumers do not develop tolerance to caffeine's pressor effects (43). Another study demonstrated that tolerance to caffeine's pressor effects persists for at least 24 hours but not longer than 3 weeks (42).

Physical dependence may require a longer period to develop than tolerance, although there is probably considerable interindividual variation. In three subjects with experimentally induced caffeine withdrawal headaches, caffeine was reintroduced for 2 weeks and then stopped again. Fewer days of headache occurred in the second withdrawal period, suggesting that 2 weeks was insufficient to establish physical dependence (69).

The caffeine withdrawal syndrome is characterized by a throbbing, diffuse headache that begins about 18–20 hours after the last ingestion of caffeine and peaks 3–6 hours thereafter (70). The headache may be accompanied by nausea, sleepiness, fatigue, laziness, and decreased vigor and alertness. It is exacerbated by exercise and exposure to bright lights (69, 70). These effects usually diminish over 5 or 6 days, but can last up to 9 days (69). The incidence of withdrawal headaches is related to daily caffeine consumption (more than 600 mg), although headaches (and other withdrawal symptoms) are not limited to heavy caffeine consumers (70). Caffeine withdrawal headaches are readily relieved by taking caffeine; dietary sources and nonprescription analgesics that contain caffeine are both effective.

Caffeine has been shown to function as a behavioral reinforcer. When subjects' intake of regular and decaffeinated coffee was monitored over a 10–17 day period (subjects were blinded to caffeine content), consumption of decaffeinated coffee was not significantly different from regular coffee. These results show that coffee drinking is a habitual behavior independent of caffeine (69).

Pregnancy

The popularity of coffee, tea, and other sources of caffeine in the diet has focused attention on its possible teratogenicity. In 1980, the FDA cautioned pregnant women to avoid caffeine or to use it sparingly (71).

Caffeine readily crosses the placenta. Three cases of fetal arrhythmia caused by excessive maternal caffeine intake (one mother consumed 10 cups of coffee just before delivery) were reported. One infant exhibited postpartum supraventricular extrasystoles (72).

Caffeine has a long half-life in women during the last 2 weeks of pregnancy (73) and in premature neonates (74). It could potentially accumulate in both mother and fetus during late pregnancy, and its effects could be protracted in neonates because of their immature metabolic pathways.

The postulated mechanisms for caffeine's alleged adverse effects on the fetus include cyclic AMP interference with fetal cell growth, a direct effect on nucleic acids resulting in chromosomal defects (caffeine is structurally similar to the purines adenine and guanine), and catecholamine release resulting in diminished blood flow to the placenta and fetal hypoxia (75).

In a prospective study, late first- or second-trimester spontaneous abortion was more likely in women who consumed moderate or large amounts of caffeine (more than 150 mg per day) than in those who consumed smaller amounts or none (75). However, maternal alcohol consumption and smoking may have affected the results. Smokers were significantly more likely to be caffeine users than nonsmokers (75), and smoking and alcohol use are risk factors for spontaneous abortion (76, 77).

Anecdotal reports of birth defects in offspring of women who consumed excessive amounts of caffeine during pregnancy have appeared in the literature (78). However, case-control studies involving large numbers of infants with various birth defects failed to show a relationship between congenital malformations and maternal caffeine intake during pregnancy (79–82).

Results of research on the effect of caffeine consumption during pregnancy on birth weight are also equivocal. A dose–response relationship between caffeine intake during pregnancy and risk of delivering a low birth weight infant has been suggested (83, 84). However, other investigations, including a large-scale analysis of more than 12,000 women (81), produced no evidence of this relationship (81, 85). Moreover, caffeine use during pregnancy was not associated with infant size (weight, length, and head circumference) at 8 months of age (86).

Caffeine has not been linked with premature birth (81, 84). The decreased birth weight observed in one study was associated with slowed growth rather than premature birth (83).

In summary, caffeine use during pregnancy has not been proven to be innocuous, so moderation in intake is advisable.

In a study of lactating women, consumption of a single beverage containing caffeine (36–335 mg) produced peak caffeine concentrations in breast milk after 1 hour (87). Caffeine appeared in breast milk within 15 minutes of ingestion and disappeared within 12 hours. The authors estimated that an average caffeine dose of 0.57 mg was available to the infants (based on an average milk intake of 90 ml every 3 hours). No caffeine or caffeine metabolites were recovered in the infants' urine, and no behavioral changes were noted. These results suggest that nursing mothers may drink an occasional caffeine-containing beverage without affecting their babies. However, moderation in caffeine use is indicated because of the potential for caffeine accumulation in infants, particularly those younger than 4 months.

The preliminary findings of an analysis of more than 6,000 pregnant women suggest a dose–response relationship between coffee consumption and self-reported difficulty in becoming pregnant (88). A study involving 104 women who had been attempting to become pregnant for 3 months also showed a dose–response relationship between intake of caffeinated beverages and impaired fertility (89). However, confounding factors, including exercise, stress, and nutritional status, may have affected the data.

Caffeine and Cancer

Epidemiologic research has examined caffeine (or coffee) use as a possible contributing factor in various malignancies. In a case-control study of 75 bladder cancer patients (and 142 controls), no statistically significant association between bladder cancer and caffeine was found (90).

Early studies found a strong association between coffee drinking and pancreatic cancer. A relative risk of 2.7 was reported for daily coffee intake of three or more cups (91). However, a more recent report indicated that the association, if any, is much less strong (92). The investigators even suggested that patients' recall of coffee consumption may have been inflated by previous reports of a link between coffee and cancer (93).

In a prospective study of more than 100,000 health maintenance organization members, no relationship was found between pancreatic cancer and use of coffee or tea (94). The same conclusion was reached by other investigators (57, 95).

Benign Breast Disease

Considerable debate has taken place about the possible role of caffeine in benign breast disease. A link between caffeine and fibrocystic breast disease has been hypothesized because elevated levels of cyclic AMP and cyclic guanosine monophosphate (cyclic GMP) are found in fibrocystic breast tissue (96).

Case-control studies have been contradictory in their conclusions (97, 98), possibly because of methodological differences (99). One study found no association between coffee consumption and benign breast disease (97). However, a positive relationship was found between caffeine intake and the occurrence of fibrocystic breast disease but not between caffeine use and fibroadenoma or other benign breast diseases (98).

Although improvement in symptoms (disappearance of pain and breast lumps) is achieved in some women with benign breast disease by complete abstinence from caffeine (96, 100), conclusive evidence of a causal role is lacking.

Fibrocystic breast disease has been identified as a risk factor for development of breast cancer (101). However, no association between caffeine and breast cancer was found in case-control studies (102).

Caffeine Metabolism and Pharmacokinetics

Caffeine is metabolized by demethylation and oxidation to theophylline, theobromine, and paraxanthine (1,7-dimethylxanthine). Further degradation yields dimethylated uric acids, monomethylxanthines, and monomethyluric acids (103). Figure 4 illustrates caffeine's metabolic pathways. Xanthine oxidase is not thought to be involved in caffeine metabolism because allopurinol (a xanthine oxidase inhibitor) does not affect caffeine kinetics (104). Caffeine does not affect uric acid formation (18) and is not contraindicated in patients with gout.

Caffeine increases the metabolism of some other drugs and may induce its own metabolism. Administration of caffeine to laboratory animals increased the drug metabolizing activity of hepatic microsomal enzymes (67).

Caffeine exhibits dose-independent kinetics at normal levels of consumption (105). The average half-life of caffeine is 3.5 hours in smokers and 6 hours in nonsmokers (106). The higher caffeine consumption observed in smokers (21) may be due (at least in part) to their higher caffeine clearance (155 ml/kg compared with 94 ml/kg for nonsmokers) (106). The difference in kinetics between smokers and nonsmokers is probably due to induction of hepatic enzymes by smoking (106). Liver disease can influence the kinetics of caffeine. A serum half-life of 96 hours was reported in an alcoholic patient with severe liver disease who consumed approximately 800 mg of caffeine a day over a 9-day hospitalization (107).

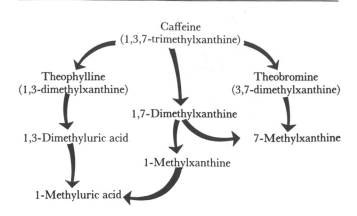

FIGURE 4   Caffeine metabolic pathways.

The half-life of caffeine was slightly prolonged in asthmatic children (3.9 hours) compared with nonsmoking adults (3.5 hours) (62). An average peak serum concentration of 13.5 mg/l occurred 1.1 hours after ingestion of 10 mg/kg (62).

Neonates cannot metabolize caffeine because of liver immaturity; caffeine's half-life in neonates is prolonged (65 hours in premature infants) (74).

Caffeine Toxicity

Caffeinism, a syndrome associated with intake in excess of 1 g a day, is characterized by dizziness, apprehension, lightheadedness, tremulousness, breathlessness, restlessness, headache, irregular heartbeat, palpitations, chest discomfort, diarrhea, and insomnia (40). It has been confused with anxiety disorders. A person suffering from headache associated with caffeinism may unknowingly aggravate the condition by self-medicating with a nonprescription analgesic that contains caffeine.

A 16-year-old adolescent survived a 6–8 g dose of caffeine (108). However, hypokalemia, hyperglycemia, tachycardia, bigeminy, agitation, respiratory alkalosis, and chest pain resulted. The elimination half-life of caffeine in this patient was 16 hours. Chest pain persisted for more than 24 hours but resolved within 45 hours.

Reports of death from caffeine poisoning are infrequent. The lethal dose of caffeine is estimated at 5–10 g in adults (109). A 27-year-old woman committed suicide by ingesting at least 6.5 g of caffeine (110). In another case, a serum caffeine concentration of 11.35 mg/l was associated with an unknown lethal oral dose in a 42-year-old woman (111). A 3-g dose was lethal in a 5-year-old child (112).

The following treatments are used to manage caffeine overdose (113):

■ Basic life support (respiratory and cardiovascular);

■ Emesis using ipecac (intubation and gastric lavage if comatose);

■ Activated charcoal;

■ Catharsis using saline cathartic (magnesium sulfate, sodium sulfate, or magnesium citrate) or sorbitol (may be given with charcoal or separately);

■ Intravenous diazepam for seizures (phenytoin or phenobarbital if diazepam fails to control seizures);

■ Intravenous fluids to replace losses;

■ Aluminum hydroxide gel for GI irritation;

■ Exchange transfusion or hemoperfusion (for extremely high serum caffeine concentrations).

Potential Interactions

Caffeine interferes with the vanillylmandelic acid (VMA) tests used to diagnose pheochromocytoma, and causes an increase in reported urinary VMA levels (114). Because caffeine also may increase urinary catecholamine excretion (through its pharmacologic effect, not a lab test interference), abstention from caffeine for at least 12 hours is recommended before testing for pheochromocytoma (30).

Caffeine can also cause false increases in serum uric acid (115).

Mechanisms of drug interactions with caffeine include induction of drug metabolizing enzymes by caffeine and inhibition by other drugs of hepatic microsomal enzymes required for caffeine metabolism. In addition, caffeine-induced reduction in liver and cerebral blood flow affects delivery of drugs to the liver and brain, which may be important for hepatically extracted and CNS drugs, respectively. Caffeine's pharmacologic effects may offset or be additive with those of other drugs such as beta-adrenergic agonists.

Both verapamil and mexiletine decrease caffeine clearance (116, 117). Clearance is decreased and both half-life and time-to-peak caffeine serum concentration are increased in women who take low-dose oral contraceptives compared with women who do not use them (118). The mechanism of these effects is unclear.

Cimetidine, disulfiram, and the quinolones ciprofloxacin, enoxacin, norfloxacin, and pipemidic acid (but not ofloxacin) all decrease the clearance of caffeine and increase its half-life (119–123). These effects are most likely mediated by inhibition of hepatic microsomal enzymes required for N-demethylation of caffeine.

The clinical significance of drug interactions with caffeine is uncertain. Caffeine use in conjunction with drugs that inhibit its metabolism could potentially allow caffeine accumulation, although tolerance develops to the pharmacologic effects of caffeine. There is some undetermined risk of acute toxicity in extreme cases. Patients who take drugs that decrease caffeine elimination may need to limit their caffeine intake to avoid adverse effects.

Caffeine can affect the disposition of other drugs. Abstinence from caffeine after heavy consumption by two patients taking lithium resulted in worsening of tremor (124). Lithium clearance decreased and serum lithium concentrations increased. Large increases or decreases in caffeine intake may affect patients stabilized on other drugs, resulting in therapeutic failure or toxicity.

SUMMARY

Patient Assessment

The pharmacist should determine the reason for stimulant product use and assess the risk of excessive caffeine intake and adverse effects. Factors to consider are total caffeine consumption, smoking, pregnancy, medical conditions, and concomitant drug therapy. The possibility that fatigue may be caused by an underlying pathology requiring medical attention should be considered.

Patient Education

The pharmacist should counsel the patient on the importance of using stimulants only occasionally and not as a substitute for sleep. The patient should be educated about the dietary and pharmaceutical sources of caffeine, particularly nonprescription analgesics. The pharmacist also should warn the patient about potential adverse effects, particularly CNS effects. The likelihood of experiencing caffeine withdrawal should be explained, and the associated symptoms should be described.

Pregnant women should be presented with the available evidence on the effects of caffeine on the fetus. The risks of caffeine accumulation in mother and fetus should be explained to women in the late stages of pregnancy.

As with all medications, the patient should be reminded to keep stimulants out of the reach of children.

Stimulant Product Use

Caffeine is generally safe to use. Attempts to link caffeine use with various cancers, diseases, and adverse effects on the fetus have yielded negative or inconclusive results. However, in the absence of proof exonerating caffeine, moderation is recommended in patients at risk (e.g., pregnant women and patients with hypercholesterolemia or cardiac rhythm disturbances).

Caffeine is not thought to cause or contribute to hypertension because tolerance develops to its pressor effect. Tolerance to the acute effects of caffeine may explain the absence of epidemiologic evidence implicating caffeine in hypertension, ischemic heart disease, arrhythmias, and other diseases.

REFERENCES

1 *Federal Register, 54,* 6814–27 (1989).

2 "The Anatomy of Sleep," Roche Laboratories, Nutley, N.J., 1966, pp. 39–59.

3 "The Nature of Sleep," G. E. W. Wolstenholme and M. O'Conner, Eds., Little, Brown and Co., Boston, Mass., 1961, pp. 86–102.

4 J. M. Krueger and M. L. Karnovsky, *Ann. N.Y. Acad. Sci.,* 1986.

5 K. L. Melmon and H. F. Morrelli, "Clinical Pharmacology—Basic Principles in Therapeutics," 2nd ed., Macmillan, New York, N.Y., 1978, pp. 886–887.

6 A. Kales et al., *Ann. Intern. Med., 106,* 582 (1987).

7 M. K. Erman, *Psychiatr. Clin. N. Am., 10,* 525 (1987).

8 "AHFS Drug Information 89," G. K. McEvoy, Ed., American Society of Hospital Pharmacists, Bethesda, Md., 1989, pp. 2–5, 16–19.

9 "The Pharmacological Basis of Therapeutics," 7th ed., A. G. Gilman et al., Eds., Macmillan, New York, N.Y., 1985, p. 686.

10 S. G. Carruthers et al., *Clin. Pharmacol. Ther., 23,* 375 (1978).

11 F. Gengo et al., *Clin. Pharmacol. Ther., 45,* 15 (1989).

12 R. S. Spector et al., *Clin. Pharmacol. Ther., 28,* 229 (1980).

13 R. H. Dreisbach, "Handbook of Poisoning," 10th ed., Lange Medical, Los Altos, Calif., 1980, p. 343.

14 C. Koppel et al., *Clin. Toxicol., 25,* 53 (1987).

15 D. Schneider-Helmert and C. L. Spinweber, *Psychopharmacology, 89,* 1 (1986).

16 *Federal Register, 53,* 6100–5 (1988).

17 E. M. Laska et al., *J. Am. Med. Assoc., 251,* 1711 (1984).

18 K. A. Nieforth and M. L. Cohen, in "Principles of Medicinal Chemistry," 3rd ed., W. O. Foye, Ed., Lea and Febiger, Philadelphia, Pa., 1989, pp. 279–282.

19 A. K. Henry and J. Feldhausen, "Drugs, Vitamins and Minerals in Pregnancy," Fisher Books, Tucson, Ariz., 1989, p. 381.

20 D. M. Graham, *Nutr. Rev., 36,* 97 (1978).

21 G. B. Schreiber et al., *Prev. Med., 17,* 295 (1988).

22 K. J. Morgan et al., *Regul. Toxicol. Pharmacol., 2,* 296 (1982).

23 H. Sholz, *J. Am. Coll. Cardiol., 4,* 389 (1984).

24 P. van Nguyen and M. G. Myers, *Clin. Pharmacol. Ther., 44,* 315 (1988).

25 C. I. Lin and M. Vassalle, *Int. J. Cardiol., 3,* 421 (1983).

26 J. Onrot et al., *N. Engl. J. Med., 313,* 549 (1985).

27 A. Sollevi et al., *Anesthesiology, 61,* 400 (1984).

28 R. W. von Borstel et al., *Life Sci., 32,* 1151 (1983).

29 D. Robertson et al., *Am. J. Med, 77,* 54 (1984).

30 L. Levi, *Acta Med. Scand., 181,* 431 (1967).

31 J. L. Izzo, Jr., et al., *Am. J. Cardiol., 52,* 769 (1983).

32 E. B. Truitt, Jr., in "Drill's Pharmacology in Medicine," 4th ed., J. R. DiPalma, Ed., McGraw-Hill, New York, N.Y., 1971, pp. 533–556.

33 B. Weiss and V. G. Laties, *Pharmacol. Rev., 14,* 1 (1962).

34 M. Bruce et al., *Br. J. Clin. Pharmacol., 22,* 81 (1986).

35 A. Goldstein et al., *J. Pharmacol. Exp. Ther., 150,* 146 (1965).

36 L. J. Dorfman and M. E. Jarvik, *Clin. Pharmacol. Ther., 11,* 869 (1970).

37 G. L. S. Pawan, *Biochem. J., 106,* 19P (1968).

38 R. B. Forney and F. W. Hughes, *Q. J. Stud. Alcohol, 26,* 206 (1965).

39 D. J. Osborne and Y. Rogers, *Aviat. Space Environ. Med., 54,* 528 (1983).

40 J. F. Greden, *Am. J. Psychiatry, 131,* 1089 (1974).

41 G. A. Pincomb et al., *Am. J. Cardiol., 56,* 119 (1985).

42 D. Robertson et al., *J. Clin. Invest., 67,* 1111 (1981).

43 G. A. Pincomb et al., *Am. J. Cardiol., 61,* 798 (1988).

44 C. France and B. Ditto, *J. Behav. Med., 11,* 473 (1988).

45 D. J. Dobmeyer et al., *N. Engl. J. Med., 308,* 814 (1983).

46 P. F. Newcombe et al., *Chest, 94,* 90 (1988).

47 M. G. Myers et al., *Am. J. Cardiol., 59,* 1024 (1987).

48 A. T. Hirsch et al., *Ann. Intern. Med., 110,* 593 (1989).

49 M. G. Myers, *Chest, 94,* 4 (1988).

50 D. S. Thelle et al., *N. Engl. J. Med., 308,* 1454 (1983).

51 P. T. Williams et al., *J. Am. Med. Assoc., 253,* 1407 (1985).

52 O. H. Førde et al., *Br. Med. J., 290,* 893 (1985).

53 S. M. Haffner et al., *Am. J. Epidemiol., 122,* 1 (1985).

54 A. Z. LaCroix et al., *N. Engl. J. Med., 315,* 977 (1986).

55 L. Rosenberg et al., *Am. J. Epidemiol., 128,* 570 (1988).

56 K. Yano et al., *N. Engl. J. Med., 316,* 946 (1987).

57 B. K. Jacobsen et al., *J. Natl. Cancer Inst., 76,* 823 (1986).

58 R. J. Mathew et al., *Br. J. Psychiatry, 143,* 604 (1983).

59 J. Onrot et al., *Clin. Pharmacol. Ther., 40,* 506 (1986).

60 A. G. Dulloo et al., *Am. J. Clin. Nutr., 49*, 44 (1989).

61 A. P. Passmore et al., *Ann. Intern. Med., 105*, 468 (1986).

62 A. B. Becker et al., *N. Engl. J. Med., 310*, 743 (1984).

63 R. Pagano et al., *Chest, 94*, 386 (1988).

64 S. Cohen and G. H. Booth, *N. Engl. J. Med., 293*, 897 (1975).

65 K. McArthur et al., *Gastroenterology, 83*, 199 (1982).

66 K. E. McArthur and M. Feldman, *Am. J. Clin. Nutr., 49*, 51 (1989).

67 C. Mitoma et al., *Arch. Biochem. Biophys., 134*, 434 (1969).

68 T. Colton et al., *Clin. Pharmacol. Ther., 9*, 31 (1968).

69 R. R. Griffiths et al., *J. Pharmacol. Exp. Ther., 239*, 416 (1986).

70 J. F. Greden et al., *Psychosomatics, 21*, 411 (1980).

71 *FDA Drug Bull., 10 (3)*, 19–20 (1980).

72 S. G. Oei et al., *Br. Med. J., 298*, 568 (1989).

73 W. D. Parsons and J. G. Pelletier, *Can. Med. Assoc. J., 127*, 377 (1982).

74 R. Gorodischer and M. Karplus, *Eur. J. Clin. Pharmacol., 22*, 47 (1982).

75 W. Srisuphan and M. B. Bracken, *Am. J. Obstet. Gynecol., 154*, 14 (1986).

76 S. Harlap and P. H. Shiono, *Lancet, 2*, 173 (1980).

77 J. Kline et al., *Lancet, 2*, 176 (1980).

78 M. F. Jacobsen et al., *Lancet, 1*, 1415 (1981).

79 K. Kurppa et al., *N. Engl. J. Med., 306*, 1548 (1982).

80 L. Rosenberg et al., *J. Am. Med. Assoc., 247*, 1429 (1982).

81 S. Linn et al., *N. Engl. J. Med., 306*, 141 (1982).

82 K. Kurppa et al., *Am. J. Public Health, 73*, 1397 (1983).

83 T. R. Martin and M. B. Bracken, *Am. J. Epidemiol., 126*, 813 (1987).

84 B. Watkinson and P. A. Fried, *Neurobehav. Toxicol. Teratol., 7*, 9 (1985).

85 O. G. Brooke et al., *Br. Med. J., 298*, 795 (1989).

86 H. M. Barr et al., *Pediatrics, 74*, 336 (1984).

87 C. M. Berlin et al., *Pediatrics, 73*, 59 (1984).

88 R. E. Christianson et al., *Lancet, 1*, 378 (1989).

89 A. Wilcox et al., *Lancet, 2*, 1453 (1988).

90 G. R. Najem et al., *Int. J. Epidemiol., 11*, 212 (1982).

91 B. MacMahon et al., *N. Engl. J. Med., 304*, 630 (1981).

92 C.-C. Hsieh et al., *N. Engl. J. Med., 315*, 587 (1986).

93 C.-C. Hsieh et al., *N. Engl. J. Med., 316*, 484 (1987).

94 R. A. Hiatt et al., *Int. J. Cancer, 41*, 794 (1988).

95 J. Cuzik and A. G. Babiker, *Int. J. Cancer, 43*, 415 (1989).

96 J. P. Minton et al., *Am. J. Obstet. Gynecol., 135*, 157 (1979).

97 F. Lubin et al., *J. Am. Med. Assoc., 253*, 2388 (1985).

98 C. A. Boyle et al., *J. Natl. Cancer Inst., 72*, 1015 (1984).

99 M. F. Jacobsen and B. F. Liebman, *J. Am. Med. Assoc., 255*, 1438 (1986).

100 J. P. Minton, *J. Am. Med. Assoc., 254*, 2408 (1985).

101 W. B. Hutchinson et al., *J. Natl. Cancer Inst., 65*, 13 (1980).

102 F. Lubin et al., *J. Natl. Cancer Inst., 74*, 569 (1985).

103 D. D. Tang-Liu et al., *J. Pharmacol. Exp. Ther., 224*, 180 (1983).

104 D. M. Grant et al., *Br. J. Clin. Pharmacol., 21*, 454 (1986).

105 M. Bonati et al., *Clin. Pharmacol. Ther., 32*, 98 (1982).

106 W. D. Parsons and A. H. Neims, *Clin. Pharmacol. Ther., 24*, 40 (1978).

107 B. E. Statland et al., *N. Engl. J. Med., 295*, 110 (1976).

108 C. L. Leson et al., *J. Toxicol. Clin. Toxicol., 26*, 407 (1988).

109 "The Pharmacological Basis of Therapeutics," 7th ed., A. G. Gilman et al., Eds., Macmillan, New York, N.Y., 1985, p. 596.

110 R. L. Alstott et al., *J. Forensic Sci., 18*, 135 (1973).

111 J. Bryant, *Arch. Pathol. Lab Med., 105*, 685 (1981).

112 V. J. M. Dimaio and J. C. Garriott, *Forensic Sci., 3*, 275 (1974).

113 "Poisindex," vol. 61, Micromedex, Inc., Englewood, Colo., (1989).

114 F. H. Meyers et al., "Review of Medical Pharmacology," 7th ed., Lange Medical Publications, Los Altos, Calif., 1980, pp. 704–705.

115 "AHFS Drug Information 89," G. K. McEvoy, Ed., American Society of Hospital Pharmacists, Bethesda, Md., 1989, pp. 1179–1182.

116 S. Nawoot et al., *Clin. Pharmacol. Ther., 43*, 148 (1988).

117 R. Joeres and E. Richter, *N. Engl. J. Med., 317*, 117 (1987).

118 D. R. Abernethy and E. L. Todd, *Eur. J. Clin. Pharmacol., 28*, 425 (1985).

119 D. C. May et al., *Clin. Pharmacol. Ther., 31*, 656 (1982).

120 L. J. Broughton and H. J. Rogers, *Br. J. Clin. Pharmacol., 12*, 155 (1981).

121 C. A. Beach et al., *Clin. Pharmacol. Ther., 39*, 265 (1986).

122 A. H. Staib et al., *Drugs, 34* (suppl. 1), 170 (1987).

123 M. Carbó et al., *Clin. Pharmacol. Ther., 45*, 234 (1989).

124 J. W. Jefferson, *J. Clin. Psychiatry, 49*, 72 (1988).

SLEEP AID PRODUCT TABLE

Product (Manufacturer)	Antihistamine	Other Ingredients
Compôz Tablets (Med-Tech)	diphenhydramine hydrochloride, 50 mg	
Dormarex Capsules (Republic)	pyrilamine maleate, 25 mg	
Dormarex 2 Tablets (Republic)	diphenhydramine hydrochloride, 50 mg	
Doxysom Tablets (Quantum Pharmics)	doxylamine succinate, 25 mg	
Excedrin PM Tablets (Bristol-Myers Products)	diphenhydramine citrate, 38 mg	acetaminophen, 500 mg
Nervine Nighttime Sleep-Aid Caplets (Miles)	diphenhydramine hydrochloride, 25 mg	
Nytol Tablets (Block)	diphenhydramine hydrochloride, 25 mg	cellulose cornstarch lactose silica stearic acid
Quiet Tabs (Commerce)	pyrilamine maleate, 25 mg	
Quiet World Tablets (Whitehall)	pyrilamine maleate, 25 mg	acetaminophen, 162 mg aspirin, 227 mg
Relax-U-Caps (Columbia Medical)	pyrilamine maleate, 25 mg	
Sleep-Eze 3 Tablets (Whitehall)	diphenhydramine hydrochloride, 25 mg	
Sleepinal (Thompson Medical)	diphenhydramine hydrochloride, 50 mg	
Sominex Pain Relief Formula Tablets (SmithKline Beecham)	diphenhydramine hydrochloride, 25 mg	acetaminophen, 500 mg
Sominex 2 Tablets (SmithKline Beecham)	diphenhydramine hydrochloride, 25 mg	
Somnicaps (Amer. Pharm.)	pyrilamine maleate, 25 mg	
Tega S-A Tablets (Ortega)	diphenhydramine hydrochloride, 50 mg	acetaminophen, 325 mg niacin, 25 mg
Twilite Caplets (Pfeiffer)	diphenhydramine hydrochloride, 50 mg	
Unisom Nighttime Sleep Aid Tablets (Leeming)	doxylamine succinate, 25 mg	

STIMULANT PRODUCT TABLE

Product (Manufacturer)	Caffeine	Other Ingredients
Caffedrine Capsules (Thompson Medical)	200 mg (timed release)	
Caffeine Capsules, Timed Release and Tablets (Various manufacturers)	100 mg (tablets) 200 mg (capsules) 250 mg (capsules)	
Citrated Caffeine (Lilly)	1 gr (equal parts caffeine and citric acid)	
Dexitac Capsules, Timed Release (Republic)	250 mg	
NoDoz Tablets (Bristol-Myers Products)	100 mg	cornstarch flavor mannitol microcrystalline cellulose stearic acid sucrose
Pep-Back (Alva Amco)	NS[a]	salicylamide
Quick-Pep Tablets (Thompson Medical)	150 mg	dextrose, 300 mg
Summit (Pfeiffer)	100 mg	acetaminophen, 325 mg
Tirend Tablets (SmithKline Beecham)	100 mg	
Valerianets Dispert (Alvin Last)		extract valerian, 50 mg
Vivarin Tablets (SmithKline Beecham)	200 mg	dextrose, 150 mg
Wakoz (Jeffrey Martin)	200 mg	

[a] Quantity not specified.

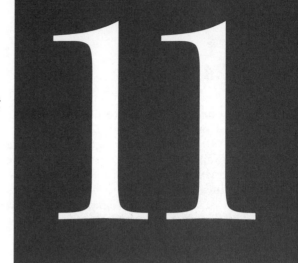

William R. Garnett

ANTACID PRODUCTS

Questions to ask in patient/consumer counseling

Can you describe the pain?

How long have you had this pain?

Where and when does the pain occur? Do you get the pain immediately after meals or several hours after meals?

Is the pain relieved by food? Do certain foods, coffee, or carbonated beverages make the pain worse?

Have you vomited blood or black material that looks like coffee grounds?

Have you noticed blood in the stool or have the stools been black or tarry?

What medications are you currently taking?

Are you taking ibuprofen, aspirin, or aspirin-containing products? Do you smoke? How much? Do you drink alcoholic beverages? How much?

Have you previously used any antacids to treat this pain? Which ones? Did they relieve the pain?

Are you on any special diet such as a low-salt diet?

Is the pain worse when you are lying down?

Are you currently under a physician's care for other medical conditions?

Do you have any medical conditions such as diabetes or kidney or heart disease?

During 1984, American manufacturers had $941 million in sales of nonprescription digestive remedies (1). The overwhelming portion of these products was antacid preparations. These products may be used without a prescription for short-term treatment of indigestion, excessive eating and drinking, heartburn, and long-term treatment of reflux esophagitis and chronic peptic ulcer disease. The pharmacist should be able to evaluate an individual's need for a medical examination before antacid therapy and should be able to select an antacid for either short-term or chronic use.

ANATOMY OF THE GASTROINTESTINAL SYSTEM

The gastrointestinal (GI) system is divided into upper and lower regions. The esophagus, stomach, duodenum, jejunum, and ileum compose the upper GI tract. Although peptic ulcer disease may occur at any site in the upper GI tract exposed to the digestive action of acid and pepsin, it usually is found in the stomach and/or duodenum (2). Gastroesophageal reflux involves the retrograde flow of gastric or duodenal contents across the gastroesophageal junction into the esophagus (3).

Esophagus

The esophagus conducts ingested materials from the mouth to the stomach. The esophagus is relaxed basally but contracts to deliver materials to the stomach. The proximal part is composed of striated muscle. The distal portion is different physiologically and ana-

243

tomically from the rest of the esophagus and is made up of smooth muscle (4, 5).

Following the ingestion and mastication of food, swallowing initiates a progressive wave of alternate contraction and relaxation (peristalsis) of the esophageal musculature to propel the food to the stomach. Gravity, to a lesser extent, also promotes the delivery of food to the stomach. Liquids are conducted without peristalsis. A region of elevated intraluminal pressure exists approximately 2–5 cm above the gastroesophageal junction. This physiologic barrier, the lower esophageal sphincter (LES), results from tonic, but variable, constriction of the muscular esophageal wall (6). It is now recognized that the LES is the major determinant of competence of the gastroesophageal barrier (7). The LES is innervated by the autonomic nervous system and becomes relaxed after either beta-adrenoreceptor stimulation or cholinergic blockage. Thus, anticholinergics or drugs that stimulate beta-receptors may predispose individuals to episodes of gastroesophageal reflux.

The LES allows the passage of food into the stomach and prevents gastric contents from refluxing up into the esophagus. This is critical because resting pressure in the esophagus is lower than that in the stomach. The LES normally prevents the retrograde flow of gastric contents up into the esophagus. It responds to the peristaltic movement of swallowing to allow ingested substances to pass into the stomach (8). The pressure can change in response to a number of stimuli. Gastrin and motilin increase pressure, and secretin, cholecystokinin, and glucagon decrease the pressure (9–13). Alcohol, smoking, and fatty foods decrease the LES pressure and increase the likelihood of reflux (14–16). However, many factors can influence the integrity of the LES, making reflux possible.

Stomach

The stomach is divided anatomically and functionally. Anatomically, the stomach consists of the cardia, fundus, body (corpus), and antrum. Functionally, the stomach is divided into proximal and distal areas concerned with gastric emptying.

Each anatomical area has a different type of mucosa and contributes different secretions to the gastric juice. The cardia, consisting of cardiac mucosa, is the smallest area of the stomach and occupies only a 0.5–3-cm strip that begins at the esophagogastric sphincter. Little is known about the function of cardiac mucosa (17).

Gastric mucosa has a total surface area of about 900 m² and contains surface mucus cells, mucus neck cells, argentaffin cells, parietal cells, and chief cells. It lines both the fundus and body and is responsible for most of the components of gastric juice. Parietal cells secrete hydrochloric acid and intrinsic factor. Chief cells secrete pepsinogen, which is activated in the presence of hydrochloric acid to the proteolytic enzyme pepsin. The mucosal cells of the epithelium protect the stomach from the acid-pepsin complex by secreting an alkaline mucus (18). Argentaffin cells are serotonin-producing cells. The pyloric mucosa and the surface mucus cells that line the antrum and the prepyloric canal secrete gastrin and a protective mucus.

The vagus nerve provides parasympathetic innervation to the stomach. The vagus fibers synapse with the intrinsic plexus and postganglionic fibers leading to the secretory glands and to muscle. However, only a small portion of the intrinsic plexus fibers, which are related to local reflexes such as secretion, synapse with the vagus (19). Thus, vagotomy by either chemical or surgical means will not totally eliminate local reflexes.

Functionally, the proximal stomach (fundus) is responsible for the emptying of liquids, and the distal stomach (antrum) is responsible for the emptying of solids (20). A pacemaker in the greater curvature initiates peristaltic waves, and the resistance of the pyloric sphincter determines the gastric emptying rate (21).

Gastric Secretion

The stomach releases secretions at different rates depending on whether it is in the basal state or has been stimulated. The three phases of gastric secretion are cephalic, gastric, and intestinal. Initiated by food, they proceed simultaneously and continue for several hours. The cephalic and gastric phases are stimulatory and synergistic. The intestinal phase is weakly stimulatory but primarily provides negative feedback (22). The general purpose of acid and pepsinogen release is believed to be the hydrolysis of protein and other foodstuffs into a liquid or semiliquid state. It is an integral part of the absorption process. However, persons with achlorhydria do not suffer from malabsorption. Therefore, the major role of acid is to kill bacteria to ensure a stable intragastric environment (23). The presence of achlorhydria or increased intragastric pH has been associated with bacterial overgrowth.

The target cell for the variety of stimuli from the three phases of gastric secretion is the parietal cell (24). The parietal cell has receptors to histamine, acetylcholine, gastrin, and other peptides. In addition, it responds to a variety of second messengers such as cyclic AMP and calcium. Within the parietal cell, the H/K ATPase proton pump is the final mediator of acid secretion. The proton pump exchanges H produced in the parietal cell for K in the gastric lumen. It offers another mechanism that pharmacologic agents can inhibit to block the secretion of gastric acid (24).

Phases of Gastric Secretion

Cephalic Phase

Only small amounts of gastric secretions are produced during the fasting state in the healthy individual. However, thought, smell, taste, chewing, and swallowing of food set off a parasympathetic response through the vagus nerve (the cephalic phase) (25). The precise site in the brain in which this occurs is uncertain because changes in acid secretion may be found when medullary, hypothalmic, limbic, or cortical areas of the brain are stimulated (26). The vagus nerve postsynaptic transmitter, acetylcholine (the "first messenger"), then stimulates the release of hydrochloric acid, pepsinogen, and gastrin (27). The exact method of stimulation is unknown but may involve activation of a second messenger such as cyclic adenosine 3':5'-monophosphate (cyclic AMP) (28). Cyclic AMP in turn may activate a protein kinase that releases gastric secretions (29). Although it is thought that cholinergic receptors as well as histamine receptors exist (30), their exact relationship is unclear (26). Vagotomy or large doses of anticholinergics may block this phase. The regulation of the cephalic phase is completely neural (31, 32).

Gastric Phase

The presence of food in the stomach stimulates secretion directly and indirectly (33). The physical presence of food distends the gastric mucosa and causes a direct release of gastric secretions that requires no intermediate mechanisms. Amino acids and peptides found in protein also cause the release of gastrin, which is a major humoral mediator for acid and pepsinogen secretion (34). The direct and indirect processes are synergistic (17). The gastric phase is also mediated by cholinergic innervation. The regulation of the gastric phase is both neural and hormonal (31, 32).

Food stimulates the release of gastrin by mechanical distention of the antrum, by vagal stimulation, and by a direct action on the G-cells of the antrum and the duodenum (35). G-cells are specialized endocrine cells that contain gastrin and respond to chemical changes. They are shaped similar to a flask, with a broad base and a narrow neck that extends to the mucosa surface. Gastrin release may also be stimulated by epinephrine and

calcium, but this process requires amounts above physiologic concentrations (36). Gastrin release is inhibited by acid, secretin, glucagon, vasoactive intestinal peptide, gastric inhibitory peptide, and calcitonin (35, 36).

There are several gastrin molecules, which vary in molecular weight, site of release, and potency (37). "Little" gastrin is secreted by the antrum and is the most potent; "big" gastrin, which has a longer half-life, is released from the duodenum; and "big-big" gastrin is released from the jejunum (38). All gastrins stimulate the same receptor. The gastric mucosa makes no distinction among the gastrins and responds by secreting hydrochloric acid and pepsinogen (35). Big-big gastrin is believed to be responsible for basal acid secretion.

Gastrin mediates physiologic functions other than acid and pepsinogen release. It may protect the stomach from the proteolytic action of acid and pepsin by stimulating gastric mucosal cell proliferation (39) and by tightening the gastric mucosal cell barrier (40). There are conflicting reports about gastrin's effect on increasing LES tone (41, 42). Because its chemical structure resembles pancreozymin and cholecystokinin, gastrin increases pancreatic enzyme secretions, bile flow, and gastric and intestinal motility (17).

The mechanism by which gastrin mediates acid and pepsinogen release is unknown (29). Gastrin may release histamine, which in turn may cause acid and pepsinogen release. Histamine receptors are classified as H_1 and H_2. H_2 receptors are responsible for acid release (43). Selective H_2 antihistamines are capable of blocking pentagastrin-mediated gastric secretion (44), suggesting that gastrin acts via histamine (45). Histamine may act by releasing cyclic AMP as a second messenger (46), which activates a protein kinase (29). Histamine may augment the release of acid by other stimuli.

Gastrin plays a crucial role in the pathogenesis of peptic ulcer disease. Peptic ulcers of Zollinger–Ellison syndrome result from an excessive secretion of gastrin that occurs in the basal state as well as in response to stimuli. In duodenal peptic ulcer patients, the basal secretional gastrin may be normal, but the regulatory feedback mechanism between gastrin secretion and gastric acid secretion is impaired. The result in duodenal peptic ulcer disease is a hypersecretion of acid. In gastric ulcer patients, the gastrin–acid feedback is appropriately regulated, and the acid secretion is normal or even low (47).

Intestinal Phase

The third phase of gastric secretion, the intestinal phase, involves both stimulation and inhibition. As long as chyme, or partly digested food, is in the intestine, there is continued gastric secretion. The mediators are big gastrin, cholecystokinin, and pancreozymin (22). Stimulation is weak, and the main function of the intestinal phase seems to be a negative feedback to further secretion. The regulation of the intestinal phase is mainly hormonal.

Inhibition is mediated by an enterogastrone, which can be any substance secreted from the small intestine that inhibits gastric secretion. An enterogastrone may inhibit gastric secretion by direct inhibition of either acid and pepsinogen release, or gastrin, or both. Cholecystokinin, pancreozymin, and glucagon inhibit gastrin release (48, 49). Gastric inhibitory peptide has been isolated from cholecystokinin. At pharmacologic doses, it acts similarly to glucagon. There is some doubt as to what it does at physiologic doses (50). Secretin blocks acid secretion and inhibits glucagon release (51, 52). Vasoactive intestinal peptide can be extracted from the gastric mucosa and has pharmacologic effects similar to secretin (50). Recently, somatostatin has been found to be a potent inhibitor of acid secretion and gastrin release (23). The stimulus for the release of enterogastrones is the presence of acid, fat, protein breakdown products, or hyperosmolar substances in the duodenum (25). Acid in the antrum also diminishes gastrin release (53).

Factors Influencing Gastric Secretion

The endogenous stimulants of gastric acid secretion are acetylcholine, gastrin, histamine, cyclic AMP, and protein kinase. The release of these endogenous substances is stimulated by exogenous substances. Amino acids and peptides are the main exogenous sources of stimuli. They are probably responsible for the increase in gastrin secretion after meals. Although digested proteins stimulate acid production, they also buffer gastric contents to decrease the fall in pH (50). Although coffee is a stimulant for gastric secretion, this effect is primarily due to its amino acid and peptide components and not to the caffeine, which is a very weak stimulant to gastric secretion (54). Calcium also promotes gastric acid secretion by stimulating gastrin release (55). Alcohol has a much greater gastric stimulatory effect in dogs than in humans (56). A model simulation demonstrated that volume-dependent gastrin secretion is of major importance in normal gastric acid regulation, whereas negative feedback by hydrogen-dependent gastrin secretion was of minor importance. This model predicts that the larger the volume of food (which requires a larger amount of acid), the greater the release of gastrin (57).

In addition to the previously described enterogastrones, a number of factors inhibit gastric secretion. A lowering of the pH in both the stomach and duodenum initiates responses that decrease gastric secretion. Acid inhibits the release of gastrin in the antrum (58) and releases enterogastrones in the duodenum. Fat, hypertonic solutions, and hyperglycemia also inhibit gastric secretion (59–62). The amount of gastric acid secreted depends on the balance of the stimulatory and inhibitory factors.

Acid and Circadian Rhythm

Acid plays a key role in the development of peptic ulcers, gastroesophageal reflux, and stress ulcers (63). Acid is required for the activation of pepsinogen to pepsin. Duodenal ulcer patients tend to be hypersecretors of acid. Gastric ulcer patients may be normosecretors or hyposecretors of acid, but acid accumulates at the site of the ulcer formation. Although local ischemia may precipitate the development of stress ulcers, it is acid that erodes the mucosa. These conditions improve when the acid is removed.

Acid secretion follows a circadian rhythm (63). The secretion of acid increases with the administration of meals. The ingestion of food buffers the intragastric pH, while the secretion of acid increases it. The peak time for the basal secretion of gastric acid is in the early morning hours, between 2 and 4 a.m., if the patient goes to bed and does not ingest food to buffer the acid secretion. This peak in acid secretion explains why patients with duodenal ulcer disease often are awakened in the middle of the night with pain. A glass of milk or small snack will often buffer the acid, relieve the pain, and allow the patient to go back to sleep. Excessive nocturnal acid may explain why patients with duodenal ulcer disease may be difficult to treat. H_2 antagonists should be dosed after dinner or at bedtime so that their onset and maximal acid suppression coincide with the peak acid secretion.

Although acid is physiologically important for the digestive process, the gastroduodenal defense mechanism is also important in protecting the mucosa from hyperacidity (63). The development of gastric disease results from an excessive imbalance of the aggressive factors dominated by acid or from a deficiency of the defensive factors that protect the mucosa.

Gastroduodenal Defense and Repair Mechanisms

The normal gastroduodenal mucosa has the ability to resist the erosive potential of gastric acid and pepsin by a combination of defensive and repair processes (64). These defenses include the mucus–bicarbonate barrier, the secretion of bicarbonate, surface epithelial cells, mucosal repair, intestinal blood flow, endogenous sulfhydryls, and prostaglandins (65).

The surface epithelial cells are important in the first line of GI defense. They are relatively impermeable to hydrogen ion and provide a physical barrier to diffusion. The phospholipids in these cells allow high lipid-soluble molecules to pass but retard water-soluble ions such as hydrogen. The surface epithelial cells also deliver mucus and transport bicarbonate ions (64).

Mucus is a thick water-insoluble glycoprotein gel that is secreted in the stomach by the goblet cells and in the duodenum by the goblet cells and Brunner's glands. Mucus forms a continuous adherent layer overlying the GI mucosa; it protects the epithelium from damage by passage of food and provides a lubricant for the movement of solid material. The ability to protect the mucosa depends on the thickness of the mucus. Mucus is decreased by mucolytic agents and is increased by prostaglandins. Mucus retards the diffusion of hydrogen ions but is not sufficient to entirely protect the GI tract (66).

Bicarbonate is secreted at a rate that is 5–10% of the maximal acid output rate. Chloride and bicarbonate ions may be exchanged either actively or passively in the stomach and the intestine.

GI blood flow delivers oxygen, nutrients, and bicarbonate to the surface epithelial cells and removes hydrogen ions. If blood flow decreases, mucosal damage increases. Mucosal damage may also result from a decreased ability to buffer the back diffusion of acid, an increased concentration of free radicals such as superoxide, or a decrease in bicarbonate. This stimulation is particularly important in stress ulcer formation because local ischemia occurs. An increased blood flow protects the mucosa from damage (6).

Endogenous sulfhydryls are naturally occurring sulfhydryl-containing amino acids that protect the mucosa from irritants. They enable the synthesis of prostaglandins and may be responsible for the mucosal defense by affecting the permeability of membranes or by preventing the release of mediators of mucosal damage.

The local generation of prostaglandins is believed to be responsible for the mucosal adaptation to irritant attack. Luminally applied prostaglandins protect the mucosa from irritants, increase the local blood flow, and help dissipate the irritant. They have also been shown to increase bicarbonate, increase the surface-active phospholipids, increase sodium and chloride transport, increase cyclic AMP, stabilize lysozomes, and maintain sulfhydryls (68).

If injured, the gastroduodenal mucosa can quickly repair itself. When a single cell is damaged, repair occurs by extrusion of the damaged cell with minimal disruption of mucosal integrity. When a large number of cells is involved, epithelial cells rapidly spread and migrate to cover the basal lamina and form "tight junctions" between epithelial cells. These regenerated cells have normal function. This repair process is usually completed within 30 minutes (65).

The defense and repair processes play a major role in determining whether peptic ulcer disease will occur. If they predominate, the mucosa remains healthy; if they are overwhelmed, there is erosion. There has been recent interest in drugs that stimulate the defense and repair processes (69). These drugs include carbenoxolone, tripotassium dicitratobismuthate, prostaglandins, and perhaps sucralfate.

Gastric Motility

The proximal stomach receives and stores ingested foods. By slow, sustained contractions, it releases its contents into the distal stomach where peristaltic contractions mix the contents with gastric juice before allowing them to pass through the pyloric sphincter into the duodenum. The contraction rate is regulated by a pacemaker under vagal control (25).

The gastric emptying rate depends on the resistance of the pyloric sphincter, which is controlled by many stimuli (21). Hormones (secretin, cholecystokinin, and motilin), hyperosmolar solutions, acid solutions, and fats delay gastric emptying; gastric distention increases the emptying rate (70). Distention is the only physiologic factor known to directly stimulate gastric emptying (71). Gastric emptying may be stimulated by pharmacologic agents, such as metoclopramide or bethanechol.

The stomach is considered to be exposed to the outside environment; it receives anything capable of entering the mouth and passing down the esophagus. The stomach must respond to and act on agents that are hot or cold, acid or alkaline, polar or nonpolar, liquid or solid, digestible or nondigestible. Occasionally, the protective mechanisms fail to cope with these agents, and inflammation occurs in the form of acute or chronic upper GI distress (72).

Heliobacter Pylori

Heliobacter pylori, formerly called *Campylobacter pylori*, are Gram-negative curved bacilli that are microaerophilic, motile, and oxidase and catalase positive. These organisms have been found in patients with chronic gastritis and in patients with peptic ulcer disease (73–84). Evidence from morphologic, serologic, and therapeutic studies implicate *H. pylori* as a causative organism in patients with gastritis. Its role in peptic ulcer disease is somewhat more elusive. The low pH induced by excess acid production seen in peptic ulcer disease, especially duodenal ulcer disease, may allow the *H. pylori* to colonize at the site of the ulcer. Inflammation and ulceration may follow. Some reports indicate that the presence of *H. pylori* is responsible for the recurrence of peptic ulcer disease. However, although *H. pylori* has been associated with gastritis and peptic ulcer disease, true cause and effect have not been shown. The most effective antiulcer medication against *H. pylori* is colloidal bismuth. However, antacids have also been reported to eradicate *H. pylori*. Future therapy may involve pharmacologic agents that promote the healing of the peptic ulcer as well as pharmacologic agents that eradicate *H. pylori* and prevent recurrence of the disease.

TYPES OF GI DISORDERS

Acute Upper GI Distress

Acute upper GI disorders develop quickly but usually are self-limiting. They usually respond quickly to symptomatic treatment with acid neutralization. With the exception of hemorrhagic gastritis, these disorders are usually not life-threatening. Chronic acid suppression is not required for treatment.

Gastroesophageal Reflux

Gastroesophageal reflux is the retrograde flow of gastric or duodenal contents across the gastroesophageal junction into the esophagus. This reflux may occur in normal persons up to 15 times a day and often goes unnoticed (3). The effects depend on the mixture of gastric acid, pepsin, bile salts, and pancreatic enzymes refluxing onto the esophageal mucosa (5). Although gastroesophageal reflux may be asymptomatic (85), the most common patient complaint is retrosternal discomfort, which radiates upward and is aggravated in the recumbent position (5). Reflux esophagitis is also aggravated by obesity, tight garments about the abdomen, and pregnancy. The patient may refer to these symptoms as "heartburn," "indigestion," or "sour stomach." The regurgitation of fluid while sleeping or bending over is conclusive evidence of gastroesophageal reflux. Other less common symptoms include painful or difficult swallowing, hemorrhage, and pulmonary complaints (7). These symptoms may also represent more serious GI disorders including carcinomas. Although gastroesophageal reflux may exist simultaneously with a hiatal hernia, the terms are not synonymous. Gastroesophageal reflux and hiatal hernia are two separate clinical entities, and one has no effect on the other (7). In fact, only about 5% of patients with hiatal hernia complain of reflux symptoms (86).

There is general agreement that dysfunction of the lower esophageal sphincter is the cause of reflux (5).

Symptoms have been associated with unexplained, inappropriate, and transient relaxation of the LES (87). However, there is no explanation for the LES dysfunction. Other factors that may be associated with reflux are disordered peristalsis and delayed gastric emptying (88, 89). Gastroesophageal reflux is related to gastric volume. Overeating, which increases gastric volume, enhances reflux; this is especially true at bedtime (90). The symptoms may vary over 24 hours. The greatest amount of reflux usually occurs during the evening, perhaps because the basal tone of the distal esophageal high-pressure zone decreases in the evening (91). Large evening meals and recumbency may also contribute to reflux.

A cycle of events occurs in which reflux causes inflammation and damage leading to esophagitis. Esophagitis could result in defective peristalsis and an incompetent LES (92).

An appropriate history and prompt relief by acid neutralization usually indicate gastroesophageal reflux. Diagnostic testing may be necessary if cardiac, biliary, or gastroduodenal disorders are suspected. The techniques used to diagnose gastroesophageal reflux include barium esophagography with fluoroscopy, esophageal endoscopy, esophageal mucosal biopsy, esophageal manometry, acid perfusion test, esophageal pH monitoring, and gastroesophageal scintiscanning (5). Acid perfusion and esophageal biopsy are the most sensitive tests. Prolonged pH monitoring may also be useful (92). The more invasive tests are used primarily in patients who have severe symptoms or who are hard to treat.

The treatment of gastroesophageal reflux is divided into three phases. Phase I involves dietary and lifestyle changes, measures to improve acid clearance, and use of antacids. Phase II uses omeprazole, H_2 antagonists, bethanechol, metoclopramide, and sucralfate. Phase III is antireflux surgery (92, 93).

Although most pharmacologic therapy is aimed at improving LES tone and/or neutralizing gastric acid, some very effective results can be obtained if the patient changes lifestyle (7). Smoking and the ingestion of fatty foods, coffee, and chocolate, which can decrease LES tone, should be discouraged. Patients should be asked if they are taking any drugs known to decrease LES tone. These drugs include theophylline, diazepam, verapamil, isoproterenol and other beta-adrenergic agonists, and anticholinergics (93). Individuals should eat slowly and not recline after meals. Carbonated beverages will also increase intragastric pressure and should be avoided. Perhaps the most effective treatment is to use gravity to diminish the gastroesophageal pressure gradient by elevating the head of the patient's bed with 6-inch (15-cm) blocks (94, 95). Weight loss is also successful in decreasing symptoms. Bethanechol, metoclopramide, and antacids have been used to increase LES competence. Alginic acid has been used to provide a physical barrier that will be neutral if refluxed, although there is controversy regarding the efficacy of this agent (88). The recent availability of omeprazole offers a unique mechanism to completely shut off acid secretion. Omeprazole has been useful in severe refractory reflux esophagitis. If nonpharmacologic measures and antacids, omeprazole, or H_2 antagonists are not effective, bethanechol or metoclopramide may be tried. However, bethanechol has the therapeutic disadvantage of increasing gastric acidity through its cholinergic action (96). It also may cause diarrhea and urinary frequency. Metoclopramide is reported to strengthen the LES and to increase the gastric emptying rate (97). Sucralfate may also be useful (98). Antireflux surgery is indicated only if other therapies fail. Antireflux surgery has the disadvantage of rendering the patient unable to vomit or belch.

Gastritis

The term "gastritis" implies an inflammation of the gastric mucosa. Acute gastritis has occurred after the ingestion of aspirin, other nonsteroidal anti-inflammatory drugs (NSAIDs), and alcohol, in uremia, following gastric freezing, during treatment with antitumor agents, during an infection, after ingestion of caustic substances, and as a complication of stress (99). The disease mechanism appears to be a break in the normal gastric mucosal barrier allowing hydrochloric acid to enter the mucosa, injure vessels, and cause inflammation, erosion, and hemorrhage (100). The lesions are usually superficial, but more severe lesions may develop (99). *H. pylori*, which has been associated with gastritis, may play a part in the etiology.

The primary manifestation of gastritis is acute GI bleeding. Acute gastritis may account for as much as 30% of all GI bleeding episodes. Radiologic examination is of no use in acute gastritis. Diagnosis is best made by endogastroscopy (72).

The process is usually self-limiting and the bleeding stops spontaneously in 2–5 days if the initiating cause is removed. Patients may require intensive antacids or H_2 antagonists for a short period of time, but chronic therapy is not required. Occasionally, lavage or surgery is required to stop the bleeding, especially in patients taking anticoagulants. If antacids or H_2 antagonists fail to relieve the symptoms quickly, the possibility of a hiatal hernia or gallbladder disease should be considered (38).

Alkaline Reflux Gastritis and Esophagitis

The reflux of duodenal contents may also cause gastritis and esophagitis (101). The composition of these contents may be bile, pancreatic enzymes, or alkali. The diagnostic features include chronic continuous epigastric pain that is exacerbated by eating, vomiting, weight loss, iron deficiency anemia, achlorhydria, and intragastric bile. There is no exact diagnostic test, and some have questioned whether alkaline reflux is a separate disease entity (102). The pathophysiology is believed to result from bile-induced mucosal damage. Therapy with antacids, H_2 antagonists, bile salt absorbants, and metoclopramide has been unsuccessful. Prostaglandins and sucralfate are now being studied (101).

Nonulcer Dyspepsia

Nonulcer dyspepsia is a commonly encountered clinical problem, whose pathophysiology is poorly understood (103). Dyspepsia is a term used loosely by patients and clinicians to include any abnormal discomfort, including retasting of food, acid regurgitation, heartburn, fullness, belching, and rumblings, as well as any signs of peptic ulceration. Many publications on dyspepsia do not contain a definition of the term. It has been described as a "wastebasket" diagnosis for conditions of intermittent upper abdominal discomfort for which the cause is not clearly defined (104). Symptoms of dyspepsia are common and may indicate that the patient has a peptic ulcer process. However, nonulcer dyspepsia (i.e., symptoms of dyspepsia without the presence of an ulcer) occurs about twice as often as peptic ulcer. There is no clear relationship between nonulcer dyspepsia and *H. pylori*, stress, emotions, diet, environmental factors, or other diseases. Chronic nonulcer dyspepsia (lasting longer than 3 months or recurrent) is often treated symptomatically, but a careful evaluation for peptic ulcer disease should be done before the patient is committed to long-term therapy for peptic ulcer disease (105).

Drug-Induced Ulceration

Alcohol, aspirin, caffeine, glucocorticosteroids, reserpine, colchicine, NSAIDs, and tobacco smoke are often reported as being ulcerogenic. The amino acids and peptides in coffee stimulate gastric secretion (106). Coffee has a greater effect on stimulating gastric secretion and on lowering esophageal sphincter pressure than an equivalent amount of caffeine. Caffeine alone produces no change or only a slight decrease in LES pressure (107). Decaffeinated and instant coffee and whole coffee beans seem equipotent (108). Increased gastrin release caused by coffee or decaffeinated coffee cannot be explained by distension, osmolarity, or calcium or amino acid content (109). Aspirin and alcohol cause breaks in the mucosal barrier, resulting in acute gastritis. This gastritis represents an erosion of mucosal cells without the occurrence of a deep penetrating ulcer crater. Corticosteriods may prevent the manifestation of the symptoms of a peptic ulcer before perforation occurs. However, they do not cause peptic ulcer disease (110). Indomethacin and other NSAIDs cause inconsistent breaks (106). In evaluating drug-induced ulcers, it must be remembered that some diseases such as rheumatoid arthritis and systemic lupus erythematosus are associated with a higher incidence of ulcers even without drug therapy.

Drugs can cause acute gastroduodenal lesions as shown by increased microbleeding and cell-shedding rates and a decrease in mucosal potential difference. These lesions may result in erosions, submucosal bleeding, gastritis, and duodenitis. However, it is unknown whether these effects will occasionally develop into peptic ulceration with continued drug intake (111). Patients with peptic ulcers have been shown to heal despite the continued administration of NSAIDs (112–116). In addition, there may be mucosal adaptation to the injury induced by aspirin. One investigator reported that submucosal hemorrhages and/or local lesions secondary to aspirin were present within 24 hours of drug intake, maximal within 3 days, and less on day 7 than day 1 (114).

Drugs may also cause ulceration in the esophagus. Doxycycline and tetracycline have been reported to cause severe ulceration. They should be taken with large volumes of water to prevent lodging.

The data on drug-induced ulcerations are often inconclusive. Furthermore, the data are usually anecdotal, retrospective, and lacking in control groups. In those studies where there appears to be an association, the patient numbers are usually too small to determine incidence data. Misoprostol, a synthetic prostaglandin analogue, has recently been approved by the Food and Drug Administration (FDA) for prophylaxis of NSAID-induced gastritis (117).

Stress Ulcer

Stress ulcers occur frequently in critically ill patients and in patients undergoing physical stress. They may be considered as a subclassification of hemorrhagic gastritis. Stress ulcers are acute ulcerations that occur mainly in the stomach but may also be found in the duodenum and esophagus. They are usually multiple, shallow, small, superficial erosions but may be associated with wider ulcers if there is bleeding. The destruction and scarring seen in peptic ulcers are lacking in stress ulcers. The real incidence is unknown because many heal as rapidly as gastritis, but they may be the most common cause of upper GI bleeding (118). The cause is usually identifiable, and stress ulcers have been associated with central nervous system (CNS) lesions, trauma, burns (Curling's ulcer), sepsis, uremia, cerebrovascular accidents, surgery, and endrocrine tumors producing gastrin (119). The greater the number of risk factors, the greater the chance of developing a stress ulcer (120).

Painless GI bleeding is the major, and often only, clinical manifestation of stress ulceration. There is usually a delay between the development of lesions and overt hemorrhage. There may be signs of subtle blood loss, such as guaiac-positive stools, nasogastric aspirates, and decreasing hemoglobin and hematocrit levels before the patient develops the signs of hemorrhagic shock. Lesions begin in the body and fundus but can progress to the antrum and duodenum. The primary method of diagnosing stress ulcerations is gastroduodenoscopy (121).

The mechanism of stress ulcers seems to depend on an interaction among acid, changes in mucosal circulation, excretion of glycoproteins in the mucus, and mitotic rate of mucosal stomach lining. Mucosal ischemia seems to be the ultimate mediator of stress ulcers (122). Cold, starvation, increased acidity, bile reflux, adrenalectomy, and hemorrhage favor ulceration. Luminal acid and pepsin are believed to be required for the development of ulceration (123). Vagotomy, anticholinergics, antacids, elemental diets, vitamin A, prevention of bile reflux, epinephrine, norepinephrine, serotonin antagonists, and immediate replacement of blood loss are inhibiting factors (124). The major treatment is removing the precipitating event; long-term antacid therapy is rarely required.

Preventing the formation of a stress ulcer is preferable to treating a stress ulcer after it has formed and begun to bleed (125–128). It is more cost effective to prevent stress ulcers than it is to treat GI hemorrhage. Prophylaxis of stress ulceration can be achieved by neutralizing gastric acid with frequent administration of antacids (every 1 to 2 hours), by blocking the secretion of gastric acid with H_2 antagonists or omeprazole, or by providing a barrier to the GI tract with sucralfate.

Early studies indicated that antacids were more effective than H_2 antagonists in preventing stress ulcers (129). These studies allowed the antacids to be titrated until a gastric aspirate with a pH greater than 3.5 was reached, however, and compared that treatment with a fixed dose of H_2 antagonist. One investigator recognized that the fixed administration of cimetidine every 6 hours resulted in a significant period of time in which the drug was below the minimum inhibitory concentration because of its short duration of action (130). In studies where the H_2 antagonist could be titrated, the efficacy of the H_2 antagonist was equal to or better than antacids with fewer side effects (125). To achieve an acceptable intragastric pH, antacids often must be given every 1 to 2 hours (126). This dosage has a significant potential to alter GI transit time. In addition to the potential for diarrhea with magnesium or constipation with aluminum, hypophosphatemia, hypermagnesemia, or hyperaluminemia may occur.

The focus in stress ulcer prophylaxis has shifted to continuous infusion of H_2 antagonists or to bolus administration of potent agents such as famotidine (127). The key to prophylaxis of stress ulceration is sufficient elevation of the intragastric pH. The pH, as measured by an aspirate from the nasogastric tube, should be at least 4.0. Higher pH values may provide additional protection (123) and may be needed if GI hemorrhage develops. For patients being mechanically ventilated and who are prone to aspiration, the administration of sucralfate may be advantageous (128) because there is a reported increase in Gram-negative pneumonias in patients with higher gastric pHs. A pharmacist may make a slurry by grinding a tablet, adding water, and stirring the mixture. A suspension dosage form is currently undergoing clinical investigation.

It should be remembered that the long-term prognosis of a patient with stress ulcer depends more on treating the underlying diseases than on the prophylaxis of the stress ulcer. It may be possible to prevent the stress ulcer but for the patient not to survive because of the underlying pathology.

Chronic Upper GI Distress

Chronic Gastritis

Chronic gastritis refers to a variety of gastric lesions that persist over long periods of time. There is a variation in effect on gastric function. In chronic superficial gastritis, gastric secretion remains normal. In atrophic gastritis there is a variable loss of function, and in gastric atrophy there is a complete loss of gastric glands. The risk of a coexisting active gastroduodenal ulcer has been correlated with the presence and grade of gastritis in the antrum and body mucosa. The risk of coexisting duodenal ulcer and gastric ulcer increases with an increase in the grade of atrophic gastritis in the antrum but decreases with an increase in the grade of atrophic gastritis of the gastric body (131).

Indirect evidence tends to corroborate the suggestion that there is a strong correlation between chronic gastritis and smoking. However, it is still not known whether smoking itself is a definite cause of chronic gastritis. In addition, it has long been suspected that heredity plays a role in the pathogenesis of chronic gastritis, because pernicious anemia, a disease associated with atrophic gastritis, tends to run in families. *H. pylori* has been associated with chronic gastritis and may play a major role in the etiology of the disease.

There are no specific symptoms associated with chronic gastritis. There may be bleeding and symptoms that correspond with deficiencies in secretion (cyanocobalamin deficiency due to deficient intrinsic factor). Although diagnosis can be made by endoscopy in severe cases, it is best made by performing multiple biopsies.

Although it is suggested that repeated attacks of acute gastritis can lead to chronic gastritis, no firm data substantiate this. An association with bile salt reflux and atrophic gastritis has been made.

Management of chronic gastritis primarily involves treating pernicious anemia if it develops and monitoring for occult blood (99).

Peptic Ulcer Disease

Peptic ulcers are chronic but may have acute exacerbations. They are most often solitary and occur at any level of the GI tract exposed to the proteolytic action of acid and pepsin. They are truly peptic. If acid and pepsin are diverted from an established ulcer, the ulcer will heal and not recur (132). In decreasing order of incidence, they occur in the duodenum, stomach (gastric), esophagus, stoma of a gastroenterostomy, Meckel's diverticulum, and jejunum (2). However, the most significant sites of peptic ulcer disease are the duodenum and stomach. Peptic ulcers are caused by an increase in acid and pepsin, a decrease in the mucosal resistance, or a combination of the two (132). Chronic peptic ulcers differ from acute gastritis or stress ulcers by the presence of fibrosis in the ulcer wall. They tend to be deep, burrowing through the mucosa and submucosa to the muscularis (133). Although they are often considered together, duodenal and gastric ulcers have different symptoms and causes. However, both types may be induced by acid and pepsin stimulation (134).

Before World War I, gastric ulcers were more common, but today, duodenal ulcers predominate (135). The incidence of both types seems to have peaked and is on the decline (136). While hospitalizations for duodenal ulcers have declined, those for gastric ulcers have not (137). Men have a higher incidence of the disease than women, but the predominance is decreasing (138). The incidence of peptic ulcer differs in different parts of the world. There are also ethnic differences in the response to antiulcer therapy.

Although there is a decline in the overall incidence of peptic ulcer disease, there has been an increase in the percentage of patients over 60 years of age who have been hospitalized for both gastric and duodenal ulcer disease (139). The incidence of complications and death is highest in individuals born around the beginning of this century, which indicates that there may be a birth cohort at greatest risk of peptic ulcer disease mortality (140–143). Ulcers may recur even after surgical removal of the diseased tissue (144). Both types have a low mortality but may cause morbidity. The disease does not occur in primitive tribes or lower primates until they live in conditions of "civilization."

Peptic ulcer disease has serious health and economic consequences for society. It is a costly disease in terms of hospitalization, physician care, and medications as well as loss of productivity caused by absenteeism (145). Cost effectiveness is an important consideration in therapy.

Gastric Ulcer

Approximately 600,000 persons in the United States experience gastric ulceration each year (146). Approximately 3,000 deaths per year are attributed to gastric ulcers (137). Gastric ulcers occur most often as single lesions along the lesser curvature and adjacent posterior wall of the antrum up to within 4 to 5 cm of the pyloric sphincter (Figure 1). They may occur occasionally in the cardia, pyloric canal, and greater curvature of the body and fundus (133). Hyperacidity is a less frequent observation in gastric ulcers than in duodenal ulcers. Gastric ulcer patients may have low or normal acid secretion. However, there are areas of higher acidity in the stomach and duodenum, and most gastric ulcers occur in areas adjacent to acid-secreting mucosa where the local pH is more acidic (147). Primary gastric ulcers are characterized by low-acid secretion; gastric ulcers secondary to duodenal ulcers are characterized by hypersecretion (148). Acid seems more important in determining where, rather than when, a gastric ulcer will occur, so that lesser curvature ulcers are frequently associated with diminished acid production. Gastric ulcers associated with duodenal ulcers are frequently associated with normal acid production, and prepyloric gastric ulcers are often associated with increased acid production. Patients with pernicious anemia and achlorhydria rarely develop gastric ulcers (149).

Etiology Several theories have been proposed for the cause of gastric ulcer disease (132, 146, 148, 150–152). Among these theories are delayed gastric emptying and distention accompanied by increased gastric secretions (153). Although this hypothesis is based on experimental and clinical observations, there are reasons to question its accuracy because some patients with gastric ulcers have normal gastric emptying times and low acid secretion in the presence of high gastrin levels (150, 154).

Many gastric ulcer patients have chronic gastritis, which may damage the mucosa and make it more susceptible to peptic ulceration. However, gastritis may persist after the ulcer heals (151). Chronic gastritis may increase back diffusion of hydrogen ions that break down the gastric mucosal barrier; this process may continue even after resolution of the ulcer (40).

One theory holds that reflux of duodenal contents, especially bile acids, is caused by pyloric sphincter dysfunction (155). Smoking, which is associated with an increased incidence of gastric ulcer, induces duodeno-gastric reflux (156). Bed rest improves ulcer healing and decreases reflux (157). Hypergastrinemia occurs in gastric ulcer patients, and gastrin has been reported to inhibit the pyloric sphincter tone (158). Pyloric sphincter dysfunction has been shown in patients with gastric ulcer, whereas control subjects and duodenal ulcer patients have normal pyloric sphincter pressure (159, 160). A reflux of bile salts may cause gastritis in the distal portion of the stomach and a break in the mucosal barrier. The damaged mucosa next to the acid-secreting mucosa is more susceptible to ulceration. Bile salts occur more frequently and in higher concentrations in the stomachs of gastric ulcer patients than in normal persons or patients with duodenal ulcers (155). As plausible as this theory is, reflux has not been shown to precede either gastritis or gastric ulceration (161). Also, bile salt reflux occurs in normal people as well as patients with gastric ulceration.

Gastric ulcers may result from an abnormality in the gastric mucosa. Normally, a relatively impermeable barrier, called the gastric mucosal barrier, prevents the back diffusion of certain ions. If the barrier is impaired and allows the back diffusion of hydrogen ions, bleeding and ulceration could occur (152).

Other factors may be involved. A genetic factor is implied by the association of gastric ulcer in patients with blood group type O and nonsecretor status (162). Smoking is associated with both gastric and duodenal ulcers (163). The use of aspirin on 4 or more days per week for at least 3 months is associated with a higher incidence of gastric but not duodenal ulcer (121). Repeated episodes of NSAID-induced gastritis may result in a gastric peptic ulcer. Unknown environmental factors may cause ulcers, or the disease may be a heterogeneous group of disorders that requires the interrelation of several factors in a predisposed individual. Gastric ulcer disease is probably a multifactorial disease. Although acid and pepsin may not be the primary causative agents, they are still necessary for the occurrence of gastric ulcers (149).

Symptoms Although gastric mucosal erosion may be asymptomatic, the most common complaints are pain and GI bleeding. Gastric ulcer pain occurs within 30–60 minutes after eating and lasts 60–90 minutes. The pain may be described as aching, nagging, cramplike, or dull. Its relationship to food intake results from distention of inflamed areas and acid release. The patient may associate the pain with eating and may stop eating, with resultant weight loss. Rhythm or chronicity associated with the pain is rare, and the pain covers a wide area of the midepigastrium. Somatic pain radiating into the back indicates penetration, perforation, or obstruction. These three conditions constitute a medical emergency and referral is indicated. If there is GI bleeding, the vomitus or stool may contain blood (the stool is black and tarry). Nausea, bloating, anorexia, vomiting, and weight loss may also occur.

Diagnosis Five to ten percent of gastric ulcers are carcinomas of the stomach; therefore definitive diagnosis is needed for chronic or recurring symptoms. Bleeding, either acute or chronic, requires medical evaluation. Although a patient history is helpful, it is not as definitive for gastric ulcers as it is for duodenal ulcers. Physical examination rarely helps to locate the ulcer. Definitive gastric ulcer diagnosis is made by endoscopy with a biopsy. Less definitive, and less used, diagnostic techniques include x-ray with radiopaque contrast media, gastric analysis for acid and cytogenic cells, and testing for blood (occult or frank) in the feces.

Prognosis The mortality from nonmalignant gastric ulcers is low, but the morbidity is high. Spontaneous healing frequently occurs in gastric peptic ulcers; this must be considered in evaluating clinical trials. The most frequent complications are bleeding and perforation (146). Gastric ulcers are less responsive to medical management than duodenal ulcers and more often require surgery. Perforation and other serious complications are more frequent in elderly patients. Many elderly patients will experience perforation as the first symptom. Emergency surgery for perforation in persons over 70 years of age has about a 30% mortality rate.

A historical prospective cohort investigation indicated that surgery for benign gastric ulcer may lead to an increased risk of gastric cancer. The rate of gastric cancer was higher in patients receiving a Billroth II subtotal gastrectomy than in patients with gastric or duodenal ulcer who did not undergo surgery (164).

Five factors have been found to be associated with the healing rate of gastric ulcers: a history of gastric ulcers, symptoms that do not disappear within 1 week of beginning therapy, an ulcer larger than 200 mm, ulcers located in the angle, and a round or oval-shaped ulcer. The greater the number of these variables, the slower the healing of the gastric ulcer (165).

Duodenal Ulcer

In the United States, about 2.4 million people experience symptoms of duodenal ulcer each year. Of these, an estimated 200,000 are new cases (166). Approximately 3,000 deaths per year are attributed to duodenal ulcer disease (137). The incidence of hospitalizations secondary to duodenal ulcer appears to be decreasing in the young population, which may reflect earlier treatment with effective antiulcer agents and emphasis on outpatient, rather than inpatient, therapy. Effective prophylactic therapy has reduced the incidence of ulcer recurrence. The relative incidence in ulcer patients has not changed. The incidence is greatest in individuals born around the turn of this century (167). Duodenal ulcers are mucosal lesions in the anterior wall of the duodenum's proximal end just beyond the pyloric channel through which gastric contents enter the duodenum (Figure 1). Ulcers also may occur distal to the duodenal bulb or spread back into the pyloric channel or antrum. These ulcers may recur frequently or infrequently, hence the term "duodenal ulcer diathesis" (168). Duodenal ulcer is caused by excessive acid and pepsin (148). The role of mucosal resistance has been incompletely evaluated (150).

Etiology Several abnormalities may explain increased acid and pepsin delivery from the stomach to the duodenum (148, 150–152). There may be an increased capacity to secrete because of a large parietal cell mass, an increased response to agents that normally stimulate secretion, an increased vagal or hormonal drive to secrete, a defective inhibition to secretion, or an increased gastric emptying rate (169–173). Conflicting data exist for each of these theories, and there is question as to whether they should be evaluated using maximal secretory capacity or physiologic secretory rates (174). There seem to be less supporting data for an increased vagal or gastrin stimulus to secrete and an impaired feedback (174, 175).

Other factors may be interrelated. Familial or genetic influence is evidenced by the threefold increase in the incidence of duodenal ulcer in first-degree or primary relatives of patients with duodenal ulcer (176). In addition, there is a higher concordance in identical than fraternal twins, and a greater incidence in those with blood type O who are nonsecretors of blood group substances (150). Persons with elevated plasma pepsinogen I are eight times as likely to experience duodenal ulceration (177). Persons who smoke cigarettes are twice as likely to have duodenal ulceration (178). With regard to smoking, this difference may be caused by a nicotine-induced decrease in pancreatic bicarbonate secretion, allowing a lower duodenal pH (179). Emotional and psychologic factors are believed to contribute to the disease but have never been documented (138). Patients with other diseases such as arthritis, chronic pancreatitis, chronic pulmonary disease, hyperthyroidism, and cirrhosis also seem to have an increased incidence of duodenal ulcers (180).

Cigarette smoking, intake of aspirin and related drugs, dietary salt, and alcohol abuse may form the etiological link of the association of peptic ulcer disease with chronic lung disease, rheumatoid arthritis, hypertensive disease, and liver cirrhosis, respectively (167).

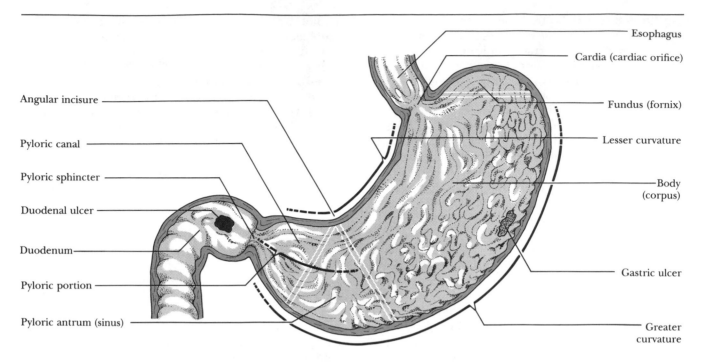

FIGURE 1   Sites of duodenal and gastric ulcers. Adapted from F. H. Netter, "The Ciba Collection of Medical Illustrations," Vol. 3, Part II, Ciba Pharmaceutical Company, New York, N.Y., 1962, pp. 49, 52.

The role of mucosal defense and repair remains poorly defined (181). It has been suggested that duodenal ulcer disease represents a mixture of disorders with different causes but a common pathologic expression that is hyperacidity (181–183).

Symptoms As in gastric ulcer, the primary symptoms of duodenal ulcer are pain and GI bleeding. However, key differences occur in the way the patient describes the symptoms (184, 185). Duodenal ulcer pain is rhythmical, periodic, and chronic. The rhythmical nature corresponds to the release of gastric acid. The pain usually begins 2 to 3 hours after meals and may continue until the next meal. It occurs when the stomach is empty and is relieved by eating. The sensation is described as gnawing, burning, pressing, aching, or resembling hunger pain. The patient is often awakened at night by the pain. It is usually located in an area in the midepigastrium between the xiphoid and the umbilicus and is so localized that the patient can indicate the locus of pain by pointing with one finger. Typically the pain does not radiate. The pain is prone to exacerbation and remission with or without therapy. Exacerbations are most common in the spring and fall and may last for days or months (168).

If there is bleeding, stool color and consistency may change. The stools become black and tarry because of the blood (melena). Other GI symptoms include retrosternal burning, alteration in bowel habits, and rarely, nausea and vomiting. The patient's appetite is good; frequently, weight gain results from the increased food intake to allay pain (180).

The major complications of duodenal ulcer are bleeding, perforation, and obstruction. Bleeding may cause anemia, iron deficiency, and hypotension. Iron deficiency anemia is characterized by weakness, fatigue, tachycardia, and dyspnea on exertion. Inflammation of the tongue (glossitis), brittleness and deformity of the nails (koilonychia), inflammation of the corners of the mouth, and stomatitis are rare complications. Perforation and obstruction are indications for acute surgical intervention and are manifested by acute changes in symptoms. Perforation is accompanied by a sudden, severe, generalized abdominal pain, prostration, abdominal rigidity, and pneumoperitoneum (air or gas in the abdominal cavity). Vomiting is the most common symptom of gastric outlet obstruction (168).

Diagnosis A good patient history is essential in recognizing duodenal ulcer. As in gastric ulcer, physical assessment helps localize the site of pain but does little to make the diagnosis. Definitive diagnosis is made by duodenoscopy. Endoscopy of either the stomach or the duodenum involves passing fiberscopes down the upper GI tract and is the most sensitive method of detecting ulcers (186, 187).

Factors Affecting Healing The risk factors that have been associated with the healing rate of duodenal ulcers have been assessed in two studies. In one study, pain radiating to the back, deep ulcers, multiple ulcers, number of cigarettes smoked per day, and male gender were associated with slower healing (163). In the other study, alcohol use, ulcer size, bleeding symptoms, a previous duodenal ulcer, and the previous use of salicylates were independently shown to delay ulcer healing (188). These risk factors suggest that the therapy for duodenal peptic ulcers should be individualized (189).

Duodenal peptic ulcers also tend to heal spontaneously. One-third to two-thirds of the patients will heal spontaneously on placebo in 4–6 weeks. Drug therapy must be compared with this. Pharmacologic intervention is used to facilitate healing and reduce the potential for complications.

PATIENT ASSESSMENT

The most valuable service that the pharmacist can provide in consulting with a patient is to help the patient decide whether the ailment is amenable to self-therapy or requires medical attention. In upper GI complaints, only acute gastritis without bleeding and gastroesophageal reflux should be treated without medical intervention. Careful patient interviewing is the only method for the pharmacist to evaluate the type, severity, and duration of patient complaint.

When recommending an antacid, the pharmacist should ascertain that the symptoms are acute in onset and can be related to overeating, dietary indiscretion, alcohol consumption, or tension. The pain of peptic ulcer disease and gastroesophageal reflux may mimic the pain of angina or a myocardial infarct. The pharmacist should elicit the relationship of the pain to exercise, the presence of pain radiating down the left axilla, or a crushing, viselike pain in the chest. Patients with these symptoms should be immediately referred to a physician. If the pain is acute but suggestive of perforation, the patient should also be referred. If the pain is chronic or resembles ulcer disease, the patient should have endoscopic evaluation (5) because symptoms of more serious diseases, such as hiatal hernia, ulcerating gastric carcinoma, duodenal neoplasm, pancreatitis, coronary artery disease, pancreatic carcinoma, and radiating pleuritic chest pain, may mimic ulcer pain (180, 186). Patients returning frequently with complaints of acute gastritis should receive a medical examination because repeated gastritis may be associated with gastric ulcer. Chronic gastroesophageal reflux should also be medically evaluated. If relief is not obtained

promptly and sustained, the pharmacist should refer the patient to a physician for evaluation.

The pharmacist should look for patient symptoms suggesting bleeding, vomiting, or obstruction that are life threatening and require immediate medical evaluation. Bleeding may be suspected in a patient complaining of black tarry stools or vomitus resembling coffee grounds. A blood loss of 50–100 ml at one time will result in black tarry stools; a blood loss of 500 ml at one time will result in systemic symptoms of anemia. Prolonged vomiting may lead to fluid and electrolyte abnormalities. If perforation or obstruction is suspected, the patient should be referred for surgical evaluation.

TREATMENT

Antacids are useful in the treatment of acute and chronic upper GI disorders. In addition, they may be useful in the prophylaxis of GI bleeding, stress ulcers, and aspiration pneumonitis. Ulcer disease is unique in that nonprescription medications are often used in its medical management. A patient may find that the physician alters only the dosage or dosing interval. In addition to the use of antacids, careful dietary habits; rest; removal from a stressful environment; cessation of smoking or alcohol ingestion; and the use of H_2-receptor antagonists, sucralfate, omeprazole, and/or anticholinergics may prevent the need for surgery.

Antacids

Antacids have been used in the treatment of GI distress for more than 2,000 years, but until the modern era of intensive antacid therapy, their use was mainly empirical and subjective (190). Only recently have the actions of antacids been evaluated closely and objectively.

Pharmacology

Antacids are compounds that raise the pH of gastric contents. Most are not classical alkalis in that they do not contain the OH radical (191). The primary action of antacids is to neutralize gastric acid, resulting in an increase in the pH in the stomach and duodenal bulb (192). They do not neutralize all of the stomach acid, nor do they bring the pH to 7.0. At a pH of 2.3, 90% of the acid has been neutralized, and at a pH of 3.3, 99%

has been neutralized (193). Because the optimal proteolytic range of pepsin is at a pH of 1.5–2.5, raising the pH inhibits the action of pepsin with resultant progressive proteolytic neutralization. Above the pH of 4.0, pepsin activity is completely inhibited (194). The main antipepsin effect of antacids is attributed to altered pH. A secondary effect may be the adsorption of pepsin by the antacid; however, this is controversial (195–197). Antacids containing aluminum are more likely to adsorb pepsin (191). The reduced concentration of pepsin in gastric aspirates of persons taking antacids containing aluminum hydroxide may be caused by a precipitation rather than an inactivation by adsorption (198).

In one study, aluminum hydroxide–magnesium hydroxide gel was shown to increase the volume of postprandial acid secretion primarily in the 2–4 hours immediately following meals. However, more than one-half of the acid secreted was neutralized, leading to a marked decrease in the net gastric acid. Neutralization was incomplete because of the formation of aluminum trichloride. Antacids did not modify the rate of postprandial gastric emptying, but increased the dilution of gastric contents expanding the intragastric volume (199). Antacids have a more pronounced effect on duodenal pH than on gastric pH and have a shorter duration of action in hypersecretors of acid than in normosecretors (200).

Antacids do not coat the mucosal lining (201). A possible protective effect is the tightening of the mucosal barrier (202). Antacids increase the LES tone; this action may be responsible for the effectiveness of antacids in esophageal reflux (heartburn) (203, 204). Raising intragastric pH leads to elevated serum gastrin levels and may explain the antacid effect on the gastric mucosa, LES, and increased volume of postprandial acid secretion. Although it has been postulated that the increase in serum gastrin is responsible for the increase in LES tone, this has been challenged and is controversial (205). The effect of antacids on gastrin release is not uniform (205). Calcium-containing antacids have the greatest effect. Many factors including alkalization, distention, vagal stimulation, and hypercalcemia are thought to be involved (206). Of the cations in antacids, only aluminum seems to delay gastric emptying time in animals (207). In humans, this effect is related to the concentration of aluminum in solution in the stomach (208). Aluminum hydroxide binds bile acids more strongly than magnesium hydroxide or aluminum phosphate (209). The affinity of aluminum hydroxide for bile salts and lysolecithin is comparable to that of cholestyramine. The strength of the binding depends on the bile salt and is independent of pH (210). The potential therapeutic benefit that may result from the binding of bile salts by antacids has not been studied, but it may be useful in gastric ulcers where a reflux of bile salts has been found. In the duodenum, calcium and magnesium cause pancreatic enzyme secretion and gallbladder emptying. This effect is believed to be mediated by an increase in the release of cholecystokinin (211).

Recently it has been suggested that antacids may have a cytoprotective effect. In rat studies, disruption of the gastric mucosa by sodium taurocholate was prevented by aluminum-containing antacids. This effect was lost if the rats were pretreated with indomethacin. The authors postulated that antacids might cause a local hyperosmolarity that would stimulate prostaglandin synthesis (212). Rat data have also shown that antacids increase the depth of the gastric mucus layer, which is considered the site of hydrochloric acid neutralization (213).

In humans, antacids may stimulate the gastroduodenal defense mechanisms (214–216). The administration of antacids results in increased prostaglandin synthesis, an increase in mucus, and an increase in local blood supply. A recent study showed an increase in mucosal prostaglandins after 3 weeks of low-dose antacid therapy, which suggested that the increase in prostaglandin synthesis was a result of an increase in prostaglandin cyclo-oxygenase. Even a single dose of antacid has been shown to cause morphologic changes and secretory stimulation in the gastric mucosa. Doses of antacid that are lower than those required to neutralize gastric acid have been shown to heal peptic ulcers. The mechanism for this healing may be a stimulation in the cytoprotective mechanisms. Additional work must be done in this area, but may lead to a reduction in the dose of antacids required for acid peptic disorders and an improvement in the side effect profile.

An ideal antacid has the following qualities:

- Efficient—Only small amounts of the drug should be required to neutralize large amounts of gastric acid.

- Effective—The drug should exert a prolonged effect without a secondary increase in gastric secretion and should not release carbon dioxide after reacting with hydrochloride.

- Safe—The drug should not interfere with electrolyte balance or blood glucose, or cause diarrhea or constipation when administered in therapeutic amounts. It should not interfere with absorption or excretion of nutrients or other drugs the patient may be taking.

- Inexpensive—Because treatment with antacids may be prolonged, they should be inexpensive.

- Palatable—Antacids must be taken frequently; therefore, compliance will be enhanced if their taste is appealing.

All antacid products contain at least one of the four primary neutralizing ingredients: sodium bicarbonate, calcium carbonate, aluminum salts, and magnesium salts.

Sodium Bicarbonate

Sodium bicarbonate is a potent, rapid-acting, effective antacid of short duration for relief of symptoms of occasional overeating or indigestion. It reacts with gastric acid to form sodium chloride, water, and carbon dioxide. This may be represented as $NaHCO_3 + HCl \rightarrow NaCl + H_2O + CO_2$ (217). The loss of carbon dioxide makes the reaction irreversible. Ingestion of sodium bicarbonate results in a base excess equivalent to the amount ingested because sodium chloride will not react with carbonate, phosphate, or hydroxide ions in the GI tract (218). It is contraindicated for chronic or prolonged therapy because large doses or prolonged therapy may lead to sodium overload or systemic alkalosis (193).

Each gram of sodium bicarbonate contains 12 mEq of sodium. This large quantity may cause problems for individuals on low-salt diets, patients receiving diuretic therapy, pregnant patients, or those with a tendency toward fluid overload. The suggested daily maximum intake is 200 mEq of sodium bicarbonate for patients under 60 years of age and 100 mEq for those 60 years of age and older (219).

Because the bicarbonate ion is readily absorbable, it can cause systemic alkalosis. Chronic administration of sodium bicarbonate with milk or calcium leads to an increase in calcium absorption and may precipitate the milk-alkali syndrome (220, 221), a possibility enhanced by a salt-losing nephropathy (222). The syndrome is characterized by hypercalcemia, renal insufficiency, and metabolic alkalosis (223). Symptoms include nausea, vomiting, headache, mental confusion, and anorexia (224). This may be particularly important in pregnancy where milk or calcium intake is emphasized (225). Symptomatic improvement and resolution of the alkalosis and hypercalcemia can be hastened by the intravenous administration of saline. This relieves volume contraction and increases calcium and bicarbonate excretion. Only rarely is hemodialysis necessary (226). The condition improves when the antacid and calcium are discontinued.

Gastric distention and flatulence leading to perforation may occur with effervescent sodium bicarbonate. A rebound gastric hypersecretion of acid has been postulated but has not been shown in humans, even with sodium bicarbonate doses of 4–8 g (227). Some commercial forms of sodium bicarbonate contain aspirin. Ingesting such products after heavy alcohol intake may lead to hematemesis and melena (228).

Calcium Carbonate

Calcium carbonate exerts rapid, prolonged, and potent neutralization of gastric acid. It reacts with gastric acid to form carbon dioxide, water, and calcium chloride. The reaction is $CaCO_3 + 2HCl \rightarrow CaCl_2 + H_2O + CO_2$ (217). However, the calcium chloride will react with carbonate or phosphate in the GI tract to form calcium carbonate or phosphate. Acid neutralization is reversible and systemic alkalosis is of a lesser magnitude than sodium bicarbonate (218). It may be used safely in small doses (0.5 g) for relief of occasional gastritis, but it is not recommended for chronic use. Constipation has been thought to be a limiting factor. A literature search indicated that calcium carbonate may not only be nonconstipating, but it may even occasionally act as a laxative. There is some evidence that the constipation seen in patients taking calcium carbonate for peptic ulcer disease may be caused by the ulcer rather than calcium (229). A recent survey of elderly antacid users revealed that males using calcium carbonate had diarrhea more frequently than control subjects (230). A recent study indicates that calcium carbonate increases fecal bulk and the fecal excretion of fatty acids and bile salts without altering GI transit time (215).

Although there has been much enthusiasm for calcium carbonate as the antacid of choice, the recognition of its systemic side effects has prompted a reevaluation of the agent. Calcium carbonate reacts with hydrochloric acid to form calcium chloride, which is highly soluble and available for absorption while in the stomach. The absorption is limited because about 90% of the calcium chloride is reconverted to insoluble calcium salts, mainly calcium carbonate, when it reaches the small intestine (231). However, enough calcium may be absorbed after several days of antacid ingestion to induce hypercalcemia, which in turn may induce neurologic symptoms, renal calculi, and decreased renal function. This uncommon side effect is most likely to occur in patients with impaired renal function (223, 232).

Although rare, the milk-alkali syndrome is more common with sodium bicarbonate, but it also occurs after calcium carbonate therapy. The risk of developing this syndrome is increased by prolonged administration of calcium carbonate or the concomitant administration of sodium bicarbonate and/or homogenized milk containing vitamin D. It is presumed that patients who absorb large amounts of calcium develop alkalosis because the net loss of hydrogen ions in the stomach is no longer balanced by the binding of bicarbonate ions in the upper small intestine by unabsorbed calcium. When marked hypercalcemia occurs, increased epigastric pain, nausea, vomiting, polyuria, alkalosis, and eventually azotemia may result. Patients with renal impairment or dehydration and electrolyte imbalance are predisposed to developing the milk-alkali syndrome.

Calcium carbonate may induce gastric hypersecretion, an action markedly enhanced by food (227, 233, 234). Gastric secretory volume and acidity were found to be greater after calcium carbonate ingestion than after aluminum hydroxide or food ingestion (235). In a study of 24 patients with chronic duodenal ulcer disease, 4–8 g of calcium carbonate induced gastric hypersecretion 3–5.5 hours after ingestion, whereas 30–60 ml of aluminum hydroxide or 4–8 g of sodium bicarbonate did not (227). This mechanism may be mediated by the calcium ion action in the GI tract.

To determine the effect of various antacids on gastric secretion, four equivalent neutralizing doses of calcium carbonate, sodium bicarbonate, and magnesium hydroxide were administered to 20 duodenal ulcer patients. The mean gastric output in the 60-minute period beginning 2 hours after the last dose of antacid and 30 minutes after the insertion of a nasogastric tube was twice as great with calcium carbonate as it was in the basal state or with the other antacids (236). Thus, calcium carbonate itself, rather than a nonspecific action of antacids, may be responsible for the effects.

Observance of increased gastric secretion after calcium infusion suggests that calcium may increase serum gastrin and that hypergastrinemia may be responsible for the hypersecretion (237). A dose as small as 0.5 g of calcium carbonate (the usual dose recommended as an antacid) may increase acid secretion in male subjects with or without duodenal ulcers (238). Although several theories have been presented to explain this acid rebound, it seems most likely that the mechanism is a local effect of calcium on the gastrin-producing cells (233).

A recent review noted that all antacids have the potential to induce hypergastrinemia and that there are methodological flaws in the studies assessing acid rebound (239). Hypergastrinemia may result from an increase in intragastric pH and is not necessarily a function of calcium or calcium carbonate. All drugs that increase the intragastric pH will cause an increase in serum gastrin. Hypergastrinemia occurs with H_2 antagonists and omeprazole. An increase in serum gastrin that tightens the LES has been postulated as a mechanism of action for antacids in gastroesophageal reflux. The infusion of an H_2 antagonist was found to block the increase in serum gastrin induced by aluminum–magnesium hydroxide. The acid rebound phenomenon is complex and elusive. Antacids may react with gastric acid in a manner similar to food; that is, they may cause an initial buffering of acid followed by an increase in acid secretion. The antacid remaining in the gut would neutralize the acid secreted, and antacids such as calcium carbonate and aluminum–magnesium hydroxide gel that remain in the gut longer than sodium bicarbonate would have a more prolonged effect. This potential hypergastrinemia suggests that antacids must be used properly to ensure adequate acid neutralization, especially if they are to be used chronically for the treatment of peptic ulcer disease. Thus, the clinical significance of antacid-induced acid rebound is questionable. There are no data that suggests calcium-containing antacids or other antacids delay ulcer healing by inducing acid rebound (240).

Aluminum

Aluminum is administered most often as the hydroxide, but also may be given as the carbonate, phosphate, or aminoacetate. Of these, aluminum hydroxide has the greatest neutralizing capacity but still less than magnesium hydroxide, calcium carbonate, or sodium bicarbonate. The reaction is $Al(OH)_3 + 3HCl \rightarrow AlCl_3 + 3H_2O$ (217). Products that contain large quantities of anhydrous aluminum oxide react too slowly to be useful as antacids. After aluminum antacids interact with gastric acid to form $AlCl_3$, a series of chlorohydroxides is formed. This, along with the formation of insoluble $AlPO_4$, reduces the anticipated neutralizing capacity to about 80% (218). Liquid preparations that lose their water content lose their neutralizing effect, and it cannot be regained by resuspending the dried powder in water (193). The drying procedure needed to convert the aluminum hydroxide gel into a powder or tablet alters the structure and results in a less reactive antacid (241).

The main side effect of aluminum antacids is constipation. Intestinal obstruction may occur in the elderly and in patients with decreased bowel motility, dehydration, or fluid restrictions (193). Impaction may be increased by agents such as sodium polystyrene sulfonate resin (Kayexalate) (242). The constipative effect may be avoided by combining aluminum with magnesium salts or by administering laxatives and stool softeners. A recent study indicated that aluminum does not alter GI transit time and may increase fecal fat and fecal bile acid excretion (215).

It was thought that aluminum was not absorbed and did not cause systemic toxicity. However, several studies reported elevated serum or bone levels of aluminum in patients receiving chronic aluminum hydroxide therapy (243–245). Systemic aluminum toxicity was postulated after elevated aluminum levels were found in brain gray matter of uremic patients who died of a neurologic syndrome of unknown cause (246). These patients had taken aluminum hydroxide as a phosphate binder for 3 years or longer. Aluminum is known to be toxic to the nervous system, and an encephalopathy was reported in an aluminum flake powder factory worker (247, 248). It was shown recently that aluminum is absorbed in small quantities and excreted readily in the urine (249). In patients with little or no renal function who chronically ingest aluminum salts, aluminum may accumulate and possibly be neurotoxic. Aluminum may also accumulate in the bone in patients with impaired renal function. The absorption of aluminum may be enhanced by citrate or orange juice and may be more significant in the elderly (250, 251). The measurement of urinary aluminum is a better gauge of changes in absorption (251). The time needed for aluminum toxicity to appear is usually longer than the treatment time of either acute gastritis or peptic ulcer.

Aluminum binds with and decreases dietary phosphate absorption in the gut. This effect is useful in patients with chronic renal failure who have hyperphosphatemia, but it can cause phosphate depletion in others. Dosages of 30 ml of aluminum hydroxide 3 times a day can have adverse effects on phosphate and calcium metabolism (252). Hypophosphatemia is manifested by anorexia, malaise, and muscle weakness (193). Phosphate depletion causes release of calcium from bone with resulting hypercalciuria leading to osteomalacia and osteoporosis (253). The hypophosphatemia induced by phosphate binders alters the metabolism of vitamin D, which may cause the osteomalacia (254). Serum phosphate levels may need to be monitored bimonthly during chronic therapy with aluminum-containing antacids (255). The syndrome may occur as early as the second week of therapy and is complicated by a low-phosphate diet, diarrhea, or restoration of renal function after a renal transplant, and is particularly likely to occur in the elderly (256–259). Alcoholics also have an increased risk (260). Effects may be reversed by aluminum phosphate or by increasing phosphate in the diet, so that 300 mg of phosphate is excreted in the urine daily (256, 261). In addition to the effects on phosphate, prolonged administration of aluminum antacids may also lead to calcium depletion (262).

Magnesium

The magnesium salts with antacid properties are the oxide, carbonate, hydroxide, and trisilicate. (Magnesium oxide is converted to hydroxide in water.) Of these, the hydroxide, carbonate, and oxide are the most potent.

Their potencies are somewhat greater than that of aluminum hydroxide but somewhat less than that of sodium bicarbonate and calcium carbonate.

Magnesium antacids react with gastric acid to form magnesium chloride and water (218). The reaction is $Mg(OH)_2 + 2HCl \rightarrow MgCl_2 + 2H_2O$ (217). Magnesium forms insoluble salts that are responsible for osmotic diarrhea, its major side effect. The diarrhea that occurs as a consequence of magnesium occurs without any changes in GI motility (263). This may cause systemic effects of fluid and electrolyte depletion (231). This side effect may lead to patient noncompliance; however, noncompliance may be minimized by using a combination of magnesium salts and aluminum salts. If this fails, alternating an aluminum–magnesium product with an

aluminum product may be of benefit.

After hydrochloric acid is neutralized by magnesium salts, magnesium chloride is formed. It is partly absorbed and is rapidly eliminated by the kidneys; but in the presence of renal disease, magnesium may accumulate, causing hypermagnesemia (231). Hypermagnesemia is manifested by hypotension, nausea, vomiting, depressed reflexes, muscle paralysis, respiratory depression, and coma (264, 265). Significant increases in magnesium levels may be seen 3–5 days after starting therapy (266). This condition may be complicated by the administration of other magnesium-containing products and may occur after renal transplant (267). Hypermagnesemia occurs primarily in patients with impaired renal function.

Magnesium is a strong CNS depressant, and toxicity may cause severe cardiac depression leading to coma and death.

Manifestations of magnesium cardiotoxicity do not usually occur until there is severe hypermagnesemia (10–15 mEq/l; normal magnesium levels are 1.8–2.4 mEq/l) in the presence of depressed renal function. However, junctional bradyarrhythmia occurred in a patient with chronic renal failure receiving 30 ml of a magnesium–aluminum combination antacid every 2 hours, although the patient's blood magnesium level never rose above 4.8 mEq/l (268).

An infrequent side effect of magnesium trisilicate is the formation of renal stones. When this antacid is taken daily for long periods (several years), silica renal stones may develop (269–271).

Caution should be used if more than 50 mEq of magnesium are given daily to a patient with renal disease (219). Magnesium should be avoided in patients with severe renal disease.

Magnesium–Aluminum Combinations

The total neutralizing capacity of magnesium and aluminum combinations appears to be roughly equivalent to the sum of the capacities of its constituents, although the pH value at which buffering occurs may be altered (272). A mixture of magnesium and aluminum hydroxide gels is a less potent acid buffer than an equal volume of magnesium hydroxide if a pH higher than 4.5 is desired. However, if a pH less than 3.5 is desired, it is a more potent buffer. One report indicated that a mixture of aluminum hydroxycarbonate gel and magnesium hydroxide failed to meet the sum of the acid neutralization of each antacid (273). It has been hypothesized that the aluminum hydroxycarbonate forms a coating on the magnesium hydroxide because of electrostatic attraction. The coating reduces the neutralizing capacity of the magnesium hydroxide (273). Because of the presence of both salts, magnesium–aluminum combinations have the potential for any of the adverse effects of either agent. They may cause hypermagnesemia in patients with chronic renal failure, hypophosphatemia, or aluminum retention.

A recent study comparing the duration of effect of an aluminum–magnesium hydroxide gel with an equal neutralizing dose of sodium bicarbonate indicated that the aluminum–magnesium hydroxide mixture had a longer duration of action. It was postulated that the water-insoluble aluminum–magnesium hydroxide mixture leaves the stomach more slowly (274).

The administration of aluminum and magnesium hydroxide does not induce an acid base disturbance. The same is true for cation exchange resins. However, when they are given together to patients with impaired renal function, a moderate to severe metabolic alkalosis may occur (275). The magnesium and aluminum ions are balanced to minimize any alteration in bowel function, but diarrhea or constipation may occur. The frequency of diarrhea may be as high as 76% and may be reduced if an anticholinergic is combined with the antacid (276).

A case of copper deficiency in a woman abusing an antacid combination that included aluminum and magnesium oxides has been reported (277).

Magaldrate is a chemical entity of aluminum and magnesium hydroxides, not a physical mixture, and has a lower neutralizing capacity than a physical mixture (278).

Additional Ingredients

Antacid preparations may contain ingredients that have no basic antacid properties but give the preparation an added basis for unique advertising claims.

Sugars   Some antacid preparations contain considerable amounts of sugars and hexitols. When taken in large quantities or for an extended period of time, these ingredients could result in various clinical problems, especially diabetes management. Ingestion of large amounts of sugars and hexitols could complicate the control of diabetes. With prolonged use, tooth decay may also be accelerated.

Simethicone   Simethicone, an inert silicon polymer, is a gastric defoaming agent. By reducing surface tension, it causes gas bubbles to be broken or coalesced into a form that can be eliminated more easily by belching or passing flatus. It has no activity as an antacid. In a randomized, double-blind, placebo-controlled trial, statistically significant improvement in symptoms treated with simethicone was measured by patients and physicians (279). The FDA considers simethicone safe and effective (219). It is rational to administer simethicone for acute symptoms that have components related to gas, but there is no indication for chronic use of simethicone in peptic ulcer disease. In addition, one report indicated that simethicone's defoaming activity was greatly reduced when combined with aluminum hydroxide. The observed low activity suggested that the defoaming agent had been adsorbed onto the antacid, rendering both substances less available (280). The combination of simethicone with aluminum-containing antacids is questionable.

Alginic Acid   Some antacid products contain alginic acid with sodium bicarbonate and other antacid ingredients. In the presence of saliva in the buccal cavity, alginic acid reacts with sodium bicarbonate to form a highly viscous solution of sodium alginate. A tablet containing alginic acid is chewed and followed by a glass of water to wash the sodium alginate into the stomach, where it floats on top of the gastric contents. If there is esophageal reflux, the esophageal mucosa comes into contact with the sodium alginate rather than the acidic gastric contents (281). It has been shown that alginic acid does not have any effect on LES pressure and that its entire effect is due to its foaming, floating, and viscous properties (282). Although one study showed no effect (95), other studies have shown a decreased exposure of the esophagus to acid (281–286). Contact was decreased by 39% in one study (281). Effectiveness of the preparation in esophageal reflux depends on the patient's remaining in a vertical position (283–285). The patient should be instructed to sleep on pillows or to elevate the head of the bed with 15-cm blocks. The FDA considers the drug safe (219). Products containing alginic acid should be restricted to treatment of esophageal reflux and hiatal hernia and should not be used for acute gastritis or peptic ulcer disease. There is insufficient bicarbonate, aluminum hydroxide, or magnesium trisilicate in the commercial preparations containing alginic acid to effectively buffer gastric acid. Alginic acid is regarded as useful in mild to moderate symptomatic disease but is probably not adequate for patients with severe disease (88).

Bismuth   Bismuth compounds have been used for gastric distress since the 1850s but have declined in popularity in recent years since they were shown to have little antacid activity (287). In addition, bismuth absorption from preparations such as the subgallate, subnitrate, or oxychloride has resulted in reversible encephalopathy, which has limited its use (288). There has been renewed interest in bismuth since the introduction in Europe of a new bismuth salt, tripotassium dicitratbismuthate, which is poorly soluble and insignificantly absorbed (289). This new stable colloidal complex acts by chelating protein and amino acids produced by necrotic ulcer tissue to form a protective layer at the site of the ulcer crater, thereby protecting the ulcer from acid-pepsin digestion (290). This is a different compound and mechanism of action from the bismuth salts available in the United States. The bismuth product available in the United States also contains salicylate. Salicylate can irritate the GI mucosa and is absorbed. The salicylate can cause its own side effects.

The effectiveness of colloidal bismuth in the treatment of both duodenal and gastric ulceration has been verified by a number of endoscopically controlled studies of 4–6 weeks' duration (291). Colloidal bismuth may help eradicate *H. pylori* (292, 293).

Colloidal bismuth is safe and is available in liquid form, but has the disadvantages of causing black stools, occasionally causing a black tongue, and having an unpleasant odor of ammonia.

Bismuth compounds available in the United States are being reviewed by the FDA advisory review panel on miscellaneous external analgesic drug products for various conditions such as overindulgence and intestinal distress. Although still under review by the FDA for treatment of intestinal distress and overindulgence, the bismuth compounds that are available in the United States are categorized as antacids and are not recognized as gastric mucosal protectants.

Evaluation

No commercially available product fulfills the criteria previously mentioned for an ideal antacid. Therefore, antacid evaluation must include the formulation, neutralizing capacity, sodium content, sugar content, intended use, palatability, and cost effectiveness.

Formulation

Antacids are available as chewing gums, tablets, lozenges, powders, and liquids. Insoluble antacids depend on particle size for acid neutralization. A smaller particle size increases the surface area; the greater surface area increases the wettability and ease of mixing with gastric contents. Therefore, an increased surface area means an increased antacid effect. Many solid dosage forms must be chewed before they will disintegrate and react with acid in the stomach. Chewable antacid tablets must be chewed thoroughly before swallowing for the patient to receive the greatest therapeutic benefit. Liquid suspensions of antacids are milled to a fine particle size and provide a greater surface area. Tablet antacids are not equal to liquid antacids on a milligram-for-milligram basis (231). Although in vitro effects of liquid and tablet antacids have been described as equal, one in vivo test showed that a chewable antacid tablet was inferior to a liquid suspension in neutralizing capacity (294, 295). Although equal neutralizing capacity can be obtained with tablets and liquids, the difference is in the extraordinarily large number of tablets needed to reach the desired neutralizing capacity (296). When

tablets and liquid antacids are given in equal neutralizing capacity doses, the tablet antacid has been found to have a longer duration of activity (297). This difference may be due to the desiccation process used in manufacturing. Tablets that do not disintegrate may lodge in the bowel and cause obstruction (298). Powders must be suspended in water before ingestion. Liquids (suspensions) generally are easier to ingest and have a greater neutralizing capacity. Tablets should be reserved for people who find liquids awkward or inconvenient and subsequently are noncompliant. However, it may be possible to achieve ulcer healing with antacid tablets. A 4-week trial achieved an 81% healing rate in duodenal ulcer patients treated with an aluminum hydroxide/magnesium carbonate antacid tablet (299). This rate was superior to placebo but not different from ranitidine.

Potency

Several in vitro comparisons showed that all antacids are not equally potent (267, 300–303). A 17-fold difference in acid-neutralizing capacity was found in commercial antacids following a standard test meal. This difference is even more pronounced with the new high-potency or concentrated antacids (296, 304). One test (the Fordtran test) correlated in vivo potency with in vitro potency; this has been used to compare the newer concentrated antacids (Table 1) and also tablet antacids (Table 2) (278, 296). The neutralizing capacities in independent tests are less than those capacities quoted by individual companies (305).

The FDA defines antacids in terms of minimal buffering capacity. To be called an antacid, the ingredient must contribute 25% of the total acid neutralization of the product. The product must neutralize at least 5 mEq of acid per recommended dose and must maintain a pH of 3.5 for 10 minutes in an in vitro test.

The potencies listed in Tables 1 and 2 are the most clinically useful guidelines to antacid neutralizing capacity. Antacids that contain calcium carbonate and concentrated antacids are the most potent. However, as previously discussed, calcium carbonate should be avoided for chronic intensive therapy. Aluminum–magnesium hydroxide gels generally offer adequate neutralizing capacity with the least toxicity potential. An initial attempt to correlate the FDA test to the Fordtran test used a limited number of antacids. The neutralizing capacity results for both tests were less than the values stated by the manufacturers. The modified FDA test closely approximated the data from the Fordtran test, but the modified FDA test was faster (306).

Neutralizing capacity will vary with the formulation of the antacid (307). The neutralizing capacity may also vary among manufacturers (308). In a recent study, one

TABLE 1 Various antacids listed in order of decreasing in vitro neutralizing capacity

Antacid[a]	Capacity (mEq/ml)	Equivalent volume[b] (ml)
Maalox TC[d]	4.2	19.0
Mylanta II[c]	4.14	19.3
Delcid[d]	4.1	19.5
Titralac[c]	3.87	20.7
Mylanta II[d]	3.6	22.2
Camalox[c]	3.59	22.3
Gelusil II[d]	3.0	26.7
Basaljel ES[d]	2.9	27.6
Aludrox[c]	2.81	28.5
Maalox[c]	2.58	31.0
Creamalin[c]	2.57	31.1
Di-Gel[c]	2.45	32.7
Mylanta[c]	2.38	33.6
Silain-Gel[c]	2.31	34.6
Maalox Plus[d]	2.3	34.8
Marblen[c]	2.28	35.1
WinGel[c]	2.25	35.6
Riopan[c]	2.21	36.2
Gelusil[d]	2.2	36.4
Amphojel[c]	1.93	41.5
Riopan Plus[d]	1.8	44.4
A.M.T.[c]	1.79	44.7
Kolantyl Gel[c]	1.69	47.3
Trisogel[c]	1.65	48.5
Robalate[c]	1.13	70.8
Phosphaljel[c]	0.42	190.5

[a]For antacid components, see product table.

[b]Based on a desired 80 mEq of neutralizing capacity. To determine the amount of antacid to use for a desired neutralizing capacity, divide the milliequivalents per milliliter capacity into the desired milliequivalents of antacid. For example, the neutralizing capacity of Maalox is 2.58 mEq/ml. To achieve 156 mEq of antacid activity, 60 ml of Maalox must be given; to achieve the same antacid potency using Trisogel, 94.5 ml must be given.

[c]A mEq of antacid is defined by the mEq of HCl that is required to keep antacid suspension at pH=3 for 2 hours in vitro (Fordtran).

[d]A mEq of antacid is defined by the mEq of HCl that is required to keep antacid suspension at pH=3 for 1 hour in vitro (Drake and Hollander).

Adapted from J. S. Fordtran et al., *N. Engl. J. Med.*, *288*, 923 (1973), and D. Drake and D. Hollander, *Ann. Intern. Med.*, *94*, 215 (1981).

TABLE 2 Various tablet antacids listed in order of decreasing in vitro neutralizing capacity

Antacid[a]	Acid neutralizing capacity	Dose equivalent in tablets[b]
Camalox	16.7	5
Basaljel	15.4	6
Mylanta II	11.0	8
Tums	10.5	8
Alka II	10.5	8
Riopan Plus	10.0	8
Titralac	9.5	9
Gelusil II	8.2	10
Rolaids	6.9	12
Maalox Plus	5.7	14
Digel	4.7	17
Amphojel	2.0	40

[a]For antacid components, see product table.

[b]Based on a desired 80 mEq of neutralizing capacity. For method of calculation, see Table 1.

Adapted from D. Drake and D. Hollander, *Ann. Intern. Med.*, *94*, 215 (1981).

Efficacy

Gastroesophageal Reflux   The treatment of gastroesophageal reflux includes bethanechol, metoclopramide, alginic acid, H_2 antagonists, and acid neutralization. Adjunctive measures such as ingestion of small meals, exclusion of individual food intolerances and cigarette smoking, a low-fat diet, weight reduction, and avoidance of tight-fitting garments can be undertaken to prevent gastroesophageal reflux. In addition, elevating the head of the bed increases the gravity factor or pressure gradient between the stomach and esophagus, thereby facilitating clearance of refluxed material and reducing the duration of reflux. Antacids have been the mainstay of self-treatment of gastroesophageal reflux. Antacids neutralize hydrogen ions present in gastric secretion, thereby reducing their concentration in the refluxed material (310). In addition to neutralizing gastric acid, antacids have been reported to increase LES pressure (5), although this observation has not been confirmed (311). Antacids appear to be a logical treatment; however, much of the data on their effectiveness in gastroesophageal reflux are empiric (88). Most proprietary antacid tablet use is in the symptomatic treatment of reflux esophagitis (312).

Subjectively, antacids appear to relieve symptoms associated with reflux esophagitis. However, recent placebo-controlled trials question the use of antacids in gastroesophageal reflux. One study reported no differ-

product did not meet the FDA guidelines to qualify as an antacid (309). This study employed a relatively easy assay technique to evaluate neutralizing capacity. Although the method described has not been correlated with in vivo neutralizing capacity, it could be used to evaluate antacids.

ence between 30-ml doses of aluminum–magnesium hydroxide and placebo in the relief of spontaneous heartburn (313). Another study treated 32 patients with chronic reflux esophagitis in a double-blind comparison of liquid antacid and placebo (314, 315). The drug treatment consisted of 15-ml (80-mEq) doses of magnesium–aluminum hydrochloride or placebo taken 1 and 3 hours after meals and at bedtime. Both groups showed improvement in the frequency and severity of heartburn, an increase in the timed Bernstein test, and an improvement in the degree of esophagitis. The natural history of the disease is to improve with either antacid or placebo. Thus antacids may provide symptomatic relief for patients who have mild symptoms or self-limiting disease (316).

In a recent double-blind, crossover study of patients with scleroderma and reflux esophagitis, cimetidine was found to be superior to antacids in relief of heartburn and endoscopic improvement in the esophageal mucosa (317). This syndrome represents a chronic condition and suggests that antacids may give acute relief but no long-term benefit. Ranitidine and famotidine have been shown to be effective in reducing reflux esophagitis (318). The recent approval of omeprazole, which is more effective than the H_2 antagonists, may supplement or even replace antacids or the H_2 antagonists in the treatment of gastroesophageal reflux. Sucralfate may also be useful.

Nonulcer Dyspepsia Antacids and H_2 antagonists are widely used for nonulcer dyspepsia. Subjectively they appear to relieve symptoms, but it is believed that patients with peptic ulcer disease have a higher response rate than those with nonulcer dyspepsia (318). Although one study reported that cimetidine was superior to antacids or placebo in relieving nausea and vomiting associated with nonulcer dyspepsia (319), most studies have failed to show that either antacids or H_2 antagonists are better than placebo in treating this condition (320, 321).

Acute Gastritis, Stress Ulceration, and Gastrointestinal Bleeding The treatment goal for acute gastritis and stress ulceration is the prevention of GI bleeding (118). Histamine H_2 antagonists, anticholinergics, vitamin A, steroids, gastric lavage, and acid neutralization have all been tried (121). The key to preventing stress ulceration is maintaining the gastric pH above 4.0. Sucralfate was also found to be as effective as antacids in preventing bleeding from stress ulcers (322).

Initially, antacids were thought to be more effective than H_2 antagonists in the prevention of stress ulcers (323). Early trials compared the efficacy of antacids with cimetidine and allowed the dose of antacids to be titrated to achieve an intragastric pH of 3.5 or greater. This required the administration of antacids every 1 to

2 hours. However, the dose of cimetidine was fixed at every 6 hours. Because cimetidine is the least potent of the currently available H_2 antagonists, it has a short duration of action. One investigator showed that if cimetidine were given every 6 hours, there was a significant period of time in which the patient did not maintain a concentration of cimetidine above the minimum inhibitory concentration (130). However, continuous infusion of cimetidine was shown to be effective in elevating the intragastric pH over 3.5 (324). When the dose of the H_2 antagonists is titrated to achieve an intragastric pH comparable to titrated antacids, the H_2 antagonists are equal to or better than antacids in preventing stress ulceration. The H_2 antagonists also have fewer side effects. The frequent administration required for the antacids often results in changes in GI motility and other side effects.

Although continuous infusion of cimetidine has been shown to be effective in preventing stress ulceration, it has also been associated with changes in mental status (325). More potent H_2 antagonists (e.g., ranitidine and famotidine) have also been effectively used in bolus doses or by continuous infusion to elevate the intragastric pH over 4.0. The use of a more potent H_2 antagonist may reduce the frequency of dosing, obviate the need for continuous infusion, and reduce costs (326, 327).

Sucralfate has also been shown to be effective in preventing stress-induced ulceration. It may be particularly effective in patients who are ventilated and are likely to aspirate (328).

If GI bleeding occurs, neither antacids nor H_2 antagonists are very effective in stopping the bleeding or preventing recurrence (329). In a study of 20 patients, sucralfate was found to be an alternative in healing bleeding peptic ulcers (330).

In an attempt to find a medical regimen that would induce sustained fasting achlorhydria, one study found that cimetidine (300 mg/6 h) raised the intragastric pH to 3.5, and antacids (30 ml/h) raised the intragastric pH to 4.6, and the combination increased the intragastric pH to 6.8. Constant intravenous (IV) infusions of cimetidine (50 mg/h) and oral antacids (0.5 ml/min) resulted in intragastric pH values of 4.3 and 5.2, respectively. When given in combination by continuous infusion, the resulting intragastric pH was 7.4 but was not sustained in all patients. Only when the dose of cimetidine infusion was doubled to 100 mg/h and concurrent antacid given by a constant infusion was sustained achlorhydria maintained in each patient (331).

Peptic Ulcer Disease Antacids have a long history of empiric use in the treatment of peptic ulcer disease. However, only in the past few years have antacids been tested for efficacy in peptic ulcer disease (332, 333). When given in adequate doses, antacids promote the healing of peptic ulcers. In one study, statistically significant improvement in healing and pain relief was reported in patients with gastric ulcers treated with calcium carbonate tablets (334). However, other studies (335–337) using small doses of liquid antacids failed to show significant improvement when compared with placebo in either healing or pain relief for gastric or duodenal ulcers. A formulation identical to Mylanta II, a liquid antacid, but containing less simethicone, was given in seven divided doses [1 and 3 hours after each meal and at bedtime (30 ml/dose, 1,008 mEq of neutralizing capacity/day)] for 28 days to patients with duodenal ulcers (338). Patients showed significant improvement in ulcer healing but no difference in symptomatic relief compared with a placebo group. An example of more recent studies shows that this intensive dosage schedule is as effective as an H_2 blocker in promoting healing (339).

There is agreement that intensive antacid therapy will promote healing of duodenal ulcer (338, 340–342). Ulcer healing has no reliable association with pain relief (343). One study showed that antacids were significantly superior to placebo in relieving pain associated with duodenal ulcer (344). Although the placebo effect is very important (345, 346), it is rational to give something for pain relief. Although it has been suggested that asymptomatic patients with an ulcer may not need treatment, ulcer complications may be prevented with therapy (343).

Although acid secretion may be diminished in gastric ulcers, antacids will reduce the diffusion of acid into vulnerable areas (342). Although the evidence supporting the efficacy of antacids in the treatment of gastric ulcer is less clear than for duodenal ulcer (340, 341), clinical experience supports the use of antacids for gastric ulcer (342). Low doses of antacids (e.g., 320 mEq of neutralizing capacity per day) were not different from placebo in promoting gastric ulcer healing. However, the antacid therapy was also not different from cimetidine, which was significantly different from placebo, in promoting healing (347). Intensive doses of antacids, given in addition to cimetidine for the treatment of gastric ulcers, did not improve the healing rate (348).

Antacids given in adequate doses are generally accepted as more effective than placebo in promoting the healing of gastric and duodenal peptic ulcers (349). The advent of H_2 antagonists and sucralfate has reduced antacid/placebo efficacy studies to comparative studies of antacids to the newer agents. These studies indicate that antacids are equally effective as H_2 antagonists and sucralfate in promoting the healing of peptic ulcers (350). Caution should be used in evaluating antacid efficacy data because studies showing efficacy as well as lack of efficacy tend to summarize all antacids in all forms when only one antacid in one form was studied.

There are no data suggesting that one antacid (e.g., magnesium hydroxide or calcium carbonate) is more efficacious than another. The choice of an antacid is often made on the basis of side effects. In evaluating all efficacy studies, the large placebo response rate and the tendency of ulcers to heal themselves should be remembered (351). The placebo response rate ranges from one-third to two-thirds of the patients treated. In using an antacid for the treatment of peptic ulcer, the frequent administration time and potential for side effects (e.g., altered bowel function) must be kept in mind.

Although antacids are no different from placebo in promoting pain relief in peptic ulcer disease, this does not contraindicate their use. It should be remembered that giving nothing definitely does not relieve pain. Although the pain relief may be a placebo response, patients often seek help because of the pain. Pain relief is one of the treatment goals in peptic ulcer disease.

Antacids may be given as needed for pain in peptic ulcer disease and may be used in this manner to supplement other therapy (e.g., H_2 antagonists or sucralfate). The dose of the antacid should be individualized, starting with 40–80 mEq of neutralizing capacity. The dose should be given as needed and the frequency of dosing recorded. The use of antacids for pain relief should diminish over the first 10–14 days.

Miscellaneous Gastrointestinal Complaints

Patients often seek antacids for a variety of miscellaneous GI complaints related to eating or excessive indulgence in alcohol or food. Although these are common complaints, they are not often the subject of controlled studies. The FDA advisory panel on OTC drugs recently reviewed digestive aid drug products and drug products for relief of symptoms associated with overindulgence in alcohol or food (352, 353). The FDA panel included antacids in a review of drugs for the relief of immediate postprandial upper abdominal distress (IPPUAD). The panel found the antacids to be safe at the doses stated earlier but that data proving efficacy were lacking (352).

In reviewing the agents useful in relieving abdominal complaints associated with a hangover, the panel endorsed the use of antacids. Although the panel noted that the cause is not hyperacidity but more likely acute gastritis, it believed that the antacids protect the mucosa from gastric acid. The panel also endorsed the combination of analgesics (e.g., aspirin or acetaminophen) with antacids (353). This is different from an earlier panel's recommendation.

Palatability

Patients frequently complain about the taste of antacids as a reason for noncompliance. They should be questioned about palatability as a guide to compliance.

Taste was recently cited as a reason why patients prefer one antacid over another of equal neutralizing capacity (354). The pharmacist should consider recommending to the physician that the patient be switched to another antacid if the patient develops a taste aversion to one particular product. Refrigerating the antacid may improve the flavor. However, care should be taken to avoid freezing suspensions. Freezing causes particles, particularly magnesium hydroxide, to become coarse and less reactive to acid (355). Mylanta II has been the most accepted antacid in taste tests, although there is much individual variation (356, 357). The newer high-potency antacids allow ingestion of a smaller volume of antacid while still achieving the same acid neutralization as the larger volume. Patient acceptance of long-term antacid therapy may be enhanced by administering a flavored antacid tablet (358). Long-term compliance with an antacid regimen is achievable (359).

Dosage Recommendations

Dosage recommendations depend on intended use (acute or chronic), antacid neutralizing capacity, dosage interval, and temporal relationship to meals. Antacids ingested in the fasting state reduce acidity for only approximately 30 minutes. This short duration of action is caused by rapid gastric emptying of the antacid. On the other hand, antacids ingested 1 hour after meals reduce gastric acidity for at least 3 hours (360). Also, the reactivity of antacids in aqueous solutions may be reduced if they are given with foods—especially protein-containing foods (361). The dose of liquid antacids is best expressed in terms of milliequivalents of neutralizing capacity. As has already been discussed, equal volumes are not equipotent.

Gastroesophageal Reflux The dosing for gastroesophageal reflux may be different from other disorders especially if the gastroesophageal reflux is chronic. In acute incidences of gastroesophageal reflux, 40–80 mEq of liquid antacid of 2–4 g of sodium bicarbonate or calcium carbonate are often effective. Acute incidences are usually self-limiting and will resolve spontaneously.

In chronic gastroesophageal reflux, more frequent treatment, ideally frequent daily dosing, is indicated. A noncalcium-containing antacid should be used because hypercalcemia may result from long-term high-dose usage, especially in patients with renal failure. It has been suggested that a dose be given immediately after each meal and be repeated in 2 hours and at bedtime (88). Because of patient intolerance, smaller, more frequent doses may be used (362). Although no studies have been done to document an effective dose, a dose of 80–160 mEq of antacid would seem appropriate. A lower dose may be used if adequate documentation is available to demonstrate that a patient is a hyposecretor of gastric acid, as may be found in many of these patients (363).

Prevention of Gastric Bleeding The treatment goal in the prophylaxis of GI bleeding is to keep the gastric pH above 3.5. Therapy may be started with 120 mEq of antacid and doubled every hour until the subsequent gastric aspirate has a pH greater than 3.5 (364).

Peptic Ulcer Disease Recommended regimens for antacids in peptic ulcer disease range from taking the antacid only when there is pain to taking as much antacid as can reasonably be tolerated (365). The latter protocol is favored for promotion of healing because objective data support it (338). Intensive antacid therapy for hospitalized patients who are not eating begins with 40 mEq per hour during waking hours for gastric ulcer patients and 80 mEq per hour for duodenal ulcer patients (231). These individuals should be closely monitored for side effects and adverse reactions.

Hourly dosing is neither practical nor necessary when the patient resumes eating. Food acts as a buffer to stomach acid for about 60 minutes, and then gastric acidity increases (366, 367). Antacids taken on an empty stomach have a duration of action of only 20–40 minutes (368). However, if they are taken 1 hour after meals, their duration of action is increased to up to 3 hours (278). For chronic therapy, antacids should be given 1 and 3 hours after meals and at bedtime.

The optimal dose of antacids in peptic ulcer disease has not been determined. It is unknown whether larger doses will promote higher healing rates than currently recommended doses. Also, it may be possible to give lower doses than those currently recommended and still promote healing. Recent studies (369–372) have used less than the usually recommended antacid regimen in duodenal ulcer therapy and found significant ulcer healing, while another study used lower doses in gastric ulcer and found that healing was not improved over placebo (373). In the absence of data, it is better to use 80 mEq of antacid for gastric ulcer and 160 mEq of antacid for duodenal ulcer given 1 and 3 hours after meals and at bedtime. Therapy should be continued for 6–8 weeks (374). The cytoprotective effect of antacids may result in use of lower doses of antacids (375). The data are encouraging but should be confirmed in larger studies. Antacids may be effectively used to relieve pain on an as-needed basis. They are best titrated to individual response by starting with a dose of 40–80 mEq administered as needed by the patient.

Special Concerns for the Elderly

The dosing of antiulcer drugs in the elderly offers a special challenge (376, 377). Elderly patients appear to have a higher risk of mortality from peptic ulcer disease, perhaps because of the existence of a birth-related cohort. The aging process also results in changes that affect the pharmacokinetics of drugs, especially the metabolism and elimination of drugs. There may be pharmacodynamic changes that increase the potential for side effects. The H_2 antagonist should be dosed carefully. If renal function is impaired, the dose of the H_2 antagonist should be reduced. The clearance of cimetidine has been shown to be reduced in the elderly. Age itself does not affect the clearance of the other H_2 antagonists, provided the renal function is normal. The elderly appear to be more likely to develop mental confusion and CNS side effects with the H_2 antagonists, particularly cimetidine, because of decreased clearance. The elderly are also more likely to develop side effects with antacids. Hypophosphatemia has been reported with aluminum–hydroxide antacids in the elderly. The elderly are already prone to changes in bowel motility, and antacids may exacerbate these changes, increasing diarrhea or constipation.

Prevention of Peptic Ulcer Disease Recurrence

Peptic ulcer disease heals in 4–6 weeks of active therapy in most patients (378). However, a dictum states that "once an ulcer, always an ulcer" because peptic ulcer disease is likely to recur. Duodenal ulcer disease recurs in 80–90% of the patients in the first 12 months if prophylactic therapy is not given. Recurrence is more likely in patients who smoke, have a previous history of ulcer disease, have significant nocturnal acid secretion, and are older. A lower but significant recurrence rate (35%) has been reported for gastric ulcers (379). The recurrence of peptic ulcer disease is independent of the type of therapy initially used to facilitate healing (380). The recurrence has been attributed to *H. pylori*. A biopsy at the time of diagnosis is not predictive of the ulcer's recurrence (381). Although some clinicians treat each acute exacerbation as an individual event, others provide prophylactic therapy, especially if the exacerbations are frequent or the patient is in a high-risk group (382). The risk of relapse is increased by age, male gender, hypersecretory states, smoking, positive family history, and disease complications.

Antacids have been shown to be more effective than placebo in preventing the recurrence of duodenal peptic ulcers, but they require frequent administration (383–387). Sucralfate is equally effective to H_2 antagonists (388, 389) but it must be given 2–4 times a day for effective prophylaxis. The H_2 antagonists are effective in preventing recurrence and are safe for long-term use. They also can be dosed once a day. It is recommended that the single daily dose be given at bedtime so that the drug's peak activity coincides with the peak in nocturnal acid secretion. The once-daily maintenance dose of the H_2 antagonists is half the usual dose given to

facilitate healing (i.e., 20 mg of famotidine, 150 mg of ranitidine, 150 mg of nizatidine, and 400 mg of cimetidine). Famotidine and ranitidine are equally effective and may be somewhat more effective than cimetidine (390–392). The duration of prophylactic therapy is not known. Relapse rates after the second year approximate the original relapse rate if the prophylactic therapy is stopped. However, in some patients the ulcer may "burn itself out," which suggests that the prophylactic therapy may be successfully withdrawn at some point.

Summary of the Use of Antacids in Acid Secretory Disorders

Antacids are effective in promoting the healing of peptic ulcers. However, in the currently recommended dosages, they must be given frequently and in large doses. Studies using moderate or small doses suggest that lower doses may be effective, but these studies need confirmation (393–395). Even in small doses, antacids require frequent administration for the promotion of healing of peptic ulcers. The advent of the H_2 antagonists, sucralfate, and omeprazole has reduced the role of antacids in peptic ulcer disease. These agents now represent the drugs of first choice. The role of antacids in peptic ulcer disease is now one of "as-needed" use for pain relief. Because the relief of pain and the rate of ulcer healing do not always coincide, it is acceptable to administer antacids as needed for pain relief. Antacids may also be used in patients who do not respond to or who cannot tolerate the first-line agents.

Antacids are available without a prescription and therefore will remain popular for short-term relief of gastroesophageal reflux. However, when the disease becomes chronic, the role of antacids is reduced. Because of their ease of use, lower incidence of GI side effects, and effectiveness, the H_2 antagonists and omeprazole are more useful chronically.

For prophylaxis of stress ulcers, antacids must be given frequently. This frequent administration of antacids may induce significant GI side effects. Again, the role of antacids is being reduced by the H_2 antagonists, sucralfate, and perhaps omeprazole.

Other Therapy for Acid Secretory Disorders

Diet

Withholding food during the acute phase of peptic ulcer disease will remove a main stimulus for acid secretion. However, some patients will continue to have pain, and fasting is obviously not a practical long-term treatment. For chronic treatment, bland diets or ulcer diets are ineffective in treating peptic ulcers (396). Conversely, there is no evidence that pepper or other spices are ulcerogenic (333). Milk increases gastric acid production and has no antacid properties. Therefore, diets that alternate milk and antacids have been or should be abandoned (397). Bland diets are monotonous and unpalatable, have a poor patient compliance, and are ineffective (398). Coffee (both caffeinated and decaffeinated), caffeine-containing beverages (such as cola), and alcohol are the only items that should be withheld from an ulcer patient. The patient should also be encouraged to stop smoking (396). Patients should be advised to have regular meals and to avoid foods known to cause symptoms. Duodenal ulcer patients on a high-fiber diet have been shown to have fewer recurrences than patients on a low-fiber diet (399). Patients on a low-carbohydrate diet reported that their symptoms were less than they were on a high-carbohydrate diet (400).

Anticholinergics

Anticholinergics are prescription ingredients that have been used to reduce acid secretion and to prolong the duration of action of antacids. If they are used, the dose of both the antacid and the anticholinergic should be individualized; side effects from the anticholinergic may occur if it is administered in fixed combination with antacids. The FDA considers fixed-dose combinations of antacids and anticholinergics unsafe (219). Anticholinergic agents should not be administered simultaneously with antacids because antacids reduce absorption of anticholinergics.

Of the controlled clinical trials that have studied the use of anticholinergics in peptic ulcer disease, most have shown no significant benefit (333), although most of these studies were done before endoscopy was available. Not all anticholinergics have been shown to reduce gastric acid (401). The benefit from these drugs seldom justifies the side effects they cause. Recent evidence suggests that the side effects have been caused by excessive dosage. Although it is customary to dose to the precipitation of side effects, some studies have reported no difference in food-stimulated acid secretion after a 15-mg dose of propantheline compared with the accepted "optimal-effective dose" of 15–90 mg (402). The smaller dose would prevent many of the side effects. This dose also augmented the effect of cimetidine to reduce gastric acid. A recent comparison of cimetidine (200 mg 3 times a day and 400 mg at bedtime), to propantheline (doses beginning at 15 mg 3 times a day and 30 mg at bedtime), showed no difference in healing rate but greater incidence of adverse reactions in the propantheline-treated group (403).The main indications for anticholinergics in peptic ulcer disease are as adjunctive therapy for duodenal ulcer patients who have persistent pain, especially nocturnal pain not responding to routine measures, for patients whose ulcers fail to heal after an adequate trial of standard therapy, and for those with a high incidence of recurrence (404). This technique has been shown to accelerate healing of duodenal ulcer (405). However, recent data with combined anticholinergic administration and a potent H_2 antagonist failed to suppress the secretion of nocturnal acid over the H_2 antagonist (famotidine) alone. The timing of the H_2 antagonist may be more important than the addition of the anticholinergic agent (406).

H_2 Antagonists

The discovery of histamine H_2 receptors and the development of H_2-receptor antagonists have done much to explain gastric physiology. The presence of an ultimate mediator has been postulated by the ability of H_2 antagonists to block the release of gastric acid from multiple stimuli (vagal stimulation, gastrin, or calcium).

Currently, four H_2 antagonists are available: cimetidine, ranitidine, famotidine, and nizatidine. They all have the same mechanism of action and block the release of gastric acid by being competitive, reversible blockers of the H_2 receptor (407, 408). Although they are competitive blockers of the H_2 receptors and result in an increase in gastrin, there is no rebound secretion of gastric acid. These drugs are all more effective than placebo in promoting the healing of duodenal and gastric ulcers (409). As with all ulcer therapies, there is a better response in duodenal ulcer than gastric ulcer and a large placebo response in both (410). None of the H_2 antagonists has been shown to be more effective than intensive antacid therapy or sucralfate in promoting ulcer healing. All are equally effective (411), and there are some treatment failures with each. They have all been shown to be effective in decreasing the recurrence of duodenal ulcer (412).

The H_2 antagonists have similar pharmacokinetic profiles in healthy normal volunteers (413, 414). They have good oral absorption and have peak concentrations around 90 minutes after administration. The half-life is approximately 2 hours. A significant amount of each drug is excreted unchanged in the urine (415–417). All H_2 antagonists have a decreased clearance in patients with impaired renal function (418). Cimetidine and ranitidine have decreased clearance in patients with impaired hepatic function. Famotidine's clearance does not appear to be affected by stable or progressive hepatic disease (419). The clearance of cimetidine is decreased in the elderly, but the clearance of famotidine is not affected by age in patients who have normal renal function for their age (420, 421).

There are significant differences in the potency of the H_2 antagonists (422). The difference in potency translates into a difference in the duration of effect of each H_2 antagonist. The greater the potency, the longer the drug concentration stays above the minimal concentration needed to suppress acid production. This may be particularly important in selecting a drug or dosing interval for stress ulcer prophylaxis. Cimetidine is the least potent, ranitidine and nizatidine are more potent than cimetidine and about equal to each other, and famotidine is the most potent of the H_2 antagonists. A recent meta analysis of studies concerning the effectiveness of the H_2 antagonists in promoting the healing of peptic ulcers showed that the increased potency of the H_2 antagonists was associated with a higher healing rate (423). There was a higher healing rate with the regimen of 40 mg of famotidine once daily followed by the regimen of 300 mg of ranitidine once daily at bedtime.

The potency and the appreciation of the significance of nocturnal acid secretion have changed the dosing interval of the H_2 antagonists. The H_2 antagonists are effective if administered once a day at bedtime (424). This allows the maximal effect during the early morning hours when the nocturnal acid secretion is greatest. A recent study suggests that the efficacy may be enhanced by giving the drug after dinner to allow the maximal effect of the H_2 antagonist during the peak of acid secretion (425, 426). The duration of effect of 40 mg of famotidine is approximately 18 hours and was initially dosed once a day. The other H_2 antagonists may also be given once a day, but the dose has to be increased to an equipotent dose. The once-a-day dose of cimetidine is 800 mg, and the once-a-day dose of ranitidine or nizatidine is 300 mg. The prophylactic dose of the H_2 antagonists should also be given in the evening to have its maximal effect of nocturnal acid secretion. The prophylactic dose is one-half of the dose given to facilitate healing.

These drugs are relatively safe for short-term administration in otherwise healthy patients (427, 428). However, cimetidine can lead to mental status changes if given in normal doses to patients with impaired hepatic and/or renal function. This effect may go unnoticed and untreated in geriatric patients. Cimetidine has an antiandrogen effect, especially when given in large doses (429). The antiandrogen effect of cimetidine is primarily of importance in patients with the Zollinger-Ellison syndrome who require large doses administered chronically. Ranitidine, nizatidine, and famotidine have a safer profile but have not had as much clinical experience. The safety of these drugs when given for prolonged periods of time is undetermined (430).

Cimetidine inhibits mixed function oxidative drug metabolism at normal doses. Therefore cimetidine may potentially interfere with drugs undergoing oxidative metabolism. Numerous drug interactions with cimetidine have been reported. They include theophylline, quinidine, phenytoin, beta-blockers, and others (431). The other H_2 antagonists have lesser or no effects on cytochrome P-450. Originally it was thought that H_2 antagonists altered hepatic blood flow and interfered with drugs undergoing first-pass metabolism. However, hepatic blood flow is not altered by any H_2 antagonist, and alterations in metabolism appear to be related to cimetidine's interference with mixed function oxidative enzymes (432). Cimetidine may compete for the tubular secretion of cationic drugs. Cimetidine interferes with procainamide and N-acetylprocainamide excretion by this mechanism (433). Ranitidine seems to have the same effect but to a lesser extent (434). No drug interactions with famotidine have been reported. All of the H_2 antagonists alter the intragastric pH and have the potential for altering the absorption of weak acids and weak bases (435).

Sucralfate

Sucralfate is a sulfated polysaccharide to which aluminum has been added. In the presence of acid, it becomes a highly condensed adhesive substance that can bind to ulcer craters as well as normal mucosa (436). By binding to proteinacious material, sucralfate forms a barrier at the ulcer site (436). It inhibits the diffusion of hydrogen ion, inhibits the action of pepsin, and neutralizes acid locally without affecting the intragastric pH. Sucralfate also binds to bile salts (436). Sucralfate has been reported to lower the density of *H. pylori* (437). The cytoprotective effect (438, 439) of sucralfate has recently been extensively discussed (440–442). Acutely, the gastroprotection effect of sucralfate is mediated by prostaglandins and sulfhydryl, protection and maintenance of blood flow, and preservation of the proliferative zone. In chronic ulcers, the healing induced by sucralfate is mediated by enhancement of the mucus and bicarbonate secretion, increased ability of the mucus to maintain a pH gradient, increased binding of epidermal growth factor, maintained blood supply, and enhanced epithelialization.

In the treatment of duodenal ulcers, sucralfate is more effective in promoting healing than placebo and is equally effective as H_2 antagonists and intensive antacid therapy. Healing rates for gastric ulcers are also similar to H_2 antagonists and antacids (436). Sucralfate also has been reported to be efficacious in esophageal reflux (443), nonerosive gastritis (444), NSAID-induced gastritis (445), and the prophylaxis of stress ulceration (446).

Only 3–5% of a dose of sucralfate is absorbed, and more than 90% is excreted unchanged. The drug may be found at the ulcer crater for up to 6 hours after administration. The frequent side effects are constipa tion (3–4%), xerostomia (1%), and skin eruptions (0.6%) (436). The administration of sucralfate may increase aluminum serum concentrations after as few as 2 days of therapy (447).

The usually recommended dose for sucralfate is 1 g 4 times a day taken on an empty stomach. However, a dose of 2 g twice a day has been shown to be effective in treating acute peptic ulcer disease (448–450) and in preventing the recurrence of peptic ulcer disease (451, 452). Drug interactions with sucralfate are not usually clinically significant. However, a recent case report suggests a significant interaction with ciprofloxacin, resulting from the chelation of the aluminum in sucralfate with the quinolone (453). This interaction is potentially very significant but requires confirmation with a carefully controlled study.

Omeprazole

Omeprazole represents a new class of drugs that act within the parietal cell to inhibit the proton pump (i.e., the $H^+ \cdot K^+$-ATPase pump) and block the secretion of acid regardless of the stimuli. In this way omeprazole blocks the final pathway to the secretion of gastric acid (454, 455).

Omeprazole is variably absorbed from the GI tract, and the rate, but not the extent of absorption, may be affected by food (456–461). Oral bioavailability is about 70% of an oral solution. Omeprazole degrades in an acidic medium; as it inhibits the secretion of gastric acid, it may promote its own absorption (456, 457). At least three metabolites have been identified (457). Most of the drug (99%) is metabolized before the inactive metabolites are excreted in the urine (458). The half-life of omeprazole is about 60 minutes after an IV dose and about 2 to 3 hours after an oral dose. The volume of distribution of omeprazole is comparable to the extracellular fluid volume. A small change in the volume of distribution of omeprazole has been reported in the elderly. The drug is 95% bound to plasma proteins. Omeprazole has been shown to produce a marked and long-lasting inhibition of acid secretion (460). A decrease in 24-hour intragastric pH has been reported after repeated daily dosing. With doses of omeprazole achieving near maximal suppression of acid secretion, the acid secretion returned to normal 4 days after discontinuing the drug (461).

Omeprazole is more effective than other therapies for treating gastroesophageal reflux, is more effective than cimetidine and ranitidine in treating duodenal peptic ulcers, is at least as effective as H_2 antagonists in treating gastric ulcers, and is the drug of choice in hypersecretory patients with Zollinger–Ellison syndrome (462–468).

Omeprazole appears to be well tolerated (469, 470). The most frequently reported side effects are nausea and diarrhea. Increases in liver function tests have been reported. Concern has been raised over the potential for omeprazole to induce carcinoid tumors and bacterial overgrowth. This potential exists with any drug that raises the intragastric pH and causes the release of gastrin (471, 472). Omeprazole will increase serum gastrin levels but not to levels that are clinically associated with the enterochromaffin-like cell proliferation of the carcinoid syndrome (473). It is unlikely that these side effects will occur with short-term use. Omeprazole will bind to cytochrome P-450, and there is the potential for omeprazole to inhibit drugs with phase I metabolism (474, 475). Omeprazole is not approved for chronic therapy.

The dose of omeprazole for peptic ulcers is 20–40 mg once daily in the morning. Patients with reflux esophagitis should receive 20 mg once daily for 4–8 weeks. Patients with Zollinger–Ellison syndrome have taken up to 360 mg per day in divided doses (476), but most patients can be successfully managed with 120 mg per day or less.

Misoprostol

Misoprostol is a synthetic prostaglandin E_1 analogue (476). Misoprostol produces a dose-related inhibition of gastric acid and pepsin secretion by a direct action on the parietal cell to reduce the formation of cyclic AMP. Misoprostol also has a separate and direct effect to enhance mucosal resistance (477). The enhancement in mucosal resistance may result from the stimulation of mucus and bicarbonate secretion, maintenance or enhancement of gastric mucosal blood flow, prevention of disruptions of the gastric mucosal barrier at tight junctions, stimulation of surface-active phospholipids, maintenance of gastric mucosal sulfhydryl compounds, and improvement in mucosal regenerative capacity (478).

Misoprostol is rapidly absorbed; a peak concentration is reached in 30 minutes (479, 480). It is rapidly metabolized to an active metabolite. This metabolite is further metabolized, and less than 1% of the drug or primary metabolite is excreted unchanged in the urine. The protein binding is approximately 85–90%. The volume of distribution of misoprostol may change in the elderly, resulting in a slightly higher area under the concentration curve. No dosage reduction is suggested for the elderly or for patients with renal impairment (481, 482).

The most frequent side effects reported with misoprostol are GI complaints (483, 484). Dose-dependent diarrhea has occurred in up to 40% of patients. The diarrhea occurs soon after starting therapy with a mean onset of 13 days. It is self-limiting and may not require the discontinuation of therapy. The diarrhea may be minimized by giving the drug after meals.

Crampy abdominal pain has also been reported in up to 20% of patients. The drug has the potential to be an abortifacient and is contraindicated in pregnant patients. Other subjective complaints have been noticed in less than 1% of the patients.

Misoprostol has been approved for the prophylaxis of NSAID-induced gastritis (117). In short-term trials, misoprostol has been more effective than cimetidine or sucralfate for preventing NSAID-induced gastritis. Misoprostol does not appear to have an advantage over, and may be less effective than, H_2 antagonists and omeprazole in the treatment of peptic ulcer disease.

The dose of misoprostol for the prevention of NSAID-induced gastritis is 200 mcg orally 4 times a day with meals and at bedtime (159). It is suggested that the misoprostol be taken for the duration of the NSAID dosage. The dose in peptic ulcer disease is 200 mcg 4 times a day or 400 mcg twice a day (485).

Combination Therapy

The benefit of combination therapy has been suggested (402, 486). One study demonstrated that intensive antacids plus one-half the dose of trimipramine or cimetidine gave comparable healing rates to full doses of trimipramine or cimetidine alone (487). The ideal combination therapy has not yet been elucidated from clinical trials. In one group of patients with inactive duodenal ulcers, the most convenient regimen was cimetidine, an anticholinergic, and antacids at the end of each meal (488). The most effective regimen was cimetidine with antacids 1 and 3 hours after meals. None of the combination regimens was more effective than cimetidine for decreasing nocturnal acid. The combination of sucralfate and cimetidine as initial therapy did not result in higher or faster healing rates than either drug alone.

Miscellaneous

Drugs under investigation for the treatment of acid secretory disorders include pirenzepine, carbenoxolone sodium, tripotassium dicitrate bismuthate, anisotropine methylbromide, anitidine, tiotidine, amylopectin, benzimidazole, prostaglandin E_2, trimipramine, sulpiride, pepstatin, zinc, and octreolide (489–500).

Drug Interactions Due to Antacids

General Mechanisms

The GI tract may be the site of clinically important drug interactions. Antacids may interfere with other drugs by forming insoluble complexes or altering GI absorption or renal elimination. Raising the gastric pH with antacids may alter disintegration, dissolution, solubility, ionization, and gastric emptying time of other drugs and as a result may either increase or decrease absorption (498, 501). Enteric coating dissolves more readily in an alkaline medium, exposing acid labile drugs to digestion and exposing the upper GI tract to irritating drugs. Weakly acidic drugs have decreased absorption because ionization is increased. Conversely, weakly basic drugs are absorbed at a faster rate.

Weakly acidic drugs include isoniazid, pentobarbital, nalidixic acid, nitrofurantoin, penicillin, sulfonamides, and salicylates. Weakly basic drugs include pseudoephedrine. Antacids may bind or adsorb other drugs in their surfaces. Magnesium trisilicate and magnesium hydroxide have the greatest adsorption potential, calcium carbonate and aluminum hydroxide have an intermediate potential, and kaolin and bismuth have the least potential (502).

Antacid-induced changes in the urinary pH may alter drug elimination (503). Readily absorbed antacids such as sodium bicarbonate have the most pronounced effect. Studies in which various doses of commercial antacids were administered 4 times a day found that aluminum hydroxide and dihydroxyaluminum aminoacetate had no effect on urinary pH. Magnesium hydroxide and calcium carbonate suspensions raised urinary pH by 0.4 and 0.5 units, respectively, and magnesium–aluminum hydroxide gel raised urinary pH by 0.9 units (504). A follow-up study revealed that both 15 and 30 ml of magnesium–aluminum hydroxide gel significantly increased the urinary pH. However, the increase resulting from 30 ml was not significantly different from the increase resulting from 15 ml. The effect on the urine persisted for 1 day after the antacid was stopped (505). The effect of antacids does not change the circadian sine-wave nature of urinary pH but does shift it in a more alkaline direction (506). The effect is enough to enhance the excretion of acidic drugs and inhibit the excretion of basic drugs (503).

Drug Interactions with Antacids

The significance of antacid drug interactions is often difficult to evaluate. There are many types of antacids and often a study is done using only one of them (e.g., aluminum–magnesium hydroxide gel). However, if a significant interaction is found, the article may indict all antacids when this may or may not be true. Further, the doses used may not represent the range of antacid doses used clinically. For example, the study may document a drug interaction using the intensive dosing schedule intended for peptic ulcer disease and not evaluate smaller, less frequent doses used for discomfort associated with food overindulgence. Conversely, the lack of an interaction using single low doses does not rule out an interaction using intensive doses. Drug interaction studies not achieving statistical significance also rarely discuss the power of the test (i.e., the probability of an interaction exists, but the sample was of insufficient size to detect it). Interaction studies rarely study the effect of staggered dosing (separating the drug and the antacid by 2 or more hours). Many of the interaction studies show an altered area under the concentration time curve (AUC) for drugs with no documented therapeutic range. Although there is a statistically significant interaction, the clinical significance is unknown. For drugs with no known therapeutic range, drug concentrations may change with no change in the therapeutic response. Finally, most of the studies evaluate a single dose of the drug; while the effect on chronic dosing of the drug may be postulated, it is unknown.

The type of interaction reported is also important. Many interactions with antacids result in a decreased rate of drug absorption, but the extent of drug absorption is unchanged. This would be more important for single doses (e.g., analgesics) or for drugs that must reach a critical peak (e.g., antibiotics). For most drugs administered chronically, the extent rather than the rate is more important (500).

The presence of a drug interaction does not mean that the two drugs cannot be used together. An interaction means that the benefit of each drug and possible alternatives must be carefully considered. Then, if the two interacting drugs are given together, there should be careful patient monitoring with consideration given to dosage adjustment. When in doubt, the administration of the antacid and the questionable drug should be separated by 1 or 2 hours.

Significant Interactions Tetracyclines exert their therapeutic effect by a bacteriostatic mechanism of action. Therefore, it is important that serum levels not fall below the minimum inhibitory concentrations. Because antacids inhibit the absorption of tetracyclines by chelation with polyvalent cations (aluminum, calcium, and magnesium), clinical response to the antibiotic would be expected to vary depending on the extent of chelation (507). Antacids incapable of causing chelates (sodium bicarbonate) may also decrease the extent of absorption of tetracycline capsules by increasing gastric pH and thereby decreasing the dissolution rate (508). The effect is not based totally on raising the gastric pH, however (509). A 90% reduction in tetracycline absorption was demonstrated in one group of patients when given concomitantly with magnesium–aluminum hydroxide gel, but there was no decrease in the rate or extent of absorption when tetracycline was given with cimetidine. Pharmacists should advise patients on appropriate spacing of doses of tetracycline when taken

with antacids, calcium-containing foods such as milk, or iron supplements (510). If antacids are indicated, they should be administered at least 3 hours after tetracycline administration. Likewise, iron salts should not be given with antacids because antacids decrease iron absorption (511).

The quinoline antibiotics (e.g., ciprofloxacin and norfloxacin) seem prone to forming chelates with antacids (512, 513). The administration of 1–3 g of aluminum hydroxide 1 hour prior to the morning dose of ciprofloxacin, again at lunch, and 2 hours after the evening dose of ciprofloxacin decreased the ciprofloxacin peak concentration in the serum and in the dialysate of uremic patients on continuous ambulatory peritoneal dialysis (514). It is recommended that the antacids be separated from the quinoline dose by at least 2 hours (515).

Digoxin and digitoxin are adsorbed to antacids in vitro (516) and in vivo (517). Because variable bioavailability of cardiac glycerides is recognized as a factor in possible therapeutic failures with these drugs, pharmacists should advise patients on the proper spacing of doses when these drugs must be taken concurrently.

The administration of a magnesium trisilicate–aluminum hydroxide antacid caused a decrease in plasma chlorpromazine levels after oral administration (518). Decreased absorption may also occur when chlorpromazine is given with magnesium-aluminum hydroxide gel (519). Antacids and chlorpromazine should not be given concurrently. Dosing at alternate times may reduce the probability of this interaction.

Antacids do not alter quinidine absorption (520); however, because quinidine excretion varies inversely with urinary pH, a potentially dangerous interaction could result through alteration of urinary pH by antacids (521). In fact, a single case report documenting quinidine toxicity due to an alteration in urinary pH has appeared in the literature (521). Concurrent use of these drugs should be avoided or monitored closely.

In vitro, indomethacin is adsorbed by magnesium trisilicate, magnesium oxide, aluminum hydroxide, bismuth oxycarbonate, calcium carbonate, and kaolin (522). In vivo, the peak concentration is delayed, and the bioavailability is reduced (523, 524). Although antacids frequently are suggested for patients taking indomethacin, concurrent dosing should be avoided. Again, alternating doses may decrease the probability of this interaction.

Buffering agents added to aspirin tablets result in a faster rate of dissolution, which results in earlier and higher peaks. However, the extent of absorption between buffered and unbuffered tablets is the same (525). The absorption rate may increase if aspirin is given in an enteric-coated form along with an antacid (526–528). Although the separate ingestion of antacids and aspirin has not been extensively studied, renal elimination of aspirin may be increased by 30–70% by an antacid-induced increase in urinary pH (528). In a small study of five uremic patients, the administration of either aluminum–magnesium hydroxide or calcium carbonate 2 hours before a dose of aspirin resulted in a decrease in the C_{max} and resulted in delayed but incomplete inhibition of thromboxane B. There was no effect on C_{max} or the inhibition of thromboxane B if the antacids and aspirin were administered simultaneously (529). If aspirin and aluminum–magnesium hydroxide gel are given together and sustained levels of aspirin/salicylate are important, as in rheumatoid arthritis and systemic lupus erythematosus, it is advisable to monitor serum levels and observe symptoms.

Levodopa absorption is increased as much as three times when antacids are taken concurrently (530). Alkalinization accelerates gastric emptying and delivers more levodopa to the small intestine, where it is more rapidly absorbed (531). There may be individual variation in response (532). The addition of antacids to a well-controlled parkinsonism patient's regimen may result in toxicity. Relapse may occur if the patient is well controlled on levodopa and antacid and the antacid is removed.

One in vivo study confirmed an in vitro interaction between magnesium trisilicate and dexamethasone. Measurement of urinary excretion of 11-hydroxycorticosteroids revealed a significant decrease in the effect of dexamethasone on 11-hydroxycorticosteroids when the steroid was given with the antacid (533). However, in seven healthy subjects, a magnesium–aluminum hydroxide antacid, when given as either tablets or liquid, had no effect on cortisone absorption (534). Conflicting reports exist on the effect of antacids on prednisone bioavailability. One study reported a decrease in the oral bioavailability of prednisone when given with aluminum hydroxide or aluminum–magnesium hydroxide, although this finding has not been confirmed (535, 536). Therefore, further studies of corticosteroid–antacid interactions are needed.

The in vitro adsorption of nitrofurantoin to magnesium trisilicate has been confirmed in vivo. Both the rate and extent of absorption were decreased. In addition, the time during which the drug concentration in the urine was above the minumum effective concentration was also significantly reduced (537).

An antacid mixture consisting of aluminum hydroxide, magnesium carbonate, magnesium hydroxide, and sorbitol decreased the bioavailability of captopril by 45% in 10 healthy volunteers. Although the AUC was decreased significantly, there was no change in the diastolic blood pressure or heart rate (538). In the same study, food reduced the captopril bioavailability by more than 50%. This decrease was reflected by decreased effects on blood pressure and heart rate (538).

Antacids have been reported to reduce the bioavailability of H$_2$ antagonists. Concomitant administration of aluminum hydroxide and cimetidine reduced peak concentrations and AUC of cimetidine (539). When the antacids were separated by 1 hour before or after the administration of cimetidine, there was no effect on cimetidine's absorption (540). An antacid containing aluminum and magnesium hydroxide has been reported to decrease the AUC of ranitidine (541–543). Aluminum phosphate decreased the peak ranitidine concentration by 40% and the AUC by 30% (544). The administration of 10 ml of a concentrated aluminum–magnesium hydroxide antacid resulted in a small but significant reduction in the C_{max} and AUC of famotidine (545). The effect could be avoided if the dosing of the antacid and famotidine was separated by 2 hours (546). It would be wise to separate the administration of antacids and H$_2$ antagonists by at least 1 hour.

The administration of antacids and sucralfate should be separated by at least 30 minutes. Sucralfate needs an acidic medium to form the viscous slurry that binds to gastric and duodenal mucosa. Antacids raise gastric pH and may prevent the dissociation of sucralfate (436). Ketoconazole requires an acidic pH for absorption. H$_2$ antagonists and antacids increase gastric pH and reduce the bioavailability of ketoconazole (547).

Potentially Significant Interactions   Isoniazid absorption is more inhibited by aluminum hydroxide than by magaldrate. The mechanism is probably due to decreased gastric emptying rate and caused primarily by aluminum. It has been reported, however, that isoniazid is adsorbed in vitro by magnesium oxide (548). Although the clinical significance is not known, isoniazid probably should be given 1 hour before the antacid (549).

A potentially significant interaction between antacids and anticoagulants can be avoided by selecting the proper anticoagulant. The absorption of a single oral dose of dicumarol was increased by 50% by 15 ml of magnesium hydroxide and 30 ml of aluminum hydroxide (550). The absorption or the effect of warfarin is not altered by antacids (551, 552). Therefore, only patients taking dicumarol should be cautioned about antacids. Patients who require both anticoagulants and antacids should be given warfarin (552).

Different antacids affect naproxen differently. Sodium bicarbonate administered with naproxen resulted in earlier and higher peak concentrations of naproxen, while magnesium oxide and aluminum hydroxide delayed absorption and decreased peak plasma concentrations. Aluminum–magnesium hydroxide gel tended to decrease the time required to reach peak plasma concentrations and slightly increased the total area under the curve (553). The clinical significance of this effect is unknown. The doses of antacids and naproxen should be separated.

Urinary excretion of amphetamine is decreased with sodium bicarbonate (554). Because of the potential for retention and subsequent intoxication caused by urinary pH alteration with all antacids, antacids and amphetamines should not be given concurrently.

Benzodiazepines react differently with antacids. When chlordiazepoxide was administered with magnesium–aluminum hydroxide gel, the absorption rate of chlordiazepoxide was slowed, but the total amount absorbed and the apparent rate of elimination remained unchanged (555). Thus, the interaction would be significant only for acute anxiety states where single doses of chlordiazepoxide are used. It would not be significant for chronic therapy. The absorption of diazepam has been reported to be increased by administration with aluminum hydroxide (556). Administration of diazepam with either aluminum–magnesium hydroxide gel or aluminum hydroxide trisilicate decreased the rate of absorption but not the extent of absorption (557).

The simultaneous administration of an unspecified antacid and phenytoin resulted in low nontherapeutic phenytoin levels in three patients. When the same dose of phenytoin was given 2 to 3 hours before the antacid, plasma levels increased two- to threefold from the levels occurring with simultaneous administration (558). Additional studies using specified doses of specific antacids have provided conflicting results. Studies showing no effect of antacids used small doses (559, 560), while studies using larger doses of antacids showed decreased bioavailability of phenytoin (561, 562). A large intersubject variability has been shown (563). The effect may be related to the dose of the antacid.

The absorption rate of pseudoephedrine was increased in the first 4 hours in six volunteers. The antacid increased the portion of the drug that was in the nonionized, more soluble form. Total absorption was not changed, and the clinical significance was unknown (563).

Administration of a single dose of aluminum hydroxide decreased the bioavailability of a simultaneously administered single dose of propranolol in four of five subjects (564). What effect the concomitant administration of antacids and propranolol will have on prolonged therapy has not been assessed. Likewise, the clinical significance of this interaction remains to be determined. The bioavailability of atenolol was reduced by an antacid containing aluminum hydroxide, magnesium hydroxide, and magnesium carbonate. This same antacid increased the bioavailability of metoprolol (565). Calcium carbonate reduced the bioavailability of atenolol by 51% in six patients (566).

Aluminum–magnesium hydroxide antacid has been shown to decrease the rate and extent of aminophylline absorption at 40 and 60 minutes. However, at later sampling times, while the rate was decreased, the extent of absorption was not significantly different. This would not be clinically significant for chronic administration (567).

The administration of single doses of valproic acid with aluminum–magnesium hydroxide, calcium carbonate, and aluminum hydroxide–magnesium trisilicate resulted in a significant increase in total absorption with aluminum–magnesium hydroxide and a trend toward increased absorption with the other two (568).

Magnesium trisilicate has been found to adsorb both estrogen and progestogen components of oral contraceptives in vitro (569). Although this interaction has not been reported in vivo, it may be important and can be avoided if patients are counseled not to take antacids and oral contraceptives concomitantly.

Sodium bicarbonate increased the renal elimination of methotrexate in 11 patients. The mechanism was believed to be by urinary alkalinization (570).

PRODUCT SELECTION GUIDELINES

The label of an antacid product as defined by the FDA may contain the following indications: "upset stomach associated with heartburn, sour stomach, or acid indigestion." The label must contain a caution if constipation or diarrhea occurs in more than 5% of the population and if the product contains more than 25 mEq of potassium, 50 mEq of magnesium, or 5 g of lactose per daily dose. If the product contains more than 0.2 mEq (5 mg) of sodium per dosage unit, the content must be on the label. Directions for time intervals between doses must be given, and a limit of 2 weeks of self-therapy is stated. A listing of the quantity of active ingredients is voluntary (219, 571).

The FDA review panel did not make specific dosage recommendations or give any comparative data. The label is an aid to product selection, but final selection and dosage must be based on individual evaluation and patient history. Antacids containing little or no sodium should be selected for individuals on low-salt diets (patients who are pregnant or who have congestive heart failure, hypertension, edema, or renal failure). Sodium content should be compared for equipotent volumes of drug to be administered. The sodium content in all antacids, except sodium bicarbonate, has been reduced in the past few years to minimize this problem. Magnesium-containing antacids should be avoided in patients with chronic renal failure. Antacids that cause constipation or diarrhea should not be given to a patient who already has these complaints. However, a magnesium antacid may be appropriate for an elderly patient who complains of chronic constipation.

The patient's current medications should be reviewed so that a product or a dosage schedule can be selected that does not interfere with any other concurrent therapy.

Although cost is not a major consideration in the initial selection of a product, there is great variability when acid-neutralizing capacity is compared. These differences are reflected in the wholesale costs of 1 month of therapy, which varies from $35 to $55 with the five most potent antacids, and from $61 to $498 with the five least effective antacids (572). Cost should be computed for equipotent, not equivolume, quantities.

PATIENT COUNSELING

The patient should be given the following specific advice:

- Antacids for relief of indigestion symptoms should not be taken longer than 2 weeks. If relief is not obtained, a physician should be contacted. If the antacid is being taken for peptic ulcer disease, it should be taken 1 and 3 hours after meals and at bedtime to provide a maximum duration of action.

- To prevent self-medication of an iatrogenic condition, the patient should understand that the antacid may cause diarrhea or constipation.

- Patients with restricted salt intake should be informed of the amount of sodium in the medications and advised of those products with a low-sodium content. Patients with medical problems that could be influenced by potassium or magnesium should be told of the content of these ions. Most antacid preparations have been reformulated to remove or reduce the sodium.

- The lesser neutralizing capacity of antacid tablets should be made clear. If liquid antacids are unacceptable, tablets should be chewed thoroughly and followed with a full glass of water to help dissolution and dispersion in the stomach. Effervescent tablets should be dissolved in water and most of the bubbles allowed to subside before the liquid is swallowed.

- Additional medication that the patient is taking should be identified to enable the pharmacist to monitor for drug interactions.

SUMMARY

Before recommending an antacid for self-therapy, the pharmacist must ensure that the use is appropriate. If the patient's history is indicative of peptic ulcer, or if there is evidence of bleeding, the patient should be referred to a physician for a medical evaluation.

Self-medication may be recommended if the history is indicative of acute gastritis, indigestion, heartburn, or upset stomach. Subjectively, any antacid will be effective, and therapy may be initiated with 40–80 mEq of a liquid antacid or 2–4 g of sodium bicarbonate or calcium carbonate. A product with simethicone should be recommended for the patient with gas. The pharmacist should caution against frequent use and monitor the patient for effectiveness and toxicity. If the discomfort is not relieved after 2 weeks or recurs frequently, medical help is indicated.

Because antacids are frequently used in peptic ulcer therapy, the pharmacist may be asked to recommend an antacid for the physician-supervised management of peptic ulcer disease. A concentrated form of aluminum–magnesium hydroxide gel is the agent of choice for initial therapy in the absence of other complications. Other agents would be more appropriate for patients with renal failure, those on low-salt diets, and those with abnormal bowel function.

All antacids are not equal. Care should be taken to select one with good buffering capacity and a taste acceptable to the patient. Equipotent volumes should be used if side effects necessitate switching to another product. Failure of antacid therapy may be caused by poor selection, too infrequent or poorly timed administration, inadequate doses, or noncompliance because of unpalatability or disagreeable side effects.

REFERENCES

1   *Generic Line*, *17*(2), 8, Charles H. Kline and Co. (1985).

2   S. L. Robbins, "Pathologic Basis of Disease," W. B. Saunders, Philadelphia, Pa., 1974.

3   B. Joelsson, *Scand. J. Gastroenterol.*, *23* (suppl. 155), 101–105 (1988).

4   R. Fisher and S. Cohen, *Med. Clin. North Am.*, *62*, 3 (1978).

5   J. Christensen, *Clin. Gastroenterol.*, *5*, 15 (1976).

6   A. C. Guyton, "Textbook of Medical Physiology," W. B. Saunders, Philadelphia, Pa., 1981.

7   Charles E. Pope, in "Gastrointestinal Disease: Pathophysiology, Diagnosis, Management," 2nd ed., M. H. Sleisenger and J. S. Fordtran, Eds., W. B. Saunders, Philadelphia, Pa., 1978, pp. 541–568.

8   J. Christensen et al., *Am. J. Physiol.*, *225*, 1265 (1973).

9   G. R. Freeland et al., *Gastroenterol.*, *71*, 570 (1976).

10   D. O. Castell and L. D. Harris, *N. Engl. J. Med.*, *282*, 886 (1970).

11   W. H. Lipshutz and S. Cohen, *Am. J. Physiol.*, *222*, 775 (1972).

12   H. Resin et al., *Gastroenterol.*, *64*, 946 (1973).

13   H. M. Jennewein et al., *Gut*, *14*, 861 (1973).

14   W. J. Hogan et al., *J. Appl. Physiol.*, *36*, 755 (1972).

15   G. W. Dennis and D. O. Castell, *N. Engl. J. Med.*, *284*, 1136 (1971).

16   O. T. Nebel and D. O. Castell, *Gut*, *14*, 270 (1973).

17   A. C. Guyton, "Textbook of Medical Physiology," W. B. Saunders, Philadelphia, Pa., 1976, p. 858.

18   "Peptic Ulcer," H. M. Spiro, Ed., Rorer, Fort Washington, Pa., 1971.

19   M. I. Grossman, in "Gastrointestinal Disease: Pathophysiology, Diagnosis, Management," 2nd ed., M. H. Sleisenger and J. S. Fordtran, Eds., W. B. Saunders, Philadelphia, Pa., 1978, pp. 640–659.

20   K. A. Kelley, "Surgery Annual," Appleton-Century-Crofts, New York, N.Y., 1974, p. 103.

21   A. M. Cooperman and S. A. Cook, *Surg. Clin. N. Am.*, *56*, 1277 (1976).

22   K. J. Ivey, *Am. J. Med.*, *58*, 389 (1975).

23   M. M. Wolfe and A. H. Soll, *N. Engl. J. Med.*, *319 (26)*, 1707–1715 (1988).

24   D. H. Malinowska and G. Sachs, *Clin. Gastroenterol.*, *13*, 309 (1984).

25   R. R. Dozois and K. A. Kelley, *Surg. Clin. N. Am.*, *56*, 1267 (1975).

26   F. P. Brooks, "Handbook of Physiology," Vol. II, Sec. 6, C. F. Code, Ed., American Physiological Society, Washington, D.C., 1967, p. 805.

27   H. T. Debas, *Am. Surg.*, *42*, 498 (1976).

28   J. H. Eichhorn et al., *Nature*, *248*, 238 (1974).

29   J. H. Wyllie, "Surgery Annals," L. M. Nyhus, Ed., Appleton-Century-Crofts, New York, N.Y., 1979, p. 207.

30   B. Schofield et al., *Gastroenterol.*, *68*, A-125 (1975).

31   C. G. Nicholl et al., *Ann. Rev. Nutr.*, *5*, 213–239 (1985).

32   M. J. Sanders and A. H. Soll, *Ann. Rev. Physiol.*, *48*, 89–101 (1986).

33   T. Scratcherd, *Clin. Gastroenterol.*, *2*, 259 (1973).

34   J. E. McGuigan, *Am. J. Dig. Dis.*, *22*, 712 (1977).

35   A. M. Ebeid and J. E. Fischer, *Surg. Clin. N. Am.*, *56*, 1249 (1976).

36   J. H. Walsh and M. I. Grossman, *N. Engl. J. Med.*, *292*, 1324 (1975).

37   J. E. McGuigan, *Gastroenterol.*, *64*, 497 (1973).

38   D. H. Stern and J. H. Walsh, *Gastroenterol.*, *64*, 363 (1973).

39   S. Cohen and W. Lipshutz, *J. Clin. Invest.*, *50*, 449 (1971).

40   M. L. Chapman et al., *Gastroenterol.*, *63*, 962 (1972).

41   I. W. McCall et al., *Br. J. Surg.*, *62*, 15 (1975).

42   W. J. Dodds et al., *Am. J. Dig. Dis.*, *20*, 201 (1976).

43   J. W. Black et al., *Nature*, *236*, 385 (1972).

44   S. J. Konturek et al., *Am. J. Dig. Dis.*, *19*, 609 (1974).

45   J. H. Wyllie et al., *Lancet*, *2*, 1117 (1972).

46   R. R. Dozois et al., *Physiologist*, *18*, 196 (1975).

47   C. B. H. W. Lamers, *Drugs*, *35* (suppl. 3), 10–16 (1988).

48   A. M. Brooks and M. I. Grossman, *Gastroenterol.*, *59*, 114 (1970).

49   D. E. Wilson et al., *Gastroenterol.*, *63*, 45 (1972).

50   E. Straus, *Med. Clin. North Am.*, *62*, 21 (1978).

51   K. G. Wormsley, *Gastroenterol.*, *62*, 156 (1972).

52   J. Hansky et al., *Gastroenterol.*, *61*, 62 (1971).

53   M. H. Wheeler, *Gut*, *15*, 420 (1974).

54   R. Cano et al., *Gastroenterol.*, *70*, 1055 (1976).

55   R. F. Barbaras, *Gastroenterol.*, *64*, 1168 (1973).

56   H. D. Becker et al., *Ann. Surg.*, *179*, 906 (1974).

57   B. Van Duijn et al., *Am. J. Physiology*, *257 (1)*, G157–G168 (1989).

58   J. H. Walsh et al., *J. Clin. Invest.*, *55*, 462 (1975).

59   R. A. Gross et al., *Gastroenterol.*, *70*, 891 (1976).

60   A. S. Ward et al., *Gut*, *10*, 1020 (1969).

61   R. K. Teichmann et al., *World J. Surg.*, *3*, 623 (1979).

62   I. L. MacGregor et al., *Gastroenterol.*, *70*, 197 (1976).

63   G. D. Kerr, *Meth. Find. Exp. Clin. Pharmacol.*, *11* (suppl. 1), 9–12 (1989).

64   J. R. Clanp and D. Ene, *Meth. Find. Exp. Clin. Pharmacol.*, *11* (suppl. 1), 19–25 (1989).

65   G. Flemstrom and L. A. Twinberg, *Clin. Gastroenterol.*, *13*, 327 (1984).

66   J. L. Wallace, *Meth. Find. Exp. Clin. Pharmacol.*, *11* (suppl. 1), 27–33 (1989).

67   B. J. R. Whittle, *Meth. Find. Exp. Clin. Pharmacol.*, *11* (suppl. 1), 35–43 (1989).

68   C. J. Hawkey, *Meth. Find. Exp. Clin. Pharmacol.*, *11* (suppl. 1), 45–51 (1989).

69   *Lancet*, *2*, 473 (1982).

70   A. R. Cooke, *Gastroenterol.*, *68*, 804 (1975).

71   S. Moberg, *Scand. J. Gastroenterol.*, *15 (80)*, 17 (1980).

72   S. H. Danovitch, in "Disorders of the Gastrointestinal Tract, Disorders of the Liver, Nutritional Disorders," J. M. Dietschy, Ed., Grune and Stratton, New York, N.Y., 1976, p. 111.

73   D. G. Colin-Jones, *J. Clin. Gastroenterol.*, *11* (suppl. 1), S30–S42 (1989).

74   D. Y. Graham, *J. Clin. Gastroenterol.*, *11* (suppl. 1), S43–S48 (1989).

75   G. N. J. Tytgat et al., *J. Clin. Gastroenterol.*, *11* (suppl. 1), S49–S53 (1989).

76   C. P. Dooley and H. Cohen, *Ann. Intern. Med.*, *108*, 70 (1988).

77   J. I. Wyatt et al., *Lancet*, *i*, 118 (1988).

78   C. S. Goodwin, *Lancet*, *ii*, 1467 (1988).

79   M. Gibaldi, *Perspectives in Clinical Pharmacy*, 7 (7), 58–60 (July 1989).

80   J. E. Ormand and N. J. Talley, *J. Clin. Gastroenterol.*, *5*, 492–495 (1989).

81   S. N. Tewari et al., *J. Clin. Gastroenterol.*, *11 (3)*, 271–277 (1989).

82   B. J. Rathbone et al., *Scand. J. Gastroenterol.*, *23* (suppl. 142),140–143 (1988).

83   M. Lopez-Brea and M. L. Jimenez, *Meth. Find. Exp. Clin. Pharmacol.*, *11* (suppl. 1), 13–17 (1989).

84   A. Berstad et al., *Gastroenterol.*, *95*, 619–624 (1988).

85   R. S. Fisher et al., *Gastroenterol.*, *70*, 301 (1976).

86   J. Behar, *Arch. Int. Med.*, *136*, 560 (1976).

87   J. Dent et al., *J. Clin. Invest.*, *65*, 256 (1980).

88   C. S. Winans, *Drug Ther.*, *10*, 33 (1980).

89   M. D. Kaye and J. P. Showalter, *J. Lab. Clin. Med.*, *83*, 198 (1974).

90   W. J. Dobbs et al., *Gastroenterol.*, *81*, 376 (1981).

91   K. Gudmundsson et al., *Scand. J. Gastroenterol.*, *23*, 75–79 (1988).

92   J. E. Richter and D. O. Castell, *Ann. Int. Med.*, *97*, 93 (1982).

93   J. L. Frazier and K. J. Fendler, *Clin. Pharm.*, *2*, 546 (1983).

94   R. S. Fisher et al., *Gastroenterol.*, *68*, 893 (1975).

95   L. F. Johnson and R. R. Demuster, *Am. J. Gastroenterol.*, *62*, 325 (1974).

96   D. W. Piper, *Gastroenterol.*, *52*, 1009 (1967).

97   R. M. Pinder et al., *Drugs*, *12*, 81–131 (1976).

98   W. S. Brooks, *Am. J. Gastroenterol.*, *80*, 206 (1985).

99   G. H. Jeffries, in "Gastrointestinal Disease: Pathophysiology, Diagnosis, Management," 2nd ed., M. H. Sleisenger and J. S. Fordtran, Eds., W. B. Saunders, Philadelphia, Pa., 1978, pp. 733–743.

100   B. S. Wolf, *J. Am. Med. Assoc.*, *235*, 1244 (1976).

101   B. J. Nath and A. L. Warshaw, *Ann. Rev. Med.*, *35*, 383 (1984).

102   W. P. Ritchie, *Gut*, *25*, 975 (1984).

103   N. J. Talley and S. F. Phillips, *Ann. Intern. Med.*, *108*, 865–879 (1988).

104   S. P. Lagarde and H. M. Spiro, *Clin. Gastroenterol.*, *13*, 437 (1984).

105   D. G. Colin-Jones, *Scand. J. Gastroenterol.*, *23* (suppl. 155), 8–11 (1988).

106   A. R. Cooke, *Am. J. Dig. Dis.*, *21*, 155 (1976).

107   G. W. Dennish and D. O. Castell, *Am. J. Dig. Dis.*, *17*, 993 (1972).

108   *Nutrition Reviews*, *34*, 167 (1976).

109   F. Acquaviva et al., *J. Clin. Gastroenterol.*, *8 (2)*, 150–153 (1986).

110   A. R. Cooke, in "Gastrointestinal Disease: Pathophysiology, Diagnosis, Management," 2nd ed., M. H. Sleisenger and J. S. Fordtran, Eds., W. B. Saunders, Philadelphia, Pa., 1978, pp. 807–826.

111   S. Domschke and W. Domschke, *Clin. Gastroenterol.*, *13*, 405 (1984).

112   J. C. O'Laughlin et al., *Arch. Int. Med.*, *141*, 781 (1981).

113   L. H. Gerber et al., *J. Clin. Gastroenterol.*, *3*, 7 (1981).

114   D. Y. Graham et al., *Dig. Dis. Sci.*, *28*, 1 (1983).

115   R. Jaszewski et al., *Dig. Dis. Sci.*, *34 (9)*, 1361–1364 (1989).

116   D. Nunes et al., *Drugs*, *38 (3)*, 451–461 (1989).

117   R. E. Garris and C. F. Kirkwood, *Clin. Pharm.*, *8 (9)*, 627–644 (1989).

118   C. E. Lucas et al., *Arch. Surg.*, *102*, 266 (1971).

119   W. C. Butterfield, *Surg. Annu.*, *7*, 261 (1975).

120   K.-H. Chan et al., *Neurosurgery*, *25 (3)*, 378–382 (1989).

121   M. Levy, *N. Engl. J. Med.*, *290*, 1158–1162 (1979).

122   W. T. Wightkin, *Am. J. Hosp. Pharm.*, *37*, 1651 (1980).

123   G. C. Marrone and W. Silen, *Clin. Gastroenterol.*, *13*, 635 (1984).

124   P. H. Guth, *Gastroenterol.*, *64*, 1187 (1973).

125   R. B. Shuman et al., *Ann. Intern. Med.*, *106 (4)*, (1987).

126   C. M. Wilcox and J. G. Spenney, *Am. J. Gastroenterol.*, *83 (11)*, 1199–1211 (1988).

127   J. K. Siepler et al., *DICP*, *23 (10)*, S40–S43 (1989).

128   M. R. Driks et al., *N. Engl. J., Med.*, *317 (22)*, 11–26 (1987).

129   J. C. Stothert et al., *Surgery*, *192*, 169–174 (1980).

130   Ostro, *Gastroenterol.*, *88 (9)*, 532–537 (1985).

131   P. Sipponen et al., *Gut*, *30*, 922–929 (1989).

132   M. I. Grossman, *Scand. J. Gastroenterol.*, *15 (58)*, 7 (1980).

133   J. E. McGuigan, in "Disorders of the Gastrointestinal Tract, Disorders of the Liver, Nutritional Disorders," J. M. Dietchy, Ed., Grune and Stratton, New York, N.Y., 1976, p. 88.

134   M. I. Grossman et al., *Gastroenterol.*, *69*, 1071 (1975).

135   M. J. S. Langman, *Clin. Gastroenterol.*, *2*, 219 (1973).

136   R. C. Brown et al., *Br. Med. J.*, *1*, 35 (1976).

137   J. H. Kurata and B. M. Haile, *Clin. Gastroenterol.*, *13*, 289 (1984).

138   R. A. L. Sturdevant, *Am. J. Epidemiol.*, *104*, 9 (1976).

139   J. D. Elashoff and M. I. Grossman, *Gastroenterol.*, *78*, 280 (1980).

140   M. Susser, *J. Chron. Dis.*, *35*, 29–40 (1982).

141   A. Sonnenberg and H. Muller, *J. Chron. Dis.*, *37 (9/10)*, 699–704 (1984).

142   A. Sonnenberg, *Gastroenterol.*, *86*, 398–401 (1984).

143   A. Sonnenberg et al., *J. Chron. Dis.*, *38 (4)*, 309–317 (1985).

144   B. E. Stabile and E. Passaro, *Gastroenterol.*, *70*, 124 (1976).

145   P. M. Jensen, *Am. J. Med.*, *77* (suppl. 5B), 8 (1983).

146   C. T. Richardson, in "Gastrointestinal Disease: Pathophysiology, Diagnosis, Management," 2nd. ed., M. H. Sleisenger and J. S. Fordtran, Eds., W. B. Saunders, Philadelphia, Pa., 1978, pp. 875–891.

147   Y. Nagamachi and S. C. Skoryna, *Am. J. Surg.*, *133*, 593 (1977).

148   L. Olbe, *Scand. J. Gastroenterol.*, *14 (55)*, 49 (1979).

149   J. Alexander-Williams and R. L. Wolverson, *Clin. Gastroenterol.*, *13*, 601 (1984).

150   M. I. Grossman et al., *Ann. Intern. Med.*, *84*, 57 (1976).

151   A. Ippoliti and J. Walsh, *Surg. Clin. N. Am.*, *56*, 1479 (1976).

152   M. L. Chapman, *Med. Clin. N. Am.*, *62*, 39 (1978).

153   L. R. Dragstedt and E. R. Woodward, *Scand. J. Gastroenterol.*, *5*(6), 243 (1970).

154   A. H. Soll, *J. Clin. Gastroenterol.*, *11* (suppl. 1), S1–S5 (1989).

155   J. Rhodes and B. Calcraft, *Clin. Gastroenterol.*, *2*, 227 (1973).

156   N. W. Read and P. Grech, *Br. Med. J.*, *3*, 313 (1973).

157   F. J. Flint and P. Grech, *Gut*, *11*, 735 (1970).

158   R. S. Fisher and G. Boden, *Gastroenterol.*, *66*, 839 (1974).

159   R. S. Fisher and S. Cohen, *N. Engl. J. Med.*, *288*, 273 (1973).

160   J. E. Valenzuela and C. Defilipi, *Am. J. Dig. Dis.*, *21*, 229 (1976).

161   R. A. Roverstad, *Am. J. Dig. Dis.*, *21*, 165 (1976).

162   J. I. Rotter and D. L. Rimoin, *Gastroenterol.*, *73*, 604 (1977).

163   S. G. Chiverton and R. H. Hunt, *J. Clin. Gastroenterol.*, *11* (suppl. 1), S29–S33 (1989).

164   C. Toftgaard, *Ann. Surg.*, *210 (2)*, 159–164 (1989).

165   M. Okada et al., *Am. J. Gastroenterol.*, *84 (5)*, 501–505 (1989).

166   R. A. L. Sturdevant and J. H. Walsh, in "Gastrointestinal Disease: Pathophysiology, Diagnosis, Management," 2nd ed., M. H. Sleisenger and J. S. Fordtran, Eds., W. B. Saunders, Philadelphia, Pa., 1978, pp. 840–860.

167   A. Sonnenberg, *Scan. J. Gastroenterol.* (suppl. 155), 119–140 (1988).

168   G. A. Hallenback, *Surg. Clin. N. Am.*, *56*, 1235 (1976).

169   A. J. Cox, *Arch. Pathol.*, *54*, 407 (1952).

170   J. I. Isenberg et al., *J. Clin. Invest.*, *55*, 330 (1975).

171   J. E. McGuigan and W. L. Trudeau, *N. Engl. J. Med.*, *228*, 64 (1973).

172   J. H. Walsh et al., *J. Clin. Invest.*, *55*, 462 (1975).

173   J. S. Fordtran and J. H. Walsh, *J. Clin. Invest.*, *52*, 645 (1973).

174   J. R. Malagelada, *Scand. J. Gastroenterol.*, *14 (55)*, 39 (1979).

175   W. Creutzfeldt and R. Arnold, *World J. Surg.*, *3*, 605 (1979).

176   J. I. Isenberg, *Postgrad. Med.*, *57*, 163 (1975).

177 J. I. Rotter et al., *N. Engl. J. Med., 300*, 66 (1979).

178 A. Harrison et al., "Surgeon General's Report on Smoking and Health," 1979.

179 W. H. Taylor and A. Walker, *J. Roy. Soc. Med., 73*, 159 (1980).

180 "Harrison's Principles of Internal Medicine," 9th ed., G. W. Thorn et al., Eds., McGraw-Hill, New York, N.Y., 1980.

181 S. K. Lam, *Clin. Gastroenterol., 13*, 447 (1984).

182 J. I. Rotter and D. L. Rimoin, *Gastroenterol., 73*, 604 (1977).

183 H. Susser, *J. Chron. Dis., 20*, 435 (1967).

184 R. Earlam, *Gastroenterol., 71*, 314 (1976).

185 E. Scapa, et al., *J. Clin. Gastroenterol., 11 (5)*, 502–506 (1989).

186 H. Colcher, *N. Eng. J. Med., 293*, 1129 (1975).

187 M. C. Sheppard et al., *Gut, 18*, 524 (1977).

188 J. C. Reynolds, *Ann. Intern. Med., 111*, 7–14 (1989).

189 S. Massarrat et al., *Gut, 29*, 291–297 (1988).

190 H. M. Pollard and N. A. Augar, *Practitioner, 201*, 139 (1968).

191 D. W. Piper and J. Kang, *Drugs, 17*, 124 (1979).

192 S. Hannibal et al., *Scand. J. Gastroenterol., 15 (58)*, 29 (1980).

193 M. D. Korenmen et al., *J. Am. Med. Assoc., 240*, 54 (1978).

194 D. W. Piper and B. H. Fenton, *Gut, 5*, 506 (1964).

195 J. T. Kuruvilla, *Gut, 12*, 897 (1971).

196 H. A. Holm, *Scand. J. Gastroenterol., 2 (42)*, 119 (1976).

197 D. W. Piper and B. H. Fenton, *Am. J. Dig. Dis., 6*, 134 (1961).

198 A. Berstad, *Scand. J. Gastroenterol., 17* (suppl. 75), 13 (1982).

199 T. B. Deering et al., *Gastroenterol., 77*, 986 (1979).

200 F. Bendtsen and S. J. Rune, *Scand. J. Gastroenterol., 23*, 935–940 (1988).

201 J. F. Morrissey et al., *Arch. Intern. Med., 119*, 510 (1967).

202 J. E. Dill, *Gastroenterol., 62*, 697 (1972).

203 R. H. Higgs et al., *N. Engl. J. Med., 291*, 486 (1974).

204 D. O. Castell and S. M. Levine, *Ann. Intern. Med., 74*, 223 (1971).

205 G. E. Feurle, *Gastroenterol., 68*, 1 (1975).

206 E. Schrumpf, *Scand. J. Gastroenterol., 15* (58), 97 (1980).

207 A. Hurwitz and M. B. Sheehan, *J. Pharmacol. Exp. Ther., 179*, 124 (1971).

208 A. Hurwitz et al., *Gastroenterol., 71*, 268 (1976).

209 J. E. Clain et al., *Gastroenterol., 73*, 556 (1977).

210 E. Kivilaakso, *Scand. J. Gastroenterol., 17* (suppl. 75), 16 (1982).

211 K. H. Holtermuller and M. Dehdaschti, *Scand. J. Gastroenterol., 17* (suppl. 75), 24 (1982).

212 S. I. Postiuss and H. Engler, *Eur. J. Pharmacol., 88*, 403 (1983).

213 S. L. James and C. Marriott, *Pharm. Acta. Helv., 57*, 265 (1982).

214 G. Preclik et al., *Gut, 30*, 148–151 (1989).

215 D. Hollander and A. Tarnawski, *Gut, 30,* 145–147 (1989).

216 D. Saunders et al., *Dig. Dis. Sci., 33 (4)*, 409–413 (1988).

217 J. R. Malagelada and G. L. Carlson, *Scand. J. Gastroenterol., 17* (suppl. 75), 10 (1982).

218 J. R. Malagelada and G. L. Carlson, *Scand. J. Gastroenterol., 14* (55), 67 (1977).

219 A. M. Schmidt, *Federal Register, 39*, 19862 (1974).

220 C. H. Barnett et al., *N. Engl. J. Med., 240*, 787 (1949).

221 C. J. Riley, *Practitioner, 205*, 657 (1970).

222 A. Ansari and J. A. Vennes, *Minn. Med., 54*, 611 (1971).

223 D. W. Piper, *Clin. Gastroenterol., 2*, 361 (1973).

224 F. W. Green et al., *Am. J. Hosp. Pharm., 32*, 425 (1975).

225 R. E. Barry, *J. Intern. Med. Res., 6* (1), 11 (1978).

226 E. S. Orwell, *Ann. Int. Med., 97*, 242 (1982).

227 J. S. Fordtran, *N. Engl. J. Med., 279*, 900 (1968).

228 *Medical Letter on Drugs and Therapeutics, 15* (8), 36 (1973).

229 J. D. Clemens and N. Feinstein, *Gastroenterol., 72*, 957 (1977).

230 R. B. Stewart et al., *Dig. Dis. Sci., 28*, 1062 (1983).

231 J. S. Fordtran, in "Gastrointestinal Disease: Pathophysiology, Diagnosis, Management," 2nd ed., M. H. Sleisenger and J. S. Fordtran, Eds., W. B. Saunders, Philadelphia, Pa., 1973, p. 718.

232 J. Stiel et al., *Gastroenterol., 53*, 900 (1967).

233 R. F. Barreras, *Gastroenterol., 64*, 1168 (1973).

234 R. M. Case, *Digestion, 8*, 269 (1973).

235 H. Breuhaus et al., *Gastroenterol., 16*, 172 (1950).

236 R. F. Barreras, *N. Engl. J. Med., 282*, 1402 (1970).

237 D. D. Reeder et al., *Ann. Surg., 172*, 540 (1970).

238 J. A. Levant et al., *N. Engl. J. Med., 289*, 555 (1973).

239 E. C. Texter, *Am. J. Gastroenterol., 84 (2)*, 97–108 (1989).

240 K. H. Holtermuller, *Hepato-gastroenterol., 29*, 135 (1982).

241 S. L. Hem, *J. Chem. Educ., 52*, 383 (1975).

242 C. M. Townsend et al., *N. Engl. J. Med., 288*, 1058 (1973).

243 E. M. Clarkson et al., *Clin. Sci., 43*, 519 (1972).

244 G. M. Berlyne et al., *Lancet, 2*, 494 (1970).

245 V. Parsons et al., *Br. Med. J., 4*, 273 (1971).

246 A. C. Alfrey et al., *N. Engl. J. Med., 294*, 184 (1976).

247 C. A. Miller and E. M. Levine, *J. Neurochem., 22*, 751 (1974).

248 A. I. McLaughlin et al., *Br. J. Ind. Med., 19*, 253 (1962).

249 W. D. Kaehny et al., *N. Engl. J. Med., 296*, 1389 (1977).

250 A. A. Bakir et al., *Clin. Nephrol., 31* (1), 40–44 (1989).

251 R. Weberg and A. Berstad, *Eur. J. of Clin. Investig., 16*, 428–432 (1986).

252 *J. Am. Med. Assoc., 238*, 1017 (1977).

253 H. Spencer and M. Lender, *Gastroenterol., 76*, 603 (1979).

254 G. J. Ward et al., *Am. J. Med., 77*, 747 (1984).

255 D. E. Abrams et al., *West. J. Med., 120*, 157 (1974).

256 H. M. Shields, *Gastroenterol., 75*, 1137 (1978).

257 M. Lotz et al., *N. Engl. J. Med., 278*, 409 (1968).

258 R. E. Chojnacki, *Ann. Intern. Med., 74*, 297 (1971).

259 K. L. Insogna et al., *J. Am. Med. Assoc., 244*, 2544 (1980).

260 A. Walan, *Scand. J. Gastroenterol., 17* (suppl. 75), 63 (1982).

261 H. Spencer and M. Lender, *Gastroenterol., 76*, 603 (1979).

262 H. Spencer and L. Kramer, *Arch. Int. Med., 143*, 657 (1983).

263 J. Erckenbrecht et al., *Digestion, 25*, 244 (1982).

264 R. E. Randall et al., *Ann. Intern. Med., 61*, 73 (1964).

265 F. J. Goodwin and F. P. Vince, *Br. J. Urol., 42*, 586 (1970).

266 S. Jameson, *Scand. J. Urol. Nephrol., 6*, 260 (1972).

267 A. C. Alfrey et al., *Ann. Intern. Med., 73*, 367 (1970).

268 A. S. Berns and K. R. Kollmeyer, *Ann. Intern. Med., 85*, 760 (1976).

269 J. R. Herman and A. S. Goldbert, *J. Am. Med. Assoc., 174*, 1206 (1960).

270 C. Lagergren, *J. Urol., 87*, 994 (1962).

271 A. M. Joekes et al., *Br. Med. J., 1*, 146 (1973).

272 F. W. Greene et al., *Am. J. Hosp. Pharm., 32*, 425 (1975).

273 R. K. Vanderlaan et al., *J. Pharm. Sci., 68*, 1498 (1979).

274 T. C. Simmons et al., *J. Clin. Gastroenterol., 8 (2)*, 146–149 (1986).

275 N. E. Madias and A. S. Levey, *Am. J. Med., 74*, 155 (1983).

276 M. Strom, *Scand. J. Gastroenterol., 17* (suppl. 75), 54 (1982).

277 P. M. VanKalmthout et al., *Dig. Dis. Sci., 27*, 859 (1982).

278 M. D. Korenmen et al., *J. Am. Med. Assoc., 240*, 54 (1978).

279 J. E. Bernstein and A. M. Kasich, *J. Clin. Pharmacol.*, *14*, 617 (1974).

280 J. A. Stead et al., *J. Pharm. Pharmacol.*, *30*, 350 (1978).

281 C. Stanciu and J. R. Bennet, *Lancet*, *1*, 109 (1974).

282 L. S. Malmud et al., *J. Nucl. Med.*, *20*, 1023 (1979).

283 M. Beeley and J. O. Warner, *Curr. Med. Res. Opin.*, *1*, 63 (1972).

284 *S. Afr. Med. J.*, *48*, 2239 (1974).

285 G. L. Beckloff et al., *J. Clin. Pharmacol.*, *12*, 11 (1972).

286 D. E. Barnardo et al., *Curr. Med. Res. Opin.*, *3*, 388 (1975).

287 *Lancet*, *1*, 1290 (1975).

288 R. Burns et al., *Br. Med. J.*, *1*, 220 (1974).

289 *Postgrad. Med. J.*, *51 (5)* (1975).

290 R. N. Brogden et al., *Drugs*, *12*, 401 (1976).

291 I. N. Marks, *Drugs*, *20*, 283 (1980).

292 E. Bayerdorffer et al., *Lancet*, *ii*, 1467 (1988).

293 G. B. Porro et al., *Gut*, *28*, 907 (1987).

294 G. Ekeved and A. Walan, *Scand. J. Gastroenterol.*, *10*, 267 (1975).

295 J. R. B. J. Brouwers and G. N. J. Tytgat, *J. Pharm. Pharmacol.*, *30*, 148 (1978).

296 D. Drake and D. Hollander, *Ann. Intern. Med.*, *94*, 215 (1981).

297 C. C. Barnett and C. T. Richardson, *Dig. Dis. Sci.*, *30 (11)*, 1049–1052 (1985).

298 D. Patyk, *N. Engl. J. Med.*, *283*, 134 (1970).

299 A. Berstad et al., *Scand. J. Gastroenterol.*, *17*, 953 (1982).

300 D. W. Piper and B. H. Fenton, *Gut*, *5*, 585 (1964).

301 E. W. Packman and A. R. Gennaro, *Am. J. Pharm.*, *145*, 162 (1973).

302 J. E. Clain et al., *S. Afr. Med. J.*, *57*, 158 (1980).

303 R. E. Barry and J. Ford, *Br. Med. J.*, *1*, 413 (1978).

304 W. L. Peterson and J. S. Fordtran, in "Gastrointestinal Disease: Pathophysiology, Diagnosis, Management," 2nd ed., M. H. Sleisenger and J. S. Fordtran, Eds., W. B. Saunders, Philadelphia, Pa., 1978.

305 M. P. Dutro and A. B. Amerson, *Colo. Pharm.*, *8*, Sept.–Oct. (1980).

306 G. D. Rudd, *Am. Intern. Med.*, *95*, 120 (1981).

307 J. Pawlaczyk et al., *Pharmazie*, *39*, 334 (1984).

308 S. L. Hem et al., *Am. J. Hosp. Pharm.*, *39*, 1925 (1982).

309 M. C. Sherrill and G. D. Rudd, *Am. J. Hosp. Pharm.*, *39*, 300 (1982).

310 S. Fox and J. Behar, *Clin. Gastroenterol.*, *8*, 37 (1979).

311 M. M. Kline et al., *Gastroenterol.*, *68*, 1137 (1975).

312 D. Y. Graham et al., *Am. J. Gastroenterol.*, *78*, 257 (1983).

313 C. Meyer et al., *Gastroenterol.*, *76*, 1201 (1979).

314 D. Y. Graham and D. J. Patterson, *Gastroenterol.*, *82*, 1072 (1982).

315 D. Y. Graham and D. J. Patterson, *Dig. Dis. Sci.*, *28*, 559 (1983).

316 J. Rhodes, *Scand. J. Gastroenterol.*, *17* (suppl. 75), 74 (1982).

317 R. J. Petrokubi and G. H. Jeffries, *Gastroenterol.*, *77*, 69 (1979).

318 M. G. Robinson, *Am. J. Med.*, *77* (suppl. 5B), 106 (1984).

319 R. Gotthard et al., *Scand. J. Gastroenterol.*, *23*, 7–18 (1988).

320 O. Nyren et al., *N. Engl. J. Med.*, *314*, 339–343 (1986).

321 H. Petersen, *Scand. J. Gastroenterol.*, *17* (suppl. 75), 77 (1982).

322 E. Burrero et al., *Am. J. Surg.*, *148*, 809 (1984).

323 S. Derrida et al., *Critical Care Medicine*, *17 (2)*, 122–125 (1989).

324 W. Frank et al., *Clin. Pharmacol. Ther.*, *46*, 234–239 (1989).

325 F. B. Cerra, *Ann. Surg.*, *196 (5)*, 565–570 (1982).

326 J. J. Schentag et al., *DICP*, *23 (10)*, S36–S39 (1989).

327 R. J. Nolly and V. A. Skoutakis, *DICP*, *23 (10)*, S23–S28 (1989).

328 L. A. Cannon et al., *Arch. Intern. Med.*, *147 (12)*, 2101–2106 (1987).

329 G. Zuckerman et al., *Am. J. Med.*, *76*, 361 (1984).

330 J. P. Goldfarb and M. J. Czaja, *Am. J. Gastroenterol.*, *80*, 5 (1985).

331 W. L. Peterson and C. T. Richardson, *Gastroenterol.*, *88*, 666 (1985).

332 E. Christensen et al., *Gastroenterol.*, *73*, 1170 (1977).

333 J. H. Meyer et al., *West. J. Med.*, *126*, 273 (1977).

334 D. Hollander and J. Harlan, *J. Am. Med. Assoc.*, *226*, 1181 (1973).

335 M. L. Butler and H. Gersh, *Am. J. Dig. Dis.*, *20*, 803 (1975).

336 R. A. L. Sturdevant et al., *Gastroenterol.*, *72*, 1 (1977).

337 A. Littman et al., *Gastroenterol.*, *73*, 6 (1977).

338 W. L. Peterson et al., *N. Engl. J. Med.*, *297*, 341 (1977).

339 R. Gotthard et al., *Scand. J. Gastroenterol.*, *17* (suppl. 75), 86 (1975).

340 M. I. Grossman, *Scand J. Gastroenterol.*, *15 (58)*, 37 (1980).

341 T. Morris and J. Rhodes, *Gut*, *20*, 538 (1979).

342 D. M. McCarthy, *Hosp. Pract.*, *14*, 52 (1979).

343 A. Ippoliti and W. Peterson, *Clin. Gastroenterol.*, *8*, 53 (1979).

344 S. J. Rune and A. Zachariassen, *Scand. J. Gastroenterol.*, *15 (58)*, 41 (1980).

345 E. Gudjonsson and H. Spiro, *Am. J. Med.*, *65*, 399 (1978).

346 H. Sarles et al., *Digestion*, *16*, 289 (1977).

347 J. I. Isenberg et al., *N. Engl. J. Med.*, *308*, 1319 (1983).

348 S. J. Rune et al., *Scand. J. Gastroenterol.*, *19*, 56 (1984).

349 A. F. Ippoliti, *Scand. J. Gastroenterol.*, *17* (suppl. 75), 82 (1982).

350 A. Walan, *Clin. Gastroenterol.*, *13*, 473 (1984).

351 H. J. B. Frederiksen et al., *Scand. J. Gastroenterol.*, *19*, 417 (1984).

352 *Federal Register*, *47*, 454 (1982).

353 *Federal Register*, *47*, 43540 (1982).

354 A. L. Blum, *Eur. J. Clin. Inv.*, *16*, 515–518 (1986).

355 J. I. Warbick and A. N. Martin in "American Pharmacy," J. B. Sprowls and H. B. Beal, Eds., J. B. Lippincott, Philadelphia, Pa., 1972, p. 176.

356 R. P. Schneider and A. C. Roach, *South. Med. J.*, *69*, 1312 (1976).

357 D. Sklar et al., *N. Engl. J. Med.*, *296*, 1007 (1977).

358 C. Marriott, *J. Clin. Hosp. Pharm.*, *8*, 69 (1983).

359 P. G. Farup et al., *Hepato-Gastroenterol.*, *33*, 260–261 (1986).

360 J. S. Fordtran and J. A. H. Collyns, *N. Engl. J. Med.*, *274*, 921 (1966).

361 F. Halter et al., *Eur. J. Clin. Inv.*, *12*, 209 (1982).

362 R. F. Barreras et al., *Gastroenterol.*, *72*, 1027 (1977).

363 S. Cohen and W. J. Snape, *Arch. Intern. Med.*, *138*, 1398 (1978).

364 H. J. Priebe et al., *N. Engl. J. Med.*, *302*, 426 (1980).

365 M. J. S. Langman, *Drugs*, *14*, 105 (1977).

366 J. S. Fordtran and J. H. Walsh, *J. Clin. Invest.*, *52*, 645 (1973).

367 J. R. Malagelada et al., *Gastroenterol.*, *70*, 203 (1976).

368 J. S. Fordtran and J. A. H. Collyns, *N. Engl. J. Med.*, *274*, 921 (1966).

369   R. Weberg et al., *Gastroenterology, 95*, 1465–1469 (1988).

370   R. Weberg and A. Berstad, *Scand. J. Gastroenterol., 23*, 237–243 (1988).

371   G. B. Porro et al., *J. Clin. Gastroenterol., 8 (2)*, 141–145 (1986).

372   A. Rydning et al., *Gastroenterol., 91*, 56–61 (1986).

373   A. Berstad, *Scand. J. Gastroenterol., 17* (suppl. 75), 97 (1982).

374   A. Littmann, *Gastroenterol., 61*, 567 (1971).

375   S. Szabo and T. E. Bynum, *Scand. J. Gastroenterol., 23*, 1–6 (1988).

376   P. R. Holt, *Am. J. Gastroenterol., 81 (6)*, 403–411 (1986).

377   S. G. Chiverton and R. H. Hunt, *Am. J. Gastroenterol., 83 (3)*, 211–215 (1988).

378   J. W. Freston, *J. Clin. Gastroenterol., 11* (suppl. 1), S34–S38 (1989).

379   J. D. Wolosin and J. I. Isenberg, *Gastroenterology, 97 (3)*, 803–804 (1989).

380   A. Ippoliti et al., *Gastroenterol., 85*, 875 (1983).

381   K. A. Jonsson et al., *Scand. J. Gastroenterol., 23*, 199–208 (1988).

382   D. W. Piper, *Drugs, 26*, 439 (1983).

383   K. D. Bardhan et al., *Gut, 29*, 1748–1754 (1988).

384   J. D. Wolosin et al., *J. Clin. Gastroenterol., 11 (1)*, 12–16 (1989).

385   J. M. Rodrigo and J. Ponce, *Meth. Find. Exp. Clin. Pharmacol., 11* (suppl. 1), 131–135 (1989).

386   R. Sainz-Samitier and F. Gomollon-Garcia, *Meth. Find. Exp. Clin. Pharmacol., 11* (suppl. 1), 137–145 (1989).

387   J. Ponce and J. M. Rodrigo, *Meth. Find. Exp. Clin. Pharmacol., 11* (suppl. 1), 123–130 (1989).

388   G. N. J. Tytgat et al., *Clin. Gastroenterol., 13*, 543 (1984).

389   G. Bresci et al., *Int. J. Tiss. Reac., 5*, 345 (1983).

390   S. E. Silvis, *J. Clin. Gastroenterol., 7*, A83 (1985).

391   K. R. Dough et al., *Lancet, 2*, 661 (1984).

392   E. C. Texter et al., *Am. J. Med., 29* (suppl. 4B), 81 (1986).

393   F. L. Lanza and C. M. Sibley, *Am. J. Gastroenterol., 82 (12)*, 1223–1241 (1987).

394   U. Becker et al., *Acta. Med. Scand., 221*, 95–101 (1987).

395   V. Garrigues-Gil, *Meth. Find. Exp. Clin. Pharmacol., 11* (suppl. 1), 73–77 (1989).

396   H. Peterson, *Scand. J. Gastroenterol 14* (55), 56 (1979).

397   J. D. Welsh, *Gastroenterol., 72*, 740 (1977).

398   H. S. Caron and H. P. Roth, *Am. J. Med. Sci., 261*, 61 (1971).

399   A. Ryding et al., *Lancet, 2*, 736 (1982).

400   J. Yudkins, *Br. Med. J., 280*, 483 (1980).

401   A. Walan, *Scand. J. Gastroenterol., 14* (55), 84 (1979).

402   M. Feldman et al., *N. Engl. J. Med., 297*, 1427 (1977).

403   H. O. Adam et al., *Dig. Dis. Sci, 27*, 388 (1982).

404   K. J. Ivey, *Gastroenterol., 68*, 154 (1975).

405   J. Bowers et al., *Gastroenterol., 72*, 1032 (1977).

406   S. Fiorucci et al., *Am. J. Gastroenterol., 83 (12)*, 1371–1375 (1988).

407   R. P. Walt, *Meth. Find. Exp. Clin. Pharmacol., 11* (suppl. 1), 97–99 (1989).

408   J. G. Mills and J. R. Wood, *Meth. Find. Exp. Clin. Pharmacol., 11* (suppl. 1), 87–95 (1989).

409   S. R. Brazer et al., *Dig. Dis. Sci., 34 (7)*, 1047–1052 (1989).

410   C. W. Legerton, *Am. J. Med., 77* (suppl. 5B), 2 (1984).

411   J. M. Thomas and G. Misiewicz, *Clin. Gastroenterol., 13*, 501 (1984).

412   M. Robinson, *Am. J. Med., 77* (suppl. 5B), 23 (1984).

413   A. Somogyi and R. Gugler, *Clin. Pharmacokinet., 8*, 463 (1983).

414   C. J. C. Roberts, *Clin. Pharmacokinet., 9*, 211 (1984).

415   S. M. Grant et al., *Drugs, 37*, 801–870 (1989).

416   H. D. Langtry et al., *Drugs, 38 (4)*, 551–590 (1989).

417   *Drugs, 36 (5)*, 521–539 (1988).

418   J. T. Callaghan et al., *J. Clin. Pharmacol., 27*, 618–624 (1987).

419   M. Y. Morgan and D. Stambuk, *Postgrad. Med. J., 62* (suppl. 2), 29–37 (1986).

420   N. Inotsume et al., *Eur. J. Clin. Pharmacol., 36*, 517–520 (1989).

421   C. E. Halstenson et al., *J. Clin. Pharmacol., 27*, 782–787 (1987).

422   H. S. Merki et al., *Gut, 29*, 81–84 (1988).

423   D. B. Jones et al., *Gut, 28*, 1120–1127 (1987).

424   A. J. McClullough et al., *Gastroenterology, 97*, 860–866 (1989).

425   P. Bauerfeind et al., *Digestion, 37*, 217–222 (1987).

426   V. Savarino et al., *Eur. J. Clin. Pharmacol., 35*, 203–207 (1988).

427   J. M. Richter et al., *Am. J. Med., 87*, 278–284 (1989).

428   M. J. S. Langman, *Drugs, 35* (suppl. 3), 17–19 (1988).

429   J. W. Freston, *Ann. Intern. Med., 97*, 728 (1982).

430   H. M. Spiro, *J. Clin. Gastroenterol., 5* (suppl. 1), 143 (1983).

431   J. R. Powell and K. H. Dunn, *Am. J. Med., 77* (suppl. 5B), 57 (1984).

432   J. R. Powell and K. H. Dunn, *J. Clin. Gastroenterol., 5* (suppl. 1), 95 (1983).

433   A. Somogyi et al., *Eur. J. Clin. Pharmacol., 25*, 339 (1983).

434   A. Somogyi et al., Abstracts of the Second World Conference on Clinical Pharmacology and Therapeutics, 110 (1983).

435   W. Kirch et al., *Clin. Pharmacokinet., 9*, 493 (1984).

436   W. R. Garnett, *Clin. Pharm., 1*, 307 (1982).

437   W. M. Hui et al., *Am. J. Med., 86* (suppl. 6A), 60 (1989).

438   R. Nagashima et al., *Scand. J. Gastroenterol., 18* (suppl. 83), 17 (1983).

439   A. Tarnawski et al., *Gastroenterol., 84*, 1331 (1983).

440   C. J. Shorrock and W. D. W. Rees, *Am. J. Med., 86* (suppl. 6A), 2 (1989).

441   C. Tasman-Jones et al., *Am. J. Med., 86* (suppl. 6A), 5 (1989).

442   S. Szabo and D. Hollander, *Am. J. Med., 86* (suppl. 6A), 23 (1989).

443   R. H. Schotborgh et al., *Am. J. Med., 86* (suppl. 6A), 77 (1989).

444   M. Guslandi, *Am. J. Med., 86* (suppl. 6A), 45 (1989).

445   H. A. Shepherd et al., *Am. J. Med., 86* (suppl. 6A), 49 (1989).

446   A. N. Laggner et al., *Am. J. Med., 86* (suppl. 6A), 81 (1989).

447   S. Pai et al., *J. Clin. Pharmacol., 27*, 213–215 (1987).

448   T. S. Schubert, *Am. J. Med., 86* (suppl. 6A), 108 (1989).

449   A. Hjortrup et al., *Am. J. Med., 86* (suppl. 6A), 113 (1989).

450   T. E. Bynum and G. G. Koch, *Am. J. Med., 86* (suppl. 6A), 127 (1989).

451   M. Paakonen et al., *Am. J. Med., 86* (suppl. 6A), 133 (1989).

452   B. May, *Meth. Find. Exp. Clin. Pharmacol., 11* (suppl. 1), 113–116 (1989).

453   J. H. Yuk et al., *J. Am. Med., Assoc., 262 (7)*, 901 (1989).

454   B. Wallmark and P. Lindberg, *ISI Atlas of Science: Pharmacol., 1*, 158–161 (1987).

455   B. Wallmark, *Meth. Find. Exp. Clin. Pharmacol., 11* (suppl. 1), 101–106 (1989).

456   C. G. Regardh, *Scand. J. Gastroenterol., 118* (suppl.), 79–94, (1985).

457 C. W. Howden et al., *Eur. J. Clin. Pharmacol.*, *26*, 641–643 (1984).

458 C. G. Regardh et al., *Scand. J. Gastroenterol.*, *108* (suppl.), 79–94 (1985).

459 J. Naesdal et al., *Clin. Pharmacol. Ther.*, *40*, 344–351 (1986).

460 P. J. Prichard et al., *Gastroenterology*, *88*, 64–69 (1985).

461 M. H. Adams et al., *Clin. Pharm.*, *7 (10)*, 725–745 (1988).

462 S. Sandmark et al., *Scand. J. Gastroenterol.*, *23*, 625–632 (1988).

463 M. Ruth et al., *Scand. J. Gastroenterol.*, *23*, 1141–1146 (1988).

464 G. Vantrappen et al., *Dig. Dis. Sci.*, *33 (5)*, 523–529 (1988).

465 A. Walan et al., *N. Engl. J. Med.*, *320 (2)*, 69–75 (1989).

466 D. J. Hetzel et al., *Gastroenterol.*, *95*, 903–912 (1988).

467 J.-C. Delchier et al., *Gut*, *30*, 1173–1178 (1989).

468 P. N. Maton et al., *Gastroenterology*, *97*, 827–36 (1989).

469 A. Walan, *Meth. Find. Exp. Clin. Pharmacol.*, *11* (suppl. 1), 107–111 (1989).

470 C. W. Howden and J. L. Reid, *Eur. J. Clin. Pharmacol.*, *26*, 639–640 (1984).

471 B. Rybert et al., *Regulatory Peptides*, *25*, 235–246 (1989).

472 C. Simoens et al., *Gastroenterology*, *97*, 837–845 (1989).

473 S. Lanzon-Miller et al., *Aliment. Pharmacol. Therap.*, *1*, 239–251 (1987).

474 P. J. Prichard et al., *Br. J. Clin. Pharmacol.*, *24*, 543–545 (1987).

475 R. Gugler and J. C. Jensen, *Gastroenterology*, *89*, 1235–1241 (1985).

476 J. P. Monk and S. P. Clissold, *Drugs*, *33*, 1–30 (1987).

477 D. E. Wilson et al., *Dig. Dis. Sci.*, *31*, 126S–129S (1986).

478 T. A. Miller, *Am. J. Physiol.*, *245*, G601–G623 (1983).

479 G. Schoenhard et al., *Dig. Dis. Sci.*, *30*, 126S–128S (1985).

480 A. Karim, *Prostaglandins*, *33* (suppl.), 40–50 (1987).

481 A. Karim and P. Nicholson, in "Treatments and Prevention of NSAID-induced Gastropathy," R. Cheli, Ed., Royal Society of Medical Services, New York, N.Y., 1989, pp. 43–54.

482 A. Karim et al., *Postgrad. Med. J.*, *64* (suppl. 1), 80 (1988).

483 R. L. Herting and G. A. Clay, *Dig. Dis. Sci.*, *30*, 185S–193S (1985).

484 R. A. Wildeman, *Clin. Invest. Med.*, *10*, 243–245 (1987).

485 P. Bright-Asare et al., *Drugs*, *35* (suppl. 3), 1–9 (1988).

486 J. H. B. Saunders et al., *Br. Med. J.*, *1*, 418 (1977).

487 A. Berstad et al., *Scand. J. Gastroenterol.*, *15* (58), 46 (1980).

488 W. L. Peterson et al., *Gastroenterol.*, *77*, 1015 (1979).

489 G. S. Wagby, *Gastroenterol.*, *74*, 7 (1978).

490 H. Abrahamsson and G. Dotevall, *Scand. J. Gastroenterol.*, *14* (55), 17 (1979).

491 K. F. R. Sewing et al., *Gut*, *21*, 750 (1980).

492 S. Kaojarern et al., *Clin. Pharmacol. Ther.*, *29*, 198 (1981).

493 *Br. Med. J.*, *3*, 95 (1980).

494 L. Olbe et al., *Scand. J. Gastroenterol.*, *14* (55), 131 (1979).

495 C. Johansson and B. Kollberg, *Scand. J. Gastroenterol.*, *14* (55), 126 (1979).

496 S. Wetterhas et al., *Scand. J. Gastroenterol.*, *14* (55), 124 (1979).

497 S. K. Lam et al., *Gastroenterol.*, *76*, 322 (1979).

498 A. Hurwitz, *Clin. Pharmacokinet.*, *2*, 269 (1977).

499 J. E. Banos and O. Bulbena, *Meth. Find. Exp. Clin. Pharmacol.*, *11* (suppl. 1), 117–122 (1989).

500 J. Christiansen et al., *Gastroenterology*, *97*, 568–74 (1989).

501 J. A. Romankiewicz, *Primary Care*, *3*, 537 (1976).

502 S. Khalil and M. Moustafa, *Pharmazie*, *28*, 116 (1973).

503 *Br. Med. J.*, *2*, 405 (1975).

504 M. Gibaldi et al., *Clin. Pharmacol. Ther.*, *16*, 520 (1974).

505 M. Gibaldi et al., *J. Pharm. Sci.*, *64*, 2003 (1975).

506 J. W. Ayers et al., *Eur. J. Clin. Pharmacol.*, *12*, 415 (1977).

507 S. K. Khalil et al., *Pharmazie*, *31*, 105 (1976).

508 W. H. Barr et al., *Clin. Pharmacol. Ther.*, 12, 779 (1971).

509 M. Garty and A. Hurwitz, *Clin. Pharmacol. Ther.*, *28*, 203 (1980).

510 "Evaluations of Drug Interactions," 2nd ed., American Pharmaceutical Association, Washington, D.C., 1976, pp. 227–230.

511 G. Ekenved et al., *Scand. J. Haematol.*, *28* (Suppl.) 65 (1976).

512 P. F. D'Arcy and J. C. McElany, *DICP*, *21*, 607–617 (1987).

513 G. K. Hoffken et al., *Eur. J. Clin. Microbiol.*, *4*, 345 (1985).

514 T. A. Golper et al., *Antimicrob. Agents Chemother.*, *31*, 1787–1790 (1987).

515 W. Bianchi et al., *Antimicrob. Agents Chemother.*, *32 (6)*, 65 (1988).

516 S. A. Khalil, *J. Pharm. Pharmacol.*, *26*, 961 (1974).

517 D. D. Brown and R. P. Juhl, *N. Engl. J. Med.*, *295*, 1034 (1976).

518 W. E. Fann et al., *J. Clin. Pharmacol.*, *13*, 388 (1973).

519 F. M. Forrest et al., *Biol. Psychiatry*, *2*, 53 (1970).

520 J. A. Romankiewicz et al., *Am. Heart J.*, *96*, 518 (1978).

521 M. B. Zinn, *Tex. Med.*, *66*, 64 (1970).

522 V. F. Naggar et al., *Pharmazie*, *31*, 461 (1976).

523 H. W. Emori et al., *Am. Rheum. Dis.*, *35*, 333 (1976).

524 R. L. Galeazzi, *Euro. J. Clin. Pharmacol.*, *12*, 65 (1977).

525 R. K. Nayak et al., *J. Pharmacokin. Biopharm.*, *5*, 597 (1977).

526 B. Strickland-Hodge et al., *Rheumatol. Rehabil.*, *15*, 148 (1976).

527 S. Feldman and B. C. Carlstedt, *J. Am. Med. Assoc.*, *227*, 660 (1974).

528 G. Levy et al., *N. Engl. J. Med.*, *293*, 323 (1975).

529 F. Gaspari et al., *Am. J. Kid. Dis.*, *11 (4)*, 338–342.

530 L. Rivera-Calimlim et al., *Euro. J. Clin. Invest.*, *1*, 313 (1971).

531 G. B. T. Pocelinko and H. M. Solomon, *Clin. Pharmacol. Ther.*, *13*, 149 (1972).

532 A. S. Leon and H. E. Spiegel, *J. Clin. Pharmacol.*, *12*, 263 (1972).

533 V. F. Naggar et al., *J. Pharm. Sci.*, *67*, 1029 (1978).

534 R. L. Galleazzi et al., *Schweiz. Mediz. Wochen.*, *103*, 1021 (1973).

535 M. Uribe et al., *Gastroenterology*, 80, 661 (1981).

536 H. Bergrem et al., *Scand. J. Urol. Nephrol.*, *64* (suppl.), 167 (1981).

537 V. F. Naggar and S. A. Khalil, *Clin. Pharmacol. Ther.*, *25*, 857 (1979).

538 R. Mantyla et al., *Int. J. Clin. Pharmacol. Ther. and Tox.*, *22*, 626 (1984).

539 R. Gugler et al., *Eur. J. Clin. Pharmacol.*, *20*, 225 (1981).

540 W. M. Steinberg et al., *N. Engl. J. Med.*, *307*, 400 (1982).

541 G. W. Mihaly et al., *Br. Med. J.*, *285*, 998 (1982).

542 F. N. Eshelman et al., *Clin. Pharmacol. Ther.*, *33*, 216 (1983).

543 K. Frislid and A. Berstad, *Br. Med. J.*, *286*, 1358 (1983).

544 H. Albin et al., *Eur. J. Clin. Pharmacol.*, *32*, 97–99 (1987).

545 J. H. Lin et al., *Br. J. Clin. Pharmacol.*, *24*, 551–553 (1987).

546 N. Barzaghi et al., *J. Clin. Pharmacol.*, *29*, 670–672 (1989).

547 J. W. M. Vandermeer et al., *J. Antimicrob. Chemo. Ther.*, *6*, 552 (1980).

548 W. H. Wu et al., *J. Pharm. Sci.*, *59*, 1234 (1970).

549 A. Hurwitz and D. L. Scholozman, *Am. Rev. Respir. Dis.*, *109*, 41 (1974).

550 J. J. Ambre and L. J. Fischer, *Clin. Pharmacol. Ther.*, *14*, 231 (1973).

551 D. S. Robinson et al., *Clin. Pharmacol. Ther.*, *12*, 491 (1971).

552 P. D. Hansten, "Drug Interactions," 4th ed., Lea & Febiger, Philadelphia, Pa., 1979, p. 36.

553 E. J. Segre et al., *N. Engl. J. Med.*, *291*, 582 (1974).

554 A. H. Beckett et al., *Lancet*, *1*, 302 (1965).

555 D. J. Greenblatt et al., *Clin. Pharmacol. Ther.*, *19*, 234 (1976).

556 S. G. Nair et al., *Br. J. Anaesth.*, *48*, 1175 (1976).

557 D. J. Greenblatt et al., *Clin. Pharmacol. Ther.*, *24*, 600 (1978).

558 H. L. Kutt, *Epilepsia*, *16*, 393 (1975).

559 D. J. Chapron et al., *Arch. Neurol.*, *36*, 436 (1979).

560 L. S. O'Brien et al., *Br. J. Clin. Pharmacol.*, *6*, 176 (1978).

561 V. K. Kulshrestha et al., *Br. J. Clin. Pharmacol.*, *6*, 177 (1978).

562 B. L. Carter et al., *Ther. Drug Monitor*, *3*, 333 (1981).

563 R. Lucarotti et al., *J. Pharm. Sci.*, *61*, 903 (1972).

564 J. H. Dobbs et al., *Curr. Ther. Res.*, *21*, 887 (1977).

565 C. G. Regardh et al., *Biopharm. Drug Dispos.*, *2*, 79 (1981).

566 W. Kirch et al., *Clin. Pharmacol. Ther.*, *30*, 429 (1981).

567 L. A. Arnold et al., *Am. J. Hosp. Pharm.*, *36*, 1059 (1979).

568 C. A. May et al., *Clin. Pharm.*, *1* (3), 244–247 (1982).

569 S. A. Khalil and M. Iwragwr, *J. Pharm. Pharmacol.*, *28*, 47 (1976).

570 T. E. Sand and S. Jacobsen, *Eur. J. Clin. Pharmacol.*, *19*, 453 (1981).

571 *FDA Consumer*, July–Aug. 1974 (DHEW Publication No. FDA-75-3003).

572 D. Drake and D. Hollander, *Ann. Intern. Med.*, *94*, 215 (1981).

ANTACID PRODUCT TABLE

Product (Manufacturer)	Dosage Form	Calcium Carbonate	Aluminum Hydroxide	Magnesium Oxide or Hydroxide	Magnesium Trisilicate	Sodium Content	Other Ingredients
Alamag (Goldline)	suspension	45 mg/ml	40 mg/ml (hydroxide)			NS[a]	mint flavor
Algenic Alka (Rugby)	liquid	6.3 mg/ml				NS[a]	magnesium carbonate, 82.4 mg/ml sodium alginate EDTA saccharin sorbitol
Algenic Alka Improved (Rugby)	chewable tablet		80 mg		20 mg	NS[a]	sodium bicarbonate butterscotch flavor
Algicon (Rorer)	chewable tablet		aluminum hydroxide and magnesium carbonate, 360 mg			5.06 mg	lemon swiss-creme flavor magnesium carbonate, 320 mg
Alka-Mints (Miles)	chewable tablet	850 mg				< 0.5 mg	sorbitol spearmint flavor
Alka-Seltzer Effervescent Antacid (Miles)	tablet					12.9 mEq	sodium bicarbonate, 958 mg citric acid, 832 mg potassium bicarbonate, 312 mg
Alka-Seltzer, Extra Strength (Miles)	effervescent tablet					588 mg	sodium bicarbonate, 1985 mg citric acid, 1000 mg aspirin, 500 mg
Alka-Seltzer, Flavored (Miles)	effervescent tablet					506 mg	sodium bicarbonate, 1710 mg citric acid, 1220 mg aspirin, 324 mg saccharin
Alka-Seltzer with Aspirin (Miles)	effervescent tablet					567 mg	sodium bicarbonate, 1916 mg citric acid, 1000 mg aspirin, 325 mg

ANTACID PRODUCT TABLE, continued

Product (Manufacturer)	Dosage Form	Calcium Carbonate	Aluminum Hydroxide	Magnesium Oxide or Hydroxide	Magnesium Trisilicate	Sodium Content	Other Ingredients
Alkets (Upjohn)	tablet	780 mg		65 mg		NS[a]	magnesium carbonate, 130 mg
Allimin (Health Care Industries)	tablet					NS[a]	garlic powder, 309 mg parsley powder
Almacone (Rugby)	chewable tablet suspension		200 mg 40 mg/ml	200 mg 40 mg/ml (hydroxide)		NS[a]	simethicone, 20 mg 4 mg/ml peppermint flavor
Almacone II (Rugby)	suspension		80 mg/ml	80 mg/ml (hydroxide)		NS[a]	simethicone, 8 mg saccharin sorbitol
Alma-Mag #4 Improved (Rugby)	chewable tablet		200 mg	200 mg (hydroxide)		NS[a]	simethicone, 25 mg sorbitol peppermint flavor
Alma-Mag, Improved (Rugby)	liquid		40 mg/ml	40 mg/ml (hydroxide)		NS[a]	simethicone, 5 mg/ml
Almora (Forest)	chewable tablet					NS[a]	magnesium gluconate, 500 mg
ALternaGel (Stuart)	suspension		120 mg/ml			0.5 mg/ml	simethicone
Alu-Cap (Riker)	capsule		475 mg			NS[a]	
Aludrox (Wyeth)	suspension		61.4 mg/ml	20.6 mg/ml (hydroxide)		0.46 mg/ml	simethicone saccharin sorbitol
Aluminum Hydroxide (Rugby)	tablet		600 mg			NS[a]	
Aluminum Hydroxide (Roxane)	tablet		608 mg (dried gel)			NS[a]	
Aluminum Hydroxide, Concentrated[b] (Roxane)	suspension		135 mg/ml			0.2-0.5 mg/ml	
Aluminum Hydroxide Gel (Various manufacturers)	suspension		64 mg/ml 120 mg/ml			NS[a]	
Alu-Tab (Riker)	tablet		600 mg			NS[a]	
Amitone (SmithKline Beecham)	tablet	350 mg				< 2 mg	mint flavor

ANTACID PRODUCT TABLE, continued

Product (Manufacturer)	Dosage Form	Calcium Carbonate	Aluminum Hydroxide	Magnesium Oxide or Hydroxide	Magnesium Trisilicate	Sodium Content	Other Ingredients
Amphojel (Wyeth-Ayerst)	tablet suspension		300 or 600 mg/ tablet 64 mg/ml			1.8 or 2.9 mg/ tablet < 2.3 mg/ 5 ml	sorbitol saccharin plain or peppermint flavor (all suspension)
Anta Gel (Halsey)	liquid		40 mg/ml	40 mg/ml (hydroxide)		NS[a]	simethicone, 4 mg/ml
Anta-Gel-II (Halsey)	liquid		80 mg/ml	80 mg/ml (hydroxide)		1.8 mg/ ml	simethicone, 6 mg/ml
Banacid (Buffington)	chewable tablet		NS[a]	NS[a] (hydroxide)	NS[a]	free	
Basaljel (Wyeth)	capsule tablet suspension		aluminum carbonate, equiv. to: 500 mg aluminum hydroxide/ capsule or tablet 80 mg aluminum hydroxide/ ml			2.8 mg/ capsule 2.8 mg/ tablet 2.9 mg/ 5 ml (suspension)	saccharin (suspension) sorbitol (suspension)
Bell/ans (C.S. Dent)	tablet					144 mg	sodium bicarbonate, 520 mg wintergreen ginger flavor
Bicalma (Ferndale)	chewable tablet	250 mg			300 mg	NS[a]	
BiSoDol (Whitehall)	tablet powder	194 mg/ tablet		178 mg/tablet		0.007 mEq/ tablet > 0.8 mEq/ tsp (powder)	sodium bicarbonate, 716 mg/tsp (powder) magnesium carbonate, 528 mg/tsp (powder) mint flavor
Bromo-Seltzer (Warner-Lambert)	granular effervescent salt					0.761 g	sodium bicarbonate, 2781 mg acetaminophen, 325 mg citric acid, 2224 mg
Calcilac (Schein)	tablet	420 mg				0.3 mg	glycine, 180 mg
Calcium Carbonate (Roxane)	tablet suspension	1250 mg/ tablet 100 mg/ml				NS[a]	
Calcium Carbonate (Various manufacturers)	tablet	500 mg 650 mg				NS[a]	

ANTACID PRODUCT TABLE, continued

Product (Manufacturer)	Dosage Form	Calcium Carbonate	Aluminum Hydroxide	Magnesium Oxide or Hydroxide	Magnesium Trisilicate	Sodium Content	Other Ingredients
Calglycine (Rugby)	chewable tablet	420 mg				NS[a]	glycine saccharin vanilla-spearmint flavor
Calglycine[b] (Rugby)	chewable tablet	420 mg				< 0.3 mg	glycine, 150 mg
Camalox (Rorer)	tablet suspension	250 mg/ tablet 50 mg/ml	225 mg/ tablet 45 mg/ml	200 mg/tablet 40 mg/ml (hydroxide)		0.04 mEq/ tablet 0.05 mEq/ ml	
Chooz (Schering-Plough)	gum tablet	500 mg				free	
Citrocarbonate (Upjohn)	granular effervescent salt					6.09 mEq/ ml	sodium bicarbonate, 200 mg/g sodium citrate anhydrous, 467 mg/g
Creamalin (Mentholatum)	tablet		248 mg	75 mg (hydroxide)		1.78 mEq	magnesium stearate cornstarch flavor mannitol sodium saccharin
Dialume (Armour)	tablet		500 mg (dried gel)			0.05 mEq	
Diatrol (Otis Clapp)	tablet	261 mg				NS[a]	pectin, 65 mg
Dicarbosil (SmithKline Beecham)	tablet	500 mg				0.12 mEq	peppermint oil
Di-Gel (Schering-Plough)	liquid		40 mg/ml (dried gel)	40 mg/ml (hydroxide)		free	simethicone, 4 mg/ml
Di-Gel, Advanced Formula (Schering-Plough)	chewable tablet	280 mg		128 mg (hydroxide)		free	simethicone, 20 mg mint or lemon/ orange flavor
Dimacid[b] (Otis Clapp)	chewable tablet	270 mg				NS[a]	magnesium carbonate, 97 mg fruit flavor
Duracid (Fielding)	chewable tablet	325 mg	aluminum hydroxide				magnesium carbonate, 175 mg
ENO (SmithKline Beecham)	powder					819 mg/ 5 ml	sodium tartrate, 1.6 g/ 5 ml sodium citrate, 1.2 g/5 ml
Equilet (Mission)	chewable tablet	500 mg				0.3 mg	

ANTACID PRODUCT TABLE, continued

Product (Manufacturer)	Dosage Form	Calcium Carbonate	Aluminum Hydroxide	Magnesium Oxide or Hydroxide	Magnesium Trisilicate	Sodium Content	Other Ingredients
Gas-X (Sandoz)						free	simethicone, 80 mg
Gas-X, Extra Strength (Sandoz)						free	simethicone, 125 mg
Gaviscon (Marion)	chewable tablet suspension		80 mg 6.3 mg/ml		20 mg	19 mg/ tablet	sodium bicarbonate, 70 mg/tablet alginic acid, 200 mg/ tablet magnesium carbonate, 27.5 mg/ml sodium alginate, 27.2 mg/ml
Gaviscon ESR (Marion)	tablet		160 mg			1.3 mEq	magnesium carbonate, 105 mg alginic acid, 200 mg
Gaviscon ESRF (Marion)	suspension		50.8 mg/ml			0.18 mEq/ ml	magnesium carbonate, 47.5 mg/ml sodium alginate, 20 mg/ ml
Gaviscon-2 (Marion)	chewable tablet		160 mg		40 mg	36.8 mg	sodium bicarbonate, 140 mg alginic acid, 400 mg
Gelusil (Parke-Davis)	chewable tablet liquid	200 mg/ tablet 40 mg/ml	200 mg/tablet 40 mg/ml (hydroxide)			free	chewable tablets: simethicone, 25 mg magnesium stearate mannitol sorbitol sugar liquid: simethicone, 5 mg/ml citric acid hydroxypropyl methylcellulose parabens sodium carboxymethyl cellulose sodium saccharin sorbitol solution xanthan gum

ANTACID PRODUCT TABLE, continued

Product (Manufacturer)	Dosage Form	Calcium Carbonate	Aluminum Hydroxide	Magnesium Oxide or Hydroxide	Magnesium Trisilicate	Sodium Content	Other Ingredients
Gelusil II (Parke-Davis)	chewable tablet liquid		400 mg/ tablet 80 mg/ml	400 mg/tablet 80 mg/ml (hydroxide)		free	chewable tablets: simethicone, 30 mg calcium stearate FD&C yellow #6 fumaric acid mannitol povidone sodium saccharin sorbitol sugar liquid: simethicone, 6 mg/ml citric acid hydroxypropyl methylcellulose sodium saccharin sorbitol solution xanthan gum
Genalac (Goldline)	chewable tablet	420 mg				NS[a]	glycine base
Glycate (Forest)	tablet	300 mg				NS[a]	glycine, 150 mg
Kessadrox (McKesson)	suspension		67 mg/ml	11 mg/ml (hydroxide)		0.08 mEq/ ml	peppermint oil sorbitol
Kolantyl (Lakeside)	gel		30 mg/ml	30 mg/ml (hydroxide)		< 5 mg/ 5 ml	alcohol, 0.2% benzyl alcohol, 0.3% citric acid flavors methylcellulose parabens saccharin sodium sodium lauryl sulfate sorbitol
Kudrox Double Strength (Schwartz Pharma Kremers Urban)	liquid		113 mg/ml	36 mg/ml (hydroxide)		≤ 15 mg/ 5 ml	
Liquid Antacid (McKesson)	liquid		67 mg/ml	11 mg/ml (hydroxide)		0.08 mEq/ ml	peppermint oil sorbitol
Losotron Plus (Dixon-Shane)	liquid					NS[a]	magaldrate, 108 mg/ml simethicone, 4 mg/ml

ANTACID PRODUCT TABLE, continued

Product (Manufacturer)	Dosage Form	Calcium Carbonate	Aluminum Hydroxide	Magnesium Oxide or Hydroxide	Magnesium Trisilicate	Sodium Content	Other Ingredients
Lowsium (Rugby)	chewable tablet suspension					< 0.5 mg/ tablet NS[a] (suspension)	magaldrate, 480 mg/ tablet 108 mg/ml simethicone, 20 mg/tablet 4 mg/ml
Lowsium Plus (Rugby)	tablet suspension					NS[a]	magaldrate, 480 mg/ tablet 108 mg/ml simethicone, 20 mg/tablet 4 mg/ml
Maalox (Rorer)	tablet suspension		200 mg/ tablet 45 mg/ml (dried gel)	200 mg/tablet 40 mg/ml (hydroxide)		0.03 mEq/ tablet 0.06 mEq/ ml	
Maalox Extra Strength (Rorer)	tablet		400 mg (dried gel)	400 mg (hydroxide)		0.06 mEq/ tablet	
Maalox Plus (Rorer)	tablet		200 mg, dried gel	200 mg (hydroxide)		0.03 mEq/ tablet	simethicone, 25 mg
Maalox Plus, Extra Strength (Rorer)	suspension		100 mg/ml	90 mg/ml (hydroxide)		0.05 mEq/ml	simethicone, 8 mg/ml
Maalox Plus, Extra Strength[b] (Rorer)	liquid		100 mg/ml	90 mg/ml (hydroxide)		1.2 mg/ 5 ml	simethicone, 8 mg/ml saccharin sorbitol
Maalox TC (Rorer)	tablet suspension		600 mg/ tablet 120 mg/ml (dried gel)	300 mg/tablet 60 mg/ml (hydroxide)		0.03 mEq/ ml 0.02 mEq/ tablet	
Magnagel (Hauck)	tablet					NS[a]	aluminum hydroxide and magnesium carbonate, 325 mg
Magna Gel (Vortech)	suspension		45 mg/ml (dried gel)	40 mg/ml (hydroxide)		NS[a]	peppermint flavor
Magnatril (Lannett)	chewable tablet suspension	16 mg/ml	260 mg/ tablet 30 mg/ml	130 mg/tablet (hydroxide)	455 mg/tablet 80 mg/ml	NS[a]	
Magnesia and Alumina Oral Suspension (Roxane)	suspension		44 mg/ml	40 mg/ml (hydroxide)		0.07 mEq/ ml	sorbitol, 15% peppermint
Mag-Ox 400 (Blaine)	tablet			400 mg (oxide)		free	
Mallamint[b] (Hauck)	chewable tablet	420 mg				< 0.1 mg	mint flavor
Maox (Kenneth Manne)	tablet			420 mg (hydroxide)		NS[a]	tartrazine

ANTACID PRODUCT TABLE, continued

Product (Manufacturer)	Dosage Form	Calcium Carbonate	Aluminum Hydroxide	Magnesium Oxide or Hydroxide	Magnesium Trisilicate	Sodium Content	Other Ingredients
Marblen (Fleming)	tablet suspension[b]	520 mg/ tablet 104 mg/ml				3.2 mg/ tablet 3 mg/ 5 ml	magnesium carbonate, 400 mg/ tablet 80 mg/ml peach-apricot flavor
Mi-Acid (Major)	liquid		40 mg/ml	40 mg/ml (hydroxide)		NS[a]	simethicone, 4 mg/ml
Milk of Magnesia (Various manufacturers)	tablet liquid			325 mg/tablet 78 mg/ml (hydroxide)		NS[a](tablet) 0.12 mg/ 5 ml (liquid)	
Mintox (Major)	suspension		45 mg/ml	40 mg/ml (hydroxide)		NS[a]	simethicone, 5 mg/ml mint flavor
Mintox Plus (Major)	liquid		45 mg/ml	40 mg/ml (hydroxide)		NS[a]	simethicone, 5 mg/ml lemon flavor
Mygel (Geneva Generics)	suspension		40 mg/ml	40 mg/ml (hydroxide)		NS[a]	simethicone, 4 mg/ml
Mylanta (Stuart)	tablet suspension	200 mg/ tablet 40 mg/ml		200 mg/tablet 40 mg/ml (hydroxide)			simethicone, 20 mg/tablet 4 mg/ml
Mylanta II (Stuart)	tablet suspension	400 mg/ tablet 80 mg/ml		400 mg/tablet 80 mg/ml (hydroxide)			simethicone, 40 mg/tablet 8 mg/ml
Mylicon (Stuart)	chewable tablet						simethicone, 40 mg calcium silicate lactose povidone saccharin
Mylicon Drops (Stuart)	drop						simethicone, 40 mg/0.6 ml carbomer 934 P citric acid red #3 hydroxypropyl methylcellulose saccharin sodium benzoate sodium citrate
Mylicon-80 (Stuart)	chewable tablet						simethicone, 80 mg cereal solids lactose mannitol povidone red #3 talc

ANTACID PRODUCT TABLE, continued

Product (Manufacturer)	Dosage Form	Calcium Carbonate	Aluminum Hydroxide	Magnesium Oxide or Hydroxide	Magnesium Trisilicate	Sodium Content	Other Ingredients
Mylicon-125 (Stuart)	chewable tablet						simethicone, 125 mg cereal solids lactose mannitol povidone red #3 talc
Nephrox[b] (Fleming)	suspension		64 mg/ml			3.3 mg/ 5 ml	mineral oil, 10% watermelon flavor
Neutralin (Dover)	tablet		NS[a]	NS[a]		free	
Noralac (Vortech)	chewable tablet	227 mg				NS[a]	magnesium carbonate, 130 mg bismuth sub-nitrate, 32 mg
Nutramag (Cenci)	suspension			NS[a]		NS[a]	aluminum oxide
Phillips' Milk of Magnesia (Glenbrook)	tablet suspension			311 mg/tablet 80 mg/ml		0.1 mEq/ tablet NS[a] (sus-pension)	
Phosphaljel[a] (Wyeth-Ayerst)	suspension		46.6 mg/ml			7 mg/ 5 ml	
Riopan (Whitehall)	chewable tablet tablet suspension					≤ 0.004 mEq/ tablet ≤ 0.004 mEq/ 5 ml	magaldrate, 480 mg/ tablet 108 mg/ml
Riopan Extra Strength (Whitehall)	liquid					< 0.3 mg/ 5 ml	magaldrate, 216 mg/ml
Riopan Plus (Whitehall)	chewable tablet suspension					≤ 0.004 mEq/ tablet ≤ 0.004 mEq/ 5 ml	simethicone, 20 mg/tablet 4 mg/ml magaldrate, 480 mg/ tablet 108 mg/ml
Riopan Plus, Extra Strength (Whitehall)	chewable tablet suspension					≤ 0.021 mEq/ tablet ≤ 0.013 mEq/5 ml	simethicone, 30 mg/tablet 6 mg/ml magaldrate, 1080 mg/ tablet 216 mg/ml
Rolaids (Warner-Lambert)	chewable tablet					53 mg	dihydroxy-aluminum sodium car-bonate, 334 mg

ANTACID PRODUCT TABLE, continued

Product (Manufacturer)	Dosage Form	Calcium Carbonate	Aluminum Hydroxide	Magnesium Oxide or Hydroxide	Magnesium Trisilicate	Sodium Content	Other Ingredients
Rolaids Calcium Rich (Warner-Lambert)	chewable tablet	550 mg				< 0.4 mg	cherry or fruit flavor
Rolaids Sodium Free (Warner-Lambert)	chewable tablet	317 mg		64 mg (hydroxide)		< 0.4 mg	
Rulox (Rugby)	suspension		45 mg/ml	40 mg/ml (hydroxide)		0.82 mg/ 5 ml	simethicone, 5 ml/ml
Rulox #1 (Rugby)	chewable tablet		200 mg	200 mg (hydroxide)		NS[a]	mint flavor
Rulox #2 (Rugby)	chewable tablet		400 mg	400 mg (hydroxide)		NS[a]	sorbitol mint flavor
Simaal Gel (Schein)	liquid		40 mg/ml	40 mg/ml (hydroxide)		NS[a]	simethicone, 4 mg/ml saccharin sorbitol
Simaal 2 Gel (Schein)	liquid		80 mg/ml	80 mg/ml (hydroxide)		NS[a]	simethicone, 6 mg/ml
Soda Mint (Various manufacturers)	tablet					NS[a]	sodium bicarbonate, 325 mg
Sodium Bicarbonate (Various manufacturers)	tablet					NS[a]	sodium bicarbonate, 325 mg 650 mg
Spastosed (Vortech)	tablet	226 mg (precipitated)				NS[a]	magnesium carbonate, 162 mg
Tempo Drops (Thompson Medical)	chewable tablet	414 mg	133 mg	81 mg		free	simethicone, 20 mg
Titracid (Trimen)	chewable tablet	420 mg				NS[a]	glycine, 180 mg mint flavor
Titralac[b] (3M Personal Care)	chewable tablet	420 mg/ tablet				< 0.3 mg	glycine, 150 mg/ tablet spearmint flavor
Titralac Plus[b] (3M Personal Care)	liquid	100 mg/ml				0.0001 mg/ ml	simethicone, 4 mg/ml
Triconsil (Geneva Generics)	chewable tablet		80 mg		80 mg	50.6 mg	sodium bicarbonate, 200 mg
Trimagel (Columbia Medical)	tablet		250 mg (dried gel)		500 mg	NS[a]	
Tums (SmithKline Beecham)	tablet	500 mg				0.12 mEq	peppermint oil

ANTACID PRODUCT TABLE, continued

Product (Manufacturer)	Dosage Form	Calcium Carbonate	Aluminum Hydroxide	Magnesium Oxide or Hydroxide	Magnesium Trisilicate	Sodium Content	Other Ingredients
Tums Extra Strength (SmithKline Beecham)	liquid	200 mg/ml				< 1 mg/ml	sorbitol peppermint flavor
Tums E-X Extra Strength (SmithKline Beecham)	chewable tablet	750 mg				≤ 2 mg	wintergreen or fruit flavor
Uro-Mag (Blaine)	capsule			140 mg (oxide)		free	
WinGel (Winthrop)	tablet suspension		180 mg/tablet 36 mg/ml	160 mg/tablet 32 mg/ml		0.1 mEq/tablet 0.02 mEq/ml	mint flavor

[a] Quantity not specified.
[b] Sugar free.
[c] Contains the dye tartrazine.

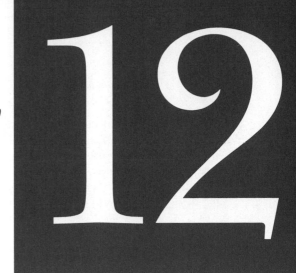

Gary M. Oderda and Barbara H. Korberly

EMETIC AND ANTIEMETIC PRODUCTS

*Q*uestions *to ask in patient/consumer counseling*

Emetics

Do you want the emetic for immediate emergency use or possible future use?

Whom is the medication for?

How old is the patient?

What substance was ingested?

How long ago did the ingestion occur?

How much was taken?

Has the patient already been given something for the ingestion?

What symptoms is the patient showing?

Antiemetics

Do you know what has caused the nausea and vomiting?

Whom is the medication for?

How old is the patient? Is the patient pregnant?

How long has the nausea or vomiting been present?

Have you noted blood in the vomitus that resembles coffee grounds?

Have you noted other symptoms such as abdominal pain, headache, or diarrhea?

What medications are currently being taken?

What other medical problems does the patient have?

Severe nausea and the realization that one is about to vomit are two of the more unpleasant symptoms an individual may have. However disagreeable the sensation, vomiting (emesis) is an important defense mechanism for ridding the body of a variety of toxins and poisons; vomiting can also be caused by travel (i.e., motion sickness) or pregnancy.

Nonprescription antiemetics have been used to prevent or control the symptoms of nausea and vomiting primarily due to motion sickness, pregnancy, and mild infectious diseases. Some nonprescription antiemetics are promoted for the relief of such vague symptoms as "upset stomach," "indigestion," and "distention" associated with excessive food indulgence, although their value in treating these complaints is not well documented.

Nonprescription emetic drugs are used to induce vomiting primarily in the treatment of poisoning.

Nausea and vomiting associated with radiation therapy, cancer chemotherapy, and serious metabolic and endocrine disorders are not appropriate conditions for self-medication and are not covered in this chapter.

THE VOMITING PROCESS

Vomiting is a complex process involving both the central nervous system (CNS) and the gastrointestinal (GI) system (Figure 1). The reflex is mediated by a "vomiting center" located in the medulla oblongata. The vomiting center itself does not carry out the function of vomiting but rather coordinates the activities of other neural structures to produce a patterned response. The vomiting center receives stimuli from peripheral areas, such as the gastric mucosa, in addition to stimuli from areas within the CNS itself, in part through the coordination of the chemoreceptor trigger zone (CTZ). Stimulation of the CTZ, which is the afferent pathway to the vomiting center, is responsible for its activation and may be involved in eliciting nausea and vomiting from a variety of causes (1, 2). Nausea is an unpleasant sensation that is vaguely associated with the epigastrium and abdomen; nausea usually precedes vomiting. Retching is a strong involuntary effort to vomit.

Centrally acting emetics work primarily by stimulating the CTZ, while centrally active antiemetics inhibit the CTZ. In addition to stimuli from the CTZ, impulses from the GI tract and the labyrinth apparatus in the ear are received at the vomiting center. Stimuli then are sent to the abdominal musculature, stomach, and esophagus to initiate vomiting. (See Chapter 3, *Antacid Products.*)

Vomiting begins with a deep inspiration, closing of the glottis, and depression of the soft palate. A forceful contraction of the diaphragm and abdominal musculature occurs, producing an increase in intrathoracic and intra-abdominal pressure that compresses the stomach and raises esophageal pressure. The body of the stomach and the esophageal musculature relax. The positive intrathoracic and intra-abdominal pressure moves stomach contents into the esophagus and mouth. Several cycles of reflux into the esophagus occur before the actual vomiting (3). Regurgitation is the casting up of stomach contents without oral expulsion. Vomitus is expelled from the esophagus by a combination of increased intrathoracic pressure and reverse peristaltic waves (4, 5). Normally, the glottis closes off the trachea

and prevents the vomitus from entering the airway. Aspiration of the vomitus may occur in some cases (for example, in patients with CNS depression).

Vomiting is a symptom produced by benign processes as well as by significant, serious illnesses. The practitioner should be aware of the possibility that patients using nonprescription antiemetics may be self-treating the early stages of a serious illness. Nausea and vomiting are common side effects of most oral medications and some parenteral and topical drugs. Knowledge of the patient's drug history is important in assessing the cause of nausea and vomiting. Nausea and vomiting may be caused by pregnancy or cancer chemotherapy or be symptoms of diverse disorders such as hypothyroidism, pyelonephritis, renal calculi, acute appendicitis, cholecystitis, migraine headache, food allergy, or radiation. Vomiting may produce complications including dehydration, aspiration, malnutrition, and electrolyte and acid–base abnormalities.

Overstimulation of the labyrinth apparatus produces the nausea and vomiting of motion sickness. The three semicircular canals on each side of the head in the inner ear (labyrinth) are responsible for maintaining equilibrium. Postural adjustments are made when the brain receives nervous impulses initiated by the movement of fluid in the semicircular canals. Some individuals are more tolerant than others to the effect of a particular type of motion, but no one is immune. Moreover, it appears that individuals can vary in their susceptibility to various kinds of motions, such as flying and boat riding (6). Motion sickness may be produced by unusual motion patterns in which the head is rotated in two axes simultaneously. Mechanisms other than the stimulation of the semicircular canals also are important. Erroneous interpretation of visual stimuli by stationary subjects watching a film taken from a roller coaster or an airplane doing aerobatics or simply extending the head upward while standing on a rotating platform can produce motion sickness. Regardless of the type of stimulus-producing event, motion sickness is much easier to prevent than to treat once it has already begun.

The mechanism of vomiting, or "morning sickness," of pregnancy has not been established. One-half of all pregnant women experience nausea, and about one-third suffer vomiting (7). Increased levels of chorionic gonadotropin have been implicated as a cause of morning sickness because levels of this hormone are highest during early pregnancy when nausea and vomiting are most common (7, 8). Other research suggests that there is no relationship between chorionic gonadotropin levels and morning sickness (9). Nausea and vomiting of pregnancy are difficult symptoms to treat, partly because no agent seems to be completely effective, but more importantly because of the concern that drug use during pregnancy should be restricted when-

STIMULI	MECHANISM	VOMITING

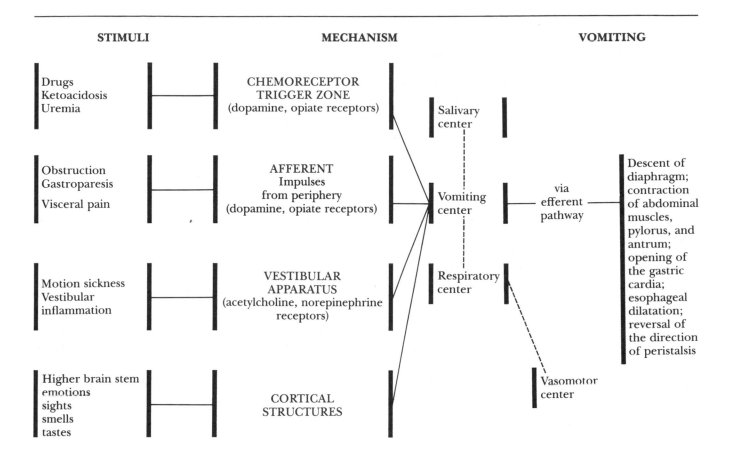

FIGURE 1   Causes, treatments, and mechanisms of vomiting. Adapted with permission from R. S. Finley, in "Applied Therapeutics: The Clinical Use of Drugs," 4th ed., L. Y. Young and M. A. Koda-Kimble, Eds., Applied Therapeutics, Vancouver, Wash., 1988, p. 86.

ever possible because of the potential for teratogenic effects (8).

Acute transient attacks of vomiting, in association with diarrhea, are very common. Fever may be slight or absent. No precise figure is available for the incidence of this "viral gastroenteritis," although this usually harmless, self-limiting disorder may affect any age group and can occur in sizable outbreaks (7).

tal poisonings occur frequently in children under 5 years of age. During 1988, 61 poison centers throughout the United States, serving a population of 155.7 million, submitted 1,368,748 cases to the American Association of Poison Control Centers data collection system (10). Included in these cases were 545 fatalities (10). Mortality data alone do not adequately describe the problem. Many additional poisonings go unreported even though they result in significant morbidity and mortality.

EMETICS

Incidence of Poisoning

Emetics are used most commonly for the treatment of poisoning, both accidental and intentional. Acciden-

Emergency Treatment with a Nonprescription Emetic

Emetics remove potentially toxic agents from the stomach. It is often difficult to decide whether a patient should be referred directly to an emergency treatment facility or should be given a nonprescription emetic and managed at home. Obtaining a reliable history, identifying the agent, and accurately assessing the patient's condition are critical in making this decision. Knowing the telephone number of the nearest poison control center is also extremely important. All ingestions where moderate to severe toxicity is expected must be referred to an emergency treatment facility. If minimal toxicity (no serious or life-threatening symptoms) is anticipated, the administration of a nonprescription emetic at home by a competent adult may be all that is necessary. Many ingestions reported to poison control centers fall into this category. For example, a child who ingests 150–300 mg/kg of aspirin can usually be treated at home by emesis induced with syrup of ipecac and appropriate follow-up.

To determine whether administration of a nonprescription emetic is appropriate or whether the patient should be referred, the following information must be obtained.

Name of Product Ingested

The ingredients and the amount of each ingredient can be determined once the name of the ingested product is known. The product label or container, if available, may list ingredients and the name of the manufacturer (11, 12). Then the potential toxicity of each ingredient must be investigated.

Amount Ingested

The amount ingested is frequently difficult to determine. For example, a child is found with an empty bottle of medication, and no one is quite sure how full the bottle was before ingestion. A parent often underestimates the amount consumed or provides unreliable information. For example, a parent reports that a child has taken two digoxin tablets. To substantiate the consumption of only two tablets, the parent may respond that the child was alone only for a short period or that the tablets had an unpleasant taste.

Drugs can be both therapeutic agents and poisons, depending on the dose. Thus, a 2-year-old who takes two children's aspirin tablets would require no treatment; the same child who takes 15 adult aspirin tablets may be severely poisoned.

Time Since Ingestion

The time since ingestion is important because an emetic is useful only if a sufficient amount of the ingested substance remains in the stomach. Thus, an emetic is not recommended after ingestion of quickly absorbed agents if several hours have elapsed. The use of an emetic may be rational several hours after ingestion of some agents that are slow to leave the stomach.

Drugs that slow gastric emptying and GI motility include anticholinergics, such as atropine and scopolamine, as well as drugs that have anticholinergic activity, such as antihistamines, antidepressants, and phenothiazines.

Symptoms

Certain symptoms contraindicate the use of emetics. For example, if CNS depression or other significant symptoms such as lethargy, ataxia, hallucinations, or seizures are present, a nonprescription emetic at home should not be used. Because of the potential for significant life-threatening toxic effects occurring in these patients, they must be referred to a physician or emergency room staff for immediate treatment.

Patient's Age and Weight

Much toxicity information is given on a dose-per-body weight basis (mg/kg). Thus, knowledge of the patient's weight is needed to determine appropriate treatment. The patient's age may help to determine the appropriateness and dose of an emetic.

Prior Treatment

Has any first aid, or other procedure, been performed? Some procedures, such as the use of salt water as an emetic, may affect the toxicity and change further recommendations.

Name and Location of Patient

If talking with the patient by phone, the pharmacist should ask for the patient's name and location in case the call is cut off and to allow for follow-up.

Appropriate information should be sought to help answer the following questions: Is an emetic indicated? Are there any contraindications to using an emetic? Can the emetic be administered safely outside an emergency treatment facility? Poison control centers are available to help pharmacists answer these questions or handle referrals. Pharmacists should be able to contact the nearest poison control center. A list of certified regional poison control centers is currently printed in the *Merck Index,* the *Physician's Desk Reference*, the *Drug Topics Red Book*, and in the appendix at the end of this chapter.

Treatment of Poisoning

The mainstay of treatment in poisoning cases is the provision of symptomatic and supportive care. Support of vital functions, especially respiratory and cardiovascular, is critical. Treatment of specific symptoms such as seizures also is important. Most patients will detoxify themselves and survive with only symptomatic and supportive care. Other specific treatments, including emptying the stomach and administering agents such as adsorbents, cathartics, or antidotes, do not replace the need for symptomatic and supportive care.

Stomach contents may be removed by administering an emetic or by lavage. Gastric lavage is a procedure in which a tube is placed into the stomach through the mouth or nose and the esophagus. Fluid then is instilled into the tube, allowed to mix with stomach contents, and removed through suction or aspiration. Emetics and lavage are most effective if used within 4 hours of ingestion of readily absorbed drugs (13).

The efficacy of ipecac treatment and lavage in removing gastric contents was compared in 20 patients, 12–20 months of age, who had ingested salicylates (14). Each patient was lavaged with a small nasogastric tube and also given syrup of ipecac, and the amount of salicylate returned was measured. Approximately one-half of the patients were lavaged first, and the others were given syrup of ipecac first. Ipecac was superior to lavage in removing salicylate. In patients who had vomited with ipecac, little more salicylate was removed by subsequent lavage.

In another study, two adult patients who had ingested aspirin were lavaged first with 3 liters of normal saline through a small (20 French, or 6.7 mm) tube 10–15 minutes after ingestion and then given syrup of ipecac (15). Twenty-five tablets from one patient and 10–15 tablets from the other patient were included in the vomitus following ipecac administration. Lavage alone would have left a toxic dose of aspirin in the stomach.

It also was shown that, under optimal conditions and immediately after ingestion, dogs given sodium salicylate returned 38% of the ingested dose after lavage and 45% after ipecac-induced emesis (16). Of greater significance were the results under delayed conditions wherein the procedure was not instituted for 30 minutes with emesis or 60 minutes with lavage. The lavage was done at approximately the same time emesis occurred. Delayed emesis recovered 39% of the administered dose, whereas delayed lavage recovered only 13% of the administered dose. In these studies, the lavage tube was considerably smaller than the 36–50 French (12.0–16.7 mm) orogastric tubes that are recommended for acute poisoning, and it is difficult to evaluate these data based on the larger tubes currently recommended. A prospective study using thiamine as a marker in overdosed patients found that lavage was superior to induced emesis (17). Eighteen fasting adult volunteers showed a mean regurgitation of 28% with ipecac and 45% with lavage using a 32 French

orogastric tube of administered cyanacobalamin (18). Concerns relating to methodology leave this issue unresolved (19). Ipecac syrup is the only method of induced emesis available for use in the home. In the hospital setting, both induced emesis and lavage are frequently used. Lavage is more frequently used on adults and induced emesis in children.

Contraindications to Emetics

CNS Depression or Seizures Efforts to induce vomiting should not be attempted in patients who are lethargic or comatose because vomiting may not be produced and, if it is, these patients are at high risk of aspirating gastric contents while vomiting. There is also a high risk of aspiration if vomiting occurs while a patient is experiencing a seizure. Emetics are generally not recommended when patients have taken agents that may produce a rapid decrease in level of consciousness (e.g., antidepressants) or agents that may rapidly produce seizures (e.g., camphor and amphetamines).

Caustic Ingestions Patients who have ingested a caustic substance should not be made to vomit. Caustic agents are strong acids and bases that can produce severe burns of the mucous membranes of the GI tract, including the mouth and esophagus. If emesis is induced, these tissues are reexposed to the caustic agent, and more damage may occur. In addition, if the esophagus is already damaged, the force of vomiting may cause esophageal or gastric perforation.

When ingestion of a caustic agent is suspected, the patient should immediately be given water or milk to drink (if the patient is conscious and able to drink) to dilute the caustic agents. Attempts to neutralize the caustic agent using an acid or base could generate heat and produce more serious injury and, therefore, must be avoided. Most patients who have ingested a caustic agent should be referred to a medical facility.

Controversial Areas

Antiemetic Drug Ingestion Emetic use in cases of undesired or excessive antiemetic drug ingestion is controversial. If an emetic is not given soon after an antiemetic has been ingested, a significant emetic failure rate may result. Two studies suggest that this is not a problem clinically (20, 21). If an emetic is given in the hospital setting and vomiting does not occur, gastric lavage may be necessary to remove the initially ingested antiemetic substance.

Hydrocarbon Ingestion Patients who have ingested aliphatic hydrocarbons (e.g., kerosene, gasoline, and furniture polish, many of which are petroleum distillates) traditionally have not been given emetics. It was thought that induced vomiting increased the likelihood of aspiration of the hydrocarbon into the lungs, leading to alveolar irritation and pneumonitis. Even though studies have shown that aspiration is not likely to occur when vomiting is induced, emptying the stomach of aliphatic hydrocarbons is generally not necessary because the systemic toxicity caused by them does not appear to be directly related to their absorption. However, when a potentially dangerous chemical such as a pesticide is dissolved in a hydrocarbon base, emptying the stomach may be necessary, and the use of syrup of ipecac is appropriate.

A retrospective study showed that of patients who had ingested petroleum distillates, a lower percentage developed aspiration pneumonitis when vomiting was induced with ipecac than with either lavage or spontaneous vomiting (22). Other research has shown that aspiration pneumonitis is less likely to occur in ipecac-treated patients than in those who were lavaged (23). The pneumonitis that developed in this study was less severe in the ipecac-treated patients than in those who were lavaged (23). Based on these findings, it was suggested that ipecac be used instead of gastric lavage for alert patients who ingested a hydrocarbon and that gastric removal is necessary.

Syrup of Ipecac

Syrup of ipecac is the emetic of choice. It is prepared from ipecac powder, a natural product derived from *Cephaelis ipecacuanha* or *acuminata*, and contains approximately 2.1 g of powdered ipecac per 30 ml. Vomiting probably is produced by both a local irritant effect on the GI mucosa and a central medullary effect (stimulation of the CTZ) (24). The central effect is probably caused by emetine and cephaeline, two alkaloids present in ipecac.

When a patient asks to purchase syrup of ipecac, the pharmacist should determine whether it is to be used immediately to treat a poison ingestion or is being purchased to keep in the home in the event an ingestion occurs. If the purchase is for immediate use, the pharmacist should determine whether that use is appropriate and if the local poison control center or other medical advisor has been contacted. If not, the pharmacist should contact the poison control center to alert it of the problem and to receive instructions on how to manage the ingestion and instruct the purchaser.

If the ipecac is being purchased for later use should an ingestion occur, the pharmacist should discuss poison prevention with the patient, distribute poison prevention materials, and provide the patient with the telephone number of the nearest poison control center. Additionally, the purchaser should be advised

that whenever possible in poisoning emergencies, syrup of ipecac should not be given without first consulting a poison control center, pharmacist, or physician.

Toxicity Toxicity following syrup of ipecac administration is rare. After therapeutic doses, diarrhea and slight CNS depression are common; mild GI upset may last for several hours following emesis. Clinical experience has shown that ingestion of 30 ml of syrup of ipecac (the largest amount available without a prescription in a single unit of purchase) is safe in children over 1 year of age. In larger doses, ipecac is cardiotoxic and may cause bradycardia, atrial fibrillation, and hypotension (25).

Fluidextract of ipecac is 14 times stronger than syrup of ipecac and should no longer be found in any pharmacy. Severe toxicity and death have occurred when fluidextract of ipecac was given by mistake (26–29).

The death of a 14-month-old child following administration of less than 30 ml of ipecac syrup given to her for an ingestion of amaryllis leaves was not a direct result of the pharmacologic effects of ipecac, but rather due to an anatomic defect (30). An additional fatality believed to be related to syrup of ipecac has been reported in an 84-year-old patient who had ingested a boric acid solution (31).

Pharmacists must be aware that syrup of ipecac is used inappropriately by some bulimic patients to remove food from the stomach and to lose weight. This practice is dangerous particularly because of electrolyte imbalance and cardiotoxicity. It is important, however, to recognize that the abuse problem does not warrant removing 1 oz bottles of syrup of ipecac from nonprescription status (32). Any person regularly buying syrup of ipecac should be questioned to be certain it is being used appropriately.

Dosages In children over 1 year of age, the recommended dose of syrup of ipecac is 15 ml (1 tbsp). Children under 1 year may be given 5–10 ml (1 to 2 tsp). Although home use of ipecac in children under 1 year of age is controversial, a recent study has shown that this practice is both safe and effective (32).

Ipecac does not work well if the stomach is nearly empty. Therefore, it is recommended that at least 6–8 oz of water be given to children and 12–16 ounces to adults immediately after the ipecac to partially distend the stomach. One study of adult volunteers given a 15-ml ipecac dose suggests that the time to induce vomiting is longer when milk is given with the ipecac than when other fluids are used (33). Another study of the time taken for vomiting to occur when overdosed children were given either milk or water with ipecac showed no difference in time for vomiting to occur (34). Use of clear fluids is preferred because administration of milk offers no advantages over the use of clear fluids and because the milk may obscure examination of the vomitus for regurgitated tablets and capsules. Vomiting should occur in 15–20 minutes. If vomiting has not occurred in 20 minutes, the initial dose of syrup of ipecac should be repeated.

The initial dose of syrup of ipecac for adolescents and adults is 15–30 ml and can be repeated once, if necessary. Syrup of ipecac is virtually 100% effective when 15 ml or more is given (35, 36). Whether the fluids are given before or after the ipecac or whether the fluids are tepid (104°F or 40°C) or cold (50°F or 10°C) does not affect the time for vomiting to occur (37, 38). Although no scientific evidence exists, patients who are ambulatory seem to vomit more quickly than those who are not. Therefore, children should be encouraged to play quietly rather than recline, and adults should be encouraged to move around. Stimulation of the posterior pharynx by inserting a finger into the throat also may help to induce vomiting, but care must be taken to avoid injury.

If the patient is to be brought to an emergency facility or physician's office, the patient should be made to vomit in a bucket or container so that the vomitus can be inspected for evidence of the poison. It is not necessary or advisable to wait for the patient to vomit before transporting. In case the patient vomits while en route for treatment, a bucket should be taken along.

Drug Interactions The only well-documented drug interaction with syrup of ipecac involves activated charcoal. Activated charcoal is used as an adsorbent in many poisoning cases. When it is administered with ipecac, the ipecac is adsorbed by the charcoal (39), and emesis is prevented. In addition, the adsorptive capacity of the charcoal is reduced. If both activated charcoal and ipecac are used, the activated charcoal must be given after successful vomiting has been induced by the ipecac.

Other Methods to Induce Emesis

Vomiting may be induced in numerous ways. Syrup of ipecac is the only safe and effective nonprescription emetic. Home remedies other than ipecac are frequently ineffective and, in some cases, dangerous.

Mechanically induced vomiting is produced by giving the patient fluids and then manually stimulating the gag reflex at the back of the throat with either a blunt object or a finger. Care must be taken not to injure the patient during this procedure. The percentage of persons who vomit following this procedure has been shown to be low, and the mean volume of vomitus is small compared with that induced by syrup of ipecac (40). However, if an emergency exists and no appropriate emetic or medical care is available, it may be a worthwhile initial effort to induce vomiting by mechanical stimulation.

Salt water is an unpalatable, unreliable, and potentially dangerous emetic. Salt water may be quite toxic because of sodium absorption; in fact, fatalities have been produced in children and adults from the use of salt as an emetic (41–45). If vomiting is not produced, severe hypernatremia may result. It is estimated that 1 tbsp of salt contains about 250 mEq of sodium. If retained and absorbed, this amount would raise the serum sodium level by 25 mEq/l in a 3-year-old child with an estimated total body water of 10 liters. Salt water should not be used under any circumstances (46).

Mustard water is an unreliable and unpalatable emetic and should not be routinely recommended.

Copper and zinc sulfate have been used as emetics and act by producing direct gastric irritation leading to reflex stimulation of the vomiting center. Copper sulfate is usually given in a dose of 150–250 mg dissolved in 30–60 ml of water. In three children who vomited soon after the administration of copper sulfate as an emetic, 54–67% of the dose was recovered in the vomitus (47). In the same study, all six children who had been given copper sulfate as an emetic had significant increases in serum copper levels (15–105 mcg/100 ml). However, no evidence of copper intoxication, such as jaundice or oliguria, was noted. Copper sulfate administered to another patient with a three-fourths gastrectomy caused renal failure and death (48). Based on the available data, copper sulfate is an effective emetic, but concerns about copper absorption and its potential toxicity preclude routine recommendation of this agent for the induction of emesis (49).

Apomorphine produces rapid emesis; however, it is available only by prescription and must be given parenterally. Apomorphine may produce or worsen CNS and respiratory depression. Naloxone can usually reverse these effects. In several cases, significant respiratory and/or CNS depression unresponsive to naloxone developed in patients who had been given apomorphine (50).

Liquid dishwashing detergent has been studied as an emetic agent (51). Although almost all patients who drank most of the administered solution vomited, many patients refused to drink any or all of the solution. The overall success rate in all patients, including those who refused the solution, was 10/15 (66.7%). Administration of liquid dishwashing solution should not replace the use of syrup of ipecac. In those situations where ipecac cannot be obtained in a timely fashion (e.g., weather, long distances) liquid dishwashing detergent can be considered. The pharmacist must be aware that the ingredients in liquid dishwashing products are subject to change and that toxic ingredients may be included in the future. For this reason, it would be appropriate to check with a poison control center or the manufacturer before recommending a given product. *It should also be noted that automatic dishwasher products and laundry detergents contain caustic ingredients and must never be used as an emetic.*

Activated Charcoal

Activated charcoal is an effective adsorbent for most drugs and chemicals. It is usually administered as a water slurry (60–100 g for adults and 15–30 g for children) in 250 ml of water. Because measuring the correct amount of charcoal is difficult, preweighed packages are available in glass or polyethylene containers. The slurry can be prepared by adding water to the container and shaking it (52). Activated charcoal preparations with a higher surface area (e.g., Superchar) have been developed; they are three times as effective as traditional charcoal (53). Products premixed with water, sorbitol, or water and carboxymethylcellulose are commercially available. When multiple doses of activated charcoal are given, a cathartic should be given only with the first dose. Pharmacists should check premixed charcoal products to see if they contain sorbitol. If they do, other cathartics should not be given and the sorbitol-containing product should be given only once. Optimally, charcoal should be given as soon as possible after ingestion; however, in some cases, it has been shown to be effective even when delayed by several hours. Although not effective for all ingestions, activated charcoal can reduce absorption of the many common causes of poisonings such as analgesics (e.g., salicylates, acetaminophen, and propoxyphene), sedative–hypnotics, and tricyclic antidepressants (Table 1). There is no systemic toxicity or maximum dose limit. Repeat doses of activated charcoal are recommended to interrupt enterohepatic recycling and to bind agents secreted into the GI tract following ingestion of some agents (e.g., phenobarbital, cyclic antidepressants, and theophylline). Contrary to popular belief, burnt toast is not a substitute for activated charcoal and is not indicated in the treatment of poisoning.

Previously, a "universal antidote" mixture of activated charcoal, magnesium oxide, and tannic acid was used. This combination is ineffective because the adsorptive capacity of the charcoal is diminished and may produce significant toxicity because of the tannic acid (54).

Following ingestion of activated charcoal, a saline cathartic such as magnesium sulfate may be administered if bowel sounds are present, to speed elimination of the charcoal–drug complex. The role of gastric emptying and activated charcoal in preventing absorption from the GI tract and toxicity is unclear. Studies have compared various combinations of gastric emptying, charcoal, and cathartics (55–57). Two of the studies used near-therapeutic doses or simulated overdoses in

TABLE 1	Compounds known to be effectively bound by activated charcoal in man or animals

Oral activated charcoal inhibits absorption of the following chemicals from the gastrointestinal tract[a]

Acetaminophen	Methyl salicylate
Aconitine	Nadolol
d-Amphetamine	Nicotine
Aspirin	Nortriptyline
Atropine	Paraquat
Barbital	Pentobarbital
Benzene	Phencyclidine
Carbamazepine	Phenobarbital
Chlordane	Phenylbutazone
Chloroquine	Phenylpropanolamine
Chlorpheniramine	Phenytoin
Chlorpromazine	Propantheline
Chlorpropamide	Propoxyphene
Digoxin	Quinine
Doxepin	Salicylamide
Ethchlorvynol	Secobarbital
Ethylene glycol	Sodium salicylate
Glutethimide	Sodium valproate
Hexachlorophene	Strychnine
Kerosene	Theophylline
Malathion	Tetracycline
Mefenamic acid	Tolbutamide
Mercuric chloride	Yohimbine

Multiple oral doses of activated charcoal accelerate body clearance of the following drugs[b]

Carbamezepine	Phenobarbital
Dapsone	Phenylbutazone
Digitoxin	Theophylline
Nadolol	

[a]Based on controlled experimental investigations in man or experimental animals.
[b]Not necessarily clinically significant.
Adapted with permission from "Medical Toxicology: Diagnosis and Treatment of Human Poisoning," 1st ed., M. Ellenhorn and D. Barceloux, Eds., Elsevier Science Publishing, New York, N.Y., 1988, p. 59.

human volunteers (55, 56). The final study was a randomized prospective study of overdose patients treated in an emergency room (57). The results of these three studies, although preliminary, suggest that using emetics in addition to the administration of activated charcoal and a cathartic may not improve efficacy at preventing absorption. In the home, activated charcoal is not a viable substitute for syrup of ipecac because it is difficult for parents to successfully administer a therapeutic dose to children (58).

ANTIEMETICS

Nausea and vomiting are symptoms common to many minor and serious disorders. The pharmacist should be cautious about recommending self-medication of these symptoms and should question the patient appropriately to determine whether physician referral is indicated.

Evaluation

The following are some of the more important considerations to determine whether an antiemetic should be used.

Age of Patient

Vomiting in newborns results from a number of serious abnormalities including obstruction of the GI tract and neuromuscular control disorders. Vomiting in newborns may lead to acid–base disturbances and dehydration. Physician referral is recommended for further work-up of any vomiting in newborns.

Nonprojectile vomiting, where milk appears to spill gently from the mouth, is common in infants. Often the causes are simple, such as overfeeding, feeding too quickly, ineffective burping, laying the infant down after feeding, and the immaturity of the esophageal sphincters.

One of the more common causes of vomiting in children is acute gastroenteritis. There are no data on the effects of nonprescription antiemetics on vomiting caused by viral gastroenteritis. Some sources question the safety of treating children with antiemetics in an acute, self-limiting disorder (51, 59). One theory suggests that vomiting in gastroenteritis is a body defense that sheds the pathogen and therefore should not be suppressed. However, recurrent or protracted vomiting can lead to dehydration and electrolyte imbalance in small children.

Other Antiemetics

Nondrug remedies such as Coca-Cola syrup and carbonated beverages have been used to help control vomiting on an empirical basis. In addition, vomiting may be produced by acidosis and dehydration secondary to severe diarrhea; rehydration may minimize this vomiting (60).

Pregnancy

Nausea and vomiting may be one of the earliest symptoms of pregnancy. A woman who notes nausea and vomiting in the early part of the day and who has no other symptoms except a missed menstrual cycle and perhaps weight gain should be referred for a pregnancy test and follow-up. Most physicians are reluctant to prescribe any drug for a pregnant woman. Nonprescription antiemetics are not indicated for nausea and vomiting of pregnancy. Some practitioners suggest eating small frequent meals to control morning sickness, although the benefits of this approach are not clear (61). Others have suggested treating morning sickness with soda crackers and cola (62). Because excessive caffeine should be avoided during pregnancy, women should consult their physician for the treatment of morning sickness. Of course, no drug should be ingested during pregnancy without the advice of a physician. (See Chapter 7, *Menstrual Products*.)

Current Drug Use

Some drugs are known to cause nausea and vomiting as a side effect or as a toxic effect. Drugs such as estrogens and the opiate analgesics may cause nausea and vomiting as side effects. Digitalis toxicity may be manifested as nausea and vomiting. In these situations, nonprescription antiemetics are not indicated and referral to a physician is appropriate.

Symptoms Requiring Physician Referral

Bulimia (binge–purge) behavior, a psychologic disorder in which patients attempt to lose weight by repeated vomiting and the chronic use of purgatives, should be referred for medical and psychologic management of the underlying problems (63). In addition, any patient who exhibits severe nausea, vomiting, and abdominal pain or who has forceful, bloody, or protracted vomiting should be referred to a physician. Adults with persistent vomiting for more than 2 days should also be referred to a physician.

Ingredients in Nonprescription Products

The available nonprescription antiemetic preparations that are classified as safe and effective are indicated for prevention and treatment of nausea, vomiting, or dizziness associated with motion sickness (64).

Motion sickness occurs when visual and vestibular stimuli are not in accord. Although no one is immune to motion sickness, some individuals are more resistant than others. The symptoms consist of pallor, yawning, restlessness, nausea, and then vomiting. Susceptibility to motion sickness appears to vary with age. Infants are generally immune to motion sickness, while young children, 2–12 years of age, are highly susceptible. In young children, motion sickness associated with car travel may be minimized by placing the child in a car seat (65). The resulting elevation is sufficient to allow vision out of the front window and may prevent motion sickness (66).

Antihistamines are the primary nonprescription agents used to prevent or control motion sickness. Cyclizine, meclizine, dimenhydrinate, and diphenhydramine are nonprescription antihistamines generally recognized as safe and effective in the prevention of motion sickness in the Food and Drug Administration (FDA) monograph on antiemetic drug products for over-the-counter (OTC) human use (64).

Some data indicate that scopolamine may be more effective than some of the currently available antihistamines (67–69). Scopolamine is currently available by prescription as a transdermal patch that can be easily applied and removed before and after travel. Side effects are minimal and may include drowsiness and some anticholinergic effects such as dry mouth. However, scopolamine can result in dry eyes, which can pose a problem for contact lens wearers.

Cyclizine, Meclizine, Dimenhydrinate, and Diphenhydramine

Cyclizine and meclizine are members of the benzhydryl piperazine group of antihistamine compounds. They are reported to depress labyrinth excitability and are safe and effective for the prevention and treatment of nausea and vomiting associated with motion sickness.

Doses of meclizine for adults are 25–50 mg once a day, administered every 24 hours. The drug has a relatively long duration of action, and studies have suggested that it provides 24-hour protection against motion sickness (64). Meclizine is not recommended for use in children under 12 years of age.

Adult doses of cyclizine are 50 mg every 4–6 hours, not to exceed 200 mg in 24 hours, and for children 6 years of age and older, 25 mg every 6–8 hours, not to exceed 75 mg in 24 hours. Cyclizine is not recommended for use in children under 6 years of age. To be effective in preventing motion sickness, the drug should be administered 30–60 minutes before departure (64). Cyclizine has a shorter duration of action when compared with meclizine.

In 1966, the FDA required that products containing meclizine and cyclizine carry a warning against their use by pregnant women. This warning was based on animal studies in several species that suggested that the drug may have teratogenic or embryolethal potential. Subsequent epidemiologic studies of many pregnant women have not shown an increase in embryo deaths or malformations in children of women who used these drugs during early pregnancy (70). The warning about the possible teratogenic effects of these agents in pregnant women is no longer required; however, these agents are not indicated for the treatment of morning sickness caused by pregnancy.

Dimenhydrinate is the 8-chlorotheophyllinate salt of the antihistamine diphenhydramine. Dimenhydrinate is safe and effective for the prevention and treatment of nausea and vomiting associated with motion sickness. The usual dosage for adults is 50–100 mg every 4–6 hours, not to exceed 400 mg in 24 hours. The dosage for children 2 to under 6 years of age is 12.5–25 mg every 6–8 hours, not to exceed 75 mg in 24 hours, and for children 6 to under 12 years of age, the dosage is 25–50 mg every 6–8 hours, not to exceed 150 mg in 24 hours (64).

Diphenhydramine is safe and effective for the prevention and treatment of motion sickness. The recommended dosage for adults is 25–50 mg every 4–6 hours, not to exceed 300 mg in 24 hours; the recommended dosage for children 6–11 years of age is 12.5–25 mg every 4–6 hours, not to exceed 150 mg in 24 hours (64).

Drowsiness with therapeutic doses of antihistamines can occur and is the most common unwanted side effect. Patients should be cautioned not to drive a car or operate hazardous machinery while using antihistamines. The effects are additive to those of other CNS depressants such as alcohol and tranquilizers. In large doses, these agents also produce anticholinergic effects, including blurred vision and dry mouth. The drugs should be used with caution in patients with asthma, narrow-angle glaucoma, obstructive disease of the GI or genitourinary tracts, or prostatic enlargement because of the potential exacerbation of symptoms.

Phosphorated Carbohydrate

Phosphorated carbohydrate solution is a mixture of levulose (fructose), dextrose (glucose), and phosphoric acid, which is added to adjust the pH to between 1.5 and 1.6. This product is promoted for nausea and vomiting associated with upset stomach caused by intestinal flu, food indiscretions, and emotional upset. Theoretically, this mixture has the potential to inhibit gastric emptying and reduce gastric tone through the high osmotic pressure exerted by the solution of simple sugars. However, because there are no studies establishing the efficacy of this product, the FDA panel on antiemetic products classified phosphorated carbohydrate as Category III (insufficient evidence to establish effectiveness) (64).

The usual adult dosage of the phosphorated carbohydrate is 15–30 ml or 1 to 2 tbsp at 15-minute intervals until vomiting ceases. Doses should be limited to five per hour. The solution should not be diluted, and the patient should not consume other liquids for 15 minutes after taking a dose. If vomiting does not cease after five doses, a physician should be contacted. Large doses of levulose may cause abdominal pain and diarrhea. Practitioners should be aware of the high glucose content and associated problems in diabetics. In addition, the product contains fructose and should not be used by individuals with hereditary fructose intolerance.

Bismuth Salts

Bismuth salts have been used for more than two centuries for various GI complaints (71). Bismuth subsalicylate is available as a nonprescription product for the relief of upset stomach associated with nausea, heartburn, and fullness caused by overindulgence in the combination of food and drink (72). The proposed mechanism of action is a coating effect of the bismuth preparation on the gastric mucosa. Bismuth salts appear to be poorly absorbed from the GI tract, although the large quantities of bismuth subsalicylate recommended in nonprescription preparations may allow for absorption of salicylate (73).

SUMMARY

Emetics are useful in cases of oral poisoning to remove gastric contents and to prevent further absorption of the ingested agent. Syrup of ipecac is the most effective and safest nonprescription emetic for this purpose. It should be kept in all homes with young children and used with the guidance of a poison control center or physician if an ingestion occurs.

Nonprescription antiemetics are useful in limited, patient-diagnosed situations, such as prevention of motion sickness. Antiemetics should always be used with caution because of the potential danger of masking the symptoms of organic disease. The pharmacist should ascertain the reason for purchasing a nonprescription antiemetic and suggest referral if necessary. Chronic unsupervised use of antiemetics, especially for an "upset stomach," should be discouraged, and the patient should be encouraged to seek additional medical help for continuous discomfort.

REFERENCES

1 H. L. Borison and S. L. Wang, *Pharmacol. Rev.*, *5*, 193–230 (1953).

2 A. J. Cummins, *Am. J. Dig. Dis.*, *3*, 710–721 (1958).

3 T. R. Hendrix, in "Medical Physiology," 14th ed., Vol. 2, V. Mountcastle, Ed., C. V. Mosby, St. Louis, Mo., 1980, p. 1336.

4 "Harrison's Principles of Internal Medicine," 9th ed., G. W. Thorn et al., Eds., McGraw-Hill, New York, N.Y., 1980, p. 194.

5 J. Kirsner, in "Pathologic Physiology: Mechanisms of Diseases," 5th ed., W. Sodeman and W. Sodeman, Jr., Eds., W. B. Saunders, Philadelphia, Pa., 1974, p. 711.

6 J. Brand and W. Perry, *Pharmacol. Rev.*, *18*, 895 (1966).

7 I. Gordon et al., in "Gastroenterologic Medicine," M. Paulson, Ed., Lea and Febiger, Philadelphia, Pa., 1969, pp. 468, 1233–1234.

8 "Williams Obstetrics," L. Hellman and J. Prichard, Eds., Meridith, New York, N.Y., 1971, pp. 343–344.

9 M. L. Soule et al., *Obstet. Gynecol.*, *55*, 696 (1980).

10 T. L. Litovitz et al., *Am. J. Emerg. Med.*, *7*, 495 (1989).

11 R. H. Dreisbach, "Handbook of Poisoning," 10th ed., Lange, Los Altos, Calif., 1980.

12 R. E. Gosselin et al., "Clinical Toxicology of Commercial Products," 4th ed., Williams and Wilkins, Baltimore, Md., 1976.

13 R. H. Dreisbach, "Handbook of Poisoning," 10th ed., Lange, Los Altos, Calif., 1980, p. 20.

14 L. Boxer et al., *J. Pediatr.*, *74*, 800 (1969).

15 L. Goldstein, *J. Am. Med. Assoc.*, *208*, 2162 (1969).

16 F. Arnold, Jr., et al., *Pediatrics*, *23*, 286 (1959).

17 P. S. Auerbach et al., *Ann. Emerg. Med.*, *15*, 692 (1986).

18 D. Tandberg et al., *Am. J. Emerg. Med.*, *4*, 205 (1986).

19 T. L. Litovitz, *Am. J. Emerg. Med.*, *4*, 294 (1986).

20 A. S. Manoguerra and E. P. Krenzelok, *Am. J. Hosp. Pharm.*, *35*, 1360 (1978).

21 M. E. Thoman and H. J. L. Verhulst, *J. Am. Med. Assoc.*, *196*, 433 (1966).

22 S. Molinas, National Clearinghouse for Poison Control Centers, U.S. Public Health Service, Washington, D.C., March-April 1966.

23 R. C. Ng et al., *Can. Med. Assoc. J.*, *111*, 537 (1974).

24 "The Pharmacological Basis of Therapeutics," 6th ed., A. G. Gilman et al., Eds., Macmillan, New York, N.Y., 1980, p. 1609.

25 J. McLeod, *N. Engl. J. Med.*, *268*, 146 (1963).

26 J. D. Speer et al., *Lancet*, *1*, 475 (1963).

27 T. Bates and E. Grunwaldt, *Am. J. Dis. Child.*, *103*, 169 (1962).

28 R. Allport, *Am. J. Dis. Child*, *98*, 786 (1959).

29 R. Smith and D. Smith, *N. Engl. J. Med.*, *265*, 23 (1964).

30 W. O. Robertson, *Vet. Human Toxicol.*, *21*, 87 (1979).

31 W. Klein-Schwartz et al., *Ann. Emergency Med.*, *13*, 1152 (1984).

32 R. J. Schift et al., *Pediatrics*, *78*, 410 (1986).

33 R. J. Varipapa and G. M. Oderda, *N. Engl. J. Med.*, *296*, 112 (1977).

34 P. A. Grbcich et al., *Vet. Hum. Toxicol.*, *28*, 499 (1986).

35 W. Robertson, *Am. J. Dis. Child*, *103*, 58 (1972).

36 W. MacLean, *J. Pediatr.*, *82*, 121 (1973).

37 D. B. Bukis et al., *Vet. Human Toxicol.*, *20* (1978).

38 R. W. Spiegel et al., *Clin. Toxicol.*, *14*, 281 (1979).

39 D. O. Cooney, *J. Pharm. Sci.*, *67*, 426 (1978).

40 I. A. Dabbous et al., *J. Pediatr.*, *66*, 952 (1965).

41 J. Barer et al., *Am. J. Dis. Child.*, *125*, 899 (1973).

42 F. DeGenaro and W. Nyhan, *J. Pediatr.*, *78*, 1048 (1971).

43 D. Ward, *Br. Med. J.*, *2*, 432 (1963).

44 B. Lawrence and B. Hopkins, *Med. J. Aust.*, *1*, 1301 (1969).

45 W. Robertson, *J. Pediatr.*, *78*, 877 (1971).

46 *Federal Register*, *42*, 31803 (1977).

47 N. Holtzman and R. Haslam, *Pediatrics*, *42*, 189 (1976).

48 R. S. Stein et al., *J. Am. Med. Assoc.*, *235*, 801 (1976).

49 W. D. Meester, *Vet. Human Toxicol.*, *22*, 225 (1980).

50 J. Schofferman, *J. Am. Coll. Emerg. Phys.*, *5*, 22 (1976).

51 O. Anderson, *Pediatrics*, *46*, 319 (1970).

52 J. Grensher et al., *J. Am. Coll. Emerg. Phys.*, *8*, 261–263 (1979).

53 D. O. Cooney, *Clin. Toxicol.*, *11,* 387 (1977).

54 "AMA Drug Evaluations," 4th ed., American Medical Association, Chicago, Ill., 1980, pp. 1438–1439.

55 R. A. Curtis et al., *Arch. Intern. Med.*, *144*, 48 (1984).

56 P. J. Neuvonen et al., *Eur. J. Clin. Pharmacol.*, *24*, 557 (1983).

57 K. Kulig et al., *Vet. Hum. Toxicol.*, *25*, 286 (1983).

58 P. A. Orbach et al., *Vet. Hum. Toxicol.*, *29,* 458 (1987).

59 M. Casteels-Van Dael et al., *Arch. Dis. Child.*, *45*, 130 (1970).

60 H. Hirschhorn and W. B. Greenough, in "Davidson's Principles and Practices of Medicine," 19th ed., A. M. Harvey, Ed., Appleton-Century-Crofts, New York, N.Y., 1976, p. 1264.

61 C. DiIorio, *Nurse Practitioner, 13*, 23–28 (1988).

62 W. A. Check, *J. Am. Med. Assoc.*, *242*, 2518 (1979).

63 P. J. Beumond et al., *Psychol. Med.*, *6*, 617 (1976).

64 *Federal Register, 52*, 15886-93 (1987).

65 E. L. Schor, *N. Engl. J. Med.*, *301*, 1066 (1979).

66 W. M. Jay et al., *N. Engl. J. Med.*, *302*, 1091 (1980).

67 S. P. Clissold and R. C. Heel, *Drugs*, *29*, 189 (1985).

68 S. Noy et al., *Aviation, Space, and Environmental Medicine, 55*, 1051 (1984).

69 E. Dahl et al., *Clinical Pharmacology and Therapeutics, 36*, 116 (1984).

70 S. Shapiro et al., *Am. J. Obstet. Gynecol.*, *128*, 480 (1977).

71 S. J. Konturek et al., *Scan. J. Gastro.*, *21*, 6–13 (1986).

72 *Federal Register, 47*, 43540-59 (1982).

73 J. R. Dipalma, *Am. Fam. Phys.*, *38*, 244–246 (1988).

APPENDIX: MAJOR POISON CONTROL CENTERS

ALABAMA

Alabama Poison Center
809 University Boulevard East
Tuscaloosa, AL 35401
Emergency numbers:
205-345-0600
800-462-0800 (Alabama only)

Children's Hospital of Alabama Regional
  Poison Control Center
1600 7th Avenue South
Birmingham, AL 35233
Emergency numbers:
205-939-9201 (Alabama only)
205-933-4050
800-292-6678

ALASKA

Anchorage Poison Control Center
3200 Providence Drive
Anchorage, AK 99519-6604
Emergency numbers:
907-261-3193
800-478-3193

ARIZONA

Arizona Poison and Drug Information Center
Health Sciences Center
Room 3204K
1501 North Campbell
Tucson, AZ 85724
Emergency numbers:
602-626-6016 (Tucson)
800-362-0101 (Arizona only)

Samaritan Regional Poison Center
Good Samaritan Medical Center
130 East McDowell, Suite A5
Phoenix, AZ 85006
Emergency number:
602-253-3334

ARKANSAS

Arkansas Poison and Drug Information Center
College of Pharmacy–UAMS
4301 West Markham Street
Slot 522
Little Rock, AR 72205
Emergency numbers:
501-666-5532
800-482-8948

University Hospital Poison Control Center
4301 West Markham
Slot 584
Little Rock, AR 72205-7199
Emergency number:
501-661-6161

CALIFORNIA

Fresno Regional Poison Control Center
Fresno Community Hospital and Medical Center
Fresno and R Streets
Fresno, CA 93715
Emergency numbers:
209-445-1222
800-346-5922

Los Angeles County Medical Association Regional
  Poison Center
1925 Wilshire Boulevard
Los Angeles, CA 90057
Emergency numbers:
213-664-2121
213-484-5151
800-777-6476

San Diego Regional Poison Center
UCSD Medical Center
25 Dickinson Street
San Diego, CA 92103-1990
Emergency numbers:
619-543-6000
800-876-4766

San Francisco Regional Poison Center
San Francisco General Hospital
1001 Potrero Avenue, Room I-E-86
San Francisco, CA 94110
Emergency numbers:
415-476-6600
800-523-2222

Santa Clara Valley Medical Center
Regional Poison Center
751 South Bascom Avenue
San Jose, CA 95128
Emergency numbers:
408-299-5112
800-662-9886

UC Davis Regional Poison Control Center
2315 Stockton Boulevard, Room 1511
Sacramento, CA 95817
Emergency numbers:
916-453-3692
800-342-9293 (northern California only)

University of California Irvine Medical Center
  Regional Poison Center
101 The City Drive
Route 78
Orange, CA 92668
Emergency numbers:
714-634-5988
800-544-4404 (southern California only)

COLORADO

Rocky Mountain Poison and Drug Center
645 Bannock Street
Denver, CO 80204-4507
Emergency number:
303-629-1123 (Colorado only)

CONNECTICUT

Connecticut Poison Control Center
University of Connecticut Health Center
Farmington Avenue
Farmington, CT 06032
Emergency number:
800-343-2722

DISTRICT OF COLUMBIA

National Capital Poison Center
Georgetown University Hospital
3800 Reservoir Road, N.W.
Washington, DC 20007
Business/Emergency numbers:
202-625-3333
202-784-4660 (TTY)

FLORIDA

Florida Poison Information Center
The Tampa General Hospital
Davis Islands
Post Office Box 1289
Tampa, FL 33601
Emergency numbers:
813-253-4444 (Tampa only)
800-282-3171 (Florida only)

St. Vincent's Medical Center
1800 Barrs Street
Jacksonville, FL 32203
Emergency number:
904-387-7500

University Hospital of Jacksonville Clinical
  Toxicology Service
655 West 8th Street
Jacksonville, FL 32209
Emergency number:
904-350-6899 (Operator will page consultant on call)

GEORGIA

Georgia Regional Poison Control Center
80 Butler Street, S.E.
Atlanta, GA 30335-3801
Emergency numbers:
404-589-4400
800-282-5846 (Georgia only)

Savannah Regional/EMS Poison Center
Memorial Medical Center, Inc.
4700 Waters Avenue
Savannah, GA 31403
Emergency number:
912-355-5228

HAWAII

Hawaii Poison Center
Kapiolani Women's & Children's Medical Center
1319 Punahou Street
Honolulu, HI 96826
Emergency number:
808-941-4411

ILLINOIS

Chicago and Northeastern Illinois Regional
  Poison Control Center
Rush-Presbyterian-St. Luke's Medical Center
1653 West Congress Parkway
Chicago, IL 60612
Emergency numbers:
312-942-5969
800-942-5969 (Illinois only)

Regional Poison Control Center for Central
  and Southern Illinois
St. John's Hospital
800 East Carpenter
Springfield, IL 62769
Emergency numbers:
217-753-3330
800-252-2022

INDIANA

Indiana Poison Center
Methodist Hospital of Indiana, Inc.
1701 North Senate Boulevard
Indianapolis, IN 46206
Emergency numbers:
317-929-2336 (TTY/TTD)
317-929-2323
800-382-9097 (Indiana only)

IOWA

St. Luke's Poison Center
St. Luke's Regional Medical Center
2720 Stone Park Boulevard
Sioux City, IA 51104
Emergency numbers:
712-277-2222
800-352-2222 (stateside WATS)

Variety Club Poison and Drug Information Center
Iowa Methodist Medical Center
1200 Pleasant Street
Des Moines, IA 50309
Emergency numbers:
515-283-6254
800-362-2327 (outside Des Moines)

KANSAS

Mid-America Poison Control Center
Kansas University Medical Center
Department of Pharmacy, Room B-400
39th and Rainbow Boulevard

Kansas City, KS 66103
Emergency numbers:
913-588-6633
800-332-6633 (Kansas only)

KENTUCKY

Kentucky Regional Poison Center of Kosair
  Children's Hospital
224 East Broadway, Suite 305
Louisville, KY 40202
Emergency numbers:
502-589-8222
800-722-5725 (Kentucky only)

LOUISIANA

Terrebone General Medical Center
936 East Main Street
Houma, LA 70360
Emergency number:
504-873-4066

MAINE

Maine Poison Control Center
Maine Medical Center
22 Bramhall Street
Portland, ME 04102
Emergency number:
800-442-6305 (Maine only)

MARYLAND

Maryland Poison Center
20 North Pine Street
Baltimore, MD 21201
Emergency numbers:
301-528-7701
800-492-2414 (Maryland only)

MASSACHUSETTS

Massachusetts Poison Control System
300 Longwood Avenue
Boston, MA 02115
Emergency numbers:
617-232-2120 (Boston area)
800-682-9211 (Massachusetts only)

MICHIGAN

Bixby Medical Center Poison Center
818 Riverside Avenue
Adrian, MI 49221
Emergency numbers:
517-263-0711

Blodgett Regional Poison Center
1840 Wealthy Street S.E.
Grand Rapids, MI 49506
Emergency number:
800-632-2727 (Michigan only)

Bronson Poison Information Center
252 East Lovell Street
Kalamazoo, MI 49007
Emergency numbers:
616-341-6409
800-442-4221 (Michigan only)

Poison Control Center
Children's Hospital of Michigan
3901 Beaubien Boulevard
Detroit, MI 48201
Emergency numbers:
313-745-5711 (Metro Detroit)
800-462-6642 (Rest of Michigan)

Saginaw Regional Poison Center
Saginaw General Hospital
1447 North Harrison
Saginaw, MI 48602
Emergency numbers:
517-755-1111
800-451-4585

University of Michigan Poison Information Center
1500 East Medical Center Drive
Ann Arbor, MI 48109
Emergency number:
313-764-7667

MINNESOTA

Hennepin Regional Poison Center
Hennepin County Medical Center
701 Park Avenue South
Minneapolis, MN 55415
Emergency number:
612-347-3141

Minnesota Regional Poison Center
St. Paul-Ramsey Medical Center
640 Jackson Street
St. Paul, MN 55101
Emergency numbers:
612-221-2113
800-222-1222 (Minnesota only)

MISSISSIPPI

Forrest General Hospital
400 South 28th Avenue
Hattiesburg, MS 39401
Emergency number:
601-288-4236

MISSOURI

Cardinal Glennon Children's Hospital Regional
  Poison Center
1465 South Grand Boulevard
St. Louis, MO 63104
Emergency numbers:
314-772-5200
800-392-9111 (Missouri only)
800-366-8888

Children's Mercy Hospital
24th at Gillham Road
Kansas City, MO 64108
Emergency number:
816-234-3000

NEBRASKA

Mid-Plains Poison Center
8301 Dodge Street
Omaha, NE 68114
Emergency numbers:
402-390-5400 (local)
800-642-9999 (Nebraska only)
800-228-9515 (surrounding states)

NEW HAMPSHIRE

New Hampshire Poison Information Center
Dartmouth-Hitchcock Medical Center
2 Maynard Street
Hanover, NH 03756
Emergency number:
800-562-8236 (New Hampshire only)

NEW JERSEY

New Jersey Poison Information and Educational System
201 Lyons Avenue
Newark, NJ 07112
Emergency numbers:
201-923-0764 (outside New Jersey)
800-962-1253 (New Jersey only)

NEW MEXICO

New Mexico Poison and Drug Information Center
University of New Mexico
Albuquerque, NM 87131
Emergency numbers:
505-843-2551
800-432-6866 (New Mexico only)

NEW YORK

Central New York Poison Control Center
750 East Adams Street
Syracuse, NY 13210
Emergency numbers:
315-476-4766
800-252-5655

Ellis Hospital Poison Control Center
1101 Nott Street
Schenectady, NY 12308
Emergency number:
518-382-4039

Finger Lakes Regional Poison Control Center at Life Line
University of Rochester Medical Center
601 Elmwood Avenue
Rochester, NY 14642
Business number:
716-423-9490

Hudson Valley Poison Center
Nyack Hospital
North Midland Avenue
Nyack, NY 10960
Emergency number:
914-358-1000

Long Island Regional Poison Control Center
2201 Hempstead Turnpike
East Meadow, NY 11554
Emergency number:
516-542-2323

New York City Poison Center
455 First Avenue, Room 123
New York, NY 10016
Emergency numbers:
212-340-4494
212-764-7667

New York State Department of Health-Injury
  Control Program
Corning Tower, Room 621
Empire State Plaza
Albany, NY 12237
Business/Emergency number:
518-473-1143

Western New York Poison Control Center at
  Children's Hospital of Buffalo
219 Bryant Street
Buffalo, NY 14222
Emergency numbers:
716-878-7654
716-878-7655

NORTH CAROLINA

Duke Regional Poison Control Center
Duke University Medical Center
Box 3007
Durham, NC 27710
Emergency number:
800-672-1697 (North Carolina only)

Poison Control Center
Catawba Memorial Hospital
810 Fairgrove Road
Hickory, NC 28602
Emergency number:
704-322-6649

Triad Poison Center
1200 North Elm Street
Greensboro, NC 27401-1020
Emergency numbers:
919-379-4105 (local)
800-722-2222 (North Carolina only)

NORTH DAKOTA

North Dakota Poison Center
720 Fourth Street North
Fargo, ND 58122
Emergency numbers:

701-234-5575
800-732-2200 (North Dakota only)

OHIO

Akron Regional Poison Center
281 Locust Street
Akron, OH 44308
216-379-8562
800-362-9922 (Ohio only)

Bethesda Poison Control Center
Bethesda Hospital
2951 Maple Avenue
Zanesville, OH 43701
Emergency number:
614-454-4221

Central Ohio Poison Center
700 Children's Drive
Columbus, OH 43205
Emergency numbers:
614-228-1323
800-682-7625

Greater Cleveland Poison Control Center
2101 Adelbert Road
Cleveland, OH 44123
Emergency number:
216-231-4455

Mahoning Valley Poison Center
St. Elizabeth Hospital Medical Center
1044 Belmont Avenue
Youngstown, OH 44501
Emergency numbers:
216-746-2222
216-746-5510 (TTY)
800-426-2348

Regional Poison Control System and Cincinnati
  Drug and Poison Information Center
231 Bethesda Avenue, M.L. #144
Cincinnati, OH 45267-0144
Emergency number:
513-558-5111

Stark County Poison Control Center
1320 Timken Mercy Drive, N.W.
Canton, OH 44708
Emergency number:
800-722-8662

Western Ohio Poison and Drug Information Center
Children's Medical Center
One Children's Plaza
Dayton, OH 45404
Emergency numbers:
513-222-2227
800-762-0727

OKLAHOMA

Oklahoma Poison Control Center
Children's Memorial Hospital

940 N.E. 13th Street
Oklahoma City, OK 73126
Emergency numbers:
405-271-5454
800-522-4611 (Oklahoma only)

OREGON

Oregon Poison Center
Oregon Health Sciences University
3181 S.W. Sam Jackson Park Road
Portland, OR 97201
Emergency numbers:
503-279-8968
800-452-7165 (Oregon only)

PENNSYLVANIA

Capital Area Poison Center
University Hospital
The Milton S. Hershey Medical Center
Hershey, PA 17033
Emergency number:
717-531-6111

Delaware Valley Regional Poison Control Center
One Children's Center
34th & Civic Center Boulevard
Philadelphia, PA 19104
Emergency number:
215-386-2100

Hamot Poison Control Center
Hamot Medical Center
201 State Street
Erie, PA 16550-0001
Emergency numbers:
814-870-6111
814-870-6112 (TDD)
800-221-5252 (Pennsylvania, Ohio, New York only)

Keystone Region Poison Center
Mercy Hospital of Altoona
2500 Seventh Avenue
Altoona, PA 16603
Emergency number:
814-946-3711

Lehigh Valley Poison Center
The Allentown Hospital Site
17th and Chew Streets
Allentown, PA 18102
Emergency number:
215-433-2311

Northwest Regional Poison Control Center
Saint Vincent Health Center
232 West 25th Street
Erie, PA 16544
Emergency number:
814-452-3232 (24-hour hotline)

Pittsburgh Poison Center
One Children's Place
3705 5th Avenue at DeSoto

Pittsburgh, PA 15213
Emergency number:
412-681-6669

St. Joseph Hospital and Health Care Center
250 College Avenue
Lancaster, PA 17604
Emergency number:
717-291-8111

Susquehanna Poison Center
Geisinger Medical Center
P.O. Box 273A
Danville, PA 17821
Emergency numbers:
717-275-6116
717-271-6116

RHODE ISLAND

Rhode Island Poison Center
593 Eddy Street
Providence, RI 02903
Emergency numbers:
401-277-5727
401-277-8062 (TDD)

SOUTH CAROLINA

Palmetto Poison Center
University of South Carolina
College of Pharmacy
Columbia, SC 29208
Emergency numbers:
803-765-7359
800-922-1117 (South Carolina only)

SOUTH DAKOTA

St. Luke's Midland Regional Medical Center
305 South State Street
Aberdeen, SD 57401
Emergency number:
605-229-3100

McKennan Poison Center
800 East 21st Street
Sioux Falls, SD 57117-5045
Emergency numbers:
800-952-0123 (South Dakota only)
800-843-0505 (Iowa, Minnesota, Nebraska, and
  North Dakota)

TENNESSEE

Middle Tennessee Regional Poison Center
1161 21st Avenue South
501 Oxford House
Nashville, TN 37232-4632
Emergency numbers:
615-322-6435
800-288-9999

Southern Poison Center, Inc.
848 Adams Avenue

Memphis, TN 38103
Emergency number:
901-528-6048

TEXAS

Medical Center Hospital
500 Medical Center Boulevard
Conroe, TX 77304
Emergency number:
409-539-7700

North Texas Poison Center
5201 Harry Hines Boulevard
Dallas, TX 75235
Emergency numbers:
214-590-5000
800-441-0040 (Texas only)

Texas State Poison Center
University of Texas Medical Branch
Galveston, TX 77550-2780
Emergency numbers:
409-765-1420 (Galveston)
713-654-1701 (Houston)
512-478-4490 (Austin)
800-392-8548 (Texas only)

UTAH

Intermountain Regional Poison Control Center
50 North Medical Drive
Building 528
Salt Lake City, UT 84132
Emergency number:
801-581-2151

VERMONT

Vermont Poison Center
Medical Center Hospital of Vermont
111 Colchester Avenue
Burlington, VT 05401
Emergency number:
802-658-3456

VIRGINIA

Blue Ridge Poison Center
Blue Ridge Hospital, Box 67
Charlottesville, VA 22901
Emergency numbers:
804-924-5543
800-451-1428 (Virginia only)

Southwest Virginia Poison Center
Roanoke Memorial Hospitals
Belleview at Jefferson Street
Roanoke, VA 24033
Emergency number:
703-981-7336

Tidewater Poison Center
DePaul Medical Center
150 Kingsley Lane

Norfolk, VA 23505
Emergency numbers:
804-489-5288
800-552-6337 (Virginia only)

WASHINGTON

Central Washington Poison Center
2811 Tieton Drive
Yakima, WA 98902
Emergency numbers:
509-248-4400
800-572-9176 (Washington only)

Mary Bridge Poison Center
317 South K Street
Tacoma, WA 98405-0987
Emergency numbers:
206-594-1420
206-594-1400

Seattle Poison Center
Children's Hospital and Medical Center
4800 Sand Point Way, N.E.
Seattle, WA 98105
Emergency numbers:
206-526-2121
206-527-4859
800-732-6985 (Washington only)

Spokane Poison Center
South 715 Cowley, Suite 132
Spokane, WA 99202
Emergency numbers:
509-747-1077
800-572-5842 (Washington only)
800-541-5624 (outside Washington)

WEST VIRGINIA

West Virginia Poison Center
3110 MacCorkle Avenue, S.E.
Charleston, WV 25304
Emergency numbers:
304-348-4211 (local)
800-642-3625 (West Virginia only)

WISCONSIN

Green Bay Poison Control Center
St. Vincent Hospital
835 South Van Buren
Green Bay, WI 54307-3508
Emergency numbers:
414-433-8100
414-433-8101

LaCrosse Area Poison Center
700 West Avenue South
LaCrosse, WI 54601
Emergency number:
608-784-0971

Milwaukee Poison Center
9000 West Wisconsin

Milwaukee, WI 53201
Emergency numbers:
414-266-2220
414-266-2222

University of Wisconsin Hospital Regional
  Poison Center
600 Highland Avenue, E5/238 CSC
Madison, WI 53792
Emergency number:
608-262-3702

CANADA

British Columbia Drug and Poison
  Information Centre
1081 Burrard Street
Vancouver, British Columbia
Canada V6Z 1Y6
Emergency number:
604-682-5050

Poison and Drug Information Services
Foothills Hospital
1403 29th Street, N.W.
Calgary, Alberta
Canada T2N 2T9
Emergency numbers:
403-270-1414 (Calgary only)
800-332-1414

NEW ZEALAND

National Toxicology Group
University of Otago Medical School
GT King Street
Dunedin, New Zealand 9003
Emergency numbers:
006-024-761-028
006-024-738-375

ANTIEMETIC PRODUCT TABLE

Product (Manufacturer)	Dosage Form	Active Ingredients	Other Ingredients
Bonine (Leeming)	chewable tablet	meclizine hydrochloride, 25 mg	
Calm-X (Republic)	tablet	dimenhydrinate, 50 mg	
Dizmiss (Jones Medical)	chewable tablet	meclizine hydrochloride, 25 mg	
Dramamine (Vicks Health Care)	chewable tablet	dimenhydrinate, 50 mg	aspartame; citric acid; FD & C yellow #5 (tartrazine); flavor; magnesium stearate; methacrylic acid copolymer; sorbitol
	tablet	dimenhydrinate, 50 mg	acacia; carboxymethylcellulose sodium; cornstarch; magnesium stearate; sodium sulfate
	liquid	dimenhydrinate, 3 mg/ml	sucrose, 54%; ethanol, 5%; cherry flavor, 0.2%; FD & C Red #40; glycerin; methylparaben; water
Emetrol (Adria)	liquid	phosphorated carbohydrate solution	color; flavors; glycerin; methylparaben; water
Marezine (Burroughs Wellcome)	tablet	cyclizine hydrochloride, 50 mg	
Marmine (Vortech)	tablet	dimenhydrinate, 50 mg	
Meclizine HCl (Various manufacturers)	chewable tablet tablet	meclizine hydrochloride, 25 mg	
Naus-A-Way (Hauck)	liquid	phosphorated carbohydrate solution	
Tega-Vert (Ortega)	capsule	dimenhydrinate, 50 mg	
Triptone Caplets (Commerce)	tablet	dimenhydrinate, 50 mg	

R. Leon Longe

13

ANTIDIARRHEAL AND OTHER GASTROINTESTINAL PRODUCTS

Questions to ask in patient/consumer counseling

How long have you had diarrhea? Was it sudden in onset? How often do you have a bowel movement?

Is the diarrhea associated with other symptoms such as fever, vomiting, or abdominal pain? Do stools contain blood?

Have you tried any antidiarrheal treatments or products? Which ones? How effective were they?

How old is the patient?

Have other family members experienced similar symptoms?

Have you changed your diet recently?

Can you relate the onset of diarrhea to a specific cause such as a particular food (milk products) or drug? Have you recently traveled to a foreign country?

Are you currently taking or have you recently taken any prescription or nonprescription medications? Which ones?

Do you have diabetes or any other chronic disease?

Diarrhea is usually characterized by increased frequency of excretion of loose, watery stools during a limited period. Abnormal, increased passage of formed stools is also considered diarrhea. The frequency of bowel movements varies with the individual. Some healthy adults may have as many as three stools a day; others may defecate once in 2 or more days (1). The mean daily fecal weight is 100–150 g. An increase to 200–300 g is interpreted as diarrhea. The major factor contributing to diarrhea is excretion of water that normally is reabsorbed from the gut. Disruption in the water absorption process, resulting in accumulation in the gut of even a few hundred milliliters of water, may cause diarrhea (2, 3).

Diarrhea is often viewed and treated as a symptom of an undiagnosed and presumed minor and transient gastrointestinal (GI) disorder. More than 50 medical conditions, including major diseases involving the kidneys, heart, liver, and thyroid and the acquired immunodeficiency syndrome (AIDS), are associated with diarrhea. Additionally, numerous drugs may induce diarrhea. Often, diarrhea is only one of many symptoms associated with a major illness (4–6).

313

PHYSIOLOGY OF DIGESTIVE SYSTEM

The small intestine is a convoluted tube, approximately 6.4 m long, made up of the duodenum, jejunum, and ileum. It originates at the pylorus and terminates at the cecum of the ascending colon (Figure 1). The small intestine is the primary site of digestion, absorption of nutrients, and retention of waste material; these activities depend on normal musculature, nerve tone, and digestive enzymes.

The alimentary tract is basically a long, hollow tube surrounded by layers of smooth muscle: a thick, circular layer on the mucosal side of the intestine; a thinner, longitudinal layer on the serosal side; and a third layer of both circular and longitudinal muscle fibers. The active contractions of the various muscles control tone, or tension, of the intestinal wall. Normally, this tone is maintained with little expenditure of energy so that the muscles remain generally free from fatigue and capable of continued performance.

A mucous layer protects and lubricates the walls of the intestine. The mucus, composed of glycoproteins and sulfated aminopolysaccharides, is released from goblet cells interspersed among the columnar epithelial cells in the intestine. Secretion of mucus is increased by local irritation from foods or cathartics and by psychic trauma, which suggests control by the autonomic nervous system. The mucus is more viscous in the upper part of the small intestine than in the colon and forms a protective physical barrier to the intestinal lining, reducing contact with irritating substances and bacteria. The alkalinity of the mucus contributes further to the protection of the intestinal lining by neutralizing acidic dietary and bacterial products.

Normal intestinal motility and peristalsis are maintained by smooth muscles and intrinsic nerves. The vagus and parasympathetic pelvic nerves stimulate intestinal motility; sympathetic innervation inhibits intestinal motility and secretion. Extrinsic autonomic innervation influences the strength and frequency of these movements and mediates reflexes by which activity in one part of the intestine influences another.

Eating causes the lumen of the intestine to distend, and the smooth muscle layers to contract. Normally, the segmental contractions of the circular muscles are accompanied by a decrease in the propulsive activity of the gut. This process retains the food in the lumen and increases the duration of its exposure to the digestive elements, enhancing digestion and absorption.

Normally, about 7 l of digestive fluid are secreted into the GI tract each day. This is made up of about 1 l of saliva, 2 l of gastric juice, 2 l of pancreatic juice, 1 l of fluid from the liver, and 1 l from the small bowel. An additional 2 l enter the GI tract with food and liquids.

Of these 9 l, 8 are reabsorbed in the small intestine. The large bowel reabsorbs about 850 ml of the remaining 1 l, leaving about 150 ml to be excreted in the stool each day.

Approximately 3 l of fluid containing electrolytes and nutrients enter the small intestine every 24 hours. Reabsorption reduces the quantity that reaches the large intestine to approximately 1,000 ml of an isotonic semiliquid substance (chyme) consisting in part of nonabsorbed, undigested food residue, nutrients, electrolytes, water, and bacteria. Chyme has an average electrolyte content of 83 mEq of sodium, 20 mEq of bicarbonate, 6 mEq of potassium, and 60 mEq of chloride (7).

The large intestine, which is about 1.5 m long, extends from the cecum to the rectum. It is composed of the cecum, ascending colon, transverse colon, descending colon, sigmoid colon, and rectum. The colon has two primary functions: absorption and storage. The first two-thirds of the colon facilitates absorption, and the remainder functions as a storage area. The proximal half (ascending and transverse parts) of the colon reduces chyme to a semisolid substance called feces, or stool. Stool is a 75% water and 25% solid material consisting of nonabsorbed food residue, bacteria, desquamated epithelial cells, unabsorbed minerals, and a small quantity of electrolytes (Table 1). Stool is generally stored in the descending colon until defecation.

The colon is structured like the small intestine with both circular and longitudinal muscles. The longitudinal muscles are shorter than the underlying colonic tissue and tend to draw the colon into sacs. The segments of the circular musculature further divide the colon into sausage-like units known as haustra. Through segmented contractions, they facilitate churning of the colonic contents and the absorption of water. Thus, a decrease in the occurrence or intensity of these segmental contractions and the predominance of the propulsive force of the longitudinal muscles may lead to diarrhea. In the absence of circular muscle contractions, mass colonic movements may occur during which the colon contracts to half its length and resembles a smooth, hollow tube devoid of segmented units. Colonic activity is increased by parasympathetic stimulation, whereas sympathetic stimulation inhibits colonic motor activity.

Normal bowel movement, or defecation, begins with the stimulation of stretch receptors in the rectum by feces. Peristaltic waves propel the feces to the anal canal where the voluntarily controlled external anal sphincter controls defecation (8).

In the colon, bacteria produce enzymes necessary for degradation of waste products, synthesize certain vitamins, and generate ammonia. *Bacteroides* and anaerobic *Lactobacillus* make up the majority of the colonic bacterial flora. Pathogenic organisms such as Entero-

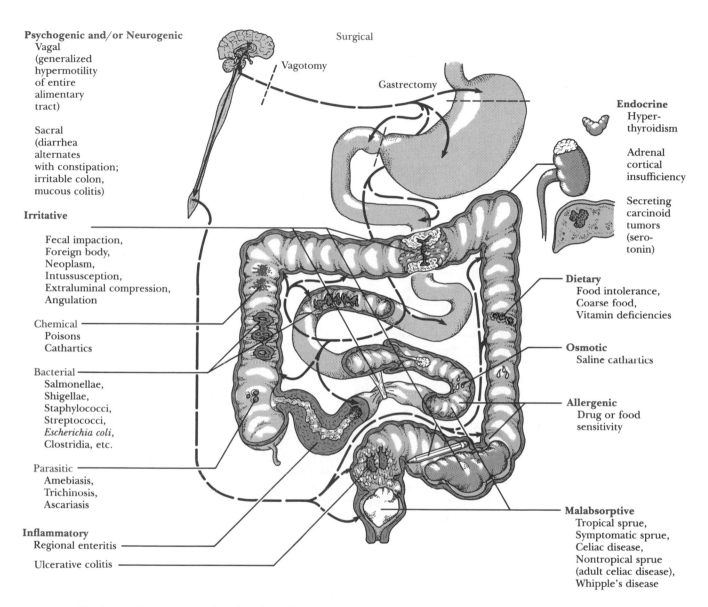

Psychogenic and/or Neurogenic
 Vagal
 (generalized
 hypermotility
 of entire
 alimentary
 tract)

 Sacral
 (diarrhea
 alternates
 with constipation;
 irritable colon,
 mucous colitis)

Irritative

 Fecal impaction,
 Foreign body,
 Neoplasm,
 Intussusception,
 Extraluminal compression,
 Angulation

 Chemical
 Poisons
 Cathartics

 Bacterial
 Salmonellae,
 Shigellae,
 Staphylococci,
 Streptococci,
 Escherichia coli,
 Clostridia, etc.

 Parasitic
 Amebiasis,
 Trichinosis,
 Ascariasis

Inflammatory
 Regional enteritis
 Ulcerative colitis

Surgical
 Vagotomy
 Gastrectomy

Endocrine
 Hyper-
 thyroidism

 Adrenal
 cortical
 insufficiency

 Secreting
 carcinoid
 tumors
 (sero-
 tonin)

Dietary
 Food intolerance,
 Coarse food,
 Vitamin deficiencies

Osmotic
 Saline cathartics

Allergenic
 Drug or food
 sensitivity

Malabsorptive
 Tropical sprue,
 Symptomatic sprue,
 Celiac disease,
 Nontropical sprue
 (adult celiac disease),
 Whipple's disease

FIGURE 1   The lower digestive tract showing the induction of diarrhea by various causes. Adapted from F. H. Netter, "The Ciba Collection of Medical Illustrations," Vol. 1, Ciba Pharmaceutical Co., New York, N.Y., 1962, p. 99.

bacteriaceae (*Escherichia coli*), hemolytic *Streptococcus*, *Clostridium*, and yeasts also are found in the colon, but represent only a small portion of the normal flora. Many factors such as diet, pH, GI disease, and drugs such as antibiotics influence the proportion of the population of these organisms. If these potential pathogens are allowed to grow uncontrolled, their increased proportion can present serious complications (9).

ETIOLOGY OF DIARRHEA

The variability in the origins of diarrhea makes identification of the pathophysiologic mechanism difficult and may require a complete physical examination, including supportive clinical laboratory tests. The etiology of diarrhea can be psychogenic, neurogenic, surgical, endocrine, irritant, osmotic, dietary, allergenic, malabsorptive, infectious, or inflammatory.

TYPES OF DIARRHEA

Acute diarrhea is characterized by a sudden onset of frequent, liquid stools accompanied by weakness, flatulence, pain, and often fever and vomiting. Chronic diarrhea is the abnormal, frequent passage of stools and usually is the result of multiple factors.

Acute Diarrhea

Acute diarrhea may be infectious, toxic, drug-induced, or dietary in origin. It may also be the result of acute or chronic illness. Infectious diarrhea is usually viral in origin.

The development of diarrhea may involve four general pathophysiologic mechanisms: decreased absorption, increased secretion, varied exudation, and motility alterations (Table 2). The gut maintains a balance between absorption and secretion of GI fluids. Historically, diarrhea has been thought of as malabsorption syndrome. However, evidence supports the theory that diarrhea, characterized by large-volume stools, is more often a hypersecretory disease (10). Hypersecretion into the intestinal lumen is a common response to infectious organisms in the gut (11). Diarrhea also may be provoked by stimulating adenyl cyclase, causing a rise in cyclic adenosine monophosphate (AMP), which leads to hypersecretion (12, 13).

Infectious Diarrhea

Although the causative agent is not readily identified in most cases of acute diarrhea, the bacterial pathogens most commonly responsible in the United States are *E. coli*, *Shigella*, *Salmonella*, *Campylobacter*, and *Staphylococcus* (14–18). Some organisms cause diarrhea through an enterotoxin (toxigenic *E. coli* and *Staphylococcus aureus*). Others (*Shigella*, *Salmonella*, and invasive *E. coli*) directly invade the mucosal epithelial cells. Patients with diarrhea caused by toxin-producing agents clinically present with a cholera-like syndrome, which primarily involves the small bowel. The patient experiences an abrupt onset of large volumes of watery stools, variable nausea, vomiting, cramps, and possibly a low-grade fever. Invasive organisms produce a dysentery-like syndrome if the large bowel is the site of attack. This type

is characterized by fever, abdominal cramps, tenesmus (straining), and frequent small-volume stools that may contain blood and pus.

When the patient is first seen, a careful history is essential in identifying a cause. For example, staphylococci grow rapidly in food (especially ham and poultry), producing a toxin. Upon ingestion, the toxin quickly (within 1–2 hours) provokes the attack of vomiting with some diarrhea. In contrast, the incubation period for *Salmonella* is 12–24 hours. Fever, malaise, muscle aches, and profound epigastric or periumbilical discomfort with severe anorexia suggest an infectious, inflammatory disease of the bowel. Severe periumbilical pain and vomiting are commonly experienced with viral gastroenteritis and are acute for 2–3 days before gradually subsiding (19).

Campylobacter jejuni is another cause of acute bacterial diarrhea. The diarrhea is usually limited to 1 week. If supportive therapy fails, erythromycin is the drug of choice. *Yersinia enterocolitica* is an isolate of bacterial diarrhea that lasts 1–3 weeks and is self-limiting.

The acute diarrhea that frequently develops among tourists visiting foreign countries with warm climates and relatively poor sanitation is usually caused by bacterial enteropathogens. However, a study conducted during the Fifth World Congress of Gastroenterology found that enterotoxigenic *E. coli* was the most common cause of traveler's diarrhea in Mexico. It results from ingestion of the causative organism found in food. Traveler's diarrhea is characterized by a sudden onset of loose stools, nausea, occasional vomiting, and abdominal cramping. Children seem particularly susceptible, and most cases develop during the first week of exposure to the new location.

Infectious diarrhea is treated with water and electrolytes. In many instances the illness is self-limiting,

TABLE 1	Electrolyte and water content of normal and diarrheal feces	
Components	**Normal**	**Diarrheal**
Bicarbonate[a]	30	30–45
Chloride[a]	15	20–40
Potassium[a]	90	35–60
Sodium[a]	40	25–50
Water[b]	0.1–0.2	3–10

[a]mEq/l; [b]l/24 hrs

Adapted from R. L. Longe and J. T. DiPiro, in "Pharmacotherapy: A Pathophysiologic Approach," Elsevier Science Publishing, New York, N.Y., 1989, p. 468, and D. E. Kohan, in "Manual of Medical Therapeutics," Little, Brown and Co., Boston, Mass., 1989, p. 54

TABLE 2	Classification of diarrhea	
Type	**Mechanism**	**Typical Causes**
Osmotic	Nonabsorbable solute	Lactase deficit, magnesium antacid
Secretory	Increased secretion of electrolytes	*E. coli* infection, ileal resection, thyroid cancer
Motility disorder	Decreased contact time	Irritable bowel syndrome, diabetic neuropathy
Exudative	Defective colonic absorption, outpouring of mucus and/or blood	Ulcerative colitis, shigellosis, leukemia

and normal function of the alimentary tract is restored with or without treatment in 24–48 hours. If the patient has a persistent infectious diarrhea, an antibiotic may be indicated.

Viral Diarrhea

Diarrhea in infants and young children is a common pediatric problem, and the etiology often is difficult to identify, although it is frequently caused by viral infection of the intestinal tract. Diet and systemic and local infections, such as otitis media, are other known etiologies of acute diarrheal episodes in children.

Rotaviruses have been implicated as the cause of about 50% of all infantile diarrhea (20, 21). Clinical features include a 12–48 hour incubation period, vomiting, watery diarrhea, and a low-grade fever. The illness usually is self-limiting, lasting 5–8 days. Generally, it requires only symptomatic therapy. Evidence has demonstrated that breast-feeding is effective in preventing viral diarrhea (22, 23). Parvoviruses also have been implicated in infantile diarrhea, with signs and symptoms resembling those of rotaviruses (24). Norwalk is the first of the parvovirus group to be isolated. Unlike rotaviruses, all age groups can be infected. The diarrhea is sudden, with fever, malaise, and abdominal cramps. The diarrhea usually lasts 2–3 days.

In children, particularly infants, acute diarrhea may cause severe, and possibly dangerous, dehydration and electrolyte imbalance. In the newborn, water may comprise 75% of the total body weight; water loss in

severe diarrhea may be 10% or more of body weight. After 8–10 bowel movements in 24 hours, a 2-month-old infant could lose enough fluid to cause circulatory collapse and renal failure. For this reason, moderate to severe diarrhea in infants should receive a physician's evaluation. The pharmacist must be cautious in recommending treatment for any pediatric patients with diarrhea (25–29).

Protozoal Diarrhea

Giardia lamblia and *Entamoeba histolytica* are protozoa associated with acute diarrhea. Giardiasis especially infests hikers, children, travelers, and institutionalized patients. Following a 1–3 day incubation, sudden onset of explosive watery stool begins along with abdominal cramps. Quinacrine, 100 mg orally 3 times a day for 7 days, is the treatment of choice (30). Metronidazole, 250 mg orally 3 times a day for 7 days, is generally effective (31, 32). The pediatric dosage for metronidazole is 15 mg/kg in 24 hours, taken by mouth for 10 days (33).

Entamoeba histolytica causes amebiasis in areas with poor sanitation, in institutionalized patients, and among travelers and migrant workers. The illness is characterized by severe crampy pain, tenesmus, and dysentery within 3–10 days. Metronidazole, 750 mg orally 3 times a day, is generally effective (34). The pediatric dosage of metronidazole for amebic dysentery is 35–50 mg/kg in 24 hours, taken by mouth for 10 days. In immunologically deficient patients, *Isospora*, *Cryptosporidium*, and *Blastocystis hominis* have been isolated.

Drug-Induced Diarrhea

Diarrhea is frequently a side effect of drug administration. All antibiotics can produce adverse GI symptoms including diarrhea, but severity depends largely on the specific antibiotic. Antibiotics that have a broad spectrum of activity against aerobic and anaerobic organisms frequently cause diarrhea. Ampicillin, clindamycin, erythromycin, lincomycin, neomycin, trimethoprim–sulfamethoxazole, the tetracyclines, and the cephalosporins are commonly prescribed broad-spectrum antibiotics (35).

Antibiotic-associated diarrhea (AAD) may be caused by overgrowth of an antibiotic-resistant bacterial or fungal strain or a toxin-producing bacterium. Intestinal microorganisms that tend to proliferate during antibiotic therapy include *Staphylococcus aureus*, *Pseudomonas aeruginosa*, *Streptococcus faecalis*, *Candida albicans*, and species of *Salmonella* and *Proteus*. AAD may be self-limiting (with antibiotic discontinuation). More severe and potentially fatal diarrhea is known as pseudomembranous colitis (PMC). *Clostridium difficile*, a toxin-producing microbe, causes pseudomembranous colitis (36). *C. difficile* produces at least two identified toxins (A and B). The stool may appear watery or mucoid. The diarrhea usually starts during antibiotic treatment, but it can begin after the antibiotic has been discontinued. The diagnosis is confirmed with a test for the toxins in the stool. The antibiotic must be discontinued and *C. difficile* eradicated. *C. difficile* is sensitive in vitro to bacitracin, erythromycin, tetracycline, and some cephalosporins. However, oral vancomycin (250 mg every 6 hours for 10 days) or oral metronidazole (250 mg 3 times daily for 10 days) are more often prescribed (36–40). Cholestyramine may also be tried in mild diarrhea, but it does not kill *C. difficile* (41). Agents that inhibit peristalsis, such as opiates, may prolong and worsen the condition.

Other drugs, such as cathartics, which irritate the intestinal mucosa, may precipitate diarrhea, as may drugs that cause the retention of salts and water in the intestinal lumen. Certain antacid preparations contain magnesium to prevent the constipating effects of aluminum and calcium. Depending on the dose taken and the individual, these types of antacid preparations may induce diarrhea. Drugs that alter autonomic control of intestinal motility also may cause diarrhea. For example, it is not uncommon for the antiadrenergic, antihypertensive agents such as guanethidine, methyldopa, and reserpine to produce diarrhea. Generalized cramping and diarrhea may follow the use of a parasympathomimetic drug, such as bethanecol, which is used as a urinary tract stimulant (42). Other drugs that frequently cause diarrhea include anticancer agents, quinidine, and colchicine.

Food-Induced Diarrhea

Food intolerance can also provoke diarrhea. It may be caused by allergy or the ingestion of foods that are excessively fatty or spicy or that contain a high degree of roughage or a large number of seeds. If diarrhea occurs in more than one person within 24 hours of ingestion of a common meal, it is likely that a toxin (food poison) has been ingested.

Food intolerance and diarrhea may be associated with disaccharidase deficiency (lactase deficiency). Carbohydrates in the diet commonly include lactose and sucrose, which are hydrolyzed to monosaccharides. Milk and ice cream may be particularly problematic because of the lactose content. These enzymatic activities are reduced in intestinal disorders such as infectious diarrhea, congenital disaccharide deficiency, and GI allergy. When disaccharides such as sucrose and lactose are not hydrolyzed, they pool in the lumen of the intestine where they ferment and produce an osmotic and pH change. The resulting osmolarity increase draws more fluid into the lumen, resulting in diarrhea.

Botulism results from ingestion of food contaminated with toxins produced by *Clostridium botulinum*. Botulism is almost always associated with poorly prepared food that is contaminated with clostridium spores. The toxin blocks the cholinergic nerves within 12–72 hours. The patient has dysarthria, dysphagia, dyspnea, and a descending paralysis. The most dangerous complication is respiratory paralysis.

Prevention is very important. All home-canned foods must be boiled for 10 minutes to kill the spores and destroy the toxin. Any pressurized container must maintain a vacuum pressure or be discarded.

Treatment consists of respiratory support and botulism antitoxin. The patient should be hospitalized in an intensive care unit. Although efficacy is not proven, the trivalent antitoxin should be administered within 24 hours of developing symptoms. The antitoxin is available from the Centers for Disease Control (CDC) in Atlanta, Ga.

Chronic Diarrhea

Chronic diarrhea is usually the result of multiple factors and therefore can be difficult to diagnose (Table 3). The condition may be defined as recurring episodes of watery stools lasting more than 2 weeks. It may be caused by a disease of the bowel or may be a secondary manifestation of a systemic disease. Some investigators differentiate chronic diarrhea into functional or organic groups (43). The pharmacist should refer patients with persistent or recurrent diarrhea to a physician. Correct causative diagnosis usually can be made only after a physician carefully studies the patient's history and performs a physical examination and appropriate laboratory tests. Chronic diarrheal illness may be caused by one of many conditions but is generally related to GI diseases.

Diagnosing chronic diarrhea can be very difficult because it does not always involve frequent daily passage of watery stools. Three categories of chronic diarrhea can be described: frequent, small, formed stools with tenesmus; large, oily, malodorus, formed stools; and frequent, voluminous, loosely formed stools. The patient may complain of weight loss, fever, anxiety or depression, nausea, vomiting, or perianal tenderness (44).

Psychogenic factors are frequent causes of chronic diarrhea. Psychogenic diarrhea is usually characterized by small, frequent stools and abdominal pain. The stools may be watery and may follow a normal bowel movement or may appear shortly after eating. Psychogenic diarrhea is related to emotional stress that may periodically increase the parasympathetic nervous system impulses to the GI tract. The diarrhea may alternate with constipation. Patients complaining of chronic diarrhea that appears to be psychogenically related

TABLE 3 Pathophysiologic classification of chronic diarrhea

Decreased absorption
Small intestine
  Generalized malabsorption
    Mucosal damage (celiac disease)
    Impaired intraluminal digestion (pancreatic insufficiency)
    Bacterial overgrowth (bile salt deconjugation and mucosal injury—scleroderma)
  Specific malabsorption
    Enzyme deficiency (disaccharidases)
    Transport defect (chloridorrhea glucose–galactose malabsorption)
    Nonabsorbable solute (magnesium, lactulose)
Colon
  Idiopathic inflammatory bowel disease
    Ulcerative colitis
    Crohn's disease
  Specific inflammatory bowel disease
    Amebiasis
    Ischemic colitis
    Radiation colitis

Increased secretion
Small intestine
  Dumping syndrome
  Gastric hypersecretion (Zollinger–Ellison syndrome)
  Endogenous secretogogues (vasoactive intestinal peptide, prostaglandins, serotonin)
Colon
  Unabsorbed fatty acids
  Bile acids (failure of ileal reabsorption)
  Unabsorbed carbohydrates (lactase deficiency)
  Fluid-secreting tumor (large villous adenoma)

Motor disturbances (decreased mixing activity)
Small intestine and colon
  Carcinoid syndrome
  Postvagotomy diarrhea
  Hyperthyroidism
  Diabetic visceral neuropathy
  Scleroderma
Colon
  Irritable bowel syndrome

Malabsorption syndromes
Failure of digestion
  Decreased pancreatic enzymes
  Impairment of bile acid micelle formation
    Bacterial overgrowth
  Inadequate mixing of food, bile, and pancreatic enzymes
    Gastrojenjunostomy
Failure of absorption
  Inadequate absorptive surface
    Intestinal bypass surgery
  Damaged absorbing surface
    Celiac disease
  Biochemical defect without anatomic alteration
    Lactase deficiency
  Infiltration of intestinal wall
    Crohn's disease
Impaired lymph and blood flow
  Developmental abnormality
  Lymphatic obstruction
    Tuberculosis
  Mesenteric vascular insufficiency

Adapted from Harvey et al., "The Principles and Practice of Medicine," 22nd ed., Appleton and Lange, San Mateo, Calif., and Norwalk, Conn., 1988, pp. 814, 823.

should be referred to a physician.

Many people believe a daily bowel movement is essential for good health. This belief may lead to laxative abuse. The abuse of laxatives is a serious health problem that can result in chronic diarrhea. In recent years, chronic abuse of purgatives for weight control has become a problem. Usually the problem is resolved only after other causes cannot be identified. Upon questioning, the patient usually denies laxative abuse. A hospitalized patient's diarrhea may stop, but reoccurs at home. To identify the abuser, a careful drug history must be taken. The pharmacist must watch for frequent laxative purchases. (See Chapter 15, *Laxative Products*.)

The laxative abuser usually complains of weight loss and diarrhea. Chronic laxative use leads to serious water and electrolyte loss, protein wasting (hypoalbuminemia), and colitis (45–48). Recovery requires laxative withdrawal, bowel training, psychologic counseling, and, in some cases, hospitalization.

Some people who suffer from persistent diarrhea are aware of the cause and can manage the condition symptomatically. For example, about 2.5% of adult diabetics and 22% of diabetics with evident neuropathy have chronic diarrhea. (See Chapter 16, *Diabetes Care Products*.) Individuals who have persistent or recurrent diarrhea and are unaware of its cause should seek prompt medical attention because conditions such as cancer of the stomach or colon or an endocrine tumor may be causing the diarrhea. One of the seven danger signals of cancer is a change in bowel habits. In both sexes, cancer of the colon and rectum is a frequently reported type of cancer. The American Cancer Society estimates that almost three of every four patients may be saved by early diagnosis and proper treatment (49). A follow-up study of patients who had been suffering from "unexplained" diarrhea revealed the risk of missing a diagnosis such as neoplasm (50).

EVALUATION

The most common complaints of patients with acute diarrhea are abrupt onset of frequent, watery, loose stools, abdominal cramping, flatulence, fever, muscle aches, vomiting, and malaise. In chronic diarrhea, the most significant finding is usually a history of previous bouts of diarrhea and complaints of anorexia, weight loss, and chronic weakness. These patients generally have histories of poor health.

In assessing the patient's complaint, the pharmacist should determine:

- The patient's age;
- Mode of onset (events coincident, past episodes, acute or chronic onset, duration);
- The character and location of the symptom;
- Factors that precipitate or aggravate the complaint;
- The medications (including laxatives) the patient is taking;
- Factors that relieve the symptom;
- Past treatment of the problem;
- Other current illness or family history of diarrhea or GI disorders.

Evaluation of patient responses should enable the pharmacist to recommend an appropriate course of action, which may include self-treatment or referral to a physician. This triage function requires that pharmacists differentiate symptoms, recognize their limitations, and make clinical judgments.

The pharmacist should obtain a history of the present illness before recommending self-treatment. The following four groups of patients with either acute or chronic diarrhea should be referred to a physician for a complete diagnostic evaluation:

- Children under 3 years of age;
- Persons over 60 years of age who have multiple medical conditions;
- Persons with a medical history of chronic illness such as asthma, peptic ulcer, diabetes, or heart disease;
- Pregnant women.

Other medical conditions that necessitate physician referral include:

- Bloody stools;
- Abdominal tenderness;
- High fever;
- Dehydration;
- Weight loss of greater than 4% of body weight;
- Diarrhea that has lasted 5–7 days.

Clinical judgment must be used in evaluating these patients. For example, access to medical treatment may not be readily available, and temporary self-treatment may be needed until a medical appointment can be arranged. When a drug is implicated as a cause of diarrhea, the pharmacist should refer the patient to a physician because the patient may need to continue taking the drug even though it is causing problems.

The medication history helps detect drug-induced diarrhea. With this background, the pharmacist should determine which self-treatments have already been tried, the patient's age, symptoms, date of onset, and characteristics of stools (number, consistency, odor, and appearance). Alcohol abuse, ankylosing spondylitis, diverticulitis, emotional problems, gastritis, irritable bowel syndrome, and ulcerative colitis or regional enteritis are some frequently reported past medical problems. Referral to a physician is the rule and not the exception in such patients.

The early signs of dehydration include sunken eyes, dry mucous membranes, and decreased skin turgor. The patient should be questioned about the nature and amount of fluid intake, occurrence of vomiting, and frequency of urination.

Stool character gives valuable information about diarrhea. For example, undigested food particles in the stool indicate small bowel irritation; black, tarry stools can indicate upper GI bleeding, and red stools suggest possible lower bowel bleeding or simply the recent ingestion of red food such as beets or drug products such as Povan. Diarrhea originating from the small bowel probably is manifested as a marked outpouring of fluid high in potassium and bicarbonate. A pastelike or semi-solid loose stool is indicative of diarrhea associated with a colon disorder.

TREATMENT

Diarrhea is a symptom, and symptomatic relief must not be interpreted as a cure for the underlying cause. Symptomatic relief generally suffices in simple functional diarrhea that is only temporary and relatively uncomplicated. More than 100 nonprescription products are available; however, the pharmacist should exercise caution in recommending their use in self-medication. Certain diseases that cause diarrhea might be serious or treated more effectively with agents specific for the underlying cause. Table 4 summarizes the causes of diarrhea and appropriate treatment. The following statement is required by the Food and Drug Administration (FDA) on all nonprescription antidiarrheal products:

> **WARNING** Do not use for more than 2 days or in the presence of high fever or in infants or children under 3 years of age unless directed by a physician.

Prophylaxis of Infectious ("Traveler's") Diarrhea

Traveler's diarrhea is usually managed with water and electrolyte replacement. Antibiotics such as trimethoprim–sulfamethoxazole, tetracycline, norfloxacin, ciprofloxacin, and trimethoprim have been used.

Many remedies have been tried to prevent traveler's diarrhea. Antibiotics are the most effective drugs available. Doxycycline (100 mg daily) has been effective in the prophylaxis of diarrhea. Trimethoprim–sulfamethoxazole (160–800 mg twice daily) has been shown to prevent this disorder when the offending organism is enterotoxigenic *E. coli* or *Shigella* (51). Norfloxacin and ciprofloxacin, 5-fluoroquinolones, are also effective in preventing diarrhea (52). Antiperistaltic agents such as diphenoxylate may prolong or enhance the severity of the symptoms of traveler's diarrhea if the patient has fever or is passing blood because of retention of the invasive bacteria in the intestine (53–56). Bismuth subsalicylate has been shown to be effective in treatment and prevention of symptoms (57, 58). The bismuth subsalicylate appears to inhibit intestinal secretions. The prophylactic dosage is 30–60 ml or 2 tablets taken 4 times a day during the first 2 weeks of travel. During acute illness, 30–60 ml should be taken every 30 minutes for a total of 8 doses (59–61).

The salicylate may be a problem if patients are taking aspirin or other salicylate-containing drugs because toxic levels of salicylate may be reached even if the patient follows label directions for each drug (62–64). Patients who are sensitive to aspirin should not use bismuth salicylate. Bismuth salicylate may interact adversely with oral anticoagulants, methotrexate, probenecid, and sulfinpyrazone or any drug that potentially interacts with aspirin. Also, serum salicylate levels may exert an antiplatelet effect.

The FDA suggests that travelers to areas where hygiene and sanitation are poor may prevent diarrhea by eating only recently peeled and thoroughly cooked foods and by drinking only boiled or bottled water, bottled carbonated soft drinks, beer, or wine. Tap water used for brushing teeth or for ice in drinks may be a source of infection.

Nondrug Treatment

Mild acute diarrhea, sometimes accompanied by vomiting, is usually self-limiting. Proper dietary measures can help replace lost fluids and electrolytes and thereby prevent dehydration. Table 5 lists oral rehydration solutions. Children under 3 years of age who have diarrhea and adults with diarrhea who lose more than 4% of their body weight should be referred to their physicians. The following dietary management of mild diarrhea for children over 3 years of age without a high fever or vomiting has been recommended as one method of treatment in cases of uncomplicated gastroenteritis (65):

- The stomach and intestines should be allowed to rest by not giving the child anything to eat for 4–6 hours.

- Pedialyte, Lytren, Rehydralyte, or Resol (available in pharmacies) at room temperature may be given to the child.

- One tsp of one of these liquids (above) should be given every 10–15 minutes for approximately 30 minutes; if the child retains this amount, 1 tbsp should be given every 15–20 minutes, followed by 2 tbsp (1 oz) every 30 minutes. If the child cannot retain the fluid, or if watery diarrhea persists, the physician should be notified.

- For the next 12 hours, ¼ cup of fluid should be given every 30 minutes; if diarrhea, vomiting, or "dry heaves" occurs at this time, the physician should be notified.

- For the next 24 hours, easily digested foods (bananas, rice, and applesauce) should be given. Sweet, clear liquid foods should be continued.

In moderate to severe diarrhea (4–12% weight loss), sodium, chloride, potassium, bicarbonate, glu-

TABLE 4   Infectious diarrheas and their treatment

Type	History	Symptoms	Treatment	Prognosis
BACTERIAL				
Salmonella	Ingestion of improperly cooked or refrigerated poultry and dairy products; homosexual	Onset of 24–48 hours, diarrhea, fever, and chills	Water and electrolytes; no antibiotics	Self-limiting
Shigella	Ingestion of contaminated vegetables or water; homosexual	Onset of 24–48 hours, nausea, vomiting, diarrhea	Water and electrolytes; antibiotics reserved (cotrimoxazole, ampicillin, ciprofloxicin/ norfloxicin)	Self-limiting
Escherichia coli Enterotoxigenic (Traveler's)	Ingestion of contaminated water, recent travel outside U.S.	Onset of 8–24 hours, watery diarrhea	Water and electrolytes; moderate or severe cases, antibiotics (cotrimoxazole, doxycycline, fluoroquinolones)	Self-limiting
Campylobacter jejuni	Ingestion of contaminated water, or fecal–oral route; homosexual	Nausea, vomiting, headache, malaise, fever, watery diarrhea	Water and electrolytes; in severe or persistent diarrhea, antibiotics (erythromycin, tetracycline, clindamycin, ciprofloxicin, aminoglycosides)	Self-limiting
Clostridium difficile	Antibiotic-associated diarrhea	Watery or mucoid diarrhea, high fever, cramping	Water and electrolytes; discontinue offending agent; oral vancomycin, oral metronidazole, bacitracin, cholestyramine	Mild to severe

(continued)

cose, and water must be given intravenously. Administering water without electrolytes is very dangerous. The normal diet should be reinstituted slowly. Milk should be avoided for 10 days. Some investigators have suggested adding milk, administered half strength, to the diet 12 hours after the patient has shown steady improvement by an appreciable reduction in number and volume of stools (66). This recommendation concerns acute infectious diarrhea in children when dehydration is not significant enough to require hospitalization. If milk intolerance occurs, infants may receive soy-based formulas such as Isomil, Soyalac, or ProSobee. Spicy and fatty foods should be avoided for 5–6 days.

Pharmacologic Agents

Some antidiarrheal drugs are directed against the symptoms of diarrhea, some against the cause, and some against the effect of the disease such as loss of nutrients or electrolytes. The categories of drugs generally used are opiates, adsorbents, astringents, electrolytes, nutrients, bulk laxatives, anti-infectives, digestive enzymes, intestinal flora modifiers, sedatives, tranquilizers, smooth muscle relaxants, and anticholinergic drugs. Many of the drugs used to combat diarrhea (opiates, anti-infectives, and sedatives) are available only by prescription.

TABLE 4 *continued*

Type	History	Symptoms	Treatment	Prognosis
Clostridium botulinum	Improper preparation or storage of food	Neurotoxin causes dysphagia, dry mouth, diplopia, dysarthria, dyspnea, paralysis	Hospitalization; respiratory support; botulism antitoxin	Severe
Staphylococcus aureus	Ingestion of improperly cooked or stored food	Enterotoxin causes nausea, vomiting, watery diarrhea	Water and electrolytes; no antibiotics	Self-limiting
PROTOZOA				
Giardia lamblia	Ingestion of water contaminated with human or animal feces; travel outside U.S.; homosexual	AIDS; chronic watery diarrhea	Quinacrine, metronidazole, furazolidone	Good, if treated
Cryptosporidia	Travel outside U.S.; AIDS; homosexual	Chronic watery diarrhea	Water and electrolytes	Self-limiting, except in AIDS or other immune deficit state
Entamoeba histolytica	Travel outside U.S.; fecal-soiled food or water; homosexual	Chronic watery diarrhea	Water and electrolytes; metronidazole; iodoquinol	Good, except for immune deficit patient
VIRUSES				
Rotaviruses	Infects infants; fecal–oral spread	Vomiting, fever, nausea, acute watery diarrhea	Vigorous water and electrolyte replacement; no antibiotics	Good to severe
Parvoviruses (Norwalk agent)	Infects all ages	"24 hour flu," vomiting, nausea, headache, myalgia, fever, watery diarrhea	Water and electrolytes; no antibiotics; bismuth subsalicylate; loperamide	Good

In 1975, the FDA advisory review panel on over-the-counter (OTC) laxative, antidiarrheal, emetic, and antiemetic drug products published its report on antidiarrheal agents. According to the panel, only opiates and polycarbophil were recognized as being safe and effective for nonprescription use. The panel concluded that "adequate and reliable scientific evidence is not available at this time to permit final classification" of other ingredients submitted, including alumina powder, attapulgite, belladonna alkaloids, bismuth salts, calcium carbonate, calcium hydroxide, carboxymethyl cellulose sodium, charcoal, kaolin, species of *Lactobacillus*, pectin, salol, and zinc phenosulfonate. Generally, the panel agreed that the agents are safe in recommended dosages but believed that there was a lack of acceptable clinical evidence to establish their effectiveness as antidiarrheal agents.

Opiates and Opiate-Like Agents

The opiates (opium powder, tincture of opium, and paregoric) are safe and effective in dosages of 15–20 mg of opium (1.5–2.0 mg of morphine) for adults and 5–10 mg of opium (0.5–1.0 mg of morphine) for children 6–12 years of age taken 1–4 times a day, not to exceed 2 days (67). Most opiate-containing nonprescription antidiarrheals contain paregoric or its equivalent in the usual dose of 1 tsp (~5.0 ml) of paregoric containing 20 mg of powdered opium (2.0 mg of morphine). Several nonprescription products incorporate

TABLE 5 Oral rehydration solutions

	WHO-ORS[a]	Lytren (Mead Johnson)	Pedialyte (Ross)	Rehydralyte (Ross)	Resol (Wyeth)
OSMOLALITY (mOsm/l)	333	220	249	304	269
CARBOHYDRATES[b] (g/l)	20	20	25	25	20
CALORIES (cal/l)	77	85	100	100	80
ELECTROLYTES (mEq/l)					
Sodium	90	50	45	75	50
Potassium	20	25	20	20	20
Chloride	80	45	35	65	50
Citrate	—	30	30	30	34
Bicarbonate	30	—	—	—	—
Calcium	—	—	—	—	4
Magnesium	—	—	—	—	4
Sulfate	—	—	—	—	—
Phosphate	—	—	—	—	5

[a] World Health Organization Oral Rehydration Solution
[b] Carbohydate is glucose
Adapted from R. L. Longe and J. T. DiPiro, in "Pharmacotherapy: A Pathophysiologic Approach," Elsevier Publications, New York, N.Y., 1989, p. 471.

paregoric or its equivalent in a mixture with other ingredients.

Because of their morphine content, paregoric-containing products exert a direct musculotropic effect to inhibit effective propulsive movements in the small intestine and colon. Thus, hyperperistaltic movements decrease, and the passage of intestinal contents slows, resulting in reabsorption of water and electrolytes. In the usual oral antidiarrheal dosages, addiction liability is low for acute diarrheal episodes because the morphine is not well absorbed orally. The low dose given produces an effective action in the GI tract without causing analgesia or euphoria. However, acute overdose or chronic use, as in ulcerative colitis, increases the risk of physical dependency (68). Paregoric alone is a Schedule III prescription-only item; in combination with antidiarrheals that contain no more than 100 mg of opium (5 tsp, or about 25 ml, of paregoric per 100 ml of mixture), it is a Schedule V item available for nonprescription purchase. Opium derivatives are central nervous system (CNS) depressants, and excessive sedation may be a problem in patients taking other CNS depressants with the diarrheal remedy.

Recently loperamide (Imodium A-D) became available without prescription. It is an elixir dosage form containing 1 mg per teaspoon. It slows intestinal motility and affects electrolyte and water movement through the gut. Like other antiperistaltic drugs, in acute diar-

rhea it should be used for only 48 hours unless clinical improvement is noted. The usual dosage is 4 mg initially, then 2 mg after each loose bowel movement.

Antiperistaltic drugs (diphenoxylate, paregoric, and loperamide) are effective in relieving cramps and stool frequency. However, they do not appear to prevent fluid loss. In addition, they may worsen the effects of invasive bacterial infection and toxic megacolon in antibiotic-induced diarrhea. Therefore, these drugs should be used with caution in patients presenting with fecal leukocytes, fever, or recent history of antibiotic use (69, 70).

Polycarbophil

Polycarbophil is a calcium salt of a synthetic polyacrylic resin that acts as an absorbent. Because of its ability to absorb 60 times its original weight in water, it has been recommended in the treatment of both diarrhea and constipation (71). Clinical studies in patients with acute diarrhea and chronic diarrhea have shown polycarbophil to be safe and effective (72–77). The frequency of bowel movements decreased, and the consistency of stools improved. Polycarbophil is metabolically inert, and no systemic toxicity has been demonstrated. Local toxicities have included epigastric pain and bloating, which are dose related. The effective adult dose is 4.0–6.0 g a day taken orally. Adults should chew two

500-mg tablets 4 times a day. Children 6–12 years of age should chew one 500-mg tablet 3 times a day, and children 3–6 years of age should chew one 500-mg tablet 2 times a day. Dosage instructions are not commercially available for children under 3 years of age.

Adsorbents

The adsorbents are the most frequently used type of drug in nonprescription antidiarrheal preparations. Because large doses generally are used, most commercially available products are formulated as flavored liquid suspensions to improve palatability. Adsorbents generally are used in the treatment of mild diarrhea. The FDA panel determined that even though adsorbents are safe, there is insufficient evidence that these agents are effective in treating diarrhea.

Adsorption is not a specific action, and when given orally, materials possessing this capability adsorb nutrients and digestive enzymes as well as toxin, bacteria, and various noxious materials in the GI tract. They also may have the effect of adsorbing drugs from the GI tract. Although the systemic absorption of a drug from the GI tract during a diarrheal episode is expected to be poor, its absorption may be further hampered by the concomitant administration of an antidiarrheal adsorbent. Thus, a judgment must be made when drugs other than the antidiarrheal preparation are to be taken by the patient, perhaps for an unrelated condition. Depending on the medication involved, its usual rate and site of absorption, and the absolute necessity of attaining specific and consistent blood levels of the drug, an alteration of the dose or the dosage regimen may be required. In some cases, it might be better to administer the drug parenterally until the diarrheal episode is over and adsorbent drugs are discontinued. A disadvantage of adsorbent agents is their interference with laboratory identification of parasites. Therefore adsorbents should not be consumed until stool specimens are collected (78).

Following the initial treatment, most antidiarrheal preparations containing adsorbents are taken after each loose bowel movement until the diarrhea is controlled. The total amount of adsorbent taken may be quite large if the diarrheal episodes occur in rapid succession and for several hours. Because there is negligible systemic absorption of the adsorbent drug, usually the only consequence is constipation.

The main GI adsorbents used are activated charcoal, aluminum hydroxide, attapulgite, bismuth subsalts, kaolin, magnesium trisilicate, and pectin. Adsorbents used with ion-exchange resins combine their individual activities in relieving gastric distress and diarrhea. These agents are relatively inert and nontoxic except for possible interference with drug and nutrient adsorption. Kaolin, which has long been used in the Far East against diarrhea and dysentery, is a native hydrated aluminum silicate. It is activated by thermal treatment and used in a finely powdered form. Although it is seldom used as an antidiarrheal today, activated charcoal, which in a single gram has a surface area of about 1,000 m², possesses excellent adsorption properties and has been used for conditions of various origin, including cholera and infantile and nervous diarrhea (79). In a study of the treatment of acute nonspecific diarrhea, 8 children, 3–11 years of age, were treated for 2 days with either kaolin–pectin concentrate (Kao-Con), kaolin suspension, pectin suspension, diphenoxylate–atropine liquid (Lomotil), or placebo. The treatments resulted in additional stool consistency, but the actual volume of water loss remained unchanged (80).

Pectin, a purified carbohydrate extracted from the rind of citrus fruit or from apple pomace, is used in the treatment of diarrhea, although its exact mechanism of action is not known. Pectin generally is found in combination with other adsorbents.

The bismuth subsalts such as subnitrates and subsalicylates are used in antidiarrheal preparations as adsorbents, astringents, and protectives. However, subnitrate may form nitrate ion in the bowel, which upon absorption may cause hypotension and methemoglobinemia. Bismuth subnitrate is contraindicated in children under 2 years of age. Stools may become dark with use of a bismuth compound. According to the FDA panel, bismuth salts are safe in amounts taken orally (0.6–2.0 g of bismuth subsalicylate every 6–8 hours). At the time of the FDA panel report, there was insufficient data to establish the effectiveness of bismuth in diarrhea; however, recent data indicate that bismuth may be effective in the treatment and prevention of symptoms of traveler's diarrhea.

Anticholinergics

The formulations of adsorbents are frequently fortified by the addition of belladonna alkaloids (anticholinergics) in concentrations that make them prescription drugs. The primary effect of anticholinergic agents is relief of cramping through the reduction of contractile activity. Their effectiveness in the reduction of diarrhea is negligible in doses typically contained in nonprescription products (81). Anticholinergics do not appear to be effective in acute infectious diarrhea. When the diarrhea is caused by increase in intestinal tone and peristalsis, belladonna alkaloids are effective when given in doses that are equivalent to 0.6–1.0 mg of atropine sulfate. However, in some available combinations of nonprescription antidiarrheal products, the usual dosage of belladonna alkaloids is less than the recognized effective dosage. When these agents are combined with adsorbents, the possibility of inactivation by adsorption must be considered. Therefore, the

FDA panel recommends that "antidiarrheal products containing anticholinergics when given in doses that are equivalent to 0.6–1.0 mg of atropine sulfate be available only by prescription."

Anticholinergics have a narrow margin of safety, especially in young children. Their containers carry the following warning statement that should be reviewed with the patient before dispensing:

> **WARNING** Not to be used by persons having glaucoma or excessive pressure within the eye, or by elderly persons (when undiagnosed glaucoma or excessive pressure in the eye occurs more frequently), or by children under 6 years of age, unless directed by physician. Discontinue use if blurring of vision, rapid pulse, or dizziness occurs. Do not exceed recommended dosage. Not for frequent or prolonged use. If dryness of the mouth occurs, decrease dosage. If eye pain occurs, discontinue use and see your physician immediately as this may indicate undiagnosed glaucoma.

Lactobacillus Preparations

One of the most controversial forms of diarrheal treatment is the use of lactobacillus organisms. The bacteriology of the intestinal tract is extremely complex, and it is difficult to explain changes in the numbers and types of microorganisms. The flora of the GI tract plays a significant role in maintaining bowel function, nutrition, and the overall well-being of the individual. Antibiotic therapy often disrupts the balance of intestinal microorganisms, resulting in abnormal intestinal and bowel function. Seeding the bowel with viable *Lactobacillus acidophilus* and *Lactobacillus bulgaricus* has been suggested as effective treatment for intestinal disturbances, including diarrhea. These microorganisms are believed to be effective in suppressing the growth of pathogenic microorganisms and in reestablishing the normal intestinal flora. A diet of milk, yogurt, or buttermilk, containing 240–400 g of lactose or dextrin, is equally effective in colonizing the intestine without supplemental lactobacilli. However, the FDA panel states that there are no controlled studies documenting the effectiveness of lactobacillus preparations in treating diarrhea.

Other Active Ingredients

Various other active ingredients are blended in antidiarrheal products. These include drugs such as zinc phenolsulfonate (zinc sulfocarbolate), carboxymethyl cellulose sodium, zinc phenol, phenyl salicylate, and various digestive enzymes. The indications are myriad. Intestinal antiseptic and astringent action has been attributed to zinc phenolsulfonate; phenyl salicylate (salol) is reported to be hydrolyzed into phenol and salicylic acid and to act as an antiseptic (82–84). Carboxymethyl cellulose sodium, a bulking agent, supposedly adds consistency to the watery diarrhea. In the small amounts in nonprescription drugs, these agents appear to be safe; however, their efficacy has not been proven.

For patients with lactase deficiency, lactase enzymes are available as Lactaid and Lactrase. These preparations are added to milk products or taken with milk at mealtimes to prevent diarrhea.

Fluid Therapy

Replacement of fluid loss and correction of electrolyte imbalance are very important. In mild to moderate diarrhea, oral fluids can be safely prescribed if the patient is not vomiting. The secretory and absorptive mechanisms appear to function separately; therefore, an oral sugar–electrolyte solution can be absorbed during severe diarrhea. This treatment has saved many lives in the third world countries (85). Glucose is essential for the absorption of electrolytes. The World Health Organization (WHO) recommends an oral replacement fluid that contains, per liter, 20 g of glucose, 90 mEq of sodium, 30 mEq of bicarbonate, and 20 mEq of potassium (86). No commercial product available fulfills WHO recommendations. The CDC recommends a homemade solution (Table 6); this mixture, however, is seldom used and if not mixed correctly is dangerous. In severe cases of diarrhea, fluid deficits must be replaced intravenously. In developed countries, commercial oral electrolyte replacement solutions are more convenient and potentially safer because they are premixed and there is less chance of error in preparation (Table 5).

TABLE 6 Home treatment of diarrhea	
Glass No. 1	**Glass No. 2**
8 oz orange, apple, or other fruit juice (rich in potassium)	8 oz tap water (boiled or carbonated if purity of source is unknown)
½ tsp honey or corn syrup (rich in glucose necessary for absorption of essential salts)	¼ tsp baking soda (sodium bicarbonate)
1 pinch of table salt (sodium chloride)	

Drink alternately from each glass. Supplement with carbonated beverages, water (boiled if necessary), tea, or coffee, as desired.
Adapted from J. J. Plorde, *Drug Ther.* (hosp. ed.), *9*, 51 (1979).

Patients with chronic conditions should be under a physician's care. Treatment is based on managing the underlying cause and avoiding the ingestion of agents that contribute to the condition. The medications prescribed may include prescription-only drugs, such as antispasmodics and anti-inflammatory agents, and nonprescription products, such as bulk formers and mucilaginous products.

Many commercial products sold as protectives are thick, viscous suspensions that probably physically protect the mucous membranes from the irritating agents. The adsorbent drugs can bind certain offending agents for short periods of time. The drug substances that form bulk or thick mucilaginous fluids within the GI tract can dilute the concentration of the irritant, act as a physical barrier between it and the GI walls, and hasten the passage of the irritant toward the bowel.

PRODUCT SELECTION GUIDELINES

The information obtained during the patient interview and from the family medication record must be assessed before product selection. Water–glucose–electrolyte products are extremely important. The treatment alternatives are an adsorbent such as attapulgite–pectin mixture, loperamide, a nonprescription opiate-containing antidiarrheal product, calcium polycarbophil, or physician referral.

The pharmacist should assess previous response to treatments and recommend a product that the patient has taken and found satisfactory. Nonprescription antidiarrheal products usually can manage mild to moderate acute diarrhea. Severe acute diarrhea usually requires diphenoxylate, loperamide, or paregoric.

Uncomplicated acute diarrhea usually improves within 24 hours. If the condition remains the same, the pharmacist should recommend continuing treatment for another 24 hours with the same or a more potent product or advise the patient to consult a physician. If control of the symptoms is not achieved within 48 hours, a physician should be consulted. Immediate physician contact is required if the patient is an infant.

The pharmacist should review the label contents to determine the appropriate dosage schedule based on the patient's age, the maximum number of doses per 24 hours, proper storage, and auxiliary administration information such as the need to shake the product before using. The patient must be informed about special precautions on the label such as contraindications to use. Adjunctive therapy includes rest, drinking appropriate fluids, and appropriate diet. Physical and GI tract rest should be encouraged by advising bed rest and discontinuation of all solid foods.

Fluid loss and electrolyte imbalance is a primary problem, especially in infants, young children, and elderly patients.

SUMMARY

Diarrhea is often treated as a simple disorder, but it can be a symptom of a more serious underlying disease. The condition is either acute or chronic. Acute diarrhea is characterized by a sudden onset of loose stools in a previously healthy patient. Chronic diarrhea is characterized by persistent or recurrent episodes accompanied by anorexia, weight loss, and chronic weakness. Simple diarrhea usually can be treated by supportive care or with a nonprescription product.

The debilitating effect of persistent diarrhea is largely caused by loss of water through excretion resulting in electrolyte imbalance. The replacement of these vital fluids and electrolytes is an integral part of diarrheal therapy, particularly in infants and children. This replacement can be accomplished by ingesting appropriate fluids or oral sugar–electrolyte formulations that provide a balanced formulation of electrolytes and carbohydrates.

Complaints of GI irritation should be evaluated for their severity and nature (acute or chronic). For relatively minor acute problems, such as food or drink intolerance, relief may be provided by nonprescription protectives containing adsorbent, bulk-forming, or mucilaginous ingredients. All severely acute, uncontrolled, or chronic GI complaints should be promptly referred to a physician. The pharmacist can contribute to better patient care by being familiar with the disease processes involved in diarrhea and other GI illnesses and by assisting in appropriate selection and use of pharmacologic agents.

REFERENCES

1 A. M. Connell et al., *Br. Med. J., 2,* 1095 (1965).

2 E. Engler, "Dealing with Diarrhea," Science and Medical, Chicago, Ill., 1974.

3 S. F. Phillips, *Postgrad. Med., 57,* 65 (1974).

4 H. L. Dupont and R. B. Hornick, "Disease a Month," Yearbook Medical, Chicago, Ill., July 1969, pp. 1–40.

5 "The Macmillan Medical Cyclopedia," W. A. R. Thomas, Ed., Macmillan, New York, N.Y., 1955, p. 244.

6 W. C. Matousek, "Manual of Differential Diagnosis," Yearbook Medical, Chicago, Ill., 1967, p. 76.

7 "Documentia Geigy: Scientific Tables," 7th ed., K. Diem and C. Lentner, Eds., Ciba-Geigy, Ltd., Basel, Switzerland, 1970, pp. 657–658.

8 A. C. Guyton, "Textbook of Medical Physiology," 5th ed., W. B. Saunders, Philadelphia, Pa., 1976, pp. 850–866.

9 "Gastroenterology," A. Bogoch, Ed., McGraw-Hill, New York, N.Y., 1973, pp. 33–38, 602–721.

10 R. A. Findlestein, *CRC Crit. Rev. Microbiol., 2*, 563 (1973).

11 "Textbook of Medicine," 15th ed., vol. 2, P. B. Beason et al., Eds., W. B. Saunders, Philadelphia, Pa., 1979, p. 1479.

12 M. Field et al., *J. Clin. Invest., 51*, 796 (1972).

13 R. A. Frizzell and S. G. Schultz, *Gastrointes. Physiol., 19*, 205 (1979).

14 L. K. Pickering et al., *Am. J. Clin. Pathol., 68*, 562 (1977).

15 R. B. Sack, *Ann. Intern. Med., 94*, 129 (1981).

16 R. B. Hornick, *Adv. Intern. Med., 21*, 349 (1976).

17 R. C. Patter, *Am. Fam. Phys., 23*, 112 (1981).

18 R. Fekety, *Rev. Infect. Dis., 5*, 246 (1983).

19 "Harrison's Principles of Internal Medicine," 8th ed., G. W. Thorn, Ed., McGraw-Hill, New York, N.Y., 1977, pp. 210–214.

20 A. Z. Kapikian, *N. Engl. J. Med., 294*, 965 (1976).

21 D. S. Schreiber, *Gastroenterology, 73*, 174 (1977).

22 A. Simhon and L. Mata, *Lancet, 1*, 39 (1978).

23 J. L. Wolf and D. S. Schreiber, *Med. Clin. N. Amer., 66*, 575 (1982).

24 J. R. Hamilton, *Can. Med. Assoc. J., 12*, 29 (1980).

25 S. M. Mellinkoff, "The Differential Diagnosis of Diarrhea," McGraw-Hill, New York, N.Y., 1964, pp. 310–325.

26 "Pediatric Therapy," 6th ed., H. C. Shirkey, Ed., C. V. Mosby, St. Louis, Mo., 1980, pp. 602–604.

27 S. Ware, *Lancet, 1*, 252 (1977).

28 *Lancet, 2*, 1126 (1976).

29 J. O. Sherman and J. D. Lloyd-Still, *Drug. Ther.* (hosp. ed.), *2*, 52 (1977).

30 J. E. Mitchell and M. M. Skelton, *Am. Fam. Phys., 37*, 195 (1988).

31 M. S. Wolf, *N. Engl. J. Med., 298*, 319 (1978).

32 E. J. Eastham et al., *Lancet, 2*, 950 (1976).

33 "Problems in Pediatric Drug Therapy," L. Pagliats and R. Levin, Eds., Drug Intelligence, Hamilton, Ill., 1979.

34 A. A. F. Machmoud and K. S. Warren, *J. Infect. Dis., 134*, 639 (1976).

35 W. L. George et al., *J. Infect. Dis., 136*, 822 (1977).

36 J. G. Bartlett, *Rev. Infect. Dis., 1*, 530 (1978).

37 *FDA Drug Bulletin, 5*, 2 (1975).

38 F. J. Tedesco et al., *Ann. Intern. Med., 81*, 429 (1974).

39 F. J. Tedesco et al., *Lancet, 2*, 226 (1978).

40 F. J. Tedesco, *Med. Clin. N. Amer., 66*, 655 (1982).

41 F. J. Tedesco, *J. Infect. Dis., 135*, 95 (1977).

42 F. J. Owens, *Primary Care, 8*, 285 (1982).

43 J. W. Matseshe and S. F. Phillips, *Med. Clin. N. Am., 62*, 141 (1978).

44 E. B. Chang and M. Field, *Drug Ther., 12*, 211 (1982).

45 J. H. Cummings et al., *Br. Med. J., 1*, 537 (1974).

46 W. D. Heizer et al., *Ann. Intern. Med., 68*, 839 (1968).

47 L. S. Basser, *Med. J. Aust., 1*, 47 (1979).

48 M. D. Rawson and M. B. Leeds, *Lancet, 2*, 1121 (1966).

49 "Cancer Facts and Figures," American Cancer Society, New York, N.Y., 1975.

50 C. F. Hawkins and R. Cockel, *Gut, 12*, 208 (1971).

51 H. L. Dupont, *Gastroenterology, 84*, 75 (1983).

52 H. E. T. Pichler et al., *Am. J. Med., 82*, S329–S332, (1987).

53 H. L. Dupont et al., *N. Engl. J. Med., 307*, 841 (1982).

54 C. D. Ericsson et al., *Ann. Intern. Med., 106*, 216 (1987).

55 P. Johnson et al., *J. Am. Med. Assoc., 255*, 757 (1986).

56 H. L. Dupont and R. B. Hornick, *J. Am. Med. Assoc., 226*, 1525 (1973).

57 C. D. Ericsson et al., *J. Infect. Dis., 136*, 693 (1977).

58 H. L. Dupont et al., *Gastroenterology, 74*, 829 (1978).

59 H. L. Dupont, *J. Am. Med. Assoc., 243*, 237 (1980).

60 H. L. Dupont, *Drug Intel. and Clin. Pharm., 21*, 687 (1987).

61 H. L. Dupont et al., *J. Am. Med. Assoc., 257*, 1347 (1987).

62 S. Feldman, *Clin. Pharmacol. Ther., 29*, 788 (1981).

63 S. Feldman et al., *Clin. Pharmacol. Ther., 29*, 788 (1981).

64 L. K. Pickering et al., *J. Pediatr., 99*, 654 (1981).

65 *Patient Care, 12(9)*, 221 (1978).

66 R. Barker, *Postgrad. Med., 65*, 173 (1979).

67 *Federal Register, 40*, 12924 (1975).

68 H. L. Dupont, *Drug Ther., 13*, 127 (1983).

69 Opium Preparations, Section 28:08, American Hospital Formulary Service, Washington, D.C., 1989.

70 R. Wheeldon and H. J. Heggarty, *Arch. Dis. Child., 46*, 562 (1971).

71 H. L. Dupont and R. B. Hornick, *J. Am. Med. Assoc., 226*, 1525 (1973).

72 B. D. Pimparker et al., *Gastroenterology, 40*, 397 (1961).

73 A. J. Grossman et al., *J. Am. Geriatr. Soc., 5*, 187 (1957).

74 M. L. Rutledge et al., *Clin. Pediatr., 2*, 61 (1963).

75 A. Winkelstein, *Curr. Ther. Res., 6*, 572 (1964).

76 J. L. A. Roth, *Am. J. Dig. Dis., 5*, 965 (1960).

77 W. S. Lacorte, *Clin. Pharmacol. Ther., 27*, 263 (1980).

78 M. L. Rutledge, *Curr. Ther. Res., 23*, 443 (1978).

79 J. A. Riese and F. Damrau, *J. Am. Geriatr. Soc., 12*, 500 (1964)

80 B. L. Portnoy et al., *J. Am. Med. Assoc., 236*, 844 (1976).

81 "AMA Drug Evaluations," 4th ed., American Medical Association, Chicago, Ill., 1980, p. 962.

82 "The Merck Index," 9th ed., M. Windholz et al., Eds., Merck, Rahway, N.J., 1976, pp. 927, 951, 1309.

83 "Clinical Toxicology of Commercial Products," 4th ed., R. E. Gosselin et al., Eds., Williams and Wilkins, Baltimore, Md., 1976, pp. 99, 138.

84 "Martindale's The Extra Pharmacopeia," 26th ed., N. W. Blacow and A. Wade, Eds., The Pharmaceutical Press, London, England, 1972, pp. 459, 582, 893, 931.

85 N. Hirschhorn, *Am. J. Clin. Nutr., 33*, 637 (1980).

86 A. Chatterjee et al., *Arch. Dis. Child., 53*, 284 (1978).

ANTIDIARRHEAL PRODUCT TABLE

Product (Manufacturer)	Dosage Form	Opiate	Adsorbent	Other Active Ingredients	Inactive Ingredients
Amogel PG[a] (Vortech)	suspension	powdered opium, 24 mg/ 30 ml	kaolin, 6 g/30 ml pectin, 142.8 mg/30 ml	hyoscyamine sulfate, 0.1037 mg/30 ml atropine sulfate, 0.0194 mg/30 ml scopolamine hydro-bromide, 0.0065 mg/ 30 ml	
Bacid (Fisons)	capsule			carboxymethylcellulose sodium, 100 mg *Lactobacillus acidophilus*	
Corrective Mixture with Paregoric[a] (Beecham Labs)	liquid	paregoric, 0.12 ml/ml	bismuth subsalicy-late, 17 mg/ml	pepsin, 9 mg/ml phenyl salicylate, 4.4 mg/ml zinc sulfocarbolate, 2 mg/ml	alcohol, 2% carminatives demulcents flavor
Devrom (Parthenon)	chewable tablet		bismuth subgal-late, 200 mg		
Diabismul[a] (Forest)	suspension	opium, 0.47 mg/ ml	kaolin, 170 mg/ml pectin, 5.3 mg/ml		parabens
DIA-quel[a] (MiLance)	liquid	paregoric, 0.15 ml/ml	pectin, 4.8 mg/ml	homatropine methyl-bromide, 0.003 mg/ ml	alcohol, 10%
Diar-Aid (Thompson Medical)	tablet		activated attapul-gite, 750 mg pectin, 150 mg		
Diarrest (Dover)	tablet		pectin	calcium carbonate	
Diasorb (O'Connor)	liquid tablet		activated attapulgite, 750 mg/5 ml 750 mg/tablet		
Diatrol (Otis Clapp)	tablet		pectin, 65 mg	calcium carbonate, 261 mg	
Digestalin (Vortech)	tablet		activated charcoal, 5.3 mg bismuth subgal-late, 3.8 mg	pepsin, 2 mg berberis, 1.2 mg papain, 1.2 mg pancreatin, 0.4 mg hydrastis, 0.08 mg	
Donnagel (Robins)	suspension		kaolin, 200 mg/ml pectin, 4.76 mg/ ml	hyoscyamine sulfate, 0.0035 mg/ml atropine sulfate, 0.0006 mg/ml scopolamine hydro-bromide, 0.0002 mg/ ml	alcohol, 3.8% sodium benzoate, 2 mg/ml
Donnagel-PG[a] (Robins)	suspension	powdered opium, 0.8 mg/ml	kaolin, 200 mg/ml pectin, 4.76 mg/ ml	hyoscyamine sulfate, 0.0035 mg/ml atropine sulfate, 0.0006 mg/ml scopolamine hydro-bromide, 0.0002 mg/ ml	alcohol, 5% sodium benzoate, 2 mg/ml

ANTIDIARRHEAL PRODUCT TABLE, continued

Product (Manufacturer)	Dosage Form	Opiate	Adsorbent	Other Active Ingredients	Inactive Ingredients
Imodium A-D (McNeil)	caplet	loperamide hydrochloride, 2 mg			lactose
Imodium A-D (McNeil)	liquid	loperamide hydrochloride, 1 mg/5 ml			alcohol, 5.25% citric acid flavor glycerin parabens
Infantol Pink[a] (Scherer)	liquid	opium, 0.5 mg/ml	pectin, 7.4 mg/ml bismuth subsalicylate, 13 mg/ml	zinc phenolsulfonate, 3.5 mg/ml	calcium carrageenan, 3.6 mg/ml saccharin sodium, 0.27 mg/ml glycerin alcohol, 2% peppermint oil
Kaodene Non-Narcotic (Pfeiffer)	suspension		kaolin, 129.6 mg/ml pectin, 6.5 mg/ml		
Kaodene with Codeine[a] (Pfeiffer)	suspension	codeine phosphate, 32.4 mg/30 ml	kaolin, 3.9 g/30 ml pectin, 194.4 mg/30 ml bismuth subsalicylate	carboxymethylcellulose sodium	
Kaodene with Paregoric[a] (Pfeiffer)	suspension	paregoric, 0.125 mg/ml	kaolin, 129.6 mg/ml pectin, 6.4 mg/ml		
Kaolin Pectin Suspension (Roxane)	suspension		kaolin, 190 mg/ml pectin, 4.34 mg/ml	carboxymethylcellulose sodium, 0.4%	glycerin, 1.75% lime/mint flavor saccharin sodium, 0.025%
Kaopectate (Upjohn)	chewable tablet tablet		attapulgite, 300 mg/chewable tablet 750 mg/tablet		
Kaopectate Concentrated (Upjohn)	suspension		attapulgite, 600 mg/15 ml		
Kao-tin (Major)	suspension		kaolin, 5.85 g/30 ml pectin, 130 mg/30 ml		
K-C (Century)	suspension		kaolin, 5.2 g/30 ml pectin, 260 mg/30 ml bismuth subcarbonate, 260 mg/30 ml		
K-P (Century)	suspension		kaolin, 5.2 g/30 ml pectin, 260 mg/30 ml		

ANTIDIARRHEAL PRODUCT TABLE, continued

Product (Manufacturer)	Dosage Form	Opiate	Adsorbent	Other Active Ingredients	Inactive Ingredients
K-Pek (Rugby)	suspension		kaolin, 5.85 g/ 30 ml pectin, 130 mg/ 30 ml		
Lactinex (Becton Dickinson)	granules tablet			*Lactobacillus acidophilus Lactobacillus bulgaricus*	
More-Dophilus (Freeda)	powder			acidophilus-carrot derivative, 4 billion units/g	
Parepectolin[a] (Rorer)	suspension	paregoric, 0.12 ml/ml	kaolin, 186 mg/ml pectin, 5.5 mg/ml		alcohol, 0.69%
Pepto-Bismol (Procter & Gamble)	chewable tablet liquid		bismuth subsalicylate, 300 mg/ tablet 525 mg/30 ml		
Percy Medicine (Merrick)	liquid		bismuth subnitrate, 959 mg/ 10 ml	calcium hydroxide, 21.9 mg/10 ml	alcohol, 5%
Quiagel (Rugby)	suspension		kaolin, 6 g/30 ml pectin, 194.4/ 30 ml	hyoscyamine sulfate, 0.1037 mg/30 ml atropine sulfate, 0.0194 mg/30 ml scopolamine hydrobromide, 0.0065 mg/30 ml	
Quiagel PG[a] (Rugby)	suspension	powdered opium, 24 mg/ 30 ml	kaolin, 6 g/30 ml pectin, 142.8 mg/ 30 ml	hyoscyamine sulfate, 0.1037 mg/30 ml atropine sulfate, 0.0194 mg/30 ml scopolamine hydrobromide, 0.0065 mg/30 ml	
Rheaban (Leeming)	tablet		activated attapulgite, 750 mg		

[a] Schedule V drug; nonprescription sale forbidden in some states.

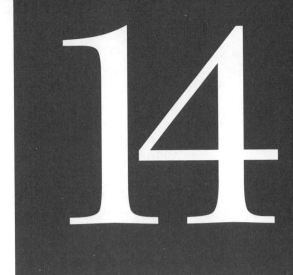

John M. Kinsella

ANTHELMINTIC PRODUCTS

Questions to ask in patient/consumer counseling

Have worms appeared in the stools?

Have you had any nausea, diarrhea, or abdominal pain recently?

Have you been bothered by itching in the anal area?

Are other members of your family or close contacts also affected?

Have you lost weight or do you become fatigued easily?

How long have the symptoms been present?

Have you seen a physician for this problem?

Has the problem occurred in the past? How was it treated? Did the treatment work?

If the patient is not an adult, what is the age and approximate weight of the patient?

Have you traveled out of the country? If so, where and when?

Anthelmintics are used to treat worm (helminth) infections. An estimated 4.5 billion humans harbor helminths. The incidence of helminth infection may exceed 90% in areas where sanitation is insufficient, economic conditions are poor, and preventive medicine practices are inadequate (1). Worm infections are a serious health problem, particularly in tropical regions, and result in a general debilitation of large populations. These infections reduce resistance to disease, physical development in children, and productivity.

Nematode (roundworm) infections endemic in the United States include enterobiasis (pinworms), ascariasis, whipworms, hookworms, anisakiasis, and trichinosis. Other worms that parasitize humans are cestodes (tapeworms) and trematodes (flukes). Table 1 lists common human helminth infections and their symptoms.

The immigration of thousands of Southeast Asian refugees has introduced an exotic element to medical practice in states such as California, New Mexico, and Montana where hookworms, whipworms, and liver flukes were not endemic (2). Fortunately, the life cycles of these worms cannot be completed in these areas, minimizing the risk of transmission and the threat to public health.

Pyrantel pamoate is now the only nonprescription anthelmintic on the market; its sole indication is for pinworms. Nevertheless, the pharmacist is often the first person called upon when a patient suspects a helminth infection. Most people find the thought of a worm infection extremely disturbing, so the pharmacist should be aware of the signs, symptoms, and life cycles of common helminths to appropriately counsel patients and refer them to a physician when indicated.

ENTEROBIASIS

Enterobiasis, or oxyuriasis, is commonly called pinworm, seatworm, or threadworm infection. The intestinal infection in humans is caused by *Enterobius vermicularis*. Unlike many helminth infections, enterobiasis is not limited to rural and poverty-stricken areas but occurs in urban communities of every economic status. *Enterobius vermicularis* is common in temperate climates and is especially prevalent among schoolchildren. The female adult worm is about 10 mm long, and the adult male is about 3 mm. The adult worms inhabit the first portion of the large intestine. The mature female usually stores eggs in her body until several thousand accumulate. She then migrates down the colon and out the anus and deposits the eggs in the perianal region. Within a few hours, infective larvae develop within the eggs. Ingestion of the eggs releases larvae in the small intestine. Within 15–43 days of ingestion, newly developed gravid females migrate to the anal area and discharge eggs, and the cycle continues.

The most common ways of transmitting pinworm infection in children are probably direct anus-to-mouth transfer of eggs by contaminated fingers and eating food that has been handled by soiled hands. Reinfection may occur readily because eggs often are found under the fingernails of infected children after scratching anal areas. The eggs may be dislodged from the perianal region into the environment and may enter the mouth via hands, food, or the swallowing of airborne eggs.

Symptoms

Slight infections of enterobiasis may be asymptomatic. The most important and most frequent symptom is usually an irritating itching in the perianal and perineal regions. This itching normally occurs at night when the gravid female deposits her eggs in these areas. Scratching to relieve the itching may lead to bacterial infection of the area. Nervousness, inability to concentrate, lack of appetite, and unusual dark circles around the eyes frequently are observed in pinworm-infected children. Worms occasionally enter the female genital

tract and become encapsulated within the uterus or fallopian tubules, or they may migrate into the peritoneal cavity, resulting in the formation of granulomas in these areas.

The physical symptoms are not the sole misery-inducing effects of pinworms. Parents are often dismayed to find worms near the anus of a child, and this psychologic trauma or "pinworm neurosis" also must be considered one of the harmful effects of enterobiasis (3). Patients need to be assured that pinworms are common and that no stigma is attached to their occurrence.

Perianal itching is a symptom of many other conditions mistakenly attributed to pinworm infection (4). Seborrheic dermatitis, atopic eczema, psoriasis, lichen planus, and neurodermatitis may produce severe itching when the perianal region is involved. An allergic or contact dermatitis may result from soaps or ointments used by the patient in an attempt to alleviate the initial mild symptoms. Ointments containing local anesthetics are well-known sensitizers and should be suspected as contributing to the problem. Other parasitic infestations that induce itching, such as scabies and pediculosis pubis, may involve the perianal skin in addition to the larger areas of the body. Monilial infection may be the cause of pruritus ani especially in patients with diabetes mellitus. Other causes of pruritus include excessive vaginal discharge and urinary incontinence in women and excessive sweating during hot weather. When mineral oil is used as a cathartic, it tends to leak and may produce increased moisture and itching unless appropriate anal hygiene is practiced.

Treatment of pinworm infection should begin with an accurate diagnosis. This can be done by either of two methods (5). One method is to cover the end of a swab or tongue depressor with scotch tape (sticky side out) and apply this end to the perianal area. The presence or absence of eggs is confirmed by examining the tape under the microscope. Collection of eggs can be done at home, but inspection and evaluation must be done in a laboratory or physician's office. Another detection method used frequently in children is to visually inspect the anal site using a flashlight an hour or so after the child has gone to bed. Female pinworms, which are 6–12 mm in length, can be seem emerging from the perianal region after depositing their eggs.

Treatment

In the past, gentian violet was the only nonprescription drug available for treatment of pinworm infections. Genetic toxicity data indicate that gentian violet interacts with deoxyribonucleic acid (DNA) in cultured cells, suggesting a potential carcinogenic ef-

TABLE 1 Human helminth infections

Class/ Genus and species	Common name	Source of infection	Symptoms
NEMATODA			
Ancylostoma duodenale, Necator americanus	Hookworm	Contact with contaminated soil; larvae are ingested or penetrate the skin on contact	Anemia caused by blood loss (0.5 ml/ worm/day); indigestion, anorexia, headache, cough, vomiting, diarrhea, weakness, urticaria at the site of entry into the skin
Ascaris lumbricoides, Ascaris suum	Roundworm	Ingestion of eggs through contact with fecally contaminated soil	Mild cases may be asymptomatic; GI discomfort, pain, diarrhea; intestinal obstruction in severe cases; occasionally, bile or pancreatic duct may be obstructed; allergic reactions
Enterobius (Oxyuris) vermicularis	Pinworm, Seatworm, Threadworm	Ingestion of eggs by fecal contamination of hands, food, clothing, and bedding; reinfection is common; the most common worm infestation in the United States, especially in schoolchildren	Indigestion, intense perianal itching, especially at night, resulting in loss of sleep; scratching may cause infection; irritability and fatigue in children
Trichinella spiralis	None	Ingestion of poorly cooked wild animal meat or pork; becoming rare in the United States	Adult worms in intestinal tract cause vomiting, nausea, diarrhea; migrating larvae cause malaise, weakness, fever, sweating, dermatitis, cardiac and respiratory distress; can be fatal
Trichuris trichiuria	Whipworm	Ingestion of eggs through contact with fecally contaminated soil	Mild cases may be asymptomatic; insomnia, loss of appetite, diarrhea, anemia; in severe cases, colitis, proctitis, prolapsed rectum
Anisakis and *Pseudoterranova*	None	Eating raw or poorly cooked fish	Tingling throat, abdominal pain, fever, nausea, vomiting, diarrhea
CESTOIDEA			
Taenia saginata	Beef tapeworm	Eating poorly cooked infected beef	No characteristic symptoms; digestive upset, diarrhea, anemia, dizziness vary with the degree of infestation
Taenia solium	Pork tapeworm	Eating poorly cooked infected pork	Similar to beef tapeworm infection; self-infection with eggs may lead to cysts in eye, brain, heart, other organs
Diphyllobothrium latum	Fish tapeworm	Eating raw or inadequately cooked fish	Similar to beef tapeworm infestation
Hymenolepis nana	Dwarf tapeworm	Eating food contaminated with human feces	Similar to beef tapeworm infestation

fect (6–8). Even though the evidence is not conclusive, the Food and Drug Administration (FDA) has declared gentian violet a "nonmonograph ingredient"; therefore it can no longer be marketed as an anthelmintic (9).

Pyrantel pamoate was first used in veterinary practice as a broad-spectrum drug for pinworms, round-worms, and hookworms. Because of its effectiveness and lack of toxicity, it became an important drug for treating certain helminth infections in humans (10). Pyrantel is a depolarizing neuromuscular agent that paralyzes helminths. This causes them to lose their hold on the intestinal wall and be eliminated from the body.

The FDA has accepted the recommendation to move pyrantel pamoate from prescription only to non-prescription status for the treatment of pinworms (9). Helminth infections other than pinworms should be treated only by a physician. During 1989–90, Pfizer has gradually replaced its prescription Antiminth oral suspension with nonprescription packaging under the same brand name. The FDA panel has recommended the following labeling for pyrantel pamoate products:

Indication

- For the treatment of pinworms.

Warnings

- If upset stomach, diarrhea, nausea, or vomiting occurs with this medication, discontinue using it and consult a physician.

- If you are pregnant or have liver disease, do not take this product unless directed by a physician.

Directions

- The recommended dose is 5 mg/lb or 11 mg/kg, not to exceed 1 g. A dosage schedule by weight will be included.

- When one individual in a household has pinworms, the entire household should be treated. Infants under 2 years of age, or children who weigh less than 25 pounds, should not be treated without first consulting a physician.

- Take only according to directions.

- Do not exceed the recommended dosage.

- If any worms other than pinworms are present before or after treatment, consult a physician.

The following additional measures are recommended to prevent reinfections (11):

- Wash bed linens, bed clothes, and underwear of entire family.

- Take a daily morning shower to remove eggs deposited in the perianal region during the night.

- Use disinfectants daily on the toilet seat and bathtub.

- Wear close-fitting shorts under one-piece pajamas to prevent scratching at night and migration of worms.

- After an infected child goes to the bathroom, scrub the child's fingers with a brush; trim the child's nails regularly.

- Wash hands frequently, especially before meals and after using the toilet.

ASCARIASIS

Ascariasis is caused by *Ascaris lumbricoides* (roundworm). The adult ascarids are 15–35 cm long and live in the small intestine. The female lays eggs that are passed in the feces and develop into infective larvae in the soil. Although mature larvae in the shell remain viable in the soil for many months, the eggs do not hatch until they are ingested by humans. Upon ingestion, the larvae are released in the small intestine. They penetrate the intestinal wall, migrate via the bloodstream to the lungs, travel up the respiratory tree to the epiglottis where they are swallowed, and develop into male and female adults in the small intestine.

Although *A. lumbricoides* has been primarily a problem of the southeastern United States, recent information has shown that swine *Ascaris*, *A. suum*, is also infective to humans and occurs in northern states such as New Hampshire, Washington, and Montana (12). *A. suum* is more common in children and usually does not develop to the egg-laying stage. Instead, the immature worm, about 15 cm long, is rejected and passes out with the stool. The use of pig manure in home gardens should be discouraged. Pharmacists should consider this type of infection if a patient mentions a large worm has been passed.

Symptoms

The larvae and adults are capable of extensive migration and therefore induce diverse symptoms involving the respiratory and gastrointestinal (GI) tracts. Although many patients are asymptomatic, the most common symptoms caused by ascarid infections are vague abdominal discomfort and abdominal colic (13). Occasionally diarrhea is present. Children characteristically have fever and may lose weight or fail to grow. The symptoms may suggest abdominal tumor or peptic ulcer disease. Migration of the worms may cause intestinal obstruction that may lead to perforation, appendicitis, and peritonitis. Light infestations may be asymptomatic; heavy infestations present symptoms that may be mistaken for a variety of respiratory and GI diseases.

Cough is produced during migration of the larvae through the lungs; the larvae may be coughed up and seen in the sputum. Fever and a pulmonary infiltrate also may accompany this pulmonary syndrome.

Allergic reactions such as asthma, hay fever, urticaria, and conjunctivitis also may result from absorption of toxins from the worm.

Treatment

There are no nonprescription drugs for treating ascarid infections. Cure rates greater than 90% are achieved with mebendazole, piperazine salts, and pyrantel pamoate, which are available only by prescription (10). Pyrantel pamoate, now available as a nonprescription drug for pinworms, may be available in the future for treating ascarid infections. Piperazine is contraindicated in the presence of convulsive disorders or impaired renal or hepatic functions. The treatment of swine ascariasis is unnecessary if the worm has already been passed, but the physician may prescribe a course of treatment for the patient's peace of mind in case more worms are present.

HOOKWORM INFECTION

In the United States, hookworm infection in humans is caused by *Necator americanus*. The adult worms, which are about 10 mm long, attach themselves to the small intestine. Their eggs are excreted in the feces, hatch in warm, moist soil, and develop into active filariform larvae. On contact with humans, the larvae rapidly penetrate the skin, enter the bloodstream, and are carried to the lungs. They then enter the alveoli, ascend the trachea to the throat, are swallowed, and pass into the small intestine, where they develop into mature adults.

Symptoms

When the larvae penetrate the exposed skin, an erythematous maculopapular rash and edema with severe itching may persist for several days. The lesions most commonly occur on the feet, particularly between the toes, and have been termed "ground itch." Dog and cat hookworm larvae may also penetrate human skin and cause a similar condition, but they do not progress to the lung or intestinal stages.

Heavy infections may produce a cough and fever when the larvae migrate through the lungs. Mild intestinal infections may be asymptomatic; moderately severe infections may result in indigestion, dizziness, headache, weakness, fatigue, nausea, and vomiting. In advanced cases, there is epigastric pain, abdominal tenderness, chronic fatigue, and alternating constipation and diarrhea. The epigastric pain is relieved by eating foods high in bulk or fiber (14). As with ascariasis, these symptoms may be mistaken for those of some respiratory and GI disorders.

A major clinical manifestation of hookworm infection is iron deficiency anemia resulting from the loss of blood (as much as 0.15 ml per worm each day), which the adult worm extracts while it is attached to the intestinal mucosa (15). Malnourished children and some menstruating women are especially prone to anemia, depending on the severity of the infection. Even people with adequate iron intake may become anemic if the hookworm infection is severe enough to cause a blood loss that the normal body erythropoietic mechanisms cannot handle.

Treatment

Mebendazole and pyrantel pamoate are the drugs of choice to treat hookworm infections.

WHIPWORM INFECTION

Whipworms, *Trichuris trichiuria*, range from 30 to 50 mm long, with a threadlike anterior end and a thick posterior end, resembling a whip. The anterior ends are burrowed into the mucosa of the ileocecal area. Eggs excreted in the feces mature in warm, shady soil in about 21 days. When swallowed, the eggs hatch in the small intestine, and the larvae enter the Lieberkühn's crypts. After molting, they reenter the lumen and migrate to the ileocecal area, maturing in about 3 months.

Symptoms

Infections of fewer than 100 worms rarely cause clinical symptoms. Trauma to the intestinal epithelium and submucosa can cause a chronic hemorrhage, resulting in anemia. Secondary bacterial infection may result in colitis, proctitis, and, in extreme cases, prolapse of the rectum. Symptoms of infection include insomnia, loss of appetite, urticaria, flatulence, and prolonged diarrhea (16).

Treatment

Mebendazole is the drug of choice for whipworms. No nonprescription drugs are available.

ANISAKIASIS

Because of the recent popularity of raw fish dishes such as sushi, previously rare anisakid infections have become a growing problem, especially on the West Coast. Larval nematodes, infective to marine mammals such as seals and sea lions, when ingested by man may cause moderate to severe intestinal problems. Pacific red snapper and Pacific salmon have a particularly high prevalence of infection with these nematodes (17).

Symptoms

Some anisakid species do not invade the intestinal mucosa but wander into the oropharynx or esophagus, causing a tingling sensation. They are often coughed up within 48 hours of ingestion, causing considerable consternation. Other species penetrate the wall of the stomach or intestine, causing symptoms mimicking diseases such as acute appendicitis, ulcer, or cancer. Because no eggs are produced, stool examination is of no use, and diagnosis may depend on endoscopic examination or even laporotomy (17).

Treatment

Anthelmintics are apparently ineffective in killing anisakid larvae. The only definitive treatment in severe cases is surgical resection of the inflamed intestine. Patients should be warned of the dangers of eating raw or poorly cooked fish, especially fish from areas where marine mammals are prevalent. Freezing fish at $-17°C$ for 24 hours will kill any larvae present (18).

TRICHINOSIS

Trichinosis is caused by a small nematode (*Trichinella spiralis*). Although pork is the principal source of infection, in recent years the percentage of cases attributed to eating wild bear meat has increased dramatically. These cases characteristically peak in December and January because of the consumption of homemade sausage during the Christmas holidays (19).

When infected meat is eaten, gastric juices free the larvae, which penetrate the wall of the small intestine and develop into sexually mature adults. After the female deposits larvae in the intestinal mucosa, the larvae are carried by the bloodstream throughout the body and enter striated muscle fibers where they become encysted. The muscles of the diaphragm, tongue, and eye, and the deltoid, pectoral, and intercostal muscles are affected most often. Larvae that reach other tissues, such as the heart and brain, disintegrate and are absorbed. Absorption can cause marked inflammation and result in myocarditis and encephalitis.

The incidence of trichinosis in the United States fell from approximately 150 cases a year in the 1970s to 57 cases in 1986 (20). This decline is directly attributed to laws requiring that garbage fed to hogs be thoroughly cooked and that meat for human consumption be stored at low temperatures. In addition, public education programs were implemented on the need to thoroughly cook pork.

Symptoms

Symptoms of trichinosis are extremely variable, depending on the severity of the infection. If the meat is heavily infected, larval invasion into the intestinal mucosa may cause nausea, vomiting, and diarrhea 1–4 days after ingestion. In some cases, no symptoms are evident. After the seventh day, migration of the larvae may produce muscle weakness, stiffness or pain, and irregular, persistent fever of 100–105°F (37.7–40.5°C). These symptoms may be accompanied by an urticarial rash and respiratory symptoms such as cough and bronchospasm. Skeletal muscle invasion produces muscular pain, tenderness, and often severe weakness. There may be pain when chewing, swallowing, breathing, or moving the eyes or limbs. Another common symptom is edema, usually manifested as a puffiness around the eyes. Once the larvae are encysted, the only symptom may be a vague aching in the muscles.

Clinical diagnosis of trichinosis is difficult because most mild infections are asymptomatic and the nature of the symptoms may vary and change. A combination of irregular fever, periorbital edema, GI disturbances, muscle soreness, and hemorrhages in the nail beds may suggest trichinosis. The pharmacist should refer patients with these symptoms to a physician for evaluation and diagnosis. Self-diagnosis is unwise, because many diseases, such as sinusitis and influenza, mimic the symptoms of trichinosis (21).

Treatment

Treatment includes mild analgesics (for pain relief), sedatives, adequate diet, and anti-inflammatory steroids. Thiabendazole has been shown to kill the larvae in animal experiments; results in humans have varied. It also has been effective in reducing the fever and relieving the muscle pain, tenderness, and edema of trichinosis (22). For severe symptoms, the current recommended therapy is corticosteroids in addition to thiabendazole (23). There are no nonprescription drugs for the mitigation of the disease.

CERCARIAL DERMATITIS

Cercarial dermatitis, or swimmer's itch, is caused by flukes of the genera *Trichobilharzia* and *Ornithobilharzia*, which are normally blood parasites of ducks and muskrats. Eggs of these worms when released into water infect various species of snails, which, in turn, release a free-swimming infective stage called a cercaria. These cercariae are capable of penetrating the skin of swimmers or waders, where they are rapidly killed by an immune reaction.

Symptoms

The inflammation resulting from the cercariae produces a local erythema, a minute macule at the site of penetration, and an intense itching. Because hundreds of cercariae may penetrate, the result is a generalized fiery rash. Cases usually occur in spring and summer both in freshwater and saltwater areas where migratory waterfowl and large snail populations are present.

Treatment

Treatment of swimmer's itch should be symptomatic because it generally subsides in 24–48 hours. Antihistamines and topical steroids will reduce the local immune response, and warm baths are helpful in combating the itching.

SUMMARY

The pharmacist should be familiar with the common helminth infections and their effects and should discourage self-diagnosis and treatment. The clinical manifestations of these parasitic diseases are so general and characteristic of so many other illnesses that attempting self-diagnosis of helminthiasis not only is difficult, but could also lead to the neglect of a more serious condition. Diagnosis should be based on clinical and laboratory evidence.

Enterobiasis is the only helminth infection that should be treated with a nonprescription drug. Self-medication should be discouraged for all other helminth infections. The availability of effective, relatively safe, easy-to-take prescription drugs that can eradicate many helminth infections in one or two doses should be reason enough to avoid self-medication. The pharmacist certainly should encourage the patient to consult a physician for treatment.

REFERENCES

1 "Foundations of Parasitology," 2nd ed., G. D. Schmidt and L. S. Roberts, Eds., C. V. Mosby, St. Louis, Mo., 1981, p. 2.

2 M. R. Skeels et al., *Am. J. Publ. Health*, 72, 57–59 (1982).

3 H. C. Wormser and H. N. Abramson, *U.S. Pharmacist*, 2, 46 (1977).

4 T. L. Schrock, in "Gastrointestinal Disease," M. H. Sleisinger and J. S. Fordtran, Eds., W. B. Saunders, Philadelphia, Pa., 1978, pp. 1882–1884.

5   *Federal Register, 45,* 59543 (1980).

6   H. R. Rosencranz and H. S. Carr, *Br. Med. J., 3,* 702 (1971).

7   W. Au et al., *Mutation Res., 58,* 269 (1978).

8   T. C. Hsu et al., *Mutation Res., 45,* 233 (1977).

9   *Federal Register, 51,* 27756 (1986).

10   "The Pharmacological Basis of Therapeutics," 7th ed., A. G. Gilman et al., Eds., Macmillan, New York, N.Y., 1985, p. 1024.

11   "Drugs of Choice 1978/1979," W. Modell, Ed., C. V. Mosby, St. Louis, Mo., 1978, p. 378.

12   W. D. Lord and W. L. Bullock, *N. Eng. J. Med., 306,* 1113 (1982).

13   L. L. Brandborg, in "Gastrointestinal Diseases," M. H. Sleisinger and J. S. Fordtran, Eds., W. B. Saunders, Philadelphia, Pa., 1978, p. 1164.

14   L. L. Brandborg, in "Gastrointestinal Diseases," M. H. Sleisinger and J. S. Fordtran, Eds., W. B. Saunders, Philadelphia, Pa., 1978, p. 1169.

15   "Foundations of Parasitology," 2nd ed., G. D. Schmidt and L. S. Roberts, Eds., C. V. Mosby, St. Louis, Mo., 1981, p. 473.

16   "Foundations of Parasitology," 2nd ed., G. D. Schmidt and L. S. Roberts, Eds., C. V. Mosby, St. Louis, Mo., 1981, p. 448.

17   J. H. McKerrow et al., *N. Eng. J. Med., 319,* 1228 (1988).

18   M. M. Kliks, *Am. J. Trop. Med. Hyg., 32,* 52 (1983).

19   *Morbid. Mortal. Weekly Rep., 29,* 482 (1980).

20   *Morbid. Mortal. Weekly Rep., 37,* 1 (1988).

21   S. E. Gould, "Trichinosis in Man and Animals," Charles C. Thomas, Ed., Springfield, Ill., 1970, pp. 307–321.

22   W. C. Campbell and A. C. Cuckler, *Tex. Rep. Biol. Med., 27 (2),* 665 (1969).

23   *Med. Lett. Drugs Ther., 30,* 15 (1988).

ANTHELMINTIC PRODUCT TABLE

Product (Manufacturer)	Dosage Form	Active Ingredients	Inactive Ingredients
Antiminth (Pfizer)	suspension	pyrantel, 250 mg/5 ml (as pamoate)	caramel-currant flavor citric acid glycerin lecithin magnesium aluminum silicate polysorbate povidone simethicone emulsion sodium benzoate sorbitol solution water
Reese's Pinworm (Reese)	liquid	pyrantel, 250 mg/5 ml (as pamoate)	

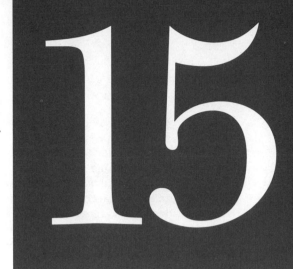

Clarence E. Curry, Jr., and
Demetris Tatum-Butler

LAXATIVE PRODUCTS

Questions to ask in patient/consumer counseling

Why do you feel you need a laxative?

Do you have any abdominal discomfort or pain, bloating, weight loss, nausea, or vomiting? What other symptoms do you have?

Are you currently being treated by a physician for any illness?

Have you recently had abdominal surgery?

Are you pregnant?

How often do you normally have a bowel movement? Have you noticed a change in frequency?

How would you describe your bowel movements? Have they recently changed in any way?

Has the appearance of your stools changed? In what way?

How long has constipation been a problem?

Have you previously used laxatives to relieve constipation?

Are you using a laxative now? How often and how long have you used a laxative?

Are you currently taking any medicine other than laxatives?

Have you attempted to relieve the constipation by eating more cereals, bread with a high fiber content, fruits, or vegetables?

How much physical exercise do you get?

How many glasses of water do you drink each day?

Are you allergic to any medicines?

Have you had any unwanted effects from laxatives, such as diarrhea?

Extensive media advertising promotes the idea that having clockwork-like bowel movements in some way enhances well-being and social acceptability. With the general increase in consumer interest in natural products, particularly products for constipation, overall sales of laxatives in chain pharmacies alone in the United States in 1988 increased 8% over the previous year and accounted for one-third of a billion dollars in sales (1). However, not all laxatives are natural products in the pharmaceutical sense, nor are "natural" products natural to normal body biochemical and physiologic processes.

Laxative products facilitate the passage and elimination of feces from the colon and rectum (2). There

343

are few recognized medical indications for the use of laxatives, but many people use these products to alleviate what they consider to be constipation. Constipation has different meanings for different patients; however, it generally is defined as a decrease in the frequency of fecal elimination characterized by the difficult passage of hard, dry stools. It usually results from the abnormally slow movement of feces through the colon with resultant accumulation in the descending colon.

CAUSES OF CONSTIPATION

Causes of constipation are numerous (Tables 1–5). Idiopathic constipation often begins in childhood or adolescence. In adults, constipation of recent origin suggests an organic or drug-induced cause (3). The main disorders of the colon, ulcerative colitis and excessive parasympathetic stimulation, and the chronic misuse of irritant laxative drugs may cause constipation or diarrhea. The etiology of colitis remains unknown. Constipation is often a problem in patients with ulcerative colitis that is limited to the rectum. In ulcerative colitis patients with diarrhea, the use of antidiarrheal agents can result in colonic dilation and the accumulation of hard stool in an area of bowel not affected by disease (4).

Constipation of organic origin may be caused by hypothyroidism, megacolon, stricture, or lesions (benign or malignant). Laxatives are contraindicated in such cases; proper diagnosis and medical treatment should be obtained.

PHYSIOLOGY OF THE GASTROINTESTINAL TRACT

The digestive and absorptive functions of the gastrointestinal (GI) system involve the intestinal smooth muscle, visceral reflexes, and GI hormones (Figure 1). (See Chapter 11, *Antacid Products*.) Nearly all absorption (>94%) occurs in the small intestine; relatively little absorption occurs in the stomach or duodenum. The function of the colon is to allow for the orderly elimination from the body of nonabsorbed food products, desquamated cells from the gut lumen, and detoxified and metabolic end products. The colon functions to conserve fluid and electrolytes so that the quantity eliminated represents about 10% presented to it in a 24-hour period. In addition to conserving fluid and electrolytes, the colon has the capacity (as does the kidney) to absorb certain electrolytes in a nonisotonic fashion (5). If approximately 6 liters of fluid per day are ingested and supplied by secretions of the GI tract, about 1.5%, or 90 ml, will be excreted with the feces (6).

Tonic contractions of the stomach churn and knead food, and large peristaltic waves start at the fundus and move food toward the duodenum. The rate at which the stomach contents are emptied into the duodenum is regulated by autonomic reflexes or a hormonal link between the duodenum and the stomach. Carbohydrates are emptied from the stomach most rapidly, proteins more slowly, and fats exhibit the slowest emptying rate. Vagotomy and fear tend to lengthen

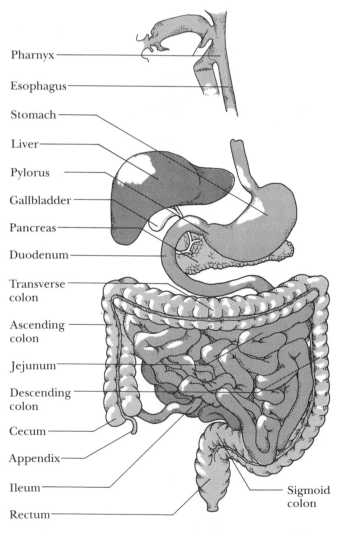

Pharnyx

Esophagus

Stomach

Liver

Pylorus

Gallbladder

Pancreas

Duodenum

Transverse colon

Ascending colon

Jejunum

Descending colon

Cecum

Appendix

Ileum

Rectum

Sigmoid colon

Note: Portion of small intestine pulled aside for clarity.

FIGURE 1   Anatomy of the digestive system.

emptying time; excitement generally shortens it. Most factors that slow the stomach emptying rate also inhibit secretion of hydrochloric acid and pepsin. When the osmotic pressure of the stomach contents is higher or lower than that of the plasma, the gastric emptying rate is slowed until isotonicity is achieved.

The mixing and passage of the contents of the small and large intestines are the result of four muscular movements: pendular, segmental, peristaltic, and vermiform. Pendular movements result from contractions of the longitudinal muscles of the intestine, which pass up and down small segments of the gut at the rate of about 10 contractions per minute. Pendular movements mix, rather than propel, the contents. Segmental movements result from contractions of the circular muscles and occur at about the same rate as pendular movements. Their primary function also is mixing. Pendular and segmental movements are caused by the intrinsic contractility of smooth muscle and occur in the absence of innervation of intestinal tissue.

Peristaltic movements propel intestinal contents by circular contractions that form behind a point of stimulation and pass along the GI tract toward the rectum. The contraction rate ranges from 2 to 20 cm per second. These contractions require an intact myenteric (Auerbach's) nerve plexus, which apparently is located in the intestinal mucosa. Peristaltic waves move the intestinal contents through the small intestine in about 3.5 hours. Vermiform (wormlike) movements occur mainly in the large intestine (colon) and are caused by the contraction of several centimeters of the colonic smooth muscle at one time. In the cecum and ascending colon, the contents retain a fluid consistency, and peristaltic and antiperistaltic waves occur frequently. However, the activity of the transverse, descending, and sigmoid segments of the colon is very irregular, and here, through further water absorption, the contents become semisolid.

Three or four times a day, a strong peristaltic wave (mass movement) propels the contents about one-third (38 cm) the length of the colon. When initiated by a meal, the mass movement is referred to as the gastrocolic reflex. This normal reflex seems to be associated with the entrance of food into the stomach. The sigmoid colon serves as a storage place for fecal matter until defecation. Except for the fauces and anus, the entire alimentary canal normally functions involuntarily as a coordinated unit (7).

The act of defecation involves multiple physiologic processes, but basically is the rectal passage of accumulated fecal material. The rectum is a passageway and a central "notification chamber" (8). The fecal material from the sigmoid colon is propelled into the rectum by a mass peristaltic movement, which usually occurs at breakfast time in normal persons with normal eating habits. This movement results in a desire to defecate

TABLE 1 Drugs inducing constipation

Analgesics
Anesthetic agents
Antacids (calcium and aluminum compounds)
Anticholinergics
Anticonvulsants
Antidepressive agents
Barium sulfate
Bismuth
Diuretics
Drugs for parkinsonism
Ganglionic blockers
Hematinics (especially iron)
Hypotensives
Laxative addiction
MAO inhibitors
Metallic intoxication (arsenic, lead, mercury, phosphorus)
Muscle paralyzers
Opiates
Psychotherapeutic drugs

Adapted with permission from "Gastrointestinal Disease," J. S. Fordtran and M. Sleisenger, Eds., W. B. Saunders, Philadelphia, Pa., 1989, pp. 336–338.

TABLE 2 Metabolic and endocrine disorders inducing constipation

Metabolic disorders

Diabetes: acidosis, neuropathy
Porphyria
Type I (Portuguese) and type II (Indiana) amyloid neuropathy; sporadic primary amyloidosis
Uremia
Hypokalemia

Endocrine disorders and changes

Panhypopituitarism
Hypothyroidism
Hypercalcemia: pseudohypoparathyroidism, hyperparathyroidism, milk-alkali syndrome, carcinomatosis
Pheochromocytoma
Enteric glucagon excess

Adapted with permission from "Gastrointestinal Disease," J. S. Fordtran and M. Sleisenger, Eds., W. B. Saunders, Philadelphia, Pa., 1989, pp. 336–338.

TABLE 3 Neurogenic constipation

Peripheral

Aganglionosis (Hirschsprung's disease)
Hypoganglionosis
Hyperganglionosis
Ganglioneuromatosis:
  Primary
  von Recklinghausen's disease
  Multiple endocrine neoplasia, type 2B
Autonomic neuropathy: paraneoplastic, pseudo-obstruction
Chagas' disease

Central medulla

Trauma to nervi erigentes
Cauda equina tumor
Meningocele (anterior or posterior)
Shy-Drager syndrome
Tabes dorsalis
Multiple sclerosis
Trauma to the medulla

Brain

Parkinson's disease
Tumors
Cerebrovascular accidents

Reprinted with permission from "Gastrointestinal Disease," J. S. Fordtran and M. Sleisenger, Eds., W. B. Saunders, Philadelphia, Pa., 1989, p. 337.

Pathophysiology of the Lower Gastrointestinal Tract

Alteration in motor activities is responsible for disorders in the small intestine. Distention or irritation of the small intestine can cause nausea and vomiting; the duodenum is most sensitive to irritation. The motility in the small intestine is intensified when the mucosa is irritated by bacterial toxins, chemical or physical irritants, and mechanical obstruction.

Pain from various causes, including gallbladder disease, appendicitis, and regional ileitis, may inhibit GI reflexes. As a result, functional obstruction often occurs in the small intestine, resulting in symptoms of acute intestinal blockage.

Often, large masses of fecal material accumulate in a greatly dilated rectum. This is especially true of older individuals. The loss of tonicity in the rectal musculature may be caused by ignoring or suppressing the urge to defecate. It also may be caused by degeneration of nerve pathways concerned with defecation reflexes.

Painful lesions of the anal canal, such as ulcers, fissures, and thrombosed hemorrhoidal veins, impede defecation by causing a spasm of the sphincter and by promoting voluntary suppression of defecation to avoid pain. (See Chapter 26, *Hemorrhoidal Products*.)

The normal rectal mucosa is relatively insensitive to cutting or burning. However, when it is inflamed, it becomes highly sensitive to all stimuli, including those acting on the receptors mediating the stretch reflex. A constant urge to defecate in the absence of appreciable material in the rectum may occur with inflamed rectal mucosa (9).

because of the initiation of somatic impulses to the defecation center in the sacral spinal cord. The defecation center then sends impulses to the internal anal sphincter, causing it to relax. This causes an increase in intra-abdominal pressure produced by tightening of the abdominal wall muscles, and a Valsalva maneuver forces the stool down. Voluntary relaxation of the external anal sphincter occurs, followed by elevation of the pelvic diaphragm, which lifts the anal sphincter over the fecal mass allowing it to be expelled. Defecation, a spinal reflex, is voluntarily inhibited by keeping the external sphincter contracted or is facilitated by relaxing the sphincter and contracting the abdominal muscles. Distention of the stomach by food initiates contractions of the rectum (gastrocolic reflex) and, frequently, a desire to defecate. Children usually defecate after meals; in adults, however, habits and cultural factors may determine the "proper" time for defecation.

Symptoms of Constipation

If constipation does occur, complex symptoms of varying degrees may develop. Typical symptoms include anorexia, dull headache, lassitude, low back pain, abdominal distention, and lower abdominal distress. Abdominal discomfort and inadequate response to increasing varieties and doses of laxatives are frequent complaints. Although only limited quantitative data are available, one study indicated that the range of bowel movement frequency in humans is from 3 times a day to 3 times a week (10). Individuals in the latter category are usually symptom free and do not have any specific abnormality related to their individual pattern of defecation. Therefore, constipation cannot be defined solely in terms of the number of bowel movements in any given period.

Patients have many different concepts of what constipation is (11) and many misconceptions concerning

TABLE 4 Diseases of the large bowel associated with constipation

Lesions of the colon
Stenotic obstructions
  Extraluminal
    Tumors
    Chronic volvulus
    Hernias
  Luminal
    Tumors
    Strictures
    Diverticulitis
    Chronic amebiasis
    Lymphogranuloma venereum
    Syphilis
    Tuberculosis
    Ischemic colitis
    Endometriosis
    Corrosive enemas
    Surgery
Muscular abnormalities
  Diverticular disease
  Segmental dilatation of the colon
  Myotonic dystrophy
  Systemic sclerosis
  Dermatomyositis

Lesions of the rectum
Tumors
Ulcerative proctitis
Rectocele
Internal rectal prolapse
Surgical stricture (EEA anastomosis)

Lesions of the pelvic floor
Descending perineum syndrome

Lesions of the anal canal
Stenosis
Anterior ectopic anus
Anal fissure
Mucosal prolapse

Reprinted with permission from "Gastrointestinal Disease," J. S. Fordtran and M. Sleisenger, Eds., W. B. Saunders, Philadelphia, Pa., 1989, p. 338.

TABLE 5 Dietary factors associated with constipation

Lack of sufficient bulk in the diet
Excessive ingestion of foods that harden stools, such as processed cheese
Inadequate fluid intake

Adapted with permission from "Gastrointestinal Disease," J. S. Fordtran and M. Sleisenger, Eds., W. B. Saunders, Philadelphia, Pa., 1978, pp. 370-373.

TREATMENT

Constipation that does not have an organic etiology can often be alleviated without the use of a laxative product. The pharmacist should stress the importance of a high-fiber diet, plentiful fluid consumption, and exercise. However, treatment may require recommendation of a laxative.

Pharmacologic Agents

The ideal laxative would be nonirritating and nontoxic, would act only on the descending and sigmoid colon, and would produce a normally formed stool within a few hours. Its action would then cease, and normal bowel activity would resume. Because a laxative that meets these criteria is not currently available, proper selection of such an agent depends on the etiology of the constipation.

Laxative drugs have been classified according to site of action, intensity of action, chemical structure, or mechanism of action. The most meaningful classification is the mechanism of action, whereby laxatives are classified as bulk forming, emollients, lubricants, saline, and stimulants (Table 6).

Bulk-Forming Laxatives

Because they most closely approximate the physiologic mechanism in promoting evacuation, bulk-forming products are the recommended choice as initial therapy for constipation. These laxatives are natural and semisynthetic polysaccharides and cellulose deriva-

normal bowel functioning (12). Indeed, various definitions of constipation were expressed by participants in a study (11). Despite that, 75% of these persons indicated that they used a laxative when they were constipated. Regardless of how the patient defines constipation, a laxative product probably will be considered for its treatment.

TABLE 6 Classification and properties of laxatives

Agent	Dosage form	Daily dosage range — Adult	Daily dosage range — Pediatric (age in years)	Site of action	Approximate time required for action	Systemic absorption
BULK-FORMING						
Methylcellulose	Solid	4-6 g	1-1.5 g (>6)	Small and large intestines	12-72 hr	No
Carboxymethyl cellulose sodium	Solid	4-6 g	1-1.5 g (>6)	Small and large intestines	12-72 hr	No (laxative) Yes (sodium)
Malt soup extract	Solid, liquid, powder	12-64 g	6-32 oz (1 mo-2 yr)	Small and large intestines	12-72 hr	—
Polycarbophil	Solid	4-6 g	0.5-1.0 g (<2) 1-1.5 g (2-5) 1.5-3.0 g (6-12)	Small and large intestines	12-72 hr	No
Plantago seeds	Solid	2.5-30 g	1.25-15 g (>6)	Small and large intestines	12-72 hr	No
EMOLLIENT						
Dioctyl calcium sulfosuccinate	Solid	0.05-0.36 g	0.025 g (<2) 0.05-0.150 g (≥2)	Small and large intestines	12-72 hr	Yes
Dioctyl sodium sulfosuccinate	Solid	0.05-0.36 g	0.02-0.05 g (<2) 0.05-0.15 g (≥2)	Small and large intestines	12-72 hr	Yes
	Liquid	50-240 mg	10-40 mg (<3) 20-60 mg (3-6) 40-120 mg (6-12)	—	—	—
Dioctyl potassium sulfosuccinate	Solid (rectal)	0.05-0.25 g	0.1 g (children)	Colon	2-15 min	—
LUBRICANT						
Mineral oil	Liquid (oral)	14-45 ml	10-15 ml (>6)	Colon	6-8 hr	Yes-minimal amount
SALINE						
Magnesium citrate	Liquid	240 ml	0.5 ml/kg	Small and large intestines	0.5-3 hr	Yes
Magnesium hydroxide	Liquid	15-40 ml	0.5 ml/kg	Small and large intestines	0.5-3 hr	
Magnesium sulfate	Solid	10-30 g	2.5-5.0 g (2-5) 5.0-10.0 g (6)	Small and large intestines	0.5-3 hr	Yes
Dibasic sodium phosphate	Solid (oral) Solid (rectal)	1.9-3.8 g 3.8 g	¼ adult dose (5-10) ½ adult dose (≥10) ½ adult dose (>2)	Small and large intestines Colon (rectal)	0.5-3 hr 2-15 min	Yes
Monobasic sodium phosphate	Solid (oral) Solid (rectal)	8.3-16.6 g 16.6 g	¼ adult dose (5-10) ½ adult dose (≥10) ½ adult dose (>2)	Small and large intestines Colon	0.5-3 hr 2-15 min	Yes
Sodium biphosphate	Solid (oral) Solid (rectal)	9.6-19.2 g 19.2 g	¼ adult dose (5-10) ½ adult dose (≥10) ½ adult dose (>2)	Small and large intestines Small and large intestines	0.5-3 hr 2-15 min	Yes —

(continued)

TABLE 6 *continued*

Agent	Dosage form	Daily dosage range		Site of action	Approximate time required for action	Systemic absorption
		Adult	**Pediatric (age in years)**			
HYPEROSMOTIC						
Glycerin	Solid (rectal)	3 g	1-1.5 g (<6)	Colon	0.25-1 hr	—
	Liquid (rectal)	Not recommended	1-1.5 g/kg or 40g/m²	—	—	—
STIMULANTS						
Anthraquinones Aloe	Solid	0.12-0.25 g	Not recommended (<6) 0.04-0.08 g (6-8)	Colon	8-12 hr	Yes
Cascara sagrada	Fluid extract Aromatic	0.5-1.5 ml		Colon	6-8 hr	Yes
	Fluid extract Bark	2-6 ml 0.3-1.0 g	¼ adult dose (<2)	—	—	—
	Extract Casanthranol	0.2-0.4 ml 0.03-0.09 ml	½ adult dose (2-12)	—	—	—
STIMULANTS						
Senna	Powder Fluid extract Syrup Fruit extract Suppository	0.5-2.0 g 2.0 ml 8.0 ml 3.4-4.0 ml 1	⅛ adult dose (>2) ¼ adult dose (1-6) ½ adult dose (6-12) ½ adult dose (children over 60 lb)	Colon	6-10 hr	Yes
Calcium salt of Sennosides A and B	Solid	12-24 mg	20 mg (≥6) at bedtime	Colon	6-10 hr	Yes
DIPHENYL METHANES						
Bisacodyl	Solid (oral) Solid (rectal)	10-30 mg 10 mg	5-10 mg (>6) 5 mg (<2) 10 mg (≥2)	Colon Colon	6-10 hr 6-10 hr	Yes Yes
Phenolphthalein	Solid	0.03-0.27 g	Not recommended (<2) 0.015-0.020 g (2-6) 0.03-0.06 g (>6)	Colon	6-8 hr	Yes
	Liquid	60-194 mg at bedtime	1 mg/kg or 30 mg/m²	—	—	—
MISCELLANEOUS						
Castor oil	Liquid	15-60 ml	1-5 ml (<2) 5-15 ml (2-12)	Small intestines	2-6 hr	Yes

tives that dissolve or swell in the intestinal fluid, forming emollient gels that facilitate the passage of the intestinal contents and stimulate peristalsis. They are usually effective in 12–24 hours but may require as long as 3 days in some individuals. This type may be indicated for people on low-residue diets that cannot be corrected as well as in postpartum patients, elderly patients, and patients with irritable bowel syndrome or diverticular disease.

Because the hydrophilic colloid laxatives are not absorbed systemically, they do not seem to interfere with the absorption of nutrients. When given as a powder or granules, they should be mixed with pleasant tasting fluids, such as fruit juice, just before ingestion and administered with a full (8 oz) glass of fluid. Most people prefer juices, sugar-free fruit drinks, or soft drinks to water because they mask the gritty, tastelessness of the bulk-forming laxatives. Failure to consume sufficient fluid with the laxative decreases drug efficacy and may result in intestinal or esophageal obstruction. These agents may be inappropriate for persons who must severely restrict their fluid intake, such as those with significant renal disease.

Esophageal obstruction has occurred in patients who have difficulty swallowing, such as those with strictures of the esophagus, when these drugs are chewed or taken in dry form. In addition, there have been reports of acute bronchospasm associated with the inhalation of dry hydrophilic mucilloid (13). Because of the danger of fecal impaction or intestinal obstruction, the bulk-forming laxatives should not be taken by individuals with intestinal ulcerations, stenosis, or disabling adhesions. When taken properly, these agents are essentially free from systemic side effects because they are not absorbed.

Bulk-forming laxatives are derived from agar, plantago (psyllium) seed, kelp (alginates), and plant gums including tragacanth, chondrus, and karaya (sterculia). The synthetic cellulose derivatives—methylcellulose and carboxymethyl cellulose sodium—are being used more frequently, and many preparations that contain these drugs also contain stimulant and/or fecal-softening laxative drugs. Although the natural product psyllium appears to be the most popular, the synthetic colloidal materials, including methylcellulose and carboxymethyl cellulose sodium, have a high degree of uniformity and can be readily compressed into tablets.

Calcium polycarbophil, the calcium salt of a synthetic polyacrylic resin, has a marked capacity for binding water. It is indicated for the treatment of constipation associated with irritable bowel syndrome and diverticular disease. The maximum calcium content of this agent is approximately 150 mg (7.6 mEq) per tablet. The ingestion of the recommended therapeutic dosages may increase the risk of hypercalcemia in susceptible patients, although the maximum daily dosage limit for calcium adopted by the Food and Drug Administration (FDA) is considerably higher than the 1,800 mg of calcium contained in the maximum daily dosage of 12 calcium polycarbophil tablets (14).

Another bulk-forming laxative is malt soup extract, which is obtained from barley and contains maltose protein and potassium as well as amylolytic enzymes. An interesting aspect of this agent is that it reduces fecal pH, which may contribute to its activity.

One study indicated that a mixture of cellulose and pectin (Phybrex) was equivalent to psyllium as a bulk laxative. The agent had the added advantage of not gelling when mixed with liquids, allowing its usage in baked foods, sauces, drinks, stews, and other recipes. Because of its wider range of methods of consumption, this agent may ensure better compliance over long periods of time (15).

Making a specific choice among the different bulk products is relatively unimportant (16). It is more important that each dose be taken with a full glass of water (at least 240 ml, or 8 oz). The dextrose content of some of the commercial products should be evaluated in patients' carbohydrate-restricted diets. The dose should be adjusted until the required effect has been obtained. In addition to being relatively safe, bulk-forming laxatives are suitable for long-term therapy (17).

Patients with symptoms of cathartic colon from stimulant laxative overuse should be warned that the use of a bulk-forming laxative can result in intestinal obstruction.

Emollient Laxatives

Docusate, formerly known as dioctyl sodium sulfosuccinate, is a surfactant which, when administered orally, increases the wetting efficiency of intestinal fluid and facilitates admixture of aqueous and fatty substances to soften the fecal mass. Docusate does not retard absorption of nutrients from the intestinal tract. In many cases of fecal impaction, a solution of docusate is added to the enema fluid.

Other fecal-softening laxatives are docusate calcium (anionic surfactant), docusate potassium (anionic surfactant), and poloxamer 188 (nonionic surfactant). Poloxamer 188 has no irritant properties and is compatible with electrolytes.

Emollient laxatives should be used only for short-term therapy (less than 1 week without physician consultation) where hard fecal masses are present: that is, either in acute perianal disease in which elimination of painful stools is desired or in which the avoidance of straining at the stool is desirable (following rectal surgery or myocardial infarct).

Orally administered emollient laxatives are of no value in treating long-term constipation, especially in elderly and debilitated patients. One study indicated that the prophylactic administration of docusate did not alter the incidence of constipation in a hospitalized geriatric population who received the drug for a 4-week period (18).

By facilitating the absorption of other poorly absorbed substances, such as mineral oil, the toxicity of mineral oil may be increased by concomitant administration of emollient laxatives (19, 20). Docusate and its congeners are claimed to be nonabsorbable, nontoxic, and pharmacologically inert. However, it has been postulated that the detergent properties of docusate facilitates transport of other substances across cell membranes (21). Consequently, the FDA advisory review panel on over-the-counter (OTC) laxative, antidiarrheal, emetic, and antiemetic drug products recommended that these laxatives carry the following warning statement: "Do not take this product if you are presently taking a prescription drug or mineral oil" (22). Reports have indicated that daily use of preparations containing docusate sodium and oxyphenisatin acetate for 8 months or longer may produce chronic active liver disease with the attendant symptoms, including jaundice (23–26). As a result of these reports and other recommendations, laxatives containing oxyphenisatin acetate are no longer commercially available (27).

Patients with abdominal hernia, severe hypertension, or cardiovascular disease should not strain to defecate; neither should patients who are immediately postpartum nor those who are about to undergo or have undergone surgery for hemorrhoids or other anorectal disorders. An emollient or fecal-softening laxative is indicated in such cases.

Lubricant Laxatives

Liquid petrolatum and certain digestible plant oils, such as olive oil, soften fecal contents by coating them and thus preventing colonic absorption of fecal water. Emulsified products are used to increase palatability. There is little difference in their cathartic efficacy, although emulsions of mineral oil penetrate and soften fecal matter more effectively than nonemulsified preparations. Liquid petrolatum is useful when it is used judiciously in cases that require the maintenance of a soft stool to avoid straining (after a hemorrhoidectomy or abdominal surgery, or in cases of hernia, aneurysm, hypertension, myocardial infarct, or cerebrovascular accident). However, routine use in these cases is probably not indicated. Stool softeners such as docusate sodium are probably better agents for these conditions.

The side effects and toxicity of mineral oil are associated with repeated and prolonged use. Significant absorption of mineral oil may occur, especially if emulsified products are used. The oil droplets may reach the mesenteric lymph nodes and may also be present in the intestinal mucosa, liver, and spleen, where they elicit a typical foreign body reaction.

Lipid pneumonia may result from the oral ingestion and subsequent aspiration of mineral oil, especially when the patient reclines. The pharynx becomes coated with the oil, and droplets gain access to the trachea and the posterior part of the lower lobes of the lungs. Because of the possibility of aspiration into the lungs, mineral oil should not be administered at bedtime or to very young, elderly, or debilitated patients (28).

The role of mineral oil in the absorption of fat-soluble nutrients is controversial, but there is apparently sufficient evidence to consider this effect significant. Absorption of vitamins A, D, E, and K may be impaired. Impaired vitamin D absorption may affect the absorption of calcium and phosphates. Mineral oil should not be given to pregnant patients because it can decrease the availability of vitamin K to the fetus.

In addition, mineral oil should not be taken with meals because it may delay gastric emptying. Patients taking oral anticoagulants should not use mineral oil for the same reason (29).

When large doses of mineral oil are taken, the oil may leak through the anal sphincter. This leakage may produce anal pruritus (pruritus ani), hemorrhoids, cryptitis, and other perianal disease and can be avoided by reducing the dose, dividing the dose, or using a stable emulsion of mineral oil. Prolonged use should be avoided. Because of the tendency of surfactants to increase the absorption of otherwise "nonabsorbable" drugs, mineral oil should not be taken with emollient fecal softeners.

Saline Laxatives

The active constituents of saline laxatives are relatively nonabsorbable cations and anions such as magnesium and sulfate ions. Sulfate salts are considered to be the most potent of this category of laxatives. The wall of the small intestine, acting as a semipermeable membrane to the magnesium, sulfate, tartrate, phosphate, and citrate ions, retains the highly osmotic ions in the gut. The presence of these ions draws water into the gut causing an increase in intraluminal pressure. The increased intraluminal pressure exerts a mechanical stimulus that increases intestinal motility. However, reports suggest that different mechanisms, independent of the osmotic effect, also are responsible for the laxative properties of the salts. Saline laxatives have a complex series of actions, both secretory and motor, on the GI tract. For example, the action of magnesium sulfate on the GI tract is similar to that of cholecystokinin-pancreozymin. There is evidence that this hormone is released from the intestinal mucosa when saline laxatives are administered (30). This release in turn favors intraluminal accumulation of fluid and electrolytes. However, attempts at measuring cholecystokinin levels in patients before and after ingestion of magnesium-containing laxatives failed to demonstrate a change in serum cholecystokinin levels (31). One report indicated that magnesium sulfate is still useful as a cathartic in emergency situations (32).

Saline laxatives are indicated for use only in acute evacuation of the bowel (preparation for endoscopic examination and elimination of drugs in suspected poisonings) and in ridding the gut of blood in conditions such as hepatic coma. Saline laxatives do not have a place in the long-term management of constipation.

In cases of food or drug poisoning, the saline laxatives are sometimes used in purging doses. Magnesium sulfate is recommended except in cases of depressed central nervous system (CNS) activity or renal dysfunction (33).

There are cases in which the unwise choice of a saline laxative results in serious side effects. As much as 20% of the administered magnesium ion may be absorbed from magnesium salts. If renal function is normal, the absorbed ion is excreted so rapidly that no change in the blood level of the ion can be detected. If the renal function is impaired, or if the patient is a newborn or is elderly, toxic concentrations of the magnesium ion could accumulate in the extracellular body fluids. In addition, hypotension, muscle weakness, and electrocardiogram (EKG) changes may indicate a toxic effect of magnesium. Magnesium exerts a depressant effect on the CNS and neuromuscular activity.

Phosphate salts are available in oral and rectal dosage forms. The normal oral dose contains 96.5 mEq of sodium and therefore should be administered with caution to patients on sodium-restricted diets. The use of phosphate salts in children under 2 years of age can result in hypocalcemia, tetany, hypernatremia dehydration, and hyperphosphatemia (34, 35). When given in an enema, up to 10% or more of the sodium content may be absorbed. The rectal use of phosphates is indicated in barium enema preparations and in elimination of fecal impaction. Cathartics that contain sodium may be toxic to individuals with edema or congestive heart disease. Because dehydration may occur from the repeated use of hypertonic solutions of saline cathartics, phosphate salts should not be used by those who cannot tolerate fluid loss. Phosphates should be followed by at least 1 full glass of water in normal patients to prevent dehydration.

Hyperosmotic Laxatives

Glycerin suppositories are available for infants and adults and usually produce a bowel movement within 30 minutes. Glycerin for many years was the main suppository used for lower bowel evacuation. In infants, the physical manipulation usually will initiate the reflex to defecate, and because of this property, adverse reactions and side effects are minimal (36). The laxative effect of glycerin suppositories is caused by the combination of glycerin's osmotic effect with the local irritant effect of sodium stearate. However, rectal irritation may occur with its use. The customary rectal dosages of glycerin considered to be safe and effective for adults and children older than 6 years are 3 g as a suppository or 5–15 ml as an enema. For infants and children under 6 years of age, the dose is 1–1.5 g as a suppository or 2–5 ml as an enema (22). Claims have been made that suppositories may be equal in effectiveness to enemas (37).

Stimulant Laxatives

A comprehensive review of stimulant laxatives has been reported, and the structure–activity relationships of the anthraquinone- or emodin-containing laxatives have been investigated (38–40). It has long been believed that stimulant laxatives act to increase the propulsive peristaltic activity of the intestine by local irritation of the mucosa or by a more selective action on the intramural nerve plexus of intestinal smooth muscle, thus increasing motility. It has now been suggested that these laxative products stimulate secretion of water and electrolytes in both the small and large intestines (41). Depending on the specific laxative, the site of action may be the small intestine, the large intestine, or both. Intensity of action is proportional to dosage, but individually effective doses vary. All stimulant laxatives produce griping, increased mucus secretion, and, in some people, excessive evacuation of fluid. Listed doses and dosage ranges are only guides to determining the correct individual dose. Stimulant laxatives should be used with caution when symptoms of appendicitis (abdominal pain, nausea, and vomiting) are present and should not be used at all when the diagnosis of appendicitis is made.

Stimulant laxatives are effective but should be recommended cautiously because they may produce undesirable and sometimes dangerous side effects (17). This property becomes more important when the agents are abused. It has been said that of all laxative products available, stimulant laxatives are the most widely abused (42). Chronic abuse can lead to "cathartic colon," a poorly functioning colon. This condition resembles ulcerative colitis.

In general, stimulant laxatives are not recommended as initial therapy in patients with constipation, and they should never be used for more than 1 week of regular treatment. The dose should be within the dosage range indicated as safe and effective (Table 6). These laxatives do not necessarily provide the stimulus for the body to return to normal function. Major hazards of stimulant laxatives are severe cramping, electrolyte and fluid deficiencies, enteric loss of protein and malabsorption resulting from excessive catharsis, and hypokalemia. Because the intensity of stimulant laxative activity is proportional to the dose employed, if the dose is large enough, any of the stimulant laxatives can produce these unwanted side effects.

Stimulant laxatives, such as castor oil and bisacodyl, often are used before radiologic examination of the GI tract and before bowel surgery. Bisacodyl also is administered orally or rectally instead of an enema for emptying the colon before proctologic examination.

Stimulant laxatives are conveniently classified according to their chemical structure, as well as their pharmacologic activity.

Anthraquinones Anthraquinone laxative agents, also called anthracene laxatives, include aloe, cascara sagrada, danthron, and rhubarb. Also included in this category are senna, aloin, casanthranol, and frangula. The drugs of choice in this group are the cascara and senna compounds. Neither rhubarb, which contains an astringent (tannin), nor aloe or aloin, which are very irritating, should be recommended. The properties of each of the anthraquinone laxatives vary, depending on the anthraquinone content and the speed of liberation of the active principles from their glycosidic combinations. The anthraquinone glycosides are hydrolyzed by colonic bacteria into active compounds. Crude drug formulations also may contain active constituents not found in extractive preparations or more highly purified compounds.

The precise mechanism by which peristalsis is increased is unknown. The cathartic activity of anthraquinones is limited primarily to the colon, which is reached by direct passage. Bacterial enzymes are partly responsible for the hydrolysis of the glycosides in the colon, making the drug more readily absorbed. Anthraquinones usually produce their action 6–12 hours after administration but may require up to 24 hours.

The active principles of anthraquinones are absorbed from the GI tract and subsequently appear in body secretions, including human milk. However, the practical significance of this finding in nursing infants is controversial. After taking a senna laxative, postpartum patients reported a brown discoloration of breast milk and subsequent catharsis of their nursing infants. A follow-up study indicated that the amount of senna laxative principles in breast milk was inadequate to stimulate defecation in the child (43). Another study with constipated postpartum breast-feeding women receiving a senna laxative reported that 17% of their infants experienced diarrhea (44).

Chrysophanic acid, a component of rhubarb and senna excreted in the urine, colors acidic urine yellowish-brown and alkaline urine reddish-violet.

The prolonged use of anthraquinone laxatives, especially cascara sagrada, can result in a melanotic pigmentation of the colonic mucosa, which is usually found on sigmoidoscopy or rectal biopsy. The shortest time observed for the appearance of melanosis coli in patients taking an anthraquinone cathartic in the presence of fecal stasis was 4 months and the longest was 13 months. In almost all cases, melanosis disappears within 5–11 months after discontinuation of the drug (45). Melanosis coli is virtually always caused by prolonged use of anthraquinone laxatives (46). Pigment-containing macrophages appear in the mucosa, but staining reactions indicate that the pigment is not melanin but has many characteristics of lipofuscin. It may be a combination of this type of pigment and either anthraquinone or one of its breakdown products. There is little evidence to suggest that laxatives other than anthraquinones lead to this pathologic feature.

The liquid preparations of cascara sagrada (fluidextracts) are more reliable than the solid dosage forms (extract and tablet). Aromatic cascara fluidextract is less active and less bitter than cascara sagrada fluidextract. This is reflected by the recommended dosages (Table 6). Magnesium oxide, used in the preparation of the aromatic cascara fluidextract, removes some of the bitter and irritating principles from the crude drug.

Preparations of senna are more potent than those of cascara and produce considerably more griping. Preparations that contain the crystalline glycosides of senna are more stable and reliable, and cause less griping than those made from the crude drug. This difference is important in making a standardized senna product the logical choice among anthracene laxatives (47).

In 1987, the FDA announced the total recall of a formerly popular drug known as danthron. Danthron (1,8–dihydroxyanthraquinone), a breakdown product of the glycosides of senna, is a free anthraquinone with actions similar to those of the natural anthraquinones. It was withdrawn from the market because of reports of its tendency to produce liver tumors in rats (48).

Diphenylmethane Laxatives

The most common diphenylmethane laxatives are bisacodyl and phenolphthalein.

Bisacodyl Bisacodyl was introduced as a cathartic as a result of structure–activity studies of phenolphthalein-related compounds. Practically insoluble in water or a saline medium, bisacodyl exerts its action in the colon on contact with the mucosal nerve plexus. Stimulation is segmented and axonal, producing contractions of the entire colon. Its action is independent of intestinal tone, and the drug is minimally absorbed systemically (approximately 5%) (49). Action on the small intestine is negligible. A soft, formed stool usually is produced 6–10 hours after oral administration and 15–60 minutes after rectal administration. Enteric-coated bisacodyl tablets prevent irritation of the gastric lining and therefore should not be broken, chewed, or administered with alkaline materials such as antacid products.

The tablet and suppository combination has been recommended for cleaning the colon before and after surgery and before X-ray examination. Bisacodyl is effective in patients with colostomies and may reduce or eliminate the need for irrigations. No systemic or adverse effects on the liver, kidney, or hematopoietic system have been observed following its administration.

Side effects occur primarily from purgative action and include metabolic acidosis or alkalosis, hypocalcemia, tetany, and loss of enteric protein and malabsorption (50). The suppository form may produce a burning sensation in the rectum.

Phenolphthalein This drug exerts its stimulating effect mainly on the colon, but the activity of the small intestine may also be increased. Its exact mechanism of action is not known but phenolphthalein appears to alter multiple steps of the absorptive process. It is usually active 6–8 hours after administration.

Phenolphthalein is effective in small doses and is tasteless, making it desirable for marketing in candy and chewing gum forms. When ingested, it passes through the stomach unchanged and is dissolved by the bile salts and the alkaline intestinal secretions. As much as 15% of the dose is absorbed, and the rest is excreted unchanged in the feces. Some of the absorbed drug appears in the urine, which is colored pink to red if it is sufficiently alkaline. Similarly, the drug excreted in the feces causes a red coloration if the feces are sufficiently alkaline (due to the use of soapsuds enemas). This effect may be alarming, so the patient should be told about this possibility.

Part of the absorbed phenolphthalein is excreted back into the intestinal tract along with the bile. The resulting enterohepatic cycle may prolong the action of phenolphthalein for 3 or 4 days. Because bile must be present for it to be effective, phenolphthalein is ineffective in relieving constipation associated with obstructive jaundice.

Phenolphthalein is usually nontoxic. However, at least two types of allergic reactions may follow the use of phenolphthalein. In susceptible individuals, a large dose may cause diarrhea, colic, cardiac and respiratory distress, or circulatory collapse. The other reaction is a polychromatic rash that ranges from pink to deep purple. The eruptions may be pinhead-sized or as large as the palm of the hand. Itching and burning may be moderate or severe. If the rash is severe, it may lead to vesication and erosion, especially around the mouth and genital areas. Patients should be advised to report any rash to the physician or the pharmacist. Other skin reactions, including toxic epidermal necrosis and bullous eruptions, may occur and are related to sunlight exposure (42).

Osteomalacia caused by impaired absorption of vitamin D and calcium is one untoward effect that has been attributed to excessive phenolphthalein ingestion (51, 52). Phenolphthalein abuse can mimic Bartter's syndrome by inducing juxtaglomerular cell hyperplasia with secondary aldosteronism. This is characterized by hypokalemic alkalosis and marked renin increase in the absence of hypertension (53).

Miscellaneous Laxative

Castor Oil Castor oil's laxative action is caused by ricinoleic acid, which is produced when castor oil is hydrolyzed in the small intestine by pancreatic lipase. Its mechanism of action is unknown. However, its laxative effect depends on cyclic adenosine monophosphate mediated fluid secretion and not from increased peristalsis caused by the irritant effect of ricinoleic acid (54).

Castor oil, a glyceride, may be absorbed from the GI tract and is probably metabolized like other fatty acids. Because the main site of action is the small intestine, its prolonged use may result in excessive loss of fluid, electrolytes, and nutrients. Castor oil is most effective when administered on an empty stomach and produces an evacuation within 2–6 hours after ingestion. Because of its unpleasant taste, it should be administered with fruit juices or carbonated beverages. Castor oil is used in situations requiring a thorough evacuation of the GI tract; it is seldom used routinely for constipation.

Dosage Forms

Laxative products are available in a wide array of dosage forms, most of them for oral use. Variety in dosage forms probably yields the most benefits in pediatric or geriatric patients. However, by no means are all of the available dosage forms necessary for effective laxative action. Many of the dosage forms enhance patient acceptability and, perhaps, make laxative use more pleasant. Laxatives available as chewing gum, effervescent granules, and chocolate tablets may not be thought of as drug products and, consequently, may be used indiscriminately.

Enemas and suppositories are dosage forms used extensively for laxative administration. Enemas are used routinely to prepare patients for surgery, child delivery, and radiologic examination and in certain cases of constipation. The enema fluid determines the mechanism by which evacuation is produced. Tap water and normal saline create bulk by an osmotic volume effect; vegetable oils lubricate, soften, and facilitate the passage of hardened fecal matter; soapsuds produce defecation by their irritant action. There have been reports of rectal irritation that has lasted as long as 3 weeks after soap enemas. In addition, there have been reports of anaphylaxis, rectal gangrene, and serious fluid loss secondary to acute colitis after soap enemas (55). Therefore, it is recommended that soap enemas not be used (56).

The popular sodium phosphate–sodium biphosphate preparations fall into the category of saline laxatives. They are usually effective evacuants in preparing patients for surgical, diagnostic, or other procedures involving the bowel. In a crossover study of healthy individuals, these drugs were more efficient and effective than tap water, soapsuds, or saline enemas (57). These agents can alter fluid and electrolyte balance significantly if they are used on a prolonged basis. Consequently, chronic use of these products is not warranted in the control of constipation.

A properly administered enema cleans only the distal colon, most nearly approximating a normal bowel movement (58). Proper administration requires that the diagnosis, the enema fluid, and the technique of administration be correct. Improperly administered, an enema can produce fluid and electrolyte imbalances. A misdirected or inadequately lubricated nozzle may cause abrasion of the anal canal and rectal wall or colonic perforation.

Patients should be advised to carefully follow all directions for the use of these products, including adherence to food and fluid intake.

Enema fluids have caused mucosal changes or spasm of the intestinal wall. Water intoxication has resulted from the use of tap water or soapsuds enemas in the presence of megacolon (59).

To properly administer an enema, the patient should be placed on the left side with knees bent or in the knee–chest position. If the patient is in a sitting position, use of an enema clears only the rectum of fecal material. The container holding the fluid should be 2.5–5 cm above the buttocks to allow free but not forcible flow of the fluid from the tube. The solution should be allowed to flow into the rectum slowly; if the patient is uncomfortable, the flow is probably too fast. One pint (500 ml) of properly introduced fluid usually causes adequate evacuation if it is retained until definite lower abdominal cramping is felt. As long as 1 hour may be needed for the entire procedure. Two or three pints of nonirritating fluid usually produce a clean bowel and a nonirritated mucosa.

Bisacodyl-, senna-, and carbon dioxide-releasing suppositories are promoted as replacements for enemas in cases where cleaning the distal colon is required. Suppositories that contain senna concentrate are advertised as effective in postsurgical and postpartum care; those that contain bisacodyl are promoted for postoperative, antepartum, and postpartum care and are adequate in the preparation for proctosigmoidoscopy. Although bisacodyl suppositories are prescribed and used more frequently than others, some clinicians still use enemas as agents for cleaning the lower bowel.

It has been suggested that the carbon dioxide-releasing suppository might replace the enema in some cases. One study reported that suppositories successfully replaced enemas in institutionalized, spastic, and mentally retarded pediatric patients. Suppositories also replaced enemas in preparing these patients for intravenous pyelograms and for instillation of rectal anesthetics (59).

Pediatric Laxative Use

Laxatives are often given to pediatric patients. Parents often administer laxatives to their children according to their own interpretation of what normal bowel habits should be, and as a result, indiscriminate use may occur. Stool patterns vary widely in children, and constipation in children can be a complex problem often difficult to detect and manage. Parents should observe the child for stool frequency, difficulty in passing stools, pain experienced during bowel movements, and the child's withholding of stools. Any deviation from the child's normal pattern should be noted. Constipation in infants who pass one to two stools a day is frequently unrecognized by the parent. Infants and children appear to show a decreasing frequency of stools with increasing age. Normally, neonates may pass more than four stools a day during the first week of life. This declines to 1.2 stools a day by 4 years of age. Infants whose stool frequency is less than average in the first weeks of life may be prone to develop chronic constipation in later years (60–64). A number of factors that can alter bowel habits in children must be considered to determine whether constipation exists. Such factors include emotional distress, family conflict, changes in diet (e.g., human to cow's milk), febrile illness, or recent travel (60, 65).

In many instances, increasing the bulk content of the child's diet may improve bowel habits and decrease frequency of constipation. Simply increasing the amount of fluid or sugar in the formula may be corrective in the first few months of life. After this age, better results are obtained by adding or increasing the amounts of cereal, vegetables, and fruits. Sugar water solutions (e.g., juice or soda) often diminish the child's appetite for solid foods and should be administered in moderation. The child should be encouraged to drink water, but excessive milk should be avoided. Unbuttered popcorn is an excellent bulk-containing snack for children (66).

In children under 4 or 5 years of age who have difficulty passing hard stools, stimulation of the rectum with a thermometer or finger dilatations may be beneficial. However, excessive anal stimulation should be avoided. If medications are required, glycerin suppositories may initiate the defecation reflex; results are usually seen within 15–60 minutes. Malt soup extract is relatively safe for infants under 2 months of age. The use of senna may be required to move hard stools in cases of more severe constipation (60, 67). Dark corn syrup (1–2 tsp per feeding) or milk of magnesia (beginning with one-half teaspoon) may be useful for fecal impaction, and bisacodyl may be used for moderate to severe constipation. In general, stimulants should probably be avoided as should excessive use of enemas (68). Enemas are not usually recommended for children under 2 years of age. Senna and mineral oil should be administered only on the advice of a physician. In cases where successful bowel evacuation cannot be achieved with oral supplementation or enemas, pediatricians may prescribe a balanced polyethylene glycol–electrolyte solution (Golytely, Colyte) to be administered orally (66). Pharmacists dispensing these solutions should inform parents that as much as 523 ml/kg may be required to effectively cleanse the bowel (66). Children may find that these solutions are more palatable if they are chilled.

A child's age should always be considered when recommending laxative products. The route of administration and the taste of oral products may be especially significant in children. The frequent use of laxatives in older children may be avoided if they are encouraged to establish a regular pattern of bowel movements and adhere to suggested dietary guidelines.

Geriatric Laxative Use

Constipation is a common complaint of many elderly persons. Frequently the problem has progressed with age. Hence, laxative use is not uncommon in this population. Many elderly persons, because of the advertising claims made for laxative products, have been laxative dependent for many years. Practitioners may find that laxative dependency is difficult to treat. Proper education about laxative products and advice on selecting a product are perhaps more crucial for the elderly patient than for the general population.

It has been suggested that the three primary causes of constipation in the elderly are failure to establish a time habit, insufficient fluid or bulk intake, and abuse of laxatives, usually the result of a patient's attempt to regulate bowel activity (69, 70). Constipation in the elderly is often associated with a prolonged transit time through the colon and a decrease in the perception of the need to defecate (71–73). Elderly patients often strain to pass hard stools. Such straining can lead to serious complications, including cardiovascular problems, hemorrhoids, and laxative abuse (71). The aging process is accompanied by physiologic changes that may affect or be affected by drug therapy. Also, geriatric patients tend to have multiple diseases and take multiple drugs (e.g., sedatives/hypnotics, antipsychotics, tricylic antidepressants, and medications with anticholinergic properties).

Laxative preparations apparently increase the rate at which other drugs pass through the GI tract by increasing GI motility. As a result, absorption of drugs may be decreased if excessive motility is produced. In patients taking several drugs, there is the likelihood that concurrent use of a laxative may pose a problem. Pharmacists should consider this factor when advising patients. Elderly patients usually have decreased fluid volumes and are particularly sensitive to shifts in fluid with the accompanying shifts in electrolytes. Use of any type of laxative that alters fluid volume, particularly saline-type laxatives, can be inappropriate for use in elderly patients.

In geriatric patients without a history of constipation, a thorough investigation should be done to determine whether acute cases of constipation have resulted from new or old diseases or from the use of medications. Many geriatric patients have an atonic colon resulting in loss of muscle tone and consequently rely on laxatives or enemas for bowel movements.

In addition, a low-residue diet, poor chewing of food, or a diet consisting mainly of soft foods because of ill-fitting dentures may cause constipation in this age group. Finally, many geriatric patients take drugs that can induce constipation. If any of these factors exists, corrective action in the patient's lifestyle or therapy should be advised instead of immediately recommending a laxative.

It has been suggested that an acute episode of constipation be treated with plain water (16 oz or less) or saline enemas (71, 72, 74). Soapsud enemas should be avoided because they can be irritating and may cause serious complications (72, 75). Sodium phosphate and biphosphate (Fleet) enemas are beneficial, but their use should be limited (76). Polyethylene glycol-electrolyte solutions (Colyte, Golytely), commonly used as bowel preparations for GI procedures, have been safely used for acute management of constipation in elderly patients suffering from cardiac and/or renal disease (71, 72, 77). Dietary fiber should be increased by including bran, fruits, and vegetables (Table 7). Pharmacists should advise patients that increasing bran in the diet may initially lead to erratic bowel habits, flatulence, and abdominal discomfort during the first few weeks. It is suggested that excess bran be avoided in patients with hypocalcemia or low serum iron and in patients confined to bed (71, 72, 74). For patients requiring laxatives, bulk-forming agents are the laxatives of choice. Onset is usually in 2–3 days. Sugar-free products (e.g., Konsyl, Serutan, SF Metamucil) are recommended for diabetic patients (72). Some physicians may recommend chronic stimulant laxative use, particularly senna products, for certain elderly patients, but such use should not be generally recommended to all persons in this age group. The use of mineral oil should be discouraged because of possible malabsorption of fat-soluble vitamins or possible aspiration (71). Glycerin suppositories and orally administered lactulose are safe and have been used successfully in the elderly (72, 77–79). Lactulose may be of particular benefit in elderly bedridden patients (72).

TABLE 7 Provisional dietary fiber table

Food	Analytical method[a]	Fiber (g) per 100 g	Calories per 100 g	Serving size	Fiber (g) per serving	Calories per serving
BREAKFAST CEREALS						
All-Bran	1	29.9	249	⅓ c (1 oz)	8.5	71
Bran Buds	1	27.7	258	⅓ c (1 oz)	7.9	73
Bran Chex	1	16.2	319	⅔ c (1 oz)	4.6	91
Cheerios-type	1	3.8	391	1¼ c (1 oz)	1.1	111
Corn Bran	1	19.0	346	⅔ c (1 oz)	5.4	98
Cornflakes	1	1.1	389	1¼ c (1 oz)	0.3	110
Cracklin' Bran	1	15.1	382	⅓ c (1 oz)	4.3	108
Crispy Wheats n' Raisins	1	4.6	349	¾ c (1 oz)	1.3	99
40% Bran-type	1	13.4	325	¾ c (1 oz)	4.0	93
Frosted-Mini Wheats	1	7.6	359	4 biscuits (1 oz)	2.1	102
Graham Crackos	1	6.1	361	¾ c (1 oz)	1.7	102
Grape-Nuts	1	4.8	357	¼ c (1 oz)	1.4	101
Heartland Natural Cereal, plain	1	4.7	434	¼ c (1 oz)	1.3	123
HoneyBran	1	11.1	341	⅞ c (1 oz)	3.1	97
Most	1	12.4	337	⅔ c (1 oz)	3.5	95
Nutri-Grain, barley	1	5.8	372	¾ c (1 oz)	1.7	106
Nutri-Grain, corn	1	6.2	381	¾ c (1 oz)	1.8	108
Nutri-Grain, rye	1	6.4	359	¾ c (1 oz)	1.8	102
Nutri-Grain, wheat	1	6.3	360	¾ c (1 oz)	1.8	102
Oatmeal, regular, quick, and instant, cooked	4,5	0.9	62	¾ c (1 oz)	1.6	108
100% Bran	1	29.6	269	½ c (1 oz)	8.4	76
100% Natural Cereal; plain	1	3.7	470	¼ c (1 oz)	1.0	133
Raisin Bran-type	1	11.3	312	¾ c (1 oz)	4.0	115
Rice Krispies	1	0.2	395	1 c (1 oz)	0.1	112
Shredded Wheat	1	9.3	359	⅔ c (1 oz)	2.6	102
Special K	1	0.8	390	1⅓ c (1 oz)	0.2	111
Sugar Smacks	1	0.9	373	¾ c (1 oz)	0.4	106
Tasteeos	1	3.5	393	1¼ c (1 oz)	1.0	111
Total	1	7.2	352	1 c (1 oz)	2.0	100
Wheat 'n' Raisin Chex	1	6.6	343	¾ c (1⅓ oz)	2.5	130
Wheat Chex	1	7.4	367	⅔ c (1⅓ oz)	2.1	104
Wheat germ	1	14.3	386	¼ c (2 oz)	3.4	108
Wheaties	1	7.0	349	1 c (1 oz)	2.0	99
FRUITS						
Apple (w/o skin)	2,3,4	2.1	57	1 med	2.7	72
Apple (w/skin)	2	2.5	59	1 med	3.5	81
Apricot (fresh)	2,3	1.7	48	3 med	1.8	51
Apricot, dried	6	8.1	238	5 halves	1.4	42
Banana	2,4	2.1	92	1 med	2.4	105
Blueberries	2	2.7	51	½ c	2.0	39
Cantaloupe	3	1.0	24	¼ melon	1.0	30
Cherries, sweet	2,3	1.2	72	10	1.2	49
Dates	3,4	7.6	275	3	1.9	68
Grapefruit	2,3,4	1.3	32	½	1.6	38
Grapes	3,4	1.3	63	20	0.6	30
Orange	2,4	2.0	47	1	2.6	62
Peach (w/skin)	4	2.1	43	1	1.9	37
Peach (w/o skin)	2,3	1.4	43	1	1.2	37
Pear (w/skin)	4	2.8	59	½ large	3.1	61
Pear (w/o skin)	2,3,4	2.3	59	½ large	2.5	61

(continued)

TABLE 7 *continued*

Food	Analytical method[a]	Fiber (g) per 100 g	Calories per 100 g	Serving size	Fiber (g) per serving	Calories per serving
Pineapple	2,3	1.4	49	½ c	1.1	39
Plums, Damsons	2,4	1.7	60	5	0.9	33
Prunes	3,4	11.9	239	3	3.0	60
Raisins	3,4	8.7	300	¼ c	3.1	108
Raspberries	3,4	5.1	57	½ c	3.1	35
Strawberries	2,3	2.0	30	1 c	3.0	45
Watermelon	2	0.3	26	1 c	0.4	42
Juices						
Apple	2	0.3	47	½ c (4 oz)	0.4	56
Grapefruit	2	0.4	41	½ c (4 oz)	0.5	51
Grape	2	0.5	51	½ c (4 oz)	0.6	64
Orange	2	0.4	45	½ c (4 oz)	0.5	56
Papaya	2	0.6	57	½ c (4 oz)	0.8	71
VEGETABLES						
Cooked						
Asparagus, cut	2,3	1.5	20	½ c	1.0	15
Beans, string, green	2,3,4	2.6	25	½ c	1.6	16
Broccoli	2,4	2.8	26	½ c	2.2	20
Brussels sprouts	2,3	3.0	36	½ c	2.3	28
Cabbage, red	4	2.0	20	½ c	1.4	15
Cabbage, white	4	2.0	20	½ c	1.4	15
Carrots	2,3,4	3.0	31	½ c	2.3	24
Cauliflower	3,4	1.7	22	½ c	1.1	14
Corn, canned	2,3	2.8	83	½ c	2.9	87
Kale leaves	3	2.6	34	½ c	1.4	22
Parsnip	3,4	3.5	66	½ c	2.7	51
Peas	2,3,4	4.5	71	½ c	3.6	57
Potato (w/o skin)	3,4	1.0	93	1 med	1.4	97
Potato (w/skin)	4	1.7	93	1 med	2.5	106
Spinach	2,4	2.3	23	½ c	2.1	21
Squash, summer	2,4	1.6	14	½ c	1.4	13
Sweet potatoes	2,3	2.4	141	½ med	1.7	80
Turnip	3,4	2.2	23	½ c	1.6	17
Zucchini	4	2.0	12	½ c	1.8	11
Raw						
Bean sprout, soy		2.6	46	½ c	1.5	13
Celery, diced	3,4	1.5	8	½ c	1.1	10
Cucumber	3,4	0.8	15	½ c	0.4	8
Lettuce, sliced	3,4	1.5	12	1 c	0.9	7
Mushrooms, sliced	3	2.5	28	½ c	0.9	10
Onions, sliced	3,4	1.3	23	½ c	0.8	33
Pepper, green, sliced	3,4	1.3	23	½ c	0.5	9
Tomato	3,4	1.5	22	1 med	1.5	20
Spinach	2	4.0	26	1 c	1.2	8
LEGUMES						
Baked beans, tomato sauce	3	7.3	121	½ c	8.8	155
Dried peas, cooked	3,4	4.7	115	½ c	4.7	115
Kidney beans, cooked	3	7.9	118	½ c	7.3	110
Lima beans, cooked/canned	2	5.4	75	½ c	4.5	64
Lentils, cooked	3	3.7	97	½ c	3.7	97
Navy beans, cooked	6,3	6.3	118	½ c	6.0	112

(continued)

TABLE 7 *continued*

Food	Analytical method[a]	Fiber (g) per 100 g	Calories per 100 g	Serving size	Fiber (g) per serving	Calories per serving
BREADS, PASTAS, AND FLOURS						
Bagels	1	1.1	264	1 bagel	0.6	145
Bran muffins	1	6.3	263	1 muffin	2.5	104
Cracked wheat	1	4.10	246	1 sl	1.0	62
Crisp bread, rye	1	14.9	376	2 crackers	2.0	50
Crisp bread, wheat	1	12.9	376	2 crackers	1.8	50
French bread	1	2.0	291	1 sl	0.7	102
Italian bread	1	1.0	278	1 sl	0.3	83
Mixed grain	1	3.7	235	1 sl	0.9	59
Oatmeal	1	2.2	253	1 sl	0.5	63
Pita bread (5″)	1	0.9	273	1 piece	0.4	123
Pumpernickel bread	1	3.2	207	1 sl	1.0	66
Raisin bread	1	2.2	267	1 sl	0.6	67
White bread	1,4	1.6	279	1 sl	0.4	78
Whole wheat bread	1,4	5.7	243	1 sl	1.4	61
Pasta and rice (cooked)						
Macaroni	1,5	0.8	111	1 c	1.0	144
Rice, brown	3,5	1.2	119	½ c	1.0	97
Rice, polished	1,4,5	0.3	109	½ c	0.2	82
Spaghetti (regular)	1,5	0.8	111	1 c	1.1	155
Spaghetti (whole wheat)	1,5	2.8	111	1 c	3.9	155
Flours and grains						
Bran, corn	4	62.2				
Bran, oat	3	27.8				
Bran, wheat	1,3,4,5	41.2				
Rolled oats	4,5	5.7				
Rye flour (72%)[b]	4	4.5	350			
Rye flour (100%)[b]	4	12.8	335			
Wheat flour:						
Brown (85%)[b]	3,4	7.3	327			
White (72%)[b]	3,4	2.9	333			
Wholemeal (100%)[b]	3,4	8.9	318			
NUTS						
Almonds	4	7.2	627	10 nuts	1.1	79
Filberts	3	6.0	634	10 nuts	0.8	90
Peanuts	3	8.1	568	10 nuts	1.4	105

Dietary fiber values are averages compiled from literature sources. Users of the table are advised to read the accompanying manuscript to understand fully the derivation and meaning of the values.

[a] The numbers in this column refer to the analytical method used to obtain the mean dietary fiber value, as follows:
1. Neutral detergent fiber
2. Neutral detergent fiber plus water-soluble fraction
3. Southgate procedure
4. Total dietary fiber procedure
5. Englyst, nonstarch polysaccharide (NSP)

[b] The number in parentheses refers to the extraction rate of the flour. White-type breads and household flour are made with 72% flour; 85% extraction flour was consumed in the United States before World War II.

Reprinted from E. Lanza and R. R. Butrum, *J. Am. Dietetic Assoc.*, *86*, 732 (1986).

Caution should be exercised in the use of magnesium-containing cathartics in the elderly because of the potential risks of hypermagnesemia in patients with renal failure and sodium overload in patients with cardiovascular disease (71).

Recommendations of laxative products for geriatric patients should be considered individually because of the elderly's vulnerability to medications in general. Even though bulk-forming agents have been successfully used in these patients, a complete and thorough history should provide the information needed to make appropriate individual recommendations (80).

Self-Medication in Pregnancy

Constipation is a common occurrence in pregnancy. One study showed a 31% incidence, with 65% of these women treating themselves with either diet or laxatives without professional advice (44). Constipation that develops during pregnancy is often attributed to compression of the colon caused by the increasing size of the uterus. However, the primary reason is probably a reduction in muscle tone, which contributes to a decrease in peristalsis (81). In addition, vitamin and mineral supplements that contain iron and calcium tend to be constipating.

Most types of laxatives appear to be effective in pregnancy. However, because of various effects such as possible loss of vitamins caused by mineral oil, premature labor brought on by the irritant effect of castor oil, or the possibility of dangerous electrolyte imbalance with osmotic agents, women should probably use only bulk-forming laxatives during pregnancy (82). Stimulant laxatives probably should be avoided during pregnancy. At least one report indicates that some stimulants may be acceptable for use during the lactation period with precautions (83). Senna and related anthraquinones have been used during breast-feeding despite a lack of information regarding their concentration in breast milk. If these products are used, the infant should be carefully observed for diarrhea. Bisacodyl appears in the breast milk in trace amounts and may not pose problems for the infant (83); however, the infant should be watched for the development of diarrhea. Saline cathartics probably should be avoided because appreciable GI absorption can occur in the mother. Toxicity occurring from a saline cathartic such as magnesium sulfate could be significant considering that such toxicity usually results in diarrhea, drowsiness, hypotonia, and respiratory difficulty.

Pregnant women should be counseled on proper diet, adequate fluid intake, and reasonable amounts of exercise (81). If these measures do not alleviate or prevent the development of constipation, the recommendation of a laxative preparation may be appropriate. The pharmacist should consult with the woman's physician, especially if any doubt exists regarding the physician's desire for the patient to have a laxative. Laxatives may also have to be administered postpartum to reestablish normal bowel function that may have been lost due to ileus secondary to colonic dilatation in a decompressed abdomen, perineal pain, laxness of the anal sphincter and abdominal musculature, and low fluid intake and the administration of enemas during labor. In addition, hemorrhoids in the period after delivery are aggravated, if not caused, by constipation (84).

Laxative Abuse

Routine use of most laxative preparations can result in laxative abuse. The pharmacist should be aware of this possibility and remember that the laxative abuser is not always elderly. For example, some college students use laxatives for weight control (85). Such abuse is often part of a pattern of "purging behavior," which also may include self-induced vomiting (86). These persons may suffer from bulimia nervosa.

Excessive use of laxatives can cause diarrhea and vomiting, leading to fluid and electrolyte losses, especially hypokalemia, in which there is a general loss of tone of smooth and striated muscle (87, 88). The clinical features of laxative abuse include (87):

- Factitious diarrhea;
- Electrolyte imbalance (hypokalemia, hypocalcemia, hypermagnesemia);
- Osteomalacia;
- Protein-losing enteropathy;
- Steatorrhea;
- Cathartic colon;
- Liver disease.

Cathartic colon, which develops after years of laxative abuse, is difficult to diagnose and may present symptoms similar to acute nephritis, diabetes insipidus, neurasthenia, ulcerative colitis, or Addison's disease. In a study of seven hospitalized female patients, 26–65 years of age, the chief admitting complaints were abdominal pain and diarrhea, the number of hospital admissions ranged from 2 to 11, and the total number of days spent in the hospital ranged from 58 to 202 (80, 87). The diagnosis of laxative abuse was difficult because the patients denied taking laxatives, and none of the colonic tissue characteristics usually associated with excessive laxative use was observed on sigmoidoscopy or radiologic examination. However, excessive laxative use was later revealed.

Diarrhea can be a serious consequence of the overuse of laxative products, especially irritant laxatives. The prolonged misuse of laxative drugs can cause morbid anatomical changes in the colon. In a study of 12 chronic laxative users, the primary anatomical changes were loss of intrinsic innervation, mucosal inflammation, atrophy of smooth muscle coats, and pigmentation of the colon (89). Most users had been taking laxatives regularly for 30–40 years; two were under 30 years of age when their colons were removed and therefore had a much shorter history. In these cases, the myenteric plexus showed many swollen, but otherwise normal, neurons. This evidence suggests that the initial action of an irritant laxative is to stimulate neurons and that prolonged and continuous stimulation causes cell death. In such cases, the transverse colon is often pendulous, the sigmoid section is highly dilated, and the muscle coats are thin and contain excess adipose tissue, indicating some tissue atrophy.

Laxative abuse can usually be classified as either habitual or surreptitious abuse. The habitual abuser often believes that a daily bowel movement is a necessity and uses a laxative to accomplish this end. Such patients may freely admit their use because, to them, it seems entirely correct and natural (41). On the other hand, surreptitious abuse is similar to other illnesses. This group of abusers tends to manifest various psychiatric disturbances (80, 90–93). Confronting this type of abuser does not usually help resolve the problem. Psychiatric help should be sought. In order to assess the abuser, the diagnostic process must include effective detection methods. Investigators have developed a sensitive procedure for screening urine samples for the presence of the most commonly used laxatives (94, 95). Once adequate substantiation of the abuse has been established, it may be possible to wean the patient off the laxative before permanent bowel damage occurs and to regularize the bowel habits with a high-fiber diet (46, 80, 96) supplemented by bulk-forming laxatives, as needed. Once an abuser is withdrawn from the laxative, several months may be required to retrain the bowel in regular unaided function. Affected patients should be educated about laxative abuse. The information provided to them should describe types of laxatives and their harmful effects. Patients should be told that constipation, weight gain, bloating, or abdominal distention may occur following the end of laxative abuse. These persons should be encouraged to exercise, increase their dietary fiber, and maintain adequate fluid intake. The pharmacist should encourage patients to discuss their attitudes about laxative abuse and should answer any questions that arise in such discussions.

PRODUCT SELECTION GUIDELINES

Consultation Information

The most useful approach in counseling the person who requests a laxative product for self-medication should first include a discussion of dietary habits, exercise, fluid intake, and general emotional well-being. It is well known that these factors may be largely responsible for problems associated with constipation. It cannot be assumed that people understand the interplay of these factors in the development of constipation. For example, one study on self-medication showed that 65% of persons questioned about their use of laxative products were unable to associate the role of diet with the development of constipation (11). This indicates the lack of understanding of constipation and the kinds of normal factors that can have a larger effect on its development. The following factors are very important in returning a person to a relatively normal state without laxative intervention (8, 97):

- Adequate fiber in the diet;
- Retraining the individual to respond to the urge to defecate;
- Physical exercise;
- Adequate fluid intake;
- Relaxation to reduce emotional stress and its effect on defecation.

A diet consisting of high-fiber foods and plenty of fluids (4–6 8-oz glasses of water a day) will help relieve chronic constipation. Caution regarding fluid intake must be used in patients on fluid restriction. Dietary fiber is that part of whole grain, vegetables, fruits, and nuts that resists digestion in the GI tract (Table 7). It is composed of carbohydrates (cellulose, hemicelluloses, polysaccharides, and pectin) and a noncarbohydrate, lignin. Food fiber content, which is expressed in terms of crude fiber residue after treatment with dilute acid and alkali, has a significant effect on bowel habits. Because fiber holds water, in persons with a higher fiber intake, stools tend to be softer, bulkier, and heavier and probably pass through the colon more rapidly.

Along with a high-fiber diet, the pharmacist may encourage regular, mild exercise such as walking, provided the patient's cardiovascular system is normal and the patient is under a physician's care. Physical activity is important in the propulsion mechanisms in the colon.

Exercise in any form improves muscle tone, but exercise using the abdominal muscles is the most beneficial in improving intestinal muscle tone (8).

The patient should learn not to ignore the urge to defecate and should allow adequate time for elimination (47). A relaxed, unhurried atmosphere can be very important in aiding elimination. The patient should be encouraged to set a regular pattern for bathroom visits. Mornings, particularly after breakfast, seem to be a good time. Having a specific time period set aside for elimination may help the body adjust itself to producing a regular stool.

The fact that normal defecation empties only the descending and sigmoid colon should be remembered when considering the use of any preparation in a suspected situation of constipation. The preparation chosen should duplicate the normal process as much as possible. Clearly, most stimulant products act more distantly to this process than other types of laxatives. Such products cause emptying of the entire colon and thereby discourage the proper return to normal function. The laxative user who is unaware of this effect may take another laxative dose on the first or second post-laxative day, thereby maintaining a completely empty colon.

In counseling the patient on laxative use, the pharmacist should stress the following points:

- Laxative agents should not be used regularly; more natural methods such as diet, exercise, and fluid intake should be used to produce regular movements.

- The use of a laxative agent in the treatment of constipation should be only a temporary measure; once regularity has returned, the laxative product should be discontinued.

Indications for self-medication with a nonprescription laxative include preparation for diagnostic procedures and acute constipation. A physician should supervise use of laxatives during treatment for perianal disease (preoperatively or postoperatively), during conditions in which straining is undesirable (e.g., postoperative, postmyocardial infarct), or for chronic constipation (98). Because defecation has been found to alter hemodynamics, straining to defecate has resulted in death from emboli, ventricular rupture, and cardiogenic shock in patients who had experienced a myocardial infarct (99).

Specific advice about laxative products should include these reminders:

- Laxatives are not designed for long-term use; if they are not effective after 1 week, a physician should be consulted.

- If a skin rash appears after the patient has taken a laxative containing phenolphthalein, the product should be discontinued and a physician should be contacted.

- Saline laxatives should not be used daily and should not be administered orally to children under 6 years of age or rectally to infants under 2 years of age.

- Mineral oil should not be given to children under 6 years of age or in conjunction with emollient laxatives; it should not be used during pregnancy and should be avoided in patients taking anticoagulants.

- Castor oil should not be used to treat constipation.

- Enemas and suppositories must be administered properly to be effective.

- Laxatives should not be used in the presence of abdominal pain, nausea, vomiting, bloating, or cramping.

- Laxatives containing phenolphthalein, rhubarb, or senna may discolor urine; laxatives containing phenolphthalein may discolor feces pink to red depending on the alkalinity.

Specific product notes for pharmacists include the following:

- Laxative products containing more than 15 mEq (345 mg) of sodium, more than 25 mEq (975 mg) of potassium, or more than 50 mEq (600 mg) of magnesium in the maximum daily dose should not be used if kidney disease or other conditions requiring sodium, potassium, or magnesium restriction are present.

- Any product containing dextrose should be used with caution in diabetic patients because of the possibility of loss of control (100).

Patient Assessment

The pharmacist should obtain as much information as possible before making any recommendations for relief of constipation. The information allows the pharmacist to make rational recommendations based on knowledge of the patient, the problem, the product, and the pharmacist's judgment and experience. Because laxative products are both widely used and abused, the pharmacist can provide a valuable service by educating patients about the appropriate use of laxatives.

The first question that the pharmacist should ask is for what purpose the patient intends to use a laxative product. Not all people purchasing a laxative are constipated. The product might be needed as a result of an upcoming X-ray examination of the bowel, or the product may be purchased for a friend or a relative. It is important to know why the patient feels that a laxative product is necessary at the present time.

The pharmacist should determine the person's symptoms and their duration. If symptoms have persisted for more than 2 weeks or have recurred after previous laxative use, the patient should be referred to a physician. Perhaps the patient has already attempted to alleviate symptoms by dietary measures such as increasing fruit and vegetable consumption. This, too, is important information for the pharmacist.

Any patient who has an established disease affecting the GI tract presents particular concern. It is quite possible that laxative products used by these patients may adversely affect their condition. The pharmacist should obtain accurate information regarding all diseases present. The patient should be referred to a physician when insufficient information or any doubt exists regarding disease states.

As previously suggested, the normal population experiences from 3 bowel movements a day to 3 bowel movements a week (8), and individuals who fall outside this range might be classed as unusual but not always abnormal. Thus, the frequency of movements may not be the most relevant concern; the consistency of the stool and accompanying symptoms are important characteristics of constipation as well (101).

When it is necessary to use a laxative for the treatment of constipation, the recommended choice is a bulk-forming product; however, the pharmacist should keep in mind the situations in which its use is inappropriate. Laxatives are not recommended to treat constipation associated with intestinal pathology or to treat constipation secondary to laxative abuse unless bowel retraining has been successful. They also are not a cure for functional constipation and therefore are of only secondary importance in its treatment.

The pharmacist should also be concerned about the patient's current and past use of laxative products. The patient already may be using one or more products, and improper use may be preventing the desired effect. The possibility of laxative abuse also should be considered. Stimulant laxatives may cause constipation in abusers because of tolerance development. An in-depth knowledge of the patient's history of laxative use provides the pharmacist with information about past patterns of drug use, effective or ineffective products, the incidence of constipation, and the use of home remedies. Depending on the pharmacist's findings, referral to a physician may be necessary.

Furthermore, all medication use by a patient is an important consideration of the pharmacist. Caution should be exercised when laxatives are recommended

for use by patients receiving prescription drug products. Laxative preparations may increase the rate at which other drugs pass through the GI tract. The resulting effect could be decreased absorption of those drugs (102, 103). Drugs with constipating side effects (calcium or aluminum antacids, narcotic analgesics, and anticholinergic-type drugs) may counteract the effects of laxatives or require their use. Recently a clinical syndrome known as the narcotic bowel syndrome (NBS) has been described. This syndrome is characterized by chronic abdominal pain, nausea and vomiting, abdominal distention, constipation, and at least one occurrence of intestinal pseudo-obstruction (104). When narcotics are discontinued and NBS does not abate, patients may be administered continuous subcutaneous infusions of metoclopramide (105). Such a condition might occur in a cancer patient or in other patients who require significant chronic administration of narcotics (106).

Some drugs, such as magnesium antacids, prostaglandins (misoprostol), and antiadrenergic-type drugs, have laxative side effects and may tend to intensify the effect of laxative ingredients. Pharmacists must investigate all drug use and provide guidance for the rational selection of appropriate laxatives.

In some cases, treatment for another ailment may relieve symptoms of constipation. In perianal disease, for example, constipation is usually the result of the patient's unwillingness to defecate because of the pain encountered. When medical and/or surgical treatment is given, the barrier to normal defecation is removed. Conditions such as hypothyroidism or depression may be responsible for a patient's complaint of constipation. Successful treatment of these disorders usually eliminates constipation.

SUMMARY

The widespread abuse of nonprescription laxatives is evidence of a greater need for professional consultation and patient education. Successful treatment of someone with constipation depends on careful identification of the cause. To determine whether referral to a physician or self-therapy is indicated, the pharmacist requires a knowledge of the case history and current symptoms. If the case history discloses a sudden change in bowel habits that has persisted for 2 weeks, the pharmacist should refer the patient to a physician. However, if the constipation can be treated without physician intervention, knowledge of the many available products is essential.

For most cases of simple constipation, proper diet, exercise, and adequate fluid intake will alleviate the condition. Therapy with any laxative product should be limited in most cases to short-term use (1 week). If no relief has been achieved after a 1-week period of proper laxative therapy, the product should be discontinued.

Pharmacists who conscientiously perform their professional responsibilities with nonprescription laxatives will promote appropriate use of these products, and they will establish themselves as important public health consultants.

REFERENCES

1 *Drug Store News, 11 (10)*, IP 27 (1989).

2 "New and Non-Official Drugs," Lippincott, Philadelphia, Pa., 1965, p. 615.

3 D. L. Elliott et al., *Postgrad. Med., 74*, 143 (1983).

4 A. Jacknowitz, *Am. J. Hosp. Pharm., 38*, 1122 (1981).

5 W. D. Carey, *Cleveland Clin., 44*, 73 (1977).

6 J. R. DiPalma, "Drill's Pharmacology in Medicine," 4th ed., McGraw-Hill, New York, N.Y., 1971, p. 747.

7 W. F. Ganong, "Review of Medical Physiology," 6th ed., Lange Medical, Los Altos, Calif., 1971, p. 357.

8 *Drug Ther., 5*, 41 (1975).

9 F. H. Netter, "The Ciba Collection of Medical Illustrations," Vol. 3, Part II, Ciba Pharmaceutical, Summit, N.J., 1962, p. 98.

10 A. M. Connell et al., *Br. Med. J., 2*, 1095 (1965).

11 D. A. Matte and W. M. McLean, *Drug Intell. Clin. Pharm., 12*, 603 (1978).

12 G. E. Sladen, *Proc. Roy. Soc. Med., 65*, 289 (1972).

13 R. Gross, *J. Am. Med. Assoc., 241*, 1573 (1979).

14 *Federal Register, 39*, 19874 (1974).

15 G. A. Spiler et al., *J. Clin. Pharmacol., 19*, 313 (1979).

16 T. P. Almy, *Ann. N.Y. Acad. Sci., 58*, 398 (1954).

17 K. Rutter and D. Maxwell, *Br. Med. J., 2*, 997 (1976).

18 J. Goodman et al., *J. Chron. Dis., 29*, 59 (1976).

19 *Med. Lett. Drugs Ther., 19*, 45 (1977).

20 K. Naess, *J. Am. Med. Assoc., 212*, 1961 (1970).

21 C. A. Dujoune et al., *J. Lab. Clin. Med., 79*, 832 (1972).

22 *Federal Register, 40*, 12907, 12911–12 (1975).

23 T. B. Reynolds et al., *N. Engl. J. Med., 285*, 813 (1971).

24 E. Gjone et al., *Scand. J. Gastroenterol., 7*, 395 (1972).

25 O. Dietrichson et al., *Scand. J. Gastroenterol., 9*, 473 (1974).

26 R. L. Willing and R. Hecker, *Med. J. Aust., 1*, 1179 (1971).

27 *J. Am. Med. Assoc., 211*, 114 (1970).

28 L. E. Nochmovitz et al., *S. Afr. Med. J., 49*, 2187 (1975).

29 E. C. Rosenow, *Ann. Intern. Med., 77*, 977–991 (1972).

30 R. R. Harvey and A. E. Reed, *Lancet, 2*, 185 (1973).

31 L. Sillin et al., *Gastroenterology, 74*, 1144 (1978).

32 D. G. Spoeke, *Am. J. Hosp. Pharm., 38*, 498 (1981).

33 "The Pharmacological Basis of Therapeutics," 7th ed., L. G. Goodman et al., Eds., Macmillan, New York, N.Y., 1985, p. 876.

34 T. H. McConnell, *J. Am. Med. Assoc., 216*, 147 (1971).

35 R. W. Chisney and P. B. Haughton, *Am. J. Dis. Child., 127*, 684 (1974).

36 J. Travel, *Ann. N.Y. Acad. Sci., 58*, 416 (1954).

37 M. R. Barnes, *Radiology, 9*, 948 (1968).

38 S. J. Loewe, *J. Pharmacol. Exp. Ther., 94*, 288 (1948).

39 L. Schmidt and E. Seeger, *Arzneim-Forsch, 6*, 22 (1965).

40 M. H. Habacher and S. Doernbert, *J. Pharm. Sci., 53*, 1067 (1964).

41 K. J. Moriarty and D. B. A. Silk, *Dig. Dis., b*, 615–629 (1988).

42 R. G. Pietrusko, *Am. J. Hosp. Pharm., 34*, 291 (1977).

43 M. W. Werthmann and S. V. Krees, *Med. Ann. D.C., 42*, 4 (1973).

44 J. O. Greenhalf and H. S. Leonard, *Practitioner, 210*, 259 (1973).

45 "Gastrointestinal Disease," 2nd ed., M. H. Sleisinger and J. S. Fordtran, Eds., W. B. Saunders, Philadelphia, Pa., 1978, p. 1862.

46 J. H. Cummings, *Gut, 15*, 758 (1975).

47 K. Goulston, *Drugs, 14*, 128 (1977).

48 W. E. Gilbertson and M. Lessing, *Military Med., 153*, 487–488 (1988).

49 "The Pharmacological Basis of Therapeutics," 7th ed., L. G. Goodman et al., Eds., Macmillan, New York, N.Y., 1985, p. 999.

50 F. Nahman and G. D. Cam, *South Med. J., 66*, 724 (1973).

51 B. Frame et al., *Arch. Intern. Med., 128*, 794 (1971).

52 B. M. Frier and R. D. M. Scott, *Br. J. Clin. Pract., 31*, 17 (1977).

53 N. Fleisher et al., *Ann. Intern. Med., 70*, 791 (1969).

54 H. J. Binder et al., *Gastroenterology, 72*, 1079 (1977).

55 B. F. Pike et al., *N. Engl. J. Med., 265*, 217 (1971).

56 "Applied Therapeutics: The Clinical Use of Drugs," 3rd ed., M. A. Koda-Kimble et al., Eds., Applied Therapeutics, San Francisco, Calif., 1983, p. 107.

57 S. G. Page et al., *J. Am. Med. Assoc., 157*, 1208 (1955).

58 *Drugs of Choice*, W. Modell, Ed., C. V. Mosby, St. Louis (1978), p. 359.

59 H. C. Shirkey, *Nebr. State Med. J., 50*, 67 (1965).

60 M. J. Pettei, *Pediatr. Ann., 16 (10)*, 796–800, 804–806, 811–813 (1987).

61 J. N. Lemoh et al., *Arch. Dis. Child., 54*, 719 (1979).

62 W. L. Nyan, *Pediatrics, 10*, 414 (1952).

63 I. J. Wolmon, "Intestinal Motility in Infancy and Childhood," Laboratory Applications in Clinical Pediatrics, McGraw-Hill, New York, N.Y., 1975.

64 L. T. Weaver et al., *Arch. Dis. Child., 59*, 649 (1984).

65 G. S. Glanden, *Br. Med. J., 1*, 515 (1976).

66 T. F. Hatch, *Pediatr. Clin. North Am., 35 (2)*, 257–280 (1988).

67 E. W. Godding, *Pharmacology, 36 (Suppl. 1)*, 230–236 (1988).

68 W. M. Liebman, *Postgrad. Med., 66*, 105 (1979).

69 S. C. Castle, *Arch. Intern. Med., 147 (10)*, 1702–1704 (1987).

70 R. S. Smith et al., in "Geriatric Medicine: Medical Care of Later Maturity," E. J. Steiglitz, Ed., J. B. Lippincott, Philadelphia, Pa., 1954, pp. 519–522.

71 L. J. Brandt, *Pract. Gastroenterol., XI (2)*, 31–36 (1987).

72 P. Rosseau, *Postgrad. Med.*, *83 (4)*, 339–340, 343–345, 349 (1988).

73 J. C. Brocklehurst et al., *Gerontol. Clin. (Basel)*, *11 (5)*, 293–300 (1969).

74 L. J. Brandt, "Gastrointestinal Disorders of the Elderly," Raven Press, New York, N.Y., 1984, pp. 261–367.

75 P. Rosseau, *Postgrad. Med.*, *83 (4)*, 352–353 (1988).

76 J. C. Brocklehurst in "Textbook of Geriatric Medicine and Gerontology," J. C. Brocklehurst, Ed., Longman (Churchill–Livingstone), New York, N.Y., 1985, pp. 534–556.

77 G. R. Davis et al., *Gastroenterol.*, *78*, 991–995 (1980).

78 A. I. Jacknowitz in "Current Geriatric Therapy," T. R. Covington and J. I. Walker, Eds., W. B. Sanders, Philadelphia, Pa., 1984, 178–238.

79 J. C. Brocklehurst, *Clin. Gastroenterol.*, *14 (4)*, 725–747 (1985).

80 H. Cummings et al., *Br. Med. J.*, *1*, 537 (1974).

81 J. S. G. Biggs and E. J. Vesey, *Drugs*, *19*, 70 (1980).

82 L. L. Hart in "Applied Therapeutics: The Clinical Use of Drugs," 4th ed., M. A. Koda-Kimble et al., Eds., Applied Therapeutics, San Francisco, Calif., 1989, p. 112.

83 S. Chaplin et al., *Adv. Drug React.*, *1*, 255 (1982).

84 L. Mundow, *Br. Med. J. Clin. Prac.*, *29*, 95 (1975).

85 J. R. Vanin and K. E. Saylor, *J. Am. Coll. Heath*, *37 (5)*, 227–230 (1989).

86 K. A. Halmi et al., *Psychol. Med.*, *11 (4)*, 697–706 (1981).

87 R. R. Babb, *West. J. Med.*, *122*, 93 (1975).

88 L. S. Basser, *Med. J. Aust.*, *1*, 47 (1979).

89 B. Smith, *Dis. Colon Rectum*, *16*, 455 (1973).

90 J. deGraeff, *Ned Tijdschr Geneesk.*, *105*, 200–202 (1961).

91 W. D. Heizer et al., *Ann. Intern. Med.*, *68*, 839–852 (1968).

92 H. P. Wolff et al., *Lancet*, *i*, 257–261 (1968).

93 N. F. Coghill et al., *Br. Med. J.*, *i*, 14–19 (1959).

94 F. A. deWolff et al., *Clin. Chem.*, *27*, 914 (1981).

95 L. Loof et al., *Ther. Drug Monit.*, *2*, 345 (1980).

96 M. D. Rawson, *Lancet*, *1*, 1121 (1966).

97 H. R. Erle, *Primary Care*, *3*, 301 (1976).

98 W. G. Thompson, *Drugs*, *19*, 49 (1980).

99 A. D. Dennison, *Am. J. Cardiol.*, *1*, 400 (1968).

100 J. Catellani and R. J. Collins, *Lancet*, *2*, 98 (1978).

101 W. G. Thompson, *Can. Med. Assoc. J.*, *114*, 927 (1976).

102 "Remington's Pharmaceutical Sciences," 17th ed., A. Osol, Ed., Mack, Easton, Pa., 1985, p. 1801.

103 "AHFS Drug Information 89," G. K. McEvoy, Ed., American Society of Hospital Pharmacists, Washington, D.C., 1989, p. 1578.

104 J. E. Sandgren et al., *Ann. Intern. Med.*, *101*, 331–334 (1984).

105 E. Bruera et al., *Cancer Treat. Rep.*, *71*, 1121–1122 (1987).

106 R. E. Enck, *Am. J. Hospice Care*, *5 (5)*, 17–19 (1988).

LAXATIVE PRODUCT TABLE

Product (Manufacturer)	Dosage Form	Stimulant	Bulk	Emollient/ Lubricant	Other Laxatives	Other Ingredients
Adlerika (Alvin Last)	liquid				magnesium sulfate	
Afko-Lube (Amer. Pharm.)	capsule syrup			docusate sodium 100 mg (capsule) 4 mg/ml (syrup)		
Afko-Lube Lax (Amer. Pharm.)	capsule	casan- thranol, 30 mg		docusate sodium, 100 mg		
Agoral (Parke-Davis)	emulsion[a]	phenol- phthalein, 0.2 g	agar tragacanth acacia	mineral oil, 4.2 g		benzoic acid egg albumin glycerin sodium, 0.98 mEq/ 15 ml citric acid
Agoral Plain (Parke-Davis)	emulsion		agar tragacanth acacia	mineral oil, 4.2 g		benzoic acid egg albumin glycerin sodium, 0.98 mEq/ 15 ml citric acid
Alophen (Parke-Davis)	tablet	phenol- phthalein, 60 mg				sodium free
Alphamul (Lannett)	emulsion	castor oil, 60%				flavor
Atrocholin (Glaxo)	tablet				dehydrocholic acid, 130 mg	
Bisacodyl (Various manufacturers)	tablet suppository	bisacodyl, 5 mg/tablet 10 mg/ suppository				
Bisco-Lax (Raway)	suppository	biscodyl, 10 mg				
Black Draught (Chattem)	tablet granules syrup	senna equi- valent 600 mg (tablet) senna equi- valent 660 mg/g (granules) casanthranol 6 mg/ml (syrup)				sucrose, 54.6% tartrazine (syrup only) alcohol, 5% (syrup only)
Caroid (Mentholatum)	tablet	cascara sagrada, 50 mg phenoph- thalein, 32.4 mg				

LAXATIVE PRODUCT TABLE, continued

Product (Manufacturer)	Dosage Form	Stimulant	Bulk	Emollient/ Lubricant	Other Laxatives	Other Ingredients
Carter's Little Pills (Carter)	tablet	bisacodyl, 5 mg				
Cascara Sagrada (Various manufacturers)	tablet	cascara sagrada, 325 mg				
Cascara Sagrada Aromatic Fluid (Various manufacturers)	liquid	cascara sagrada				alcohol, 18%
Castor Oil (Various manufacturers)	liquid	castor oil				
Ceo-Two (Beutlich)	suppository					sodium bicarbonate potassium bitartrate
Cholan-HMB (Fisons)	tablet				dehydrocholic acid, 250 mg	
Cillium (Whiteworth)	powder		psyllium seed husks, 4.94 g			
Citrate of Magnesia (Various manufacturers)	solution				magnesium citrate	
Citroma (Century)	solution				magnesium citrate	
Citro-Nesia (Century)	solution				magnesium citrate	
Citrucel (Lakeside)	powder		methylcellulose, 2 g/tbsp			flavor sodium, 3 mg
Colace (Mead Johnson)	capsule liquid[a] syrup			docusate sodium, 50 and 100 mg/ capsule, 10 mg/ml (liquid), 4 mg/ml (syrup)		citric acid sucrose, 600 mg/ml (syrup) sodium, 0.11 mEq/ 50 mg (capsule), 0.015 mEq/ml alcohol (syrup)
Colax (Rugby)	tablet	phenophthalein, 65 mg		docusate sodium, 100 mg		
Cologel (Lilly)	liquid		methylcellulose, 96 mg/ml			alcohol, 5% saccharin
Concentrated Milk of Magnesia (Roxane)	suspension				magnesium hydroxide, 0.233 g/ml	glycerin, 2.5% sorbitol, 29% sugar, 8% lemon sodium, 0.09 mEq/ml

LAXATIVE PRODUCT TABLE, continued

Product (Manufacturer)	Dosage Form	Stimulant	Bulk	Emollient/ Lubricant	Other Laxatives	Other Ingredients
Constiban (Columbia Medical)	capsule	casanthranol, 30 mg		docusate sodium, 100 mg		
Correctol (Schering-Plough)	tablet	yellow phenolphthalein, 65 mg		docusate sodium, 100 mg		sodium, 0.34 mEq
Dacodyl (Major)	tablet suppository	bisacodyl, 5 mg/tablet 10 mg/ suppository				
DC 240 (Goldline)	capsule			docusate calcium, 240 mg		
Dialose (Stuart)	capsule			docusate potassium, 100 mg		sodium free
Dialose Plus (Stuart)	capsule	casanthranol, 30 mg		docusate potassium, 100 mg		sodium free
Diocto (Various manufactures)	liquid syrup			docusate sodium, 10 mg/ml (liquid) 4 mg/ml (syrup)		
Diocto C (Various manufacturers)	syrup	casanthranol, 2 mg/ml		docusate sodium, 4 mg/ml		
Diocto-K (Rugby)	capsule			docusate potassium, 100 mg		
Diocto-K Plus (Rugby)	capsule	casanthranol, 30 mg		docusate potassium, 100 mg		
Dioctolose (Goldline)	capsule			docusate potassium, 100 mg		
Dioctolose Plus (Goldline)	capsule	casanthranol, 30 mg		docusate potassium, 100 mg		
Dioeze (Century)	capsule			docusate sodium, 250 mg		
Di-Sosul Forte (Drug Industries)	tablet	casanthranol, 30 mg		docusate sodium, 100 mg		
Dio-Sul (Vortech)	capsule			docusate sodium, 100 mg		
Diothron (Vortech)	capsule	casanthranol, 30 mg		docusate sodium, 100 mg		
Disanthrol (Lannett)	capsule	casanthranol, 30 mg		docusate sodium, 100 mg		

LAXATIVE PRODUCT TABLE, continued

Product (Manufacturer)	Dosage Form	Stimulant	Bulk	Emollient/ Lubricant	Other Laxatives	Other Ingredients
Disolan (Lannett)	capsule	phenol- phthalein, 65 mg		docusate sodium, 100 mg		
Disolan Forte (Lannett)	capsule	casan- thranol, 30 mg	carboxymethyl cellulose sodium, 400 mg	docusate sodium, 100 mg		
Disonate (Lannett)	capsule liquid syrup			docusate sodium, 100 and 240 mg/ capsule 10 mg/ml (liquid) 4 mg/ml (syrup)		
Disoplex (Lannett)	capsule		carboxymethyl cellulose sodium, 400 mg	docusate sodium, 100 mg		
Docusate Calcium (Various manufacturers)	capsule			docusate cal- cium, 240 mg		
Docusate Potassium w/ Casanthranol (Various manufacturers)	capsule	casan- thranol, 30 mg		docusate potas- sium, 100 mg		
Docusate Sodium (Roxane)	capsule syrup			docusate sodium, 50 mg (capsule) 100 mg (cap- sule and tablet) 250 mg (capsule) 3.33 mg/ml (syrup) 4 mg/ml (syrup)		propylene glycol 20% (syrup) sucrose, 55% (syrup) sodium, 0.06 mEq/ml
Docusate w/ Casanthranol (Various manufacturers)	capsule syrup	casan- thranol, 30 mg (capsule) 2 mg/ml (syrup)		docusate sodium, 100 mg (capsule) 4 mg/ml (syrup)		
DOK (Major)	capsule liquid			docusate sodium, 100 mg 250 mg (capsules) 10 mg/ml (liquid)		
Doss (My-K Labs)	syrup			docusate sodium, 4 mg/ml		

LAXATIVE PRODUCT TABLE, continued

Product (Manufacturer)	Dosage Form	Stimulant	Bulk	Emollient/ Lubricant	Other Laxatives	Other Ingredients
Doxidan (Hoechst-Roussel)	capsule	phenol-phthalein, 65 mg		docusate calcium, 60 mg		
Doxinate (Hoechst-Roussel)	capsule solution[a]			docusate sodium, 240 mg (capsule) 50 mg/ml (sol.)		sodium, 0.13 mEq/ 60 mg 0.53 mEq/ 240 mg 1.1 mEq/dose (sol.) alcohol, 5% (sol.)
Dr. Caldwell's Senna Laxative (Gebauer)	liquid	senna, 33.3 mg/ml				alcohol, 4.9% sodium free
DSMC Plus (Geneva Generics)	capsule	casan-thranol, 30 mg		docusate potassium, 100 mg		sodium free
Dulcolax (Boehringer Ingelheim)	tablet suppository	bisacodyl, 5 mg/tablet 10 mg/ suppository				sodium free
Duosol (Kirkman)	capsule			docusate sodium, 100 mg 250 mg		
D-S-S (Warner-Chilcott)	capsule			docusate sodium, 100 mg		
D-S-S Plus (Warner-Chilcott)	capsule	casan-thranol, 30 mg		docusate sodium, 100 mg		
Effersyllium (Stuart)	powder		psyllium, hydrocolloid, 3 g/tsp			sodium < 5 mg/ tsp sucrose flavor
Emulsoil (Paddock)	instant-mix liquid[a]	castor oil, 95%				flavor
Epsom Salt (Various manufacturers)	granules				magnesium sulfate, ≈ 40 mEq/ 5 mg	
Equalactin (Pfizer)	tablet		calcium polycarbophil, 625 mg			flavor povidone
Espotabs (Combe)	tablet	yellow phenolphthalein, 97.2 mg				

LAXATIVE PRODUCT TABLE, continued

Product (Manufacturer)	Dosage Form	Stimulant	Bulk	Emollient/ Lubricant	Other Laxatives	Other Ingredients
Evac-Q-Kit (Adria)	liquid tablet suppository	phenolphthalein, 130 mg (tablet)			magnesium citrate (liquid), 300 ml carbon dioxide releasing suppository	sodium, 0.84 mEq/dose (liq.) trace (tablet) 7.63 mEq/ suppos.
Evac-Q-Kwik (Adria)	liquid tablet suppository	phenolphthalein, 130 mg (tablet)			magnesium citrate (liquid), 300 ml bisacodyl, 10 mg (suppository)	sodium, 0.84 mEq/dose (liq.), trace (tablet) trace (suppos.)
Evac-U-Gen (Walker)	chewable tablet	yellow phenolphthalein, 97.2 mg				sodium, 0.004 mEq
Evac-U-Lax (Hauck)	chewable tablet	phenolphthalein, 80 mg				
Ex-Lax (Sandoz Pharm.)	chocolated tablet unflavored pill	yellow phenolphthalein, 90 mg	acacia (unflavored)			
Ex-Lax Extra Gentle (Sandoz Pharm.)	sugar coated tablet	yellow phenolphthalein, 65 mg	acacia	docusate sodium, 75 mg		
Feen-A-Mint (Schering-Plough)	chewing gum mint tablet	yellow phenolphthalein, 97.2 mg (gum and mint) 65 mg (tablet)		docusate sodium, 100 mg (tablet)		flavor
Feen-A-Mint Pills (Schering-Plough)	tablet	yellow phenolphthalein, 65 mg		docusate sodium, 100 mg		sodium, 0.34 mEq
Femilax (G & W Labs)	tablet	phenolphthalein, 65 mg		docusate sodium, 100 mg		
Fiberall (CIBA Consumer)	tablet		calcium polycarbophil, 1250 mg			crospovidone, dextrose, flavors, magnesium stearate
Fiberall, Natural (CIBA Consumer)	powder[a]		psyllium hydrophilic mucilloid, 3.4 g			citric acid, flavor
Fiberall, Oatmeal Raisin or Fruit & Nut (CIBA Consumer)	wafer		psyllium hydrophilic mucilloid, 3.4 g			wheat bran, glycerin, lecithin

LAXATIVE PRODUCT TABLE, continued

Product (Manufacturer)	Dosage Form	Stimulant	Bulk	Emollient/ Lubricant	Other Laxatives	Other Ingredients
Fiberall, Orange (CIBA Consumer)	powder[a]		psyllium hydrophilic mucilloid, 3.4 g			wheat bran, citric acid, flavor, saccharin
FiberCon (Lederle)	tablet		calcium polycarbophil, 625 mg			sodium free
Fleet Babylax (Fleet)	liquid				glycerin, 4 ml	
Fleet Bagenema (Fleet)	enema				liquid castile soap, 19.7 ml	
Fleet Bagenema #1105 (Fleet)	enema	bisacodyl, 10 mg				
Fleet Bisacodyl (Fleet)	enema tablet suppository	bisacodyl, 10 mg 5 mg/tablet 10 mg/ suppository				
Fleet Castor Oil Stimulant (Fleet)	emulsion	castor oil, 67%				
Fleet Enema (Fleet)	enema				sodium biphosphate, 0.16 g/ml sodium phosphate, 0.06 g/ml	
Fleet Mineral Oil (Fleet)	enema			mineral oil, 120 ml		
Fleet Pediatric Enema (Fleet)	enema				sodium biphosphate, 0.16 g/ml sodium phosphate, 0.06 g/ml	sodium, 96 mEq/60 ml
Fletcher's Castoria for Children (Mentholatum)	liquid	senna, 6.5%				alcohol, 3.5%
Garfields Tea (Alvin Last)	cut and sifted botanical	senna				mixed botanicals
Genasoft (Goldline)	capsule			docusate sodium, 100 mg		
Genasoft Plus (Goldline)	capsule	casanthranol, 30 mg		docusate sodium, 100 mg		
Genna (Goldline)	tablet	senna concentrate, 217 mg				

LAXATIVE PRODUCT TABLE, continued

Product (Manufacturer)	Dosage Form	Stimulant	Bulk	Emollient/ Lubricant	Other Laxatives	Other Ingredients
Gentlax S (Blair)	tablet	senna concentrate, 187 mg		docusate sodium, 50 mg		
Gentle Nature (Sandoz)		sennosides A & B, 20 mg				
Glycerin, USP (Various manufacturers)	suppository				glycerin	sodium stearate
Haley's M-O (Glenbrook)	emulsion[a]			mineral oil, 25%	magnesium hydroxide, 6%	
Hydrocil Instant (Rowell)	powder[a]		psyllium, 95%			povidone
Innerclean Herbal Laxative (Alvin Last)	cut and sifted botanical	senna leaves buckthorn bark	psyllium seed husks			anise seed fennel seed
Innerclean Herbal Laxative (Alvin Last)	tablet	senna leaves buckthorn bark	psyllium seed husks			anise seed fennel seed
Kasof (Stuart)	capsules			docusate potassium, 240 mg		sodium free
Kellogg's Tasteless Castor Oil (SmithKline Beecham)	liquid	castor oil, 100%				sodium free
Kondremul (Fisons)	microemulsion[a]		chondrus	mineral oil, 55%		sodium, 0.09 mEq/ 15 ml
Kondremul with Cascara (Fisons)	microemulsion[a]	cascara	chondrus	mineral oil, 55%		sodium, 0.07 mEq/ 15 ml
Kondremul with Phenolphthalein (Fisons)	microemulsion	phenolphthalein	chondrus	mineral oil, 55%		sodium, 0.10 mEq/ 15 ml
Konsyl (Lafayette)	powder[a]		psyllium mucilloid, 100%			sodium, < 4 mg
Konsyl-D (Lafayette)	powder		psyllium hydrophilic mucilloid, 50%			dextrose, 50% sodium, < 4 mg
L.A. Formula (Burton, Parsons)	powder		psyllium mucilloid, 50%			dextrose, 50%
Lane's Pills (Alvin Last)	tablet	casanthranol, 45 mg				
Laxcaps (Glenbrook)	capsule	phenolphthalein, 90 mg		docusate sodium, 83 mg		

LAXATIVE PRODUCT TABLE, continued

Product (Manufacturer)	Dosage Form	Stimulant	Bulk	Emollient/ Lubricant	Other Laxatives	Other Ingredients
Laxinate 100 (Hauck)	capsule			docusate sodium, 100 mg		
Lax-Pills (G & W)	tablet	phenol-phthalein, 90 mg				
Liqui-Doss (Ferndale)	emulsion			docusate sodium, 2 mg/ml mineral oil		
Mag-Ox 400 (Blaine Co.)	tablet				magnesium oxide, 400 mg	
Maltsupex (Wallace)	tablet liquid powder		malt soup extract, 750 mg/tablet 16 g/tbsp (liquid & powder)			tartrazine (tablet)
Metamucil (Proctor & Gamble)	powder		psyllium mucilloid, 3.4 g			potassium, 31 mg sucrose, 13.5 g sodium, 1 mg
Metamucil Instant Mix, Lemon Lime Flavor (Procter & Gamble)	powder in single-dose packets[a]		psyllium mucilloid, 3.4 g/ packet			calcium carbonate sodium, 1 mg sucrose citric acid potassium, 290 mg sodium aspartame
Metamucil, Orange Flavor (Procter & Gamble)	powder		psyllium mucilloid, 3.4 g			potassium, 31 mg sucrose, 7.1 g sodium, 1 mg
Metamucil, Orange Flavor, Instant Mix (Procter & Gamble)	powder[a]		psyllium mucilloid, 3.4 g/ packet			aspartame citric acid sodium bicarbonate sodium, 1 mg potassium, 290 mg
Milk of Magnesia (Various manufacturers)	liquid				magnesium hydroxide, ≈ 80 mEq magnesium/ 30 ml	
Milk of Magnesia USP (Roxane)	suspension				magnesium hydroxide, 0.078 g/ml	sodium, 0.03 mEq/ 15 ml
Milk of Magnesia-Cascara Suspension, Concentrated (Roxane)	suspension	cascara sagrada (equiv. to 5 ml USP fluidextract)			magnesium hydroxide, 0.078 g/ml	sodium, 0.12 mEq/ 15 ml

LAXATIVE PRODUCT TABLE, continued

Product (Manufacturer)	Dosage Form	Stimulant	Bulk	Emollient/ Lubricant	Other Laxatives	Other Ingredients
Milk of Magnesia, Concentrated (Roxane)	liquid				magnesium hydroxide	
Mineral Oil (Various manufacturers)	liquid			mineral oil		
Mitrolan (A.H. Robins)	chewable tablet		calcium polycarbophil			sodium, 0.02 mEq
Modane (Adria)	tablet	phenol-phthalein 130 mg				
Modane Bulk (Adria)	powder		psyllium hydro-philic mucil-loid, 50%			dextrose, 50% sodium, 2 mg/tsp
Modane Mild (Adria)	tablet	phenol-phthalein, 60 mg				
Modane Plus (Adria)	tablet	phenol-phthalein, 60 mg		docusate sodium, 100 mg		
Modane Soft (Adria)	capsule			docusate sodium, 100 mg		sodium, 0.27 mEq/dose
Modane Versabran (Adria)	powder		psyllium, 3.4 g			saccharin
Naturacil (Bristol-Myers)	chewable pieces		psyllium, 3.4 g			sodium, 11 mg flavor
Natural Vegetable (Various manufacturers)	powder		psyllium mucil-loid, 3.4 g			sodium, < 10 mg dextrose
Nature's Remedy (SmithKline Beecham)	tablet	aloe, 100 mg cascara sagrada, 150 mg				
Neo-Cultol (Fisons)	suspension			refined mineral oil jelly		sodium, 0.03 mEq/ 15 ml chocolate flavor
Neoloid (Lederle)	emulsion	castor oil, 36.4%				saccharin flavor
Perdiem (Rorer)	granule	senna, 18%	psyllium, 82%			
Perdiem Fiber (Rorer)	granule		psyllium, 100%			
Peri-Colace (Mead Johnson)	capsule syrup	casan-thranol, 30 mg/ capsule, 2 mg/ml		docusate sodium, 100 mg/ capsule, 4 mg/ml		alcohol, 10% (syrup)

LAXATIVE PRODUCT TABLE, continued

Product (Manufacturer)	Dosage Form	Stimulant	Bulk	Emollient/ Lubricant	Other Laxatives	Other Ingredients
Peri-Dos (Goldline)	capsule	casanthranol, 30 mg		docusate sodium, 100 mg		
Phenolax (Upjohn)	chewable wafer	phenolphthalein, 64.8 mg				tartrazine
Phillips' LaxCaps (Glenbrook)	capsule	phenolphthalein, 90 mg		docusate sodium, 83 mg		
Phillip's Milk of Magnesia (Glenbrook)	suspension tablet				magnesium hydroxide, 80 mg/ml 311 mg/ tablet	peppermint oil, 0.038 mg/ml, 1.166 mg/ tablet sodium, 0.004 mEq/ml, (unflavored) 0.007 mEq/ml, (flavored) 0.13 mEq/ tablet
Phospho-Soda (Fleet)	liquid				sodium biphosphate, 0.48 g/ml sodium phosphate, 0.18 g/ml	sodium, 96.4 mEq/ 20 ml flavors
Pro-Cal-Sof (Vangard)	capsule			docusate calcium, 240 mg		
Pro-Sof (Vangard)	capsule syrup			docusate sodium, 100 mg 250 mg 4 mg/ml		
Pro-Sof Plus (Vangard)	capsule	casanthranol, 30 mg		docusate sodium, 100 mg		
Prulet (Mission)	chewable tablet	phenolphthalein, 60 mg				flavor
Purge Evacuant (Fleming)	liquid	castor oil, 95%				
Regulace (Republic)	capsule	casanthranol, 30 mg		docusate sodium, 100 mg		
Regulax SS (Republic)	capsule			docusate sodium, 100 mg 200 mg		
Reguloid, Orange (Rugby)	powder		psyllium mucilloid, 3.4 g			sucrose, 70% flavor
Reguloid, Natural (Rugby)	powder		psyllium hydrophilic mucilloid, 50%			dextrose, 50%

LAXATIVE PRODUCT TABLE, continued

Product (Manufacturer)	Dosage Form	Stimulant	Bulk	Emollient/ Lubricant	Other Laxatives	Other Ingredients
Regutol (Schering-Plough)	tablet			docusate sodium, 100 mg		sodium, 0.34 mEq
Sani-Supp (G & W Labs)	suppository				glycerin	sodium stearate
Senexon (Rugby)	tablet	senna concentrate, 187 mg				
Senna-Gen (Goldline)	tablet	senna concentrate, 217 mg				
Senokot (Purdue Frederick)	granules tablet suppository syrup	senna concentrate, 326 mg/tsp (granules), 187 mg/ tablet, 652 mg/ suppository, 50 mg extract/ml (syrup)				alcohol, 7% (syrup) sodium, 0.06 mEq/dose (granules) 0.007 mEq dose (tablet)
Senokot-S (Purdue Frederick)	tablet	senna concentrate, 187 mg		docusate sodium, 50 mg		sodium, 0.15 mEq
Senokot-X-tra (Purdue Frederick)	tablet	senna concentrate, 374 mg				sodium, 0.014 mEq/ dose
Senolax (Schein)	tablet	senna concentrate, 217 mg				
Serutan (SmithKline Beecham)	powder granules		psyllium, 3.4 g (powder) 2.5 g (granules)			saccharin (granules) sodium, < 0.1 g (powder) < 0.3 g (granules) flavor
Siblin (Parke-Davis)	granules		psyllium seed husks, 2.5 g			sucrose, 2.4 g
Sodium Phosphates Oral Solution USP (Roxane)	solution[a]				sodium biphosphate, 0.48 g/ml sodium phosphate, 0.18 g/ml	saccharin, 0.265% sodium, 0.055 mEq/ml
Softenex (Alval Amco)	drops			docusate sodium		vitamin B$_6$ fructose
Sulfalax Calcium (Major)	capsule			docusate calcium, 240 mg		
Surfak (Hoechst-Roussel)	capsule			docusate calcium, 50 and 240 mg		sodium free alcohol, 1.3% (50 mg) 3% (240 mg)

LAXATIVE PRODUCT TABLE, continued

Product (Manufacturer)	Dosage Form	Stimulant	Bulk	Emollient/ Lubricant	Other Laxatives	Other Ingredients
Swiss Kriss (Modern Product)	powder tablet	senna, 52.5%	oat bran psyllium seed husks			sodium free
Syllact (Wallace)	powder		psyllium seed husks, 50%			dextrose, 50%
Syllamalt (Wallace)	powder		malt soup extract, 50% psyllium seed husks, 50%			
Therac Plus (Jones Medical)	enema			docusate sodium, 283 mg	glycerin	benzocaine, 20 mg PEG-400
Therevac-SB (Jones Medical)	enema			docusate sodium, 283 mg	glycerin	PEG-400
Unilax (B.F. Ascher)	tablet	yellow phenolphthalein, 130 mg		docusate sodium, 230 mg		
Uro-Mag (Blaine Co.)	capsule				magnesium oxide, 140 mg	
V-Lax (Century)	powder		psyllium hydrophilic muciloid, 50%			dextrose, 50%
Zymenol (Houser)	emulsion[a]			mineral oil, 50%		sorbitol saccharin

[a] Sugar free.

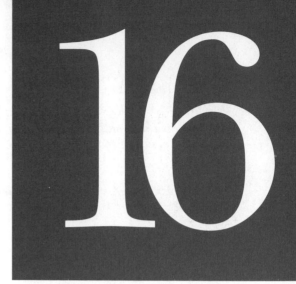

*L. M. Evenson-St. Amand
and R. Keith Campbell*

DIABETES CARE PRODUCTS

*Q*uestions to ask in patient/consumer counseling

Is there a history of diabetes in your family?
———

When were you last tested for diabetes? What were the results of those tests?
———

How long have you had diabetes?
———

How do you feel about having diabetes? Do members of your family understand the condition and the factors that affect control?
———

Do you belong to the local diabetes association?
———

How long has it been since you discussed your diabetes treatment program with your physician?
———

Do you use insulin? What type of insulin do you use? What brand of insulin do you use? How do you store your insulin?
———

If you use insulin, where do you inject it? How much do you inject? Do you rotate the sites of injection? How often do you rotate sites?
———

What drugs have been prescribed for you? Are you taking medications for diabetes?
———

Are you taking other medications, such as pain killers or cough medicines?
———

Are you allergic to sulfa drugs? Are you allergic to beef or pork insulin?
———

Do you test your blood glucose? If so, how often do you do the testing? Do you read the strips visually or use a meter? Do you keep track of all blood glucose readings? Do you show your blood glucose records to your physician?
———

Do you test your urine for glucose at home? If so, which test do you use? How often do you do the testing? Do you keep track of all urine glucose readings? Do you report urine glucose test results of 2+ or more to your physician?
———

Do you test your urine for ketones? If so, which test do you use? How often do you do the testing? Do you keep track of all urine ketone readings? Do you report all positive urine ketone tests to your physician?
———

Explain how you test your urine using TesTape, Clinitest tablets, Diastix, or Clinistix.
———

What kind of diet has your physician prescribed? Do you have any trouble following the prescribed diet?
———

Have you worked with a dietitian to help plan meals and snacks?
———

Do you have a regular schedule for exercise? Do you check your blood glucose before and after exercise? What do you do if your blood glucose is low?
———

Do you follow any of the popular "fad" diets? If so, who recommended the diet to you?
———

How much alcohol (including wine and beer) do you drink in a week?
———

Do you visit an ophthalmologist regularly? When was your last eye examination? What did the doctor tell you?

Do you visit a dentist regularly? When was your last checkup?

Do you ever see a podiatrist? Do you examine your feet daily? What foot care products do you use regularly?

What do you think has affected the control of your diabetes? Are you eating differently? Are you exercising more or less? Have you had any infections? Is there anything that is emotionally upsetting you?

Successful management of diabetes mellitus requires the combined efforts of a total health care team: physician, dietitian, diabetes nurse specialist, physical therapist, podiatrist, and pharmacist. The physician must accurately diagnose the condition, properly classify the type of diabetes, and motivate the patient to learn to control and monitor the condition. Dietitians explain the importance of diet control, the glycemic index, and good nutrition. Diabetes nurse specialists help patients develop a positive attitude and learn to perform laboratory tests, monitor the effectiveness of management efforts, inject insulin, and keep records of the factors that affect control of diabetes. Physical therapists teach patients to incorporate exercise into their daily lives, develop strategies to avoid the complications of exercise, and instruct patients in the benefits of regular physical exercise and good health. The pharmacist's access to the patient offers a unique opportunity to help the patient maintain a proper therapeutic regimen. The pharmacist can answer the patient's questions about the disease; urine and blood testing; drug therapy; diet; and proper oral, skin, and foot care. In addition, the pharmacist can stress the importance of complying with the instructions of the physician, dietitian, nurse specialist, podiatrist, and physical therapist; be a positive re-

Editor's Note: Frequently, the term "patients with diabetes" and its acronym "PWD" are currently used in professional and scientific literature on diabetes when referring to persons who have diabetes. However, because the terms "asthmatics" and "bronchitics" are used in certain chapters of this edition of the Handbook, the term "diabetics" has also been retained in the interest of consistency.

inforcement of those instructions; and monitor the control of diabetic patients, particularly in relation to the use of drugs (1, 2).

Approximately 7 million diabetics are currently being treated in the United States, another 5 million have undiagnosed diabetes (mild symptoms or asymptomatic) (3), and an additional 5 million will develop diabetes sometime during their lives. Diabetes currently affects approximately 5% of the U.S. population. Roughly 25% of the population (50 million people) either have diabetes, will develop diabetes, or have a relative with diabetes (4).

The incidence of diabetes is increasing at an annual rate of 6% (5). It is now the number one cause of new blindness in the United States; more than one-half of the heart attacks that occur are related to diabetes; diabetic kidney disease is common and often fatal; neurologic complications occur frequently; and complications of pregnancy caused by diabetes are well recognized. More than 40,000 amputations a year are performed because of diabetes-related complications in the feet and legs (6). Diabetes and its associated complications are the third leading cause of death and are responsible for approximately 8% of hospital admissions (7, 8). Diabetes kills nearly 40,000 people each year in the United States, and about 300,000 more die of its complications (9). Coronary artery disease is seven times more prevalent in diabetic women than in unaffected women (10). Women are 50% more likely to have diabetes than men; nonwhites are 20% more likely to have it than whites; people with low incomes (less than $5,000 a year) are three times more likely to have it than those in middle- and upper-income groups; and the chances of developing it doubles with every 20% of excess weight and with every decade of life (11). Approximately 40% of the diabetic population is over 65 years of age (12).

This increase in the number of diabetics has been attributed to three primary factors: a sharp increase in the geriatric population (who are more prone to develop the disease); more sophisticated methods of screening and diagnosis; and third-generation diabetics who may not have been born if insulin had not been discovered (10).

It is estimated that in 1987 diabetics generated total costs of $20.4 billion (13). Economic costs are 13% higher for insulin-dependent diabetics than for noninsulin-dependent diabetics (14). The average cost for diabetes care products is estimated to be $4 per day (12). Frequently, the diabetic is neglected by manufacturers of pharmaceuticals, health and beauty aids, food, drinks, and candy. The diabetic is offered a bewildering selection of products that are improperly formulated or poorly labeled and often does not receive adequate patient education or comprehensive instructions in self-care (15, 16). The pharmacist has an excellent opportunity to help these patients by reiterating instructions and warning signs, by assessing the patient's ability to carry out self-help measures, and by providing education related to those self-help measures. The pharmacist also can be a consultant to both physician and patient concerning the disease and the drugs and devices used in its treatment (17).

CLASSIFICATION OF DIABETES

Diabetes mellitus is a difficult condition to define because it is really a variety of conditions; hyperglycemia is the common physiologic problem that must be brought under control. Several types of diabetes have been identified; all have different etiologies, clinical courses, and methods of treatment. However, chronic hyperglycemia is the common denominator and often leads to the symptoms and complications of the disease. Table 1 summarizes the new system for classifying the various types of diabetes and compares it with the old methods. Approximately 10% of the diabetics in the United States are classified as Type I (insulin dependent); the remaining 90% are Type II (noninsulin dependent) (20). Table 2 further defines Type I and Type II diabetes according to the distinguishing features. However, a diabetic may present with mixed characteristics (18). A clinical classification of diabetes to aid physicians and pharmacists in developing treatment protocols is also shown in Table 2 (19).

There are two distinct categories of patients in the Type II classification group. About 10% of patients with Type II diabetes are nonobese, and the other 90% are obese. Nonobese Type II diabetes often occurs in patients during youth, is often inherited in an autosomal dominant pattern, and is called maturity onset diabetes of the young (20). Obese Type II diabetes frequently occurs in adults who are over 40 years of age.

TABLE 1 Classification of diabetes and glucose intolerance

New names	Old names
CLINICAL CATEGORIES	
Type I: Insulin-dependent diabetes mellitus (IDDM)	Juvenile diabetes Juvenile-onset diabetes Ketosis-prone diabetes Growth-onset diabetes Brittle diabetes

Type II: Noninsulin-dependent diabetes mellitus (NIDDM)
    Type a: nonobese
    Type b: obese
	Adult-onset diabetes
	Maturity-onset diabetes
	Ketosis-resistant diabetes
	Stable diabetes
	Maturity-onset diabetes of youth

Diabetes mellitus associated with other conditions or syndromes	Secondary diabetes (drug-induced diabetes; impaired glucose tolerance due to other hormonal irregularities)
Impaired glucose tolerance (IGT)	Asymptomatic diabetes Chemical diabetes Subclinical diabetes Borderline diabetes Latent diabetes
Gestational diabetes	Gestational diabetes
STATISTICAL RISK	
Previous abnormality of glucose tolerance	Latent diabetes Prediabetes
Potential abnormality of glucose tolerance	Potential diabetes Prediabetes

Reprinted with permission from *Diabetes, 28 (12),* 1039 (1979).

TABLE 2 Distinguishing features of two major types of diabetes mellitus

	Insulin-dependent Type I (IDDM)	Noninsulin-dependent Type II (NIDDM)
Age of onset	Usually, but not always, during childhood or puberty	Frequently over 35
Type of onset	Abrupt	Usually gradual
Prevalence	0.5%	2–4%
Incidence	<10%	>75%
Family history of diabetes	Frequently negative	Commonly positive
Primary cause	Pancreatic beta-cell deficiency	End organ (insulin receptors) unresponsiveness to insulin action
Nutritional status at time of onset	Usually undernourished	Obesity usually present
Postglucose plasma or serum insulin[a], μU/ml	Absent	>100 at 2 hours
Symptoms	Polydipsia, polyphagia, and polyuria	Maybe none
Hepatomegaly	Rather common	Uncommon
Stability	Blood sugar fluctuates widely in response to small changes in insulin dose, exercise, and infection	Blood sugar fluctuations are less marked
Possible etiologic factors include: Inheritance	Associated with specific HLA tissue types, but only 40–50% concordance in twins	95–100% concordance in twins, but not associated with specific HLA tissue types
Autoimmune disease	50–80% circulating islet-cell antibodies	Negative; <10% circulating islet-cell antibodies
Viral infections	Coxsackie, mumps, influenza	No evidence
Proneness to ketosis	Frequent, especially if treatment program is insufficient in food and/or insulin	Uncommon except in the presence of unusual stress or moderate to severe sepsis
Insulin defect	Defect in secretion; secretion is impaired early in disease; secretion may be totally absent late in disease	Insulin deficiency present in some patients; others are insulin resistant
		Insulin deficiency—in most patients, insulin secretion fails to keep pace with inordinate demands caused by obesity; this defect may appear initially as a failure to respond to glucose alone, suggesting an impairment in the glucoreceptor of the pancreatic beta-cell
		Insulin resistance—in some patients, there is a defect in tissue responsiveness to insulin and evidence of hyperinsulinemia, in such patients, insulin resistance may be mediated by decreased number of insulin receptors in target cells
		Increased hepatic glucose production in response to altered cellular glucose uptake

(continued)

TABLE 2 *continued*

	Insulin-dependent Type I (IDDM)	Noninsulin-dependent Type II (NIDDM)
Plasma insulin (endogenous)	Negligible to zero	Plasma insulin response may be either adequate but delayed so that postprandial hypoglycemia may be present when diabetes is discovered or diminished but not absent
Vascular complications of diabetes and degenerative changes	Infrequent until diabetes has been present for ~5 years	Frequent
Usual causes of death	Degenerative complications in target organs (e.g., renal failure due to diabetic nephropathy)	Accelerated atherosclerosis (e.g., myocardial infarct); to lesser extent, microangiopathic changes in target tissues (e.g., renal failure)
Diet	Mandatory in all patients	If diet is used fully, hypoglycemic therapy may not be needed
Insulin	Necessary for all patients	Necessary for 20–30% of patients
Oral agents	Rarely efficacious	Often efficacious

[a]Normal response is between 50 and 135μU/ml at 60 minutes and less than 100 μU/ml at 120 minutes after 100 g of oral glucose.

ETIOLOGY

The most common predisposing factors for diabetes are heredity, obesity, age, stress, hormonal imbalance, vasculitis of the vessels supplying the beta-cells of the pancreas, and viruses that affect the autoimmune responses (1, 21).

Type I diabetes is characterized by an absence of functioning insulin-secreting pancreatic islet cells. The abnormal cells may be affected by many intrinsic factors. For example, genetic defects in the production of certain macromolecules may interfere with proper insulin synthesis, packaging, or release, or the beta-cells may not recognize glucose signals or may not replicate normally (22). Extrinsic factors that affect beta-cell function include damage caused by viruses (e.g., mumps or Coxsackie B4), by destructive cytotoxins and antibodies released by sensitized lymphocytes, or by autodigestion in the course of an inflammatory disorder involving the adjacent exocrine pancreas. Cells have many antigen types. Specific histocompatibility locus antigen (HLA) genes may increase susceptibility to a diabetogenic virus, or certain immune-response genes may predispose patients to a destructive autoimmune response against their own islet cells. In the severe form of Type I diabetes, circulating islet-cell antibodies have been detected in as many as 80% of the cases tested in the first few weeks of the diabetes onset (6, 22, 23). In Type II diabetics, as in severe Type I diabetics, the patient may inherit a response to a viral infection that causes a beta-cell defect as a consequence of viral stress.

In Type II diabetics who have excess insulin and are obese, hyperinsulinism and insulin resistance may be correlated with a decrease in insulin receptors (6, 24, 25). Moreover, studies have shown that the tissues of insulin-resistant, obese patients exhibit reduced insulin binding. The reduced number of insulin receptors is the basic, and often reversible, defect present in insulin-resistant patients (6, 24, 25).

Resistance to insulin's action also appears to be a result of an impairment in the target cell's response to insulin, caused by a defect in postreceptor binding. In Type II patients with severe hyperglycemia, it appears that both a decreased number of insulin receptors and a postreceptor defect exist in combination (25).

Normal Carbohydrate Metabolism

Under normal conditions, the body maintains a balance of glucose, fatty acids, and ketone bodies in the tissue cells and blood to keep plasma glucose levels within a narrow range and provide adequate glucose to the central nervous system (CNS) through a combination of continuous basal insulin release and bolus release (26). Insulin is stored in pancreatic beta-cells in granules and is released in response to changes in the concentration of plasma glucose (27). An initial rapid insulin release in response to an increase in plasma glucose is followed by a lower sustained release, which gradually increases over time (28, 29). Insulin stimulates glucose uptake and utilization, increases muscle and liver glycogen levels, decreases hepatic glucose output, increases the synthesis of fatty acids and triglycerides, decreases lipolysis and the production of ketone bodies, and enhances incorporation of amino acids into proteins. Insulin is rapidly cleared by the liver, which allows changes in insulin secretion to compensate for fluctuations in blood glucose levels. Insulin, in concert with glucagon, somatostatin, growth hormone, corticosteroids, epinephrine, and other chemicals, maintains the blood glucose between 50–150 mg/100 ml (mg %) at all times. Any increase or decrease in the hormones or other chemicals that affect insulin activity (e.g., drug therapy), can cause a nondiabetic to become diabetic or cause a diabetic to lose control of the disease.

because of the lack of insulin and signal the person to eat (polyphagia), which increases the blood glucose level even further.

Insulin has a direct inhibitory effect on the enzyme lipoprotein lipase, which mobilizes body fat (lipolysis). Other hormones such as glucocorticoids and epinephrine enhance lipolysis. The lack of insulin results in enhanced lipase activity, and fat is converted to free fatty acids, which circulate through the blood. Because fats rather than carbohydrates are being metabolized, weight loss occurs with time. The acidic ketone bodies that result from the breakdown of free fatty acids eventually lead to a metabolic acidosis. This ketoacidosis can lead to deep and labored breathing, sometimes called "air hunger" or Kussmaul's breathing. The breath will have a fruity acetone odor. Ketones can also depress the CNS, resulting in coma and death if insulin is not administered. The presence of ketones in the urine may indicate ketoacidosis.

Figure 1 shows the clinical manifestations that occur in an untreated Type I diabetic. The signs of insulin deficiency will result in abnormal urine and blood values that can be monitored for and used to determine how well the diabetes is being controlled.

Diabetic Carbohydrate Metabolism

Type I Diabetes

In Type I (insulin-dependent) diabetes, no release of insulin occurs in response to increased blood glucose levels after a meal or a snack. Hyperglycemia results as insulin is required to facilitate glucose transport into the fat or muscle tissue. In an attempt to provide glucose to the glucose-deficient tissue, amino acids are converted into glucose by hepatic gluconeogenesis, and liver glycogen is converted to glucose by glycogenolysis. However, without insulin, the tissues cannot use this glucose either, and the hyperglycemia becomes even more pronounced.

The blood glucose level at which glucose first appears in the urine is clinically referred to as the renal threshold for glucose. Normally, glucose does not spill into the urine until the venous blood glucose reaches 180 mg/100 ml. In diabetics, the threshold level for glucose may increase to 250 mg/100 ml or more. The threshold level will also increase with pregnancy and advancing age (6, 30).

The increased osmotic load in the kidney draws body water with it and is responsible for the excretion of large amounts of urine (polyuria), loss of fluid, and dehydration. The osmotic diuresis and water loss may initially cause dry mouth and progress to significant hypovolemia, electrolyte loss, and cellular dehydration. A compensatory increase in thirst (polydipsia) occurs. The tissue cells cannot use the circulating blood glucose

Type II Diabetes

Type I diabetes typically has a rapid onset with the usual signs and symptoms of polyuria, polyphagia, polydipsia, weakness, weight loss, dry mouth, and ketonuria or ketoacidosis; Type II (noninsulin-dependent) diabetes, however, is frequently asymptomatic (6, 31, 32). Type II diabetes (Figure 2) most often is detected when glucose is found in the urine or when elevated blood glucose is found on a routine examination. Careful study of the older, obese group of diabetics reveals glucosuria, proteinuria, postprandial hyperglycemia, microaneurisms, and even retinal exudates (30, 32).

Nonobese Type II diabetics may have low, normal, or high blood insulin levels (33). Obese Type II diabetics usually have normal or elevated blood insulin levels. Glucose is transported into muscle and fat cells and, therefore, these patients are not ketosis prone and seldom develop ketoacidosis except during periods of significant stress. However, because of their high blood glucose levels, they may develop nonketotic hyperglycemic coma. Obesity in patients may cause hyperinsulinemia, resulting in fewer insulin receptors and thus producing the clinical finding of hyperglycemia. Weight reduction to an ideal body weight often allows the blood glucose levels of many obese Type II diabetics to return to normal (31, 32). Dietary therapy is frequently the only treatment needed for nonobese Type II diabetics (33).

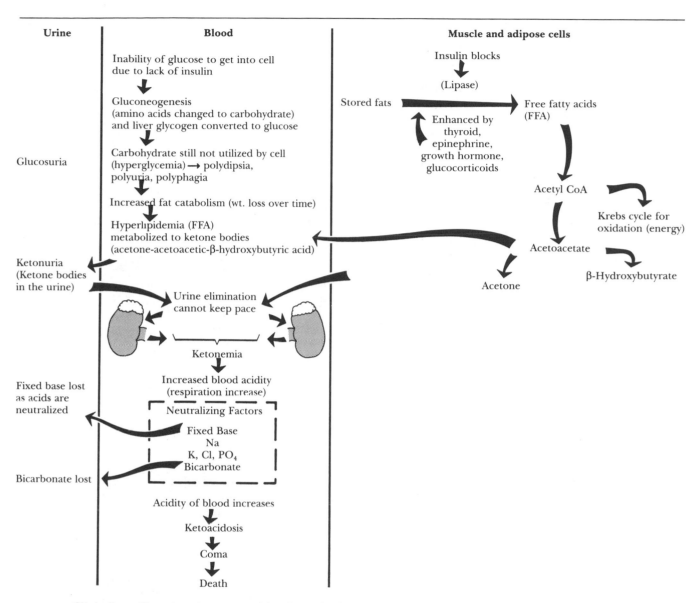

Urine	Blood	Muscle and adipose cells

FIGURE 1   Clinical manifestations in untreated insulinopenic diabetics.

CONSEQUENCES OF DIABETES

All major physiologic systems are affected by chronic hyperglycemia (34) (Tables 3 and 4). Diabetics frequently develop kidney failure (nephropathy), lesions of the eye (retinopathy), and lesions in the peripheral nerves (neuropathy). The molecular mechanisms leading to these late complications of diabetes have not been conclusively established, although capillary basement membrane thickening appears to be the basic pathologic change (35, 36). The direct cause of this thickening is unknown; however, because basement membranes are composed of collagen-like glycoproteins whose synthesis is controlled by both post-transcriptional and genetic factors, environmental influences could be important. Advanced glycosylation end products may be partly responsible because they can form covalent bonds with amino groups on other proteins, resulting in cross-linking, and can accumulate in the basement membrane (37). It has been shown that microvascular complications, including peripheral vascular disease, occur because hyperglycemia results in increased nonenzymatic protein glycosylation, accelerated atherosclerosis, and inadequate metabolic control, resulting in increased glucose metabolism by the polyol pathway (6, 32, 33, 38–40). The enzymes not normally

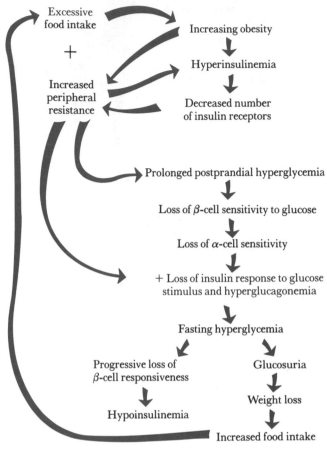

FIGURE 2   Pathogenesis of insulinoplethoric diabetes mellitus.

involved in glucose metabolism pathways, such as the polyol pathway, metabolize the excess glucose, thus increasing sorbitol levels. Aldose reductase and sorbitol dehydrogenase are two enzymes used in the noninsulin-dependent pathway of metabolizing glucose that produce abnormally high amounts of sorbitol and fructose.

Both sorbitol and fructose have been found in increased amounts in the lenses and nerves of hyperglycemic diabetic animals. The accumulation of these polyols could produce osmotic injury to the lens (with precipitation of proteins) and the nerve. It has been demonstrated that the elimination of hyperglycemia by insulin prevents or delays the development of diabetic neuropathy and cataracts in experimental diabetic animals. In addition, it has been clinically demonstrated that when acutely elevated blood glucose levels in diabetics were normalized, symptoms of neuropathy were more severe but then disappeared (35, 36, 41). Sorbinil (Pfizer) and Tolrestat (Ayerst) are aldose reductase inhibitors that hold much promise to help prevent or reduce the severity of several diabetic complications

that result from excess sorbitol. These agents are being evaluated in clinical trials.

Abnormalities of glycoprotein metabolism have been found in both Type I and Type II diabetics. These findings include increased levels of a minor hemoglobin component, hemoglobin A_{1c}, which is used clinically to monitor diabetes control (36). Hemoglobin A_{1c} levels reflect mean blood glucose concentration over a period of weeks and are useful in assessing chronic control of hyperglycemia (42).

There is substantial evidence that the microvascular complications of diabetes are decreased by minimizing hyperglycemia (33, 38, 43). Because of these findings, there is a renewed emphasis on strict, but reasonable, control of blood glucose to prevent severe diabetic complications (39, 44–47).

Atherosclerotic lesions in the diabetic appear to be the same as those in the nondiabetic, but they develop earlier, occur more often, and generally are more severe (48). Atherosclerosis contributes to the twofold increase in cardiovascular mortality and morbidity that occurs in diabetics, although it is questionable how much it contributes to the development of microvascular disease (41). Hyperglycemia results in damage to the intimal cells of the arteries and is probably the initial lesion in atherosclerosis. It has been suggested that lower than normal levels of plasma high-density lipoprotein cholesterol and elevated low-density lipoprotein cholesterol result in cholesterol deposition and plaque formation (49–56). Atherosclerotic lesions produce symptoms in various areas (41, 55). Diabetics suffer from occlusive vascular changes in the lower extremities as a result of both atherosclerosis and damage to smaller arteries (microangiopathy). Peripheral le-

TABLE 3   Harmful effects of hyperglycemia (blood glucose over 150 mg/dl)
Increased capillary basement membrane thickening
Glucose metabolized via polyol pathway, leading to increased levels of sorbitol
Increased platelet adhesiveness
Faulty lipid metabolism leading to higher levels of fat and possibly accelerating atherosclerosis
Abnormally high levels of minor (glycosylated) hemoglobins
Impairment of phagocytosis (ability to fight infection)
Increased neonatal morbidity and mortality
From *Am. Pharm.*, Module 4, NS26 (5), 7 (1986).

TABLE 4 Complications of diabetes mellitus and their treatment

Body Location	Description	Treatment
Eyes	Retinopathy, cataract formation, glaucoma, and periodic visual disturbances due to microvascular disease and other metabolic complications such as increased sorbitol. Leading cause of new blindness	Strict control of blood glucose to avoid need for treatment via laser photocoagulation, vitrectomy
Mouth	Gingivitis, increased incidence of dental cavities and periodontal disease	Strict control and daily hygiene. See dentist often
Reproductive system (Pregnancy)	Increased incidence of large babies, stillbirths, miscarriages, neonatal deaths, and congenital defects due to metabolic abnormalities	Strict control of blood glucose before and during pregnancy
Nervous system	Motor, sensory and autonomic neuropathy leading to impotence, neurogenic bladder, parathesias, gangrene, altered gastrointestinal motility and cardiovascular problems	Strict control, daily foot care, surgery, and antidepressants and phenothiazines
Vascular system	Large vessel disease resulting in atherosclerosis and microvascular disease leading to retinopathy, nephropathy and decreased peripheral perfusion	Strict blood glucose control, artery bypass surgery
Skin	Numerous infections and specific lesions such as skin spots, diabetic bullae, lipodystrophies, and necrobiosis lipoidica diabeticorum due to small vessel disease, increased lipids in blood, and pruritus	Strict control, daily hygiene
Kidneys	Diabetic glomerulosclerosis causing nephropathy	Strict control; eventually, diet low in proteins. Prednisone, dialysis, and renal transplantation
Reticuloendothelial system (infections)	Cystitis, tuberculosis, skin infections, difficulty in overcoming infections, and moniliasis in diabetic women	Strict control and aggressive anti-infective therapy

From *Am. Pharm.*, Module 4 NS26 (5), 8 (1986).

sions, alone or in combination with hemorrheologic factors, may cause intermittent claudication, gangrene, and impotence. Widespread disease of small vessels is common. Cardiomyopathy, cardiovascular disease, neuropathy, and silent myocardial infarct may also occur in diabetics (6, 47, 54). Most chronic adverse conditions in the diabetic can be traced to an inadequate blood supply to the affected area. Besides the vascular and nerve changes that can result from prolonged hyperglycemia, diabetics frequently experience difficulty in eradicating bacterial infections (47, 57). Hyperglycemia may impair the phagocytic activity of the body's white blood cells. Because glucose levels in saliva are increased in uncontrolled diabetes, these patients have a higher incidence of dental cavities and gum dis-

ease. Pharmacists should encourage good oral hygiene and regular dental examinations. (See Chapter 23, *Oral Health Products*.)

SCREENING FOR DIABETES

The pharmacist's role in promoting and supporting diabetes detection programs cannot be overstressed. Within a 3-week period, the pharmacist may see up to 70% of the community residents; this contact provides an excellent opportunity to screen patients for diabetes. If all pharmacists set aside 1 day each month to screen patients for diabetes, they would have a substantial impact on detecting the more than 5 million undiagnosed diabetics in the United States. Possible diabetics could then be referred to physicians for a complete physical examination, medical history, and laboratory analysis (58). Patients known to have diabetes could be interviewed for compliance and monitored for blood glucose control. During the screening program, as well as at other times, the pharmacist should be able to answer questions that patients may have about diabetes.

The screening requires blood test strips, alcohol swabs, lancets, literature, and an analyzing machine to test the strips' color changes. One screening program involves taking a blood sample from the subject's finger or earlobe. The blood is then analyzed, using a blood glucose analyzer. In some states, only licensed medical technicians, registered nurses, or physicians may legally draw blood from patients. In such cases, contact with a volunteer nurses' association may be of value in launching a screening program (58). A highly sensitive, simple, and fast urine dip stick screening test (Biotel/Diabetes by American Diagnostics) is available to provide early detection of glucosuria. Pharmacists interested in diabetes-screening programs or in diabetic patient education can contact the sources listed in Appendix 1, Information for Pharmacists, for assistance.

The pharmacist can use several criteria to select patients for a screening program. Patients with all types of cardiac problems, including high blood pressure, stroke, congestive heart failure, and angina, have a higher incidence of diabetes. Diabetes is also more common in patients who have suffered from hyperthyroidism, Addison's disease, Cushing's syndrome or who have been on long-term steroid therapy. At least 75% of all diabetics have relatives with diabetes. Approximately 80% of diabetics 40–65 years of age are overweight (57). Approximately 40% of the diabetic population is over 65 years of age (12).

Symptoms

The pharmacist should obtain a careful patient history before attempting an evaluation. In addition to the more common symptoms of diabetes (polydipsia, polyphagia, and polyuria), several other symptoms such as weight loss, recurrent monilial infections, gout, prolonged wound healing, and visual disturbances should be considered when interviewing potential diabetics and when monitoring diagnosed diabetics for blood glucose control. Pharmacists who detect these medical problems should refer patients to their family physician or a physician who specializes in treating diabetes.

Weight Loss

Weight loss associated with normal or increased calorie intake may be a sign of diabetes. In diabetics, the pharmacist must evaluate diet restriction verses loss of blood glucose control as the reason for weight loss. Other conditions that cause weight loss are hyperthyroidism, cancer, anorexia nervosa, and other chronic diseases and uncommon genetic disorders.

Recurrent Monilial Infections

Monilial infections are common in diabetics, especially fungal infections of the vulva and anus in women. Recurrent monilial vaginal infections may be the first indicator of increased blood glucose levels in females. Chronic skin infections, carbuncles, furuncles, and eczema are also common in diabetics. Any recurrent infections should be assessed by a physician to determine their cause. Diabetics require close monitoring whenever they have infections because they may experience loss of blood glucose control.

Gout

The percentage of patients with gout who have diabetes (5–10%) is higher than the norm. Patients with gout are at higher risk of developing diabetes and, therefore, should be screened for diabetes.

Prolonged Wound Healing

Minor cuts and scratches may take twice as long to heal in a diabetic. Wounds are also more likely to become infected if not cared for properly. All people at risk of having diabetes should be instructed in proper wound care; wounds that do not heal promptly or that become infected should be assessed by a physician.

Visual Disturbances

Visual disturbances may be the only early symptoms of diabetes; patients who wear glasses may notice that increasingly stronger lenses are required at relatively short intervals. As such, ophthalmologists detect a large number of diabetics (59). Cataracts and open-angle glaucoma in older diabetics are common. Research suggests that an increased level of sorbitol may result in the increased frequency of cataracts in diabetics (34, 39, 41). Sorbitol is the intermediate in the metabolism of glucose to fructose by the polyol pathway. When hyperglycemia is present, sorbitol cannot diffuse out of the cell and accumulates in certain tissues. Cataract formation occurs because of the high sugar alcohol concentration in the lens, which causes an influx of water and eventual disruption of lens fiber membranes and protein deposits.

Psychologic Changes

Some of the first symptoms of hypoglycemia affecting the nervous system are irritability, nervousness, and anxiety. Generalized fatigue and depression occur more often in diabetics. Frequent emotional flare-ups may signal an abnormality in the body's biochemistry possibly resulting from diabetes.

Laboratory Diagnosis

If a patient has glucose in the urine, higher than normal glucose in the blood, or presents with one or more of the signs and symptoms of diabetes, the physician should administer an appropriate screening test. Patients with borderline oral glucose tolerance tests should be rechecked periodically, especially when they become symptomatic. One or two fasting blood sugar (FBS) levels greater than 140 mg/dl would be considered diagnostic.

Diagnostic or screening tests for diabetes include the FBS, the 2-hour postprandial blood glucose test, and the hemoglobin A_{1c}.

Nondiabetic causes of glucose intolerance include liver disease, prolonged physical inactivity, acute stress, fever, trauma, surgery, heart attack, starvation, hypokalemia, some renal and endocrine diseases, and drug therapy (Table 5). A positive test for glucose in the urine is not necessarily diagnostic for diabetes, but indicates the need for more definitive testing. Glucosuria generally occurs when the blood glucose level is approximately 180 mg/dl although studies have shown it to occur from 54 to 180 mg/dl (mean of 130 mg/dl) (60). The renal threshold for glucose may rise to more than 300–400 mg/dl with aging and decreased renal function; therefore, older diabetics may not demonstrate glucosuria despite high blood glucose levels (30, 60). Glucosuria without hyperglycemia may occur in pregnancy or with impaired renal function.

TREATMENT

The objectives of diabetic treatment in order of importance are relief and prevention of diabetic symptoms (polyuria, polydipsia, polyphagia, weight loss, fatigue, recurrent infections, ketoacidosis, or hyperosmolar nonketotic episodes); prevention of hypoglycemic reactions; maintenance of optimal weight; maintenance of blood glucose levels close to euglycemia (50–150 mg/dl) to prevent or slow progression of chronic complications; promotion of normal growth and development in children; elimination or minimization of all other cardiovascular risk factors; and integration of the diabetic into health care through intensive education (5, 60, 61). These objectives can be met only through the combined efforts of the physician, nurse specialist, dietitian, physical therapist, podiatrist, pharmacist, and patient. Treatment of all types of diabetics involves the five DEEDS: diet, exercise, education, drugs, and self-monitoring. Sulfonylureas, insulin, diet, and exercise are used to control hyperglycemia, and nonprescription products formulated especially for use by the diabetic are helpful. Diet, exercise, and insulin are all part of the treatment plan and must be delicately balanced in Type I diabetics; caloric restrictions and increased physical activity when possible are usually the essential components of treatment in Type II diabetics. Intensive insulin therapy using multiple injections or an insulin infusion pump improves control with fewer complications. Self-monitoring of urine and blood glucose has made it possible for the diabetic to carefully adjust medication, diet, and exercise to maintain blood glucose levels near euglycemia. Strict control of blood glucose levels may delay or decrease the severity of late complications of diabetes (52, 57, 62–66).

Diabetes Medications

The medications used to treat diabetes fall into two broad categories: oral hypoglycemic agents and insulin. The use of oral hypoglycemic agents has been controversial from the standpoint of effectiveness and long-term side effects. However, when used properly, they are both safe and effective. The pharmacist can use diabetic patient monitoring checklists (Figures 3 and 4) to monitor all aspects of a diabetic's treatment.

Although insulin must be initially prescribed by a physician, pharmacists frequently are the health care professionals consulted about problems. Therefore, pharmacists should be familiar with the various strengths and sources of insulin and with different onsets and durations of action.

Oral Hypoglycemic Agents

The mechanism by which sulfonylureas correct defects in insulin action is not completely understood. It is known that sulfonylureas initially stimulate insulin secretion by the pancreas and possibly increase the number of insulin receptors on target tissues. It is also believed that the sulfonylureas decrease liver glycogen conversion to glucose and somehow correct or improve the postreceptor defect. The six products used in the

TABLE 5 Drugs that may cause hypoglycemia or hyperglycemia

Hypoglycemia	Hyperglycemia
Acetaminophen	Acetazolamide
Amitriptyline	Albuterol
Anabolic steroids	Amiodarone
Beta-blockers	Amoxapine
Biguanides	Antimicrobial (pentamidine, rifampin, sulfasalazine, nalidixic acid)
Chloroquine	Asparaginase
Chlorpromazin	Caffeine
Clofibrate	Calcium channel blockers
Disopyramide	Chlorpromazine
Ethanol	Clorthalidone
Fenfluramine	Corticosteroids
Fluphenazine	Cyclosporine
Haloperidol	Diazoxide
Imipramine	Encainide
Insulin	Epinephrine-like drugs (phenylephrine, phenylpropanolamine, and
Lithium	psuedoephedrine)
MAO inhibitors	Estrogens
Norfloxacin	Ethacrynic acid
Oxytetracycline	Droperidol
Pentamidine	Fentanyl/Furosemide
Perphenazine/Amitriptyline	Guanethidine
Phenobarbital	Indapamide
Prazosin	Indomethacin
Propoxyphene	Interferon alpha
Quinine	Lactulose
Salicylates in large doses	Levadopa
Sulfonamide antibiotics	Loxapine
Sulfonylurea agents	Morphine
Tetrahydrocannabinol	Niacin and nicotinic acid
	Nicotine
	Nifedipine
	Oral contraceptives
	Phenytoin
	Probenecid
	Sugars (dextrose, fructose, mannitol, sorbitol, sucrose)
	Sympathomimetic amines
	Terbutaline
	Theophylline
	Thiazide diuretics
	Thyroid preparations
	Tricyclic antidepressants

United States are summarized in Table 6. The differences in metabolism of each sulfonylurea account for clinical differences in the onset and duration of action.

Hypoglycemia is the most common side effect of the sulfonylureas. Frequent "drug–drug" interactions resulting in enhanced hypoglycemia or interference with diabetes control by causing hyperglycemia are well documented (18, 60, 67–70). Table 5 lists drugs that are known to increase or decrease blood glucose levels by themselves or by interacting with sulfonylureas to enhance or decrease the effect of oral hypoglycemic agents.

Chlorpropamide is the longest acting sulfonylurea in use in the United States. It has the highest incidence of side effects (5–8%); tolbutamide may have the lowest incidence (34). Chlorpropamide is not recommended as the drug of choice in elderly patients and patients with renal failure because these patients may suffer severe hypoglycemia resulting from decreased elimination and accumulation. In Type II diabetes, diet is the main

Patient	
Name	Home Phone ( )
Present address (street, city, zip)	

History

Is there diabetes in your family? ☐ Yes ☐ No Relationship   What type?

When was the last time the nondiabetic members of your family were tested?

How long have you had diabetes?

How do you feel about having diabetes?

Do members of your family understand the conditions and factors that affect control? ☐ Yes ☐ No

Is there anything that is emotionally upsetting you? ☐ Yes ☐ No

Do you belong to the local diabetes association? ☐ Yes ☐ No

Other diabetes associations? ☐ Yes ☐ No

Physician/Laboratory Test Results

When was your last glucose tolerance test?	What were the results of those tests?

Medication

Are you taking anything for diabetes? ☐ Yes ☐ No If "Yes," what?	Are you taking drugs prescribed by physician(s) other than the one treating you for diabetes? ☐ Yes ☐ No If "Yes," what are they? Who prescribed them?
Do you take insulin? ☐ Yes ☐ No If "Yes," what kind?	Are you taking any drugs for pain? ☐ Yes ☐ No If "Yes," what?
Where do you inject your insulin? Do you rotate injection sites?	Are you allergic to sulfa drugs? ☐ Yes ☐ No Are you allergic to any other drugs? ☐ Yes ☐ No If "Yes," which one(s)?
How much do you inject? How often?	Do you routinely take "OTC" drug products? ☐ Yes ☐ No If "Yes," which one(s)?
What other drugs have been prescribed for you? List:	

Personal Observation   Complications

What do you think has affected the control of your diabetes?

Have you had any infections? ☐ Yes ☐ No

Any other problems?

Diet   Exercise

What kind of diet has your doctor prescribed?

Do you have a regular schedule for exercise?
☐ Yes ☐ No

Do you use "fad" diets? ☐ Yes ☐ No
If "Yes," which one(s)?

Are you exercising more or less?
☐ More ☐ Less

Do you use alcohol? ☐ Yes ☐ No How much?

Are you eating differently? ☐ Yes ☐ No

Testing

Do you test your urine? ☐ Yes ☐ No If "Yes," how?   Which product?   How often?

What do you test for? ☐ Sugar ☐ Ketones ☐ Protein

Do you test your own blood for glucose? ☐ Yes ☐ No If "Yes," how?

Which product?   How often?

FIGURE 3   Suggested diabetic condition analysis form. From *Am. Pharm.*, *Module 4, NS26 (5)*, 10, 11 (1986).

Adverse Episodes   **Dates**   **Severity—Outcome**

Hypoglycemia   ☐   _____

Hyperglycemia (Glucosuria) ☐   _____

Ketoacidosis   ☐   _____

Drug Interaction Guide

Can Potentiate Sulfonylureas
phenylbutazone
nonsteroidal anti-inflammatory agents
salicylates
sulfonamides
chloramphenicol
probenecid
coumarins
monoamine oxidase inhibitors
beta-adrenergic blocking agents
propranolol
alcohol (acute)

Can Inhibit Sulfonylureas

diuretics	calcium channel blockers
corticosteroids	sympathomimetics
phenothiazines	thyroid products
thyroid products	isoniazid
estrogens	alcohol (chronic)
oral contraceptives	
phenytoin	
nicotinic aid	

Prescription Drugs Taken

Medication	
Date	
Rx #	
Prescriber	
Directions	
Route	
Quantity	
Refills	
Price	
Comments	

Over-the-Counter Drugs (taken on a regular basis)   ☐ None

Category	Name of Product	How Often Used
1.		
2.		
3.		
4.		

Patient Education

Date	
Subject	

FIGURE 3 *continued*

TABLE 6 Basic biopharmaceutics and pharmacokinetics of the oral hypoglycemics

Drug	Equivalent therapeutic dose (mg)	Usual minimum and maximum daily dose	Mean half-life	Duration of activity	Metabolism and excretion
FIRST-GENERATION SULFONYLUREAS					
Acetohexamide (Dymelor)	500	0.25–1.5 g single or divided doses	1.5 hr, parent; 6 hr, metabolites	12–18+ hr	Metabolite's activity greater than parent drug. Metabolite excreted, in part, via kidney.
Chlorpropamide (Diabinese)	250	0.1–0.5 g single dose	35 hr	24–72 hr	Extensive metabolism to compounds with unknown activity. 20% excreted unchanged (may vary widely).
Tolazamide (Tolinase)	250	0.1–1.0 g single or divided doses	7 hr	10–16+ hr	Some metabolites have weak activity; excreted via kidney.
Tolbutamide (Orinase)	1,000	0.5–3.0 g divided doses	7 hr	6–12 hr	Totally metabolized to compounds with negligible activity.
SECOND-GENERATION SULFONYLUREAS					
Glyburide (DiaBeta) (Micronase)	5	1.25–20 mg single (or divided dose)	10 hr	24 hr	Metabolized to compounds one of which may be weakly active.
Glipizide (Glucotrol)	5	2.5–40 mg single or divided doses	4 hr	16–24 hr	Metabolized to inactive compounds.

method of treatment, accompanied by regular exercise whenever possible; sulfonylureas should be used only when diet and exercise fail.

Patients who are not candidates for oral agents and conditions that usually contradict oral antidiabetic agents include the following (68):

- Diabetics under 30 years of age;
- Gestational diabetics;
- Diabetics who are pregnant or lactating;
- Ketosis-prone patients;
- Diabetics prone to or with symptoms of acidosis;
- Type I patients;
- Patients needing rapid control of their blood glucose levels;
- Type II patients in whom diet control has not been tried;
- Diabetics with severe infections;
- Diabetics undergoing major surgery (during and immediately after);
- Diabetics who are allergic to sulfa or sulfonylurea compounds.

Use of oral antidiabetic agents is controversial for underweight Type II patients and patients with heart disease (68).

No treatment plan will succeed if the patient has not been thoroughly educated about the importance of all aspects of therapy including self-monitoring (68). Pharmacists dispensing sulfonylureas should explain to the patient the brand and generic name of the drug, that the medication is used to treat diabetes, and that it is important to take the medication regularly and exactly as prescribed by the physician. If the patient develops adverse drug reactions to the sulfonylureas, such as hypoglycemia (blood glucose less than 50–70 mg/dl), sore throat, fever, mouth sores, water retention, or dark-colored urine, the physician should be contacted. The pharmacist should advise the patient to avoid the use of alcoholic beverages and drugs containing salicylates or use them cautiously (71–73). It is important to stress the necessity of using the oral hypoglycemic agent in conjunction with the prescribed diet and exercise. The secondary failure rate ranges from 3 to 30%. This failure rate tends to increase each year for patients experiencing initial satisfactory control. Thus, only 20–30% of diabetics started on oral agents maintain satisfactory control (74). Failures occurring after initial response may evolve as the patient develops a type of tolerance to the drug. Patients who have decreased con-

Patient's Name _____

☐ Insulin-dependent
☐ Non-insulin-dependent

Year of
onset _____

Address _____ Tel. # _____ Date of Birth _____

_____

Insurance _____

Physician _____ Tel. # _____

Physician _____ Tel. # _____

Responsible Person/ _____ Tel. # _____
Emergency

Relationship
to patient _____

HISTORY

Known Allergies/Sensitivities

	Causative Agent	Occurrence Date	Treatment	Outcome
1.				
2.				

	Concurrent Diseases	Date Diagnosed	Treatment
1.			
2.			
3.			

ANTIDIABETES THERAPY

Diet: Calories _____ Sweetener _____

Oral: Sulfonylureas

Agent _____

Date						
Strength						
Frequency						

Insulin

Type _____

Date						
Units						
Frequency						

Type _____

Date						
Units						
Frequency						

Syringe size _____ Needle size _____

Monitoring   Urine ☐   Ketones ☐   Blood glucose ☐

Test or Kit   _____   _____   _____

FIGURE 4   Diabetic patient record form. From *Am. Pharm., Module 4, NS26 (5)*, 9 (1986).

trol with a first-generation agent may benefit from a change to a second-generation agent (73). The second-generation sulfonylureas are more potent, have fewer side effects and fewer drug interactions, and can usually be given once a day.

The University Group Diabetes Program cooperative study concluded that tolbutamide was no more effective than diet alone in the treatment of diabetes. Patients treated with tolbutamide had a significantly higher rate of cardiac deaths than control subjects. The validity of the study has been extensively questioned. Despite the reported findings, many physicians continue to advocate the use of tolbutamide. The oral sulfonylureas also are possible teratogens; they should not be used in the early stages of pregnancy and are absolutely contraindicated in the late stages of pregnancy because they may cause prolonged and severe hypoglycemia in the newborn (72).

Insulin

Type I diabetics must be treated with exogenous insulin. Generally, persons who initially require insulin tend to be younger than 30 years of age at the time of diagnosis, lean, prone to developing ketoacidosis, and markedly hyperglycemic even in the fasting state (31). Insulin is also indicated for Type II diabetics who do not respond to diet and exercise therapy alone or combined with oral hypoglycemic drugs (22, 60, 75). Insulin therapy is necessary in some Type II diabetics who are subject to stresses such as infections, pregnancy, or surgery.

In Type II diabetics, doses of 10–20 units of intermediate-acting insulins are occasionally needed to bring hyperglycemia under control. Type II diabetics must receive additional education concerning diet when started on insulin. Increased hunger and resultant weight gain are major problems for these patients. Insulin is also used in gestational diabetes when diet and exercise alone do not adequately control blood glucose levels. Patients who are receiving parenteral nutrition, who require high calorie supplements to meet increased energy needs, or who have drug-induced diabetes may require exogenous insulin on a short-term or intermittent basis to maintain normal glucose levels. In some very difficult to control Type II diabetics, insulin in combination with glyburide or glipizide has reduced blood glucose levels; however, combination therapies in a large population of patients have not been adequately studied. By combining the appropriate modification of diet, exercise, and variable mixtures of short-acting and longer acting insulins with self-monitoring, acceptable control of blood glucose has been achieved (22, 60). To normalize blood glucose, intensified insulin regimens using multiple injections or insulin pumps are usually required.

All classes of diabetics should be trained to inject themselves with insulin. Diabetic children should begin administering their own injections at 6–9 years of age; parents should administer one or two injections a week to stay in practice and should inject in areas difficult for the child to reach (76, 77).

Use in Ketoacidosis Diabetic ketoacidosis (DKA) constitutes an acute medical emergency, necessitating immediate diagnosis and therapy. It accounts for less than 1% of the deaths occurring in the diabetic population; however, the mortality associated with these acute episodes is 5–15%, indicating the need for strict attention to detail and management (77). The physician can rapidly diagnose DKA by assessing urinary glucose and ketones, arterial blood pH and blood gases, and serum ketone and glucose values. Pharmacists should refer patients with high blood glucose levels and urine glucose and ketones to their physicians for immediate evaluation and treatment.

Shock and cerebral edema are among the complications encountered in DKA. Shock generally develops as a consequence of life-threatening stress such as sepsis, myocardial infarct, or acute pancreatitis (78). Treatment is directed at plasma volume expansion and electrolyte replacement, correction of hypotension, reversal of acidosis and severe ketosis, and control of plasma glucose levels (75). Low-dose intravenous (IV) insulin regimens are recommended to treat DKA and nonketotic hyperosmolar coma (6, 60, 78).

Insulin Preparations Currently, 38 insulin products are available in the United States. The insulins are categorized into five types of products, which are divided into three groups according to promptness, duration, and intensity of action following subcutaneous (SC) injection. Rapid- or short-acting insulins include Semilente and regular insulin. Intermediate-acting insulins include Neutral Protamine Hagedorn (NPH), Lente, and new Humulin Ultralente insulin suspensions. The long-acting insulins include protamine zinc and animal-derived Ultralente insulin suspensions. Lente insulin is a combination of 70% Ultralente and 30% Semilente insulin as a suspension. The NPH insulin is a combination of two parts regular insulin and one part protamine zinc insulin as a suspension. Fixed-dose mixtures of insulin, at a ratio of 70% NPH and 30% regular (Mixtard, Novolin, and Humulin 70/30) are also available.

In March 1980, the Food and Drug Administration (FDA) decertified U-80 insulin, leaving two strengths of insulin available for diabetic patients: U-40 and U-100. Some patients who use small insulin doses still prefer U-40 insulin (less than 2%), but manufacturers, the FDA, and the American Diabetes Association with the support of the American Pharmaceutical Association are attempting to convert all patients to U-100 insulins

(79). Standardizing the strengths should help eliminate errors resulting from the use of incorrectly calibrated syringes and reduce confusion in mixing insulins. In non-English-speaking countries, the available insulin is usually the U-40 strength; patients traveling abroad should be encouraged to carry extra insulin and corresponding insulin syringes to prevent problems or errors (79). U-500 insulin is available from Eli Lilly as a legend product for patients who use more than 100–200 units per injection.

Methods to increase the duration of action of regular insulin include the addition of zinc and protein molecules. NPH and protamine zinc are examples of insulins to which protamine and zinc have been added. Protamine is a fish protein that slows insulin absorption from the site of injection. The amount of excess protamine and zinc content differs among insulin products. The Lente insulins result in longer or shorter acting types of insulin when the amount of zinc added to the insulin is varied. The types of preservatives used in the different insulins also varies (79).

All insulins are at a neutral pH of 7.4. Regular insulin is a clear solution. If it looks cloudy or has become tinted, it may be contaminated and should not be dispensed or used. All other available insulins are cloudy suspensions that will settle out after standing. If the suspension clumps or discolors, it may be contaminated and should not be dispensed or used. If a crystal-like glaze or frost forms on the sides of the vial or a white flocculation develops in any of the insulins, the insulin should not be dispensed or used.

The debate continues concerning which insulin patients should inject, where patients should inject insulin for most reliable absorption, how to store insulin, what causes insulin to frost, what are the consequences of mixing various insulins at various ratios, and how often patients should self-monitor (79). Changing attitudes concerning the administration of insulin (i.e., once-a-day versus multiple daily injections, or multiple intermittent injections versus continuous infusions by pump) and which insulin to use have created confusion. Table 7 summarizes the factors that can be used to compare insulins.

Clinical Considerations in Insulin Use The source from which the insulin is derived and its antigenicity can influence its effect on blood glucose control and insulin resistance and sensitivity (79–83). Commercially available animal-derived insulins are beef, pork, or a mixture of beef and pork. Beef insulin has greater antigenicity because its structure differs from human insulin by three amino acids; pork differs by only one amino acid (81–83). Lilly has developed a biosynthetic human insulin through recombinant deoxyribonucleic acid (DNA) technology, and Nordisk and Squibb-Novo have developed a semisynthetic human insulin by con-

---

TABLE 7 Factors considered in comparing insulins

Onset and duration of action: short vs. intermediate vs. long acting (this can be complicated also by insulin antibodies)

Species source: human is < (less immunogenic, i.e., les likely to confer immunity) pork < mixed beef and pork < beef

Strength of regular insulin: U-40 vs. U-100 vs. U-500

Method of achieving long action, preservatives, buffers (the two prolongation additives used in insulin manufacture are protamine and zinc)

Purity: as defined in parts per million of proinsulin

Mixing compatibility

Cost

Indications

From *Practical Diabetol.*, 15–17 (Jan.-Feb. 1988).

---

verting pork insulin into a human insulin using an enzyme-controlled reaction, transpeptidation, at position 30 of the B chain with substitution of threonine for alanine (80–83). All three of the human insulin preparations are less antigenic than other sources of insulin. Almost all of the patients with persistent local allergy to beef or mixed beef–pork insulin improve if treated with pure pork insulin or human insulin.

Newer methods of purification now ensure that all commercially available insulins are highly purified. The average content of certain minor components of insulin, such as proinsulin, desamino insulin, arginine insulin, esterified insulin, and glucagon has been decreased, resulting in fewer insulin sensitivity reactions. Highly purified pork and semisynthetic human insulins are clinically important in reducing insulin allergy, lipoatrophy (SC concavities caused by a wasting of the lipid tissue), and insulin-binding capacity of serum, but only occasionally in adjusting the dose. All insulin preparations available in the United States are now relatively highly purified (see Insulin Preparations Product Table) and contain between 0 and 10 parts per million (ppm) of proinsulin (84). The purity of insulin is based on the ppm of proinsulin in 1 cc. Humulin has 0 ppm of proinsulin. Squibb-Novo's human insulin (Novolin) and Nordisk's human insulin (Velosulin, Insulatard) have less than 1 ppm of proinsulin. The purified pork insulins have 1 ppm; beef and beef–pork insulins have 10 ppm of proinsulin (84). One study showed that the purified type of insulin produced less antigenicity and allowed a 15% decrease in the dose required by the average patient (85).

Diabetics who demonstrate a sensitivity to insulin usually develop redness at the injection site. When diabetics were initially treated with pork or beef insulin, insulin-sensitivity reactions were common and occurred over several weeks, then gradually subsided. These reactions were treated with diphenhydramine or hydroxyzine (75). New diabetics are now started on human insulin; therefore, insulin-sensitivity reactions are very rare.

Insulin resistance, a state requiring more than 200 units per day of insulin for more than 2 days in the absence of ketoacidosis or acute infection, occurs in about 0.001% of diabetics. These patients almost invariably have high titers of insulin-neutralizing immunoglobulin G (IgG) antibodies. Glucocorticoids are indicated (60–80 mg of prednisone per day) (86), human insulin is also recommended.

Another factor that can affect the clinical use of insulin preparations is how they are administered parenterally (87). Regular insulin injected intramuscularly (IM) provides faster insulin absorption with a greater drop in plasma glucose than when injected subcutaneously. Intravenous regular insulin produces the highest pharmacologic level of insulin in the least time and is the route of choice in patients suffering from DKA. Insulin suspension preparations should never be administered IM or IV.

Insulin absorption is affected by exercise. Leg exercise accelerates insulin absorption from the leg. Arm or abdominal injections prevent accelerated absorption during leg exercise and reduce exercise-induced hypoglycemia (84, 88). Therefore, a diabetic whose day includes a hard game of tennis should inject that day's insulin into the abdomen rather than into the arm or leg (61, 84, 89, 90). If more than 60 units of insulin are injected at one site, there is potential for erratic absorption. Thus, patients receiving large doses of insulin should split the doses and inject in two different sites and should be monitored closely (91).

The insulin regimen should be part of the overall treatment plan agreed to by the physician and patient. Different insulin regimens are part of the several different levels of intensity of therapy as suggested by the American Diabetes Association's guide to physicians (92). Pharmacists should be familiar with the different types of insulin regimens commonly prescribed by diabetologists and general practitioners.

Diabetics who choose intensified insulin therapy to help maintain blood glucose levels that approximate euglycemia have two options: multiple insulin injections or the use of an insulin infusion pump. Several products are being promoted to ambulatory diabetics to try to normalize blood glucose using intensified insulin therapy. These products achieve normalization of blood glucose while allowing the patient to continue daily activities without interrupting lifestyle. In fact, some of these intensive programs actually increase lifestyle flex-

ibility. For example, pump patients can more easily adjust insulin dosages to accommodate any changes in daily activities. Infusion pumps are discussed in more detail later in this chapter.

Diabetics willing to use multiple injections can use various combinations of insulins depending on the individual's response pattern (Figure 5). For example, regular insulin can be injected before meals and an intermediate-acting insulin can be injected at bedtime to cover blood glucose levels while sleeping. Another alternative is to inject a long-acting (Ultralente) and regular insulin before breakfast, regular insulin before lunch, and regular and Ultralente again before dinner. The pain and inconvenience of multiple injections may be reduced by using the Button infuser or the Teflon catheter

Relationship between insulin and glucose.

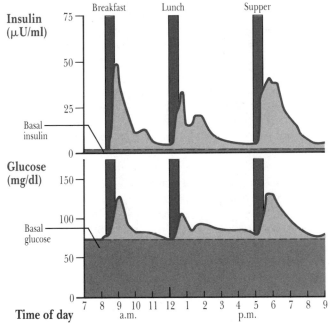

Intensive insulin therapy regimens

	7 a.m.	11 a.m.	4-5 p.m.	H.S.
1. 2 doses, Intermediate	X		X	
2. 2 doses, Regular and Intermediate	Reg. & Intermed.		Reg. & Intermed.	
3. 3 doses, Regular or Regular and Intermediate	Reg. & Intermed.	Reg.	Reg. & Intermed.	
4. 4 doses, Regular and Long Acting	Reg.	Reg.	Reg.	Long Acting

Note: Many other regimens are used as "intensive" therapy plans. The therapy is individualized to the responses of the diabetic patient.

FIGURE 5 Relationship between insulin and glucose. Adapted with permission from *U.S. Pharmacist, 13 (11)* (suppl.), 41 (1988).

(Insuflow), which is a flexible catheter that is inserted SC and through which doses of insulin are injected. Blood glucose monitoring at least 4 times a day is essential for these patients.

Another potential complication of insulin therapy is insulin lipodystrophy. Lipodystrophy occurs in two forms: lipoatrophy (the breakdown of SC fatty tissue, leaving hollow areas under the skin) and lipohypertrophy (the hyperdevelopment of fatty tissue, causing bulges under the skin) (93). Lipodystrophic changes usually are unattractive and may be difficult for the patient to accept. Lipoatrophy improves in most patients when human insulin is substituted because it may be caused by an immune response to more antigenic insulin preparations (94, 95). Lipohypertrophy is generally seen in patients who use the same sites for repeated insulin injections. It may decrease insulin absorption from the affected site. Lipohypertrophy does not respond when human insulin is used; in fact, it may be worsened because of human insulin's lipogenic action. This condition provides one of the main reasons for educating patients to rotate their injection sites.

Mixing and Storage   As the purity of insulins has improved, the problem of stability in mixing insulins has decreased. Regular insulin may be mixed with NPH or Lente insulin in any proportion desired. However, Lente–regular combinations are stable for only 5 minutes (60, 91). There is in vitro binding of the regular insulin if the mixtures are allowed to stand. This can significantly change blood glucose control because the action of the regular insulin may be blunted or slowed (84). If the Lente–regular mixtures cannot be used immediately, they should be discarded and a new dose prepared (60, 73).

NPH–regular mixtures of insulin are now available from the manufacturer in premixed formulations that are 70% NPH insulin and 30% regular insulin. A combination insulin that is 50% NPH insulin and 50% regular insulin will soon be available. NPH–regular combinations are stable and are absorbed as if injected separately. The NPH–regular mixture is stable for approximately 1 month at room temperature and 3 months when refrigerated.

Insulin manufacturers will not guarantee the sterility of prefilled syringes prepared by the pharmacist or in the home; patients should be given the smallest number of prefilled syringes possible at any one time. Binding can be prevented by administering the dose immediately after preparation (56, 60). Velosulin by Nordisk and Humulin-BR by Lilly should not be mixed with any Lente preparation (84).

Regular insulin may be added to protamine zinc insulin. However, because of the excess protamine in protamine zinc insulin, mixtures in a ratio of less than 1:1 have the same activity as protamine zinc insulin

alone. As the proportion of regular to protamine zinc insulin approaches 2:1, a time–activity curve approximating that of NPH insulin is obtained. When the ratio exceeds 2:1 (i.e., when the amount of regular insulin is increased further), the time–activity of the mixture approaches that of a regular–NPH combination. Mixtures of regular and protamine zinc insulin have unpredictable stability and should be used immediately or given as separate injections (60, 84).

Semilente, Lente, and Ultralente insulins may be combined in any ratio at any time. Mixtures are stable in any proportion for 18 months if refrigerated, although sterility cannot be guaranteed (73, 84).

Regular insulin may be mixed in any proportion with normal saline if necessary for dilution or for use in older infusion pumps; however, the combination should be used within 2 or 3 hours after mixing because pH changes and dilution of buffer may affect stability (60). Regular insulin may be mixed with Lilly's Insulin Dilution Fluid in any proportion and will be stable indefinitely. Diabetics using older insulin infusion pumps may dilute the insulin with either normal saline or Lilly's Insulin Dilution Fluid, which provides a more stable mixture. New insulin pumps do not require diluted insulin preparations. Regular insulin may form crystal deposits in the catheter tubing of insulin pumps. Humulin-BR and Velosulin contain phosphate buffers to limit or prevent this reaction. A white frosting or flocculation in the bottle has been reported to occur with regular human insulin when less than 3 ml remain. This effect has been associated with a loss of potency. Patients should be instructed to inspect every vial of insulin before each use. The vial of insulin should not be used if it appears to have crystals, frostings, flocculation, or discloration. A new vial of insulin should be selected and the old vial discarded or returned. Insulin manufacturers will replace any bottles of insulin that appear to have degraded (84).

Because insulin is a heat-labile protein, care must be exercised in storing all preparations so that potency and maximum stability are maintained. Regular insulin's potency may decline as much as 1.5% a month if stored at room temperature (59–85° F or 15–30° C), although other studies have indicated that all commercially available insulins are stable for several months at room temperature (60, 73, 84). Color changes may be associated with denaturation of protein and should be interpreted as evidence of potency loss. With regular insulin, the rate of potency loss increases as the temperature increases. At 100° F or 38° C, all insulins lose a significant amount of potency within 1 or 2 months (60). Lente insulins retain their potency when stored at room temperature for 24 months, but signs of potency loss such as discoloration and clumping may occur after 30 months. With NPH and protamine zinc insulins, loss of potency does not occur at room temperature for up to 36 months. Thus, many of the insulins are stable unrefrigerated for long periods; however, the pharmacist should advise patients to keep extra bottles of insulin in the refrigerator (36–46° F or 2–8° C). Insulin should not be stored in the freezer; freezing insulin may cause aggregation, precipitation, and clumping but does not necessarily affect potency (96). Vials of insulin currently in use may be kept out of the refrigerator because they contain bacteriostatic agents but should be used in 1 or 2 months (73). Insulin should be stored in a cool area, away from radiators or sunny windows. Patients traveling in warm climates should keep insulin in a insulated container with ice, "blue ice," or some other cooling agent; in a Medicool Insulin Protector; or between several layers of clothing in a suitcase (97–99). Insulin should never be stored in glove compartments or trunks of motor vehicles or in uninsulated backpacks or cycle bags.

Higher temperatures may also cause the insulin suspensions to aggregate, precipitate, or clump. Potency may not necessarily be lost, but there is a problem in drawing up the correct dose when clumping has occurred. Injection of insulin at room temperature is recommended because refrigerator-temperature insulin produces more pain.

Mixing Insulins in the Syringe   It is important for the diabetic to understand how to mix insulin properly in the syringe. The technique generally recommended is as follows:

- Inspect vials for signs of possible contamination or degradation.

- Wash hands with soap and water.

- Make sure that the proper equipment is used (correct insulin in the correct strength from the source normally used).

- Agitate all insulins, except regular insulin, before withdrawing from the vial. The vials should be gently rolled between the palms of the hands or inverted several times until the suspension is evenly distributed (60). To avoid generating air bubbles in the insulin, the vials should not be shaken. New, unused vials may require vigorous agitation to loosen the sediment on the bottom. Vials should not be used until any foam that may have formed during agitation of the insulin has subsided.

- Wipe off the top of the vials with a cotton ball moistened in alcohol or with an alcohol swab; make sure that no cotton or cloth fibers remain on the rubber stopper of the vials.

- Remove a clean syringe from storage. Touch only the hub of the plunger and the barrel of the syringe. Avoid touching the hub of the needle.

- If necessary, remove any excess water or alcohol from the syringe by pushing the plunger back and forth a few times. If any liquid is left in the syringe, it will cause an error in measuring the insulin. This step can be skipped when using disposable, single-use syringes.

- Pull the plunger back to the prescribed number of units of intermediate- or long-acting insulin on the barrel.

- Observing aseptic technique, put the needle (with the beveled edge up) through the rubber cap on the first vial of intermediate- or long-acting insulin and push the plunger down to inject into the vial a volume of air equal to the dose. Withdraw the needle without withdrawing the dose.

- With the vial of regular or short-acting insulin, inject air equal to the dose; turn the vial upside down and pull the plunger back slowly to the prescribed number of units (the barrel of the syringe should be held at eye level to ensure accurate reading of the syringe). This will withdraw the proper dose of regular or short-acting insulin. If air bubbles appear in the syringe, hold the vial up straight and push the plunger down to force the air back into the vial. It may be necessary to tap the barrel of the syringe briskly with the fingers to help remove some of the air bubbles.

- When the correct number of units of regular insulin (without air bubbles) has been measured, withdraw the needle.

- Turn the vial of intermediate- or long-acting insulin upside down, insert the needle, and slowly pull the plunger back the prescribed number of units; this will withdraw the dose of this insulin into the syringe containing the regular insulin. Remove the needle from the vial.

- Holding the syringe with the needle pointing up, draw an air bubble into the syringe, invert the syringe, and roll the bubble through the syringe to mix the insulins.

- Tap the barrel of the syringe briskly 2 or 3 times to remove any tiny air bubbles.

- Expel the air bubble and recap the needle or lay the syringe on a flat surface such as a table or shelf with the needle over the edge to avoid contamination.

- Check the intended injection site and administer the insulin to the patient in the usual manner.

- Some insulins may also be premixed in a vial in the proper short-, intermediate-, and long-acting insulin proportions.

Injection Technique Pharmacists should make sure that diabetics know the correct manner of injecting insulin. The following procedure is recommended:

- After properly preparing the insulin dose, check the record to determine where insulin was injected previously. Injection sites should be rotated (Figure 6A and B).

- Clean the injection site with an alcohol swab or a cotton ball moistened with alcohol.

- Pinch a fold of skin with one hand. With the other hand, hold the syringe as a pencil, place the needle on the skin with the beveled edge up, and push the needle quickly through the fold of skin at a 45–90°

angle, depending on the degree of obesity. Before injecting the insulin, draw back slightly on the plunger (aspirate) to be sure a blood vessel has not been hit. If blood appears in the syringe barrel, withdraw the needle and repeat the injection in another site (Figure 7).

- Inject the insulin by pressing the plunger in as far as it will go.

- Withdraw the needle quickly and press on the injection site with the alcohol swab or the cotton ball moistened with alcohol.

- Record the injection site.

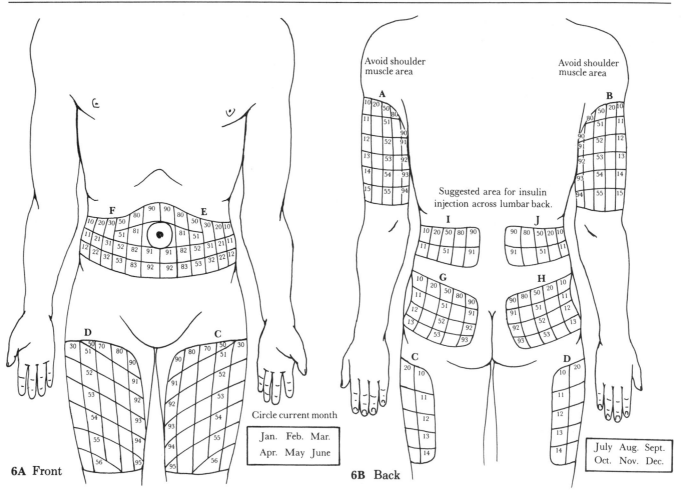

6A Front   **6B** Back

FIGURE 6   A and B. Record of insulin injection sites. This body map is designed to systematically record insulin injection sites. The diagram is for both hospital and home use: The numbers printed in the squares are mainly for hospital recording of insulin injection sites on each patient's chart. The numbers may be used at home, but a simpler method of recording would be to write the date of each injection in the corresponding square on the map at the time of injection. With continued use, this diagram will facilitate the rotation of insulin injection sites over the entire body and thereby avoid injection too often in a single location.

"The Body Map," adapted with permission from the Baptist Hospitals Foundation, Birmingham, Ala.

■ When finished using the syringe, discard the syringe and needle, and break disposable needles to prevent reuse.

Patients should be taught that insulin is to be injected deep into SC tissue. Properly injected insulin leaves only the needle puncture dot to show the injection site. The technique for injection may need to be altered with each individual, depending on the amount of SC fat present. For many patients, a 60° angle or more with the skin stretched accomplishes the necessary deep SC injection (Figure 7). For a thin person, a 45° angle with the skin pinched up may be best to avoid penetrating the muscle. The purpose of pinching is to lift the fat off the muscle and avoid IM or IV injection, which may result in rapid onset of action and severe hypoglycemia.

Pharmacists should stress to diabetic patients the importance of rotating injection sites in preventing local irritation, tissue reactions, and lipodystrophy. Injection sites include the arms, thighs, hips, and abdomen (Figure 6A and B). The absorption of insulin depends on many factors. The site of injection can result in variance of absorption and degree: from greatest to lowest, abdomen > deltoid > thigh > hip. Massaging or exercising the area of injection will increase the rate of absorption from that site. Diabetics who exercise regularly should be advised to avoid injecting into the thigh on days when they will be running or working their legs excessively and to avoid the arm on days when they will be playing tennis, lifting weights, digging, or shoveling (60, 61). Diabetics who experience erratic control should confine injection site rotation to a specific area of the body, such as the abdomen. Injection into a site where the SC tissue has atrophied or thickened will produce erratic absorption. Fibrosis and atrophy can be prevented by injection in the same site at no less than 14-day intervals. Deep IM injections will produce a much more rapid onset of action because of the increased rate of absorption. Fever, exercise, extremely hot weather, or a sauna or jacuzzi can increase blood flow, which speeds insulin absorption (60). Conversely, cold packs, cold extremities, or a hypothermia blanket may slow onset of action because of decreased absorption from the injection site.

If insulin leaks through the puncture in the skin, a longer needle should be used and the needle should be inserted at a right angle to the skin.

Adverse Reactions to Insulin Therapy The most common complication of insulin therapy is hypoglycemia. Factors predisposing the patient to insulin reactions include insufficient food intake (skipping meals, vomiting, or diarrhea), excessive exercise, inaccurate measurement of insulin, concomitant intake of hypoglycemic drugs, very tight euglycemic control, or termina-

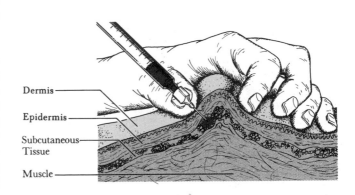

FIGURE 7   Correct method of insulin injection. Avoid areas already fibrotic or atrophic. Prevent fibrosis or atrophy by injecting in one site at no less than 10-day intervals. Properly injected insulin leaves only the needle puncture dot to show the injection site. Several techniques are good; the one illustrated serves well because the needle penetrates the skin at its thinnest area (dimple) and must enter the subcutaneous space. The needle angle should be 45° or more.

tion of diabetogenic conditions. In diabetics, the counterregulatory hormones—glucagon, epinephrine, cortisone, and growth hormone—that protect people from hypoglycemia may not respond appropriately to the hypoglycemic stimuli (100). Symptoms include ataxia and blurred vision, parasympathetic response (nausea, hunger, or flatulence), diminished cerebral function (confusion, agitation, lethargy, or personality changes), sympathetic responses (tachycardia, sweating, or tremor), coma, and convulsions, although every patient may present with slight variations (101).

Patients using intensive insulin therapy who have altered counterregulatory hormone response to hypoglycemia are at high risk for undetected severe hypoglycemic reactions (102). They no longer experience the warning signs that normally occur in response to hypoglycemia. A pattern of hyperglycemia in the morning (Somogyi phenomenon) has been shown to be a result of asymptomatic nocturnal hypoglycemia in patients who were otherwise well controlled on current intensive insulin regimens (103).

In elderly patients who have decreased nerve function, diabetes with advanced neuropathy, or patients who are receiving beta-blockers, the symptoms of hypoglycemia are sometimes lacking, and the reaction may go undetected and untreated. These patients may present with hyperglycemia, confusion, or loss of consciousness without any other signs or symptoms of hypoglycemia, and appropriate therapy may not be administered (4, 103). If their normal hormonal defenses do not respond and increase blood glucose, they will continue to be hypoglycemic until the injected insulin dissipates (41). These patients must monitor their blood glucose levels at least 4 times a day and occasionally between 2 and 3 a.m. to ensure euglycemia and record the results along with any changes in diet and activities. They may also require a reduction in insulin dosage (it has been suggested that the Somogyi phenomenon is a result of overinsulinization). They should be instructed in interpreting the results and responding with adjustments in their therapy to maintain euglycemia. All manifestations of hypoglycemia are rapidly relieved by glucose administration.

Because of the potential danger of insulin reactions progressing to hypoglycemic coma, the diabetic should always carry packets or cubes of table sugar, a candy roll, or glucose tablets. The patient should eat 2 tsp or 2 cubes of sugar, 5 or 6 pieces of Lifesavers, or 2 glucose tablets at the onset of hypoglycemic symptoms (60). Patients may also drink at least ½ cup of orange juice, ⅓ cup of apple juice, or 6–12 oz of any sugar-containing carbonated beverage (60, 104). The treatment may be repeated in 15 minutes if glucose concentration remains below 60 mg/dl (60). A snack consisting of 1 or 2 cups of milk, a piece of fruit, or cheese and soda crackers is generally enough to treat mild hypoglycemia if it will be more than 30–60 minutes until meal time (60, 75). Blood glucose should be monitored frequently to ensure adequate levels and prevent recurrent hypoglycemia (75).

A glucagon emergency kit containing an ampule of glucagon (1 mg), and a syringe of diluent should be provided to every insulin-dependent diabetic to be mixed and injected by family or friends in case the diabetic loses consciousness. The kit should contain clearly illustrated instructions, and pharmacists should be familiar with the mixing technique for glucagon and be able to instruct patients. Glucagon should be reconstituted with the accompanying solvent, and 0.25–1.0 mg should be administered in the same manner as insulin (75). Normally, the patient will regain consciousness within 5–10 minutes and be able to swallow some sweetened water. If there is no response after 5–10 minutes, a second injection should be given. Glucagon injections may cause nausea and vomiting within 2–4 hours; steps should be taken to prevent aspiration of gastric contents (75, 105). If the response is still insufficient, more intensive treatment is indicated. The patient should be taken to an emergency room or physician immediately (106).

If a hypoglycemic person is mistakenly thought to be hyperglycemic and given insulin, severe hypoglycemia and subsequent brain damage may result. When there is doubt whether a diabetic is hypoglycemic or hyperglycemic, sugar should be given initially until the condition can be evaluated accurately.

Nondrug Therapy

One objective of diabetic control is maintaining normal weight. The pharmacist should stress the importance of proper exercise and diet. Patients who need help adjusting diet or complying with the exercise program prescribed should be referred to a dietitian or physical therapist who deals with diabetics.

Exercise

Although exercise is nearly always recommended by physicians as part of the treatment of diabetes, in the past it was rarely prescribed or considered a vital part of the treatment. However, with the advent of specialized exercise training for diabetes management and the certification of physical therapists as diabetes educators, more physicians are referring diabetics for exercise training. The physical therapist can work with the patient, physician, and dietitian to develop an exercise program that is tailored to the patient's age, activity level, disability, response of blood glucose to exercise, and daily glucose variations. Individualized exercise schedules help ensure compliance and decrease the risk of hypoglycemia (Table 8) (107).

Daily aerobic exercise as prescribed by the physical therapist helps to lower blood glucose levels by allowing the glucose to penetrate the muscle cell and be metabolized without the assistance of insulin. Exercise also improves circulatory function, an important factor in diabetic management; helps maintain ideal body weight; aids in breathing, digestion, and metabolism; and improves the individual's cardiovascular endurance. Exercise has varying effects on plasma glucose levels. It may cause hyperglycemia if inadequate insulin is available when the patient begins to exercise; it may cause hypoglycemia if the patient's blood glucose concentration is normal or low just before exercise and the diabetic does not take the proper precautions (60).

Patients are encouraged to participate in activities that use the large muscle groups at submaximal levels; swimming, running, and biking are highly recommended. Activities such as weight lifting are discouraged because of the possible damage to the smaller optic capillaries.

Consistency with exercise is a key component; patients must maintain a daily exercise program to complement the insulin dose and to avoid extremes in blood glucose levels. Consistent exercise is more difficult for the juvenile diabetic; thus, parents play an integral role in their children's programs.

Patients must be trained to monitor blood glucose levels before, during, and after exercise and to adjust diet and insulin injections accordingly. Patients who monitor their own blood glucose are often motivated to exercise because they easily see the beneficial effects of

TABLE 8   Exercise in patients with diabetes

1. Test blood glucose concentrations before, during, and after exercise.

2. For moderate exercise (e.g., bicycling or jogging for 30–45 minutes), decrease the preceding dose of regular insulin by 30–50%. If glucose concentration is normal or low before exercise, supplement the diet with a snack containing 10–15 g of carbohydrate.

3. To avoid increased absorption of regular insulin by exercise, inject into the abdomen or exercise 30 minutes to 1 hour following injection.

4. Use caution in the case of individuals with low glycogen stores who may be predisposed to the hypoglycemic effects of exercise. These individuals include alcoholics, fasting individuals, and patients on diets that are extremely hypocaloric (fewer than 800 calories) and low carbohydrate (fewer than 10 g per day).

5. Patients taking insulin are more susceptible to hypoglycemia than those taking sulfonylureas. Patients with Type II diabetes treated with diet are unlikely to develop hypoglycemia.

6. Watch for postexercise hypoglycemia. Individuals who have been exercising during the day (e.g., skiing) should increase their carbohydrate intake and test their blood glucose concentration during the night to detect nocturnal hypoglycemia. Hypoglycemia can occur 8–15 hours following exercise.

7. Do not exercise if the glucose concentration exceeds 240–300 mg/dl. This level indicates severe insulin deficiency. These patients are predisposed to hyperglycemia secondary to exercise.

8. Patients with severe proliferative retinopathy or retinal hemorrhage should avoid jarring exercise or exercise that involves moving the head below the waist.

From "Applied Therapeutics," Applied Therapeutics, Inc., Vancouver, Wash., 1988, p. 1697.

exercise on maintaining good blood glucose and weight control. An exercise log may help the patient maintain a regular daily schedule. The pharmacist can encourage the patient to follow the prescribed exercise plan as part of the total treatment of their diabetes and to monitor their blood glucose log to ensure that hypoglycemia is not occurring. If it appears there is a problem, the pharmacist should check with the patient to ensure that carbohydrates are not ingested before exercise, that insulin is injected in nonexercised sites, and that the prescribed physical activities take place at the appropriate time of day with regard to insulin peak activity and food intake.

It is also important for patients to recognize the symptoms of hypoglycemia, carry a sugar source and a glucagon emergency kit, and wear a medical identification necklace or bracelet. The pharmacist should explain to patients that if they experience a hypoglycemic event while exercising and are unable to treat themselves, others must know what is happening so they can provide appropriate treatment as quickly as possible. Because some diabetics are embarrassed about the disease, they may need to be encouraged to tell friends, teachers, or neighbors about their condition.

Diet

Diet is the most critical treatment in Type II diabetes and, in combination with exercise and insulin, is a necessary treatment for Type I diabetes as well (108). However, diet therapy often fails and creates feelings of frustration, pessimism, failure, and anger, which in turn result in poorly informed and inadequately motivated patients (109, 110). The pharmacist can provide increased patient education on proper diet and nutrition, assist the patient in understanding the need to follow the prescribed diet, and help the patient monitor diet and blood glucose levels. The pharmacist can also refer the patient to a registered dietitian for training on basic nutrition, food selection and preparation, daily food plans, and plans for meals during holidays and when traveling or eating out (111).

Factors in Dietary Control   Successful diet programs require education, dietary goals, and behavior modification. Diabetics may benefit from a referral to a registered dietitian who is trained in diet management and who can help develop an individualized diet for the patient. Whenever possible, a team approach of education, counseling, and planning should be used. The team must include the diabetic as an integral member. Diabetics should discuss the reasons for the diet, set dietary goals, actively participate in developing the meal plan to fit their lifestyles, and include foods that are acceptable to them and that meet the nutritional and caloric needs. Failure to consider patient food preferences, ethnic or religious restraints, and lifestyle factors may cause diet therapy failure. The dietitian can also provide information to the patient about eating patterns, food exchanges, and variations on meal plans to meet social needs such as parties, eating out, and holidays. Dietary education and counseling must be a continuing process conducted in an understanding and nonjudgmental manner. Psychologic, physical, and socioeconomic factors must be considered in developing the individual's daily food plan to ensure that specific changes in food intake and eating behaviors occur. If patients have a role in planning and selecting their diets and understand the importance of the diets in the overall treatment of their diabetes, and if the diets are tailored as much as possible to meet the patients' needs, diet therapy may be more successful than in the past.

To help diabetics modify their eating behaviors, they should be encouraged to keep a diet log similar to the exercise log. They should record (for 4–10 days) each time they eat, how much they eat, and why they eat (i.e., whether food ingestion was because of social pressure, loneliness, depression, nervousness, or the time of day, or whether the patient truly needed nourishment). Once eating patterns are defined and understood, modifications can be made and dietary behaviors changed (112).

When diet therapy is begun, the dietitian and physician must consider the patient's activity level and medication doses. All three components (diet, activity, and medication) must be used rationally to prevent hypoglycemic episodes and help ensure a positive therapeutic outcome. Insulin or oral agent overtreatment is probably the most common cause of inadequate diabetic control and weight gain (113). Diabetics should be evaluated to determine whether they are consuming an appropriate amount of food in relation to the amount of insulin present. Insulin causes an increased uptake of free fatty acids and conversion to triglycerides, causing an increased hunger and weight gain in some patients. In patients using insulin, it is important to time the peak insulin action to food intake and activity levels; any adjustment in medication timing must correlate with activity and meal changes. Patients who are using multiple daily insulin injections and using a more liberal time schedule for eating must be sure that they use their insulin properly to avoid periods of hyperglycemia or hypoglycemia. These patients should monitor their blood glucose levels more frequently and must be reminded of the hazards of quick snacks that may enable them to delay a meal but also may add significant calories not accounted for in their basic meal plan.

Goals of Diet Therapy   One goal of dietary treatment in diabetes is to improve the overall health of diabetics by controlling their weight, lipid levels, and blood glucose levels while attaining and maintaining optimal nutrition. Diet therapy may prevent the development and progression of vascular complications. The dietary treatment prescribed should provide for the normal physical growth of children as well as meet the needs of pregnant and lactating women (111, 114). It is also important to maintain consistency in the timing of meals and snacks to prevent swings in blood glucose levels for diabetics using medication as part of the treatment plan (114). Because about 75% of the deaths among diabetics are caused by cardiovascular disease (compared with 50% of deaths in the general population), diabetics should avoid dietary risk factors such as animal fats, which have been shown to be associated with increased atherosclerosis and cardiovascular disease (111, 114, 115).

Nutritional recommendations for diabetics outlined in a position statement by the American Diabetes Association are similar to those of the American Heart Association, the National Cancer Institute (American Cancer Society), the Nutritional Committee for Recommendations for Children with Diabetes of the American Academy of Pediatrics, and the 1985 U.S. Dietary Guidelines (114). The American Diabetes Association has recommended a diet that contains 55–60% carbohydrates, 10–15% protein (or 0.8 g/kg of the patient's weight), no more than 30% fat, and calories that will achieve and maintain a desirable body weight (114). Cholesterol is also restricted to less than 300 mg per day (110, 114). Sodium intake should not exceed 1,000 mg/1,000 kcal or 3,000 mg per day (114). Simple and refined sugars are also contraindicated for all diabetics because of the stress put on the patient (22). Complex carbohydrates are recommended because carbohydrates require utilization of smaller quantities of insulin. Simple carbohydrates produce a rapid increase in blood glucose and stress on the pancreas. The "glycemic index" concept is shedding new light on which carbohydrates cause blood glucose levels to increase rapidly.

Many diabetics believe that because diabetes results in increased blood glucose levels, carbohydrates in general should be avoided. One long-term clinical trial showed that an increased proportion of complex dietary carbohydrates (bread, potatoes, or rice and not simple sugars) did not cause deterioration of diabetic control provided that the total caloric intake was limited to maintain or achieve ideal body weight (22).

A high-fiber diet is valuable to the diabetic. Studies have indicated that increased proportions of dietary carbohydrates that are high in fiber, especially soluble fiber (whole grain cereals, oat bran, whole fruits and vegetables, lentils, and soluble-fiber supplements) rather than more highly refined carbohydrates appear to improve carbohydrate metabolism, lower total cholesterol and low-density lipoprotein cholesterol, and have other beneficial effects (114). Insoluble fibers (e.g., wheat bran) may not have these beneficial effects. Adequate dietary roughage reduces intraluminal pressure in the bowel and decreases the absorption rate of saccharides (108). When guar and pectin, components of dietary fiber, were added to a carbohydrate meal, the postprandial rise of blood glucose was delayed significantly (116). Fiber does not have miraculous weight-controlling properties and appears to be most effective when the dietary calories are derived from at least 50% carbohydrates (114); however, fiber makes it easier for a person to consume fewer calories without feeling hungry. Patients changing to a high-fiber diet should be warned to do so gradually. A sudden large increase may cause temporary flatulence and bloating (114, 117). The amount of dietary fiber necessary to achieve a maximum benefit has not been determined, but a maximum daily intake of 50 g appears to be reasonable (114). (See Chapter 15, *Laxative Products*.)

Diabetics who follow their diet therapy and maintain near euglycemic blood glucose levels are able to keep their triglyceride and serum cholesterol levels within a normal range (22). Several companies are investigating sucrose polyesters that make up an indigestible artificial fat that may eventually replace a significant amount of oils and fats now used in food preparation. It appears the indigestible fat will be used in cooking and in frozen desserts that now rely heavily on animal or vegetable oils and fats. Diarrhea is the only major side effect of consuming large quantities of indigestible fat. All diabetic patients are advised to restrict saturated fats and avoid pies, sugar, syrup, candy, alcoholic beverages, sweetened soft drinks, and cakes to help maintain ideal body weight, control blood glucose levels, and decrease the occurrence or progression of complications associated with hyperglycemia.

Use of Alternative Sweeteners In general, food for the diabetic may be adapted or prepared in two ways: by restricting the sugar content, or by restricting both the sugar content and caloric value (118). In preparing special foods, sucrose is omitted, and other sweetening agents may be substituted. The American Diabetes Association indicates that the use of various nutritive and nonnutritive sweeteners is accepted in the management of diabetes (114). The safety of some of these substitutes often has been questioned. The term "alternative sweeteners" has been substituted for the old term "artificial sweeteners" because some of the agents now used are derived from natural sources. The FDA classifies sweeteners as nonnutritive and nutritive. The term "nonnutritive" refers to a sweetener without calories, such as saccharin or cyclamates. "Nutritive" refers to sweeteners with calories, such as aspartame, fructose, sorbitol, and mannitol. Saccharin, which is 400 times sweeter than sucrose, is a common sucrose substitute in the United States. Because it has been implicated in causing malignant tumors in rats, the FDA requires a warning on all products containing saccharin. The FDA also requires all retail establishments selling saccharin-containing products to display a warning statement.

The use of sorbitol and fructose is discouraged because their caloric contribution is significant and may undermine efforts to control weight and blood glucose levels (114). Sorbitol is a glucose alcohol that is 60% as sweet as sugar. It is absorbed slowly from the gut with little effect on the blood glucose levels. Sorbitol generally is without side effects; if large quantities are taken, osmotic effects may cause diarrhea and abdominal discomfort. Sorbitol is converted to glucose and metabolized, and its energy value as calories (4 cal/g) must be counted by patients for whom weight control is necessary. Sorbitol is one of the end products of the polyol pathway of glucose metabolism that results in some of the late complications of diabetes. However, the amount of sorbitol in foods is not considered to be a risk factor to diabetics unless very large amounts are consumed. There is no evidence that small amounts of ingested sorbitol contribute to the complications of diabetes. Sorbitol is the most frequently used alcohol added to food products, but foods containing sorbitol are frequently labeled "not for weight control purposes" because they may have more calories than similar products containing other sweeteners.

Fructose is another sucrose substitute that is found in fruits and honey. It is also an end product of glucose metabolism by insulin-independent pathways and thus has a potential for adding to the late complications of diabetes (118). The American Diabetes Association warns diabetic patients that fructose has the same caloric content as table sugar (119). Diabetics planning to use fructose as a substitute sweetener should first consult with their physician or dietitian (119). The American Diabetes Association's summary statement on the use of fructose, sorbitol, and xylitol as sugar substitutes concludes: "The day-long quantitative reduction of hyperglycemia that may result from substantial substitution of these sweeteners for glucose and sucrose in the diabetic diet, and the long-term effectiveness and safety when they are ingested in substantial quantities and mixed meals, has not been established" (119).

The G. D. Searle Company manufactures aspartame. Aspartame is a combination of two naturally occurring amino acids. It is classified as a nutritive sweetener by the FDA because, technically, it provides calories. Aspartame is 200 times sweeter than sugar and yields only one-tenth of a calorie per teaspoon. Because of this, the American Diabetes Association Task Force on Nutrition has classified aspartame as a noncaloric sweetener (115). It is commonly used as a sweetener in diet soft drinks, other drink mixes, candies, and cereals, and is available in a crystal form. It is heat labile and cannot be used in cooking. Some physicians do not recommend its use in very young children.

Hoechst-Roussel Pharmaceuticals, Inc., has received FDA approval to market a new artificial sweetener, acesulfame potassium or (Sunette), for use in gum and dry food products and for sale in packets and tablets. Sunette is similar to saccharin in that it has no calories, but differs in that it has no aftertaste and does not lose potency after heating or long-term storage. Hoechst-Roussel is also seeking FDA approval to market Sunette for use in candies, liquid food products, and baked goods.

Any diabetic with an excessive intake of any sweetener requires nutritional counseling and assessment of needs (114). Although most diabetics are advised to limit their use of sweeteners, intake should be individualized, the use of other sweeteners considered, and the overall diet and nutritional adequacy considered (114).

The pharmacist has a supportive and educational role in all phases of diet therapy. Pharmacists should encourage diabetics to follow the prescribed diet and should discourage prolonged fasting or fad diets. Pharmacists can also educate the patient about the importance of diet therapy in the overall treatment plan and help arrange a self-monitoring program that allows the patient to see the effect of food intake on blood glucose control. This program should begin in the "initial or survival" phase and continue through the rest of the training and adjustment period. Patients should be encouraged to obtain dietitian or physician approval for any change in dietary habits. The pharmacist should advise the diabetic to read the labels of all foods marked "dietetic" because the foods may not be sugarless or intended for diabetics. Better labeling is needed to inform diabetics about the specific individual sweeteners and the amounts (mg or g) contained per serving (114). Some dietetic foods actually have more calories than regular foods. Pharmacists should be familiar with all products they carry that are directed at diet therapy. They should know which ingredients are acceptable for use in the diabetic, how much fat the product will contribute to the diet, and which products should be avoided by diabetic patients and why, in order to help the patient select the right products for their needs (61).

Consumption of Alcohol and Alcohol-Containing Products The American Diabetes Association recommends that diabetic patients avoid alcohol use (including alcoholic beverages and medications containing alcohol) because it may cause specific problems with hypoglycemia, neuropathy, glycemic control, obesity, and hyperlipidemia (114). Alcohol is metabolized similarly to fat; alters insulin response; changes the synthesis, storage, and release of glycogen; and can impair judgment. However, avoidance is not always possible or desired, and diabetics should be assessed individually to determine whether the presumed advantages of alcohol (e.g., reducing emotional tension, relieving anxiety, and stimulating appetite) outweigh its potential adverse effect on blood glucose control (120, 121). Consumption of alcohol such as dry wine in moderate quantities (i.e., no more than 2 equivalents of an alcoholic beverage once or twice a week) has been advocated by some diabetologists as part of diabetes therapy and is part of the American Diabetes Association's recommendations for alcohol use (114, 122).

Either hyperglycemia or hypoglycemia may develop in diabetics who ingest alcohol. Hypoglycemia is the most common effect. The hypoglycemic effect of alcohol is believed to be caused either by increased early endogenous insulin response to glucose or by inhibition of hepatic gluconeogenesis. Relatively small quantities of alcohol (48 ml of 100 proof) may cause this effect. If a diabetic patient is fasting and consumes alcohol, hypoglycemia may be severe. Alcohol has a less significant effect if a diabetic has adequate amounts of glucose in the blood (121).

Although tolbutamide and chlorpropamide have been reported to interact with alcohol, resulting in a "disulfiram-like" reaction, the other available sulfonylureas are not as likely to cause this reaction (121).

The additive hypoglycemic effects of alcohol with insulin have produced severe hypoglycemia resulting in coma, brain damage, and even death. Diabetics who are well fed and drinking alcoholic beverages with a high level of carbohydrates eventually develop hyperglycemia. Alcohol is a readily oxidizable food substance and, unlike sugar, can be readily metabolized without insulin participation. Several studies have shown that diabetics who are on a diabetic diet alone or taking insulin or a sulfonylurea can consume up to 2 oz (60 ml) of dry wine without any significant alteration in the blood glucose values (121, 122). The data available concerning diabetics' consumption of strong forms of alcohol, such as distilled liquors, are different. Ketosis may arise if strong alcohol is consumed in excess, but there is little evidence to demonstrate concern over consumption of small amounts of hard liquor.

One equivalent, or 1 oz of liquor, is equal to the amount of alcohol in a 1.5-oz shot of distilled beverage, 4 oz of wine, or 12 oz of beer. A typical 4-oz serving of dry table wine contains 90–100 calories with an average sugar content of 400 mg. Rosé wines tend to be sweeter; a 4-oz serving contains about 1.3 g of sugar. Champagne contains about 1.4 g of sugar. Sweeter white wines may contain as much as 5 g of glucose per 4-oz serving. The caloric intake for fortified wines is about twice as much as for an equal volume of dry wine, and the sugar content of sweet sherries, ports, and muscatels may be as high as 6 g per 2 oz serving. Light beer and dry wine may be better choices because of the lower carbohydrate and calorie content than regular beer or wine. Alcoholic beverages should always be consumed with food (114). Four ounces of dry wine could be consumed with the evening meal without difficulty, so long as no food is omitted from the Type I diabetic's meal plan and there are no other contraindications for use (114, 122). For Type II diabetics, alcohol may be substituted for fat exchanges because it is metabolized similarly to fat (1 oz equals 2 fat exchanges) (114). Diabetics at risk of alcohol abuse should be discouraged from using alcohol at any time (114).

More individualized guidelines for alcohol use in diabetics have been established. Alcohol is generally contraindicated in Type I diabetics who are prone to hypoglycemia, patients with neuropathies, gestational or pregnant Type I diabetics, Type II diabetics who have experienced the chlorpropamide–alcohol flush, patients with alcoholism, and patients suffering from proliferative retinopathy (34). Guidelines for alcohol use in diabetics include discussing the use of alcohol with the physician to ensure that no contraindications exist; drinking in moderation; eating first and spacing drinks; avoiding mixes that contain sugar; drinking only dry wines and avoiding beer, ale, cordials, and sweet wines; calculating the alcohol in the diet schedule and decreasing fat intake accordingly; and considering that alcohol promotes hypoglycemia the "morning after" (34). Patients who are alcoholic, overweight, or pregnant and patients whose diabetic control is unstable should not drink.

Consumption of Caffeine Consuming large amounts of caffeine-containing products such as coffee, tea, and soft drinks may increase blood glucose because of increased liver glycogen breakdown. Large amounts of caffeine can also alter the patient's perception of hyperglycemia and affect management. The response to caffeine is highly variable among patients. Caffeine intake should be considered in patients who tend to have hyperglycemic episodes at specific times of the day that cannot be attributed to other factors. (See Chapter 10, *Sleep Aid, Sedative, and Stimulant Products*.)

Consumption of Vitamins and Minerals The diet of a diabetic should meet the recommended requirements for vitamins and minerals (114). There is no evidence that indicates diabetics should supplement intake of all or specific vitamins or minerals above the recommended daily allowance unless the patient is on a very low-calorie diet or unless other special circumstances exist (114). Recent studies have shown that diabetics have low serum ascorbic acid levels and that a daily supplement may be needed. Supplementation of calcium may be necessary under special circumstances including pregnancy, lactation, and calcium-poor diets (114). (See Chapter 17, *Nutritional Supplement, Mineral, and Vitamin Products*.)

PREVENTING COMPLICATIONS

The complications of diabetes include microangiopathy, macroangiopathy, dermopathy, retinopathy, neuropathy, nephropathy, and a decreased ability to overcome infections. The prevention of complications through good diabetic control is the ultimate goal. Patients who include self-monitoring as part of their overall therapy plan are usually able to normalize blood glucose levels and maintain good diabetic control. Diabetics must be careful in using products that influence their diabetes. For instance, the ingestion of large quantities of aspirin or even ascorbic acid may influence urine tests and affect diabetic control. Nasal sprays, asthma, allergy and hay fever medications, decongestants, and cold and cough preparations that contain sympathomimetic amines should also be used with caution, especially in poorly controlled diabetic patients. Diabetics should avoid medications containing sugar or alcohol. Antihistamines or other products that produce drowsiness may cause the patient to skip insulin doses.

Diabetics have an increased occurrence of atherosclerosis that is detected earlier in life than atherosclerosis in nondiabetics, appears to progress at an accelerated rate, and is more extreme (48). Patients considering the use of niacin or nicotinic acid to control or prevent hypercholesterolemia without their physician's knowledge should be warned of the many adverse effects of the drug (123); self-medicating should be discouraged.

Diabetic patients must take specific measures to prevent problems that require special attention; these measures include giving special consideration to general hygiene, foot care, dental care, eye care, and prevention of hypoglycemic episodes.

General Hygiene

Diabetics are more susceptible to bacterial infection, particularly monilial infection, than the general population (120). The most easily infected part of the body is the skin. Infections heal slowly in diabetics with vascular disease or hyperglycemia. Minor cuts and scratches should be cleansed thoroughly with soap and water. Diabetic patients with serious cuts, burns, or punctures should see their physicians immediately.

Monilial infections of the vagina and anus are much more common in patients with glycosuria. A product containing 3 parts Amphogel, 1 part kaolin powder and 1 part Unibase is useful in treating pruritus ani. Application of this mixture to the anal area reduces itching and irritation. Daily bathing with thorough drying is also recommended for diabetic patients. Diabetics should use mild soaps and avoid all harsh chemicals including caustic powders, iodine preparations, astringents, and any other products that may produce or exacerbate vascular or neurologic complications.

Diabetics should inspect their bodies daily, starting at the top of their heads and working down to the feet and toes. They should check for any signs of dry or cracked skin, infections or injuries, areas of chafing or irritation, and areas that may be altered by increased pressure from clothing or shoes. Patients should also ensure that any problem areas already identified are being cared for and are healing properly. Any new complications or any old ones that are not healing properly should be brought to the attention of the physician as soon as possible.

Pharmacists should be able to discuss the appropriate use of nonprescription topical antimicrobial products and recommend whether the diabetic should seek medical attention. Pharmacists should know which products the physicians in their area prefer to use or avoid and why. This provides a better working relationship among the pharmacist, the diabetic, and the physician. (See Chapter 28, *Topical Anti-infective Products*.)

Foot Care

Gangrene has been reported to be 50 times more frequent in diabetics over 40 years of age than in nondiabetics of the same age (124). Before the advent of antibiotics, amputations of the leg were performed in 9 out of 10 diabetics undergoing surgery for gangrene of the foot. Even with the discovery of antibiotics, approximately 50% (40,000 per year) of major leg amputations are performed on diabetics (6, 124). Diabetics are predisposed to infection because of vascular changes resulting in poor blood supply, as well as neuropathy in the lower extremities. If feet are exposed to minor trauma or infection, the thick-walled vessels become obliterated more easily, resulting in decreased perfusion of the tissue and tissue hypoxia, decreased delivery of immune system components to the area, decreased removal of cellular waste, and an increased risk of severe ulcerations, gangrene, osteomyelitis, and systemic infections (124).

Control of diabetes is the first step in foot care. To prevent foot problems, diabetic patients must be educated to care properly for their feet. Widespread application of good foot care and patient education dealing with the problems of diabetic foot could markedly reduce the amputation rate (125). Measures, in addition to the procedures described in Chapter 37, *Foot Care Products*, include the following:

- Inspect feet and lower legs daily using a mirror (especially between toes and pressure areas).

- Rub feet thoroughly with vegetable oil, lanolin, or an appropriate commercial product to keep them soft and prevent dryness. Excessively dry skin may crack and fissure, allowing infection to enter.

- If feet become too soft and tender, they should be rubbed with alcohol once a week (22). Feet that are too soft and overly moist are more susceptible to skin infections such as athlete's foot.

- Never treat athlete's foot with acidic or astringent preparations.

- Avoid bruises, cuts, and skin irritations, and avoid burning or freezing the skin of the feet.

- Avoid going barefoot.

- Toenails should be cut or filed straight across, not shorter than the underlying soft tissue of the toe; never cut the corner of the nails.

- Never cut corns or calluses.

- Avoid corn medications because they contain keratolytic agents.

- Prevent callus formation under the ball of the foot. While exercising, finish each step on the toes and not on the ball of the foot; wear shoes that fit well and do not have excessively high heels.

- Avoid extremes in temperatures and never apply heat of any kind to the feet (77).

- Never step into a bathtub before checking the temperature of the water.

- Change shoes often and inspect shoes daily (inside and out).

- Never wear tight stockings.

- Have feet inspected at every clinic or office visit.

- Do not sit with legs crossed because this posture constricts circulation and promotes nerve pressure.

- Select a podiatrist who is familiar with diabetic foot problems.

- Have shoes professionally fitted, and break new shoes in slowly.

Patients with any type of foot problem should immediately see a physician or podiatrist. All diabetic patients should examine their feet daily for cuts, scratches, and color changes (57, 126). It is also recommended that diabetic patients abstain from the use of tobacco, which can cause vasoconstriction in the extremities and is an important risk factor in the development of coronary artery disease.

The pharmacist can screen for patients at risk of diabetic foot ulcers by asking about any neuropathic symptoms, history of claudication or resting pain, history of prior orthopedic foot problems or surgeries, and social history (smoking habits and alcohol intake). Patients who are overweight, especially men, also have a higher risk of foot problems (126). Patients with any of these risk factors should be instructed in the appropriate care of their feet and monitored closely. All diabetic patients should be encouraged to have their feet examined regularly by their physicians; patients with identifiable risk factors should insist on examination of the feet. Pharmacists should also know which foot care products are not recommended for use by diabetics and help patients make appropriate decisions in choosing foot care products and in seeking additional medical attention.

Dental Care

Gingivitis and dental caries occur at an increased rate in diabetics. Hidden abscesses of the teeth are common in hyperglycemic patients and may contribute to poor blood glucose control. Diabetics should have their teeth checked at least twice a year. Diabetics should brush and floss their teeth at least twice a day, and the gums should be massaged with a brush, Water Pik, or fingers. At the first sign of abnormal conditions of the gums, the diabetic should consult a dentist because uncontrolled diabetes seems to accentuate periodontal disease. Diabetics should inform their dentists that they have diabetes and discuss the appropriate dental care products with them.

Pharmacists should ensure that patients use sugar-free and alcohol-free dental products, know which toothbrush has been recommended, and know how to floss appropriately. Diabetics should be monitored closely for changes in oral care or complaints of problems and should be immediately referred to their dentists. (See Chapter 23, *Oral Health Products*.)

Eye Care

Diabetes is the leading cause of blindness in the United States. Some of those cases can be avoided or their severity significantly reduced if retinopathy is detected early (and the retina photocoagulated with laser therapy) and if glaucoma is detected and treated early. Pharmacists should encourage diabetics to evaluate the status of their vision and to have their eyes examined at least once a year. Pharmacists can also educate diabetics about the importance of blood glucose control in maintaining good vision. As mentioned earlier, glucose is metabolized to sorbitol during hyperglycemic episodes. Sorbitol accumulates in the lenses and other tissues, resulting in water influx into the lenses and swelling or precipitation of protein, which may lead to cataract formation (127). Pharmacists should also monitor medications of diabetics to help them avoid drugs that affect the retina, optic nerve, pupil, and ciliary muscle

(128). Parasympatholytic drugs including anticholinergics, antidepressants, antihistamines, and ganglionic blockers can alter the pupil and ciliary muscle and result in blurred vision. Diabetics should be discouraged from using any topical ophthalmic preparations, especially those that contain antihistamines, unless recommended or prescribed by their physician or ophthalmologist. Patients who note any change in vision or irritation of the eyes should see their doctors immediately. (See Chapter 20, *Ophthalmic Products*, and Chapter 21, *Contact Lenses and Lens Care Products*.)

Because pharmacists have the major role in monitoring drug use in diabetics, they should be familiar with drugs that may affect blood glucose control by themselves or by interacting with sulfonylureas or insulin and know which drugs could cause or exacerbate peripheral neuropathy, retinopathy, and nephropathy (Tables 9–11) (34).

PRODUCT SELECTION GUIDELINES

Pharmacists should be able to advise the diabetic about the purchase of proper equipment. Injection aids are available for patients with a fear of needles or for those with disabilities such as impaired vision (129–131). Several types of syringes are available, including those using prefilled and premixed cartridges and insulin pumps that provide high-intensity dosing of insulin without multiple injections (129–131). There are also many different methods for monitoring blood and urine glucose (129–131). Special products have recently been made available for diabetics who travel and must carry insulin with them (129–131).

The pharmacist should be aware of any effects that other nonprescription and prescription products may have on the diabetic as well as which drugs will interfere with urine or blood glucose testing. Because diabetic patients are more susceptible to infections (particularly monilial infections), the pharmacist should recommend that appropriate products be kept on hand, encourage strict hygiene measures, and advise additional medical attention when necessary.

Syringes and Needles

Pharmacists must ensure that the diabetic purchases the proper type of insulin and the syringe that corresponds to the strength of insulin used. Problems with insulin dosage occur when patients use the wrong

TABLE 9 Drugs of abuse that impair diabetes management

Alcohol

Impairs judgment

Is metabolized similarly to fat and alters insulin response when taken with carbohydrates

Promotes hypoglycemic attacks

Impairs the manufacture, storage, and release of glycogen

Interacts with other drugs (e.g., chlorpropamide)

Can cause precipitous drop in blood glucose in alcoholic persons who have stopped eating

Can increase blood glucose when used with sugar-containing mixers or in "sweet drinks"

Nicotine (smoking)

Is a potent vasoconstrictor

Causes a 1 to 2°F drop in skin temperature with one cigarette

Significantly alters oral and IV glucose tolerance tests

Is a risk factor in etiology of diabetic nephropathy

May decrease SC absorption of insulin

May increase insulin requirements by as much as 15–20%

Caffeine (coffee, tea, colas)

In large amounts, increases blood glucose levels

Marijuana

Alters time perception, which may affect control

May cause "munchies"

Impairs short-term memory in intoxicated state

Causes a highly dose-related effect, which is dangerous because patient may not know tetrahydrocannabinol content

Yields profound impairment when used with alcohol

With heavy use, impairs glucose tolerance, causing hyperglycemia

CNS stimulants (amphetamines, sympathomimetics, decongestants, anorectics, cocaine, and psychedelics)

Increase blood glucose levels

Increase liver glycogen breakdown, which causes hyperglycemia

Alter time perception, which may affect management steps

May cause anorexia, which increases blood glucose levels

Sedatives and hypnotics

Impair thinking and thus self-control

Opiates (heroin, morphine)

Causes euphoria, which may affect management and increase blood glucose levels

From *Am. Pharm.*, Module 4, NS26 (5), 4 (1986).

TABLE 10 Drugs that could cause peripheral neuropathies

Antimicrobials	Nitrofurantoin, ethambutol, isoniazid, colistin, streptomycin, metronidazole, amphotericin B
Anticonvulsants	Phenytoin
Antirheumatics	Indomethacin, colchicine, penicillamine, gold compounds
Cytotoxics	Vincristine, procarbazine, cytarabine, chlorambucil
Cardiovascular drugs	Hydralzine, clofibrate, disopyramide
Miscellaneous agents	Cimetidine, ergotamine, methysergide, amitriptyline, amphetamines
Nitroglycerin	Can cause postural hypotension in diabetics with autonomic neuropathy

From *Am. Pharm.*, Module 4, NS26 (5), 4 (1986).

TABLE 11 Drugs that induce nephropathies

Penicillamine, gold salts, nonsteroidal analgesics (large doses over time)

Aminoglycoside antibiotics (neomycin, kanamycin, gentamicin, tobramycin)

Cephaloridine, rifampin, cyclophosphamide, heroin, methotrexate, and methysergide

From *Am. Pharm.*, Module 4, NS26 (5), 4 (1986).

insulin or the wrong syringe. Problems caused by administering the wrong insulin, either from the wrong source or the wrong type (e.g., NPH versus Ultralente), have already been discussed. Insulin is administered in units and not in milliliters; therefore, syringes are calibrated in units (58, 60). The calibration of the syringe should correspond to the concentration of the insulin used (e.g., U-40 syringes should be used only with U-40 insulin, U-100 syringes with U-100 insulin).

Two types of syringes are available: glass (reusable) and plastic (disposable). Most diabetics use plastic insulin syringes. However, plastic syringes are more expensive than glass. The advantages of disposable syringes and needles include assured sterility and ease of penetration provided by 25% less angle in the cut, side bevels, thinner metal and a wide bore, and silicone coating (131). The needles are finer (27, 28, and 29 gauge), sharper, and lubricated for ease of insertion. Needles are available in ½-in. and ⅝-in. lengths; the longer needle is used when back leakage of insulin occurs and by obese patients (60, 130, 131). There is less pain associated with the smaller, 27-, 28-, or 29-gauge needles. The disposable syringes have virtually no "dead space," the measurable space in the needle and at the hub of the needle and syringe (60). This dead space is a potential source of error when two different fluids are drawn, measured, and mixed in the same syringe, and it also wastes insulin.

New disposable syringes with capacities of 0.3 cc (30 U) and 0.5 cc (50 U), called low-dose syringes, and 1.0 cc (100 U) may be used only with U-100 insulin. The low-dose syringes have a smaller caliber barrel so that the highly concentrated U-100 insulin can be measured more accurately, allowing patients to measure insulin in 1-unit increments (60, 131). It is important to make the distinction among the types of syringes because the 1.0-ml syringes are graduated in 2-unit increments and the low-dose syringes are graduated in 1-unit increments (60). Diabetics who require fewer than 30–50 U of U-100 insulin per injection may use the low-dose sy-

ringes to measure the dose more accurately. The 1.0-ml syringes resemble tuberculin syringes, but should not be interchanged because of differences in labeling.

Reuse of disposable insulin syringes has been reported by several researchers (132–134). One study showed that disposable syringes can be reused for at least 3 days with safety and patient satisfaction; while another study indicated that diabetics reused disposable syringes for an average of 4 days and that needle dullness was a major reason for changing to a new syringe (132, 133). Patients have been reported to place transparent tape over the barrel of the syringe to keep the numbers from rubbing off, refrigerate their syringes between uses, and wipe their needles with alcohol before reusing (60, 133). There have been no reports of increased rate of infection at the site of injection in patients who reuse disposable syringes, but there have not been any large, long-term prospective studies to ensure that this is the case; therefore, reusing syringes is not actively recommended (135). Diabetics who have been following this practice without problems for several years should probably not be discouraged (60). It is important to ensure that diabetics who reuse disposable syringes and needles pay close attention to aseptic technique and carefully replace the cap over the needle without touching the needle with their hands (131). Wiping the needle with alcohol is not recommended because it may remove the silicone coating from the needle, making skin penetration more painful.

Injection Aids for the Visually Impaired

The pharmacist should be familiar with the many products available to assist the diabetic in filling the syringe and administering injections, how they differ, and their disadvantages. Pharmacists should also be aware of the type and amount of product training that is available to them and the diabetic. The pharmacist must also be aware of any special adaptor or product needs that are associated with the specific aids. For example, "drawing aids" hold the syringe and vial and align the needle, which may be preset to aid in drawing up the correct dose (130, 131). Magnifiers enlarge the calibrations on an insulin syringe to twice their actual size (131). There are several "dose gauges" that allow doses to be dialed in, have audible dose selectors, come in Braille, or have prefilled syringes that are disposable after multiple dose use (130, 131). Jordan's Count-a-Dose holds two vials of insulin for those who need to mix doses (131).

Several insulin injection devices or automatic injectors have been designed to help diabetics who are bothered by taking shots (131). These products include insertion aids, insulin pens, jet injectors, and infusers (130, 131). An insertion aid is a jacket that fits over a filled syringe, is spring-loaded, and guides the needle into the skin. The needle and injection site may or may not be visible to the patient depending on type. Some aids allow the patient to adjust depth and angle of skin penetration (130, 131). The size of the automatic injectors varies depending on type. The syringe may be filled and carried in the jacket until the patient is ready to use it. The insulin pens look like writing pens, use disposable cartridges filled with 150 U of human insulin (regular, NPH, or 70/30 mix), may deliver preset or dial-in doses depending on the type, and require only one hand for injection (130, 131).

Needleless injectors, called jet injectors, deliver insulin as a tiny liquid stream forced through the skin under pressure. The injected insulin disperses in a very thin spray as it enters the SC tissue. Patients who use this type of device for the first time may have to adjust the insulin dose because increased tissue contact may cause it to be absorbed faster (130, 131). Diabetics who do not have enough fat tissue may actually inject insulin into the muscle tissue, which will affect absorption (131). These devices cause less lipoatrophy and inflammation than customary needle administration. The jet injector also facilitates reaching and rotating the injection sites (130). All of these devices have maximum-dose delivery limitations that must be considered when advising a patient.

A small flexible catheter, called the Button infuser or the Insuflow, is available for patients who use a syringe and needle but dislike injecting themselves. The infuser is inserted subcutaneously, usually in the abdomen, and anchored at the site. It allows the patient to give multiple doses of insulin by simply attaching a syringe to the portal and injecting. The syringe is then disconnected from the SC catheter portal and the catheter portal is "plugged" until the next dose is administered (136). The catheter can remain in place for 24–72 hours, and the patient may inject insulin several times a day through the catheter (130, 131, 136). The Button infuser is not as complicated as an insulin pump and is frequently more acceptable than individual needle and syringe use to patients requiring multiple daily injections. The patient must be instructed in preparing the site before insertion and caring for the site and the portal while the catheter is in place to prevent infections (136). Improper use of these devices may result in an improper dose being drawn or injected; improper injection technique may deliver the insulin intramuscularly or intravenously, or may inject none or only part of the dose.

A number of other adaptor and injector devices are being tested, including a new needle design called the "sprinkler" needle. This needle has a sealed end-hole and 14 small holes in the side walls to allow insulin to be sprinkled into the SC tissue instead of being depoted. This method is reported to lead to more rapid absorption of the short-acting insulin, allowing diabetics to inject themselves immediately before eating (bolus) as opposed to 30 minutes before eating (137).

Insulin Infusion Pumps

Portable, battery-driven, open-loop infusion pumps have gained some support for the administration of insulin to a small number of Type I diabetics. Intensified insulin therapy to achieve tight blood sugar control requires either multiple daily injections or insulin pump infusion, which allows the continuous SC infusion of a small (basal infusion) amount of insulin (usually 0.1 U per hour) and a bolus injection of insulin before meals and snacks (131, 138, 139). These devices are referred to as open-loop devices because the regulation of insulin is not automatically regulated by the blood glucose level and because they are not an artificial pancreas. The patient must self-monitor blood glucose at least 4 times a day to determine when and how much insulin should be injected. Some pumps can be programmed to automatically change basal rates at different times of the day; this tailors the therapy to fit the patient's lifestyle and prevents the early morning rise in blood sugar. When insulin infusion pumps are programmed to meet the individual's needs and are used in conjunction with home monitoring of blood glucose, the patient can maintain almost normal blood glucose levels. Many diabetologists and diabetic patients support the idea that tight control and close monitoring of blood glucose will help prevent the late complications of diabetes mellitus.

The objectives of insulin pump therapy include:

- Normalization of blood glucose values (i.e., 70–140 mg/dl);

- Maintenance of blood glucose values of less than 200 mg/dl;

- Normalization of glycosylated hemoglobin values;

- Prevention or reversal of diabetic complications;

- Maintenance of daily activities;

- Increased lifestyle flexibility (pump patients can more easily adjust to eating, sleeping, and exercise schedules);

- Avoidance of weight gain by maintenance of a well-planned diabetic diet;

- Avoidance of infection and complications with pump procedures;

■ Achievement of a sense of well being.

Numerous pumps are available to administer insulin SC. Some pumps have electronic control systems, but most are basically microcomputers with rechargeable batteries. All pumps currently available sound an alarm when the battery is running low. Most of the pumps use a syringe filled with regular insulin and a motorized device in the pump that is programmed to push the plunger of the syringe a set distance forward, forcing the insulin dose through a plastic tube (infusion line). This tube is attached to a 27-gauge, ⅝-in. needle or flexible cannula, which is inserted SC and taped in place. Some pumps have special storage containers or reservoirs that contain insulin; various types of pumps use different pumping mechanisms to push the insulin through the infusion line. The infusion line can be disconnected from the syringe when the diabetic is involved in swimming, showering, or intimate activities or when the infusion line is occluded. The pumps will sound an alarm if the infusion line is occluded. Most patients change the infusion line and cannula sites every 2 days to prevent soreness and infection. The pumps will also sound an alarm when they are empty or almost empty. Syringes or reservoirs must be replaced when they are empty. Some pumps still have "runaway" alarms; however, most manufacturers believe that runaways (uncontrolled infusions) are so unlikely that this alarm is not necessary (131).

The pump is programmed to provide an individualized, continuous basal amount of insulin SC throughout a 24-hour period, and will handle fluctuations in blood glucose when the patient is not eating. Guidelines for adjusting doses to account for food, exercise, and the results of self-monitoring of blood glucose are established at the time the patient begins using the pump. Before eating, the patient pushes several buttons on the pump to provide a predetermined bolus amount of insulin to handle what the diabetic consumes during the meal. Problems at the SC site include the variability in absorption of insulin, local skin reactions, and possible infection.

The pumps differ in size, alarm systems, need for insulin dilution, simplicity of dosing, supplementary dosing features, accumulative dose, manufacturer dependability, cost, life of the battery, durability, water resistance, and availability of syringes, reservoirs, and infusion sets (cannulas and tubing) that are used with the pump. Today's pumps are much smaller, lighter, and more sophisticated with improved alarm systems and simplicity of use. The smallest pump is about the size of a credit card and half an inch thick. Other pumps are about the size of a deck of cards or larger. Diabetics using insulin infusion devices can purchase many types of auxiliary pump equipment, including infusion tubing (12–42 in.), batteries and battery rechargers, syringes or reservoirs that fit specific pumps, tape (Micropore, Ensure, Tagaderm OpSite), surgical soap to wash the insertion site, tape adhesive remover, skin conditioner, diluting fluid for insulin, blood testing supplies, and log books (140).

Blood glucose self-monitoring is essential for pump users, and many studies have shown that normalization of a variety of metabolic parameters can be achieved using insulin pumps (140). Most problems in pump use are related to three primary factors: A patient could go into a ketotic phase within a matter of hours if the flow of insulin is interrupted, a patient may not experience the normal symptoms of hypoglycemia, and infections can occur at the injection site if it is not carefully monitored.

Not all diabetics are candidates for insulin pump therapy. Type II diabetics and diabetic children are not encouraged to use insulin pumps. Candidates for insulin pump therapy include the following:

■ Pregnant diabetics;

■ Diabetics experiencing complications;

■ Diabetics who have undergone renal transplant;

■ Brittle diabetics;

■ Highly motivated Type I diabetics.

Success in the use of insulin infusion devices is directly correlated with proper patient selection (141). Patients selected for insulin pump therapy must be highly motivated, capable of being educated, responsible for keeping records and following specific procedures, willing to perform and log blood tests daily, and willing to be hospitalized for 1 or 2 days for instruction and monitoring if necessary. The role of these open-loop systems in delivering insulin to the diabetic will be significant in the next few years.

Closed-loop systems are also being studied and are in initial clinical trials as an investigational method for insulin delivery. Unlike the open-loop systems, closed-loop systems can monitor serum glucose levels and deliver programmed amounts of insulin in response to a particular amount of serum glucose. Such systems include implantable devices and the artificial pancreas. The implantable pumps being tested are primarily constant-rate, vapor-powered Infusaid devices that deliver insulin intravenously or intraperitoneally (142). The programmable implantable medication system, which allows remote programming and interrogation by radio telemetry or telephone communication, is also being investigated (142). The implantable pumps have had several problems, including flow stoppage caused by tissue blockage and formation of insoluble aggregates of insulin in the pump reservoirs caused by prolonged exposure to body heat and movement (142–144). The implantable glucose sensors have also not worked well. An alternative route for insulin delivery is nasal mucosal absorption (137). Pharmacists should closely review the literature to remain current with the new products available.

Blood and Urine Testing and Record Keeping

The pharmacist's role in emphasizing the importance of urine and blood glucose testing and in keeping records of urine and blood glucose levels, medication, dose, diet, and exercise is significant in improving the patient's diabetic control (145). Urine testing is still important in controlling diabetes, although to a lesser extent than blood glucose monitoring. The pharmacist should assist the patient in selecting and using urine glucose and ketone test kits. The pharmacist should be able to explain the use of urine testing kits (glucose oxidase methods versus copper reductase reaction), how to interpret the color changes, and the importance of keeping accurate records. The pharmacist should be able to discuss concurrent drug interferences with each urine testing method. Pharmacists should assist the patient in selecting and using blood testing equipment. In addition, samples of testing products should be available in the pharmacy's diabetic center so that patients may practice techniques and demonstrate their ability to properly test their urine or blood for glucose and ketones. Pharmacists should also encourage diabetic patients to bring in their records of blood or urine tests, weight, activities, diet, and medication use, to monitor how well the patient's diabetes is being controlled.

Proper urine or blood testing for glucose and ketones, as well as adequate records of daily control, is essential for diabetics. Blood glucose testing lets the diabetic know whether the treatment program is successful. Measuring the blood glucose at certain points allows the diabetic to see what effect exercise, various foods, various medications, illness, and emotional stress have on blood glucose levels. Urine testing gives the diabetic an idea of what the blood glucose levels have been in the past several hours. It is not an indicator of the current blood glucose level. Changes in urine glucose or ketone results may signal the diabetic to increase the frequency of blood glucose monitoring, especially when the results go from negative to positive (60). Ketones in the urine and an elevated blood glucose are the first indicators of DKA. Pharmacists should monitor patients' drug therapy for drugs that interfere with either the copper reduction or glucose oxidase testing methods.

Factors in Selection

Proper blood and urine testing is especially important to the diabetic who is using insulin and must adjust the daily insulin dose according to test results (61, 73). Several studies have indicated that many diabetics either do not perform glucose tests properly or do not interpret the color changes properly (146–149). As a rule, insulin doses should never be adjusted according to urine glucose test results because the test only indicates whether there has been a blood glucose increase (but not a decrease) in the past, by virtue of sugar accumulation in the urine when blood glucose exceeds the renal threshold (73). One study demonstrated that the unpredictability of Clinitest in the critically ill was caused not only by error, but also by a changing rate of renal glucose reabsorption (148). It was concluded that blood glucose values are essential to rational dosing of insulin in the critically ill patient. Blood glucose monitoring using available home blood glucose tests is a more reliable indicator of diabetes control and, when used alone or in combination with urine glucose and ketone testing, should provide the patient with the information needed to make decisions concerning therapy changes and improve the overall control of blood sugars.

In ambulatory diabetics who have a relatively normal renal threshold for glucose (160–200 mg/100 ml), urine glucose testing is one means of determining diabetic control. The renal glucose threshold varies among individuals. In older patients, renal glucose thresholds increase. Conditions other than diabetes that may cause glucosuria are pheochromocytoma, acute pancreatitis, ingestion of very large amounts of glucose and other reducing sugars (fructose, lactose, and galactose), acromegaly, and Cushing's syndrome. Other factors that may cause unreliable urine glucose determinations include residual urine (prostate hypertrophy) and neurogenic bladder, which is a complication of diabetes that prevents the collection of urine specimens at the correct time. Urine glucose testing as the sole method of self-monitoring is recommended only for patients who cannot or will not perform blood glucose monitoring. This includes individuals who refuse to lance themselves, cannot be taught proper technique, or who are otherwise unreliable and noncompliant (61).

Blood glucose monitoring is considered by many to be the most accurate way for ambulatory diabetics to determine diabetic control. The tests are not dependent on renal glucose threshold, can be performed relatively easily, and indicate the blood glucose level at the point when the test is performed. It must be remembered that blood glucose levels are approximately 15% lower than whole blood levels reported by laboratories (61).

Routine testing for urine ketones is advised for all diabetics who use insulin. The urine should be tested for ketones whenever the blood glucose levels are greater than 200–250 mg/dl and during periods of illness or stress (61). The presence of ketones on two or more consecutive urine ketone tests should be reported to the physician.

Numerous factors should be considered in selecting a product to test the urine or blood of a diabetic. (See Chapter 4, *In-Home Diagnostic Products*.)

Diabetes Category

The type of diabetes is a major factor in determining which method of blood glucose self-monitoring to recommend. Brittle patients obviously need to test more often than stable Type II patients.

Patient Ability and Motivation

Patients unable to perform the more complex tests should be assisted or instructed in the use of one of the less complex tests, even though they are not as quantitative. The patient's willingness to learn and perform the more complicated test (Clinitest rather than TesTape or Diastix) should also be considered. The patient's willingness and ability to learn and perform the tasks associated with using strips and a monitor are also factors in the selection of home blood glucose tests.

Physical Handicaps

Patients with poor vision, which is common with diabetes, may be unable to see the Clinitest drops and therefore would have difficulty performing the tests. Special kits are available for visually impaired diabetics. Patients with trembling hands cannot perform the Clinitest test correctly (145). Not only is there a problem in the accuracy of the test results with these patients, but the tablets contain sodium hydroxide, and the test solution could be caustic if it were accidentally splashed on the skin. Patients with poor vision may also have problems interpreting the color changes on the visually read blood glucose monitoring strips. A recent study indicated that very few diabetics were able to accurately match the strips to the corresponding color chart, especially if the lighting was poor. Diabetics who performed the color match using single-source direct lighting (table lamp) were more accurate (149). Patients who are visually impaired may be able to use blood glucose meters that have audio components.

Patients who are prone to ketosis should be taught to test their urine for glucose and ketones as well as to test their blood. Patients who show positive results for glucose in urine and blood tests should also test their urine for ketones. All diabetics should periodically test their urine for protein as a warning of nephropathy. Protein in the urine can be easily tested by using Albustix, Combistix, Chemstrip GP, or Uristix.

Blood Glucose Tests

The ability to achieve and maintain normal blood glucose levels helps to prevent or delay the complications of diabetes, particularly retinopathy and nephropathy, and is the major objective of blood glucose monitoring (150). The speculations concerning the benefits of tight control are supported by research with patients using daily self-monitoring of blood glucose (150–153).

Evaluations of patients who monitor their own blood glucose have shown the following (154, 155):

- Patients were motivated to maintain their blood glucose within normal range by frequently checking blood glucose at home. Consequently, they became eager to regulate their daily lives. This positive attitude was observed in all cases.

- The method encouraged patients to become more involved in dietary control.

- Because blood glucose and urine glucose were checked simultaneously, the relationship between the two became obvious. The renal threshold for blood glucose could be demonstrated.

- Because the patient checked blood glucose daily instead of occasionally, more information on diabetic control became available, which facilitated proper insulin dosage. Adjustment of insulin dosage could be made with confidence.

- The metabolic disorder could be normalized quickly.

Maintenance of blood glucose control is impossible without measurement, and because it is convenient and less costly for the patient, self-monitoring of blood glucose is highly recommended for all types of diabetics. Even though a few diabetics are not candidates for self-monitoring of blood glucose, others enthusiastically follow protocol if sophisticated, intelligent training is provided. Eventually, most diabetics will test their blood glucose levels. Proper education of the diabetic concerning self-monitoring methods and the differences between individual meters, the importance of multiple daily tests, and interpretation of test results may motivate more patients to routinely self-monitor their blood glucose levels. The following types of diabetics should be strongly encouraged to self-monitor their blood glucose levels:

- Patients with abnormal or unstable renal thresholds;

- Patients with renal failure;

- Unstable, Type I diabetics;

- Patients with impaired color vision;

- Patients who have trouble with urine testing;

- Patients who have difficulty recognizing the symptoms of true hypoglycemia;

- Pregnant diabetics;

- Patients using nontraditional methods of injecting insulin;

- Patients who prefer self-monitoring of their own blood glucose (155).

Blood glucose monitoring is the most accurate test a patient can perform to determine the level of management of the diabetic condition.

Calibrated Blood Glucose Tests

Most blood glucose monitoring systems use reagent strips that are impregnated with glucose oxidase, which reacts with glucose and produces H_2O_2. This reaction produces a colorimetric reaction that quantitates the concentration of glucose. There are no medications that cause false readings of the glucose oxidase reagent strips. The strips can be divided into two types: visually read and meter-read. The first type is read visually. The patient places a drop of blood on the reagent strip and waits 30–60 seconds before wiping or washing off the blood, then waits an additional period of time, usually 1 minute, and either compares the color on the strip to the color chart on the side of the bottle containing the strips or uses a color meter chart (the Match Maker). The color strip must be compared with the chart immediately because the reliability of the test strip color decreases rapidly. If the test is conducted properly, a highly accurate result can easily be achieved. Visually read strips are listed in the product reference tables.

The second method of self-monitoring of blood glucose uses strips in conjunction with a blood glucose meter. Several strips can be placed into a corresponding meter with a resulting visual (or audio) readout of the blood glucose. Two monitoring systems use an amperometric measurement system that uses strips but does not require the blood to be removed from the strip before the glucose level can be determined.

A new system has been developed that uses a blood glucose sensor rather than strips. The sensor is part of the meter itself and is changed once every 30 days; patients may self-monitor blood glucose several times a day for the entire month. A drop of blood is placed on the sensor, resulting in a visual readout. Only one meter using this technology is currently available.

Several diabetics have reported that they prefer knowing the specific blood glucose level rather than the range that is obtained with visually read strips. Many patients who begin by reading visually and then go to a meter may find that their ability to read visually was not good and prefer the meters (149). All of the available meters provide a digital readout of the blood glucose; several have memories for later recall of recent blood glucose levels and may or may not give a printout of the retained data. The meters can be compared with reference to size, timing devices, calibration, accuracy, ease of use, memory or data management, printout features, battery types, need for cleaning, accessories required, audio capabilities, training or teaching materials, price, and manufacturer's dependability and availability.

Any blood glucose monitoring method that is recommended to the patient must be flexible and easily incorporated into the patient's daily lifestyle or routine. If the meter selected is too complex or requires more dexterity than the patient is capable of, it will not be useful. Patients should be encouraged to try several meters before selecting one for home use.

When the blood glucose equipment is used properly, calibrated frequently, and interpreted correctly, the accuracy is stated to be approximately plus or minus 10% (155). Test strips should be stored at room temperature. Bottle caps should be replaced immediately and tightly after a strip has been removed.

In addition to these test devices, patients also should purchase alcohol swabs or cotton balls and alcohol, blood lancets and lancet holders, and other accessory items (see product selection table). Cost may be a factor for some patients. Most insurance companies, under provisions of major medical plans, will reimburse patients for all or part of the cost of home glucose monitoring devices (4). Pharmacists should ensure that diabetics using blood glucose monitoring devices are properly trained initially and should occasionally have the patient demonstrate technique to ensure accuracy and proficiency. Pharmacists who become distributors for the blood glucose testing devices should contact the manufacturer to receive the necessary training to assist diabetics in the use of the devices.

Urine Glucose Tests

There are two methods of testing for glucose in the urine: copper reduction tests (Clinitest), and glucose oxidase tests (dip-and-read tests). In the copper reduction tests, cupric sulfate (blue) in the presence of glucose yields cuprous oxide (green to orange). Copper reduction tests are not specific for glucose and may detect the presence of other reducing substances in the urine. Care must be exercised when using the copper reduction test materials because the tablets and solutions are very caustic, and handling or splashing should be avoided. The tablets can be very dangerous if accidentally ingested and must be kept out of the reach of children. This method of testing has a "pass through phenomenon," which may result in improper interpretation of the results. The patient must watch the reaction develop because if the urine contains more than 2% glucose, the reaction may go "past" green to orange very quickly and then fade back to brown, which may be erroneously interpreted as less than 2%.

A second method is based on the enzyme glucose oxidase. Glucose in the urine in the presence of glucose oxidase yields gluconic acid and peroxide (H_2O_2), which, in the presence of *o*-toluidine, results in a color change and is the basis of glucose oxidase tests. The glucose oxidase test is more convenient and less expensive than the copper reduction test, although the test strips can be affected by humidity and are not as easily read. Patients must be specifically trained to use any of the urine testing products, and the pharmacist should occasionally have the patient demonstrate technique to ensure accuracy and proficiency. Patients must consider the accuracy, sensitivity, range, ease of testing and timing, availability of tests, multitest kits versus individual test kits, and cost when purchasing urine test kits.

Patients who are taking drugs that can interfere with urine glucose testing methods should be instructed to test their urine using both the copper reduction methods and glucose oxidase methods (Tables 12–15). If the test results differ, there is a strong possibility that a drug is interfering with the test results. Table 16 summarizes the disadvantages of urine glucose testing compared with blood glucose monitoring.

TABLE 13 Minimal concentrations of chemicals that produce false glucose oxidase reactions

Chemical	Concentration in urine (mg/ml)	False-positive or false-negative
Homogentisic acid	0.05	False-negative
L-Dopamine	0.6	False-negative
Levodopa	2.5	False-negative
Methyldopa	5.0	False-negative
5-Hydroxytryptophan	1.0	False-negative
5-Hydroxytryptamine	1.0	False-negative
Cysteine	9.0	False-negative
Glutathione	9.0	False-negative
Sodium bisulfate	5.0	False-negative
Glucuronic acid conjugates	20	False-negative
Glucose hypochlorite		False-positive
Chlorine		False-positive
Peroxide		False-positive
Hydrogen peroxide		False-positive
Ascorbic acid	0.08	False-negative
Gentisic acid	0.05	False-negative
5-Hydroxyindole acetic acid	0.25	False-negative

From *Contemp. Pharm. Prac.*, *3*, 224–225 (1980).

TABLE 12 Substances interfering with glucose oxidase tests

FALSE-POSITIVE

Chloride	Hydrogen peroxide
Glucose hypochlorite	Peroxide

FALSE-NEGATIVE

Alcaptonuria	5-Hydroxyindole acetic acid
Ascorbic acid	5-Hydroxytryptamine
Aspirin	5-Hydroxytryptophan
Bilirubin	L-Dopamine
Catalase	Levodopa
Catechols	Meralluride injection
Cysteine	Methyldopa (Aldomet)
3,4-Dihydroxyphenyl-acetic acid	Sodium bisulfate
	Sodium fluoride
Epinephrine	Tetracycline (Tetracyn, Achromycin) with vitamin C
Ferrous sulfate (Feosol)	
Gentisic acid	
Glutathione	Uric acid
Homogentisic acid	

From *Contemp. Pharm. Prac.*, *3*, 224–225 (1980).

TABLE 14 Substances interfering with copper-reduction tests that give false-positive results

FALSE-POSITIVE

Ascorbic acid	Levodopa
Cephaloridine	Metaxalone (Skelaxin)
Cephalothin	metabolite
Dilute urine	Methyldopa
Gentisic acid (aspirin)	Penicillin
Glucuronic acid conjugates	Probenecid (Benemide)
Homogentisic acid	Reducing sugars
Isoniazid	Salicylates
Lactose in pregnant women	Streptomycin

From *Contemp. Pharm. Prac.*, *3*, 224–225 (1980).

TABLE 15	Minimal concentrations of chemicals that produce false copper reduction reactions	
Chemical	**Concentration in urine (mg/ml)**	**False-negative or false-positive**
Isoniazid	5	False-positive
Streptomycin	5	False-positive
Cephaloridine	5	False-positive
Cephalothin	5	False-positive
Fructose	10	False-positive
Galactose	10	False-positive
Lactose	10	False-positive
Maltose	10	False-positive
Penicillin	10,000 U/ml	False-positive

From *Contemp. Pharm. Prac.*, *3*, 224–225 (1980).

TABLE 16   Disadvantages of urine glucose tests

1. Inability to detect low blood sugar (hypoglycemia)
2. Many possible drug interferences
3. Patient variance with reference to renal threshold for glucose
4. Urine retention in bladder
5. Lack of correlation between urine and blood glucose levels
6. In some patients, difficulty in reading and performing tests
7. More privacy than blood testing
8. Inability to detect how high blood glucose really is

Tests for Urinary Ketones

Because ketones in the blood overflow into the urine, urinary ketone levels can be tested to detect whether ketoacidosis is occurring. All diabetics should be counseled on the proper testing for ketones in the urine. The basis for the test is that sodium nitroprusside alkali turns lavender in the presence of acetone or acetoacetic acid.

Acetest reagent tablets are specific for acetoacetic acid and acetone. Acetest will not react with beta-hydroxybutyric acid/100 ml in urine. In serum plasma or whole blood, Acetest will detect 10 mg of acetoacetic acid/100 ml.

Ketostix, Chemstrip K, and others will detect 5–10 mg of acetoacetic acid/100 ml of urine. The test is easier than Acetest to perform, and no dropper is required (156). The new improved Ketostix only tests for acetoacetic acid and thus shows a false-negative result if the patient produces acetone or beta-hydroxybutyric acid. It is also difficult to find a substance at home to test the reliability of the Ketostix. Acetest can be tested for reliability by using nail polish remover that contains acetone.

Biotel/Diabetes Home Screening Test (American Diagnostics) is an extremely sensitive test used to detect glucose in the urine. It is a screening test for the presence of glucose in the urine, but is not a conclusive test for diabetes. Patients are instructed to report positive results to their physicians. The detection of glucose is based on the glucose oxidase–peroxidase–chromogen reaction. The test strips contain a control pad that should not change color and a test pad. Color fields on the container correspond to ranges of glucose con-

centrations. The primary source of error for this test is when a large amount of ascorbic acid is present in the urine; antibiotics may lead to lower or false-negative results. False-positive results may be caused by a residue of cleansing agents containing peroxide.

Tests for Other Chemicals

Several products are available that test urine for pH, protein, glucose, acetone, bilirubin, blood, and urobilinogen. Although these multiple tests are more commonly used in physicians' offices, diabetics may be instructed to use one of these reagents to test for various chemicals in the urine that may indicate the degree of diabetic control. Fresh urine is required in all tests. Urine may be refrigerated for a short time (up to 4 hours before testing) but the actual test must be performed with the urine at room temperature.

Identification Tags

All diabetics should wear identification bracelets, necklaces, or tags, or carry identification cards. This identification may be lifesaving if hypoglycemia or ketoacidosis occurs. If a diabetic becomes unconscious through an accident or hypoglycemic or hyperglycemic coma, medications regularly taken by the patient may be missed. A hypoglycemic (insulin) reaction may be confused with drunkenness; there have been reports of diabetics being jailed rather than given medical care (120).

An identification tag that can be seen easily on any diabetic should indicate that the person is diabetic and receiving medication. A diabetic identification card should include the person's name, address, and telephone number, the amount and type of medication used, the name of the patient's physician, and how the physician can be contacted.

The MedicAlert Identification bracelet may be obtained from MedicAlert Foundation, P.O. Box 1009, Turlock, Calif. 95380.

Recommendations for Travel

Diabetic patients should always take enough supplies for the entire trip plus one week. Patients should always carry an extra vial of insulin to ensure they have insulin derived from the same protein source. If traveling abroad, diabetic patients should ensure they have an adequate number of syringes because U-40 syringes are the most common type available in foreign countries. Diabetics should control their diets carefully, allow time for physical activity, and also carry candy or sugar to combat possible hypoglycemic attacks. Patients should not travel with prefilled syringes as they may be accidentally jarred and the dose wasted; they should also carry one or two glucagon kits and instructions for use.

All diabetics, and especially those who travel, should carry an identification card or wear an identification bracelet that indicates they have diabetes and are not intoxicated in the event that a hypoglycemic attack occurs. Many organizations recommend that diabetics traveling in countries where English is not the dominant language carry the names of English-speaking physicians in each city they will be visiting (157). Organizations that help locate physicians abroad for diabetics are listed in Appendix 1. Diabetics traveling to foreign countries must be able to communicate their medical needs. Although most metropolitan hotels have English-speaking employees, it is recommended that diabetics carry cards with some key phrases, such as "I am a diabetic," "Please get me a doctor," and "Sugar or orange juice, please," written in the dominant language of the countries to be visited (157). They should also carry a letter from a physician stating that they have diabetes, as well as stating other major medical problems, current medications by both brand and generic names, any problems; and information concerning medical insurance.

Diabetics changing time zones should carefully plan diet, exercise, and insulin adjustment. As a rule, changes in times zones of 2 hours or more will require adjustments of the insulin dose. The American Diabetic Association suggests that the diabetic traveler heading west use this formula to make a one-time adjustment: New NPH/Lente dose = usual NPH/Lente dose $\times$ (1 + number of time zones crossed/24). If headed east, the formula is New NPH/Lente dose = usual NPH/Lente dose $\times$ (1 − number of time zones crossed/24). Patients using a mixture of insulins or intensive therapy may not be able to use these formulas. Blood glucose monitoring frequency should be increased to ensure control (157, 158).

Diabetics should keep their insulin and syringes with them along with a glucagon kit rather than placing them in their luggage. Not only is this good practice in case luggage is lost, but also avoids exposing insulin and glucagon to extreme temperature changes in the luggage compartments of airplanes (157, 158).

Because the diabetic will probably need to increase the frequency of blood glucose monitoring as a result of changes in diet, activity, and meal schedules, they should also take extra batteries for the glucose meter, extra strips for the meter, a bottle of strips that can be read visually, alcohol wipes, cotton balls, and lancets. Even if the diabetic does not usually monitor the urine for ketones, it is advisable to do so while traveling.

The sale of syringes in various states differs. Some states have no regulations governing the sale of insulin syringes. In others, the sale of syringes must be made by a pharmacist. Certain states require a prescription for the purchase of syringes and needles. The diabetic should be aware that procedures may be different and take the appropriate precautions.

Nonprescription Products Affecting Diabetes

Reading the label on all food and drug products is essential to maintaining diabetic control. Patients should develop this habit early to avoid potential adverse effects.

Sugar-Containing Products

A list of sugar-free pharmaceutical preparations is useful so that the pharmacist may suggest a suitable sugar-free product for diabetic patients. (See Appendix 2, Sugar-free Preparations by Therapeutic Category.) For instance, cough preparations that contain simple syrup could have a clinically significant effect on a brittle insulinopenic diabetic. However, the amount of extra sugar ingested to relieve a cough would not be significant in most well-controlled diabetics. To put this in perspective, the difference between a large and small orange could include more sugar than would be found in 2 tsp of most cough syrups. Although sugar-containing medications may affect control in some diabetics, those who are properly educated to monitor their condition should have no clinically significant problem.

Many companies are promoting a number of products that are sugar-free and contain aspartame. These products are usually low in calories and fat. Each product must be evaluated individually, and if patients choose to include it in the diet, it must be accounted for in the overall meal plan.

Diabetics should read labels carefully to ensure that the dietetic product will fit into their diet plan. Many dietetic products cost much more than their nondietetic counterparts and actually have as many, if not more, calories.

Sympathomimetic Amines

Ephedrine, pseudoephedrine, phenylpropanolamine, phenylephrine, and epinephrine increase blood glucose and cause increased blood pressure by vasoconstriction. These substances should be used cautiously in diabetic patients. Sympathomimetic amines do not have as potent an effect on blood glucose as does epinephrine, which can stimulate glycogenolysis. Hyperglycemia, acetonuria, and glycosuria have been reported in three nondiabetic children who received therapeutic oral doses of phenylephrine (159–161). The major problem would occur in unstable Type I diabetics.

Salicylates

Aspirin products do not bear a warning statement for diabetics. However, aspirin in diabetics may cause hypoglycemia, possibly by stimulation of general cellular metabolism. In Type I diabetics, the degree of hypoglycemia resulting from large doses of aspirin (5 or 6 g) could stimulate a hypoglycemic reaction (59). However, the clinical significance of aspirin is questionable if a diabetic patient is monitoring for diabetes control. In addition, aspirin may cause misleading results in urine tests for glucose, but it is a dose-related phenomenon. False-negative glucose oxidase readings have been associated with doses of aspirin of approximately 2.5 g. Similar doses of aspirin can also cause false-positive glucosuria readings when the copper reduction test method is used.

DIABETIC PATIENT MONITORING

The therapeutic goal of diabetes treatment (drug, diet, exercise, education, and self-monitoring) is to control the patient's blood glucose. Diabetic patients vary considerably in their responses to therapy and in their adherence to prescribed instructions. The pharmacist can assist the patient in adhering to the prescribed regimen and in monitoring medications that may impair thinking, increase or decrease blood glucose levels, interfere with urine testing, or induce or contribute to complications. The pharmacist can also determine whether the patient has been thoroughly educated in self-care and self-monitoring. Because diabetic patients frequently see the pharmacist more often than any other health care professional, the pharmacist may be the "gate-keeper" for the rest of the medical community. The pharmacist may be the first health care professional to detect a problem related to an aspect of the diabetic patient's care and is frequently the one who refers the patients to other health care professionals for treatment and follow-up. The pharmacist is in an ideal position to develop a network of health care professionals whose specialty is diabetes.

Hoechst-Roussel Pharmaceuticals, Inc., has developed a three-page diabetic patient record form and diabetes condition analysis form to help the pharmacist monitor diabetic patients (Figures 3 and 4). The form is a patient profile checklist designed to monitor the drug therapy of the diabetic patient. The checklist enables the pharmacist to gather pertinent information about the patient, such as blood and urine glucose test results; blood pressure readings; prescribed therapy (special diet and therapy for concurrent diseases); and the patient's drug therapy, including a special section for recording insulin types, dosage, and dosage changes. The checklist may be used as the sole patient profile, or it may be used in conjunction with existing profiles.

Behavioral and Psychosocial Issues in Diabetes

Despite continuing gains in understanding diabetes, the state of knowledge remains insufficient to prevent the disease, cure it, or provide diabetic patients with optimally effective treatment. The search for a means of prevention and cure continues. However, there is a need to focus energies on easing the emotional burdens and improving the quality of life for diabetics and their families.

There is still hope for a cure; for a better way to control blood glucose; for a food that tastes great and is noncaloric; for an alternative sweetener that is safe; and for a health team that understands the varied emotional states of the diabetic patient and cares enough to provide honest, helpful, and informed information.

To be successful in the treatment program of diabetics, each health team member must be sensitive to the emotional problems encountered by patients.

Anxiety and depression are major emotions experienced by diabetic patients. This can be partially overcome by empathetic teachers in a well-planned educational program. After being exposed to the many aspects of diabetic education, the patient may feel confused and anxious. In a several-hour or even several-day program, the patient is exposed to a learning process that includes the causes and complications of diabetes, food types, diet exchanges, urine testing, blood testing, effects of exercise, insulin mixing and injection, rotation of injection sites, foot care, treatment of insulin reactions, travel tips, what to do during sick days, and miscellaneous ancillary products. The patient may have a high level of anxiety with reference to understanding the treatment aspects of diabetes and the daily regimen to be followed to keep diabetes under control.

Many diabetics live with fear because of the serious implications of the disease. Fear of an early death, the thought of suffering from diabetic complications, and the embarrassment of strange behavior or possibly convulsions during an insulin reaction may strongly affect behavior and decrease good diabetic control. For instance, patients who have suffered a serious insulin reaction often keep their blood glucose high to avoid a repeat episode.

Some diabetics try to "beat the odds" or "live each day to the fullest" and do not fully comply with the treatment regimen. Some patients may overindulge themselves and rationalize that having a chocolate shake, for example, will not cause a medical emergency, pain, or any other acute symptom. However, bad habits such as overeating are easily formed and difficult to break, leading to poor diabetic control. Often, diabetics feel guilty when they are noncompliant with the prescribed treatment protocol. However, if the treatment protocol is too stringent, it can cause frustration; there is seldom positive feedback as to whether the diabetic is following the proper procedures to maintain control and avoid complications. Blood glucose self-monitoring is one of the most significant advances in diabetes care in the past 40 years. With proper patient education, blood glucose self-testing allows the diabetic to tightly monitor blood glucose and regulate diet, exercise, and medications.

Living with the fear of complications, in addition to the daily demands of a rigorous medical regimen, is very stressful, not only for the diabetic but for the entire family. Many diabetics are subject to powerful, unpredictable mood and behavioral changes caused by metabolic imbalance (162). Moreover, chronic, nonmetabolic stresses associated with the disease include the need for diet management, rigid meal schedules, blood testing, various daily therapeutic decisions, insulin injections if required, and alterations in lifestyle. These stresses frequently result in significant emotional disequilibrium and occasionally in clinical psychiatric disorders. Impaired self-esteem is common (163). Denial, anxiety, hostility, and depression also occur and may impair interpersonal relationships at various levels.

Patient Education

Patient education is the key to success in controlling diabetes. Some diabetologists insist that the patient know as much about diabetes from the practical management aspect as the physician (164).

Education, periodic reeducation, and support systems from friends and family members are essential in fighting the burdens accompanying diabetes. Because diabetes is a particularly difficult disease for children and adolescents, it is especially important that positive steps be taken to help them understand their emotions. Diabetes is the only disease in which the young patient and the parents are expected to make independent therapeutic decisions based on daily clinical observations. Although this day-to-day control of the disease depends on the efforts of the patient and family members, it has been repeatedly demonstrated that an understanding of the disease and mastery of the necessary skills required are inadequate in a large proportion of diabetics and their families (163). Although improved understanding leads to improved care and outcome, there continues to be a need for accessible and well-designed education programs. These issues affect not only the patient but also the family, friends, teachers, employers, and the entire community of the diabetic. Clearly the emotional, social, economic, and public health problems of diabetes are enormous. The pharmacist plays a significant role in helping to overcome some of these problems.

Diabetic patients live with their disease 24 hours a day, so it is essential that they understand the condition and know when they are in trouble and need to call for help. Every diabetic patient should know the following:

- What diabetes is and why treatment is necessary;
- How to select the proper foods at each meal;
- How to test urine for sugar and acetone;
- How to test blood for glucose;
- How to administer and store insulin;
- The symptoms of uncontrolled diabetes and ketosis;
- The symptoms of hypoglycemia;
- The emergency treatment for hypoglycemia;
- When to return for follow-up;
- How to contact the attending physician, pharmacist, or emergency department;
- Precautionary measures while traveling;
- How to modify treatment for exercise or illness;
- How to care for the feet;

■ The dosage and time of administration of oral agents, if appropriate.

A team approach to patient education is essential. The physician explains the disease and the treatment objectives to the patient. The dietitian emphasizes the importance and methods of reaching and maintaining an ideal body weight. The diabetic nurse specialist usually trains the patient in using syringes and needles, mixing insulins, and injecting insulin subcutaneously; the nurse also gives advice on proper personal hygiene, foot care, urine testing techniques, and record keeping. The physical therapist teaches the patients to incorporate exercise into their daily lives, develops strategies to avoid the complications of exercise, and instructs the patients in the many benefits related to regular physical exercise.

Pharmacists play a special role in patient education with regard to mixing, storing, and injecting insulin. They also should be able to answer questions about the disease, blood and urine testing, record keeping, foot care, diet, treatment of cuts and scratches, the use of antihistamines and decongestants, products safe to use in weight control, and the alcohol and sugar content of both prescription and nonprescription drugs.

The pharmacist's role in patient education is significant. The challenge of understanding diabetic products and teaching patients how to use them properly has many benefits. Diabetic patient education methods have been summarized in some excellent articles available from major manufacturers (87, 108, 163, 165–172). Additional diabetes information sources for pharmacists and their patients are listed in Appendix 1. With the aid of this information, pharmacists should be prepared to discuss with patients any of the following topics:

■ The relationship among diet, exercise, and insulin;

■ The strength, dose, times of administration, and types of insulin;

■ The correct use of insulin syringes, needles, and dead space;

■ Diabetic diet and the prescribed caloric level;

■ Injection sites and proper site rotation;

■ Syringe preparation technique (insulin withdrawal and mixture);

■ Oral hypoglycemic agents (i.e., dosage and times of administration);

■ The availability and use of insulin infusion devices;

■ Blood and urine testing methods and techniques;

■ Urine testing times (Type I versus Type II diabetes);

■ Proper interpretation of testing results and record keeping;

■ Symptoms of possible hypoglycemic and hyperglycemic reactions;

■ Appropriate treatment of hypoglycemic and hyperglycemic reactions;

■ Proper identification, including diabetic information card and MedicAlert emblems;

■ Skin care, foot care, and personal hygiene.

Pharmacists who are interested in giving special care to diabetic patients can use a number of educational techniques.

Diabetic Care Center

To emphasize to diabetic patients that the pharmacist is truly concerned and interested in serving their needs, a clearly identified section may be established in the pharmacy. This diabetic care center should include a complete line of diabetic products: sugar-free food and drink products, nonprescription products safe for use by diabetics (sugar-free cough syrup), booklets about diabetes, and information about available diabetic services. An area also may be set up in which patients can practice testing their urine or blood and using syringes properly. Appendix 1 lists several publications that provide information to pharmacists interested in developing a diabetes care center.

Diabetic Detection Programs

Free diabetes testing kits may be distributed to pharmacy patrons. The American Diabetes Association may be helpful in providing information on how to set up a detection program. Some pharmacists set aside 1 or 2 days each month when patrons can be tested for diabetes in the pharmacy.

Diabetic "Hotline"

Pharmacists who are knowledgeable about diabetes may advise persons with questions concerning diabetes and diabetic products to call them for information.

Communication

Team effort and coordination are vital in patient education, and communication must be part of that effort. Pharmacists concerned about diabetes control should become involved in their local diabetes association or local Juvenile Diabetes Foundation. In addition, they should become familiar with community internal medicine specialists, family physicians, and pediatricians who treat diabetes and should develop a working relationship with them.

A system for communicating with diabetic patients may be developed. Using a diabetic patient drug monitoring checklist or merely a series of questions allows the pharmacist to show concern for the patient and gather information that may be helpful in monitoring the condition.

SUMMARY

Diabetes control requires team effort on the part of the physician, dietitian, nurse specialist, physical therapist, podiatrist, pharmacist, and patient. The pharmacist may play an important role by monitoring patient therapy and being informed about all aspects of the disease. Patient consultation should reinforce the patient's understanding of diabetes and should emphasize the importance of controlling blood glucose levels, testing blood and urine glucose levels, eating properly, exercising, and keeping accurate records.

Concerned pharmacists should join their local diabetes associations and consult recent literature to keep their knowledge up to date.

REFERENCES

1 R. A. Kerr, *New Environ. Pharm., 3 (2)*, 9 (1976).

2 A. R. VonSon, *Wellcome Trends Hosp. Pharm., 5 (3)*, 1 (1977).

3 L. Garrelts, *U.S. Pharmacist, 13 (11)* (suppl.), 4 (1988).

4 R. K. Campbell, "Current Concepts in the Treatment of Diabetes Mellitus," a continuing education program sponsored by the Washington State University College of Pharmacy and published by The Ames Company, Elkhart, Ind., 1980, p. 23.

5 "1977 Fact Sheet," Juvenile Diabetes Foundation, New York, N.Y., 1977.

6 "1985 Annual Report of the National Diabetes Advisory Board," Pub. No. (NIH)85-1587, U.S. Department of Health and Human Services, Rockville, Md., 1985.

7 "Diabetes in America," M. I. Harris and R. F. Hamman, Eds., Pub. No. (NIH)85-1468, U.S. Department of Health and Human Services, Rockville, Md., 1985.

8 D. W. Foster, in "Harrison's Principles of Internal Medicine," 11th ed., E. Braunwald et al., Eds., McGraw-Hill, New York, N.Y., 1987, pp. 1778–1796.

9 *Am. Drug., 176 (3)*, 54 (1977).

10 M. Ellenberg, *Pharm. Times, 40 (6)*, 56 (1974).

11 "1976 Fact Sheet," Juvenile Diabetes Foundation, New York, N.Y., 1976.

12 C. Kilo and J. Dudley, *Pharm. Times, 51 (10)*, 33 (1986).

13 R. K. Campbell, *U.S. Pharmacist, 13 (11)* (suppl.), 4 (1988).

14 R. Bonheim, *Diabetes Forecast, 38 (3)*, 32 (1985).

15 "1985 Fact Sheet," Juvenile Diabetes Foundation, New York, N.Y., 1985.

16 S. Leichter, *Diabetes Care, 5,* 126 (1982).

17 M. A. Kimble, *J. Am. Pharm. Assoc., NS14,* 80 (1974).

18 National Diabetes Data Group, *Diabetes, 28,* 1039–1057 (1979).

19 P. H. Forsham, in "Diabetes Rounds," Medcom, New York, N.Y., 1973, p. 8.

20 L. J. Melton et al., *Diabetes Care, 6,* 75–86 (1983).

21 J. Palmer, "Diabetes Update," Vol. 1, Diabetes Education Center, Deaconess Hospital, Spokane, Wash., 1977, p. 1.

22 J. H. Karam, in "Current Medical Diagnosis and Treatment," M. A. Krumpp and M. J. Chatton, Eds., Lange Medical, Los Altos, Calif., 1980, p. 749.

23 R. W. Bennett, *U.S. Pharmacist, 13 (11)* (suppl.), 6 (1988).

24 K. D. Hepp, *Diabetologia, 13,* 177 (1977).

25 O. G. Kolterman et al., *J. Clin. Invest., 68,* 957 (1981).

26 D. Porte and J. B. Halter, in "Textbook of Endocrinology," 6th ed., W. B. Saunders, Philadelphia, Pa., 1981, pp. 716–843.

27 J. E. Gerich et al., *Annual Rev. Physiol., 38,* 353 (1976).

28 G. M. Grodsky, *J. Clin. Invest., 51,* 2047 (1972).

29 D. Porte and A. A. Pupo, *J. Clin. Invest., 48,* 2309 (1969).

30 J. E. Morley et al., *Am. J. Med., 83,* 533 (1987).

31 T. G. Skillman and M. Tzagournis, "Diabetes Mellitus," Upjohn, Kalamazoo, Mich., 1977, pp. 3, 14.

32 P. Hollander, *Postgrad. Med., 85 (4)*, 211 (1989).

33 W. E. Winter et al., *N. Engl. J. Med., 316 (6)*, 285–291 (1987).

34 R. K. Campbell, *Am. Pharm., Module 4, NS26 (5)*, 7–8 (1986).

35 J. E. Gerich, *Am. Fam. Physician, 16,* 85 (1977).

36 J. Skyler, *Diabetes Care, 2 (6)*, 499 (1979).

37 M. Brownlee et al., *N. Engl. J. Med., 318, (20)*, 1315 (1988).

38 N. Baumslag et al., *Diabetes, 19,* 664 (1970).

39 K. E. Sussman, *Pharm. Times,* 42 (Oct. 1987).

40 E. A. Vandervein, *Postgrad. Med. J., 64* (suppl. 3), 5–9 (1988).

41 M. E. Molitch, *Postgrad. Med. J., 85,* 4, 182 (1989).

42 C. R. Shulman, "The New Diabetic," American Family Physician—Monograph (Apr. 1979).

43 R. H. Ungar, *Med. Clin. North Am., 66 (6)*, 1317 (1982).

44 R. Bressler, *Drugs, 17,* 461 (1979).

45 M. B. Davidson, "Diabetes Mellitus Diagnosis and Treatment," John Wiley and Sons, New York, N.Y., 1981.

46 M. S. Torre et al., *Drug Intell. Clin. Pharm., 15,* 175 (1981).

47 V. Calamia and E. Quattrocchi, *U.S. Pharmacist, 12 (11)*, 58–74 (1987).

48 J. A. Colwell et al., *Metabolism, 34 (12)* (suppl. 1), 1 (1985).

49 J. A. Colwell et al., *Am. J. Med., 30,* 67–80 (1983).

50 S. M. Grundy, *J. Am. Med. Assoc., 256,* 2849–2858 (1986).

51 R. Ross, *N. Engl. J. Med., 314,* 400–500 (1986).

52 J. D. Ward, *Drugs, 36,* 279–286 (1986).

53 T. Koschinsky et al., *Diabet. Metab., 12,* 318–325 (1987).

54 M. R. Taskinen et al., in "Diabetes Complications: Early Diagnosis and Treatment," D. Andreani et al., Eds., John Wiley, Chichester, Mass., 1987, pp. 25–35.

55 G. Crepaldi and E. Manzato, *Postgrad. Med. J., 64* (suppl. 3), 10–12 (1988).

56 D. J. Betteridge, *Br. Med. Bull., 45 (1)*, 285–311 (1989).

Beiersdorf, Inc.
Medical Division, Beiersdorf AG
BDF Plaza
P.O. Box 5529
Norwalk, CT 06856-5526
203-853-8008

Numerous publications on diabetes management.

Boehringer Mannheim Diagnostics
9115 Hague Road
Indianapolis, IN 46250
800-858-8072

Numerous publications on diabetes management.

Eli Lilly and Company
Lilly Corporate Center
Indianapolis, IN 46285

Numerous publications on diabetes management.

Hoechst-Roussel Pharmaceuticals, Inc.
Pharmacy Affairs
Route 202-206 North
Somerville, NJ 08876
201-231-3128

Numerous publications on diabetes education.

Home Diagnostics, Inc.
6 Industrial Way West
Eatontown, NJ 07723
800-342-7226

Numerous publications on diabetes management.

International Diabetes Center
Park Nicollet Medical Foundation
5000 West 39th Street
Minneapolis, MN 55416
(in conjunction with: DCI Publishing
Diabetes Center, Inc.
Post Office 739
Wayzata, MN 55391)

Numerous publications on diabetes management and education.

The Joslin Diabetes Center
One Joslin Place
Boston, MA 02215

Numerous publications on diabetes education.

The Juvenile Diabetes Foundation
432 Park Avenue South
New York, NY 10016-8013

Numerous publications on diabetes education.

Lifescan, Inc.
A Johnson & Johnson Company
1051 South Milpitas Boulevard
Milpitas, CA 95035

"Blood Glucose Monitoring: For the Phases of Your Life," published for LifeScan, Inc., by Health Education Technologies.

Monoject, Division of Sherwood Medical
Dept. T.I., 1831 Olive Street
St. Louis, MO 63103

"Professional Outline: Diabetes and Pregnancy," Garvey.

The National Diabetes Information Clearing House
Westwood Building, Room 603
Box NDIC
Bethesda, MD 20205

Numerous publications on diabetes and diabetes education.

Novo-Nordisk Pharmaceuticals Inc.
100 Overlook Center, Suite 200
Princeton, NJ 08540
800-223-0872

Numerous publications on diabetes and diabetes education.

Pfizer Laboratories Division
Division of Pfizer Incorporated
2355 East 42nd Street
New York, NY 10017

Numerous publications on diabetes education and management.

A. H. Robins Company
1407 Cummings Drive
Richmond, VA 23261-6609
804-257-2000

"Self-Care Consulting Guide," a ten-section, 20-hour continuing pharmacy education program, 1988.

Squibb-Novo, Inc.
E. R. Squibb & Sons (Parent)
211 Carnegie Center
Princeton, NJ 08540-6213
206-987-5800

Terumo Medical Corp.
Terumo Consumer Products
P.O. Box 5589
Elkton, MD 21921
301-392-7274

U.S. Pharmacist
Jobson Publishing Corporation
352 Park Avenue South
New York, NY 10010
212-685-4848

"U.S. Pharmacist's Guide to Diabetes Management," *U.S. Pharmacist, 13 (11)* (suppl.), 1988.
"U.S. Pharmacist's Diabetes Supplement," *U.S. Pharmacist, 14 (11)* (suppl.), 1989.

The Upjohn Company
Kalamazoo, MI 49001

Numerous publications on diabetes education.

Washington State Department of Social and Health Services
Diabetes Control Program
LK-13
Olympia, WA 98594
206-586-2708

Numerous publications on diabetes education.

INFORMATION FOR PATIENTS

American Diabetes Association, Inc.
1660 Duke Street
Alexandria, VA 22314

Numerous publications on diabetes education. Monthly magazine for members.

Diabetes Care and Education
A practice group of the American Dietetic Association
208 South LaSalle Street
Suite 1100
Chicago, IL 60604-1003

Numerous publications on diabetes education.

American Pharmaceutical Association
2215 Constitution Avenue, N.W.
Washington, DC 20037
202-429-7524

"Eye Care for the Diabetic Patient," R. K. Campbell, 1980.
"Diabetic Self-Monitoring Checklist," R. K. Campbell, 1982.

The Ames Company
Division of the Miles Laboratories, Inc.
P.O. Box 70
Elkhart, IN 46514

Numerous publications on diabetes management.

Becton Dickinson
Becton Dickinson Consumer Products
Becton Dickinson and Company
One Becton Drive
Franklin Lakes, NJ 07417-1883

Diabetes I.D. Card
Insulin Reaction Wallet Card
Numerous publications on diabetes education and management.

Boehringer Mannheim Diagnostics
9115 Hague Road
Indianapolis, IN 46250

Numerous publications on diabetes.

Diabetes Self-Management
Subscription Department
42-15 Crescent Street
Long Island City, NY 10016-8013

Monthly publication.

DCI Publishing
Diabetes Center, Inc.
P.O. Box 739
Wayzata, MN 55391

Numerous publications, including slides and audio cassettes, on diabetes education and management.

Eli Lilly and Company
Lilly Corporate Center
Indianapolis, IN 46285

Numerous publications on diabetes management.

Herc, Inc.
P.O. Box 30090
Lincoln, NE 68503

"Diabetes—Living and Learning," a book for the adult with Type I or Type II diabetes, 1988.
"Diabetes—Stuff and More Stuff," a book for children with diabetes and their parents, 1988.

Hoechst-Roussel Pharmaceuticals, Inc.
Pharmacy Affairs
Route 202-206 North
Somerville, NJ 08876
201-231-3128

Numerous publications on diabetes education.

The Joslin Diabetes Center
One Joslin Place
Boston, MA 02215

Numerous publications on diabetes management.

The Juvenile Diabetes Foundation
432 Park Avenue South
New York, NY 10016-8013

"What You Should Know About Juvenile (Insulin-Dependent) Diabetes," plus numerous other brochures on subjects relevant to Type I diabetics.
"Having Children—A Guide for the Diabetic Woman," R. Hausknecht.
"What You Should Know about Insulin," C. Nechemias, 1984.

Kilo Diabetes & Vascular Research Foundation
777 South New Ballas Road
Ste. 321E
St. Louis, MO 63141

"Self Blood Glucose Monitoring for the Person with Diabetes Mellitus," C. Kilo, 1984.

LifeScan, Inc.
Mountain View, CA 94043

"Blood Glucose Monitoring: For the Phases of Your Life," published for LifeScan, Inc., by Health Education Technologies.

Medic Alert Foundation, International
P.O. Box 1009
Turlock, CA 95381

Medic Alert Emergency Medical Identification necklace or bracelet engraved with the patient's specific health problem and a wallet card. The patient's medical history is computerized and is available to emergency personnel 24 hours a day via a collect phone call to the Medic Alert Foundation.

Monoject, Division of Sherwood Medical
Department T.I., 1831 Olive Street
St. Louis, MO 63103

Numerous publications on diabetes education.

The National Diabetes Information Clearing House
Westwood Building, Room 603
Box NDIC
Bethesda, MD 20205

"Resource Directory for People with Diabetes," NIH Pub. No. 81-2158, 1981.
"The Diabetes Directory."

National Institute of Child
  Health and Human Development
Bldg. 31, Room 2A32
9000 Rockville Pike
Bethesda, MD 20205

"Understanding Gestational Diabetes: A Practical Guide to a Healthy Pregnancy," D. Thomas-Doberson et al., 1989.

Novo-Nordisk Pharmaceuticals Inc.
100 Overlook Center, Suite 200
Princeton, NJ 08540
800-223-0872

Numerous publications on diabetes management.

Pfizer Laboratories Division
Division of Pfizer Incorporated
2355 E. 42nd Street
New York, NY 10017

"Learning to Live with Diabetes (noninsulin-dependent)," published for Pfizer Pharmaceutical Division by Medicine in the Public Interest.

Squibb-Novo, Inc.
120 Alexander Street
Princeton, NJ 08540

"Love Your Feet," 1986.

The Upjohn Company
Kalamazoo, MI 49001

Numerous publications on diabetes.

USP Convention Incorporated
USP-DI
12601 Twinbrook Parkway
Rockville, MD 20852

"A Guide to the Use of Oral Antidiabetic Medicines," 1980.
"A Guide to the Use of Insulin," 1980.
"A Guide to the Use of Glucagon," 1980.
"About Your Medicines," 1989.

ADDITIONAL SUGGESTED READING

The pharmacist should contact the local diabetes association for brochures to provide to diabetics with information concerning membership and activities.

General Information about Diabetes

"Diabetes: A Practical New Guide to Healthy Living," featuring the HCF Diet Program, J. W. Anderson, Arco Publishing, New York, N.Y., 1981.

"The Diabetic's Book. All Your Questions Answered," J. Biermann and B. Toohey, J. P. Tarcher, Los Angeles, Ca., 1981.

"The Diabetic's Total Health Book," J. Biermann and B. Toohey, J. P. Tarcher, Los Angeles, Ca., 1980.

"Diabetes—A New and Complete Guide to Healthier Living for Parents, Children and Young Adults Who Have Insulin-Dependent Diabetes," L. Ducat and S. S. Cohen, Harper and Row, New York, N.Y., 1983.

"Contemporary Issues in Nutrition: Diabetes Mellitus," L. Jovanovic and C. M. Peterson, Alan Liss, New York, N.Y., 1985.

"Joslin Diabetes Manual," 11th ed., L. P. Krall, Ed., Lea and Febiger, Philadelphia, Pa., 1978.

"The Diabetes Self-Care Method," L. Jovanovic and C. M. Peterson, Simon and Schuster, New York, N.Y., 1984.

"Joslin Diabetes Manual," L. Krall, Ed., Lea and Febiger, Philadelphia, Pa., 1978.

"A Diabetic Doctor Looks at Diabetes, His and Yours," P. Lodewick, RMI Corporation, Cambridge, Mass., 1982.

"Diabetes Mellitus . . . What's It All About?" S. Milchovich et al., Anaheim Memorial Hospital, California Community Health Education Center, Anaheim, Ca., 1982.

"Diabetes: Controlling It the Easy Way," S. Mirsky and J. R. Heilman, Random House, New York, N.Y., 1981.

"Juvenile Diabetes—Adjustment and Emotional Problems," New Jersey State Department of Health, Diabetic Control Program, P.O. Box 1540, Trenton, N.J. 08625. Single copies free.

"Journey of a Diabetic," L. M. Pray and R. Evans, Simon and Schuster, New York, N.Y., 1983.

"Taking Charge of Your Diabetes," C. M. Peterson, Just Mailings, P.O. Box 802, South Bend, Ind. 46624.

"Diabetes: Reach for Health and Freedom," D. F. Sims, C. V. Mosby, St. Louis, Mo., 1984.

"Living with Diabetes," G. J. Subal-Sharpe et al., Doubleday, Garden City, N.J., 1985.

"An Instructional Aid on Insulin-Dependent Diabetes Mellitus," L. Travis, American Diabetes Association Texas Affiliate, Inc., P. O. Box 14926, Austin, Tex. 78761, 1985.

Cookbooks for Diabetics

"More Calculated Cooking," J. Jones, 101 Productions, San Francisco, Ca., 1981.

"Sugar Free . . . That's Me!" J. Majors, Ballantine Books, New York, N.Y., 1980.

"Exchanges for all Occasions. Meeting the Challenge of Diabetes," F. Marion, Park Nicollet Medical Foundation, 4959 Excelsior Boulevard, Minneapolis, Minn. 55416, 1983.

"The Art of Cooking for the Diabetic," K. Middleton and M. A. Hess, Signet Books, New York, N.Y., 1979.

Exercise for the Diabetic Patient

"Fit or Fat?" C. Bailey, Houghton Mifflin, 1978.

"The Diabetic's Sports and Exercise Book," J. Biermann and B. Toohey, J. B. Lippincott, Philadelphia, PA, 1977.

"Diabetes and Exercise," M. Franz, International Diabetes Center, 1984.

"Complete Book of Exercise Walking," G. D. Yanker, Contemporary Books, 1983.

Pregnancy and Diabetes

"Diabetes and Pregnancy," J. Brooks et al., Media Library, The University of Michigan Medical Center, R4440 Kresge 3, Ann Arbor, Mich. 48109-0518, 1986.

"Treatment of Hypoglycemic Reactions During Pregnancy," M. T. Burkhart et al., Medical Library, Media Library, The University of Michigan Medical Center, R4440 Kresge 3, Ann Arbor, Mich. 48109-0518, 1986.

"Your Guide to a Healthy, Happy Pregnancy," L. Jovanovic, Biodynamics, Indianapolis, Ind., 1986.

New information is constantly being published to help diabetic patients control their condition. Pharmacists should ask the representatives of major pharmaceutical companies what information is available for them and their diabetic patients.

APPENDIX 2: SUGAR-FREE PREPARATIONS BY THERAPEUTIC CATEGORY

The following list of sugar-free preparations by therapeutic category was compiled by reviewing all of the preparations listed in the latest edition of *Drug Facts & Comparisons* (St. Louis: Facts & Comparisons, 1988). In addition, recent "sugar-free" lists were reviewed, and labels of most of the compiled products were checked.

It is very important that each health care provider using this list realize that the manufacturers of these products frequently change the ingredients. It is thus *critical* that patients be instructed to read labels carefully and not assume that a product that was once sugar free will always be sugar free. In addition, patients should be instructed to look for sugar substitutes that are calorigenic. Just because a product is labeled as "dietetic" or "sugar free" does not mean that it is intended for use by a patient with diabetes. Many dietetic products are free of sucrose but contain dextrose, fructose, or sorbitol. Patients should also read labels of products to check for alcohol content.

Patients with diabetes who are ill are usually under stress and thus should be instructed to monitor their blood glucose levels more frequently. While the amount of sugar in a given dose of most medication is not enough to significantly change the treatment protocol, the following list contains sugar-free over-the-counter (roman type) and prescription (italic type) medications that are less likely to affect blood glucose levels.

Concentrated Aluminum Hydroxide Suspension, Roxane
Di-Gel Liquid, Plough
ENO Powder, Beecham Products
Gaviscon Liquid, Marion
Gelucil Liquid, Robins
Gelucil-M Liquid, Robins
Gelucil-M Tablets, Robins
Gelucil Tablets, Robins
Gelucil-II Liquid, Robins
Gelucil-II Tablets, Robins
Kolantyl Wafers, Lakeside Pharmaceuticals
Maalox Plus Suspension, Rorer
Maalox Plus Tablets, Rorer
Maalox Suspension, Rorer
Maalox TC Suspension, Rorer
Mallamint Chewable Tablets, Mallard
Marblen Tablets, Fleming
Mylanta Liquid, Stuart
Mylanta Tablets, Stuart
Mylanta-II Liquid, Stuart
Mylicon Drops, Stuart
Nephrox Suspension, Fleming
Phosphaljel Suspension, Wyeth
Riopan Plus Suspension, Ayerst
Riopan Suspension, Ayerst
Silain-Gel Liquid, Robins
Simeco Suspension, Wyeth
Tritracid Tablets, Trimen
Tritralac Liquid, 3M Personal Care Products
Tritralac Tablets, 3M Personal Care Products
WinGel Liquid, Winthrop-Breon
WinGel Tablets, Winthrop-Breon

ANALGESICS

Over-the-Counter
Buffaprin Tablets, Buffington
Buffinol Tablets, Otis Clapp
Children's Myapap, My-K Labs
Children's Panadol Drops, Glenbrook
Children's Panadol Liquid, Glenbrook
Children's Panadol Tablets, Glenbrook
Dolanex Elixir, Lannett
Myapap Drops, My-K Labs
St Joseph's Aspirin-Free Infant Drops, Plough
St Joseph's Aspirin-Free Elixir for Children, Plough
St Joseph's Aspirin-Free Liquid for Children, Plough
Tempra Tablets, Mead Johnson
Prescription
Meperidine HCL Syrup, Roxane
Morphine Sulfate Oral Solution, Roxane

ANTACIDS/ANTIFLATULENTS

Over-the-Counter
Alamag Suspension, Goldline
Aludrox Suspension, Wyeth
Calglycine Tablets, Rugby
Camalox Suspension, Rorer
Citrocarbonate Effervescent Granules, Upjohn

ANTIASTHMATICS/BRONCHODILATORS

Over-the-Counter
Tedral Elixir, Parke-Davis
Prescription
Aeroate Liquid, Fleming
Elixicon Suspension, Berlex
Elixophylline-GG Liquid, Forest
Lixolin Elixir, Mallard
Quibron Liquid, Bristol-Myers
Quibron Plus Elixir, Bristol-Myers
Slo-Phylline GG Capsules, Rorer
Slo-Phylline GG Syrup, Rorer
Theo-Organidin Elixir, Wallace
Theophylline Oral Solution, Roxane

ANTIDIARRHEALS

Over-the-Counter
Diasorb Liquid, Schering
Diasorb Tablets, Schering
More-Dophilus Powder, Freeda
Pepto-Bismol Chewable Tablets, Procter & Gamble
Pepto-Bismol Suspension, Procter & Gamble
Prescription
Antrocol Elixir, Poythress
Corrective Mixture w/Paregoric, Beecham Labs

Lomotil Liquid, Searle
Parepectolin Suspension, Rorer
Spasmophen Elixir, Lannett

ANTI-INFECTIVES

Prescription
Augmentin Oral Suspension, Beecham Products
Furadantin Oral Suspension, Norwich Eaton
Furoxone Liquid, Norwich Eaton
NegGram Suspension, Winthrop-Breon
Uticillin Tablets, Upjohn
Uticillin VK Tablets, Upjohn

CALCIUM PRODUCTS

Over-the-Counter
Biocal Chewable Tablets, Miles Labs
Biocal Tablets, Miles Labs
Calel-D Tablets, USV
Cal-Sup Instant 1000 Powder, 3M Personal Care Products
Cal-Sup Tablets, 3M Personal Care Products
Caltrate 600 Plus Iron Tablets, Lederle
Caltrate 600 Tablets, Lederle
De-Cal Tablets, Vortech
Oyst-Cal 500 Tablets, Goldline
Oystercal 500 Tablets, Nature's Bounty
Scooby-Doo Chewable Calcium Tablets, Vita-Fresh
Super Calcicaps Tablets, Nion
Super Calcium 1200 Capsules, Schiff

COUGH PREPARATIONS

Over-the-Counter
Anatuss Syrup, Mayrand
Breonesin Capsules, Winthrop-Breon
Cerose-DM Liquid, Wyeth
Codimal DM Syrup, Central
Colrex Cough Syrup, Reid-Rowell
Colrex Expectorant Syrup, Reid-Rowell
Conar Expectorant Syrup, Beecham Labs
Conar Syrup, Beecham Labs
Contact Jr. Liquid, SmithKline Consumer
Dexafed Cough Syrup, Hauck
Hytuss Tablets, Hyrex
Hytex 2X Capsules, Hyrex
Lanatuss Expectorant Liquid, Lannett
Naldecon-DX Adult Liquid, Bristol Labs
Naldecon-DX Pediatric Drops, Bristol Labs
Naldecon-EX Syrup, Bristol Labs
Nortuss II Expectorant Liquid, Vortech
Phanatuss Syrup, Pharmakon Labs
Scot-Tussin DM Liquid, Scot-Tussin
Scot-Tussin Syrup, Scot-Tussin
Silexin Cough Syrup, Clapp
Tolu-Sed DM Liquid, Scherer
Tricodene Liquid, Pfeiffer
Trimedine Liquid, Trimen
Trind DM Liquid, Mead Johnson

Prescription
Anatuss w/Codeine Syrup, Mayrand
Codiclear DH Syrup, Central
Colrex Compound Elixir, Reid Rowell
Dimetane-DX Cough Syrup, Robins
Entuss Expectorant Liquid, Hauck
Entuss Tablets, Hauck
Hycodan Syrup, DuPont
Hycomine Pediatric Syrup, DuPont
Hycomine Syrup, DuPont
Hycotuss Expectorant Liquid, DuPont
Kwelcof Liquid, BF Ascher
Potassium Iodide Solution, Roxane
Prunicodeine Liquid, Lilly
Ryna-C Liquid, Wallace
Ryna-CX Liquid, Wallace
Tolu-Sed Cough Syrup, Scherer
Tussadon Liquid, Rugby
Tussar-FX Cough Syrup, USV
Tussi-Organidin Liquid, Wallace
Tussirex Sugar-Free Liquid, Scot-Tussin
Tussi-R-Gen Expectorant Liquid, Goldline
Tuss-Ornade Liquid, SKF

DECONGESTANTS/ANTIHISTAMINES

Over-the-Counter
Alamine Liquid, Vortech
Belix Elixir, Halsey
Bromatap Elixir, Goldline
Chlorafed Liquid, Hauck
Chlor-Trimeton Tablets, Schering
Coryban-D Cold Capsules, Leeming Pacquin
Dimetane Decongestant Elixir, Robins
Dimetapp Elixir, Robins
Myhistine Elixir, My-K Labs
Novahistine Elixir, Lakeside Pharmaceuticals
Prenhist Elixir, Rugby
Ryna Liquid, Wallace
Sinutab Maximum Strength Nighttime Liquid, Warner-Lambert
Trind Liquid, Mead Johnson
Prescription
Anamine Syrup, Mayrand
Bromophen Elixir, Rugby
Midatapp Elixir, Vangard

FISH OIL PRODUCTS

Over-the-Counter
Marine 500 Capsules, Murdock
Marine 1000 Capsules, Murdock
Proto-Chol Capsules, Squibb
Sea-Omega 50 Capsules, Rugby

FLUORIDE PREPARATIONS

Prescription
Fluorinse Topical Rinse, Oral-B
Flura-Drops, Kirkman
Flura-Drops Topical Rinse, Kirkman
Flura-Loz Tablets, Kirkman
Flura Tablets, Kirkman
Gel-Kam Topical Gel, Scherer
Karidium Drops, Lorvic
Karidium Tablets, Lorvic
Karigel-N Topical Gel, Lorvic
Karigel Topical Gel, Lorvic
Luride Drops, Colgate-Hoyt
Luride Lozi-Tabs, Colgate-Hoyt
Phos-Flur Liquid, Colgate-Hoyt
Stop Topical Gel, Oral-B

GASTROINTESTINAL PRODUCTS

Over-the-Counter
Digestex Tablets, Pasadena
Hi-Vegi-Lip Tablets, Freeda
Prescription
Reglan Syrup, Robins

IRON PRODUCTS

Over-the-Counter
Beminal Stress Plus Tablets w/Iron, Ayerst
Centrafree Tablets, Nature's Bounty
Freedavite Tablets, Freeda
Geritol Complete Tablets, Beecham Products
K-Dec Tablets, Schein
Kovitonic Liquid, Freeda
LifeStage Stress Tablets for Women, Vicks Health Care
Monocaps Tablets, Freeda
Niferex Elixir, Central
Nu-Iron Elixir, Mayrand
Parview Tablets, Freeda
Vita-Plus H Liquid, Scot-Tussin
Yelets Tablets, Freeda
Prescription
Hemo-Vite Liquid, Drug Industries
Niferex Forta Elixir, Central
Nu-Iron Plus Elixir, Mayrand

LAXATIVES

Over-the-Counter
Agoral Emulsion, Parke-Davis
Colece Liquid, Bristol-Myers
Cologel Liquid, Lilly
Correctol Powder, Plough
Disonate Liquid, Lannett
Doxinate Solution, Hoechst-Roussel
Emusoil Emulsion, Paddock
Evac-Q-Kit, Adria
Evac-Q-Kwik, Adria
Fiberall Natural Flavor Powder, Rydelle Labs
Fiberall Orange Flavor Powder, Rydelle Labs

Haley's M-O Emulsion, Winthrop-Breon
Hydrocil Instant Powder, Reid-Rowell
Kondremul Plain Emulsion, Fisons
Kondremul w/Casara Emulsion, Fisons
Konsyl Powder, Lafayette
Metamucil Orange Flavor Effervescent Powder, Procter & Gamble
Metamucil Lemon Lime Effervescent Powder, Procter & Gamble
Metamucil Sugar-Free Orange Flavor Powder, Procter & Gamble
Metamucil Sugar-Free Powder, Procter & Gamble
Milkinol Emulsion, Kremers-Urban
Neoloid Emulsion, Lederle
Sodium Phosphate Solution, Roxane
Zymenol Emulsion, Houser

MISCELLANEOUS DRUG PREPARATIONS

Over-the-Counter
Chlorophyll Tablets, Freeda
Lipomul Liquid, Upjohn
PDP Liquid Protein, Wesley
Prescription
Bilivist Capsules, Berlex
Cabalith-S Syrup, Ciba
Chloral Hydrate Syrup, Pharmaceutical Associates
Pediapred Oral Liquid, Fisons
Mysoline Oral Suspension, Ayerst
Nicorette Gum, Merrell Dow
Serentil Concentrate, Boehringer Ingleheim

POTASSIUM PRODUCTS

Prescription
Cena-K Liquid, Century Pharmaceuticals
EM-K-10% Liquid, Econo Med
Gen-K Powder, Goldline
Kaochlor-Eff Effervescent Tablets, Adria
Kaochlor S-F Liquid, Adria
Kaon-Ol 20% Liquid, Adria
Kaon Liquid, Adria
Kay Ciel Liquid, Forest
Kay Ciel Powder, Forest
Kolyum Liquid, Pennwalt
Kolyum Powder, Pennwalt
Klor-10% Liquid, Upsher-Smith
Klor-Con/EF Effervescent Tabs, Upsher-Smith
Klor-Con Powder, Upsher-Smith
Klor-Con/25 Powder, Upsher-Smith
Klorvess Effervescent Tablets, Sandoz
*Potachlor 10% w/3.8% Alcohol, My-K Labs**
Potachlor 10% w/5% Alcohol, My-K Labs
Potachlor 20% Liquid, My-K Labs
Potasalan Liquid, Lannett
Potassine Liquid, Recseil
Potassine 10% Liquid, Recseil
Rum-K Liquid, Fleming
Tri-K Liquid, Century Liquid
Trikates Liquid, Lilly

SYSTEMIC ALKALINIZERS

Prescription
Bicitra Solution, Willen
Polycitra-K Solution, Willen
Polycitra-LC Solution, Willen

TOPICAL ORAL PRODUCTS

Over-the-Counter
Anbesol Gel, Whitehall
Anbesol Liquid, Whitehall
Babee Teething Lotion, Pfeiffer
Baby Orajel, Commerce
Chloraseptic Mouthwash & Gargle, Vicks Health Care
Choraseptic Throat Spray, Vicks Health Care
Larylgan Throat Spray, Ayerst
Moi-Stir Solution, Kingswood Labs
Moi-Stir Swabsticks, Kingswood Labs
Moi-Stir 10 Solution, Kingswood Labs
Mycinettes Lozenges, Pfeiffer
N-Ice Lozenges, Beecham Labs
Oracin Cherry Lozenges, Vicks Health Care
Oracin Lozenges, Vicks Health Care
Ora-Fresh Mouthwash, AVP
Orajel Brace-Aid Gel, Commerce
Orajel Brace-Aid Rinse, Commerce
Orajel/D, Commerce
Orajel Mouth-Aid Gel, Commerce
Phenaseptic Mouthwash & Gargle, Barre
Rid-A-Pain Gel, Pfeiffer
Rid-A-Pain Drops, Pfeiffer
Salivart Solution, Westport
Sucrets Maximum Strength Mouthwash & Gargle, Beecham
  Labs
Tanac Liquid, Commerce
Tanac Roll-On Stick, Commerce
Xero-Lube Solution, Scherer

URINARY TRACT PRODUCTS

Prescription
Bicitra Liquid, Willen
Polycitra-K Syrup, Willen
Polycitra-LC Syrup, Willen

VITAMINS AND MINERALS

Over-the-Counter
Anti-Oxidant Capsules, Murdock
Arcobee w/C Capsules, Nature's Bounty
Ascorbic Acid Tablets, Approved Pharm.
Ascorbin/II Tablets, Pasadena Research
B-100 Tablets, Nature's Bounty
Bugs Bunny Chewable Vitamin and Mineral Tablets, Miles
  Labs
Bugs Bunny Children's Chewable Tablets, Miles Labs
Bugs Bunny Children's Chewable Tablets w/Extra C, Miles
  Labs
Bugs Bunny Tablets Plus Iron, Miles Labs

Calcium Ascorbate Powder, Freeda
Calcium Ascorbate Tablets, Freeda
Calcium Pantothenate Tablets, Freeda
Cal-Prenal Improved Tablets, Vortech
Ceebevim Capsules, Nature's Bounty
Chelated Magnesium Tablets, Freeda
C Speridin Tablets, Marlyn
Daily-Vite w/Iron & Minerals Tablets, Rugby
Dayalets Filmtabs, Abbott
Dayalets Plus Iron Filmtabs, Abbott
Delta-D Tablets, Freeda
Dull-C Powder, Freeda
Flavons 500 Tablets, Freeda
Flintstones Children's Chewable Tablets, Miles Labs
Flintstones Children's Chewable Tablets w/Extra C, Miles
  Labs
Flintstones Complete Chewable Tablets, Miles Labs
Flintstones Tablets Plus Iron, Miles Labs
Hi-Po-Vites Tablets, Nature's Bounty
Ibex Therapeutic Tablets, Freeda
Liponol Capsules, Rugby
LKV Drops, Freeda
Marbec Tablets, Marlyn
Mega-B Tablets, Arco
Megadose Tablets, Arco
Multi-Thera Tablets, Nature's Bounty
Multi-Thera-M Tablets, Nature's Bounty
Multi-Vita Drops, My-K Labs
Multi-Vita Drops w/Iron, My-K Labs
Neo Vadrin B Complex "50" Tablets, Scherer
Neo Vadrin B Complex "100" Tablets, Scherer
Nova-Dec Tablets, Rugby
Nu-Thera Capsules, Kirkman
One-A-Day Essential Tablets, Miles Labs
One-A-Day Plus Extra C Tablets, Miles Labs
One-A-Day Stressgard Tablets, Miles Labs
Optivite Tablets for Women, Optimox
Poly-Vi Sol Infants' Drops, Mead Johnson
Poly-Vi-Sol w/Iron Drops, Mead Johnson
Polyvitamin Drops w/Iron, Rugby
Prenavite Tablets, Rugby
Quintab Tablets, Freeda
Quintabs-M Tablets, Freeda
Scooby-Doo Children's Chewable Tablets, Vita-Fresh
Scooby-Doo Children's Chewable Tablets Plus Iron, Vita-
  Fresh
Scooby-Doo Children's Chewable Tablets w/Extra C, Vita-
  Fresh
Scooby-Doo Children's Complete Formula Tablets, Vita-
  Fresh
Sodium Ascorbate Crystals, Freeda
Sodium Ascorbate Powder, Freeda
Sodium Ascorbate Tablets, Freeda
Span-C Tablets, Freeda
Spider-Man Children's Chewable Tablets, Nature's Bounty
Spider-Man Tablets Plus Iron, Nature's Bounty
Stress-Bee Capsules, Rugby
Surbu-Gen-T Tablets, Goldline
Super-C Tablets, Goldline
Theragran Jr. Children's Chewable Tablets w/Extra C,
  Squibb

Theravim Tablets, Nature's Bounty
Triple Vita Drops, My-K Labs
T-Vites Tablets, Freeda
Ultra B-50 Tablets, Nature's Bounty
Ultra B-100 Tablets, Nature's Bounty
Ultra-Freeda Tablets, Freeda
Unicap Capsules and Tablets, Upjohn
Unicap-M Tablets, Upjohn
Unicap Senior Tablets, Upjohn
Unicap-T Tablets, Upjohn
Variplex-C Tablets, Nature's Bounty
Vi-Daylin ADC Drops, Ross
Vi-Daylin ADC Vitamins Plus Iron Drops, Ross
Vi-Daylin Multivitamin Drops, Ross
Vi-Daylin Multivitamin Plus Iron Drops, Ross
Vita-Bob Capsules, Scot-Tussin
Vita-C Crystals, Freeda
Vital B-50 Tablets, Goldline
Vitamin B2 Tablets, Freeda
Vitamin B2 Tablets, Nature's Bounty
Vitamin D3 Tablets, Freeda
Vita-Plus E Capsules, Scot-Tussin
Vita-Plus G Capsules, Scot-Tussin
Vita-Plus H Capsules, Scot-Tussin
Within Tablets, Miles Labs
Ze Caps Capsules, Everett
Prescription
DHT Intensol Solution, Roxane
DHT Oral Solution, Roxane
Multi-Vita Drops w/Fluoride, My-K Labs
Polyvite w/Fluoride Drops, Geneva Generics
Triple-Vita-Flor Drops, My-K Labs
Vi-Daylin/F ADC Drops, Ross
Vi-Daylin/F ADC Plus Iron Drops, Ross
Vi-Daylin/F Drops, Ross
Vi-Daylin/F Plus Iron Drops, Ross

---

*Potachlor 10% Liquid with 3.8% Alcohol, My-K Labs, is also
available in a preparation containing sugar.

INSULIN PREPARATIONS PRODUCT TABLE

Product[a] (Manu-facturer)	Spe-cies[b] Source	Onset[c] (hrs.)	Peak[c] (hrs.)	Dura-tion[c] (hrs.)	pH	Buffer	Pre-serva-tive	Purity[d] ppm of Proin-sulin	Stabil-ity at Room Temp.[c] (mos.)	Zinc Content (mg/ 100 U)	Pro-tein (mg/ 100 U)
Rapid Acting											
Beef Regular Iletin II (Lilly)	B	0.5	2-4	6-8	neutral		meta-cresol	< 10	10-18	0.01-0.04	none
Humulin R (Lilly)	H	0.5	2-4	6-8	neutral		meta-cresol	NS[f]	NS[f]	0.01-0.04	none
Humulin BR[g] (Lilly)	H	0.5	2.4	6-8	neutral		meta-cresol	NS[f]	NS[f]	0.01-0.04	none
Insulin Velosulin (Novo-Nordisk)	P	0.5	1-3	8	7.3	sodium phos-phate, 2.4 mg/ml	meta-cresol, 0.3%	< 1	18	0.01-0.04	none
Novolin R Human Insulin (Novo-Nordisk)	H	0.5	2.5-5	6-8	neutral	none	phenol	≤ 1	24	none[h]	none
Novolin 70/30 (Novo-Nordisk)	H	0.5	2-12	24	neutral	phos-phate	phenol/meta-cresol	NS	NS	0.02	0.25
Pork Regular Iletin II (Lilly)	P	0.5	2-4	6-8	neutral		meta-cresol	< 10	10-18	0.01-0.04	none
Regular Iletin I (Lilly)	B, P	0.5	2-4	6-8	neutral		meta-cresol	< 50		0.01-0.04	none
Regular Insulin (Novo-Nordisk)	P	0.5	2.5-5	8	neutral	none	phenol	< 10	24	none[h]	none
Regular Puri-fied Insulin (Novo-Nordisk)	P	0.5	2.5-5	8	neutral	none	phenol	< 1	24	none[h]	none
Semi-lente Iletin I (Lilly)	B, P	1-2	3-8	10-16	neutral	acetate	methyl-para-ben	< 50	24	0.12-0.25	none
Semi-lente Insulin (Novo-Nordisk)	B	1.5	5-10	16	neutral	acetate	methyl-para-ben	< 10	24	0.15	none

INSULIN PREPARATIONS PRODUCT TABLE, continued

Product[a] (Manufacturer)	Species[b] Source	Onset[c] (hrs.)	Peak[c] (hrs.)	Duration[c] (hrs.)	pH	Buffer	Preservative	Purity[d] ppm of Proinsulin	Stability at Room Temp.[e] (mos.)	Zinc Content (mg/ 100 U)	Protein (mg/ 100 U)
Semilente Purified Insulin Zinc Suspension (Novo-Nordisk)	P	1.5	5-10	16	neutral	acetate	methyl-paraben	< 1	24	0.15	none
Intermediate Acting											
Beef Lente Iletin II[i] (Lilly)	B	1-3	6-12	18-36	neutral	acetate	methyl-paraben	< 10	24-30	0.12-0.25	none
Beef NPH Iletin II[j] (Lilly)	B	1-2	6-12	18-36	neutral	phosphate	phenol, meta-cresol	< 10	36	0.01-0.04	protamine, 0.3-0.5
Humulin N (Lilly)	H	1-2	6-12	18-24	neutral	phosphate	phenol/ meta-cresol	NS[f]	NS[f]	0.01-0.04	0.3-0.5
Humulin L (Lilly)	H	1-3	6-12	18-24	neutral	acetate	methyl-para-ben	NS[f]	NS[f]	0.12-0.25	none
Insulatard NPH (Novo-Nordisk)	P	1.5	4-12	24	7.3	sodium phosphate, 2.4 mg/ml	meta-cresol, 0.15% phenol, 0.06%	< 1	20	0.01-0.04	protamine, 0.32-0.36
Lente Iletin I[i] (Lilly)	B,P	1-3	6-12	18-36	neutral	acetate	methyl-paraben	< 50	18-20	0.12-0.25	none
Lente Iletin II (Lilly)	P	1-3	6-12	18-36	neutral	acetate	methyl-paraben	< 10	24+	0.12-0.25	none
Lente Insulin[i] (Novo-Nordisk)	B	2.5	7-15	24	neutral	acetate	methyl-paraben	< 10	24	0.15	none
Lente Purified Pork Insulin Zinc Suspension (Novo-Nordisk)	P	2.5	7-15	22	neutral	acetate	methyl-paraben	< 1	24	0.15	none

INSULIN PREPARATIONS PRODUCT TABLE, continued

Product[a] (Manu-facturer)	Spe-cies[b] Source	Onset[c] (hrs.)	Peak[c] (hrs.)	Dura-tion[c] (hrs.)	pH	Buffer	Pre-serva-tive	Purity[d] ppm of Proin-sulin	Stabil-ity at Room Temp.[e] (mos.)	Zinc Content (mg/ 100 U)	Pro-tein (mg/ 100 U)
Mixtard, NPH + Regular Insulin (Novo-Nordisk)	P	0.5	4-8	24	7.3	sodium phos-phate, 2.4 mg/ ml	meta-cresol, 0.15% phenol, 0.06%	< 1	20	0.01-0.04	pro-tamine, 0.22-0.25
Novolin L Human Insulin Zinc Suspension (Novo-Nordisk)	H	2.5	7-15	22	neutral	acetate	methyl-para-ben	≤ 1	24	0.15	none
Novolin N Human Insulin Isophane Suspension (Novo-Nordisk)	H	1.5	4-12	24	neutral	phos-phate	phenol, meta-cresol	≤ 1	24	0.02	pro-tamine, 0.35
NPH Iletin I[j] (Lilly)	B,P	1-2	6-12	18-36	neutral	phos-phate	phenol, meta-cresol	< 50	36	0.01-0.04	pro-tamine, 0.3-0.5
NPH Iletin II (Lilly)	P	1-2	6-12	18-36	neutral	phos-phate	phenol, meta-cresol	< 10	36	0.01-0.04	pro-tamine, 0.3-0.5
NPH (Isophane) Insulin[j] (Novo-Nordisk)	B	1.5	4-12	24	neutral	phos-phate	phenol, meta-cresol	< 10	24	0.02	pro-tamine, 0.43
NPH Puri-fied Pork Isophane Insulin Suspension (Novo-Nordisk)	P	1.5	4-12	24	neutral	phos-phate	phenol, meta-cresol	< 1	24	0.02	pro-tamine, 0.35
Sterile Diluting Fluid for Dilution of NPH Iletin (Lilly)			.		neutral	10% hydro-chloric acid and/or 10% sodium hydroxide	phenol, meta-cresol		36		

INSULIN PREPARATIONS PRODUCT TABLE, continued

Product[a] (Manufacturer)	Species[b] Source	Onset[c] (hrs.)	Peak[c] (hrs.)	Duration[c] (hrs.)	pH	Buffer	Preservative	Purity[d] ppm of Proinsulin	Stability at Room Temp.[e] (mos.)	Zinc Content (mg/ 100 U)	Protein (mg/ 100 U)
Long Acting											
Beef Protamine[k] **Zinc Iletin II** (Lilly)	B	4-6	14-24	26-36	neutral	phosphate	phenol	< 10	36	0.15-0.25	protamine, 1-1.5
Humulin U (Lilly)	H	4-6	8-20	24-28	neutral	acetate	methylparaben	NS[f]	NS[f]	0.12-0.25	none
Protamine Zinc Iletin I[k] (Lilly)	B,P	4-6	14-24	26-36	neutral	phosphate	phenol	< 50	36	0.15-0.25	protamine, 1-1.5
Protamine Zinc Iletin II (Lilly)	P	4-6	14-24	26-36	neutral	phosphate	phenol	< 10	36	0.15-0.25	protamine, 1-1.5
Ultralente Iletin I (Lilly)	B,P	4-6	14-24	28-36	neutral	acetate	methylparaben	< 50	24-30	0.12-0.25	none
Ultralente Insulin Zinc Suspension (Novo-Nordisk)	B	4	10-30	36	neutral	acetate	methylparaben	< 10	24	0.15	none
Ultralente Purified Beef Insulin Zinc Suspension (Novo-Nordisk)	B	4	10-30	36	neutral	acetate	methylparaben	< 1	24	0.15	none

INSULIN PREPARATIONS PRODUCT TABLE, continued

Miscellaneous	Description
B-D Glucose (Becton, Dickinson)	Tablets, chewable: glucose, 5 g. For the treatment of hypoglycemia.
Glucagon for Injection (Rx) (Lilly)	Used parenterally (subcutaneously, intramuscular, or intravenously) for treatment of hypoglycemia. Stimulates the conversion of liver glycogen to glucose. Intravenous glucose is drug of choice in hypoglycemia if available. To use, lyophilized glucagon is dissolved using accompanying solution and then injected.
Gluctose (Paddock)	(Paddock Laboratories, 3101 Louisiana Ave. North, Minneapolis, MN 55427.) Oral glucose (40% dextrose) solution used to treat insulin reaction (hypoglycemia) before unconsciousness occurs.
Insta-Glucose (ICN Pharmaceuticals, Inc.)	Liquid glucose (40% dextrose). A convenient plastic tube of carbohydrate gel for use by diabetics to treat hypoglycemic symptoms. Cherry flavor.
Instant Glucose	Oral glucose gel used to treat insulin reaction. Contains 30.8 grams liquid glucose in convenient plastic tube. Available from the Diabetes Association of Greater Cleveland, 2022 Lee Road, Cleveland, OH 44118.
Monoject (Sherwood)	Liquid glucose (40% dextrose). For the treatment of hypoglycemia. Lime flavor.

[a] Most insulins are available in U-40 (coded red) and U-100 (coded orange). The ultra-pure insulins by Novo-Nordisk and the Iletin II by Lilly are only available in U-100 strengths. Lilly also manufacturers a regular (concentrated) Iletin (prescription only) containing 500 units of pork insulin/ml; used in patients with marked insulin resistance.

[b] Insulins with a combination of beef and pork contain 70% beef and 30% pork; B, beef and P, pork; H, semisynthetic human insulin that is identical in structure to that produced by the human pancreas.

[c] Biologic response varies greatly in different individuals, so times are approximate.

[d] Purity of insulins is judged on a number of factors, but primarily on the parts per million of proinsulin. Conventional USP insulin can have 20-40,000 ppm. The single-peak insulins that were manufactured in the United States after 1975 contain between 300 and 3,000 ppm. The improved single-peak insulins available in the United States after 1980 contain approximately 50 ppm of proinsulin. The purified pork insulins from Novo-Nordisk and Lilly contain less than 10 ppm of proinsulin.

[e] Mix regular with NPH in any proportion; stable for 5 minutes only. With protamine zinc insulin, use at least twice as much regular. Intermix lentes in any proportion. Stable for long periods. Lente plus regular, use within 5 minutes.

[f] Not specified.

[g] For use with external insulin pump only.

[h] May contain traces of naturally occurring zinc in extracted pork insulin.

[i] Lente can be mixed with semilente or ultralente in any proportion and is stable for 2-3 months.

[j] NPH plus regular. Mix in any proportion; stable for 5 minutes only.

[k] One part protamine zinc insulin to two parts regular equals NPH, Ultralente 70% plus semilente 30% yields lente. Lentes mix in any proportion, stable for 2-3 months.

INSULIN SYRINGES AND RELATED PRODUCTS TABLE

Product (Manufacturer or Supplier)	Sizes Available or Description	Comments
SYRINGES		
Auto-Syringe AS 6C U-100 Insulin Infusion Pump (Auto-Syringes, Inc.)	9.5 oz battery-operated infusion pump is small enough to be inconspicuous and uses a 3 cc syringe available from the same company. Requires other equipment also available from the same company.	portable insulin delivery system. Pump may be programmed to operate as an open-loop insulin delivery system for control of diabetes. An adjustable control allows for a constant rate of infused insulin throughout the day. A push button allows a bolus of insulin before meals. This product is recommended for Type I diabetics.
Busher Auto Injector (Becton Dickinson)	connects to short-type reusable insulin syringe or with an adaptor to long type. Provides quick automatic insertion of the needle at proper depth and angle.	used in past to help patients overcome needle fear. Patients should be trained to overcome emotional factors.
CPI/Lilly Insulin Infusion Pump-Model 9200 (Betatron)	5.75 oz battery-operated insulin infusion pump that provides a constant infusion of insulin to the patient. Bolus doses can be given before meals and snacks. Syringes and infusion sets are provided by CPI.	small, easy to use. Does not require mixing of insulin with diluting fluid. Has several functions not provided by other pumps. Excellent alarm system, high quality. It provides a summary of insulin units given over a period of time. Manufacturer dependability and support is excellent.
Insulin Syringe, Single Use Lo-Dose (Becton Dickinson)	0.5 cc with 28 G½″ needle. 30/package and 100/package.	cannot change needle size. Used for patients taking less than 50 units of U-100 insulin. Larger print of calibration allows more accurate dosing. Can be used up to 3 times.
Medi-Jector (Derata Corp)	high-quality needleless jet injector. Can deliver from 1 to 100 units per injection.	powered by a series of springs. Somewhat cumbersome in design. Bottle of insulin attaches to the device and once the dose is selected, it can be easily used by visually impaired diabetics. Dose changes can be made in increments of 1 unit.
Mill Hill Infuser Insulin Pump (Harvard Apparatus)	10 ½ oz battery-operated lightweight insulin infusion pump that uses a 6-ml Monoject disposable syringe. Catheters, needles, battery chargers and other equipment are also available from the company.	pump designed to administer insulin continuously throughout the day. A bolus of insulin is injected before each meal. Insulin provided by infusion pumps must be diluted and the patient needs to check his/her own blood glucose levels periodically. Somewhat larger than competition's product. Recommended for Type I diabetics.
Monoject Insulin Syringe (Kendall-Futuro)	1 cc with self-contained 27 G½″ needle. U-40 and U-100. 30/package or 100/package. 27 G⅝″ available in U-100. 0.5 cc for patients using 50 units or less of U-100 insulin.	bold numbers, preferred needle gauge, virtually no dead space, sterile. New "A" level needle point, electropolished with a polymer coating.
Novolin Pen (Novo-Nordisk)	lightweight dial-a-dose insulin delivery device, made from durable plastic polymer. Designed to resemble a fountain pen, it is 6 ½″ in length and 5 oz in weight. It utilizes a 1.5-ml cartridge of human insulin, delivering 2 to 36 units of insulin in 2-unit increments by a push button/plunger mechanism. The mean dosage accuracy is 99.5% and the coefficient of variation is 2.5% for a single dose.	

INSULIN SYRINGES AND RELATED PRODUCTS TABLE, continued

Product (Manufacturer or Supplier)	Sizes Available or Description	Comments
NovoPen (Novo-Nordisk)	made of nickel and chromium plated brass, is 6″ in length and 7 oz in weight. Designed to resemble a fountain pen, it utilizes a replaceable 1.5-ml cartridge of human insulin, delivering 2 or more units by a push-button mechanism. The standard deviation for a dose is 0.1 units.	
PenNeedle (Novo-Nordisk)	beveled and siliconized throughout its length to ensure minimal friction with the skin. Each *PenNeedle* is 27 gauge, one-half (½) inch, (12.5 mm) in length and is intended for single use only. The disposable needles are specifically designed for use with the *NovolinPen* Insulin Delivery System. The self-contained disposable single-use needle consists of a protective plastic outer cap, a smooth plastic needle cap and a protective tab. The needle should not be used if the protective tab is missing or damaged.	
Plastipak Self Contained Insulin Syringe (Becton Dickinson)	1 cc with 28 G½″ in U-40 and U-100. 1 cc with 27 G½″.	no dead space. Excellent for travel. More expensive than reusable but sterile and convenient. Less pain with 27½ G. Can be reused up to 3 times.
Single Use, Long Type (Becton Dickinson)	2 cc U-10, 30/package, detachable needles.	2 cc useful for patients taking large doses. Detachable needles produce clinically significant dead space if insulin mixing is needed.
Stylex Insulin Syringe (Pharmaseal)	1 cc U-40 and U-100 syringes with 25 G⅝″ needles.	needles pop off. Significant dead space. Lettering rubs off easily.
Syrijet Mark IV (Mizzy, Inc.)	high-quality jet injector. Up to 34 units/injection.	easy to use but requires education program and physician monitoring. Can be used up to 4 times/day to improve control. Should be used with home blood glucose monitoring. Dosage adjustments in 2-unit increments. Comparatively inexpensive.
Yale Glass Insulin Reusable Short Type Luer Tip Syringe (Becton Dickinson)	1 cc U-40 red scale, 2 cc U-40 red scale.	can use with reusable or disposable needles. Preferred over Luer-Lok. Less expensive. Dual scale yields dose errors. Encourage patients to switch to U-100 disposable.
Yale 0.35 cc Special Insulin Syringe (Becton Dickinson)	0.35 cc, calibrated up to 35 units.	available for patients using small doses of U-100 insulin.

AIDS FOR VISUALLY IMPAIRED PATIENTS

C-Better Syringe Magnifier (Tri County Rehabilitation Center, Stuart, Fla.)	snap-on magnifier.	magnifies two times. Plastic. Fits different type syringes.
Cemco Syringe Magnifier (Cemco)	unbreakable stainless steel magnifier.	easy to snap on and off. Magnifies bubbles and calibrations on syringe. Not for the totally blind.
Char-Mag Syringe Magnifier (Char-Mag Company)	magnifier made of optical quality plastic.	easy to snap on and off. Magnifies bubbles and calibrations on syringe. Not for the totally blind.
Cornwall, Becton Dickinson Adjustable Positive Stop (American Foundation for the Blind)	metal, complicated device that covers most of syringe. Dose set with plunger springs.	large and bulky. Use only with U-100 glass syringe. Accurate but expensive.

INSULIN SYRINGES AND RELATED PRODUCTS TABLE, continued

Product (Manufacturer or Supplier)	Sizes Available or Description	Comments
Dos-Aid (American Foundation for the Blind)	plastic tray that adjusts to hold syringe and insulin bottle. Plunger is pulled back to a plunger stop.	uses all types of disposable syringes. Simple to teach, accurate. Can't mix insulins
HoldEase (Meditec, Inc.)	a plastic guide device that holds both the insulin and syringe. Guide can be compressed, causing the needle to be inserted in vial.	useful in getting needle into vial. Other less expensive products are available.
Insulgage (Meditec, Inc.)	small plastic gauge that attaches to B-D long or ½ cc disposable syringes. Gauge and plunger are pulled back until gauge drops into place between plunger end and barrel.	accurate, inexpensive, simple to teach, can be used with mixed insulins. Available for U-100 disposable syringes.
Insulin-Aid (Seabee Enterprises)	device made of plexiglass that magnetically attaches to a metal surface and holds any insulin bottle inverted to make it easier to withdraw insulin into syringe.	useful if one needs an extra hand to withdraw insulin into syringe.
Insulin Needle Guide (MES 168) (American Foundation for the Blind)	round aluminum cap to fit the top of an insulin bottle. The inner contour is funnel shaped and guides the needle into rubber cap.	used for Lilly insulin bottles only. It is small, sturdy and inexpensive.
Insulin Syringe MES 260 (American Foundation for the Blind)	precision device consisting of a glass barrel inside a 3½″ metal casing. Units drawn up determined by an audible click.	used only with U-40. Syringe expensive but accurate.
Templet Insulin Measuring Device (Greater Detroit Society for the Blind)	directions for making a gauge which sets along the plunger between the barrel and the plunger end. Materials are staples and tape.	can be constructed to desired dose and is simple to use, easy to handle, accurate and inexpensive.

MISCELLANEOUS

Product (Manufacturer or Supplier)	Sizes Available or Description	Comments
Alcohol Swabs and Alcohol Wipes (Becton Dickinson, Kendall-Futuro)	70% isopropyl alcohol for single use.	unit dose of alcohol swabs. More expensive but good for travel.
Becton, Dickinson Insulin Travel Kit (Becton Dickinson)	plastic carrying case for vial of insulin and disposable syringes.	useful for travel.
Isopropyl Alcohol, 91% (Various manufacturers)	used for sterilizing needles and syringes and for cleansing skin before injections. Preferred to rubbing alcohol due to less water and not denatured; therefore, safer with insulin.	
Ster-Inge (Ster-Inge)	device to sterilize glass syringes and disposable or reusable needles.	simple to operate. Recommended for patients who do not use disposable syringes.
Syringe and Needle Destroyers (B-D's Destruclip) (Becton Dickinson)	device to destroy disposable needles after use. Cuts off needle and cuts syringe into parts.	useful in hospitals and nursing homes where large number of syringes are used.

URINE AND BLOOD GLUCOSE/KETONE TEST PRODUCT TABLE

Product (Manufacturer)	Product Formulation and Sizes	Active Ingredients	Indication of Product Deterioration	Time Required to Evaluate (seconds)	Drug Interference	Comments[a]
Acetest (Miles)	tablets: 100's, 250's	nitroprusside	darkened brown tablet	30 seconds (urine), 2 minutes (plasma), 10 minutes (whole blood)	false (+) possible but rare (levodopa)	tests for acetone and acetoacetic acid; useful in determining whether or not a diabetic is developing ketoacidosis; patient with 2% or more glucose should test for ketones
Chemstrip bG (Boehringer Mannheim)	strip: 25's	glucose, oxidase, peroxidase, o-tolidine, tetramethyl-benzidine	darkening of test area	120-180	no false (+), possibly some false (–)	product can easily be used by patients to test glucose in whole blood; required drop of blood on both zones of the test strip; requires cotton ball to wipe off blood after 60 seconds; tests are reliable but not as accurate as those read by a machine
Chemstrip 8 (Boehringer Mannheim)	strip: 50's	glucose oxidase, peroxidase, o-tolidine, sodium nitroferricyanide	discoloration of test area	0-60 (dip and read)	no false (+) (glucose)	tests for glucose, protein, pH, blood, ketones, bilirubin, urobilinogen and leukocytes; error potential is great; specific individual tests recommended
Chemstrip G (Boehringer Mannheim)	strip: 100's	glucose oxidase, peroxidase, o-tolidine	discoloration of test area	60	no false (+), possibly some false (–)	inexpensive; convenient for Type II diabetics; not quantitative
Chemstrip GK (Boehringer Mannheim)	strip: 100's	glucose oxidase, peroxidase, sodium nitroferricyanide	discoloration of test area	60	for ketones: false (+) possible but rare, for glucose: no false (+), some possible false (–)	this product is similar to Keto-Diastix in that it is useful to monitor glucose and ketones in the urine
Clinistix (Miles)	strip: 50's	glucose, oxidase, peroxide, o-tolidine	tan or dark test area	10	no false (+), some false (–) (levodopa, ascorbic acid, aspirin)	inexpensive, convenient for Type II diabetics; not quantitative

URINE AND BLOOD GLUCOSE/KETONE TEST PRODUCT TABLE, continued

Product (Manufacturer)	Product Formulation and Sizes	Active Ingredients	Indication of Product Deterioration	Time Required to Evaluate (seconds)	Drug Interference	Comments[a]
Clinitest (Miles) *5-drop method* *2-drop method*	tablets: 36's, 100's, 250's, 1000's foilwrap: 24's and 500's tablets: 36's	copper reduction	deep blue tablet	15, then shake gently	false (+) in presence of reducing agents, no false (−)	2-drop most reliable at high glucose levels; use for "sliding scale"; use for Type I; inexpensive but inconvenient (requires water dropper and test tube); not specific for glucose; only difference in 2-drop and 5-drop method is the amount of urine used
Combistix (Miles)	strip: 100's	glucose oxidase	discoloration of test area	30-60 (dip and read)	no false (+) (glucose), some false (−)	test for glucose, protein and pH
Dextrostix (Miles)	strip: 25's, 100's	glucose oxidase, peroxidase, o-tolidine	test area does not resemble "O" on color chart	60 (test for blood glucose)	no false (+), some false (−)	useful in screening; accurate if read by Dextrometer; can use to correlate blood and urine glucose levels; home use improves control; requires a drop of blood
Diastix (Miles)	strip: 50's, 100's	glucose oxidase, peroxidase, potassium iodide, chromogen	variation from light blue or "neg" on color chart	30 (dip, remove excess urine and read)	no false (+), some complete false (−) (see Clinistix)	easy to read; relatively expensive; more accurate than Tes Tape but less than Clinitest; under reading possible at high glucose levels; for use by both Type I and Type II
Keto-Diastix (Miles)	strip: 50's, 100's	glucose oxidase, nitroprusside	glucose area green; ketone area darkened	15-30 (dip and read)	no false (+) (glucose), some false (−)	useful combination product for glucose and ketones. No need to use this test often, only when passing 4+ glucose often
Ketostix (Miles)	strip: 50's, 100's	nitroprusside	tan or brown	15	false (+) possible but rare (levodopa)	test for acetoacetic acid; useful in determining whether or not a diabetic is developing ketoacidosis; patient with 2% or more glucose should test for ketones

URINE AND BLOOD GLUCOSE/KETONE TEST PRODUCT TABLE, continued

Product (Manu-facturer)	Product Formula-tion and Sizes	Active Ingredients	Indication of Product Deteriora-tion	Time Required to Evaluate (seconds)	Drug Inter-ference	Comments[a]
Labstix (Miles)	strip: 100's	glucose oxidase, nitroprusside	discoloration of test area	30-60 (dip and read)	no false (+) (glucose), some false(−)	test for blood, pH, glucose, ketones and protein; amount of use does not warrant expense for individual patient
Multistix (Miles)	strip: 100's	glucose oxidase, peroxidase, o-tolidine, sodium nitro-ferricyanide	discoloration of test area	0-60 (dip and read)	no false (+) (glucose)	same as N-Multistix but does not test for nitrite
N-Multistix (Miles)	strip: 100's	glucose oxidase, peroxidase, o-tolidine, sodium nitro-ferricyanide	discoloration of test area	0-60 (dip and read)	no false (+) (glucose)	tests for glucose, protein, pH, blood, ketones, bilirubin, urobi-linogen and nitrite; error potential is great; specific individual tests recommended
Stat Tek Test Strips (Boehringer Mannheim)	strip: 25's	glucose oxidase, peroxidase, o-tolidine	test area does not resemble "O" on color chart	120	no false (+), some false (−)	strips can be used only with Stat Tek Colorimeter; use-ful in monitoring blood glucose lev-els; requires a drop of blood
TesTape (Lilly)	strip: 100's	glucose oxidase, peroxidase, o-tolidine, yellow dye	brown color or doesn't resemble "O" on test with dis-tilled water	60	no false (+), some partial false (−) (see Clinistix)	most inexpensive test; convenient for home and travel; accuracy adequate if all 3+ read as 4+; not as quantitative as Diastix or Clinitest
Uristix (Miles)	strip: 100's	glucose oxidase	discoloration of test area	30-60 (dip and read)	no false (+) (glucose), some false (−)	test for glucose and protein; useful to determine if protein is in urine (diabetic nephropathy)

[a] Protect all products from heat, light and moisture.

MISCELLANEOUS DIABETES PRODUCTS TABLE

Product (Manu- facturer)	Description
Autolet (Ulster Scientific Inc.)	a plastic, push-button device connected to a lancet and platform that is used to prick the finger and makes it easier for diabetics to obtain a drop of blood for testing with Dextrostix, Chemstrip bG and Stat Tek Strips.
Clinilog (Miles)	a diary for diabetics to record date, urine sugars, urine acetone and remarks plus a glossary of terms for diabetic patients, plus diet information. Patient should keep track of weight, changes in medication, exercise, diet, infections or emotional stress.
Glucometer (Miles)	a battery-powered reflectance photometer with digital display and built-in timer. Used with Dextrostix. Less expensive and smaller than a Dextrometer. Easier to calibrate and use.
Injectomatic (Monoject) (Kendall Futuro)	an aluminum device that assists the patient in giving his daily injection of insulin. Patient places a filled syringe in Injectomatic, then cocks it, places on injection site and is automatically injected into the skin. Patient completes injection by pushing plunger. Helps eliminate apprehension associated with insulin injections; increases injection sites.
Monojector (Monoject) (Kendall Futuro)	a plastic device in which a lancet is inserted through a platform that allows the patient to stick his finger and obtain a drop of blood. Device is used with Monolets.
Monolets (Kendall Futuro)	a plastic-covered lance that is used with the Monojector or by itself to assist diabetic patients in getting a drop of blood for blood glucose self-monitoring.
Stat Tek Twin Beam Electronic Photometer (Boehringer Mannheim)	a meter used with Stat Tek Strips that provides accurate blood glucose determinations. Larger and more expensive than the Dextrometer. Useful for home blood glucose monitoring in appropriate diabetic patients.
Urine Specimen Jars	pharmacists should keep available for diabetic patients and encourage patients to take urine specimens when seeing their physicians.

Marianne Ivey and Gary Elmer

NUTRITIONAL SUPPLEMENT, MINERAL, AND VITAMIN PRODUCTS

17

*Q*uestions to ask in patient/consumer counseling

What are your age and weight?

Do you have any chronic illnesses (diabetes, peptic ulcer disease, ulcerative colitis, or epilepsy)?

Do you donate blood? How often?

Are you currently taking any medications (prescription or nonprescription)?

Do you smoke or are you around smokers daily?

Do you eat meats, fruits and vegetables, dairy products, and grain products every day? Are you dieting or do you have any type of dietary restrictions?

Are you menstruating now? Are you pregnant? Do you take oral contraceptives (birth control pills)?

How much alcohol do you drink in a day?

Do you participate regularly in sports or do you have a job requiring physical activity?

Why do you think you need a nutritional supplement, vitamin, or mineral?

What are your symptoms? Have they appeared suddenly or gradually?

Are you taking now or have you recently taken any nutritional supplements, vitamins, or minerals?

American consumers, convinced that they need more and better nutrients than their diets provide, spend about $3 billion a year on vitamin and nutritional products (1, 2). The health science professions frequently have associated good health with good nutrition. There is much to learn about adequate nutrition. Much that has been learned has not been communicated effectively to the public. In most cases, the average American diet does not need supplementation (3). Misconceptions about the value of supplementation abound, and marketing practices may further confuse the issue.

The label "organic" is misleading because all foods are organic. "Organically grown" foods are those that are grown without the use of agricultural chemicals and are processed without chemicals or additives. However, no laws exist that enforce the label, "organically grown," to comply with the definition. There is no evidence that organically grown foods are more nutritious than foods grown using chemical fertilizers (4).

Frequently, "natural" vitamins are supplemented with the synthetic vitamin. For example, the amount of ascorbic acid acquired from rose hips (the fleshy fruit of a rose) is relatively small, and synthetic ascorbic acid is added to prevent an unwieldy tablet size (5). However, this addition is not noted on the label, and the price of such products often is considerably higher than for the synthetic, equally effective vitamin.

The pharmacist should be aware that one of the greatest dangers of food fads and high-potency supplements is that they are sometimes used in place of sound medical care. The false hope of superior health or freedom from disease may attract individuals with cancer,

TABLE 1	Food and Nutrition Board, National Academy of Sciences–National Research Council Recommended Dietary Allowances,[a] Revised 1989

		Weight[b]		Height[b]		Protein	Fat-soluble vitamins					
Category	Age (years) or condition	(kg)	(lb)	(cm)	(in)	(g)	Vita-min A (mcg RE)[c]	Vita-min D (mcg)[d]	Vita-min E (mg α-TE)[e]	Vita-min K (mcg)	Vita-min C (mg)	Thia-min (mg)
Infants	0.0–0.5	6	13	60	24	13	375	7.5	3	5	30	0.3
	0.5–1.0	9	20	71	28	14	375	10	4	10	35	0.4
Children	1–3	13	29	90	35	16	400	10	6	15	40	0.7
	4–6	20	44	112	44	24	500	10	7	20	45	0.9
	7–10	28	62	132	52	28	700	10	7	30	45	1.0
Males	11–14	45	99	157	62	45	1,000	10	10	45	50	1.3
	15–18	66	145	176	69	59	1,000	10	10	65	60	1.5
	19–24	72	160	177	70	58	1,000	10	10	70	60	1.5
	25–50	79	174	176	70	63	1,000	5	10	80	60	1.5
	51+	77	170	173	68	63	1,000	5	10	80	60	1.2
Females	11–14	46	101	157	62	46	800	10	8	45	50	1.1
	15–18	55	120	163	64	44	800	10	8	55	60	1.1
	19–24	58	128	164	65	46	800	10	8	60	60	1.1
	25–50	63	138	163	64	50	800	5	8	65	60	1.1
	51+	65	143	160	63	50	800	5	8	65	60	1.0
Pregnant						60	800	10	10	65	70	1.5
Lactating	1st 6 months					65	1,300	10	12	65	95	1.6
	2nd 6 months					62	1,200	10	11	65	90	1.6

[a]The allowances, expressed as average daily intakes over time, are intended to provide for individual variations among most normal persons as they live in the United States under usual environmental stresses. Diets should be based on a variety of common foods in order to provide other nutrients for which human requirements have been less well defined.

[b]The use of these figures does not imply that the height-to-weight ratios are ideal.

[c]Retinol equivalents. 1 retinol equivalent = 1 mcg retinol or 6 mcg β-carotene.

heart disease, arthritis, or other serious illnesses, and the pharmacist should be aware of the limited therapeutic value, if any, of these fads.

Some vitamins and minerals are potentially toxic if consumed in amounts greater than the recommended dietary allowance (RDA) established by the National Research Council. The Food and Drug Administration (FDA), however, classifies vitamins and minerals—in product forms that are offered for their "nutritional" value—as "dietary supplements," which means they are considered as foods and are not subject to the efficacy regulations required to market nonprescription drugs. The FDA does regulate the manufacturing and safety of supplement ingredients and controls product labeling but not the quantities of ingredients in these preparations. The FDA's attempt to define maximum and minimum quantities of allowable ingredients in supplements

and to restrict certain high-potency preparations to prescription-only status was defeated in the courts in the 1970s. Unfortunately there are no restrictions on the availability of even toxic potencies of vitamins and minerals. Pharmacists should be sure that their clients are aware of the risks of high-potency products in spite of the lack of warning labels.

There is nearly universal agreement by nutrition experts (including the National Research Council Committee on Diet and Health) that foods, rather than supplements, are the preferred source of nutrients and that most individuals can easily meet their vitamin and mineral requirements by eating a balanced diet. There is less agreement about the extent to which the population consumes a balanced diet that provides these nutrients and, therefore, the extent of need for supplement use. On one side, there are those who believe that most

Water-soluble vitamins					Minerals						
Ribo-flavin (mg)	Niacin (mg NE)[f]	Vita-min B$_6$ (mg)	Folic Acid (mcg)	Vitamin B$_{12}$ (mcg)	Cal-cium (mg)	Phos-phorus (mg)	Mag-nesium (mg)	Iron (mg)	Zinc (mg)	Iodine (mcg)	Sele-nium (mcg)
0.4	5	0.3	25	0.3	400	300	40	6	5	40	10
0.5	6	0.6	35	0.5	600	500	60	10	5	50	15
0.8	9	1.0	50	0.7	800	800	80	10	10	70	20
1.1	12	1.1	75	1.0	800	800	120	10	10	90	20
1.2	13	1.4	100	1.4	800	800	170	10	10	120	30
1.5	17	1.7	150	2.0	1,200	1,200	270	12	15	150	40
1.8	20	2.0	200	2.0	1,200	1,200	400	12	15	150	50
1.7	19	2.0	200	2.0	1,200	1,200	350	10	15	150	70
1.7	19	2.0	200	2.0	800	800	350	10	15	150	70
1.4	15	2.0	200	2.0	800	800	350	10	15	150	70
1.3	15	1.4	150	2.0	1,200	1,200	280	15	12	150	45
1.3	15	1.5	180	2.0	1,200	1,200	300	15	12	150	50
1.3	15	1.6	180	2.0	1,200	1,200	280	15	12	150	55
1.3	15	1.6	180	2.0	800	800	280	15	12	150	55
1.2	13	1.6	180	2.0	800	800	280	10	12	150	55
1.6	17	2.2	400	2.2	1,200	1,200	320	30	15	175	65
1.8	20	2.1	280	2.6	1,200	1,200	355	15	19	200	75
1.7	20	2.1	260	2.6	1.200	1,200	340	15	16	200	75

[d]As cholecalciferol. 10 mcg cholecalciferol = 400 IU of vitamin D.

[e]Alpha-Tocopherol equivalents. 1 mg D-α tocopherol = 1 α-TE.

[f]NE (niacin equivalent) is equal to 1 mg of niacin or 60 mg of dietary tryptophan.

Adapted with permission from Food and Nutrition Board, National Research Council, National Academy of Sciences, "Recommended Dietary Allowances," 10th ed., National Academy Press, Washington, D.C., 1989.

of the population receives adequate levels of vitamins and minerals from the usual diet and that there is little evidence that low-dose supplementation is beneficial. The lack of vitamin and mineral deficiency symptoms in the population is cited to support this position. The National Research Council Committee on Diet and Health generally takes this position (6), as do many nutrition experts. Others, however, point to surveys that show many segments of society (e.g., the elderly, smokers, nursing home patients, teenagers) do not consume the RDA levels of all vitamins and minerals. The issue of who would benefit from vitamin and mineral supplements is complex. Primary attention should be directed toward an improvement in the diet, ideally with the help of a dietitian. Under some circumstances, a supplement may be appropriate. This chapter will provide information to help the pharmacist in deciding whether to recommend a supplement and in choosing a supplement if warranted.

OPTIMUM NUTRITION

Guidelines for optimum nutrition are provided by two organizations—the Food and Nutrition Board of the National Academy of Sciences–National Research Council and the FDA. The Food and Nutrition Board provides RDA values for essential nutrients based on sex, age, weight, and height (Table 1). The RDA values are estimates of the amounts that will meet the needs of the majority of individuals in a population. The RDA values are periodically updated, based on new information, and are set high enough to allow for variations in individual requirements caused by minor illnesses. In the Food and Nutrition Board recommendations, an "estimated safe and adequate daily dietary intake" of other nutrients for which human requirements are not quantitatively known has been promulgated (Table 2). These data should be used merely as guidelines for nutritional assessment.

The FDA publishes a less comprehensive set of RDA values to be used for labeling purposes. These values, known as the U.S. Recommended Daily Allowances (U.S. RDAs), are based on the 1968 RDA values (Table 3). Pharmacists will find U.S. RDA values to be the most useful for patient discussions, because all vitamin and mineral product potencies are expressed as percentages of the adult U.S. RDA values.

NUTRITIONAL SUPPLEMENTS

Often, persons who request a nutritional supplement have self-diagnosed their condition. By careful evaluation the pharmacist can estimate the person's nutritional status. If the evidence indicates the presence of a nutritional deficiency or any serious illness, the pharmacist should refer the patient to a physician for diagnosis and treatment. Persons purchasing a nonprescription dietary supplement should be instructed as to its use, storage, and possible side effects.

Determining Nutritional Status

The assessment of nutritional status is very difficult in the ambulatory environment. Clinical impressions about nutrition are often erroneous because the stages between the well-nourished and the poorly nourished states are not very evident to an observer. Clinical impressions are reliable only when emaciation from disease, economics, or climatic conditions is obvious.

There are guidelines, however, by which the pharmacist can gain a more objective impression of a patient's nutritional status. Pharmacists should know the population groups that are most often poorly nourished, exercise good observational skills, and know what questions may yield helpful information. Undernourished groups in the United States frequently include infants, preschool children, lactating or pregnant women, the elderly, alcoholics, the homeless, and the impoverished.

Other populations at risk are people on restricted diets, people with intestinal disease that lead to malabsorption of nutrients, people who neglect their nutritional needs (particularly people living alone), people taking certain drugs that may affect absorption of nutri-

---

TABLE 2 Estimated safe and adequate daily dietary intakes of selected vitamins and minerals[a]

Category	Age (years)	Vitamins		Trace elements				
		Biotin (mcg)	Pantothenic acid (mg)	Copper (mg)	Manganese (mg)	Fluoride (mg)	Chromium (mcg)	Molybdenum (mcg)
Infants	0–0.5	10	3	0.4–0.6	0.3–0.6	0.1–0.5	10–40	15–30
	0.5–1	15	3	0.6–0.7	0.6–1.0	0.2–1.0	20–60	20–40
Children and	1–3	20	3	0.7–1.0	1.0–1.5	0.5–1.5	20–80	25–50
adolescents	4–6	25	3–4	1.0–1.5	1.5–2.0	1.0–2.5	30–120	30–75
	7–10	30	4–5	1.0–2.0	2.0–3.0	1.5–2.5	50–200	50–150
	11+	30–100	4–7	1.5–2.5	2.0–5.0	1.5–2.5	50–200	75–250
Adults		30–100	4–7	1.5–3.0	2.0–5.0	1.5–4.0	50–200	75–250

[a]Because there is less information on which to base allowances, these figures are not given in the main table of RDA and are provided here in the form of ranges of recommended intakes.

[b]Because the toxic levels for many trace elements may be only several times usual intakes, the upper levels for the trace elements given in this table should not be habitually exceeded.

Adapted with permission from Food and Nutrition Board, National Research Council, National Academy of Sciences, "Recommended Dietary Allowances," 10th ed., National Academy Press, Washington, D.C., 1989, p. 284.

TABLE 3   U.S. Recommended Daily Allowances (U.S. RDA) for labeling purposes

	Unit	Infants	Children under 4 years of age	Adults and children 4 or more years of age	Pregnant and lactating women
Vitamin A	IU	1,500	2,500	5,000	8,000
Vitamin D	IU	400	400	400	400
Vitamin E	IU	5	10	30	30
Ascorbic acid	mg	35	40	60	60
Folic acid	mg	0.1	0.2	0.4	0.8
Thiamine	mg	0.5	0.7	1.5	1.7
Riboflavin	mg	0.6	0.8	1.7	2.0
Niacin	mg	8	9	20	20
Pyridoxine	mg	0.4	0.7	2	2.5
Cyanocobalamin	mcg	2	3	6	8
Biotin	mg	0.05	0.15	0.3	0.3
Pantothenic acid	mg	3	5	10	10
Calcium	g	0.6	0.8	1.0	1.3
Phosphorus	g	0.5	0.8	1.0	1.3
Iodine	mcg	45	70	150	150
Iron	mg	15	10	18	18
Magnesium	mg	70	200	400	450
Manganese[a]	mg	0.5	1.0	4.0	4.0
Copper	mg	0.6	1.0	2.0	2.0
Zinc	mg	5	8	15	15
Protein	g		20(28)[b]	45(65)[b]	

[a]Proposed U.S. RDA.

[b]Values in parentheses are U.S. RDAs when protein efficiency ratio (PER) is less than that of casein; the other values are used when PER is equal to or greater than that of casein. No claim may be made for a protein with a PER equal to or less than 20% that of casein.

ents or nutrient interaction, and women of childbearing age who have regular blood loss. Epidemiologic surveys have shown that schoolchildren, factory workers, businesspersons, and farmers are less likely to be poorly nourished.

The pharmacist should observe the patient's physical condition but realize that only severe dietary deficiencies are likely to be reflected physically. The texture, amount, and appearance of the hair may indicate the patient's nutritional status. The eyes, particularly the conjunctivae, may indicate vitamin A and iron deficiencies, and the mouth may show stomatitis, glossitis, or hypertrophic or pale gums. The number and general condition of the teeth may reflect the patient's choice of food. Visible goiter, skin color and texture, obesity or thinness relative to bone structure, and the presence of edema also may be indications of malnutrition. The edematous patient often looks well nourished but in fact may be severely protein malnourished. This is a common problem in the hospital, particularly among surgical patients or patients with edema due to liver, kidney, or heart disease.

The more specific the information obtained from the patient is, the more helpful the pharmacist can be in determining the need for nutritional supplementation. Questions regarding foods generally not included in the diet may give the pharmacist more information. Previous treatment for similar symptoms also may be important.

Although nutritional deficiencies may lead to disease, disease may lead to nutritional deficiencies. It is the pharmacist's responsibility to refer patients with a suspected serious illness to a physician for a definitive assessment. Guidelines for the clinical appraisal of nutritional status include evaluation of medical and dietary history; growth, development, and fitness; signs consistent with deficiencies; and biochemical assessment. Rarely in the United States do pharmacists encounter patients with severe deficiencies resulting in diseases such as scurvy (ascorbic acid deficiency), pellagra (niacin deficiency), or kwashiorkor (protein deficiency). Milder forms of malnutrition are more frequently seen, often involving simultaneous deficiencies of more than one nutrient.

Protein and Calorie (Energy) Deficiency

In the United States, protein–calorie malnutrition (marasmus) is uncommon, except as a consequence of certain diseases; in fact, an excess intake of protein and calories is more common. The U.S. RDA for protein is 45 g, or 1,600–3,100 cal, for adults. In most cases, excess protein intake (to as much as 300 g) does not lead to disease conditions. Excess caloric intake, however, leads to obesity, with resulting increased risk for coronary, vascular, and other diseases.

Protein–calorie malnutrition can be caused by either food shortage or disease. In the United States, protein–calorie malnutrition is more commonly caused by conditions such as Crohn's disease; malabsorption syndromes; short-bowel syndromes caused by surgery, trauma, or radiation; severe burns; jaw fractures; neoplastic diseases; renal disease; and psychiatric conditions such as depression and anorexia nervosa. Protein and calorie intake in some very active people, such as athletes, dancers, and manual laborers may not be adequate to meet their needs. However, in the United States, high activity levels are not common for much of the population.

For complaints of weight loss or failure to gain weight in a highly active, otherwise healthy individual, a high-protein diet or a product with a high protein and calorie concentration may be recommended. Persons with a history of weight loss without apparent cause should be referred to a physician because of the possibility of conditions such as diabetes or cancer.

Types of Formulas

Supplemental protein/calorie formula products are used as dietary adjuncts to a regular diet; they should not be used as the sole dietary product because they are not nutritionally complete. Some products (Mull-Soy and Nutramigen) are milk-free and can be used by individuals who have milk allergy disease as well as by patients with lactose malabsorption, which results in distention and diarrhea. (See Chapter 18, *Infant Formula Products*.) One product (Controlyte) with a low protein and electrolyte content is appropriate for patients with acute or chronic renal failure, whose diet must be carefully controlled. Many supplementary formula products may be combined with special recipes to make desserts, malts, and shakes that still maintain the controlled intake.

Complete formulas can be used orally or as tube feedings, and they may be used as the sole dietary intake if the patient's electrolytes are monitored (7). They also may be used as supplementation to a regular diet. The complete formulas contain various ingredients that make them appropriate for special needs. Several products (Instant Breakfast, Sustacal, and Meritene) are milk based; others (Compleat-B and Gerber Meat Base Formula) have a mixed food base. A third type provides a synthetic source of protein and carbohydrate. This type supplies the protein in the form of crystalline amino acids or protein hydrolysate, the carbohydrate in the form of oligosaccharides or disaccharides, and the vitamins and minerals in the form of individual chemicals. These are chemically defined diets known as "elemental diets"; examples include Vivonex and Jejunal. Some other complete products (Precision LR, Flexical, and Portagen) are only partly chemically defined.

Nearly all chemically defined (elemental) diets have a very low fat content and contain electrolytes, minerals, trace elements, and water-soluble and fat-soluble vitamins. All the chemically based products require little or no digestion, are absorbed over a short distance in the small intestine, and have low residue, which reduces the number and volume of the stools, making these products appropriate for patients with ileostomies or colostomies who wish also to decrease fecal output. (See Chapter 24, *Ostomy Care Products*.) The low-residue products also may be appropriate to facilitate care for elderly patients with stool incontinence or for patients with brain damage from strokes, congenital defects, or retardation. Because of the ease of absorption and low fecal residues, they are often used in postoperative care, in gastrointestinal (GI) diseases, and in neoplastic disease where tissue breakdown is extensive.

Formulation and Dosage

Supplementary and complete formulas are available in several forms: powders that must be diluted with water or milk, liquids that must be diluted, and liquids that are ready to use. The extent of dilution is based on the amount of nutrients needed and the amount that can be tolerated. Most often, adults will not tolerate preparations of more than 25% weight per volume (w/v), which generally delivers 1.0 cal/ml; the maximum concentration for infants is 12% w/v, which generally delivers 0.5 cal/ml. (Infants should be started on a concentration of 7–7.5% w/v, increasing to 12% over 4 to 5 days.) For children over 10 months of age, 15% w/v may be initiated, with gradual increases to 25%. Higher concentrations may cause osmotic diarrhea because of the sugar.

If the preparations are taken orally, 100–150 ml should be ingested at one time. Over the course of a day, 2,000 ml (about 2 qt) of most preparations provide about 2,000 cal. If the product is tube fed, 40–60 ml per hour may be given initially. The opened container should be kept cold to prevent bacterial growth, and all prepared products remaining after 24 hours should be discarded. The tubing should be rinsed 3 times a day with water. If diarrhea, nausea, or distention occurs, the diet should be withheld for 24 hours, then gradually resumed. In elderly or unconscious patients or patients who recently have had surgery, elevating the head of the bed is advisable during administration of the preparation to avoid aspiration.

Cautions

Pharmacists should store supplemental formula products at temperatures under 75°F (23.8°C) and should check expiration dates before dispensing.

Because all formulas are excellent media for bacterial growth, they should be prepared each day and refrigerated until used. They may cause diarrhea if they become bacterially contaminated. Diarrhea also may occur from the osmotic carbohydrate load, especially simple sugars, or from fat intolerance. However, some elemental diets are fat free.

Patients must be monitored to detect biochemical abnormalities of electrolyte values and to ensure adequate nutrition and hydration. Urine and blood glucose concentrations should be measured; diabetics may require increased insulin doses. Edema may be precipitated or aggravated in patients with protein–calorie malnutrition or cardiac, renal, or hepatic disease because of the relatively high sodium content of the chemically defined diets. Some commercially available nutritional products (Ensure and Ensure Plus) are a source of vitamin K supplementation, which may interfere with oral anticoagulant therapy (8). Tube feedings have also been shown to interfere with the absorption of phenytoin when the phenytoin is also given to the patient via the tube. This interaction can be avoided by flushing the tube with saline (or water) before and after phenytoin and waiting 15 minutes both before and after the phenytoin is given. Shutting off the tube feeding for this amount of time generally does not cause a problem for the patient (9). Frequently, hospital dietitians prepare formulas so that the electrolytes may be tailored to the individual patient. In many hospitals, these solutions are prepared by pharmacy services.

MINERALS

Trace mineral nutrition research continues to receive considerable attention. Deficiency states in humans are being noted and biologic functions are being defined in animal systems, providing data that may apply generally to humans.

Unlike vitamins, the mineral content of plants varies according to the composition of the soil in which the plant is grown. This in turn affects the mineral content of the grazing domestic livestock. Mineral intake varies considerably from region to region, although the use of foods delivered from diverse geographic locations tends to minimize intake variations. Marginal deficiencies of minerals have been reported only in certain segments of the population, but the increasing use of highly refined foods, which are low in minerals, may contribute to the problem.

Optimal mineral intake values for humans are still imprecise. The RDA values for calcium, phosphorus, iodine, iron, magnesium, selenium, and zinc are available (Table 1). However, only estimated ranges thought to be safe and adequate are published for chromium, fluoride, copper, manganese, and molybdenum (Table 2). These ranges are based on the content of the "average" diet. Similarly, the possible adverse effects of long-term ingestion of high-dose mineral supplements are unknown, and high doses of one mineral can decrease the bioavailability of other minerals and even vitamins (10, 11). Pharmacists should encourage the consumer to achieve balanced mineral intake through attention to a proper diet, if possible, rather than dependence on the use of mineral supplements.

Iron

Iron deficiency anemia is still a widespread problem. Although it causes few deaths, it contributes to the poor health and suboptimal performance of many people. Furthermore, it is possible that less severe iron deficiencies (those not resulting in frank anemia but rather more subtle clinical manifestations) may be quite common. Iron plays an important role in oxygen and electron transport. In the body it is either functional or stored. Functional iron is found in hemoglobin, myoglobin, heme enzymes, and cofactor and transport iron. Although functional in nature, the hemoglobin of the red blood cells also represents the major body store of iron, containing 60–70% of total body iron. The rest is stored in the form of ferritin and hemosiderin. Ferritin is a micelle of ferric hydroxyphosphate surrounded by 24 identical protein units. Hemosiderin consists of aggregated ferritin molecules and additional components. The storage sites of ferritin and hemosiderin are the intestinal mucosa, liver, spleen, and bone marrow.

Normally, adult males have iron stores of about 50 mg of iron per kg; females have about 35 mg/kg (12). Hemoglobin is about 0.34% iron. The normal hemoglobin level in adult males is about 14–17 g/100 ml of blood and in adult females, it is 12–14 g/100 ml. The RDA for iron varies from 5 to 6 mg, depending on age and sex (Table 1). The RDA for pregnant women increases to 30 mg.

Dietary iron is available in two forms. Heme iron is found in meats and is reasonably well absorbed. Nonheme iron, which constitutes most of the dietary iron, is poorly absorbed. Therefore, the published values of the iron content of foods are misleading because the amount absorbed depends on the nature of the iron in the diet in question. To gain an accurate assessment of the iron available in a meal, its composition must be considered in detail. About half of the iron in meats is heme iron, which is about 25% absorbed. The amount of absorbable nonheme iron contributed by vegetables and grains in the diet varies greatly. The presence in the diet of meat and certain organic acids, such as ascorbic acid, enhances the absorption of iron up to twofold (13, 14). Furthermore, the presence of meat or ascorbic acid may increase the amount of nonheme iron absorbed 1.5–2 times, depending on the patient's relative need for iron.

Nutrition experts believe that with a low-availability meal (containing less than 30 g of meat and 25 mg of ascorbic acid), as little as 3% of the iron is absorbed. In contrast, a high-availability meal (containing more than 90 g of meat and 75 mg of ascorbic acid) results in as much as 8% of the nonheme iron being absorbed (15). Most authorities calculate the available iron content of foods by assuming that, on the average, 10% of the total iron (heme plus nonheme) is absorbable. Another variable to consider is that in the iron-deficient state, iron absorption improves so that as much as 20% may be utilized from an "average" diet.

As may be surmised from this discussion, an accurate calculation of the absorbable iron content from foods is a complicated and inexact process. As Americans move toward consumption of less red meat, it will be important to monitor the population for iron status.

There has been concern that vegetarians may be at risk for iron deficiencies because of the lack of easily absorbed heme iron in their diets. Although intakes have been reported as marginally low, there is no evidence of deficiency (16, 17). The inherent high intake of ascorbic acid may lead to improved absorption of nonheme iron in vegetarian diets.

Ingested iron, mostly in the form of ferric hydroxide, is solubilized in gastric juice to ferric chloride and then reduced to the ferrous form. It is then chelated to substances such as ascorbic acid, sugars, and amino acids. These chelates have a low molecular weight and can be solubilized and absorbed before they reach the alkaline medium of the distal portion of the small intestine where precipitation occurs. In the plasma, iron is oxidized to the ferric state and bound to transferrin, the transport form of iron. Once released at the spleen, liver, bone marrow, and other iron storage sites, the iron is combined with apoferritin to form ferritin or a ferritin complex called hemosiderin. Iron is utilized in all cells of the body; however, most is incorporated into the hemoglobin of red blood cells. Iron is lost from the body by the sloughing of skin cells and GI mucosal cells; in the urine, sweat, and feces; by hemorrhagic loss; and by menstruation.

Etiology of Iron Deficiency

Iron deficiency results from inadequate diet, malabsorption, pregnancy and lactation, or blood loss. Because the amount of normal excretion of iron through the urine, feces, and skin is very small, iron deficiency caused by poor diet or malabsorption may develop very slowly and manifest itself only after several years. The differential diagnosis of iron deficiency in an adult male or postmenopausal female should rule out an iron deficiency due to excess blood loss. Blood loss occurs with conditions such as hiatus hernia, peptic ulcers, esophageal varices, diverticulitis, intestinal parasites (especially hookworm), regional enteritis, ulcerative colitis, and cancer. The pharmacist should be aware that anemia may be an indication of an illness more serious than iron deficiency.

Blood loss may also occur from drug ingestion. Many drugs directly irritate the gastric mucosa or have an indirect effect on the GI tract. These drugs include the salicylates, analgesic/anti-inflammatory drugs such as aspirin and the nonsteroidal anti-inflammatory agents, reserpine, steroids, and most drugs used in the treatment of neoplasms, such as fluorouracil, mithramycin, and dactinomycin.

Menstrual blood loss is a common reason for iron deficiency. (See Chapter 7, *Menstrual Products*.) Normally, the blood lost during a menstrual period is 60–80 ml; in 95% of women, this represents about 1.4 mg or less of iron lost due to normal losses plus menstrual loss (18). The iron loss due to menses, in addition to that normally lost by excretion and skin shedding, indicates a total daily requirement of absorbed iron of 0.7–2.3 mg. Although average U.S. diets contain about 5–7 mg of iron per 1,000 cal, only 10% of iron in food is absorbed. Therefore, women on restricted diets may need supplemental iron. Some women who consider their menses normal actually lose between 100 and 200 ml of blood per period. To make up this loss would require as much as 40 mg of iron per day in the diet, assuming about 10% of food iron is absorbed. Clearly, supplemental iron is desirable for these women. Despite fortification of flour and educational efforts, iron deficiency remains a problem for certain segments of the population, especially inner-city children (19) and menstruating and pregnant women (20, 21).

Formulation of a convenient diet to provide the excess iron demand during pregnancy would be difficult; therefore, supplements are recommended as a component of prenatal care.

Another source of blood loss is donation of blood. A donation is usually about 500 ml of blood. If the hemoglobin is normal, about 250 mg of iron are lost. This is not a significant problem in a healthy, well-nourished adult with adequate iron stores; however, some blood donors, especially multiple or frequent donors, may benefit from short-term iron replacement following blood donation.

Iron deficiency may be caused by not eating enough animal protein and cereal food made with iron-fortified flour. Clay eating (geophagia or pica) interferes with iron absorption by the chelation or precipitation of iron in the gut (18, 22). Achlorhydria and partial or total gastrectomy or intestinal resection cause decreased iron absorption.

Evaluation

Early symptoms of iron deficiency frequently are vague and are similar to other disease states. Easy fatigability, weakness, and lassitude cannot be related easily to iron deficiency. Often, patients without obvious symptoms have iron deficiency anemia, discovered during a routine medical examination. Other symptoms of anemia include pallor, split or "spoon-shaped" nails, sore tongue, angular stomatitis, dyspnea on exertion, palpitation, and a feeling of exhaustion. Coldness and numbness of extremities may be reported.

The pharmacist may ascertain the cause of the patient's disease by consulting the medication record. The patient might have been treated for ulcers or hemorrhoids, conditions that could cause blood loss. Checking the medication record for previous use of drugs such as phenylbutazone, reserpine, or warfarin might yield another reason for blood loss. Medications, such as aspirin or ibuprofen, that may cause blood loss are bought without a prescription and often are not included on a medication record. In these cases the pharmacist must question the patient. A patient who reports blood loss should be referred to a physician immediately. Abnormal blood loss may be indicated by any of the following symptoms:

- Vomiting blood ("coffee ground" vomitus);

- Bright red blood in the stool or black, tarry stools;

- Large clots or an abnormally large flow during the menstrual period;

- Cloudy or pink/red urine (ruling out dyes in drugs that may cause urine discoloration).

Blood loss, particularly through the stool, is not always obvious to the patient. Therefore, even when abnormal blood loss occurs, the patient may not notice it, with the result that the blood loss is not reported.

Other questions may be asked for indications of iron deficiency:

- Do you eat balanced meals on a regular basis?

- Do you have cravings for clay or ice (23)?

- Have you given blood recently?

The pharmacist should ascertain the chronicity of the patient's problem, whether self-treatment has been previously tried, and whether medical care has been sought. However, the pharmacist should remember that the presence of anemia in patients other than those who are pregnant, lactating, menstruating, or on a restricted diet may be a symptom of a more serious disorder, and these individuals should be strongly encouraged to seek medical diagnosis.

Treatment

If iron supplementation can be suggested safely, the pharmacist must determine which iron product is best. The choice of an iron preparation should be based on how well it is absorbed, how well it is tolerated in therapeutic doses, and price. Because ferrous salts are more soluble than ferric salts, it seems reasonable to choose an iron product of the ferrous group. Ferrous sulfate has been the standard against which other salts of iron—ferrous succinate, ferrous lactate, ferrous fumarate, ferrous glycine sulfate, ferrous glutamate, and ferrous gluconate—have been compared. All are absorbed about as well as ferrous sulfate. Ferrous citrate, ferrous tartrate, ferrous pyrophosphate, and some ferric salts are not absorbed as well (24).

Ferrous salts have been given in combination with ascorbic acid. At a ratio of 200 mg of ascorbic acid to 30 mg of elemental iron, the increased amount of iron absorbed validated this practice (24). Most investigators believe that the cost of iron–ascorbic acid combinations does not warrant its use for the moderate increase in iron absorption. As an economy measure, ascorbic acid tablets in relatively large doses may be given concurrently with an iron supplement. This type of therapy is probably more appropriate for people who have difficulty in absorbing adequate quantities of iron (infants and young children with severe anemia) (25). Other dietary factors that have been shown to increase absorption are sugars, amino acids, and soft drinks containing citric acid. On the other hand, phosphates in eggs, phytates in cereals, carbonates, oxalates, and tannins may decrease absorption.

In a 320-mg hydrated ferrous sulfate tablet, 20% (about 60 mg) is elemental iron. In patients with iron deficiencies, 20% of the elemental iron may be absorbed. If three 320-mg tablets are taken per day, 36 mg of iron may be absorbed. Between 36 and 48 mg of iron

Recently calcium intake has been correlated with changes in blood pressure. Ingestion of a high-calcium milk product (51) or calcium supplements (52–54) has been reported to lower blood pressure in both normotensive and hypertensive subjects. More research is needed to define the role of calcium in the therapy of hypertension, but these findings imply that adult men may also need to be concerned about their calcium intakes.

The most common calcium salts available without a prescription are the carbonate, citrate, lactate, gluconate, and phosphate salts. These salts vary in the amount of calcium contained per gram from 9% for the gluconate to 40% for the carbonate. Calcium carbonate and calcium phosphate salts are insoluble, and absorption depends on a low pH in the stomach. These insoluble salts should be taken with meals to enhance absorption (55). Patients requiring supplementation who have low levels of gastric hydrochloric acid (achlorhydria) should probably take a soluble salt (e.g., calcium citrate, calcium lactate, calcium gluconate). Good absorption was obtained in achlorhydria patients when a soluble calcium salt was used (50). In the same study, normal absorption of insoluble calcium carbonate was obtained if the supplement was given with meals. Bone meal (mostly a calcium phosphate matrix) and oyster shell products (calcium carbonate matrix) are insoluble and also require an acid pH for absorption. Additionally, some of these products have been reported to contain traces of heavy metal contaminants.

Calcium can be toxic. Large amounts taken as dietary supplementation or as antacids can lead to high levels of calcium in the urine and to renal stones. The latter may result in renal damage. Hypercalcemia, with associated anorexia, nausea, vomiting, constipation, and polyuria, is also possible, particularly in patients taking high-dose vitamin D preparations.

Phosphorus

Phosphorus is essential for most metabolic processes. As a phosphate, it serves as an integral structural component of the bone matrix (as calcium phosphate) and as a functional component of phospholipids, carbohydrates, nucleoproteins, and high-energy nucleotides. Accordingly, plasma phosphate levels are under tight biologic control involving the parathyroid hormone, calcitonin, and vitamin D.

There is a reciprocal relationship between calcium and phosphorus. Both minerals are regulated partially by parathyroid hormone. Secretion of parathyroid hormone stimulates an increase in calcium levels through increased bone resorption, gut absorption, and reabsorption in renal tubules. Parathyroid hormone causes a decrease in resorption of phosphate by the kidney tubules. Thus, when serum calcium is high, serum phosphate is generally low and the reverse is also true.

Phosphorus deficiencies are relatively uncommon. However, in patients with diabetic ketoacidosis, phosphorus deficiency can result from increased tissue catabolism, impaired glucose utilization and cellular phosphorus uptake, and increased renal excretion of phosphorus caused by metabolic acidosis (56).

Chronic use of antacids can also result in a deficiency because of the formation of insoluble and poorly absorbed dietary phosphates. Symptoms and associated findings include weakness, anorexia, bone demineralization, and hypocalcemia.

The opposite situation, hyperphosphatemia (along with hypocalcemia and hypermagnesemia), is usually present in acute renal failure. Hyperphosphatemia results from decreased renal phosphorus elimination in the face of continued release of phosphorus from the tissues (57).

The RDA values for phosphorus are identical to those of calcium except that infants over 6 months of age are estimated to require 500 mg a day and infants under 6 months, 300 mg a day. Dietary sources of phosphorus are diverse because of the importance of this element in all living systems. Rich sources include seeds, nuts, eggs, meats, fish, and dairy products. Sodium and potassium phosphate salts are available without a prescription for those requiring supplements. In addition to being used to alleviate the deficiency state, phosphates have been used to increase tissue calcium uptake in osteomalacia and to decrease serum calcium levels in hypercalcemia.

Iodine

Iodine is required to synthesize thyroxine and triiodothyronine; in its absence, thyroid hypertrophy ensues. This condition results in the classical goiter that used to be prevalent in the Midwest, where soils are iodine poor. The supplementation of iodized table salt with 0.01% potassium iodide and the consumption of foods from diverse sources have essentially eliminated goiter as a health problem in the United States.

The iodine content of typical diets in the United States has been slowly declining but is still well above the RDA value of 0.15 mg for adults (58). These findings suggest that consumption of iodine supplements is unwarranted for most individuals.

Magnesium

Magnesium, the fourth most abundant cation in the body, is required for bone structure. It is also essential for the functioning of a number of critical enzymes, including enzymes involved with adenosine triphosphatase-dependent phosphorylation, protein synthesis, and carbohydrate metabolism. Magnesium tends to mimic calcium in terms of effects on the central nervous system (CNS) and skeletal muscle. In fact, the normal response of the parathyroid glands to hypocalcemia is blunted by magnesium deficiency. Tetany due to lack of calcium cannot be corrected with calcium unless the magnesium deficiency is also corrected. Magnesium deficiency causes apathy, depression, increased CNS stimulation, delirium, and convulsions. Although muscle excitability is increased in hypomagnesemia, excess magnesium has a direct depressive effect on skeletal muscle. Advantage is taken of this activity in the use of magnesium sulfate to block the seizures of eclampsia. Excess magnesium intake will also decrease bone decalcification.

Magnesium deficiencies are rarely noted in the normal adult population because magnesium is present in most foods. Special situations, however, predispose toward suboptimal levels of magnesium (and other elements). Deficiencies have been observed in individuals with alcoholism, diabetes, chronic diarrhea, and renal tubular damage, and in patients with long-term intravenous feedings without magnesium supplementation. Hypermagnesemia is characterized by muscle weakness, CNS depression, hypotension, and confusion and can occur with overzealous use of magnesium sulfate (Epsom salts) as a cathartic or even magnesium-containing antacids in patients with severe renal failure.

The RDA values of magnesium for men and women over 18 years of age are 350 and 280 mg a day, respectively (Table 1).

Zinc

Zinc is an essential constituent of a large number of metaloenzymes. Deficiencies adversely affect deoxyribonucleic acid (DNA), ribonucleic acid (RNA), carbohydrate, and protein metabolism. In humans, zinc deficiencies have long been known to result in an impairment in healing, in taste and smell acuity, and in growth. In the Middle East, low soil zinc levels coupled with the use of unleavened whole-grain breads, rich in phytic acid (which binds zinc), have been associated with dwarfism and hypogonadism. This condition is relieved by supplemental zinc. Although zinc deficiencies are not widespread in the United States, marginally low values have been noted in certain population groups and have been associated with growth retardation in children, slow wound healing in adults, birth defects, and problems in childbirth (59–62). High-fiber diets rich in phytate, in addition to malabsorption syndromes, infection, myocardial infarct, major surgery,

alcoholism, liver cirrhosis, pregnancy, and lactation, predispose an individual to a suboptimal zinc status. Iron supplements are known to decrease zinc absorption and vice versa, probably because these minerals compete for the same transport site (63–65). If these minerals are taken with a meal, the interaction is less pronounced (58). Vegetarian diets, despite their high fiber content, did not result in low plasma zinc levels (36, 37).

Several studies (61, 66, 67) have demonstrated that oral zinc sulfate supplementation (200 mg, 3 times a day) hastened healing in zinc-deficient patients; zinc did not appear to benefit those who had adequate zinc stores. In the case of patients with impaired wound healing who seem to be zinc deficient, the addition of zinc to their diets seems to be indicated. However, the addition of extra zinc to the diets of patients who have normal serum zinc concentrations is not warranted (68).

Zinc supplementation may be necessary in patients with large abdominal fluid losses because of surgical drains, ileostomies, vomiting, or diarrhea. Zinc deficiency may lead to a decrease in nitrogen retention (69). Patients with large GI losses of zinc were found to have significantly lower insulin and higher glucose levels (and lower lactate and pyruvate levels) than patients with normal GI loss (67).

Zinc is necessary to maintain normal levels of vitamin A in plasma. Cirrhotic patients have been reported to have abnormal dark adaptation that does not respond to supplemental vitamin A (70). One study investigated the role that zinc deficiency may play in causing abnormal dark adaptation in cirrhotic patients. Administration of oral zinc corrected the abnormal adaptation (71). The study findings indicate that the improvement in dark adaptation by zinc may be caused by the enhanced activity of previously depressed retinol dehydrogenase. Zinc is also needed for normal functioning of the immune system.

Zinc is not without toxicity, although the emetic effect that occurs after consumption of large amounts of zinc minimizes the problems of accidental overdoses (66). Reported signs of zinc toxicity in humans, in addition to vomiting, include dehydration, muscle incoordination, dizziness, and abdominal pain (66). Decreased levels of high-density lipoprotein (HDL) cholesterol have been associated with zinc supplements taken by exercising subjects (72), and one school of thought suggests that consumption of a high zinc-to-copper ratio increases the risk for atherosclerosis (73). As stated earlier, it is best to achieve mineral balance through dietary means rather than through the use of supplements in order to avoid complex mineral interactions.

The zinc RDA is 12 mg for women and 15 mg for men. The value for infants is 5 mg and for children, 10 mg. Typical Western diets supply 10–15 mg of zinc per day. Zinc is only absorbed from the GI tract to the extent of 10–40%. Therefore, ingestion of a 220-mg tablet of zinc sulfate (50 mg of elemental zinc) will supply an absolute intake of only 5–20 mg of zinc.

Trace Elements

Trace elements, present in minute quantities in plant and animal tissues, are considered essential for physiologic processes. The RDA for selenium is established. The requirements for the other trace elements are not accurately known. Based on the amount in the average diet, a range of intake values for the elements thought to be safe and adequate has been published by the Food and Nutrition Board, National Academy of Sciences (Table 2).

Copper

A major role for copper in iron metabolism has been elucidated, and one of the prominent features of a copper deficiency is impaired iron absorption. This is most likely caused by loss of activity of the copper metaloenzymes, ferroxidase and ceruloplasmin, which result in hypochromic anemia (69). The ceruloplasmin is especially important in the conversion of absorbed ferrous iron to transported ferric iron. Other copper-containing enzymes are cytochrome-C oxidase, dopamine beta-hydroxylase, superoxide dismutase, tyrosinase, and lysyl oxidase. The latter enzyme is involved in cross-linking of collagen and elastin. In copper-deficient animals, bone cortices are fragile and thin due to failure of collagen cross-linking; spontaneous rupture of major vessels is also observed. Copper is essential for structure and function of the CNS and for development and pigmentation of hair.

Copper deficiencies have been observed in small premature infants whose hepatic copper stores are low, in severely malnourished infants fed milk-based, low-copper diets, and in patients receiving total parenteral nutrition with inadequate copper (74). Dietary analyses have revealed that contemporary diets provide about 0.9 mg per day for females and 1.2 mg per day for males (58, 75), which is somewhat less than the "estimated safe and adequate" range of 1.5–3.0 mg (Table 2). One report has linked copper deficiencies to high cholesterol levels and possibly coronary vascular disease (76). Copper requirements for humans are worthy of further research.

Wilson's disease is an inborn error of metabolism with failure to eliminate copper, resulting in CNS, kidney, and liver damage. Acute copper toxicity symptoms include nausea, vomiting, diarrhea, hemolysis, convul-sions, and GI bleeding. Symptoms respond to treatment with penicillamine.

Oral contraceptives have been shown to increase serum copper at the expense of tissue levels. The consequences of this effect are uncertain (77).

Manganese

Manganese is required for synthesis of the mucopolysaccharides of cartilage, for glucose utilization, for steroid biosynthesis, and for the activity of pyruvate carboxylase. Psychiatric abnormalities and neurologic disorders have been reported in occupational exposure to manganese oxide. Manganese miners in Chile were reported to manifest toxic symptoms very similar to parkinsonism. This mineral can therefore be considered potentially toxic at high levels.

Manganese deficiencies in animal experiments result in impaired reproduction and abnormalities in the offspring of deficient mothers. The presence of manganese is widespread in foods, and a manganese deficiency in humans is extremely rare. A range of 2–5 mg per day is considered safe and adequate (Table 2).

Fluorine

Fluorine is present in the soil and water, but the content varies widely from region to region. Conflicting results have been obtained in determining the necessity for fluorides in animals; no deficiency state has been found in humans. The pharmacist's interest in this element relates to its demonstrated efficacy in helping to prevent dental caries. Most municipal water supplies are brought to 1 mg/l (1 ppm) of fluoride, a level that has been shown to be safe and to reduce caries in children by about 50%. (See Chapter 23, *Oral Health Products*.) Fluoride supplements should be routinely administered to children who consume water low in fluoride ion. The safe and adequate estimated range for children is 0.5–2.5 mg per day (Table 2).

Excess fluoride can lead to toxicity, which can be either chronic or acute. Chronic toxicity is manifest as changes in the structure of bones and teeth. Bones become more dense, causing, in its most severe form, a disabling disease. The enamel of teeth acquires a mottled appearance consisting of white, patchy plaques, occurring with pitting brown stains. Prolonged ingestion of water containing more than 2 mg/l (2 ppm) has resulted in a significant incidence of mottling. Acute toxicity can be life threatening. The GI and CNS systems are affected. Symptoms include salivation, abdominal pain, nausea, vomiting, and diarrhea. Because of the calcium-binding effect of fluoride, symptoms of calcium deficiency, including tetany, are seen. The patient may show mental irritability. Eventually, respiratory and cardiac failure may occur. The dose causing acute toxicity in adults is 5 g. Death has occurred after ingestion of as little as 2 g, but much larger doses have been treated successfully. In children, as little as 0.5 g of sodium fluoride may be fatal. Treatment includes precipitation of the fluoride by using gastric lavage with 0.15% calcium hydroxide solution, intravenous glucose and saline for hydration, and calcium to prevent tetany (78).

Recently there has been interest in treating women with osteoporosis with high doses of fluoride (50 mg a day) (79). This approach has the potential for adverse effects caused by excessive fluoride, so patients should be carefully monitored.

Chromium

The only defined function for chromium is in maintaining normal glucose utilization. Chromium is a component of glucose tolerance factor, a dietary organic chromium complex that appears to facilitate glucose utilization. In genetically diabetic mice, glucose tolerance factor administration (but not chromium itself) normalizes blood glucose levels (80). In humans, experimental administration of brewer's yeast, a rich source of the as yet undefined glucose tolerance factor, has resulted in significant improvement of glucose utilization and a decrease in insulin requirements in some diabetics. Other studies have given inconsistent results (77, 81–83), perhaps because chromium intake was normal. More effort is warranted to define the therapeutic utility of chromium in diabetics. Chromium has also been reported to elevate glucose values of patients with low blood sugar (84).

One patient, receiving total intravenous feeding, developed a chromium deficiency that led to glucose intolerance and neuropathy. These symptoms were reversed after chromium supplementation (85).

The richest source of glucose tolerance factor chromium is brewer's yeast. Smaller but significant amounts are present in liver, fish, whole grains, and milk. There is concern that the increasing consumption of refined foods will eventually lead to a marginal chromium deficiency in the population. Chromium intake in the United States is low (about 0.05 mg per day) compared with other countries (Egypt, 0.129 mg per day), but adverse effects have yet to be established. The estimated safe and adequate dietary intake for adults has been set at 0.05–0.20 mg per day. Chromium has a relatively high margin of safety.

Selenium

Selenium has been identified as an essential trace element in humans (86, 87). Selenium deficiencies are not common in the general population. Selenium deficiency has been reported in patients on long-term parenteral nutrition and in a child ingesting an inadequate diet (88–90). Selenium deficiencies are endemic in certain regions of China (91). The above deficiencies are characterized by cardiomyopathy. Selenium deficiency has also been reported in patients with alcoholic cirrhosis, probably because of an insufficient diet or altered metabolism of selenium involving increased urinary or fecal output and resultant loss of the element (92). There appears to be an association between selenium deficiency and protein malnutrition disease (kwashiorkor) (93, 94). Epidemiologic studies suggest that cancer and heart disease are more common in areas of low ambient selenium availability (95, 96). A statistically significant inverse relationship was found between blood selenium levels in adult males and the total cancer mortality in 10 U.S. cities (97, 98). In the United States, the mortality in women with breast cancer is lower in areas in which grain and forage crops are high in selenium (99). In 110 cancer patients, lower serum selenium levels were usually associated with distant metastases, multiple tumors, multiple recurrences, and a shorter survival time (100). As selenium levels reached or exceeded the mean value for the carcinoma group, the tumor was usually confined to the region of origin, distant metastases occurred less frequently, and multiple primary lesions and recurrences appeared rarely.

The relationship between dietary selenium and cancer incidence is under intense investigation. In laboratory animals it is known that doses of selenium required for maximum inhibitory effects in cancer prevention are considerably higher than those required for nutrition adequacy. Further, selenium has inhibitory effects in viral-induced, chemically induced, and transplantable tumors (101, 102). Glutathione peroxidase is a seleno-enzyme that functions intracellularly. Together with vitamin E, it protects against peroxidative damage to vital cell membranes. Whether this function relates to the mechanism of action of selenium in cancer and how the results of animal studies can be extended to human cancer, remain important issues. Prospective chemoprevention trials are underway testing the ability of selenium in 50–200-mg doses to reduce cancer in high-risk populations (103). The adult RDA value has been set at 55–70 mg a day, depending on age and sex (Table 1). The selenium content of foods is highly variable and depends on the content of the soils in which they were grown. Seafoods generally contain ample selenium, as do liver and some whole grains. Fruits and vegetables are usually low. Selenium is included in some but not all multivitamin and mineral preparations.

Excess selenium does not produce the same signs in humans as those observed in animals. However, excess selenium does produce growth retardation, muscular weakness, infertility, focal hepatic necrosis, dysphagia, dysphonia, bronchopneumonia, and respiratory failure (104, 105). Consumption by 13 individuals of improperly formulated selenium tablets that contained

27 mg per tablet (182 times the labeled amount of 150 mcg) resulted in signs of selenium toxicity, including nail and hair changes, peripheral neuropathy, fatigue, abdominal pain, and diarrhea (106). A 27-year-old female developed hair loss, streaking of fingernails, discharge from fingernails, nausea, vomiting, and a sour-milk breath 11 days after she began taking the mislabeled product (101).

Other Trace Elements

Molybdenum Xanthine oxidase is a molybdenum-containing enzyme; no deficiency state has been observed in humans.

Cobalt Cobalt is a component of vitamin B_{12}, but ingested cyanocobalamin is metabolized in vivo to form the B_{12} coenzymes. No deficiency state is reported to exist.

Silicon, Tin, Nickel, and Vanadium Deficiency states involving silicon, tin, nickel, and vanadium have been produced in animals only under stringent experimental conditions. These elements are presumed essential for humans but are obtained in small but adequate amounts in the diet.

VITAMINS

Vitamins may be defined as chemically unrelated organic substances that are essential in small amounts for the maintenance of normal metabolic functions but that are not synthesized within the body and, therefore, must be furnished from exogenous sources (107). Amino acids, proteins, fats, carbohydrates, and minerals are excluded from this definition (108).

It is generally agreed that a diet that contains ample quantities of the four basic food groups (i.e., grains, meats, dairy products, and fruits and vegetables) will provide ample quantities of vitamins and minerals. The important question is what percentage of the population consumes this adequate diet. There is far from uniform agreement on the extent to which ingestion of vitamins and minerals falls below the RDA values. It may be substantial, and the increasing reliance on "fast foods," highly processed foods, and caloric restriction for weight control is a trend that will only increase the problem.

In evaluating population groups whose dietary intake may be below the RDA, it is important to remember that the RDA is not a minimum value, but rather an estimate of intake that would meet the requirements of nearly all healthy individuals. It is not necessary to meet the RDA value each day, but over time the average intake should approximate this value. Furthermore, because the value is a generous estimate, frank symptoms of vitamin deficiencies are rare in developed countries even though some of the population's dietary intake does not reach the RDA. Nevertheless, there may be substantial segments of the population that are ingesting less than optimal levels of vitamins and minerals because of poor diets and other factors, and this may have adverse consequences on health. The pharmacist can help to detect physical, environmental, and social conditions that may lead to inadequate vitamin intake. Emphasis should be placed on alleviating these situations by improving the diet so that nutritional requirements are met through food. If a supplement is also needed, the pharmacist can recommend a product that will provide appropriate levels of the needed vitamins at a reasonable price.

Fat-Soluble Vitamins

Vitamins A, D, E, and K are fat soluble and are absorbed in association with lipids; therefore, conditions that impair fat absorption, such as biliary cirrhosis, cholecystitis, and celiac disease can lead to a deficiency of these vitamins. Similarly, drugs that affect lipid absorption, such as cholestyramine (binds bile acids thereby hindering lipid emulsification) and mineral oil (increases fecal elimination of lipids), may precipitate a deficiency of one or more fat-soluble vitamins.

Vitamin A

Vitamin A is needed to prevent night blindness and xerosis (drying) of the conjunctivae, which are early symptoms of vitamin A deficiency. Drying of the epithelium on other sites of the body, nerve lesions, and increased pressure in the cerebrospinal fluid also may occur. Pregnant women must have an adequate vitamin A intake to avoid malformation of the fetus. Preformed vitamin A (retinol) is obtained from animals, and carotenoids (provitamin A), the most active of which is beta-carotene, are found in plants.

The term "vitamin A" designates several biologically active compounds. Retinol is the major naturally occurring form. Because vitamin A and carotenoids are fat soluble, they are found mainly in fatty foods. Good sources are fish, butter, cream, eggs, milk, and organ meats. Four ounces of liver contain 37,000 units of vitamin A, a week's supply for the average adult. Carotenoids are the yellow-orange pigments of carrots, squash, and pumpkin; they are also present in many dark, leafy vegetables. Deficiencies of vitamin A rarely occur in well-nourished populations, and when they do occur, they develop slowly because the body stores fat-soluble vitamins. Serum levels usually remain normal until the liver reserve becomes very small.

Vitamin A deficiency has several etiologies. Conditions such as cancer, tuberculosis, pneumonia, chronic nephritis, urinary tract infections, and prostatic diseases may cause excessive excretion of vitamin A (109). Conditions in which there is fat malabsorption, such as celiac disease, obstructive jaundice, cystic fibrosis, and cirrhosis of the liver, may impair vitamin A absorption. Neomycin or cholestyramine may cause significant malabsorption of vitamin A and other fat-soluble vitamins and precipitate deficiencies with long-term use. In the United States, vitamin A deficiency occurs more frequently because of diseases of fat malabsorption than because of malnutrition.

One of the earliest symptoms of vitamin A deficiency is night blindness, caused by a failure of the retina to obtain adequate supplies of retinol for the formation of rhodopsin. If the lesion is not reversed, it may be rapidly followed by structural changes in the retina and xerosis of the conjunctiva. Bitot spots (small patches of bubbles that resemble tiny drops of meringue) may appear. The conjunctiva may look dry and opaque, and photophobia may occur. If the deficiency continues, xerosis of the cornea occurs, followed by corneal distortion. The loss of continuity of the surface epithelium, with the formation of a noninflammatory ulcer and infiltration of the stoma, can lead to softening of the cornea, perforation prolapse of the iris, and permanent loss of vision (110).

Vitamin A deficiencies are a leading cause of blindness worldwide. The problem is mainly confined to third world nations. Measles and perhaps other infectious diseases exacerbate the problem. The World Health Organization has initiated a program in 34 countries to combat vitamin A deficiencies, which result in blindness and other health problems (111, 112). One report showed a 39% decrease in mortality among preschool children receiving a high-dose capsule of vitamin A (200,000 IU) every 6 months compared with a neighboring village whose preschool children received no vitamin A supplements (113).

Other features of vitamin A deficiency may be complicated by concurrent deficiencies of other nutrients. Notable, however, is the drying and hyperkeratinization of the skin, which predisposes patients to infections. The integrity of epithelial tissues depends on vitamin A activity.

The RDA values published by the Food and Nutrition Board, National Academy of Sciences, expresses potency of vitamin A in terms of a retinol equivalent (RE). This value compares the activity of all carotenoids and other retinol derivatives with that of retinol. The RDA still retains the international unit (IU) as a measure of potency. The RDA for adults is 5,000 IU, which is equivalent to 1,000 RE. This is increased to 8,000 IU for pregnant and lactating women and decreased to 1,500 IU for infants and 2,500 IU for children. If the pharmacist establishes that a vitamin A supplement would be appropriate, a nonprescription multiple vitamin that contains no more than the RDA of vitamin A should be recommended. Patients with corneal lesions caused by hypovitaminosis A are treated with 50,000–200,000 IU per day of a water-dispersible vitamin A preparation. In children under 5 years of age, 50,000 IU have been reported to be effective (114). High-dose vitamin A therapy should be undertaken only with close medical supervision.

Vitamin A is appreciably stored; high doses can lead to a toxic syndrome known as hypervitaminosis A. The incidence of hypervitaminosis A is increasing because of publicity regarding the potential application of vitamin A in cancer and for skin disorders. Toxicity in the form of bulging fontanel or hydrocephalus has occurred in infants given doses 10 times the RDA for several weeks (114). Fatigue, malaise, and lethargy are also common signs. Abdominal upset, bone and joint pain, throbbing headaches, insomnia, restlessness, night sweats, loss of body hair, brittle nails, exophthalmus, rough and scaly skin, peripheral edema, and mouth fissures may also occur. Severe constipation, menstrual irregularity, and emotional lability have been reported in some cases (115, 116). A single dose (2,000,000 IU or 400,000 RE) may precipitate acute toxicity 4–8 hours after ingestion. Headache is a predominant symptom, but it may be accompanied by diplopia, nausea, vomiting, vertigo, hypercalcemia, or drowsiness (117). Chronic ingestion of 25,000 IU of vitamin A, a dose readily available to the public, has resulted in toxic signs in children (118). Treatment consists of discontinuing vitamin A supplementation. The prognosis is good. Because of the dangers of high-dose vitamin A therapy, the FDA had ruled that products containing more than 10,000 IU of vitamin A per dose could not be sold without a prescription; however, this ruling was reversed in a court decision. Carotene does not produce vitamin toxicity because the rate of conversion of carotene to vitamin A is slow.

One of the most promising developments in vitamin research has been the discovery that vitamin A analogs show potential in the prevention and treatment of certain cancers and in the treatment of certain skin disorders. It has been long known that vitamin A deficiency in animals leads to hyperkeratosis and metaplasia (preneoplastic conditions) of epithelial tissues. Systemic administration of high doses of vitamin A can retard the development of these preneoplastic lesions (119, 120). Simultaneous administration of vitamin A with a carcinogen has been shown to block or delay carcinogenesis in laboratory animals (121). The disadvantage of this approach, which has direct significance to the pharmacist, is that the high doses of vitamin A required to demonstrate antitumor or chemoprevention effects are sufficient to cause toxicity.

Recent research has been directed toward the development of analogs of retinoic acid with the goal of improving the therapeutic index of vitamin A. Although retinoic acid has activity in promoting normal epithelial differentiation, it is not stored and does not share other activities of retinol such as effects on vision and fertility. Certain aromatic retinoic acid derivatives, such as 13-*cis*-retinoic acid, show particular promise (122–124) and have shown therapeutic and preventive activity against several tumors in experimental animals. Dietary surveys have shown a lower incidence of lung cancer in smokers whose diets were high in vitamin A (125, 126). Human studies now indicate that dietary beta-carotene, not vitamin A, may be the protective factor (127).

The application of retinoids in cancer therapy is still under investigation. Meanwhile, pharmacists should stay abreast of developments in order to accurately answer patients' questions. It behooves everyone to attempt to consume a diet that provides the U.S. RDA for each vitamin. Persons with an elevated cancer risk (including smokers, familial polyposis patients, and individuals whose occupations expose them to carcinogens) should pay particular attention to their intake of vitamin A and beta-carotene. The pharmacist, however, should emphasize the dangers of megadose vitamin A therapy, including the fact that vitamin A and retinoids are teratogenic in high doses. Does higher than 10,000 IU (2 times the U.S. RDA) should not be recommended. Patients taking higher doses must be under close medical supervision.

Experimental results also show promise for systemic retinoids in the treatment of acne, psoriasis, and other skin conditions characterized by hyperkeratosis (128–130). Topical retinoic acid and systemic isotretinoin are currently used to treat acne vulgaris, and therapy has proved to be quite successful. (See Chapter 29, *Acne Products*.)

Vitamin D

Vitamin D is a collective name for several structurally similar chemicals and their metabolites—ergocalciferol (vitamin D_2), derived from ergosterol; cholecalciferol (vitamin D_3), derived from cholesterol; and dihydrotachysterol, a synthetic reduction product of tachysterol. Cholecalciferol (vitamin D_3) is the natural form of vitamin D. It is synthesized in the skin from endogenous or dietary cholesterol on exposure to ultraviolet radiation (sunlight). Ergocalciferol, which differs structurally only slightly from cholecalciferol, is of dietary importance. This is sometimes called synthetic vitamin D, a misnomer, because it is obtained by ultraviolet irradiation of ergosterol, a steroid found in plants and some fungi. Ergocalciferol and cholecalciferol are equipotent.

Studies have demonstrated that vitamin D requires activation involving both the liver and kidney. One metabolite, 25-hydroxycholecalciferol, is formed by the liver and is in turn hydroxylated to its most active form, 1,25-dihydroxycholecalciferol by the kidney (131). These findings explain the observation of hypocalcemia in patients with renal failure and the failure of some of these patients to respond to even massive doses of vitamin D_3 (lowered kidney hydroxylation activity). Administration of 1,25-dihydroxycholecalciferol (available as calcitriol) to these patients has proved to be successful (132).

Vitamin D is needed to stimulate calcium absorption from the small intestine and to mobilize bone calcium. It is closely involved with parathyroid hormone, phosphate, and calcitonin in the hemostasis of serum calcium.

Vitamin D has properties of both hormones and vitamins. If exposure to sunlight is sufficient, sterol in the skin is irradiated and vitamin D is synthesized. If sun exposure is not sufficient, preformed vitamin D must be obtained from the diet.

The signs and symptoms of vitamin D deficiency diseases are reflected as calcium abnormalities, specifically those involved with the formation of bone. As serum calcium and inorganic phosphate decrease, compensatory mechanisms attempt to increase the calcium. Parathyroid hormone secretion increases, possibly leading to secondary hyperparathyroidism. If physiologic mechanisms fail to make the appropriate adjustments in levels of calcium and phosphorus, demineralization of bone will ensue to maintain essential plasma calcium levels. During growth, demineralization leads to rickets; in adults it may lead to severe osteomalacia. Rickets is a failure of bone matrix mineralization. The epiphyseal plate may widen because of the failure of calcification combined with weight load on the softened structures. As a result, rickets is manifested by soft bones and deformed joints. The diagnosis is made radiologically by observing the bone deformities. The lack of adequate calcium in muscle tissue results in tetany.

Milk and milk products are the major source of preformed vitamin D in the United States because milk is routinely supplemented with 400 IU/qt. Eggs are also a good source, and because the vitamin is stored in the liver, animal livers are rich in this vitamin. Because ultraviolet radiation is filtered out by water, fish synthesize their own vitamin D and are also a rich source of the vitamin.

Although the incidence of rickets in the United States is still low, the increasing popularity of vegetarian diets has led to rickets in children who abstain from milk and in infants breast-fed by mothers who did not drink milk or take prenatal vitamins (133, 134).

Vitamin D deficiencies caused by renal disease, malabsorption syndromes, short-bowel syndromes, hypoparathyroidism, and familial hypophosphatemia are relatively common. The clinical significance of the decreased vitamin D levels noted in patients on long-term anticonvulsant drugs is still an important clinical question (135). Some clinicians recommend giving 50,000 IU of vitamin D per day until serum calcium is normal and then giving 800–2,000 IU per day prophylactically to adult patients who are on continuous anticonvulsant therapy (136).

Large doses of vitamin D (1,000–4,000 IU) are prescribed for rickets (137). For adults with osteomalacia caused by renal disease, 0.25–1.0 mcg of calcitriol is often prescribed. Dihydrotachysterol, a synthetic analog that does not require kidney activation, may also be used.

The monitoring procedure for therapy, regardless of the particular vitamin D entity used, is extremely important. Urine and blood calcium levels must be checked to avoid hypercalcemia resulting from bone turnover and intestinal absorption. Because phosphate binds with calcium and may be deposited in soft tissue such as the brain, eyes, heart, and kidneys, phosphate in the serum should also be regulated. However, in vitamin D intoxication, the serum phosphate will usually be normal or slightly elevated.

Concurrent drug therapy must be closely monitored. Phosphate in chronically used drugs, such as certain laxatives, may lower the calcium level and contribute to a vitamin D deficiency. Patients who have vitamin D deficiency caused by renal problems should use caution in taking antacids. The pharmacist should point out to patients with renal problems that antacids should be chosen for the specific ingredients they contain; aluminum antacids may be chosen because they bind phosphates, while magnesium antacids should be avoided because of their toxicity in renal disease. A calcium antacid may be used to help increase serum calcium levels. (See Chapter 11, *Antacid Products*.)

Vitamin D is toxic when taken in large doses for long periods. In general, adults should limit doses to 400 IU per day. Doses of 50,000–100,000 IU per day (1,250–2,500 mcg cholecalciferol) are dangerous to adults and children. In infants, as little as 1,800 IU per day may inhibit growth (137). Doses of 1,380–2,370 IU have not been shown to be detrimental to children, but doses exceeding 400 IU (25 mcg cholecalciferol) are not advisable (138, 139).

The symptoms of hypervitaminosis D are anorexia, nausea, weakness, weight loss, polyuria, constipation, vague aches, stiffness, soft tissue calcification, nephrocalcinosis, hypertension, anemia, hypercalcemia, acidosis, and irreversible renal failure. The pharmacist should check the medication profile for a possible cause of the problem. For example, if a patient complained of bone pain and stiffness and the medication record showed therapy with vitamin D, the pharmacist might suspect hypervitaminosis. If a recent blood test has not been taken to measure serum calcium, a physician should be consulted.

Most persons obtain the RDA of vitamin D in dietary sources and by exposure to sunlight. If a patient asks for a vitamin D supplement and the pharmacist determines that the need is based on poor dietary intake or indoor confinement, a multivitamin supplement containing no more than 100 IU of vitamin D may be recommended. Patients who request therapeutic doses of vitamin D should be referred to a physician. Liquid preparations that contain vitamin D should be measured carefully, particularly when given to infants. Patients using prescription vitamin D products should be encouraged to see a physician regularly.

Vitamin D is included in most multivitamin preparations and is available alone in various strengths for purchase by consumers. Two active metabolites, 25-hydroxycholecalciferol [calcifediol (Calderol)] and 1,25-dihydroxycholecalciferol [calcitriol (Rocaltrol)], are available by prescription for use in patients with hypocalcemia associated with renal failure. The former compound has the advantage of having a longer half-life but is less potent. Dihydrotachysterol, a vitamin D analog, available by prescription, is also useful in renal failure because it does not require metabolic activation by the kidneys.

Vitamin E

Vitamin E refers to a series of eight cyclic compounds, each containing a C-16 isopreneoid side chain. Alpha-tocopherol is the most active in the series and the one used to calculate the vitamin E content of food. Plant oils contain considerable amounts of gamma-tocopherol, and although less than 10% as potent as alpha-1-tocopherol, it may contribute as much as 20% of ingested vitamin E activity. The Food and Nutrition Board of the National Academy of Sciences lists RDA values for vitamin E potency in terms of tocopherol equivalents; 1 mg of *d*-alpha-tocopherol is equivalent to about 1.5 IU. The RDA values for alpha-tocopherol are 10 mg for adult men and 8 mg for women (Table 1). The RDA values are still expressed in terms of IU.

In spite of the seeming lack of a defined deficiency state in adults, vitamin E has received considerable interest through claims of its therapeutic efficacy for a variety of disorders. A deficiency syndrome involving premature infants fed a vitamin E-depleted formula was noted in the late 1960s. Symptoms found were edema, hemolytic anemia, reticulocytosis, and thrombocytosis, which cleared upon supplementation with the vitamin

(140). Earlier studies on adults revealed that chronic ingestion of a vitamin E-depleted diet resulted only in an increased propensity for erythrocyte hemolysis induced by hydrogen peroxide in vitro (141). Evidence for deposition of ceroid (age) pigments, creatinuria, altered erythropoiesis, and occurrence of a myopathy was found in a group of patients with vitamin E deficiency secondary to steatorrhea (142). More recently, neuropathologic abnormalities responsive to supplemental vitamin E have been reported in some patients with biliary disease, cystic fibrosis, and abetalipoproteinemia, conditions that lead to low vitamin E absorption or transport (143–146). Patients with these conditions should receive vitamin E supplements. In contrast to humans, most animals develop a characteristic and severe deficiency state. Just why humans are not so adversely affected by vitamin E depletion is unknown. It must be recognized that some of the claims for megavitamin use of vitamin E stem from deficiency symptoms noted in animals (muscular dystrophy, coronary diseases, sterility). The rationale for this type of vitamin E use is tenuous at best.

Most investigators now believe that vitamin E serves with selenium as a cellular antioxidant, protecting vital membranes from peroxidative damage. It may also have a more specific coenzyme role in heme biosynthesis, steroid metabolism, and collagen formation, but much remains to be learned relative to its molecular function.

It is unlikely that pharmacists will see a nutritional vitamin E deficiency in infants now that infant formulas are supplemented with the vitamin. Much interest centers on the pharmacologic activity of megadoses of the vitamin. Although most claims for the vitamin are unfounded, pharmacists are urged to keep an open mind on the therapeutic applications of vitamin E. Vitamin E does appear to have some utility for certain circulatory conditions and remains inadequately tested for other pathologies. Studies in Canada and Sweden showed a significant improvement in walking distance and in leg arterial flow in patients with intermittent claudication (147, 148). The treatments required at least 400 mg a day for at least 3 months. Relief of a related circulatory problem, nocturnal leg cramps, has also been reported using vitamin E (149).

There have also been claims that vitamin E is useful in coronary diseases, particularly angina (150). Numerous conflicting reports have been published on the value of tocopherols in this disease. Two randomized double-blind studies, however, failed to find any significant benefit of vitamin E in the treatment of angina (151, 152). Careful studies have also failed to show that this vitamin is useful in improving athletic and sexual performance (153–155).

Other popular claims of the beneficial effects of vitamin E therapy have not been adequately investigated. Vitamin E is considered to be essentially nontoxic (6), although the hazards of long-term high-dose therapy are unknown. One study failed to demonstrate any adverse effects in 28 volunteers ingesting 100–800 IU per day (67–536 alpha-tocopherol equivalents) for an average of 3 years (156). Nevertheless, the enhancement of warfarin anticoagulation has been reported, and the pharmacist should caution patients taking anticoagulants to avoid vitamin E megadoses (157).

The antioxidant and free radical scavenging properties of vitamin E have led to its use in conditions resulting from inadequate protection from oxidative stress. High doses of vitamin E have been reported to be beneficial in reducing the cardiotoxicity of doxorubicin, in the treatment of glutathione peroxidase deficiency (a selenium enzyme), and in hemolysis associated with glucose-6-phosphate dehydrogenase deficiency (158–160).

Retrolental fibroplasia, which may lead to blindness, occurs in some premature infants receiving oxygen to assist ventilation. Because of the low vitamin E status of these infants and its antioxidant properties, vitamin E has been evaluated for this disorder. The low incidence of retrolental fibroplasia has made it difficult to show a statistically significant effect; nevertheless, clinical trials of vitamin E indicate it to be of some benefit, particularly in decreasing the severity (161, 162). Whether vitamin E will be of help in another oxygen-related problem in premature infants, bronchopulmonary dysplasia, needs further evaluation.

The safety of vitamin E in premature infants is open to question. A number of deaths in 1984 were associated with the intravenous use of a vitamin E product, E-Ferol. It remains unclear whether the problem lies with the formulation of this particular product or with an inherent toxicity of vitamin E in these premature infants.

The successful use of vitamin E to relieve fibrocystic breast disease (mammary dysplasia) has been reported (163), but a subsequent study did not confirm the earlier findings (164).

Requirements for vitamin E vary in proportion to the amount of polyunsaturated fatty acids in the diet. Although the polyunsaturated fatty acid content of the U.S. diet has increased in recent years, the plant oils responsible for the increase are rich in tocopherol. It has been theorized that with the increasing oxidant insult in the environment in the form of atmospheric pollutants, the intake of vitamin E should be increased. However, the lack of evidence of deficiency at the present intake supports the current RDA of 8–10 mg. Until more information is available, however, intake at the higher end of the RDA range seems appropriate for alpha-tocopherol.

Foods rich in vitamin E activity include margarines (made from plant oils), green vegetables, and whole grains. Refining of grains to produce white flour removes most of the vitamin, and bleaching further depletes it. Meats, fruits, and milk contain very little vitamin E.

If vitamin E has been prescribed, iron should not be taken at the same time. Studies with supplementation of infant formulas containing iron and vitamin E show that blood tocopherol levels do not increase (165). The relative merits of both agents must be weighed before deciding which should be employed first.

Vitamin K

Vitamin K is a fat-soluble vitamin commonly found in green leafy vegetables and found in a smaller amount in dairy products and fruits. A major amount of vitamin K required by humans is produced in the intestines by microbes.

Only a small number of available nonprescription products contain vitamin K. The new RDA values include vitamin K for the first time: 65 mcg for adult women and 80 mcg for men (Table 1). Normal U.S. mixed diets contain 300–500 mcg of vitamin K daily, so there is a low incidence of deficiency in healthy individuals. Because the absorption of vitamin K requires bile in the small intestine, anything that interferes with bile production or secretion may cause a deficiency, for example, malabsorption syndromes and bowel resections. Liver disease may also cause symptoms of vitamin K deficiency because hepatic production of prothrombin clotting factor is decreased.

In addition to agents that interfere with all fat-soluble vitamins, such as cholestyramine resins and mineral oil, the oral anticoagulants are antagonists of vitamin K. Dietary amounts of vitamin K (near the RDA value) do not usually interfere with the coumarin anticoagulant activity. An interaction with the 5-mg therapeutic dose (available only by prescription) will be significant. On the other hand, 2.5–25 mg of oral or parenteral vitamin K may be used to counteract an overdose of the coumarin anticoagulant. Although antibiotics may potentially initiate a vitamin K deficiency by decreasing gut flora synthesis of the vitamin, this interaction is not usually seen if dietary intake is normal. Hypoprothrombinemias, however, have been observed with the use of some potent third-generation cephalosporins.

Vitamin K deficiencies are almost always associated with severe pathologic conditions in which the patient is receiving intensive medical care. Hemorrhage is the most common deficiency symptom. For minor bleeding, 1–5 mg of vitamin K are given, and for major hemorrhage, 20 mg are given. The cause of the deficiency will determine whether the oral route of administration is adequate. Vitamin K (phytonadione) is routinely given to neonates at birth (one dose of 1 mg) to prevent hemorrhaging. This is necessary because placental transport of vitamin K is low and the neonate has yet to acquire the intestinal microflora that produce vitamin K.

Water-Soluble Vitamins

Ascorbic Acid (Vitamin C)

As a nutrient, ascorbic acid (vitamin C) is necessary to form collagen and to serve as a water-soluble antioxidant. Only humans and a few other species must consume ascorbic acid because it is not produced by the body. Today, scurvy is rare in the United States and develops only when psychiatric illness, alcoholism, age, GI disease, food fads, poverty, or ignorance cause inadequate nutritional consumption. Infants who are fed artificial formulas without vitamin supplements also may develop scurvy. In adults, scurvy occurs 3–5 months after all ascorbic acid consumption is stopped.

Ascorbic acid is necessary for biosynthesis of hydroxyproline, a precursor of collagen, osteoid, and dentin. A deficiency causes impairment of wound healing and reopening of old wounds. Early manifestations include anorexia, weakness, neurasthenia, and joint and muscle aches. Another early sign is prominent hair follicles on the thighs and buttocks because of plugging with keratin. The hair is coiled in the hair follicle and resembles a corkscrew, or it may be fragmented after it erupts. Bleeding abnormalities, such as hemorrhaging in the skin, muscles, joints, GI mucosa, and major organs, also occur. The gingivae become swollen, hemorrhagic, infected, and possibly necrotic; if left untreated, the teeth will fall out. Death may occur suddenly in untreated scurvy. In infants, ascorbic acid deficiency may cause retarded growth and development, skin and gum hemorrhaging, impaired bone development, and anemia.

Pharmacists are rarely confronted with overt symptoms of ascorbic acid deficiency. Only 10 mg per day of ascorbic acid prevents scurvy; a normal diet containing fresh fruits and vegetables contains many times more than this. The apparent average daily intake of vitamin C in the United States is about 77 mg for women and 109 mg for men (6), although losses during cooking may decrease the actual amount of vitamin C ingested. About 200 mg per day will saturate the body so that most of a dose above this level will be excreted. Most multivitamin supplements contain 60–100 mg of ascorbic acid, an appropriate level to consume if supplements are required. Doses over 200 mg are rarely indicated. In patients with a severe vitamin C deficiency, as evidenced by clinical signs of deficiency and laboratory determinations of plasma or leukocyte ascorbate concentrations, 300 mg of ascorbic acid per day with dietary modification to increase intake are recommended to replenish body stores. Infants who do not have ascorbic acid supplements in their formula should receive 35–50 mg per day; those who are breast-fed by well-nourished mothers will receive a sufficient amount.

Ascorbic acid has been promoted for prevention and amelioration of the common cold (166, 167). The claims of ascorbic acid advocates are primarily based on personal experience and on the results of early trials of ascorbic acid for the common cold (168–170) that have been criticized on the basis of scope and experimental design (171). The claims have not been substantiated by the randomized, well-designed, double-blind clinical trials conducted since 1970 (172–175). The results appear to depend on age, sex, and perhaps subjective factors. Positive findings could not be repeated in subsequent trials by the same investigator (172, 173). At best, megadoses resulted in only a small reduction in severity of cold symptoms. No consistent decrease in the incidence of colds in subjects taking prophylactic megadoses was found. One study found that both natural and synthetic orange juice (the latter supplemented with ascorbic acid) containing 80 mg of ascorbic acid had the same effect (14–21% total reduction in symptoms) on the common cold as has been reported using megadoses (1–10 g) (176).

One valuable finding from these trials (which now involve more than 7,000 human subjects) has been the seeming lack of toxicity of ascorbic acid. Megadoses of ascorbic acid, however, may be harmful in certain circumstances. The pharmacist must consider the risks when advising patients on ascorbic acid supplements. Isolated reports of toxicity have included increased risk of oxalate urinary tract stone formation, possible ascorbate-mediated destruction of dietary vitamin B_{12}, an interaction of ascorbate and warfarin, and rebound scurvy upon sudden withdrawal of ascorbic acid. This latter effect was detected in infants whose mothers took megadoses during pregnancy.

Urine glucose tests are affected by large quantities of ascorbic acid in the urine. The TesTape and Clinistix tests may give false-negative readings while Benedict's solutions and Clinitest tablets may give false-positive readings (177, 178). The pharmacist should instruct the patient on the procedure to modify the technique and minimize the interaction between tape tests and ascorbic acid. TesTape can be dipped in urine and the color inspection made at the moving front of the liquid because different diffusion rates allow the glucose to be chromatographically separated from the ascorbic acid. (See Chapter 16, *Diabetes Care Products*.)

Ascorbic acid (0.5–2 g every 4 hours) has been used to acidify the urine in patients taking methenamine compounds for urinary tract infections. The lower pH of the urine facilitates hydrolysis of methenamine to the antibacterial product, formaldehyde. A drug interaction may result from use of high doses of ascorbic acid. When the urine is acidified, acidic drugs are reabsorbed more readily from the tubules, resulting in higher blood levels (179). Basic drugs, such as tricyclic antidepressants and amphetamines, may be excreted more rapidly from acidified urine and their effect reduced by ascorbic acid therapy (180–182).

Additionally, crystalluria may be potentially caused by simultaneous administration of sulfonamides and ascorbic acid caused by decreased solubility in the acidified urine. The clinical significance of ascorbic acid effects on the solubility and elimination of acidic and basic drugs is controversial because the decrease in urine pH has been shown to be less than 0.25 units (183, 184). It is well to remember that pH is a logarithmic scale and a small change in pH value represents a much larger change in hydrogen ion concentration. Urinary formaldehyde concentrations were shown to be significantly higher in patients receiving methenamine with ascorbic acid (1 g 4 times a day) than in those receiving methenamine alone. There was very little difference in urinary pH values between the two groups (183). Patients should be monitored if they are on acidic or basic medications and they initiate megadose ascorbic acid therapy.

Several other uses of ascorbic acid are worthy of mention. Marginal ascorbic acid deficiencies have been reported in institutionalized elderly patients; some studies have shown that ascorbic acid supplementation in these patients resulted in measurable improvement in general health and well-being (185). Lower than normal levels of ascorbic acid (and several other vitamins) have been noted in smokers and in women taking oral contraceptives. The most recent report of the Food and Nutrition Board of the National Academy of Sciences recommends that smokers ingest at least 100 mg of vitamin C per day (6) to compensate for increased ascorbic acid metabolism with resulting lower levels in the body. There is no evidence of scurvy in these individuals, but the pharmacist may reasonably suggest an improvement in diet and cessation of smoking. If a supplement is warranted, a multivitamin product containing 60–100 mg of ascorbic acid may be recommended. Ascorbic acid can also be used to increase iron absorption by virtue of its ability to form a soluble iron-chelate and by inhibiting the oxidation of ferrous to ferric iron.

As discussed previously, ascorbic acid is necessary for collagen synthesis and has been used to promote healing following surgery, trauma, and fractures. Although there is not universal agreement on the value of this approach, some studies indicate it may be beneficial. For example, decreased recovery time from cold sores, an increased healing rate of pressure sores, and a decreased incidence of rectal polyps have been reported following administration of ascorbic acid (186–189).

Conflicting data exist concerning the ability of ascorbic acid to lower cholesterol levels in non-ascorbatic, hypercholesterolemic patients (190, 191). Much publicity was afforded an uncontrolled study that indicated a prolongation of survival of terminal cancer patients given ascorbic acid megadoses (192). However, two subsequent double-blind controlled trials, the latter involving cancer patients who had not received chemotherapy and therefore were not immunocompromised, clearly demonstrated that ascorbic acid was of no benefit in terminal cancer survival (193, 194). It is incumbent upon investigators not to promote a treatment or prevention modality until they have demonstrated, via a well-designed trial, that it is successful. Otherwise false hopes are raised and unknown therapies may be tried in place of beneficial conventional treatment regimens.

The pharmacist is urged to weigh the relative risks and benefits of ascorbic acid therapy. Short-term use to promote healing, for example, or for serious disorders such as rectal polyps, may warrant a trial of ascorbic acid with medical supervision. On the other hand, the expense and potential risks of long-term ingestion of large quantities of ascorbic acid may be questionable for a seemingly minor beneficial effect on the common cold, a self-limiting condition.

The RDA of ascorbic acid for adults is 60 mg. Ascorbic acid tablets should be stored in a sealed container and kept away from heat and moisture to maintain potency.

Ascorbic acid tablets and liquid concentrations are available in many sizes as ascorbic acid and sodium ascorbate. Sodium ascorbate is the soluble salt for parenteral use.

Thiamine Hydrochloride (Vitamin B₁)

Thiamine hydrochloride (vitamin B₁) is necessary for several critical functions in carbohydrate metabolism, and the amount of vitamin required increases with increased caloric consumption. Additionally, thiamine is essential in neurologic function; however, this mechanism is not completely understood. A thiamine deficiency can be diagnosed on the basis of impaired carbohydrate utilization with a resulting build-up of pyruvic acid or more commonly by analyzing the activity of erythrocyte transketolase, a thiamine-dependent enzyme.

The most familiar natural thiamine source is the hull of rice grains. Other good sources are pork, beef, fresh peas, and beans. It was in animals and humans whose diets consisted largely of polished rice that thiamine-deficiency disease (beriberi) was first observed. Today, beriberi caused by nutritional deficiency rarely occurs in the Western world, unless it is precipitated by economic or medical conditions.

Symptoms of thiamine deficiency can become evident 3 weeks after thiamine intake is stopped. The abnormalities center in the cardiovascular and neurologic systems. The deficiency causes cardiac failure, possibly accompanied by edema, tachycardia on only minimal exertion, enlarged heart, and electrocardiographic abnormalities. The patient may have pain in the precordial or epigastric areas. The neuromuscular symptoms are paresthesia of the extremities of maximal use, weakness, and atrophy. Beriberi literally means "I cannot," stemming from the fact that people affected have difficulty walking.

Individuals subsisting on a diet of 0.2–0.3 mg of thiamine per 1,000 calories (slightly less than the thiamine requirement) may gradually become depleted of thiamine and develop peripheral neuropathy. If the patient has been subsisting on substantially less than 0.2 mg of thiamine per 1,000 calories, deficiency will be more severe. In addition to neurologic manifestations, cardiovascular symptoms will be more apparent (195).

Beriberi may develop in infants whose mothers are on a polished rice diet in regions where thiamine hydrochloride supplements are not used. The symptoms of infantile beriberi also are neurologic. Aphonia, or silent crying, may occur, and the signs of meningitis may be mimicked. Death will ensue if thiamine treatment is not initiated.

The dosage of thiamine for the treatment of the symptoms of heart failure caused by this deficiency is 5–10 mg 3 times a day. At this dosage, the failure is rapidly corrected, but the neurologic signs correct much more slowly. The dosage of thiamine for neurologic deficits is 30–100 mg given parenterally for several days or until an oral diet can be started.

Alcoholics represent a special population in which thiamine deficiency is common. The diet of the alcoholic is often nutritionally imbalanced, and alcohol may impair thiamine transport across the intestine (196, 197). A more severe metabolic condition caused by a thiamine deficiency (Wernicke–Korsakoff syndrome) may also be seen in alcoholics (198). This syndrome may also occur in other patients who have been vomiting for extended periods or who are given glucose solutions without supplemental thiamine.

The neurologic signs (Wernicke's encephalopathy) are particularly evident. Nystagmus occurs when the patient is asked to gaze up and down along a vertical plane or from side to side along a horizontal plane. Death is common if treatment is withheld. Damage to the cerebral cortex may occur in patients who survive, and it can lead to Korsakoff's psychosis. The symptoms of the psychosis are impaired retentive memory and cognitive function; the patient commonly confabulates when given a piece of information or when asked a question.

Wernicke–Korsakoff syndrome has a high morbidity and some mortality. Irreversible neurologic damage may ensue if the condition is left untreated, necessitating institutionalization of the patient. Fortification of alcoholic beverages with thiamine has been suggested as a means of preventing this disorder (199). Thiamine is commonly given to patients who are admitted for alcohol detoxification and treatment. A vitamin supplement containing thiamine is often prescribed for the alcoholic patient.

Several genetic diseases respond to administration of thiamine. These fall in the category of "vitamin-responsive inborn errors of metabolism" and generally are attributable to a defect in the binding of enzyme and cofactor. Large doses of vitamin (5–100 mg in the case of thiamine) saturate the enzyme and usually obviate the pathology. Examples of thiamine-responsive inborn errors are lactic acidosis (defective pyruvate carboxylase), branched-chain aminoacidopathy (defective branched-chain amino acid decarboxylase), and some cases of the Wernicke–Korsakoff syndrome (defective transketolase) (200–202). These diseases are relatively rare and constitute a rational but uncommon use for megadose thiamine therapy.

Thiamine is sometimes used as a mosquito repellent. Some sportspersons claim that a dosage of 100 mg 3 times daily for 3 days before and during an outing will largely prevent mosquito bites, but published studies do not substantiate these claims (203, 204). (See Chapter 36, *Insect Sting and Bite Products*.)

Thiamine is considered to be nontoxic when taken orally. Excess vitamin is rapidly eliminated in the urine. A few reports of itching, tingling, pain, and rare anaphylactic reactions have been noted upon parenteral thiamine administration.

The RDA for adults is 1.5 mg for men and 1.1 mg for women.

Thiamine is available as an elixir, an injectable solution, and a tablet. If it is mixed in a solution, the solution should be acidic because thiamine is labile at an alkaline pH.

Riboflavin (Vitamin B₂)

Riboflavin (vitamin B$_2$), a constitutent of two coenzymes, flavin adenine dinucleotide (FAD) and flavin mononucleotide (FMN), is involved in numerous oxidation and reduction reactions. Riboflavin-dependent enzymes are called flavoproteins because the riboflavin is intimately associated with the enzyme. There are at least 40 flavoproteins in the body, including the cytochrome P-450 reductase enzyme involved in drug metabolism. Cellular growth cannot occur without riboflavin.

The RDA for riboflavin is 1.7 mg for adult males and 1.3 mg for females (Table 1). It seems that the need for riboflavin increases during periods of increased cell growth, such as during pregnancy and wound healing. Surveys have revealed lower than anticipated riboflavin levels in women taking oral contraceptives, although the pathologic consequences are unknown as yet (205). Levels of pyridoxine, folic acid, and ascorbic acid are also somewhat lower in oral contraceptive users. Marginal riboflavin deficiencies have also been detected in inner-city youths, some vegetarians, and alcoholics (206–208). It usually accompanies other vitamin deficiencies attributable to an inadequate diet. Milk is a common source of dietary riboflavin; low-riboflavin levels in some urban teenagers have been correlated with low milk consumption (206). The same may be true for strict vegetarians (vegans). Other rich dietary sources are eggs, meat, fish, liver, and whole grains.

Because of the importance of riboflavin in metabolism, it is surprising that the deficiency state is not more severe. Initial symptoms are mainly cheilosis, angular stomatitis, glossitis, corneal vascularization, and a dermatitis evident in the genital region and over the joints. Symptoms of later stages of the deficiency are seborrheic dermatitis of the face and a generalized dermatitis over the rest of the body. Photophobia may occur, and the eyes may itch and burn. The symptoms of riboflavin deficiency may be indicative of other serious conditions, such as blood dyscrasias.

Riboflavin is not very soluble. If oral absorption is a problem, 25 mg of the soluble riboflavin salt may be given intramuscularly. Riboflavin is also given intravenously as a component of injectable multivitamins, but the dosage is relatively low (about 10 mg per dose). Intravenous doses of 50 mg of riboflavin can decrease pulse rates in adults. Excess riboflavin is excreted in the urine and has a yellow fluorescense.

Niacin (Nicotinic Acid)

Niacin and niacinamide (nicotinic acid amide) are constituents of the coenzymes nicotinamide adenine dinucleotide (NAD) and nicotinamide adenine dinucleotide phosphate (NADP). The coenzymes are electron transfer agents (they accept or donate hydrogen in the respiratory mechanism of all body cells). Niacin is unusual as a vitamin because humans can synthesize it from dietary tryptophan. Most individuals receive about half of their niacin requirement from tryptophan-containing proteins and the rest as preformed niacin or niacinamide. Both niacin and niacinamide are effective in treating the niacin deficiency state (pellagra). Niacin, in high doses, will lower triglycerides and cholesterol by mechanisms unrelated to its function as an essential micronutrient. Niacinamide, however, does not produce the flushing associated with therapeutic doses of niacin nor does it have an effect on plasma lipids.

The RDA of niacin is 19 mg for adult males and 15 mg for adult females. Foods rich in niacin include lean meats, liver, kidney, fish, whole grains, legumes (peas and beans), and green vegetables.

Niacin requirements are increased under the following conditions:

- During periods when caloric expenditure is substantially increased;

- During acute illness and convalescence after severe injury, infection, or burns;

- When the caloric intake of the diet is substantially increased;

- If the patient has a low tryptophan intake (e.g., low-protein diet or high intake of corn as a staple in the diet).

Pellagra is rare, occurring most frequently in alcoholics, the elderly, and individuals on bizarre diets. It also occurs in areas where much corn is eaten because the niacin in corn is bound to indigestible constituents, making it unavailable. The main body systems affected are the nervous system, the skin, and the GI tract. Symptoms affecting the nervous system are peripheral neuropathy, myelopathy, and encephalopathy. Mania may occur, and seizures and coma precede death. Before the cause was discovered, many psychiatric admissions were due to the symptoms of niacin deficiency. There is a characteristic rash in niacin-deficient patients. Skin over the face and on pressure points may be thickened and hyperpigmented, or may appear as a severe burn and become secondarily infected. The entire GI tract is affected, including angular fissures around the mouth, atrophy of the epithelium and a beefy-red color of the tongue, and hypertrophy of the papillae. Inflammation of the small intestine may be associated with episodes of occult bleeding and/or diarrhea. A summary of the symptoms of niacin deficiency in the various systems is characterized as "three Ds"—diarrhea, dementia, and dermatitis.

The niacin status of an individual is estimated by measuring the urinary levels of niacin metabolites. Low values together with symptoms point to a diagnosis of pellagra. Treatment involves the ingestion of 300–500 mg of niacinamide daily in divided doses. Because other nutritional deficiencies may be present, treatment may include the other B vitamins, vitamin A, and iron.

Niacin has been used in daily doses of 100 mg to 3 g for hyperlipidemias and hypercholesterolemia. This modality has been carefully evaluated by the Coronary Drug Project (209). Niacin treatment increases HDL cholesterol and decreases triglycerides, total cholesterol, and low-density lipoprotein (LDL) cholesterol. In the Coronary Drug Project, niacin treatment showed a decrease in nonfatal recurrent myocardial infarct (209)

and, upon long-term follow-up (mean of 15 years), a decrease of 11% in mortality from all causes (210). This beneficial effect was evident 9 years after stopping the study and the niacin. Beneficial effects of niacin in combination with cholesterol on coronary atherosclerosis have been reported (211). The adverse reactions experienced by the volunteers were significant and included GI irritation, elevated serum enzymes, and increased arrhythmias. Niacin treatment of hyperlipidermis requires close medical supervision. Niacinamide does not have an effect on plasma lipids. Niacin is also used for patients with peripheral vascular disease, but there has been no agreement on the value of this approach. Dosages suggested by the manufacturer for these conditions are 150 mg per day in divided doses. Niacin and niacinamide, in doses of 3 g or more per day, have been used in megavitamin therapy for schizophrenia. Controlled studies do not show significantly different results when compared with placebo (212–214).

High doses of niacin may cause significant and potentially serious side effects. Because of the effects on the GI tract, high doses of niacin are contraindicated in patients with gastritis or peptic ulcer. Niacin can release histamine, and its use in patients with asthma should be undertaken carefully. It also can impair liver function, as evidenced by cholestatic jaundice, and can disturb glucose tolerance and cause hyperuricemia. If niacin and niacinamide are used in high doses, laboratory parameters, suggested by the potential side effects, should be followed. The flushing reaction experienced by many people taking niacin, especially upon initiation of therapy, may be diminished by taking 300 mg of aspirin 30 minutes before the niacin (215).

Niacin and niacinamide are available as tablets and capsules of many strengths, as injectable solutions, and as elixirs (50 mg/5 ml). Doses of niacin in supplemental products usually are 10–20 mg (prenatal multivitamins contain 20 mg of niacin).

Pyridoxine Hydrochloride (Vitamin B₆)

Pyridoxine hydrochloride (vitamin B_6), pyridoxal hydrochloride, and pyridoxamine are all equally effective in nutrition. Pyridoxine hydrochloride is the form most frequently used in vitamin formulations.

The RDA is 2 mg for adult males and 1.6 mg for adult females. The adult requirement should be increased to 2.2 mg during pregnancy and 2.1 mg during lactation. Foods rich in pyridoxine hydrochloride are meats, cereals, lentils, nuts, and some fruits and vegetables such as bananas, avocados, and potatoes. Cooking destroys some of the vitamin. The average U.S. diet provides slightly less than the RDA; certain restricted diets and haphazard diets may result in low pyridoxine intake. Artificial infant formulas are required to contain pyridoxine hydrochloride.

The symptoms of pyridoxine deficiency in infants are convulsive disorders and irritability. Treatment with pyridoxine hydrochloride (2 mg daily for infants) brings the encephalogram back to normal and resolves clinical symptoms. Symptoms in adults whose diets are deficient in pyridoxine or who have been given a pyridoxine antagonist are difficult to distinguish from those of niacin and riboflavin deficiencies. They include pellagra-like dermatitis, scaliness around the nose, mouth, and eyes, oral lesions, peripheral neuropathy, and dulling of mentation. Other conditions or circumstances may also be related to pyridoxine requirements. Treatment of sideroblastic anemia requires 50–200 mg per day of pyridoxine hydrochloride to aid in the production of hemoglobin and erythrocytes.

Several drugs affect pyridoxine utilization. Isoniazid and cycloserine (antitubercular drugs) antagonize pyridoxine (216). Hydralazine appears to have this effect as well (217). Perioral numbness resulting from peripheral neuropathy is a clinical manifestation of this antagonism, occurring most frequently in patients with poor diets. Psychotic behavior and seizures, both produced by cycloserine, may sometimes be prevented with increased pyridoxine intake. To overcome the antagonism, 50 mg per day of pyridoxine hydrochloride with isoniazid and as much as 200 mg per day with cycloserine should be used. Another recommended dosage is 10 mg pyridoxine per 100 mg isoniazid (218). Penicillamine may bind with pyridoxine hydrochloride, causing pyridoxine-responsive neurotoxicity.

Pyridoxine is intimately involved in all amino acid metabolism, particularly tryptophan metabolism. Low pyridoxine levels result in the appearance of excess xanthurenic acid, a tryptophan metabolite, in the urine. Pyridoxine status can be assessed by quantitation of urinary xanthurenic acid following administration of a loading dose of tryptophan. Estrogens seem to significantly increase xanthurenic acid production, and women taking oral contraceptives show laboratory signs of pyridoxine deficiency (219–221). Supplementation with pyridoxine (2–40 mg) returns the tryptophan metabolic pattern to normal. The pathologic consequences of these events are not known, although a depressive syndrome occasionally experienced by women on oral contraceptives has responded to pyridoxine supplementation (20–100 mg) in those women who showed signs of a marginal deficiency (219, 222, 223). Levels of other vitamins are marginally lower in some oral contraceptive users. An improved diet should be considered by women taking oral contraceptives. For some, a multivitamin supplement may be indicated.

At least five pyridoxine-dependent inborn errors of metabolism have been shown to respond to large doses of pyridoxine (224, 225). Pyridoxine (100 mg 3 times a day) for at least 11 weeks has also been reported to relieve the paresthesia and the pain in the hands of patients with carpal tunnel syndrome (226).

Pyridoxine hydrochloride acts as an antagonist of the therapeutic action of levodopa, a drug used in treating parkinsonism, because it facilitates the transformation of levodopa to dopamine before the former can cross into the CNS. The pharmacist should inform patients taking levodopa of the interaction and should advise the patients to avoid supplemental pyridoxine hydrochloride. However, it may be useful in the treatment of patients who have overdosed on levodopa. A vitamin product (Larobec) that does not contain pyridoxine hydrochloride has been formulated for parkinsonian patients taking levodopa. A combination product containing carbidopa and levodopa, a peripherally acting dopa decarboxylase inhibitor, is not affected by the concurrent administration of pyridoxine hydrochloride.

Pyridoxine is toxic in high doses. A severe sensory neuropathy, similar to that observed with the deficiency state, has been noted in 7 women taking gram quantities for relief of premenstrual syndrome (PMS) (227). Four of the affected were severely disabled. Recovery occurred upon withdrawal but was slow. Similar symptoms have been reported in women taking doses as little as 50 mg a day for PMS (228). These findings point out that the common misconception of the safety of water-soluble vitamins; they can lead to rather serious consequences. The safety of long-term megadose vitamin therapy has not been established for any vitamin.

High doses of pyridoxine (200–600 mg) have been shown to inhibit prolactin (229, 230). Prenatal vitamins contain 1–10 mg and would therefore not appear to have a significant antiprolactin effect. Large doses of pyridoxine also increase the activity of plasma aminotransferase enzymes, the consequences of which are unknown.

Pyridoxine hydrochloride is available as a tablet in varying strengths and as an injectable solution (50 mg/ml and 100 mg/ml).

Cyanocobalamin (Vitamin B₁₂)

Cyanocobalamin (vitamin B_{12}) participates in methylation reactions and hence cell division, usually in concert with folic acid. Vitamin B_{12} is necessary for metabolism of folates; therefore a folate deficiency is observed as a feature of a vitamin B_{12} deficiency. It is also necessary for metabolism of lipids, for maintenance of sulfhydryl groups in the reduced state, and in the formation of myelin.

Cyanocobalamin, the common pharmaceutical form of the vitamin, is chemically stable and is generated as part of the isolation scheme for vitamin B_{12} from natural sources. In vivo, the cyanide moiety is metabolically removed to form the active coenzyme forms of the vitamin (methyl cobalamin and 5-deoxyadenosylcobalamin). The term "vitamin B_{12}" refers to all cobalamins that have vitamin activity in humans.

The RDA for vitamin B_{12} is 2 mcg for adults. Requirements increase to 2.2 mcg during pregnancy and to 2.6 mcg during lactation. Vitamin B_{12} is produced almost exclusively by microorganisms, hence its presence in animal protein. It may also be found in small amounts in the root nodules of legumes, again because of the presence of microorganisms.

In healthy individuals who have not restricted their diets, vitamin B_{12} levels are maintained by the body. Vitamin B_{12} deficiency may be caused by poor absorption, or utilization, or an increased requirement or excretion of this vitamin (231). Because vitamin B_{12} is well conserved by the body through enterohepatic cycling and liver storage, it requires approximately 3 years for the deficiency to develop. In patients whose deficiency is related to malabsorption (ileal diseases or resection), the reabsorption phase of the enterohepatic cycle is affected, and the deficiency may occur much earlier. Some people lack the glycoprotein (intrinsic factor) necessary for the absorption of vitamin B_{12}, resulting in pernicious anemia. Because of the lack of vitamin B_{12} in vegetables, vegetarians who consume absolutely no animal products are at risk for developing a deficiency (232). Several cases of a vitamin B_{12} deficiency have been reported in infants breast-fed by vegetarian mothers (233, 234). Strict vegetarians should consider taking vitamin B_{12} supplements or adjust their diet to consume fermented foods, such as soy sauce, that contain vitamin B_{12}.

Because vitamin B_{12} is important for metabolism of folate to be used in cell production, the symptoms of a B_{12} deficiency mimic that of a folate deficiency and are manifested in organ systems with rapidly duplicating cells. Thus, an effect on the hematopoietic system results in macrocytic anemia. The GI tract is also affected, with glossitis and epithelial changes occurring along the entire tract. Because of the importance of vitamin B_{12} in the maintenance of myelin, deficiency states cause many neurologic symptoms, such as paresthesia (manifested as tingling and numbness in the hands and feet), progressing to unsteadiness, poor muscular coordination, mental slowness, confusion, agitation, optic atrophy, hallucinations, and overt psychosis.

Pernicious anemia is the term used to describe the manifestations of a vitamin B_{12} deficiency caused by a lack of intrinsic factor (i.e., a macrocytic anemia due to impaired folate metabolism as well as neural disturbances). High doses of folate will reverse the hemotologic abnormalities but not the neurologic degeneration. This is the reasoning for restricting high doses of folate (over 0.8 mg) to prescription status. Surgical removal of portions of the stomach and small intestine often result in vitamin B_{12} deficiency. Regional enteritis, tropical sprue, idiopathic steatorrhea, and celiac disease impair the absorption of vitamin B_{12}.

Certain drugs may cause poor absorption of vitamin B_{12}. Neomycin reduces the absorption, and the absorption is further decreased if colchicine is also a part of therapy (235, 236).

Past treatment of vitamin B_{12} deficiency involved crude liver extracts administered orally and parenterally. Crystalline vitamin B_{12} is now available; the parenteral vitamin form is preferred. Treatment of pernicious anemia or permanent gastric or ileal damage with injectable vitamin B_{12} is lifelong.

Vitamin B_{12} is available in tablet and injectable dosage forms. Oral forms can be used if the deficiency is nutritionally based; intramuscular or subcutaneous administration is necessary for deficiencies caused by malabsorption. Hydroxycobalamin is a longer acting form equal in hematopoietic effect to cyanocobalamin. Because it is more extensively bound to blood proteins, it remains in the body for a longer period. Vitamin B_{12} has no therapeutic value beyond that of correcting vitamin B_{12} deficiencies. A deficiency can be corrected with 3 mcg of oral vitamin B_{12} daily for adults or a minimum of 100 mcg given parenterally each month. Doses larger than needed do not cause toxicity because excretion through the urine and bile occurs once tissue and plasma binding sites are saturated.

The pharmacist should caution patients that an accurate diagnosis of the causes of a suspected anemia is essential for effective treatment. For example, folic acid deficiency anemia should be treated with folic acid, pernicious anemia with vitamin B_{12}, and iron deficiency anemia with iron. The use of "shotgun" antianemia preparations containing multiple hematinic factors should be discouraged.

Folic Acid

Folic acid is pteroylglutamic acid, the pharmaceutical form of the vitamin. In foods, folic acid exists as conjugated pteroylpolyglutamates, which are readily cleaved by intestinal conjugates to the monoglutamic acid derivatives. The terms "folate" and "folacin" refer to all folic acid derivatives with vitamin activity, and the vitamin content of foods is calculated after hydrolysis of polyglutamates to the monoglutamic acid derivatives. In its function in the body, folic acid is closely related to vitamin B_{12}. Folates are reduced in vivo to tetrahydrofolic acid (THFA) through a complex process involving dihydrofolate reductase. Tetrahydrofolic acid is involved in the transfer of one carbon unit in the biosynthesis of purine, pyrimidine, serine, methionine, and choline. Several methylated folate intermediates exist and are interconvertible. Vitamin B_{12} is necessary for metabolism and recycling of folic acid. Thus a folic acid deficiency can occur as a consequence of a vitamin B_{12} deficiency.

The RDA for folic acid is 200 mcg for adult men and 180 mcg for adult women (Table 1). The RDA is increased to 400 mcg during pregnancy.

The folic acid content of food is subject to destruction depending on how it is processed. Canning, long exposure to heat, and extensive refining may destroy 50–100% of the folic acid. Generally, foods richest in folic acid are fresh green vegetables. Yeast, liver, and other organ meats also contain folic acid.

The requirements for folic acid are related to metabolic rate and cell turnover. Thus, increased amounts of folic acid are needed during pregnancy (especially with multiple fetuses); during infections; in hemolytic anemias and blood loss where red blood cell production must be increased to replenish blood supply; in infancy; and in cases of increased metabolic rates such as in hyperthyroidism. Rheumatoid arthritis, perhaps because of the proliferation of synovial membranes or the possible salicylate-induced folic acid loss, also increases folic acid requirements. Certain hematopoietic malignancies also cause an increased need for folic acid.

Folic acid deficiency may occur readily, particularly if fresh vegetables and fruits are not eaten. The symptoms of deficiency are much the same as those of vitamin B_{12} deficiency—sore mouth, diarrhea, and CNS symptoms such as irritability and forgetfulness. The most common feature of folic acid deficiency is megaloblastic anemia.

The causes of folic acid deficiency are similar to those of B vitamin deficiencies, for example, poor diet and alcoholism. The diet should include some foods that need little cooking because folates are heat labile. Conditions that cause rapid cell turnover may induce potentially life-threatening folic acid deficiency.

Several drugs taken chronically may increase the need for folic acid. Phenytoin and possibly other related anticonvulsants may inhibit folic acid absorption, leading to megaloblastic anemia (236). This problem is further complicated by the fact that folic acid supplementation may decrease serum phenytoin levels, decreasing seizure control (237). The pharmacist should keep this in mind when dispensing folic acid to patients whose medication records indicate concurrent phenytoin use. The pharmacist should ask whether seizure activity is controlled. Another possible drug interaction occurs with oral contraceptive drugs, which may cause low folic acid levels (238). This effect is extremely rare and probably is not a significant side effect (239–241). Trimethoprim may act as a weak folic acid antagonist in humans. Megaloblastic anemia may be precipitated in patients who had a relatively low folic acid level at the onset of trimethoprim therapy; folic acid deficiency, however, is not a problem experienced by most patients using trimethoprim. Pyrimethamine, which is related to

trimethoprim, in large doses may induce megaloblastic anemia. Folic acid may be given to reverse the anemia because the mechanism of pyrimethamine's folic acid antagonism is inhibition of active tetrahydrofolate production (242). Methotrexate also causes folic acid antagonism; this effect is used in treatment of neoplastic diseases, and the toxicity produced in normal cells is controlled by the administration of a reduced folate (folinic acid) in a procedure called leucovorin rescue.

Because vitamin B_{12} is essential for metabolism of folates, a megaloblastic anemia responsive to folic acid administration is a feature of pernicious anemia. Folic acid given without vitamin B_{12} to patients with pernicious anemia will correct the anemia but will have no effect on the more insidious damage to the nervous system. The symptoms of the damage include lack of coordination, impaired sense of position, and a spectrum of mental disturbances. Because of the potential for folic acid to mask the signs of pernicious anemia, products containing greater than 0.8 mg per dose are available only by prescription (243). The inclusion of vitamin B_{12} in oral preparations will not be helpful if the patient has a malabsorption syndrome; parenteral therapy is generally required.

The dose of folic acid for correction of a deficiency is usually 1 mg, particularly if the deficiency occurs with conditions that may increase the folate requirement or suppress red blood cell formation (pregnancy, hypermetabolic states, alcoholism, hemolytic anemia). Doses larger than 1 mg are not necessary, except in some life-threatening hematologic diseases. Maintenance therapy for deficiencies may be stopped after 1–4 months if the diet contains at least one fresh fruit or vegetable daily (244). For chronic malabsorption diseases, folic acid treatment may be lifelong and parenteral doses are usually needed. Folic acid toxicity is nearly nonexistent because of its water solubility and rapid excretion—15 mg can be given daily without toxic effect.

Pharmacists should refer all patients with suspected anemias for medical consultation.

Pantothenic Acid

Pantothenic acid is a precursor to coenzyme A, a product active in many biologic reactions in the body. It is contained in many foods, and deficiency states are rare except under experimental conditions. The RDA for pantothenic acid is 3 mg for infants, 5 mg for children under 4 years of age, and 10 mg for all adults and children 4 or more years of age. The Food and Nutrition Board of the National Academy of Sciences does not list an RDA value for this vitamin but estimates a safe and adequate intake to be 2–3 mg for infants and 4–7 mg for adults.

Pantothenic acid deficiency is very hard to detect. In malabsorption syndromes, it is difficult to separate pantothenic acid deficiency symptoms from many other ones. Pantothenic acid has been withheld experimentally, and the resulting symptoms are abdominal pain, vomiting, and cramps. Later, muscle tenderness, weakness, paresthesia, and insomnia occur. Administration of pharmacologic doses of pantothenic acid reverses these symptoms.

Pantothenic acid is not known to have any therapeutic use. It has gained some notoriety in recent years as an "antistress" formula and as a supplement that prevents gray hair. These claims are not supported by experimental evidence. It frequently is incorporated into oral multivitamin preparations. As much as 20 g have been administered, and the toxicity, which is minimal, appears as diarrhea (245).

Biotin

Although biotin is known to be necessary for carboxylation reactions in the body, knowledge as to the nutritional requirements for this member of the B-complex is imprecise. Biotin is widely distributed in animal tissue and appears necessary for the metabolism of certain amino acids. In rats, biotin also seems necessary for the appropriate utilization of glucose, and some of its effects are similar to those of insulin. In humans, biotin is synthesized by gut flora. Biotin deficiency in humans can be caused by the ingestion of a large number of egg whites, which contain avidin, a protein that binds biotin, preventing its absorption. Avidin causes a dermatitis, a grayish color of the skin, anorexia, anemia, hypercholesterolemia, and lassitude (246). Biotin deficiency symptoms have also been noted in patients on total parenteral nutrition without biotin supplements. In pregnant women, blood biotin levels decrease as gestation progresses.

In rats, a combination of oxytetracycline and succinylsulfathiazole inhibited the intestinal synthesis of biotin. A similar effect might be expected in humans after using gut-sterilizing antibiotics, but it has not been reported. The Food and Nutrition Board of the National Academy of Sciences does not list an RDA value for biotin, although 30–100 mg per day are listed as safe and effective for adults (Table 3). The RDA values are 0.05 mg for infants, 0.15 mg for children under 4 years of age, and 0.30 mg for all adults and children 4 or more years of age.

Biotin has been included in several multivitamin preparations. It has been used in infants and children to treat seborrheic dermatitis and propionic aciduria. There was slight improvement in muscle tone with oral dosages (5–10 mg for 5 days) (247).

Bioflavonoids

The term "bioflavonoids" has been used to designate flavones and flavonols. Bioflavonoids were called

vitamin P (for permeability), but this designation is no longer used because no vitamin activity has been documented and no therapeutic use proven (248, 249).

Choline

Choline is a precursor in the biosynthesis of acetylcholine and is an important donator of methyl groups used in the biochemical formation of other substances in vivo. It can be biosynthesized in humans by donation of methyl groups from methionine to ethanolamine. It is a component of phosphatidyl choline, commonly known as lecithin, and several other phospholipids found in cell membranes. Choline and inositol are considered as lipotropic agents (agents involved in mobilization of lipids). They have been used in the treatment of fatty liver and disturbed fat metabolism, but their efficacy has not been established.

No choline deficiency disease in humans has been reported. Rats, hamsters, dogs, chickens, and pigs develop choline deficiency diseases including fatty liver, cirrhosis, anemia, renal lesions, and hypertension. These findings have been the basis for treating alcoholics with choline, although the literature reports no therapeutic value. Although choline is found in egg yolks, cereal, fish, and meat, it is also synthesized in the body; therefore, it is doubtful that it is a vitamin. Choline is available as a tablet and powder and in combination with other nutritional ingredients.

Inositol

Inositol is a hexitol found in large amounts in muscle and brain tissues. It is widely distributed in nature and is synthesized in the body. In cell culture, inositol seems to be necessary for amino acid transport and for the movement of potassium and sodium. It is approximately one-third as effective as glucose in correcting diabetic ketosis. Inositol is available as a tablet or powder, but its value in human nutrition has not been documented. Like choline, it is considered a lipotropic agent but of unproven therapeutic value.

β-Aminoethanesulfonate (Taurine)

β-Aminoethanesulfonate (taurine) is of importance in many metabolic activities of tissues and is an essential component of taurine bile salts, but it is normally biosynthesized in adequate amounts. Formula-fed infants, however, may be at risk of deficiency, especially if born prematurely. Essentiality has not been fully established, and therefore no RDA has been established.

L-Carnitine

L-Carnitine is required to transport long-chain fatty acids in mitochondria prerequisite to their beta-oxidation and maintenance of energy production. Although carnitine is biosynthesized adequately by adults, newborns have low capacity for carnitine synthesis from lysine and methionine and may be further compromised if fed soy formulas or maintained on total parenteral nutrition with no supplemental carnitine.

Human carnitine deficiency has been documented, but no RDA has been established (250).

Essential Fatty Acids (Vitamin F)

Linoleic and linolenic acids (vitamin F) are essential in human nutrition but do not meet the definition of a vitamin because they are required in large amounts (macronutrients). The Western diet, with its heavy use of polyunsaturated fats and oils, provides ample quantities of these essential fatty acids.

Pangamic Acid (Vitamin B$_{15}$)

Pangamic acid (vitamin B$_{15}$) has no nutritional or therapeutic value.

Laetrile (Vitamin B$_{17}$)

Laetrile (vitamin B$_{17}$) has no nutritional or therapeutic value. Furthermore, cyanide poisoning may occur with some laetrile products.

Multivitamins

Health authorities agree that attention to a balanced diet and adequate caloric intake obviates the necessity for supplemental vitamins for most individuals. Certain segments of the population, however, are known to be at risk for at least marginal vitamin deficiencies unless special attention is paid to diet or vitamin supplements are used. Multivitamin supplements and better attention to a balanced diet may be indicated in the following situations:

■ Iatrogenic situations—oral contraceptive and estrogen users, patients on prolonged broad-spectrum antibiotics, patients receiving isoniazid, or patients on prolonged total parenteral nutrition;

■ Inadequate dietary intake conditions—alcoholics, the impoverished, the aged, or patients on severe caloric-restricted diets or fad diets;

■ Increased metabolic requirements—pregnant or lactating women, infants, or patients with severe injury, trauma, major surgery, or severe infection;

■ Poor absorption—the aged, or patients with such conditions as prolonged diarrhea, severe GI disorders and malignancy, surgical removal of sections of the GI tract, celiac disease, obstructive jaundice, or cystic fibrosis.

The pharmacist should be available to counsel patients on appropriate multivitamin selection. In general, an inexpensive supplemental multivitamin preparation that supplies close to 100% of the RDA for each vitamin will meet the needs of most patients requiring or desiring supplements. The need for expensive high-potency, therapeutic vitamins is rare. Synthetic vitamins are absorbed and utilized to the same extent as the more expensive natural vitamins.

PATIENT INFORMATION

The following information may be helpful to patients (251):

■ Read the labels on all vitamin or vitamin and mineral preparations before you take them. Compare the contents and the amounts of vitamins and minerals with the RDAs.

■ Take vitamins or vitamin and mineral supplements with meals. Iron supplements may cause less stomach upset if taken with meals.

■ Do not take high doses of vitamins or minerals; high doses may be dangerous. It is best not to exceed the RDA. Follow label directions.

■ Do not self-medicate a vitamin deficiency. If you believe that you are vitamin deficient, consult your physician or pharmacist.

■ For proper nutrition, eat foods from all the basic food groups (meats, fruits and vegetables, dairy products, and grains). Vitamin supplements are not a substitute for a well-balanced diet.

■ Liquid vitamin and mineral supplements may be mixed with food (fruit juice, milk, baby formula, or cereal).

■ Iron supplements or vitamins with iron may turn stools black.

■ Some vitamin supplements have a special coating and should be swallowed whole. Ask your physician or pharmacist if your medicine must be swallowed whole.

- Vitamin and combination vitamin and mineral supplements, like any medicine, should be stored out of the reach of children. This is especially important if the product contains iron.

- Children's vitamins are not candy. Children should be taught that they are drugs and cannot be taken indiscriminately.

- Niacin-containing products may cause a flushing sensation.

- Riboflavin-containing products may cause a yellow fluorescence in the urine.

- Doses higher than 10,000 IU of vitamin A should not be taken without close medical supervision. Vitamin A is toxic and teratogenic.

SUMMARY

By being familiar with recommended dietary daily allowances of the various vitamins and minerals and knowing which natural sources provide these RDAs, the pharmacist can supply a valuable service. In addition, the pharmacist should be able to recognize nonspecific symptoms of vitamin and mineral deficiencies; prompt physician referral often is crucial in these cases. A person's cultural or socioeconomic background and physical condition are guidelines in helping the pharmacist determine nutritional status. Pregnant and lactating women require more nutrients than other normal healthy adults.

Supplementary formula products should be used as adjuncts to a regular diet and not as substitutes for food. Although dietary products can be obtained without a prescription, they are complex agents with specific indications. Medical assessment must precede their use. The pharmacist should review dilution, preparation technique, storage, and administration of these products with the patient and should offer to discuss with the patient unusual effects, such as diarrhea, that may be caused by the formulas. An antidiarrheal product may be indicated or merely a change in administration or storage procedures of the formulas. The pharmacist should not be reluctant to consult a dietitian or physician (especially a gastroenterologist, oncologist, or surgeon, who often deals with nutrition problems) concerning nutritional supplementation and should refer patients when necessary.

As the pharmacist is well aware, health authorities and the public tend to become polarized over vitamin issues. Some argue that vitamin supplements are unnecessary and that megavitamin therapy is dangerous. Others claim that everyone would benefit from supplements and that megavitamins are the answer to most health problems. The truth probably lies close to the first claim. Some segments of the population (elderly, alcoholics, dieters, patients with chronic diseases or recent trauma, and pregnant and lactating women) may benefit from supplemental multivitamins. Most others, provided that a balanced and varied diet is consumed, do not need supplements. There are specific situations where high doses of specific vitamins have been reported to be of therapeutic benefit, but for the most part the exaggerated claims of the megavitamin enthusiasts have not been confirmed. Furthermore, prolonged ingestions of vitamins at therapeutic levels have not been tested for safety; some vitamins, such as vitamins A, D, niacin, and pyridoxine, are known to be toxic in high doses. There is much to learn concerning the efficacy and safety of vitamin and vitamin analogs in therapy. The consumer should be cautioned against initiating self-medication with vitamin remedies. The chronic ingestion of large doses of any drug, including vitamins, for relief of a relatively mild and self-limiting condition such as the common cold usually should be discouraged.

REFERENCES

1 *Drug Topics*, 170 (Feb. 4, 1985).

2 *Drug Merchandising*, *62*, 23–26 (1981).

3 D. Coldsmith, *Mod. Med.*, *43*, 121 (1975).

4 *Nutrition Reviews Supplement*, *32*, 53 (1974).

5 A. Kamil, *J. Nutr.*, *4*, 92 (1972).

6 Food and Nutrition Board, National Research Council, National Academy of Sciences, "Recommended Dietary Allowances," 10th ed., 1989, p. 178.

7 R. M. Kark, *J. Am. Diet. Assoc.*, *64*, 476 (1974).

8 R. O'Reilly and D. Rytand, *N. Engl. J. Med.*, *303*, 160 (1980).

9 L. A. Bauer, *Neurol.* (NY), *32*, 570 (1982).

10 B. Sandstrom et al., *J. Nutr.*, *115*, 411 (1985).

11 M. K. Yadrick et al., *Am. J. Clin. Nutr.*, *49*, 145 (1989).

12 Committee on Iron Deficiency, *J. Am. Med. Assoc.*, *203*, 407 (1968).

13 J. D. Cook and E. R. Mansen, *Am. J. Clin. Nutr.*, *29*, 859 (1976).

14 M. Gillooly et al., *Br. J. Nutr.*, *49*, 331 (1983).

15 E. R. Monsen et al., *Am. J. Clin. Nutr.*, *31*, 134 (1978).

16 B. M. Anderson et al., *Am. J. Clin. Nutr.*, *34*, 1042 (1981).

17 L. S. McEndrec et al., *Nutr. Rep. Internat.*, *27*, 199 (1983).

18 L. Hallberg et al., "Iron Deficiency Pathogenesis, Clinical Aspects, Therapy," Academic Press, New York, N.Y., 1970, p. 169.

19 P. Vazquez-Seoane et al., *N. Engl. J. Med.*, *313*, 1239 (1985).

20 Expert Scientific Working Group, *Am. J. Clin. Nutr.*, *42*, 1318 (1985).

21 H. Pastides, *Yale J. Biol. Med.*, *54*, 265 (1981).

22 V. Minnich et al., *Am. J. Clin. Nutr.*, *21*, 78 (1968).

23 W. H. Crosby, *J. Am. Med. Assoc.*, *235*, 2765 (1976).

24 H. Brise and L. Hallberg, *Acta Med. Scand.* (suppl.), *376*, 23 (1962).

25 "Evaluations of Drug Interactions," 2nd ed., American Pharmaceutical Association, Washington, D.C., 1976, p. 74.

26 *Med. Lett. Drugs Ther.*, *20*, 46 (1978).

27 G. J. L. Hall and A. E. Davis, *Med. J. Aust.*, *2*, 95 (1969).

28 P. J. Neuvonen et al., *Br. Med. J.*, *4*, 532 (1970).

29 "Evaluations of Drug Interactions," 2nd ed., American Pharmaceutical Association, Washington, D.C., 1976, p. 231.

30 H. W. Cann and H. L. Verhulst, *Am. J. Dis. Child.*, *99*, 688 (1980).

31 *J. Pediatr.*, *77*, 117 (1970).

32 M. N. Gleason et al., "Clinical Toxicology of Commercial Products," 3rd ed., Williams and Wilkins, Baltimore, Md., 1969, p. 108.

33 S. Margen and D. H. Calloway, *Fed. Proc.*, *26*, 629 (1967).

34 R. M. Walker and H. M. Linkswiler, *J. Nutr.*, *102*, 1297 (1972).

35 A. D. Adinoff and J. R. Hollister, *N. Engl. J. Med.*, *309*, 265 (1983).

36 D. J. Baylink, *N. Engl. J. Med.*, *309*, 306 (1983).

37 H. Spencer et al., *Am. J. Clin. Nutr.*, *36*, 32 (1982).

38 "Modern Nutrition in Health and Disease," 6th ed., Lea and Febiger, Philadelphia, Pa., 1980, p. 300.

39 A. A. Albanese et al., *Nutr. Rep. Internat.*, *31*, 741 (1985).

40 J. M. Burnell et al., *Calcified Tissue Internat.*, *38*, 187 (1986).

41 J. A. Cauley et al., *J. Am. Med. Assoc.*, *260*, 3150 (1988).

42 G. S. Gordon and C. Vaughn, *J. Nutr.*, *116*, 319 (1986).

43 B. Riis et al., *N. Engl. J. Med.*, *316*, 173 (1987).

44 B. Ettinger et al., *Ann. Intern. Med.*, *106*, 40 (1987).

45 H. Spencer and L. Kramer, *J. Nutr.*, *116*, 316 (1986).

46 Editorial, *Lancet*, 1370 (June 15, 1985).

47 A. A. Albanese et al., *Nutr. Rep. Internat.*, *31*, 1093 (1985).

48 A. M. Parfitt, *Lancet*, *2*, 1181 (1983).

49 C. J. Lee et al., *Am. J. Clin. Nutr.*, *34*, 819–823 (1981).

50 T. L. Holbrook et al., *Lancet*, *2*, 1046 (1988).

51 M. L. Bierenbaum et al., *Nutr. Rep. Internat.*, *36*, 1147 (1987).

52 D. E. Grobbee and A. Hofman, *Lancet*, *2*, 703 (1986).

53 N. E. Johnson, *Am. J. Clin. Nutr.*, *42*, 12 (1985).

54 R. M. Lyle et al., *J. Am. Med. Assoc.*, *257*, 1772 (1987).

55 R. R. Recker, *N. Engl. J. Med.*, *313*, 70 (1985).

56 R. Kreisberg, *Ann. Intern. Med.*, *88*, 681 (1978).

57 "Harrison's Principles of Internal Medicine," 9th ed., G. W. Thorn et al., Eds., McGraw-Hill, New York, N.Y., 1980, p. 1296.

58 J. A. T. Pennington et al., *J. Am. Diet. Assoc.*, *89*, 659 (1989).

59 K. M. Hambridge et al., *Pediatr. Res.*, *6*, 868 (1972).

60 T. Hallbröök and E. L. Lanner, *Lancet*, *2*, 780 (1972).

61 K. Haeger and E. Lanner, *J. Vas. Dis.*, *3*, 77 (1974).

62 F. F. Cherry et al., *Am. J. Clin. Nutr.*, *34*, 2367 (1981).

63 B. B. Sandstrom et al., *J. Nutr.*, *115*, 411 (1985).

64 N. W. Solomons, *J. Nutr.*, *116*, 927 (1986).

65 M. K. Yadrick et al., *Am. J. Clin. Nutr.*, *49*, 145 (1989).

66 A. S. Prasad, in "Trace Elements in Human Health and Disease," A. S. Prasad and D. Oberleas, Eds., Academic Press, New York, N.Y., 1976, p. 15.

67 S. L. Wolman et al., *Gastroenterology*, *76*, 458 (1979).

68 K. Hambridge and B. Nichols, "Zinc and Copper in Clinical Medicine," S. P. Medical, New York, N.Y., 1978, p. 22.

69 G. R. Lee et al., in "Trace Elements in Human Health and Disease," Vol. I, A. S. Prasad and D. Oberleas, Eds., Academic Press, New York, N.Y., 1976, pp. 373–390.

70 A. J. Patek and C. Haig, *J. Clin. Invest.*, *18*, 609 (1939).

71 I. Morrison et al., *Am. J. Clin. Nutr.*, *31*, 276 (1978).

72 J. S. Goodman et al., *Metabolism*, *34*, 519 (1985).

73 L. M. Klevay, *Perspec. Biol. Med.*, *20*, 186 (1977).

74 M. F. Ivey et al., *Am. J. Hosp. Pharm.*, *32*, 1032 (1975).

75 L. M. Klevay et al., *Am. J. Clin. Nutr.*, *33*, 45 (1980).

76 L. M. Klevay, in "Metabolism of Trace Metals in Man," Vol. 1, O. M. Rennert and W. Y. Chan, Eds., CRC Press, Boca Raton, Fla., 1984.

77 S. C. Vir and A. H. G. Love, *Am. J. Clin. Nutr.*, *34*, 1479 (1981).

78 "The Pharmacological Basis of Therapeutics," 6th ed., A. G. Gilman et al., Eds., Macmillan, New York, N.Y., 1980, p. 1546.

79 C. Y. C. Pak et al., *J. Clin. Endocrinol. Metab.*, *68*, 150 (1989).

80 R. J. Doisy et al., *Excerpta Med. Found. Int. Cong. Ser.*, *280*, 155 (1973).

81 R. J. Doisy et al., in "Trace Elements in Human Health and Disease," Vol. 2, A. S. Prasad and D. Oberleas, Eds., Academic Press, New York, N.Y., 1976, p. 84.

82 R. A. Anderson et al., *Metabolism*, *32*, 894 (1983).

83 M. I. J. Uusitupa et al., *Am. J. Clin. Nutr.*, *38*, 404 (1983).

84 R. A. Anderson et al., *Metabolism*, *36*, 351 (1987).

85 K. N. Jeejeebhoy et al., *Am. J. Clin. Nutr.*, *30*, 531 (1977).

86 H. A. Schroeder et al., *J. Chron. Dis.*, *23*, 227 (1970).

87 H. A. Schroeder and A. D. Nason, *Clin. Chem.*, *17*, 461 (1971).

88 R. A. Johnson et al., *N. Engl. J. Med.*, *304*, 1210–1211 (1981).

89 W. W. King et al., *N. Engl. J. Med.*, *304*, 1305 (1981).

90 P. J. Collipp and S. Y. Chen, *N. Engl. J. Med.*, *304*, 1309 (1981).

91 *Lancet*, *2*, 889–890 (1979).

92 J. Aaseth et al., *N. Engl. J. Med.*, *303*, 944 (1980).

93 K. Schwartz, *Fed. Proc.*, *20*, Part 1, 665 (1961).

94 J. Wilstrom et al., *Acta Neurol. Scand.*, *54*, 287 (1976).

95 W. C. Willett et al., *Lancet*, 130 (July 16, 1983).

96 L. C. Clark, *Fed. Proc.*, *44*, 2584 (1985).

97 R. J. Shamberger and D. V. Frost, *Can. Med. Assoc. J.*, *100*, 682 (1969).

98 G. N. Schrauzer et al., *Bioinorg. Chem.*, *7*, 23 (1977).

99 G. N. Schrauzer and D. Ishmael, *Ann. Clin. Lab. Sci.*, *4*, 441 (1974).

100 W. L. Broghamer et al., *Cancer*, *37*, 1384 (1976).

101 J. A. Milner, *Fed. Proc.*, *44*, 2568 (1985).

102 I. P. Clement, *Fed. Proc.*, *44*, 2573 (1985).

103 L. C. Clark and G. F. Combs, *J. Nutr.*, *116*, 170 (1986).

104 R. S. Shakman, *Arch. Environ. Health*, *28*, 105 (1974).

105 A. W. Kilness and F. H. Hockberg, *J. Am. Med. Assoc.*, *237*, 2843 (1977).

106 K. Helzlsover et al., *Fed. Proc.*, *44*, 1670 (1985).

107 *Federal Register*, *44*, 16139 (1979).

108 *J. Am. Med. Assoc.*, *233*, 550 (1975).

109 T. Moore, "Vitamin A," Elsevier, Amsterdam, Netherlands, 1957, p. 355.

110 "Modern Nutrition in Health and Disease," 6th ed., R. Goodhart and M. Shils, Eds., Lea and Febiger, Philadelphia, Pa., 1980, p. 153.

111 *Lancet*, *2*, 961 (1985).

112 *Lancet*, *1*, 1067 (1987).

113 A. Sommer, *Lancet, 8*, 1169 (1986).

114 A. Pirie and P. Ambunataham, *Am. J. Clin. Nutr.*, *34*, 34–40 (1981).

115 K. J. Hofman et al., *S. Afr. Med.*, *54*, 579–580 (1978).

116 "Modern Nutrition in Health and Disease," 6th ed., R. S. Goodhart and M. E. Shils, Eds., Lea and Febiger, Philadelphia, Pa., 1980, p. 154.

117 K. J. Hofman et al., *S. Afr. Med. J.*, *54*, 579 (1978).

118 P. Patel et al., *Can. Med. Assoc. J.*, *139*, 755 (1988).

119 U. Saffiotti et al., *Cancer*, *20*, 857 (1967).

120 E. W. Chu and R. A. Malmgren, *Cancer Res.*, *25*, 884 (1965).

121 M. B. Sporn et al., *Fed. Proc.*, *35*, 1332 (1976).

122 H. Mayer et al., *Experientia*, *340*, 1105 (1978).

123 P. M. Newberne and V. Suphakarm, *Cancer*, *40*, 2553 (1977).

124 C. J. Grubbs et al., *Cancer Res.*, *37*, 599 (1977).

125 E. Bjilke, *Int. J. Cancer*, *15*, 561 (1975).

126 C. Mettlin et al., *J. Nat. Cancer Inst.*, *62*, 1435 (1979).

127 N. J. Temple and T. K. Basu, *Nutr. Res.*, *8*, 685 (1988).

128 G. L. Peck et al., *N. Engl. J. Med.*, *300*, 329 (1979).

129 G. Heidbreder and E. Christopers, *Arch. Dermatol. Res.*, *264*, 331 (1979).

130 R. P. Haydey et al., *N. Engl. J. Med.*, *303*, 560 (1980).

131 H. K. Schnoes and H. F. DeLuca, *Fed. Proc.*, *39*, 2723 (1980).

132 A. S. Brickman et al., *Ann. Intern. Med.*, *80*, 161 (1974).

133 S. Bachrack et al., *Pediatrics*, *64*, 871 (1979).

134 J. T. Dwyer, *Am. J. Dis. Child.*, *133*, 134 (1979).

135 S. Livingstone et al., *J. Am. Med. Assoc.*, *224*, 1634 (1973).

136 "The Medical Manual of Therapeutics," 22nd ed., N. V. Costrini and W. M. Thomas, Eds., Little, Brown and Co., Boston, Mass., 1977, p. 308.

137 "The Pharmacological Basis of Therapeutics," 6th ed., A. G. Gilman et al., Eds., Macmillan, New York, N.Y., 1980, pp. 1544–1545.

138 S. Fomon et al., *J. Nutr.*, *89*, 345 (1966).

139 D. Fraser and R. Slater, *Pediatr. Clin. North Am.*, *5*, 417 (1958).

140 J. H. Ritchie et al., *N. Engl. J. Med.*, *279*, 1185 (1968).

141 M. K. Horwitt et al., *Am. J. Clin. Nutr.*, *12*, 99 (1963).

142 H. J. Binder et al., *N. Engl. J. Med.*, *273*, 1289 (1965).

143 D. P. R. Muller et al., *Arch. Dis. Child.*, *52*, 209 (1977).

144 E. Elias et al., *Lancet*, *2*, 1319 (1981).

145 L. G. Tomasi, *Neurology*, *29*, 1182 (1979).

146 D. P. R. Muller et al., *Lancet*, *1*, 225 (1983).

147 K. Haeger, *Am. J. Clin. Nutr.*, *27*, 1179 (1974).

148 H. T. G. Williams et al., *Surg. Gynecol. Obstet.*, *132*, 662 (1971).

149 S. Ayres and R. Mihan, *South. Med. J.*, *67*, 1308 (1974).

150 W. E. Shute, "Vitamin E for Ailing and Healthy Hearts," Pyramid, New York, N.Y., 1972.

151 T. W. Anderson and D. B. Reid, *Am. J. Clin. Nutr.*, *27*, 1174 (1974).

152 R. E. Gillilan and B. Modell, *Am. Heart J.*, *93*, 444 (1977).

153 I. M. Sharman et al., *J. Sports Med.*, *16*, 215 (1976).

154 I. M. Sharman et al., *Br. J. Nutr.*, *26*, 265 (1971).

155 E. Herold et al., *Arch. Sex. Behav.*, *8*, 397 (1979).

156 P. M. Farrel and J. G. Bieri, *Am. J. Clin. Nutr.*, *28*, 181 (1975).

157 J. J. Shrogie, *J. Am. Med. Assoc.*, *232*, 19 (1975).

158 P. Sonneveld, *Cancer Treat. Rep.*, *62*, 1033 (1978).

159 L. A. Boxer et al., *N. Engl. J. Med.*, *301*, 901 (1979).

160 L. Corash et al., *N. Engl. J. Med.*, *303*, 416 (1980).

161 D. L. Phelps, *Pediatrics*, *70*, 420 (1982).

162 N. N. Finer et al., *Lancet*, *1*, 1087 (1982).

163 R. S. London et al., *Cancer Res.*, *41*, 3811 (1981).

164 R. S. London et al., *Obstet. Gynecol.*, *65*, 104 (1985).

165 L. A. Barness et al., *Am. J. Clin. Nutr.*, *21*, 40 (1968).

166 L. Pauling, "Vitamin C and the Common Cold," W. H. Freeman, San Francisco, Calif., 1970.

167 L. Pauling, "Vitamin C, the Common Cold and the Flu," W. H. Freeman, San Francisco, Calif., 1976.

168 G. Ritzel, *Helv. Med. Acta*, *28*, 63 (1961).

169 D. W. Cowen et al., *J. Am. Med. Assoc.*, *120*, 1267 (1942).

170 W. L. Franz et al., *J. Am. Med. Assoc.*, *162*, 1224 (1956).

171 M. H. M. Dykes and P. Meier, *J. Am. Med. Assoc.*, *231*, 1073 (1975).

172 T. W. Anderson et al., *Can. Med. Assoc. J.*, *107*, 503 (1972).

173 T. W. Anderson et al., *Can. Med. Assoc. J.*, *111*, 31 (1974).

174 J. C. Miller et al., *J. Am. Med. Assoc.*, *237*, 248 (1977).

175 H. A. Pitt and A. M. Costrini, *J. Am. Med. Assoc.*, *241*, 908 (1979).

176 I. M. Baird et al., *Am. J. Clin. Nutr.*, *32*, 1686 (1979).

177 J. Feldman et al., *Diabetes*, *19*, 337 (1970).

178 J. Mayson et al., *Am. J. Clin. Pathol.*, *58*, 297 (1972).

179 G. Levy and J. Leonards, *J. Am. Med. Assoc.*, *217*, 81 (1971).

180 F. Sioquist, *Clin. Pharmacol. Ther.*, *10*, 826 (1969).

181 L. Gram et al., *Clin. Pharmacol. Ther.*, *12*, 239 (1971).

182 M. Rowland, *J. Pharm. Sci.*, *58*, 508 (1969).

183 M. C. Nakata et al., *Am. J. Hosp. Pharm.*, *34*, 1234 (1977).

184 D. V. Naccarto, *J. Am. Geriatr. Soc.*, *27*, 34 (1979).

185 C. J. Schorah et al., *Lancet*, *1*, 403 (1979).

186 G. T. Terezhalmy et al., *Oral Surg.*, *45*, 56 (1978).

187 T. V. Taylor et al., *Lancet*, *2*, 544 (1974).

188 J. J. DeCosse, *Surgery*, *78*, 608 (1975).

189 J. J. DeCosse et al., *Cancer*, *40*, 2549 (1977).

190 C. R. Spittle, *Lancet*, *2*, 1280 (1971).

191 R. E. Hughes, *Proc. Roy. Soc. Med.*, *70*, 86 (1977).

192 E. Cameron and L. Pauling, *Proc. Natl. Acad. Sci., U.S.A.*, *73*, 3685 (1976).

193 E. T. Creagan et al., *N. Engl. J. Med.*, *301*, 687 (1979).

194 C. G. Moertel et al., *N. Engl. J. Med.*, *312*, 137 (1985).

195 "Modern Nutrition in Health and Disease," 6th ed., R. Goodhart and M. Shils, Eds., Lea and Febiger, Philadelphia, Pa., 1980, p. 686.

196 A. M. Hoyumpa et al., *J. Lab. Clin. Med.*, *86*, 803 (1975).

197 A. M. Hoyumpa et al., *Gastroenterology*, *68*, 1218 (1975).

198 M. Victor, *Contemp. Neurol. Ser.*, *7*, 1–206 (1971).

199 B. S. Centerwald and M. H. Criqui, *N. Engl. J. Med.*, *299*, 285 (1978).

200 S. H. Mudd, *Fed. Proc.*, *30*, 970 (1971).

201 C. R. Scriver, *Metabolism*, *22*, 1319 (1973).

202 J. P. Blass and G. F. Gilson, *N. Engl. J. Med.*, *247*, 1367 (1977).

203 W. G. Strauss et al., *Am. J. Trop. Med. Hyg.*, *17*, 411 (1968).

204 C. N. Smith, *Public Entomol. Soc. Am.*, *7*, 99 (1970).

205 L. J. Neuman et al., *Am. J. Clin. Nutr.*, *31*, 247 (1978).

206 R. Lopez et al., *Am. J. Clin. Nutr.*, *33*, 1283 (1980).

207 J. G. Bergan and P. T. Brown, *Am. J. Diet. Assoc.*, *76*, 151 (1980).

208 R. S. Rivlin, *Nutr. Rev.*, *37*, 241 (1979).

209 The Coronary Drug Research Group, *J. Am. Med. Assoc.*, *231*, 360 (1975).

210 P. L. Conner et al., *J. Am. Coll. Cardiol.*, *8*, 1245 (1986).

211 D. H. Blankenhorn et al., *J. Am. Med. Assoc.*, *257*, 3233 (1987).

212 T. A. Ban and H. E. Lehman, *Can. J. Psychiatry*, *15*, 499 (1970).

213 J. F. Vallely et al., *Can. J. Psychiatry*, *16*, 433 (1971).

214 T. A. Ban and H. E. Lehman, *Can. J. Psychiatry*, *20*, 103 (1975).

215 J. K. Wilkin et al., *Clin. Pharmacol. Ther.*, *31*, 478 (1982).

216 "Evaluations of Drug Interactions," 2nd ed., American Pharmaceutical Association, Washington, D.C., 1976, p. 118.

217 N. H. Raskin, *N. Engl. J. Med.*, *273*, 1182 (1965).

218 "Applied Therapeutics for Clinical Pharmacists," 2nd ed., Applied Therapeutics, San Francisco, Calif., 1978, p. 337.

219 M. Baumblatt and F. Winston, *Lancet*, *1*, 832 (1970).

220 A. Lubby et al., *Lancet*, *2*, 1083 (1970).

221 A. Lubby et al., *Am. J. Clin. Nutr.*, *24*, 684 (1971).

222 P. W. Adams et al., *Lancet*, *1*, 897 (1973).

223 P. W. Adams et al., *Lancet*, *2*, 516 (1974).

224 S. H. Mudd, *Fed. Proc.*, *30*, 970 (1971).

225 C. R. Scrivor, *Metabolism*, *22*, 1319 (1973).

226 J. M. Ellis et al., *Am. J. Clin. Nutr.*, *32*, 2040 (1979).

227 H. Schaumburg et al., *N. Engl. J. Med.*, *309*, 445 (1983).

228 K. Dalton and M. J. T. Dalton, *Acta Neurol. Scand.*, *76*, 8 (1987).

229 L. B. Greentree, *N. Engl. J. Med.*, *300*, 141 (1979).

230 M. D. Foulkas, *Br. J. Obstet. Gynecol.*, *80*, 718 (1973).

231 "Modern Nutrition in Health and Disease," 6th ed., R. S. Goodhart and M. E. Shils, Eds., Lea and Febiger, Philadelphia, Pa., 1980, p. 235.

232 J. D. Hines, *Am. J. Clin. Nutr.*, *19*, 260 (1966).

233 M. C. Higginbottom et al., *N. Engl. J. Med.*, *299*, 317 (1978).

234 J. Trader et al., *N. Engl. J. Med.*, *299*, 1319 (1978).

235 W. Faloon and R. Chodos, *Gastroenterology*, *56*, 1251 (1969).

236 C. Gerson, *Gastroenterology*, *63*, 246 (1972).

237 H. Kutt et al., *Arch. Neurol. (Chicago)*, *14*, 489 (1966).

238 T. Necheles and L. Snyder, *N. Engl. J. Med.*, *282*, 858 (1970).

239 N. Elgee, *Ann. Intern. Med.*, *72*, 409 (1970).

240 R. Swerdloff et al., *West J. Med.*, *122*, 22 (1975).

241 A. Bingel and P. Benoit, *J. Pharm. Sci.*, *62*, 179 (1973).

242 "The Pharmacological Basis of Therapeutics," 5th ed., L. S. Goodman and A. Gilman, Eds., Macmillan, New York, N.Y., 1975, p. 1058.

243 *Federal Register*, *41*, 46172 (1976).

244 "Modern Nutrition in Health and Disease," 6th ed., R. S. Goodhart and M. E. Shils, Eds., Lea and Febiger, Philadelphia, Pa., 1980, p. 254.

245 "Modern Nutrition in Health and Disease," 6th ed., R. S. Goodhart and M. E. Shils, Eds., Lea and Febiger, Philadelphia, Pa., 1980, p. 214.

246 V. Sydenstricker et al., *J. Am. Med. Assoc.*, *118*, 1199 (1942).

247 N. Barnes et al., *Lancet*, *2*, 244 (1970).

248 E. Foldi-Borcsok and M. Foldi, *Am. J. Clin. Nutr.*, *26*, 185 (1973).

249 R. Eastham et al., *Br. Med. J.*, *4*, 491 (1972).

250 Food and Nutrition Board, National Research Council, National Academy of Sciences, "Recommended Dietary Allowances," 10th ed., National Academy Press, Washington, D.C., 1989, p. 266.

251 D. L. Smith, "Medication Guide for Patient Counseling," Lea and Febiger, Philadelphia, Pa., 1977, pp. 413–414.

FOOD SUPPLEMENT PRODUCT TABLE

Product (Manufacturer)	Dosage Form[a]	Calories (per ml)	Protein (g)	Carbohydrate (g)	Fat (g)	Vitamins, Minerals	Indicated Use
Amin-Aid Instant Drink (Kendall-McGaw)	powder	2	19	366	46		enteral nutrition. For acute or chronic renal failure.
Attain (Sherwood)	liquid	1	40	120	40	various[b,c,d]	enteral nutrition. Lactose free.
Citrotein (Sandoz)	powder	0.66	41	122	1.6	various[b,c]	enteral nutrition. Lactose, cholesterol and gluten free.
Complete Modified Formula (Sandoz)	liquid	1.07	43	141	37	various[b,c,d]	enteral nutrition. Lactose and gluten free.
Complete Regular Formula (Sandoz)	liquid	1.07	43	128	43	various[b,c,d]	enteral nutrition. Milk base.
Comply (Sherwood)	liquid	1.5	60	180	60	various[b,c,d]	enteral nutrition. Lactose free.
Criticare HN (Mead Johnson)	liquid	1.06	38	222	3	various[b,c,d]	enteral nutrition. Lactose free.
Enrich w/Fiber (Ross)	liquid	1.1	39.1	159.3	36.6	various[b,c,d]	enteral nutrition. Lactose free.
Ensure (Ross)	liquid	1.06	36.6	142.6	36.6	various[b,c,d]	enteral nutrition. Lactose free.
Ensure HN (Ross)	liquid	1.06	43.6	138.9	34.9	various[b,c,d]	enteral nutrition. Lactose free.
Ensure Plus (Ross)	liquid	1.5	54	197.7	52.4	various[b,c,d]	enteral nutrition. Lactose free.
Ensure Plus HN (Ross)	liquid	1.5	61.5	196.7	49	various[b,c,d]	enteral nutrition. Lactose free.
Entrition (Biosearch)	liquid	1	35	136	35	various[b,c]	enteral nutrition. Lactose free.
Entrition HN (Biosearch)	liquid	1	44	114	41	various[b,c,d]	enteral nutrition. Lactose free.
Forta Cereal Mix[e] (Ross)	cereal	140[e]	6	23	3	various[b,c,d]	enteral nutrition. Lactose free.
Forta Drink[e] (Ross)	powder	85[e]	5	15	< 1	various[b,c,d]	enteral nutrition. Lactose free.
Forta Pudding Mix[e] (Ross)	pudding	250[e]	9	34	9	various[b,c,d]	enteral nutrition. Lactose free.
Forta Shake[e] (Ross)	powder	140[e]	9	26	< 1	various[b,c,d]	enteral nutrition. Milk base.
Forta Soup Mix[e] (Ross)	powder	250[e]	9	33	9	various[b]	enteral nutrition. Milk base.
Hepatic-Aid II Instant Drink (Kendall-McGaw)	powder	1.2	44	168	36		enteral nutrition. For chronic liver disease.

FOOD SUPPLEMENT PRODUCT TABLE, continued

Product (Manufacturer)	Dosage Form[a]	Calories (per ml)	Protein (g)	Carbohydrate (g)	Fat (g)	Vitamins, Minerals	Indicated Use
Isocal (Mead Johnson)	liquid	1.06	34	133	44	various[b,c,d]	enteral nutrition. Lactose free.
Isocal HCN (Mead Johnson)	liquid	2	75	200	102	various[b,c,d]	enteral nutrition. Lactose free.
Isotein HN (Sandoz)	powder	1.2	68	156	34	various[b,c,d]	enteral nutrition. Lactose, purine and gluten free.
Jevity (Ross)	liquid	1.06	43.7	149	36.1	various[b,c,d]	enteral nutrition. Lactose free.
Lonalac (Mead Johnson)	powder	1.01	53.7	75.5	55.7	vitamin A, B_1, B_2, B_3, Ca, Cl, Mg, P	enteral nutrition. Milk base.
Magnacal (Sherwood)	liquid	2	70	250	80	various[b,c,d]	enteral nutrition. Lactose free.
Meritene (Sandoz)	liquid	0.96	57.6	110	32	various[b,c,d]	enteral nutrition. Milk base.
Meritene (Sandoz)	powder	1	69	119	34	various[b,c,d]	enteral nutrition. Milk base.
Nutren 1.0 (Clintec)	liquid	1	40	127.2	38	various[b,c,d]	enteral nutrition. Lactose, cholesterol and gluten free.
Nutren 1.5 (Clintec)	liquid	1.5	60	170	67.6	various[b,c,d]	enteral nutrition. Lactose, cholesterol and gluten free.
Nutren 2.0 (Clintec)	liquid	2	80	196	106	various[b,c,d]	enteral nutrition. Lactose, cholesterol and gluten free.
Osmolite (Ross)	liquid	1.06	36.6	142.6	37.8	various[b,c,d]	enteral nutrition. Lactose free.
Osmolite HN (Ross)	liquid	1.06	44.4	138.9	36.1	various[b,c,d]	enteral nutrition. Lactose free.
Peptamen (Clintec)	liquid	1	40	127	39	various[b,c,d]	enteral nutrition. Lactose, cholesterol and gluten free.
Pepti-2000 (Sherwood)	powder	1	40	189	10	various[b,c,d]	enteral nutrition. For GI conditions.
Portagen (Mead Johnson)	powder	1	35.3	114.4	47.6	various[b,c,d]	enteral nutrition. Lactose free.
Pre-Attain (Sherwood)	liquid	0.5	20	60	20	various[b,c]	enteral nutrition. Lactose free.
Precision High Nitrogen Diet (Sandoz)	powder	1.05	43.9	216	1.3	various[b,c,d]	enteral nutrition. Lactose, cholesterol and gluten free.
Precision Isotonic Diet (Sandoz)	powder	1	29	144	30	various[b,c]	enteral nutrition. Lactose, cholesterol, purine and gluten free.

FOOD SUPPLEMENT PRODUCT TABLE, continued

Product (Manufacturer)	Dosage Form[a]	Calories (per ml)	Protein (g)	Carbohydrate (g)	Fat (g)	Vitamins, Minerals	Indicated Use
Precision LR Diet (Sandoz)	powder	1.6	26	248	1.6	various[b,c,d]	enteral nutrition. Lactose, cholesterol and gluten free.
Profiber (Sherwood)	liquid	1	40	132	40	various[b,c,d]	enteral nutrition. Lactose free.
Pulmocare (Ross)	liquid	1.5	61.5	104	90.6	various[b,c,d]	enteral nutrition. For pulmonary patients.
Replete (Clintec)	liquid	1	62.4	112.8	33.2	various[b,c,d]	enteral nutrition. Lactose, cholesterol and gluten free.
Resource (Sandoz)	powder	1.06	37.2	145	37.2	various[b,c,d]	enteral nutrition. Lactose free.
Stresstein (Sandoz)	powder	1.2	70	170	28	various[b,c,d]	enteral nutrition. For severe metabolic stress and trauma.
Sustacal (Mead Johnson)	liquid	1	61	140	23	various[b,c,d]	enteral nutrition. Lactose free.
Sustacal (Mead Johnson)	powder	1	60	139.4	23.3	various[b,c,d]	enteral nutrition. Milk base.
Sustacal (Mead Johnson)	pudding	1.7	6.8[e]	32[e]	9.5[e]	various[b,c,d]	enteral nutrition. Milk base.
Sustacal HC (Mead Johnson)	liquid	1.5	61	190	58	various[b,c,d]	enteral nutrition. Lactose free.
Sustagen (Mead Johnson)	powder	1.7	113	317	16.8	various[b,c,d]	enteral nutrition. Milk base.
Tolerex (Norwich Eaton)	powder	1	20.6	226.3	1.45	various[b,c,d]	enteral nutrition. Lactose free.
TraumaCal (Mead Johnson)	liquid	1.5	83	142	68	various[b,c,d]	enteral nutrition. For trauma and moderate to severe burns.
Traum-Aid HBC (Kendall-McGaw)	powder	1	66.6	197.5	14.7	various[b,c,d]	enteral nutrition. For trauma and sepsis.
Travasorb Hepatic (Clintec)	powder	1.1	29.4	215	14.7	various[b,c,d]	enteral nutrition. For liver failure.
Travasorb HN (Clintec)	powder	1	45	175	13.5	various[b,c,d]	enteral nutrition. Lactose and gluten free.
Travasorb MCT (Clintec)	powder	1	49	123	33	various[b,c]	enteral nutrition. Lactose free.
Travasorb Renal (Clintec)	powder	1.35	22.9	271	17.7	vitamin B_1, B_2, B_3, B_5, B_6, C, FA, biotin, choline	enteral nutrition. For renal failure.

FOOD SUPPLEMENT PRODUCT TABLE, continued

Product (Manu-facturer)	Dosage Form[a]	Calories (per ml)	Protein (g)	Carbo-hydrate (g)	Fat (g)	Vitamins, Minerals	Indicated Use
Travasorb STD (Clintec)	powder	1	30	190	13.5	various[b,c,d]	enteral nutrition. Lactose and gluten free.
Vital High Nitrogen (Ross)	powder	1	41.2	182.8	10.7	various[b,c,d]	enteral nutrition. Lactose free.
Vitaneed (Sherwood)	liquid	1	40	128	40	various[b,c,d]	enteral nutrition. Lactose free.
Vivonex T.E.N. (Norwich Eaton)	powder	1	38.2	206	2.77	various[b,c,d]	enteral nutrition. Lactose free.

[a] Content given in gram per liter. Powder must be added to liquid as package directs.
[b] Includes vitamins A, D, E, ascorbic acid, thiamine, riboflavin, niacin, pyridoxine hydrochloride, cyanocobalamin, and/or various other substances having vitamin activity.
[c] Includes iron, calcium, phosphorus, iodine, magnesium, copper, zinc, potassium, sodium, manganese, chromium, selenium and/or molybdenum.
[d] Includes choline, biotin, inositol and/or folic acid.
[e] Content given per serving.

IRON PRODUCT TABLE

Product (Manufacturer)	Iron (elemental)	Vitamins	Other Ingredients
Allbee C-800 Plus Iron Tablets (Robins)	27 mg (as ferrous fumarate)	vitamin E, 45 IU vitamin B_1, 15 mg vitamin B_2, 17 mg niacin, 100 mg pantothenic acid, 25 mg vitamin B_6, 25 mg vitamin B_{12}, 12 mcg vitamin C, 800 mg	folic acid, 0.4 mg
Beminal Stress Plus with Iron Tablets[a] (Whitehall)	27 mg (as ferrous fumarate)	vitamin E, 45 IU vitamin B_1, 25 mg vitamin B_2, 12.5 mg niacin, 100 mg pantothenic acid, 20 mg vitamin B_6, 10 mg vitamin B_{12}, 25 mcg vitamin C, 700 mg	folic acid, 0.4 mg
Chel-Iron Liquid and Tablets (Kinney)	50 mg/5 ml 40 mg/tablet (as ferrocholinate)		
Chel-Iron Pediatric Drops (Kinney)	25 mg/ml (as ferrocholinate)		
Femiron (SmithKline Beecham)	20 mg (as ferrous fumarate)		
Feosol Capsules, Tablets and Elixir (SmithKline)	50 mg/capsule 65 mg/tablet 44 mg/5 ml (elixir) (as ferrous sulfate)		alcohol, 5%
Feostat Chewable Tablets, Drops and Suspension (Forest)	33 mg/chewable tablet 15 mg/0.6 ml (drops) 33 mg/5 ml (susp) (as ferrous fumarate)		flavor
Ferancee (Stuart)	67 mg (as ferrous fumarate)	sodium ascorbate, 101 mg ascorbic acid, 49 mg	sodium, 0.52 mEq
Ferancee-HP (Stuart)	110 mg (as ferrous fumarate)	sodium ascorbate, 250 mg ascorbic acid, 350 mg	sodium, 1.56 mEq
Fergon Elixir and Tablets (Winthrop)	35 mg/5 ml 37 mg/tablet (as ferrous gluconate)		
Fergon Plus Caplets (Winthrop)	58 mg (as ferrous gluconate)	ascorbic acid, 75 mg vitamin B_{12}, ½ unit	
Fer-In-Sol Capsules, Drops and Syrup (Mead Johnson)	60 mg/capsule 15 mg/0.6 ml (drops) 18 mg/5 ml (syrup) (as ferrous sulfate)		alcohol, 0.02% (drops) 5% (syrup)
Fer-Iron Drops (Various manufacturers)	25 mg/5 ml (as ferrous sulfate)		
Fermalox Tablets (Rorer)	40 mg (as ferrous sulfate)		magnesium hydroxide, 100 mg aluminum hydroxide gel, dried, 100 mg
Fero-Grad-500 Tablets (Abbott)	105 mg (as ferrous sulfate)	sodium ascorbate, 500 mg	
Fero-Gradumet Tablets (Abbott)	105 mg (as ferrous sulfate)		

IRON PRODUCT TABLE, continued

Product (Manufacturer)	Iron (elemental)	Vitamins	Other Ingredients
Ferralyn Lanacaps (Lannett)	50 mg (as ferrous sulfate)		
Ferra-TD Capsules (Goldline)	50 mg (as ferrous sulfate)		
Ferro-Dok TR Capsules (Major)	50 mg (as ferrous fumarate)		docusate sodium, 100 mg
Ferro-Sequels (Lederle)	50 mg (as ferrous fumarate)		docusate sodium, 100 mg
Ferrous Fumarate Tablets (Various manufacturers)	106 mg (as ferrous fumarate)		
Ferrous Gluconate Capsules and Tablets (Various manufacturers)	35 mg/tablet 38 mg/capsule and tablet (as ferrous gluconate)		
Ferrous-S.Q.L. Capsules (Goldline)	50 mg (as ferrous fumarate)		docusate sodium, 100 mg
Ferrous Sulfate Capsules, Tablets and Elixir (Various manufacturers)	30 mg/capsule 50 mg/capsule 60 mg/tablet 65 mg/tablet 44 mg/5 ml (elixir) (as ferrous sulfate)		
Fumaral Elixir and Spancaps (Vortech)	ferrous sulfate, 45 mg/ml 108 mg/capsule (as ferrous fumarate)	ascorbic acid, 200 mg/capsule	alcohol, 5% (elixir)
Generet-500 Tablets (Goldline)	105 mg (as ferrous sulfate)	vitamin B_1, 6 mg vitamin B_2, 6 mg niacin, 30 mg pantothenic acid, 10 mg vitamin B_6, 5 mg vitamin B_{12}, 25 mcg sodium ascorbate, 500 mg	
Geriamic Tablets (Vortech)	50 mg (as ferrous sulfate)	vitamin B_1, 5 mg vitamin B_2, 5 mg niacin, 30 mg pantothenic acid, 2 mg vitamin B_6, 0.5 mg vitamin B_{12}, 3 mcg sodium ascorbate, 75 mg	
Geriot Tablets (Goldline)	50 mg (as ferrous sulfate)	vitamin B_1, 5 mg vitamin B_2, 5 mg niacin, 30 mg pantothenic acid, 2 mg vitamin B_6, 0.5 mg vitamin B_{12}, 3 mcg sodium ascorbate, 75 mg	
Hytinic Capsules and Elixir (Hyrex)	150 mg/capsule 20 mg/ml (elixir) (as polysaccharide-iron complex)		sodium, 0.2 mEq/capsules 0.13 mEq/ml (elixir)

IRON PRODUCT TABLE, continued

Product (Manufacturer)	Iron (elemental)	Vitamins	Other Ingredients
Stuartinic Tablets (Stuart)	100 mg (as ferrous fumarate)	vitamin B_1, 4.9 mg vitamin B_2, 6 mg niacin, 20 mg pantothenic acid, 9.2 mg vitamin B_6, 0.8 mg vitamin B_{12}, 25 mcg sodium ascorbate, 500 mg	
Surbex-750 with Iron Filmtabs (Abbott)	27 mg (as ferrous sulfate)	vitamin E, 30 IU vitamin B_1, 15 mg vitamin B_2, 15 mg niacin, 100 mg pantothenic acid, 20 mg vitamin B_6, 25 mg vitamin B_{12}, 12 mcg vitamin C, 750 mg	folic acid, 0.4 mg
Theragran Stress Formula Tablets (Squibb)	27 mg (as ferrous fumarate)	vitamin E, 30 IU vitamin B_1, 15 mg vitamin B_2, 15 mg niacin, 100 mg pantothenic acid, 20 mg vitamin B_6, 5 mg vitamin B_{12}, 12 mcg vitamin C, 600 mg	folic acid, 0.4 mg biotin, 45 mcg
Troph-Iron Liquid (SmithKline)	20 mg/5 ml (as ferric pyrophosphate)	vitamin B_1, 10 mg/5 ml vitamin B_{12}, 25 mcg/5 ml	saccharin parabens cherry flavor
Vitron-C (Fisons)	66 mg (as ferrous fumarate)	ascorbic acid, 125 mg	
Vitron-C Plus (Fisons)	132 mg (as ferrous fumarate)	ascorbic acid, 250 mg	tartrazine
Zentinic Pulvule Capsules (Lilly)	100 mg (as ferrous fumarate)	vitamin B_1, 7.5 mg vitamin B_2, 7.5 mg niacin, 30 mg pantothenic acid, 15 mg vitamin B_6, 7.5 mg vitamin B_{12}, 50 mcg vitamin C, 200 mg	folic acid, 0.05 mg
Zentron Liquid (Lilly)	60 mg/15 ml (as ferrous sulfate)	vitamin B_1, 3 mg/15 ml vitamin B_2, 3 mg/15 ml niacin, 15 mg/15 ml pantothenic acid, 3 mg/15 ml vitamin B_6, 3 mg/15 ml vitamin B_{12}, 15 mcg/15 ml vitamin C, 300 mg	alcohol, 2%

[a] Sugar free.

CALCIUM PRODUCT TABLE

Product (Manufacturer)	Dosage Form	Calcium[a]	Vitamin D	Other Ingredients
Biocal 250[b] (Miles)	chewable tablet	250 mg (from calcium carbonate)		
Biocal 500[b,c] (Miles)	tablet	500 mg (from calcium carbonate)		
Bone Meal with Vitamin D[b] (Nature's Bounty)		220 mg	100 IU	phosphorus, 100 mg iron, 0.45 mg copper, 3.25 mg zinc, 20 mcg manganese, 2.75 mg magnesium, 0.925 mg
Cal-Bid (Geriatric Pharm)	tablet	250 mg	125 IU	vitamin C, 100 mg
Calcet (Mission)	tablet	153 mg	100 IU	
Calcicaps (Nion)	tablet	125 mg	67 IU	phosphorus, 60 mg
Calcicaps with Iron (Nion)	tablet	125 mg	67 IU	phosphorus, 60 mg iron, 7 mg tartrazine
Calci-Chew (R&D)	chewable tablet	500 mg (from calcium carbonate)		
Calciday-667 (Nature's Bounty)	tablet	266.8 mg (from calcium carbonate)		
Calcium Carbonate (Various manufacturers)	tablet	260 mg (from calcium carbonate)		
Calcium Carbonate (Roxane)	tablet oral suspension	500 mg (from calcium carbonate) 500 mg/5 ml (from calcium carbonate)		
Calcium Gluconate (Various manufacturers)	tablet	45 mg (from calcium gluconate) 58.5 mg (from calcium gluconate) 87.75 mg (from calcium gluconate) 90 mg (from calcium gluconate)		
Calcium Lactate (Various manufacturers)	tablet	42.25 mg (from calcium lactate) 84.5 mg (from calcium lactate)		
Calcium Oyster Shell (Schein)	tablet	250 mg	125 IU	tartrazine
Calcium 600 (Schein)	tablet	600 mg (from calcium carbonate)		
Calcium 600 + D (Nature's Bounty)	tablet	600 mg	125 IU	
Calcium with Vitamin D (Schein)	tablet	600 mg	125 IU	
Calel D[c] (Rorer)	tablet	500 mg	200 IU	

CALCIUM PRODUCT TABLE, continued

Product (Manufacturer)	Dosage Form	Calcium[a]	Vitamin D	Other Ingredients
Cal-Sup[b,c] (3M Personal Care)	tablet	300 mg (from calcium carbonate)		
Caltrate[b,c] (Lederle)	tablet	600 mg (from calcium carbonate)		
Caltrate, Jr. (Lederle)	tablet	300 mg (from calcium carbonate)	60 IU	
Caltrate 600 + D[b,c] (Lederle)	tablet	600 mg (from calcium carbonate)	125 IU	
Caltrate 600 + Iron[b,c] (Lederle)	tablet	600 mg (from calcium carbonate	125 IU	iron, 18 mg
Caltro (Geneva Generics)	tablet	250 mg	125 IU	
Citracal[c,d] (Mission)	tablet	200 mg (from calcium citrate)		
Citracal 1500 + D (Mission)	tablet	315 mg	200 IU	
De-Cal[b] (Vortech)	tablet	250 mg	125 IU	
Dibasic Calcium Phosphate (Lilly)	tablet	112 mg (from dibasic calcium phosphate dihydrate)		
Dibasic Calcium Phosphate with Vitamin D (Lilly)	pulvule	116 mg	33 IU	phosphorus, 90 mg
Dical (Rugby)	caplet	116 mg	133 IU	phosphorus, 90 mg
Dical-D (Abbott)	tablet	117 mg	133 IU	phosphorus, 90 mg
	chewable wafer	232 mg	200 IU	phosphorus, 180 mg sucrose dextrose
Diostate D (Upjohn)	tablet	114 mg	133 IU	phosphorus, 88 mg tartrazine
FemCal Plus (Murdock)	tablet	250 mg		magnesium, 100 mg manganese, 1 mg copper, 0.5 mg zinc, 3.75 mg
Fergon Iron Plus Calcium Caplets (Winthrop)	caplet	600 mg	125 IU	iron, 18 mg
Florical (Mericon)	capsule	145.6 mg (from calcium carbonate)	·	sodium fluoride, 8.3 mg
Gencalc 600 (Goldline)	tablet	600 mg (from calcium carbonate)		
Neo-Calglucon (Sandoz)	syrup	115 mg/5 ml (from calcium glubionate)		
NeoVadrin Calcium 600 with Vitamin D (Mission)	tablet	600 mg	100 IU	

CALCIUM PRODUCT TABLE, continued

Product (Manufacturer)	Dosage Form	Calcium[a]	Vitamin D	Other Ingredients
NeoVadrin Oyster-shell Calcium 250 with Vitamin D (Mission)	tablet	250 mg	120 IU	tartrazine
NeoVadrin + Iron + Vitamin D (Mission)	tablet	600 mg	100 IU	iron, 18 mg
Nephro-Calci (R & D)	tablet	600 mg (from calcium carbonate)		
Os-Cal 250 + D (Marion)	tablet	250 mg	125 IU	
Os-Cal 500 (Marion)	tablet	500 mg (from calcium carbonate)		
	chewable tablet	500 mg (from calcium carbonate)		
Os-Cal 500 + D (Marion)	tablet	500 mg	125 IU	
Osteon-D (Pasadena)	tablet	100 mg	67 IU	phosphorus, 67 mg magnesium, 40 mg
Oysco 'D' (Rugby)	tablet	250 mg	125 IU	
Oysco 500 (Rugby)	chewable tablet	500 mg (from calcium carbonate)		
Oyst-Cal 500[b,c] (Goldline)	tablet	500 mg (from calcium carbonate)		
Oyst-Cal-D (Goldline)	tablet	250 mg	125 IU	tartrazine
Oyster Calcium[b] (Nature's Bounty)	tablet	375 mg	200 IU	vitamin A, 800 IU
Oystercal 500[b] (Nature's Bounty)	tablet	500 mg (from calcium carbonate)		
Oystercal-D 250[b] (Nature's Bounty)	tablet	250 mg	125 IU	
Posture (Whitehall)	tablet	600 mg (as phosphate)		
Posture D (Whitehall)	tablet	600 mg (as phosphate)	125 IU	
Scooby-Doo Calcium Chewable[b] (Vita-Fresh)	chewable tablet	300 mg	133 IU	vitamin E, 10 IU aspartame
Super CalciCaps[b] (Nion)	tablet	400 mg	133 IU	phosphorus, 42 mg
Super Calcium 1200[b,c,d] (Schiff)	soft gel capsule	600 mg (from calcium carbonate)		
Suplical (Parke-Davis)	chewy square	600 mg (from calcium carbonate)		sorbitol

[a] Expressed in mg of elemental calcium, unless specified otherwise.
[b] Sugar free.
[c] Sodium free.
[d] Dye free.

MULTIPLE VITAMIN PRODUCT TABLE

Product (Manufacturer)	Vitamin A (IU)	Vitamin D (IU)	Vitamin E (IU)	Ascorbic Acid (C) (mg)	Thiamine (B₁) (mg)	Riboflavin (B₂) (mg)	Niacin (mg)
A.C.N. Tablets (Person & Covey)	25,000			250			25
Albee C-800 Tablets (Robins)			45	800	15	17	100
Allbee C-800 Plus Iron Tablets (Robins)			45	800	15	17	100
Albee-T Tablets (Robins)				500	15.5	10	100
Albee with C Caplets (Robins)				300	15	10.2	50
Arbon (Forest)	5000	400	30	60	1.5	1.7	20
Avail Tablets (Beecham)	5000	400	30 (mg)	90	2.25	2.55	20
B•C•E & Zinc Tablets (Schein)			45 (mg)	600	15	10.2	100
Becotin Pulvules (Dista)					10	10	50
Becotin with C Pulvules (Dista)				150	10	10	50
Beelith Tablets (Beach)							
Bee-T-Vites Tablets (Rugby)				300	15	10	100
Bee-Zee Tablets (Rugby)			45 (mg)	600	15	10.2	100
Beminal-500 Tablets (Whitehall)				500	25	12.5	100
Beminal Stress Plus with Zinc Tablets (Whitehall)			45 (mg)	700	25	12.5	100
Bo-Cal Tablets[b] (Fibertone)		100					
Brewers Yeast Tablets (Nature's Bounty)					0.08	0.025	0.22
Bugs Bunny Children's Chewable Tablets[b] (Miles)	2500	400	15 (mg)	60	1.05	1.2	13.5

Pyridox-ine Hydro-chloride (B₆)(mg)	Cyanoco-balamin (B₁₂)(mcg)	Folic Acid (mg)	Panto-thenic Acid (mg)	Iron (mg)	Calcium (mg)	Phos-phorus (mg)	Magne-sium (mg)	Other Ingredients
25	12		25					
25	12	0.4	25	27				
8.2	5		23					lactose desiccated liver
5			10					saccharin lactose
2	6	0.4	22	18	100	80	100	copper, 2 mg zinc, 15 mg iodine, 150 mcg
3	9	0.4		18	NS[a]		NS[a]	chromium iodine selenium zinc, 22.5 mg
10	6		25					zinc, 22.5 mg tartrazine
4.1	1		25					
4	1		25					
20							600	
5	4		20					
10	6		25					zinc, 22.5 mg
10	5		20					lactose
10	25		20					zinc, 45 mg
					250		125	boron, 0.75 mg
1.05	4.5	0.3						sorbitol aspartame xylitol flavor

MULTIPLE VITAMIN PRODUCT TABLE, continued

Product (Manufacturer)	Vitamin A (IU)	Vitamin D (IU)	Vitamin E (IU)	Ascorbic Acid (C) (mg)	Thiamine (B₁) (mg)	Riboflavin (B₂) (mg)	Niacin (mg)
Bugs Bunny Plus Iron Chewable Tablets[b] (Miles)	2500	400	15	60	1.05	1.2	13.5
Bugs Bunny Vitamins and Minerals Chewable Tablets[b] (Miles)	5000	400	30 (mg)	60	1.5	1.7	20
Bugs Bunny with Extra C Children's Chewable Tablets[b] (Miles)	2500	400	15	250	1.05	1.2	13.5
C & E Capsules[b] (Nature's Bounty)			400	500			
Calfos-D Tablets (Pal-Pak)		100					
Cal-Prenal Improved Tablets[b] (Vortech)	4000	400		50	2	2	10
Centrovite Jr. Tablets (Rugby)	5000	400	15	60	1.5	1.7	20
Centrum (Lederle)	5000	400	30	60	1.5	17	20
Centrum Jr. Plus Iron Tablets (Lederle)	5000	400	30	60	1.5	1.7	20
Chelated Calcium Magnesium Tablets[b] (Nature's Bounty)							

Pyridox-ine Hydro-chloride (B6)(mg)	Cyanoco-balamin (B12)(mcg)	Folic Acid (mg)	Panto-thenic Acid (mg)	Iron (mg)	Calcium (mg)	Phos-phorus (mg)	Magne-sium (mg)	Other Ingredients
1.05	4.5	0.3		15				sorbitol flavor
2	6	0.4	10	18	100	NS[a]	NS[a]	copper iodine zinc, 15 mg biotin, 40 mcg
1.05	4.5	0.3						sorbitol aspartame xylitol flavor
					116	90		
1	2	0.4		49.3	230			iodine
2	6	0.4	10	18			NS[a]	copper iodine zinc
2	6	0.4	10	18	162	125	100	biotin, 30 mcg iodine, 150 mcg copper, 2 mg zinc, 15 mg manganese, 2.5 mg potassium, 40 mg chloride, 36.3 mg chromium, 25 mcg molybdenum, 25 mcg selenium, 25 mcg vitamin K, 25 mcg nickel, 5 mcg tin, 10 mcg silicon, 10 mcg vanadium, 10 mcg
2	6	0.4	10	18	NS[a]	NS[a]	NS[a]	chromium copper iodine manganese molybdenum zinc, 15 mg biotin, 45 mcg vitamin K, 10 mcg
					500		250	

MULTIPLE VITAMIN PRODUCT TABLE, continued

Product (Manufacturer)	Vitamin A (IU)	Vitamin D (IU)	Vitamin E (IU)	Ascorbic Acid (C) (mg)	Thiamine (B₁) (mg)	Riboflavin (B₂) (mg)	Niacin (mg)
Chelated Calcium Magnesium Zinc Tablets[b] (Nature's Bounty)							
Chew-Vites Chewable Tablets (Vortech)	2500	400	15	60	1.05	1.2	13.5
Clusivol Syrup (Whitehall)	2500	400		15	1	1	5
Cod Liver Oil Concentrate Capsules (Schering)	10,000	400					
Cod Liver Oil Concentrate Tablets (Schering)	4000	200					
Cod Liver Oil Concentrate Tablets with Vitamin C (Schering)	4000	200		50			
Daily-Vite with Iron & Minerals Tablets[b] (Rugby)	5000	400	30	60	1.5	1.7	20
Dayalets Filmtabs (Abbott)	5000	400	30 (mg)	60	1.5	1.7	20
Daylets Plus Iron Filmtabs[b] (Abbott)	5000	400	30 (mg)	60	1.5	1.7	20
Decagen Tablets (Goldline)	9000	400	30 (mg)	90	10	10	20
Dolomite Tablets[b] (Nature's Bounty)							

Pyridoxine Hydrochloride (B6)(mg)	Cyanocobalamin (B12)(mcg)	Folic Acid (mg)	Pantothenic Acid (mg)	Iron (mg)	Calcium (mg)	Phosphorus (mg)	Magnesium (mg)	Other Ingredients
					333		133	zinc, 8.3 mg
1.05	4.5	0.3						
0.6	2		3				3	manganese, 0.5 mg zinc, 0.5 mg
2	6	0.4	10	18	NS[a]	NS[a]	NS[a]	chlorine chromium copper iodine potassium manganese molybdenum selenium zinc, 15 mg biotin, 30 mcg vitamin K, 50 mcg
2	6	0.4						
2	6	0.4		18				
5	10	0.4	20	30	NS[a]	NS[a]	NS[a]	chromium copper iodine potassium manganese molybdenum selenium zinc, 15 mg vitamin K, 25 mcg biotin, 45 mcg
					130		78	

MULTIPLE VITAMIN PRODUCT TABLE, continued

Product (Manufacturer)	Vitamin A (IU)	Vitamin D (IU)	Vitamin E (IU)	Ascorbic Acid (C) (mg)	Thiamine (B₁) (mg)	Riboflavin (B₂) (mg)	Niacin (mg)
Ecee Plus Tablets (Edwards)			165 (mg)	100			
Econo B & C Caplets (Vangard)				300	15	10.2	50
En-Cebrin Pulvules (Lilly)	4000	400		50	3	2	10
Engran-HP Tablets (Squibb)	4000	200	15 (mg)	30	0.85	1	10
Femiron Tablets (Beecham)	5000	400	15	60	1.5	1.7	20
Filibon Tablets (Lederle)	5000	400	30 (mg)	60	1.5	1.7	20
Flintstones Children's Chewable Tablets (Miles)	2500	400	15 (mg)	60	1.05	1.2	13.5
Flintstones Complete Chewable Tablets[b] (Miles)	5000	400	30	60	1.5	1.7	20
Flintstones Plus Iron Chewable Tablets (Miles)	2500	400	15	60	1.05	1.2	13.5
Flintstones with Extra C Children's Chewable Tablets (Miles)	2500	400	15	250	1.05	1.2	13.5
Fruity Chews Chewable Tablets (Goldline)	2500	400	15 (mg)	60	1.05	1.2	13.5
Fruity Chews with Iron Chewable Tablets (Goldline)	2500	400	15 (mg)	60	1.05	1.2	13.5
Gen-bee with C Caplets[b] (Goldline)				300	15	10.2	50
Generix-T Tablets (Goldline)	10,000	400	5.5	150	15	10	100
Geravite Elixir (Hauck)					1/15 ml	1.2/15 ml	100/15 ml

Pyridox-ine Hydro-chloride (B6)(mg)	Cyanoco-balamin (B12)(mcg)	Folic Acid (mg)	Panto-thenic Acid (mg)	Iron (mg)	Calcium (mg)	Phos-phorus (mg)	Magne-sium (mg)	Other Ingredients
							70	zinc sulfate, 80 mg
5			10					tartrazine
1.7	5		5	30	250		NS[a]	copper iodine manganese zinc, 1.5 mg
1.25	4	0.4		9	325		NS[a]	iodine tartrazine
2	6	0.4	10	20				
2	6	0.4		18	125		NS[a]	iodine
1.05	4.5	0.3						sucrose
2	6	0.4	10	18	NS[a]	NS[a]	NS[a]	sorbitol copper iodine zinc, 15 mg biotin, 40 mcg
1.05	4.5	0.3		15				sucrose
1.05	4.5	0.3						sucrose fructose
1.05	4.5	0.3						
1.05	4.5	0.3		12				zinc, 8 mg copper, 0.8 mg
5			10					
2	7.5		10	15			NS[a]	copper iodine manganese zinc, 1.5 mg
	10/15 ml							alcohol, 15% l-lysine, 150 mg/ 15 ml

MULTIPLE VITAMIN PRODUCT TABLE, continued

Product (Manufacturer)	Vitamin A (IU)	Vitamin D (IU)	Vitamin E (IU)	Ascorbic Acid (C) (mg)	Thiamine (B₁) (mg)	Riboflavin (B₂) (mg)	Niacin (mg)
Geriplex-FS Kapseals (Parke-Davis)	5000		5 (mg)	50	5	5	15
Geriplex-FS Liquid (Parke-Davis)					0.2/5 ml	0.28/5 ml	2.5/5 ml
Geritol Complete Tablets (SmithKline Beecham)	5000	400	30	60	1.5	1.7	20
Geritol Liquid (SmithKline Beecham)					2.5/15 ml	2.5/15 ml	50/15 ml
Gevrabon Liquid (Lederle)					0.83/5 ml	0.42/5 ml	8.3/5 ml
Gevral Protein (Lederle)	2167	217	4.3	22	2.2	2.2	6.5
Gevral T Tablets (Lederle)	5000	400	45	90	2.25	2.6	30
Gevral Tablets (Lederle)	5000		30 (mg)	60	1.5	1.7	20

Pyridox-ine Hydro-chloride (B$_6$)(mg)	Cyanoco-balamin (B$_{12}$)(mcg)	Folic Acid (mg)	Panto-thenic Acid (mg)	Iron (mg)	Calcium (mg)	Phos-phorus (mg)	Magne-sium (mg)	Other Ingredients
	2			6	59			zinc, 0.5 mg choline, 20 mg copper manganese docusate sodium, 100 mg aspergillus oryzea enzymes, 162.5 mg
0.17/5 ml	0.83/5 ml			2.5/5 ml				alcohol, 18% sorbitol saccharin
2	6	0.4	10	50	162	125	100	biotin, 300 mcg iodine, 150 mcg copper, 2 mg manganese, 100 mg potassium, 7.7 mg chloride, 7 mg chromium, 15 mg molybdenum, 15 mcg selenium, 15 mcg zinc, 15 mg nickel, 5 mcg silicon, 10 mcg tin, 10 mcg vanadium, 10 mcg
0.5/15 ml	0.75/15 ml		2/15 ml	50/15 ml				methionine, 25 mg/oz choline bitartrate, 50 mg/15 ml
0.17/5 ml	0.17/5 ml		1.67/5 ml	2.5/5 ml			NS[a]	choline, 16.7 mg/ 5 ml iodine, 16.7 mcg/ 5 ml manganese zinc alcohol, 18% sucrose flavor
0.22	0.87		2.2	4.3	267	52.8	0.4	choline, 21 mg inositol, 22 mg lysine mono-hydrate, 1.1 g iodine, 40 mcg copper, 400 mcg zinc, 220 mcg manganese, 400 mcg potassium, 13 mg
3	9	0.4		27	162	125	100	iodine, 225 mcg copper, 1.5 mg zinc, 22.5 mg
2	6	0.4		18	NS[a]	NS[a]	NS[a]	iodine sucrose

MULTIPLE VITAMIN PRODUCT TABLE, continued

Product (Manufacturer)	Vitamin A (IU)	Vitamin D (IU)	Vitamin E (IU)	Ascorbic Acid (C) (mg)	Thiamine (B₁) (mg)	Riboflavin (B₂) (mg)	Niacin (mg)
Gevrite (Lederle)	5000			60	1.5	1.7	20
Hep-Forte Capsules (Marlyn)	1200		6.7 (mg)	10	1	1	10
Hepicebrin Tablets (Lilly)	5000	400		75	2	3	20
Herbal Cellulex Tablets[b] (Nature's Bounty)				83			
Hexavitamin Capsules and Tablets (Various manufacturers)	5000	400		75	2	3	20
Homicebrin Liquid (Lilly)	2500/5 ml	400/5 ml		60/5 ml	1/5 ml	1.2/5 ml	10/5 ml
Ibex Therapeutic Tablets[b,c] (Freeda)				150	25	25	100
KLB6 Complete Tablets[b] (Nature's Bounty)	833.3	66.7	5	10	0.25	0.28	3.3
KLB6 Softgels Capsules[b] (Nature's Bounty)							
Lanoplex Elixir (Lannett)					0.67/5 ml	1/5 ml	6.7/5 ml

Pyridox-ine Hydro-chloride (B_6)(mg)	Cyanoco-balamin (B_{12})(mcg)	Folic Acid (mg)	Panto-thenic Acid (mg)	Iron (mg)	Calcium (mg)	Phos-phorus (mg)	Magne-sium (mg)	Other Ingredients
2				18	230			
0.5	1	0.06	2					desiccated liver, 194.4 mg; liver concentrate, 64.8 mg; liver fraction number 2, 64.8 mg; lecithin; zinc, 2 mg; choline, 21 mg; inositol, 10 mg; biotin, 3.3 mg; dl-methionine, 10 mg; dried yeast, 64.8 mg
								sucrose; sodium bisulfite
				9				potassium, 33 mg
0.8/5 ml	3/5 ml							alcohol, 5%; sorbitol; saccharin; glucose
25	12	0.1	50	16.5				choline, 50 mg; inositol, 50 mg; biotin, 25 mcg; PABA, 25 mg; diastase, 65 mg; betaine, 10 mg
8.3	1	0.067						soya lecithin, 200 mg; kelp, 25 mg; cider vinegar, 40 mg; wheat bran, 83.3 mg; biotin, 0.05 mg
3.5								soya lecithin, 100 mg; kelp, 25 mg; cider vinegar, 40 mg
0.33/5 ml								alcohol, 11%; flavor

MULTIPLE VITAMIN PRODUCT TABLE, continued

Product (Manufacturer)	Vitamin A (IU)	Vitamin D (IU)	Vitamin E (IU)	Ascorbic Acid (C) (mg)	Thiamine (B₁) (mg)	Riboflavin (B₂) (mg)	Niacin (mg)
Lederplex Capsules and Tablets (Lederle)					2.25	2.6	30
Lederplex Liquid (Lederle)					1.13/5 ml	1.3/5 ml	15/5 ml
Lipovite Capsules (Rugby)					0.3	0.3	3.3
Mag-Cal Tablets[b] (Fibertone)		66.7					
Mediplex Tabules Tablets (US Pharm)			60 (mg)	300	25	10	100
Mi-Cebrin Tablets (Dista)	10,000	400	5.5	100	10	5	30
Mi-Cebrin T Tablets (Dista)	10,000	400	5.5	150	15	10	100
Mucoplex Tablets (ICN)						1.5	
Multi Vit Drops[d] (Barre-National)	1500/ml	400/ml	4.13 (mg)/ml	35/ml	0.5/ml	0.6/ml	8/ml
Multicebrin Tablets (Lilly)	10,000	400	6.6 (mg)	75	3	3	25
Multilex Tablets (Rugby)	10,000	400	5.5	100	10	5	30
Multilex-T & M Tablets (Rugby)	10,000	400	5.5 (mg)	150	15	10	100
Multi-Mineral Tablets[b] (Nature's Bounty)							
Multi-Vita-Drops[b,d] (PBI)	1500/ml	400/ml	5/ml	35/ml	0.5/ml	0.6/ml	8/ml

Pyridox- ine Hydro- chloride (B$_6$)(mg)	Cyanoco- balamin (B$_{12}$)(mcg)	Folic Acid (mg)	Panto- thenic Acid (mg)	Iron (mg)	Calcium (mg)	Phos- phorus (mg)	Magne- sium (mg)	Other Ingredients
3	9		15					
1.5/5 ml	4.5/5 ml		7.5/5 ml					sucrose honey flavor
0.3	1.67		1.67					choline bitartrate, 111 mg
					416.7 (carbonate) 166.7 (elemental)		83.3	copper, 0.167 mg manganese, 0.83 mg potassium, 1.67 mg zinc, 0.167 mg
10	25		25				NS[a]	zinc, 18.4 mg copper manganese
1.7	3		10	15			NS[a]	copper iodine manganese zinc, 1.5 mg sucrose
2	7.5		10	15			NS[a]	copper iodine manganese zinc, 1.5 mg sucrose
	5							liver fraction, 750 mg
0.4/ml	2/ml							flavor
1.2	3		5					
1.7	3		10	15			NS[a]	copper iodine manganese zinc, 1.5 mg
2	7.5		10	15			NS[a]	copper iodine manganese zinc
				3	166.7	75.7	66.7	iodine, 25 mcg copper, 0.33 mg zinc, 2.5 mg potassium, 12.5 mg manganese, 8.3 mg
0.4/ml	2/ml							

MULTIPLE VITAMIN PRODUCT TABLE, continued

Product (Manufacturer)	Vitamin A (IU)	Vitamin D (IU)	Vitamin E (IU)	Ascorbic Acid (C) (mg)	Thiamine (B₁) (mg)	Riboflavin (B₂) (mg)	Niacin (mg)
Multi-Vita Drops with Iron[b] (PBI)	1500/ml	400/ml	5/ml	35/ml	0.5/ml	0.6/ml	8/ml
Myadec Tablets (Parke-Davis)	9000	400	30 (mg)	90	10	10	20
Natabec Kapseals (Parke-Davis)	4000	400		50	3	2	10
Natabec FA Capsules (Parke-Davis)	4000	400		50	3	2	10
Natalins Tablets (Mead Johnson)	5000	400	30 (mg)	90	1.7	2	20
NeoVadrin B-Complex "100" Tablets[b] (Mission)					100	100	100
NeoVadrin B-Complex "50" Tablets[b] (Mission)					50	50	50
NeoVadrin Children's Chewable Tablets with Iron (Mission)	2500	400	15 (mg)	60	1.05	1.2	13.5
NeoVadrin Prenatal Tablets (Mission)	8000	400	30	60	1.7	2	20
Norlac Tablets (Reid-Rowell)	8000	400	30 (mg)	90	2	2	20
Nova-Dec Tablets[b] (Rugby)	10,000	400	30	250	10	10	100
One-A-Day Essential Tablets[b] (Miles)	5000	400	30 (mg)	60	1.5	1.7	20

Pyridox-ine Hydro-chloride (B₆)(mg)	Cyanoco-balamin (B₁₂)(mcg)	Folic Acid (mg)	Panto-thenic Acid (mg)	Iron (mg)	Calcium (mg)	Phos-phorus (mg)	Magne-sium (mg)	Other Ingredients
0.4/ml				10/ml				
5	10	0.4	20	30	NSᵃ	NSᵃ	NSᵃ	chromium copper iodine potassium manganese molybdenum selenium zinc, 15 mg vitamin K, 25 mcg biotin, 45 mcg
3	5			30	240			
3	5	0.1		30	240		NSᵃ	bisulfites
4	8	0.8		45	200		NSᵃ	iodine
100	100	0.4	100					PABA, 100 mg inositol, 100 mg biotin, 100 mcg choline bitartrate, 100 mg
50	50	0.4	50					PABA, 50 mg inositol, 50 mg biotin, 50 mcg choline bitartrate, 50 mg
1.05	4.5	0.3		15				flavor
2.5	8	0.8		60	250		NSᵃ	zinc, 20 mg
4	8	0.4		60	200		NSᵃ	copper iodine zinc, 15 mg
5	6	0.4	20	20			NSᵃ	copper iodine manganese zinc, 20 mg
2	6	0.4	10					

MULTIPLE VITAMIN PRODUCT TABLE, continued

Product (Manufacturer)	Vitamin A (IU)	Vitamin D (IU)	Vitamin E (IU)	Ascorbic Acid (C) (mg)	Thiamine (B₁) (mg)	Riboflavin (B₂) (mg)	Niacin (mg)
One-A-Day Maximum Formula Tablets (Miles)	1500	400	30 (mg)	60	1.5	1.7	20
One-A-Day Plus Extra C Tablets[b] (Miles)	5000	400	30 (mg)	300	1.5	1.7	20
One-A-Day Stressgard Tablets[b] (Miles)	2500	400	30 (mg)	600	15	10	100
One-Tablet-Daily Tablets (Various manufacturers)	5000	400	30 (mg)	60	1.5	1.7	20
One-Tablet-Daily with Iron Tablets[b] (Various manufacturers)	5000	400	30 (mg)	60	1.5	1.7	20
Optilets-500 Filmtabs (Abbott)	10,000	400	30 (mg)	500	15	10	100
Optilets-M-500 Filmtabs (Abbott)	10,000	400	30	500	15	10	100
Optivite for Women Tablets[b] (Optimox)	2083	16.7	14 (mg)	250	4.2	4.2	4.2
Orexin Softab Tablets (Stuart)					8.1		

Pyridox-ine Hydro-chloride (B6)(mg)	Cyanoco-balamin (B12)(mcg)	Folic Acid (mg)	Panto-thenic Acid (mg)	Iron (mg)	Calcium (mg)	Phos-phorus (mg)	Magne-sium (mg)	Other Ingredients
2	6	0.4	10	18	NS[a]	NS[a]	NS[a]	chlorine chromium copper iodine potassium manganese molybdenum selenium zinc, 15 mg biotin, 30 mcg beta carotene, 5000 IU
2	6	0.4	10					
5	12	0.4	20	18				copper zinc, 15 mg beta carotene, 2500 IU
2	6	0.4	10					
2	6	0.4	10	18				
5	12		20					
5	12		20	20			NS[a]	copper iodine manganese zinc, 1.5 mg
50	10.4	0.03	4.2	2.5	NS[a]		NS[a]	zinc, 4.2 mg choline, 52 mg inositol chromium copper iodine potassium manganese selenium citrus bioflavonoids betaine PABA rutin pancreatin biotin
4.1	25							

MULTIPLE VITAMIN PRODUCT TABLE, continued

Product (Manufacturer)	Vitamin A (IU)	Vitamin D (IU)	Vitamin E (IU)	Ascorbic Acid (C) (mg)	Thiamine (B₁) (mg)	Riboflavin (B₂) (mg)	Niacin (mg)
Os-Cal Forte Tablets (Marion)	1668	125	0.7 (mg)	50	1.7	1.7	15
Os-Cal Plus Tablets (Marion)	1666	125		33	0.5	0.66	3.3
Oxi-Freeda Tablets[b] (Freeda)	5000		150	100	20	20	40
Poly-Vi-Sol Chewable Tablets (Mead Johnson)	2500	400	15	60	1.05	1.2	13.5
Poly-Vi-Sol Infants' Drops (Mead Johnson)	1500/ml	400/ml	5/ml	35/ml	0.5/ml	0.6/ml	8/ml
Poly-Vi-Sol with Iron Chewable Tablets (Mead Johnson)	2500	400	15 (mg)	60	1.05	1.2	13.5
Poly-Vi-Sol with Iron Drops (Mead Johnson)	1500/ml	400/ml	5/ml	35/ml	0.5/ml	0.6/ml	8/ml
Polyvitamin Drops with Iron (Rugby)	1500/ml	400/ml	5 (mg)/ml	35/ml	0.5/ml	0.6/ml	8/ml
Prenatal with Folic Acid Tablets (Geneva Generics)	8000	400	30 (mg)	60	1.7	2	20
Prenatal-S Tablets (Goldline)	4000		11	100	1.5	1.7	18
Prenavite Tablets[b,c] (Rugby)	8000	400	30	60	1.7	2	20
Probec-T Tablets (Stuart)				600	12.2	10	100
Ru-lets 500 Tablets (Rugby)	10,000	400	30 (mg)	500	15	10	100
Secran Liquid (Scherer)					10		10
Sigtab Tablets (Upjohn)	5000	400	15 (mg)	333	10.3	10	100
Simron Plus Capsules (Merrell Dow)				50			

Pyridox- ine Hydro- chloride (B₆)(mg)	Cyanoco- balamin (B₁₂)(mcg)	Folic Acid (mg)	Panto- thenic Acid (mg)	Iron (mg)	Calcium (mg)	Phos- phorus (mg)	Magne- sium (mg)	Other Ingredients
2	1.6			5	250		NS[a]	manganese zinc, 0.5 mg
0.5				16.6	250			manganese zinc, 0.75 mg
20	10		20					chelated zinc, 15 mg selenium, 50 mcg glutathione, 40 mg L-cysteine, 75 mg
1.05	4.5	0.3						sucrose flavor
0.4/ml	2/ml							flavor
1.05	4.5	0.3		12				copper zinc, 8 mg
0.4/ml				10/ml				
0.4/ml				10/ml				
4	8	0.8		60	200		NS[a]	iodine
2.6	4							zinc, 25 mg
4	8	0.8		60	200		NS[a]	iodine
4.1	5		18.4					
5	12		20					
	25							alcohol, 17%
6	18	0.4	20					sucrose
1	3.33	0.1		10				

MULTIPLE VITAMIN PRODUCT TABLE, continued

Product (Manufacturer)	Vitamin A (IU)	Vitamin D (IU)	Vitamin E (IU)	Ascorbic Acid (C) (mg)	Thiamine (B₁) (mg)	Riboflavin (B₂) (mg)	Niacin (mg)
Spartus Tablets (Lederle)	5000	400	30 (mg)	300	7.5	8.5	100
Stress Formula 600 Plus Zinc Tablets (Schein)			30 (mg)	600	20	10	100
Stress Formula Vitamins Capsules and Tablets (Various manufacturers)			30	600	15	15	100
Stress-Bee Capsules[b,c] (Rugby)				300	10	10	100
Stresscaps Capsules (Lederle)				300	10	10	100
Stressgard Tablets (Miles)	5000	400	30	600	15	10	100
Stresstabs 600 Advanced Formula Tablets (Lederle)			30 (mg)	600	15	10	100
Stresstabs 600 with Zinc Tablets (Lederle)			30 (mg)	600	15	10	100
Stuart Prenatal Tablets (Stuart)	4000	400	11 (mg)	100	1.5	1.7	18
Stuart Formula Tablets (Stuart)	5000	400	15	60	1.2	1.7	20
Sunkist Multis Regular (Ciba)	2500	400	15	60	1.05	1.2	13.5
Sunkist Multis Plus C (Ciba)	2500	400	15	250	1.05	1.2	13.5
Sunkist Multis Plus Iron (Ciba)	2500	400	15	60	1.05	1.2	13.5

Pyridox-ine Hydro-chloride (B$_6$)(mg)	Cyanoco-balamin (B$_{12}$)(mcg)	Folic Acid (mg)	Panto-thenic Acid (mg)	Iron (mg)	Calcium (mg)	Phos-phorus (mg)	Magne-sium (mg)	Other Ingredients
10	30	0.4	25		NS[a]	NS[a]	NS[a]	zinc, 15 mg chlorine chromium copper iodine potassium manganese molybdenum selenium biotin, 45 mcg
5	12	0.4	25				NS[a]	zinc, 23.9 mg copper biotin, 45 mcg
5	12	0.4	20					biotin, 45 mcg
2	6		20					
2	6		20					
5	12	0.4	20	18				zinc, 15 mg copper, 2 mg
5	12	0.4	20					biotin, 45 mcg
5	12	0.4	20					zinc, 23.9 mg copper biotin, 45 mcg
2.5	4	0.8		60	200			zinc, 25 mg
2	6	0.4		18	160	125	100	iodine, 150 mcg
1.05	4.5	0.3						K$_1$, 5 mcg
1.05	4.5	0.3						K$_1$, 5 mcg
1.05	4.5	0.3		15				K$_1$, 5 mcg

MULTIPLE VITAMIN PRODUCT TABLE, continued

Product (Manufacturer)	Vitamin A (IU)	Vitamin D (IU)	Vitamin E (IU)	Ascorbic Acid (C) (mg)	Thiamine (B₁) (mg)	Riboflavin (B₂) (mg)	Niacin (mg)
Sunkist Multis Complete (Ciba)	5000	400	30	60	1.5	1.7	20
Surbex Filmtabs (Abbott)					6	6	30
Surbex-750 with Iron Filmtabs (Abbott)			30	750	15	15	100
Surbex-750 with Zinc Filmtabs (Abbott)			30 (mg)	750	15	15	100
Surbex-T Filmtabs (Abbott)				500	15	10	100
Surbex with C Filmtabs (Abbott)				250	6	6	30
Surbu-Gen-T Tablets[b] (Goldline)				500	15	10	100
Syrvite Liquid (Various manufacturers)	2500/5 ml	400/5 ml	15 (mg)/5 ml	60/5 ml	1.05/5 ml	1.2/5 ml	13.5/5 ml
Thera Multi-vitamin Liquid (Major)	10,000/ 5 ml	400/5 ml		200/5 ml	10/5 ml	10/5 ml	100/5 ml
Thera-Combex H-P Kapseals (Parke-Davis)				500	2.5	15	100
Theragenerix Tablets[b] (Goldline)	5500	400	30 (mg)	120	3	3.4	30
Theragenerix-M Tablets (Goldline)	5000	400	30 (mg)	120	3	3.4	30
Theragran Jr. Children's Chewable Tablets[b] (Squibb)	5000	400	30 (mg)	60	1.5	1.7	20

Pyridox-ine Hydro-chloride (B$_6$)(mg)	Cyanoco-balamin (B$_{12}$)(mcg)	Folic Acid (mg)	Panto-thenic Acid (mg)	Iron (mg)	Calcium (mg)	Phos-phorus (mg)	Magne-sium (mg)	Other Ingredients
2	6	0.4	10	18	100	78	20	biotin, 40 mcg; K$_1$, 10 mcg; iodine, 150 mcg; zinc, 10 mg; mang-anese, 1 mg; copper, 2 mg
2.5	5		10					
25	12	0.4	20	27				
20	12	0.4	20					zinc, 22.5 mg
5	10		20					
2.5	5		10					
5	10		20					
1.05/5 ml	4.5/5 ml							
4.1/5 ml	5/5ml		21.4/5 ml					sugar
10	5		20					bisulfites
3	9	0.4	10					biotin, 15 mcg beta carotene, 2500 IU
3	9	0.4	10	27	NS[a]	NS[a]	NS[a]	chlorine chromium copper iodine potassium biotin, 15 mcg manganese molybdenum selenium zinc, 15 mg beta carotene, 2500 IU
2	6	0.4						sorbitol mannitol

MULTIPLE VITAMIN PRODUCT TABLE, continued

Product (Manufacturer)	Vitamin A (IU)	Vitamin D (IU)	Vitamin E (IU)	Ascorbic Acid (C) (mg)	Thiamine (B₁) (mg)	Riboflavin (B₂) (mg)	Niacin (mg)
Theragran Jr. Children's Chewable Tablets with Extra Vitamin C[b] (Squibb)	5000	400	30 (mg)	250	1.5	1.7	20
Theragran Jr. with Iron Chewable Tablets[b] (Squibb)	5000	400	30 (mg)	60	1.5	1.7	20
Theragran Liquid (Squibb)	10,000/5 ml	400/5 ml		200/5 ml	10/5 ml	10/5 ml	100/5 ml
Theragran-M Tablets (Squibb)	5500	400	30 (mg)	120	3	3.4	30
Theragran Stress Formula (Squibb)			30	600	15	15	100
Theragran Tablets (Squibb)	5000	400	30 (mg)	90	3	3.4	30
Theravee Tablets (Vangard)	5500	400	30 (mg)	120	3	3.4	30
Theravee-M Tablets (Vangard)	5500	400	30	120	3	3.4	30
Therems Tablets (Rugby)	5500	400	30 (mg)	120	3	3.4	30
Therems-M Tablets (Rugby)	5500	400	30	120	3	3.4	30

Pyridox-ine Hydro-chloride (B₆)(mg)	Cyanoco-balamin (B₁₂)(mcg)	Folic Acid (mg)	Panto-thenic Acid (mg)	Iron (mg)	Calcium (mg)	Phos-phorus (mg)	Magne-sium (mg)	Other Ingredients
2	6	0.4						sorbitol mannitol
2	6	0.4		18				sorbitol
4.1/5 ml	5/5 ml		21.4/5 ml					sugar
3	9	0.4	10	27	40	NS[a]	NS[a]	chlorine chromium copper iodine potassium manganese molybdenum selenium zinc, 15 mg biotin, 15 mcg
25	12	0.4	20	27				biotin, 45 mcg
3	9	0.4	10					biotin, 35 mcg beta carotene, 1250 IU sucrose
3	9	0.4	10					biotin, 15 mcg
3	9	0.4	10	27	NS[a]	NS[a]	NS[a]	chlorine chromium copper potassium iodine manganese molybdenum selenium zinc biotin, 15 mcg
3	9	0.4	10					biotin, 15 mcg
3	9	0.4	10	27			NS[a]	chlorine chromium copper iodine potassium manganese molybdenum selenium zinc, 15 mg biotin, 15 mcg

MULTIPLE VITAMIN PRODUCT TABLE, continued

Product (Manufacturer)	Vitamin A (IU)	Vitamin D (IU)	Vitamin E (IU)	Ascorbic Acid (C) (mg)	Thiamine (B₁) (mg)	Riboflavin (B₂) (mg)	Niacin (mg)
ThexForte Caplets (Medtech)				500	25	15	100
Triasyn B Capsules and Tablets (Lannett)					2	3	20
Tri-Vi-Sol Drops (Mead Johnson)	1500/ml	400/ml		35/ml			
Tri-Vi-Sol with Iron Drops[b] (Mead Johnson)	1500/ml	400/ml		35/ml			
Trophite Liquid (SmithKline)					10/5 ml		
Ultra Freeda Tablets[b] (Freeda)	3333	133	66.6	333	16.7	16.7	33
Ultra KLB6 Tablets (Nature's Bounty)							
Unicap Capsules and Tablets (Upjohn)	5000	400	30 (mg) (capsules) 15 (mg) (tablets)	60	1.5	1.7	20
Unicap Jr. Chewable Tablets (Upjohn)	5000	400	15 (mg)	60	1.5	1.7	20
Unicap M Tablets[b] (Upjohn)	5000	400	30 (mg)	60	1.5	1.7	20
Unicap Plus Iron Tablets[b] (Upjohn)	5000	400	30	60	1.5	1.7	20
Unicap Senior Tablets[b] (Upjohn)	5000	200	15 (mg)	60	1.2	1.4	16

TIPLE VITAMIN PRODUCT TABLE, continued

ct (facturer)	Vitamin A (IU)	Vitamin D (IU)	Vitamin E (IU)	Ascorbic Acid (C) (mg)	Thiamine (B$_1$) (mg)	Riboflavin (B$_2$) (mg)	Niacin (mg)
T	5000	400	30 (mg)	500	10	10	100
plex M	5000	400	15 (mg)	60	1.5	1.7	20
plex ablets	5000	400	15 (mg)	300	10	10	100
s				300	20	10	100
lus s	4000		50	150	10	5	25
n ADC s Plus ps[b]	1500/ml	400/ml		35/ml			
n e Tablets	2500	400	15 (mg)	60	1.05	1.2	13.5
n Multi- Drops[b]	1500/ml	400/ml	4.13 (mg)/ml	35/ml	0.5/ml	0.6/ml	8/ml
n Multi- Liquid	2500/5 ml	400/5 ml	11 (mg)/5 ml	60/5 ml	1.05/5 ml	1.2/5 ml	13.5/5 ml
Multi- Plus wable	2500	400	15 (mg)	60	1.05	1.2	13.5
Multi- lus ps[b]	1500/ml	400/ml	4.1 (mg)/ml	35/ml	0.5/ml	0.6/ml	8/ml
Plus wable	2500	400	15 (mg)	60	1.05	1.2	13.5
Plus id	2500/5 ml	400/5 ml	11 (mg)/5 ml	60/5 ml	1.05/5 ml	1.2/5 ml	13.5/5 ml

MU

Pyridox-ine Hydro-chloride (B$_6$)(mg)	Cyanoco-balamin (B$_{12}$)(mcg)	Folic Acid (mg)	Panto-thenic Acid (mg)	Iron (mg)	Calcium (mg)	Phos-phorus (mg)	Prod (Man
5			10				Unica Table (Upjoh
							Unico Table (Rugby
				10/ml			Unico T&M (Rugby
	25/5 ml						
16.7	33	0.27	33	5	66.7		Vicon Capsu (Russ)
							Vicon Capsu (Russ)
							Vi-Day Vitami Iron D (Ross)
							Vi-Day Chewa (Ross)
16.7							Vi-Day vitamin (Ross)
2	6	0.4					Vi-Day vitamin (Ross)
2	6	0.4					Vi-Day vitamin Iron Ch Tablets (Ross)
2	6	0.4	10	18	NS[a]	NS[a]	Vi-Day vitamin Iron D (Ross)
2	6	0.4	10	22.5	NS[a]		Vi-Day Iron Ch Tablets (Ross)
2.2	3	0.4	10	10	NS[a]	NS[a]	Vi-Day Iron Liq (Ross)

Pyridox-ine Hydro-chloride (B₆)(mg)	Cyanoco-balamin (B₁₂)(mcg)	Folic Acid (mg)	Panto-thenic Acid (mg)	Iron (mg)	Calcium (mg)	Phos-phorus (mg)	Magne-sium (mg)	Other Ingredients
6	18	0.4	25	18				tartrazine copper iodine potassium manganese selenium zinc, 15 mg
2	6	0.4	10	18	NSᵃ			copper iodine potassium manganese zinc
2	4	0.4	20	10	NSᵃ		NSᵃ	copper iodine potassium manganese
5			20				70	zinc, 50 mg
2			10				NSᵃ	zinc, 18.4 mg manganese
				10/ml				flavor
1.05	4.5	0.3						sucrose flavor
0.4/ml	1.5/ml							alcohol, < 0.5% flavor
1.05/5 ml	4.5/5 ml							alcohol, ≤ 0.5% glucose sucrose flavor
1.05	4.5	0.3		12				sucrose flavor
0.4/ml				10/ml				alcohol, < 0.5% flavor
1.05	4.5	0.3		12				sucrose flavor
1.05/5 ml	4.5/5 ml			10/5 ml				alcohol, < 0.5% flavor

MULTIPLE VITAMIN PRODUCT TABLE, continued

Product (Manufacturer)	Vitamin A (IU)	Vitamin D (IU)	Vitamin E (IU)	Ascorbic Acid (C) (mg)	Thiamine (B₁) (mg)	Riboflavin (B₂) (mg)	Niacin (mg)
Vigortol Liquid (Rugby)					2.5/15 ml	1.25/15 ml	25/15 ml
Vigran Tablets (Squibb)	5000	400	30 (mg)	60	1.5	1.7	20
Vio-Bec Capsules (Reid-Rowell)				500	25	25	100
Vio-Bec Forte Tablets (Reid-Rowell)			30 (mg)	500	25	25	100
Viogen-C Capsules (Goldline)				300	20	10	100
Vita Bee C-800 Tablets (Rugby)			45	800	15	17	100
Vita-bee with C Captabs (Rugby)				300	15	10.2	50
Vitagett Tablets (Vortech)	5000	400	2.2 (mg)	50	3	2.5	20
Vita-Kaps Filmtabs (Abbott)	5000	400		50	3	2.5	20
Vita-Kaps-M Tablets (Abbott)	5000	400		50	3	2.5	20
Vital B-50 Tablets[b] (Goldine)					50	50	50
Vitamin B Complex Elixir (Lilly)					2.7/5 ml	1.35/5 ml	6.8/5 ml
Vitamin B Complex Pulvules (Lilly)					1	2	10

Pyridox-ine Hydro-chloride (B6)(mg)	Cyanoco-balamin (B12)(mcg)	Folic Acid (mg)	Panto-thenic Acid (mg)	Iron (mg)	Calcium (mg)	Phos-phorus (mg)	Magne-sium (mg)	Other Ingredients
0.5/15 ml	0.5/15 ml		5/15 ml	10/15 ml			NS[a]	zinc, 1 mg/15 ml choline, 50 mg/ 15 ml inositol, 50 mg/ 15 ml iodine potassium manganese alcohol, 18%
2	6	0.4						
25			40					
25	5	0.5	40					zinc, 25 mg copper
5			20				50	tartrazine zinc, 50 mg
25	12		25					
5			10					tartrazine
1.5	2.5		5	13.4	215	NS[a]	NS[a]	potassium manganese zinc, 1.4 mg
1	3							
1	3			10				copper iodine manganese zinc, 7.5 mg
50	50	0.1	50					d-biotin, 50 mcg PABA, 50 mg choline bitartrate, 50 mg inositol, 50 mg bromelain, 20 mg
0.55/5 ml	3/5 ml		2.7/5 ml					soluble liver fraction, 500 mg/ 5 ml alcohol, 17% saccharin
0.4	1		3.33					

MULTIPLE VITAMIN PRODUCT TABLE, continued

Product (Manufacturer)	Vitamin A (IU)	Vitamin D (IU)	Vitamin E (IU)	Ascorbic Acid (C) (mg)	Thiamine (B₁) (mg)	Riboflavin (B₂) (mg)	Niacin (mg)
Vitamin-Mineral-Supplement Liquid (PBI)					0.83/5 ml	0.42/5 ml	8.3/5 ml
Vi-Zac Capsules (Russ)	5000		50	500			
Within Tablets[b,c] (Miles)	5000	400	30 (mg)	60	1.5	1.7	20
Z-Bec Tablets (Robins)			45 (mg)	600	15	10.2	100
Ze Caps Capsules[b,c] (Everett)			200 (mg)				
Z-gen Tablets (Goldline)			45 (mg)	600	15	10.2	100
Zymacap Capsules (Upjohn)	5000	400	15 (mg)	90	2.25	2.6	30

[a] Quantity not specified.
[b] Sugar free.
[c] Sodium free.
[d] Alcohol free.

Pyridox-ine Hydro-chloride (B₆)(mg)	Cyanoco-balamin (B₁₂)(mcg)	Folic Acid (mg)	Panto-thenic Acid (mg)	Iron (mg)	Calcium (mg)	Phos-phorus (mg)	Magne-sium (mg)	Other Ingredients
0.17/5 ml	0.17/5 ml		1.67/5 ml	2.5/5 ml			0.33/5 ml	iodine, 16.67 mcg/ 5 ml zinc, 0.33 mg/5 ml manganese, 0.33 mg/5 ml choline, 16.67 mg/ 5 ml alcohol, 18%
								zinc, 18.4 mg
2	6	0.4	10	27	450			zinc, 15 mg tartrazine
10	6		25					zinc, 22.5
								zinc, 9.6 mg (as gluconate)
10	6		25					zinc, 22.5 mg tartrazine
3	9	0.4	15					

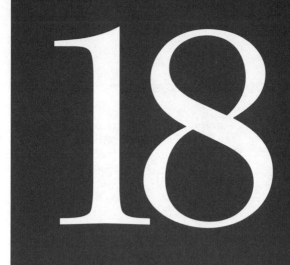

Michael W. McKenzie, Kenneth J. Bender,
and A. Jeanece Seals

INFANT FORMULA PRODUCTS

Questions to ask in patient/consumer counseling

What is your child's age and weight?

Is your child under a physician's care?

Are you breast-feeding the child or has your pediatrician recommended a formula?

Is the child allergic or sensitive to milk? Are there other dietary restrictions or health problems?

Are you using an iron-fortified formula?

Are you using a multivitamin with minerals formulation for your baby? Was it recommended by your pediatrician?

Is your baby receiving fluoride supplementation?

Does your baby have diarrhea, constipation, or vomiting?

Does your child have a fever, dry mucous membranes, or a loss of appetite?

Do you understand the method for mixing infant formula?

Milk, alone or in a mixture, is an infant's most important food. Before the 20th century, few infants not suckled by mothers or wet nurses survived their first year of life. Substitute feedings for breast milk were made possible by discoveries in biology and medicine in the late 19th century. The starting point of all modern studies on infant metabolism began with the calorimetric feeding method, which made it possible to feed infants according to their caloric (energy) requirements (1).

The modern era of infant formulas began in 1915 with the development of an artificial milk based on the fat content of human milk (2). Homogenized vegetable and animal fats and oils were added to skim cow milk to approximate the fatty acid content of human milk. The first formula was named SMA, for synthetic milk adapted. Modifications of this basic formula produced many of the current infant formulas.

Evaporated milk was the most commonly used infant food before the development of current infant formulas. Evaporated milk gained acceptance because it was inexpensive, convenient, readily available, and required no refrigeration.

By 1960, an estimated 80% of formula-fed infants in the United States were given either evaporated milk or a milk preparation marketed in evaporated form (1). By 1970, only 3% of infants were fed evaporated milk, and 75% of infants received a commercially prepared infant formula (3, 4). In the 1970s, a greater acceptance of breast-feeding resulted in a dramatic change in feeding patterns for infants. In 1984, 61% of infants were breast-fed, 45% received a prepared formula, and only 0.2% received evaporated milk (3, 4).

Advances in the uniformity, convenience, nutritional quality, and safety of infant formulas over the years established their effectiveness in infant feeding. The composition of commercial infant formulas conforms with guidelines generated from extensive assessment of infant nutritional needs. Formula variations allow a parent to select a product that is acceptable to a particular infant's nutritional needs and satisfies special nutritional requirements. However, these variations have produced differences in palatability, digestibility, and convenience of administration. The pharmacist, in consultation with the infant's physician, should be able to evaluate indications and advise on the selection of infant formulas.

PHYSIOLOGIC CONSIDERATIONS IN INFANT NUTRITION

The physiologic capabilities of the infant's gastrointestinal (GI) and renal systems are considered in the development of formulas that can adequately substitute for human milk. In early infancy, food must be liquid until coordination between complex tongue movements and mature swallowing reflexes develops. Frequent feedings are necessary because the stomach capacity is small (10–20 ml at birth and 200 ml by 12 months of age).

The newborn can digest fats, proteins, and carbohydrates. Intestinal enzymes, lactase, sucrase, maltase, isomaltase, and glucomylase are sufficiently mature in the full-term infant (38–42 weeks gestational period and birth weight > 2,500 g) to permit absorption of carbohydrates (5). Sucrase, maltase, and isomaltase are usually fully active even in preterm infants (gestational period < 38 weeks), but lactase activity may be low (5). Mature levels of pancreatic amylase activity and glucose transport occur after birth and are low in both full-term and preterm infants (5). Clinical lactose intolerance is uncommon in infants because of postnatal adaptive responses to ingested carbohydrates. Colonic flora, through fermentation of carbohydrates to hydrogen gas and short-chain fatty acids, recovers inadequately absorbed carbohydrates (5).

Protein and fat are digested mainly in the infant's small intestine. Newborn infants have low levels of lipase for breakdown of triglyceride and bile acids for emulsification of fat before and during lipolysis. Lingual and gastric lipases promote intragastric lipolysis to compensate for low levels of pancreatic lipase. In addition, the products of lipolysis, fatty acids, and monoglycerides offset the low-bile salt levels by emulsifying the lipid mixture (6, 7). In the breast-fed infant, an additional compensatory mechanism, bile-salt stimulated lipase, ensures adequate dietary fat intake (6, 7). Absorption of fat improves as the infant matures. Long-chain saturated fatty acids (butterfat) are not absorbed as well as unsaturated fatty acids (vegetable oils) (8).

Protein digestion does not differ appreciably between infants and adults, even though infants have less active trypsin and chymotrypsin (9, 10). Amino acids from protein digestion are absorbed by active transport mechanisms.

The excess ingestion of electrolytes and minerals and the metabolic end-products from protein metabolism constitute the renal solute load. A simple, direct relationship between renal solute loads and dietary concentrations of protein and minerals does not exist. Significant amounts of minerals and protein waste products are excreted through the skin (sweat), lungs (water vapor), and GI tract. In addition, amino acids from protein digestion are used in protein anabolism for tissues. When metabolized, the carbohydrates present in formulas yield essentially no solutes for renal excretion (11).

However, the renal solute load is important because it determines the quantity of water excreted through the kidney. Young infants have less ability than older infants, children, and adults to concentrate or dilute renal solute loads (10–13). Under normal conditions, infant formulas in proper concentration provide enough water (1.5 ml/kcal per day) for all routes of water loss, including urinary excretion. If decreased water intake or excessive water loss occurs, diets with high renal solute loads may stress the limited capacity of the kidney's reabsorptive system (11).

CONTENT OF MILK AND FORMULAS

The initial comparison to be considered is that between mature human milk and cow milk, which is used as the protein base for most commercial preparations. The initial milk from the breast is referred to as colostrum. Within 1 week the milk changes in composition and is referred to as transitional milk. After about 3 weeks the milk produced in the breasts is considered mature and is the standard with which most commercially prepared infant formulas are compared.

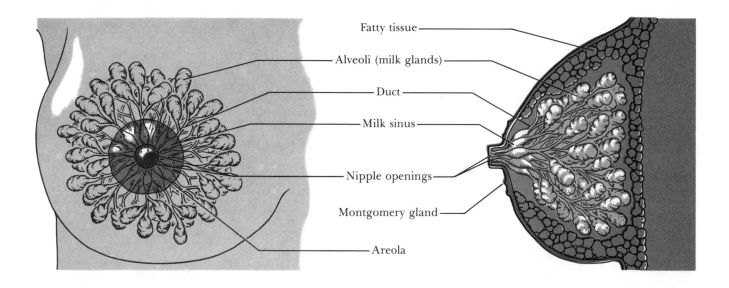

Fatty tissue

Alveoli (milk glands)

Duct

Milk sinus

Nipple openings

Montgomery gland

Areola

FIGURE 1 Anatomy of the breast.

The human breast anatomy is depicted in Figure 1, with those anatomical features identified that are principally involved in milk production and collection.

Human Milk: Standard of Comparison

Both human milk and cow milk are intricate liquids that contain more than 200 ingredients in the fat-soluble and water-soluble fractions. Table 1 lists average nutrients contained in pooled human milk and minimum federal standards for homogenized milk (14). The two types of milk differ significantly in the quantity and availability of the nutrients. Mature human milk is more effective than cow milk in meeting the nutritional requirements of the human infant. The differences in composition reflect the different needs of the human infant and the calf. Although certain conditions in the infant may necessitate therapeutic formulas, human milk is the most appropriate diet for most infants.

Both milks provide similar amounts of water and approximately the same quantity of energy. However, the nutrient sources of energy (i.e., calories) are different: protein supplies about 7% of the calories in human milk and 20% of the calories in cow milk; the carbohydrate lactose supplies about 42% of the calories in hu-

man milk and 20% of the calories in cow milk (14). The percentage of calories provided by fat is similar in both milks.

Protein

Cow milk contains more than three times the ash and protein normally found in human milk (3.5 g/100 ml of protein in cow milk and 0.9 g/100 ml of protein in human milk) (14). This difference reflects the calf's more rapid growth rate and proportionate demand for protein and minerals. The urea formed from protein nitrogen combines with the mineral residue (ash) to create a higher renal solute load for the infant ingesting cow milk. Although cow milk usually is diluted with water and carbohydrates, the solute load requiring renal excretion generally remains greater than the load from human milk.

Not only does cow milk contain a higher percentage of protein than human milk, but the protein differs in composition. The difference in protein composition alters digestibility and may create a milk "sensitivity," which may induce problems in digestion of a milk-based formula, or it may elicit an allergic response to milk protein. Breast milk proteins are defined broadly as either whey or casein protein with an approximate ratio of 60:40 of whey to caseins, respectively (15). The casein protein contains a mixture of alpha-, beta-, gamma-, and kappa-caseins; the whey protein contains alpha-lactalbumin, beta-lactoglobulin, lactoferrin, serum albumin, lysozyme, and immunoglobulins A, G, and M (IgA, IgG, and IgM). Casein is relatively insoluble and occurs in milk as a "tough" curd; whey protein is highly soluble (15).

Cow milk contains a greater amount of casein (six to seven times as much casein) than human milk, with a ratio of 80:20 of casein to whey, respectively. The large amount of casein in cow milk mixes with hydrochloric acid during digestion in the stomach to produce curds. This slows the gastric emptying rate and may cause GI distress. Processing cow milk (acidification, boiling, and treatment with enzymes) reduces the curd tension and makes it more digestible. Because of the lower casein content, human milk forms a soft, flocculent, easy-to-digest curd in the infant's stomach.

Sensitivity to cow milk differs from milk allergy. Sensitivity to cow milk may be relieved by altering the casein to lactalbumin ratio; however, an allergic reaction requires that all animal milk protein be eliminated. Although heating cow milk may increase digestibility by reducing curd tension, it will not alter its antigen activity in allergic infants.

Amino Acid Content

The amino acid content of cow milk is inappropriate for the neonate's immature enyzme system. The newborn has a limited ability to metabolize phenylalanine to tyrosine; human milk has low concentrations of these amino acids. Taurine and cystine are present in higher concentrations in human milk than in cow milk. In addition, cystathionase, an enzyme necessary for the transulfuration of methionine to cystine, is present in low concentrations in the neonate (14).

Growth Modulators

Human milk also contains a number of substances that are categorized as growth modulators: taurine, ethanolamine, phosphoethanolamine, epidermal growth factor (EGF), nerve growth factor (NGF), enzymes, and interferons (16). The biological and clinical significance of growth modulators awaits further clarification. However, evidence from animal and cell culture models suggests that they are physiologically important. The major growth modulator identified using cell culture and immunologic assays is EGF (17). EGF could promote the maturation of immature GI epithelium, or it could support the rapid growth and differentiation of epithelial cells in other tissues such as the liver (16). NGF may be involved in the arborization of the sympathetic neurons of the gut or in the maturation of sensory neurons (16). Taurine is involved in the maintenance of the structural and functional integrity of cell membranes (18). Several milk enzymes have charac-

TABLE 1 Composition of mature human milk and cow milk

Composition	Human milk	Cow milk
WATER (ml/100 ml)	87.1%	87.2%
ENERGY (kcal/100 ml)	69	66
PROTEIN (g/100 ml)	0.9	3.5
(% of protein)		
Lactalbumin	60%	18%
Casein	40%	82%
Lactoglobulin	0.2%	0.2%
Beta-lactoglobulin	–	+
Lactoferrin	+	–
Secretory IgA	+	–
FAT (g/100 ml)	4.0	3.8
(% of fat)		
Unsaturated	51%	66%
Saturated	49%	66%
CARBOHYDRATE (g/100 ml)		
Lactose	6.8	3.9
ELECTROLYTES (per liter)		
Calcium (mg)	340	1,200
Phosphorus (mg)	150	920
Calcium/phosphorus	2:1	1.2:1
Sodium (mg)	160	506
Potassium (mg)	530	1,570
Chloride (mg)	400	1,028
Magnesium (mg)	41	120
Sulfur (mg)	140	300
MINERALS (per liter)		
Chromium (mcg)	4	2
Manganese (mcg)	4	20–40
Copper (mcg)	60	110
Zinc (mg)	0.5	3–5
Iodine (mcg)	200	80
Selenium (mcg)	20	5–50
Iron (mg)	0.5	0.5
VITAMINS (per liter)		
Vitamin A (IU)	1,898	1,025
Thiamine (mcg)	150	370
Riboflavin (mcg)	380	1,700
Niacin (mcg)	1,700	900
Pyridoxine (mcg)	130	460
Pantothenate (mg)	1.8	3.5
Folic acid (mcg)	85	68
Vitamin B_{12} (mcg)	0.5	4
Vitamin C (mg)	43	11
Vitamin D (IU)	40	14
Vitamin E (mg)	3.2	0.4
Vitamin K (mcg)	34	170

Key: + means substance present; – means substance absent.

Adapted from P. Pipes, "Nutrition in Infancy and Childhood," 4th ed., Times Mirror/Mosby College Publishing, St. Louis, Mo., 1989, p. 89.

teristics similar to those of other milk proteins shown to be active in the GI tract, for example, secretory IgA and lactoferrin. These milk enzymes may function in the milk, in the GI tract to alter the mucous diffusion barrier, or in intestinal tissue, or they may be absorbed in the small intestine and transported to other organs (16).

Fat

Human milk and cow milk contain a similar total fat content. Human milk contains 3.0–4.5% fat that consists of triglycerides (98–99% of total milk fat), phospholipids, and cholesterol (19). Milk fat composition changes during lactation: the triglyceride level rises, and the phospholipid and cholesterol concentrations decrease during the transition from colostrum to mature milk (7). Mature milk maintains a constant fat composition.

Linoleic acid supplies an average of 4% of the calories of human milk, but only 1% of the calories in cow milk. The cholesterol content varies in both milks: 20–47 mg/100 ml in human milk and 7–25 mg/100 ml in cow milk (19).

The fat in cow milk differs from that in human milk in two ways. The triglycerides in cow milk contain primarily short- and long-chain fatty acids (butyric and caproic). Human milk fat includes medium-chain fatty acids (capric and lauric) but not the short-chain group. In addition, human milk contains a majority of monosaturated fatty acids, and cow milk butterfat consists primarily of saturated fatty acids. Commercial milk-based formulas incorporate the highly digestible, unsaturated, medium-chain triglycerides (MCTs) by replacing butterfat with vegetable oil and special MCT oils.

Human milk lipase functions to digest fat in the stomach because luminal bile acid concentration and pancreatic lipase are naturally low in infants under 6 months of age (6). Cow milk does not contain this necessary lipase. However, infants fed milk-based formula efficiently digest fat from vegetable oil because of gastric enzyme activity.

Carbohydrates

The carbohydrate percentage in cow milk is lower than the percentage in human milk, and carbohydrate supplementation is therefore necessary for milk-based formulas. Honey and other unrefined foods are poor choices for carbohydrate supplementation because they may contain spores of *Clostridium botulinum*. Lactose is the carbohydrate source in both cow milk and human milk. Lactose is absorbed into the brush border of the small intestine and cleaved by the enzyme lactase into galactose and glucose. These sugars are then absorbed actively against concentration gradients.

Electrolytes and Minerals

The mineral content of cow milk is several times greater than that of human milk. Cow milk and human milk differ in absolute and proportionate amounts of calcium and phosphorus. The ratio of calcium and phosphorus is 1.2:1 in cow milk compared with 2.0:1 in human milk. The effect of this difference on calcium absorption is not clear because of the interrelation of additional factors such as vitamin D, fat absorption, and active transport. The iron content of human milk decreases from 0.5 to 0.3 mg/100 ml when the infant is between 2 weeks and 5 months of age (20). Levels of iron in cow milk remain at 0.5 mg/100 ml. The iron in human milk is absorbed to a greater extent by infants; 50% of iron is absorbed from human milk, and only 10% of iron from cow milk (20).

The zinc content of human milk is lower than that of cow milk, but it is more bioavailable (a bioavailability of about 59% compared with 43–51%, respectively) (21). Zinc binds strongly to casein in cow milk; zinc binding in human milk is minimal.

Cow milk also contains more sodium, potassium, and chloride than human milk. These higher electrolyte and mineral concentrations, when combined with the high protein content of cow milk, result in a smaller margin of safety against hyperosmolar dehydration. The greater renal solute load ingested from cow milk, in combination with higher environmental temperatures, fever, vomiting, or diarrhea, can place an infant at risk for severe dehydration.

Anti-infective Substances

Human milk contains immunoglobulins, enzymes, and other factors that are absent or present in only minute quantities in cow milk. Lactoferrin and secretory IgA are present in human milk in greater quantities than in cow milk, and lysozyme is found in human milk but not in cow milk. Lactoferrin increases the bioavailability of iron; lactoferrin, lysozyme, and IgA may protect against enteric infection (22).

Evaporated Milk

The concentrations of protein, fat, carbohydrate, and major minerals are standardized in evaporated milk. Evaporated milk is sterile, convenient, and produces a smaller and softer curd. Evaporated milk formulas and unmodified cow milk fail to meet current recommendations for ascorbic acid (vitamin C), vitamin E, and essential fatty acids (23–25). (See Chapter 17, *Nutritional Supplement, Mineral, and Vitamin Products*.)

Skim Milk and Two-Percent Fresh Pasteurized Milk

Skim milk, from which fat has been removed by centrifugation, generally contains 0.1% fat and does not contain acceptable protein, fat, or carbohydrate ratios. Skim milk is generally not recommended for infants under 1 year of age. Skim milk has been used in an attempt to prevent obesity and perhaps to aid in preventing atherosclerosis. These proposed benefits have not been proved and remain controversial.

Infants fed skim milk gain less weight and slightly, but not significantly, more length than infants fed whole milk (26). Although this result may seem desirable, considerations of energy balance offer cause for concern. Infants fed skim milk use more of their stores of body fat. Over an extended period, once body fat stores have been depleted, the infant's ability to respond adequately to a major illness may be compromised (27).

Infants receiving a major percentage of their caloric intake from skim milk may receive exceedingly high protein intake, low fat intake, and an inadequate intake of essential fatty acids. The maximum concentration of protein allowed in infant formulas is 4.5 g per 100 kcal, but skim milk provides about 10 g of protein per 100 kcal.

It is important to recognize that, per unit volume, skim milk provides a slightly greater renal solute load than does whole cow milk. The solute concentration is further increased by water loss during boiling (28). Thus, skim milk is also not recommended for the treatment of diarrhea because of the possibility of hypertonic dehydration.

Two-percent milk is made from fresh whole and skim milk combined to contain 2% fat. Fat-free milk solids, vitamins, and minerals can be added to this pasteurized and homogenized milk formulation. A disadvantage of using 2% milk as the only dietary source is the unbalanced percentage of calories supplied from protein, fat, and carbohydrates. Two-percent milk supplies about 7 g of protein per 100 kcal and, therefore, exceeds the recommended amount for infants. For the normal, healthy infant, the high volumes required of low energy milks may result in sufficient amounts of water for renal excretion. However, if an infant has fever, diarrhea, and/or vomiting and concurrently experiences a decrease in milk intake, the infant has a greater potential for water imbalance because of the increased renal solute load resulting from the higher concentration of protein in these products. (See Chapter 13, *Antidiarrheal and Other Gastrointestinal Products.*)

The Committee on Nutrition of the American Academy of Pediatrics (CON/AAP) does not recommend skim milk or 2% milk during infancy (first 12 months of life) (25).

Whole Cow Milk

The appropriate age to introduce unheated, whole cow milk (WCM) into the infant diet is still controversial. Because the concentration and bioavailability of iron in WCM are low, the consumption of excessive amounts of WCM has been associated with iron-deficiency anemia (29–32). Through unknown mechanisms, WCM can also cause occult bleeding from the GI tract (33). Milk-protein intolerance and/or allergy (estimated at 0.4–7.5% of the infant population in the first 2 years of life) poses another potential complication for the use of WCM (34). However, there is no convincing evidence that feeding WCM after 6 months of age is detrimental if adequate additional feedings are given (35).

More research is needed to establish a time frame for the introduction of WCM. The CON/AAP currently endorses breast-feeding with appropriate supplementation for infants 6–12 months of age (35). WCM may be instituted if breast-feeding has been completely discontinued and infants are consuming at least one-third of their calories as supplemental foods consisting of a balanced mixture of cereal, vegetables, fruits, and other foods (thereby assuring ample sources of both iron and vitamin C) (35). Infants should be fed no more than 1 liter of WCM a day. Most infants who are not breast-fed should be ingesting a representative portion of their calories from supplemental foods after they are 6 months of age. An iron-fortified formula should be given to infants who are not consuming a significant portion of their calories from supplemental foods (35).

Goat Milk

Goat milk is commercially available in powdered and evaporated forms. It contains primarily medium- and short-chain fatty acids and may be more readily digested than cow milk. Unfortified goat milk is deficient in folates and low in iron and vitamin D. The evaporated form of Meyenberg Goat Milk is supplemented with vitamin D and folic acid. The powder formulation of Meyenberg Goat Milk is supplemented with folic acid only and is recommended by the manufacturer for use in babies over 1 year of age. Because the powder formulation is not a complete formula for infants, the manufacturer recommends supplementation with vitamins.

BREAST-FEEDING CONSIDERATIONS

Although not bacteriologically sterile, human milk and breast-feeding provide certain advantages over the use of cow milk, goat milk, and infant formulas. However, caution is needed against issuing dire warnings to mothers who cannot or do not wish to breast-feed. Normal growth and development are possible without it. When breast-feeding is unsuccessful, inappropriate, or ceased early, infant formulas provide the best alternative for meeting nutritional needs during the first year (25).

Not all of the claimed advantages of breast-feeding have been documented through scientific investigations. A review of the literature identifies several studies that present conflicting data about the proposed benefits of breast-feeding (36).

Postnatal Mortality

No studies within the past 50 years have investigated an association of lower postnatal mortality with breast-fed infants. Studies on sudden infant death syndrome (SIDS) could not detect an association between bottle-feeding and SIDS to support the hypothesis that cow milk intolerance or allergy was a causal factor (37, 38). A review of the literature from the 1970s concluded that breast-feeding does not protect against SIDS (39). There is no evidence from time trends that high rates of breast-feeding are associated with low postnatal mortality (36).

Infectious Disease Specific Morbidity

Because of the lack of opportunity for contamination and the abundance of "host-resistant factors" (including bifidus factor, lactoferrin, lymphocytes, lysozymes, macrophages, and immunoglobulins), breast-feeding theoretically protects against infections such as GI illness, respiratory infection, and otitis media.

L-Bifidus factor promotes the growth of *Lactobacillus* in the GI tract. These organisms produce acetic and lactic acids that create an environment that interferes with the growth of *Escherichia coli* and *Shigella* (40–45). Also, the acidic environment provides a medium in which lysozymes are stable so that they may exert a destructive effect on bacterial cell membranes. Breast milk contains immunoglobulins against many types of microorganisms: *Bordetella*, *Staphylococcus*, *E. coli*, and *Salmonella* (43). Lactoferrin exerts a bacteriostatic effect by depriving bacteria of an iron-containing environment necessary for their normal cell growth.

Most studies suggest an association between breast-feeding and decreased rates of GI illness (44–48). Studies have shown that infants who were breast-fed have fewer incidences of gastroenteritis, fewer episodes of diarrhea, and infrequent hospitalizations for GI illness.

Conflicting results have been reported with regard to breast-feeding and a low rate of respiratory infection. In those studies that found an association between breast-feeding and decreased risk of respiratory infection, confounding variables (socioeconomic status, maternal smoking, presence of older siblings) may account for the findings (49–53). However, several studies that found no difference in rates of respiratory illness did not compare infants who were exclusively bottle-fed and infants who were exclusively breast-fed.

Studies do not provide definitive evidence that breast-feeding is protective against otitis media (52–57). One well-designed study controlled for confounding variables of age and birth weight still demonstrated a protective effect (54). No study has examined whether a protective effect was a direct result of breast-feeding or of differences in position during feeding. The practice of bottle-feeding an infant in a supine position, which allows reflux of nasopharyngeal contents into the eustachian tube, may contribute to a higher incidence of otitis media. The more erect position required for breast-feeding may provide a protective effect against reflux of nasopharyngeal secretions into the eustachian tube.

Many questions about the apparent protective effect of breast-feeding remain to be answered. What is the duration of protection after discontinuation? What effect does change in age have on the protective effect? How great is the interactive effect of social and demographic variables? How does the addition of solid foods to the diet of a breast-fed infant influence the protective effect? What consequence does partial bottle-feeding have on the protective effect of breast-feeding? Better designed studies are needed to answer these questions and to document the advantages of breast-feeding against a variety of infections.

Allergic Disease

Breast-feeding has been postulated to protect against allergic diseases by supplying IgA, which prevents infection and blocks absorption of intact allergens through the GI tract, and by circumventing exposure in early infancy to significant amounts of foreign protein present in cow milk, which could stimulate immunoglobulin E (IgE) production and precipitate allergic symptoms. Studies have examined the protective effect of breast-feeding for allergic diseases such as eczema, asthma, allergic rhinitis, and food allergy (38, 58–63). Many of these studies found no protective effect (38, 58, 60, 61, 63). In other studies, confounding factors could account for the findings. Based on available studies, it cannot be concluded whether breast milk is protective or whether one or more of the alternative feeding regimens is allergenic.

Obesity

If fat babies become fat adults, then prevention of obesity in infants may be an effective strategy against morbidity in adults. Unfortunately, the questions of whether infant obesity is associated with adult obesity or whether infant feeding is associated with adult obesity remain unresolved. Data on whether breast-feeding versus bottle-feeding versus early introduction of solid foods affect optimal weight gain or health status are so muddled that no rational conclusions can be expressed (64). However, one well-designed study showed that weight gain at 1 year of age in bottle-fed infants was similar to that of breast-fed infants (65). No obesity or malnutrition was found in any of the infants.

Anemia

Iron deficiency anemia is the most common nutrition-related deficiency among children in the United States (36). Iron deficiency rarely develops in breast-fed infants before 4–6 months of age because neonatal iron stores can supply the major portion of iron needs during this period. Infants absorb iron from breast milk in greater amounts than iron from cow milk formulas. Even though breast milk contains a small amount of iron, about 50% of the iron in breast milk is absorbed, compared with 10% from unfortified cow milk formula (20).

Absorption of iron from breast milk averages about 0.15 mg a day, based on consumption of a liter of breast milk with a concentration of approximately 0.3 mg/l (66). This amount is significantly less than the 0.6 to 0.7 mg of iron needed daily to ensure adequate iron nutritional status (67).

A prospective study of iron nutritional status of breast-fed infants indicates that without iron supplementation a substantial proportion of such infants become iron deficient by 9 months of age (68). Therefore, the CON/AAP recommends adding iron-fortified cereal to the diet of breast-fed infants after 6 months of age (69). Glass jars of wet-packed cereal and fruit combinations with ferrous sulfate as the iron supplement have been recommended over iron-fortified dry cereal because of the reduced chance for oxidative rancidity of iron with oxygen (66).

Psychologic and Intellectual Development

The literature on psychologic and intellectual development factors of breast-feeding does not distinguish definitively between the effects of the breast-feeding mechanism and other factors that influence the feeding experience (36). The evidence is too limited to recommend breast-feeding based on the possible link between breast-feeding and a beneficial psychologic outcome (36). Studies do not demonstrate a universal phenomenon in which one method of infant feeding is superior to another in all instances, and they do not support making a mother feel that she is doing psychologic harm to her child if she is unable or unwilling to breast-feed (36).

Hyperbilirubinemia

One minor problem associated with human milk is the presence of increased levels of nonesterified fatty acid (70). Abnormal lipolytic activity in the breast milk of some women causes increased levels of nonesterified fatty acid. This results in the inhibition of UDPglucuronyl transferase and leads to a prolonged unconjugated hyperbilirubinemia in infants. Breast-feeding need not be stopped in most cases of breast milk jaundice (71). The jaundice eventually subsides even if breast-feeding is continued. If the infant appears in danger from hyperbilirubinemia itself, a temporary pause in breast-feeding for 1–4 days usually reduces the bilirubin to a safe level. Breast-feeding can then be resumed.

Medications

The need for adequate contraception by the mother of a breast-feeding infant can create concern about the use of oral contraceptive drugs. Reviews of the literature on the use of oral contraceptive drugs during lactation have produced confusing recommendations (72–75). Advances in oral contraceptive drug practices are ahead of studies of their possible influence on breast-feeding.

Most studies of the use of combined estrogen–progestin contraceptive drugs (usually containing 30–50 mcg of ethinyl estradiol or 50–100 mcg of mestranol) demonstrate that lactation is not inhibited after the immediate postpartum period. Some dose-related suppression of the quantity of milk produced and the duration of lactation is found with extended use (74, 76–79). Use of oral contraceptive drugs during lactation has not clearly been related to changes in the composition of milk. Studies with progestin-only contraceptives indicate no consistent alteration of breast milk composition or substantial reduction of milk production or the duration of lactation (74, 76, 80–83). A well-designed study on the effects of two oral contraceptive combination drugs (one containing 250 mcg of *d*-norgestrel and 50 mcg of ethinyl estradiol; the other containing 150 mcg of *d*-norgestrel and 30 mcg of ethinyl estradiol) and one progestin-only oral contraceptive pill (containing 30 mcg of *d*-norgestrel) noted that the volume and composition of breast milk vary considerably in the absence of steroidal contraception (84). Changes in these values tend to remain within the normal ranges during oral contraceptive use.

Several studies indicate that an infant consuming 600 ml of breast milk containing 50 mcg of ethinyl estradiol probably receives a daily dose of about 10 ng of the drug (85, 86). Mothers who do not use oral contraceptive drugs produce natural estradiol, so infants who consume a similar amount of breast milk receive about 3–6 ng of estradiol during anovulatory cycles and 6–12 ng during ovulatory cycles (86). Estrogen-containing or progestin-only oral contraceptive drugs do not exhibit any consistent long-term adverse effects on the growth and development of children (77, 78).

Many other drugs taken by the lactating woman may be found in her milk. The ingestion of drugs through breast milk has been the subject of extensive review (87–92).

The degree of drug transfer across the membrane between plasma and milk is influenced by the drug's solubility in lipids and water; by its pKa or degree of ionization, degree of plasma protein binding, and degree of milk protein binding; and by selective transport mechanisms. The pH of milk is less than that of plasma; consequently, milk may act as an "ion trap" for basic compounds. Conversely, acidic drugs tend to be inhibited from entering milk.

Table 2 summarizes recommendations for drugs to be avoided in breast-feeding (88). The recommendations are based on probable steady-state plasma concentrations, which may result in the infant's impaired clearance relative to the plasma concentration of an adult. This approach assumes that there should be no problems associated with breast-feeding provided the drug concentration in the infant is well below the maternal concentration. Therefore, it also assumes that these drugs have dose-related, predictable toxicity, which is not always valid (e.g., glucose-6-phosphate dehydrogenase deficiency from drugs such as acetylsalicylic acid, chloramphenicol, chlorpromazine, nitrofu-

rantoin, sulfonamides, pyrimethamine, and phenazopyridine) (88). These drugs should be avoided by the breast-feeding mother; however, there are few actual reported cases of hemolysis in breast-fed infants.

Doses of social drugs (nicotine, alcohol, caffeine, and theobromine) ingested by the mother vary. Heavy usage of these or any illegal drugs and excessive uncontrolled usage of any drug should mitigate against breast-feeding (88). It is unwise to expose an infant to even low concentrations of highly toxic drugs such as chloramphenicol, cytotoxic agents, iodine, bromides, and ergotamine (88). Other authorities recommend that the breast-feeding mother avoid diazepam, androgens, phenolphthalein, phenelzine, phenindione, bromocriptine, calciferol, clindamycin, clonidine, diphenoxylate, isotretinoin, lincomycin, lindane, lithium, methapyrolon, moxalactam, phenylbutazone, phencyclidine, propoxyphene, reserpine, sulfonamides, tetracycline, and tolbutamide, and radioactive chemicals (gallium 64, iodide 125, iodine 131, technetium) (93–96).

Certainly, duration of drug exposure is an important factor in evaluating potential drug toxicity to a

TABLE 2 Drugs to avoid while breast-feeding*

Avoid totally at all ages
Phenobarbital
Propylthiouracil

Avoid at < 52 weeks postconceptional age

Amidarone	Isoniazid
Carbimazole	Metronidazole
Ethosuximide	Theophylline

Avoid at < 44 weeks postconceptional age

Atenolol	Metoclopramide
Ethanol	Theobromine
Methimazole	Tolbutamide

Avoid at < 34 weeks postconceptional age or when unusually large doses are used

Acyclovir	Disopyramide
Amphetamine	Gold
Baclofen	Hexamine
Caffeine	Iodine
Chloramphenicol	Nadolol
Cimetidine	Paracetamol
Clemastine	Phenytoin
Clonidine	Piroxicam
Codeine	Sulfapyridine
Dapsone	

*These recommendations are based on likely plasma concentrations in the infant after breast-feeding within the indicated time periods of growth and development.

From H. C. Atkinson et al., *Clin. Pharm., 14*, 217 (1988).

nursing infant. If a mother who is breast-feeding must take a medication, she should take it shortly after she breast-feeds to allow as much time as possible for the drug to clear the maternal blood and achieve a relatively low concentration before the next feeding.

COMMERCIAL INFANT FORMULAS

Recommendations to standardize the nutrient composition of infant formulas were first published by the CON/AAP in 1967 (97). These recommendations were adopted by the Food and Drug Administration (FDA) in 1971, and were revised in 1976 by the AAP task force at the request of the FDA. Furthermore, the FDA published rules concerning the provision of nutrient content of infant formulas in 1985 (Table 3) (98).

In 1980, the U.S. Congress passed an amendment to the Federal Food, Drug, and Cosmetic Act (Infant Formula Act of 1980) stipulating new regulations giving the FDA the authority to establish quality control procedures for infant formula manufacturing, to establish recall procedures, to require adequate labeling, and to revise nutrient levels (99, 100).

The manufacturer may alter a formulation in response to changes in availability of ingredients or modifications in recommended allowances. For example, the fat source of Similac was modified by adding soy oil to corn oil in response to the decreased availability and rising cost of corn oil. Accurate listing of current ingredients and quantities may be obtained by direct communication with the manufacturer.

Physical Characteristics

All infant formulas are emulsions of edible oils in aqueous solutions. Separation of fat rarely occurs in infant formulas. If separation occurs, the fat can be redispersed by shaking the container. However, if separation of fat has occurred because of the lack of stabilizers or with storage beyond shelf life, redispersion by normal shaking may not be possible.

Protein agglomeration may occur if the storage time is excessive. This agglomeration may range from slight, grainy development through increased viscosity and formation of gels to eventual precipitation of protein (101). Protein agglomeration and fat separation do not affect the safety or nutritional adequacy of the formulas; however, the objectionable appearance and the greater viscosity are deterrents to their use.

TABLE 3 Infant nutritional recommendations for full-term infants (per 100 kcal)

Nutrient	FDA Regulations	
	Minimum	Maximum
PROTEIN (g)	1.8	4.5
FAT		
(g)	3.3	6.0
(% calories)	30.0	–
ESSENTIAL FATTY ACIDS		
Linoleic acid (g)	0.3	–
VITAMINS		
Vitamin A (IU)	250.0	750.0
Vitamin D (IU)	40.0	100.0
Vitamin K (g)	4.0	–
Vitamin E (IU)	0.7	–
Vitamin C (mg)	40.0	–
B_1 (thiamine) (mcg)	40.0	–
B_2 (riboflavin) (mcg)	60.0	–
B_6 (pyridoxine) (mcg)	35.0	–
B_{12} (mcg)	0.15	–
Niacin (mcg) [a]	2.5	–
Folic acid (mcg)	4.0	–
Pantothenic acid (mcg)	300.0	–
Biotin (mcg) [b]	1.5	–
Choline (mg) [b]	7.0	–
Inositol (mg)	4.0	–
MINERALS		
Calcium (mg)	60.0	–
Phosphorus (mg)	30.0	–
Magnesium (mg)	6.0	–
Iron (mg)	0.15	3.0
Iodine (mcg)	5.0	7.5
Zinc (mg)	0.5	–
Copper (mcg)	60.0	75.0
Manganese (mcg)	5.0	–
Sodium (mg)	20.0	60.0
Potassium (mg)	80.0	200.0
Chloride (mg)	55.0	150.0

[a] Includes nicotinic acid and niacinamide.
[b] Required only for nonmilk-based infant formulas.

Reprinted from the *Federal Register, 50,* 45106 (1985).

Liquid infant formulas contain thickening and stabilizing agents to provide uniform consistency and to prolong stability. Carrageenan is a stabilizing agent in many infant formulas. The use of guar gum, locust bean gum, distarch phosphate, acetylated distarch phosphate, phosphated distarch phosphate, hydroxypropyl starch, carrageenan, lecithin, and monoglycerides and diglycerides as stabilizers, thickening agents, and emulsifiers is covered by FDA's food additive regulations, and these agents are generally recognized as safe (102). Infant formulas may contain one or more of these substances; no one formula contains all of them.

Microbiologic Safety

Guidelines by the Infant Formula Council (a voluntary, nonprofit, trade association composed of companies engaged in the manufacture and marketing of infant formulas) require liquid formulations to be free of all viable pathogens and their spores and other organisms that may cause product degradation (103). Microbiologic contamination may alter the nutritional quality of formulas and result in diarrhea and subsequent fluid and electrolyte imbalances. The quality control measures at every stage of formulation and production provide a sterile product free of microbial effects as long as the container remains intact. Powdered formulas are essentially free of microorganisms, and the required heating during final preparation (as indicated on label directions) destroys most microorganisms introduced during preparation.

Digestibility

Milk produces a precipitate or curd when it comes in contact with hydrochloric acid in the stomach. Curds contain most of the casein and calcium of milk. The whey of milk contains proteins and lactose in the watery portion. Unprocessed milk produces tough curds that are difficult for infants to digest. Human milk contains less casein than cow milk and produces more digestible curds in the stomach. Homogenization, evaporation, boiling, and drying reduce the curd tension of cow milk. Infant formulas containing cow milk are processed to avoid problems with curd production.

Physical and Chemical Properties

Caloric Density

The metabolic calorie [large calorie or kilocalorie (kcal)] is the amount of heat required to raise the temperature of 1,000 g of water from 15° C to 16° C. The recommended daily dietary allowance (RDA) is 108 kcal/kg per day for infants from birth to 6 months of

age and 98 kcal/kg per day from 6 months to 1 year (104).

A full-term infant should have no difficulty in consuming enough diluted infant formula (20 kcal/30 ml or 67 kcal/100 ml) to meet these needs, but a preterm or low-birth-weight (LBW) (<2,500 g) infant has a higher caloric need and may require as much as 130 kcal/kg per day (105). An infant recovering from illness or malnutrition also requires more calories (24). Infant formulas with caloric densities significantly lower or higher than 67 kcal/100 ml are regarded as therapeutic formulas for management of special clinical conditions and should be used only under medical supervision.

Osmolarity and Osmolality of Infant Formulas

Osmolarity is the concentration of a solute in a solution per unit of total volume of solution (mOsm per liter of formula). Osmolarity of human milk is approximately 273 mOsm/l. The CON/AAP recommends that formulas for normal infants may have concentrations of no greater than 400 mOsm/l without a warning statement on the label (105). Hyperosmolar formulas have been implicated in causing necrotizing enterocolitis (106, 107).

Osmolality is the solute concentration in a solution per unit of solvent (mOsm per kilogram of water). The osmolality of a formula is directly related to the concentration of molecular or ionic particles in solution and is inversely proportional to the concentration of water (108). The osmolality of human milk is approximately 300 mOsm/kg. Osmolality is related to the carbohydrate and mineral content of the formula.

For dilute solutions, there is little difference in osmolality and osmolarity. However, because infant formulas are relatively concentrated solutions, osmolarity may be only 80% of the osmolality (108). Osmolality is the preferred term to report osmotic activities of infant formulas because osmotic activity is a function of a solute–solvent relationship. Manufacturers report both osmolality and osmolarity.

The relationship between osmolality and caloric density is reasonably linear in formulas having a caloric density of 44–90 kcal/100 ml, the range of caloric concentrations usually fed to infants (108). If the osmolality of a 67 kcal/100 ml formula is known, the osmolality of a formula with a calorie density of 44–90 kcal/100 ml can be calculated assuming a direct proportion between osmolality and caloric density.

The osmolality of a given formula increases with increasing caloric content. There is no meaningful difference in the osmolalities of the commonly used ready-to-feed formulas that provide 67 kcal/100 ml. The osmolalities of reconstituted concentrated products when diluted to provide 67 kcal/100 ml are not considerably different from the osmolalities of the corresponding ready-to-feed products.

Directions for diluting concentrated formulas must be followed exactly to prevent hyperosmolal states, such as diarrhea and dehydration, that could harm the infant. The soy-protein formulas have lower osmolalities than the milk-based formulas because of their different carbohydrate sources (milk-based formulas usually contain lactose; soy-protein formulas contain sucrose or corn syrup solids).

Infant formulas with 67 kcal/100 ml or 80 kcal/100 ml that are routinely used to feed preterm infants have osmolalities similar to breast milk and pose no apparent increased risk of GI mucosal injury (109). Products for preterm infants (Similac 24 LBW, Enfamil Preterm Formula, Similac Special Care, Similac 60/40) have osmolalities less than 400 mOsm/kg.

Renal Solute Load

Renal solute load is related to the protein (urea) and mineral content of the formula. It represents the total amount of water-soluble substances that must be removed from the body by the kidneys. The renal solute loads of human milk and cow milk are approximately 79 and 228 mOsm/l, respectively (103). Renal solute loads can be calculated from the sum of milliequivalents for sodium, potassium, and chloride plus 4 mOsm of urea per gram of protein in a liter of formula or milk (108).

Nutritional Requirements

Growth Patterns

The human body exhibits characteristic growth and development patterns that are basically the same in all individuals. Growth denotes change in size caused by an increase in the number and size of cells of the body. Development indicates maturation of organs and systems, acquisition of physical skills (gross motor and fine motor), and formation of psychologic competence (adjustment to stress, acceptance of responsibility, and achievement of creative expression) (110).

Growth rate is usually more meaningful than actual size. Height and weight data must be considered in relation to the variability within a certain age. Individual data on height and weight should be expressed in terms of percentiles for a particular age.

Serial measurements of growth are significant indicators of health and should be used to determine the pattern of growth in comparison with normal standards. Parents can use growth charts (available from pediatricians or pharmacists) that depict percentile data

for height, weight, and head circumference to maintain an accurate personal record of their child's growth.

Several general characteristics can be used to ascertain a sense of normal growth. Birth length is doubled by approximately age 4 and tripled by age 13 years. The average child grows approximately 20 inches in the 9 months prior to birth, 10 inches in the first year of life, 5 inches in the second, 3 to 4 inches in the third, and approximately 2 to 3 inches per year until the growth spurt of puberty occurs (110).

The average birth weight is 7 lb, 5 oz (3,333 g) (105). Within the first few days of life, up to 10% of the birth weight may be lost because of passage of meconium and urine, less intake, and physiologic edema. By 10 days of age, the infant has regained the birth weight. Infants gain weight in an average increment of approximately 1 oz (30 g) per day during the early months of life. The average weight in pounds of infants 3–12 months of age is equal to the age in months plus 11. Birth weight is doubled between the fourth and fifth months of age, tripled by the end of the first year, and quadrupled by the end of the second year. Between 2 and 9 years of age, the annual increment in weight averages about 5 lb per year.

Body weight is probably the best index of nutrition and growth. In response to nutritional deficiency, changes in height occur more slowly than changes in weight. Because of the rapid growth rate in infants during the first year of life, the nutritional adequacy of an infant's diet is very important.

Nutritional Standards

Three basic nutritional principles should be considered in evaluating an infant formula:

- It should contain adequate, but not excessive, amounts of all essential nutrients.

- It should be readily digestible.

- It should have a reasonable distribution of calories derived from protein, fat, and carbohydrate.

Metabolic studies suggest that 7–16% of the calories should be derived from protein, 30–55% from fat, and 35–65% from carbohydrates (111). Human milk provides 7%, 55%, and 38% of its calories from protein, fat, and carbohydrates, respectively. Corresponding figures for whole cow milk are 20%, 50%, and 30%.

The Food and Nutrition Board of the National Research Council established RDAs that meet the needs of most healthy infants (Table 4) (112). (See Chapter 17, *Nutritional Supplement, Mineral, and Vitamin Products.*) The FDA has established standards for formulas prepared for healthy infants from birth (2.5–4.0 kg) to 12 months of age (8–10 kg) (Table 3) (98).

TABLE 4 Recommended daily allowances of nutrients for full-term infants	
Nutrient	**RDA (0–6 mo)**
ENERGY (kcal/kg/day)	108
PROTEIN (g)	13
ESSENTIAL FATTY ACIDS	
Linoleic acid (% of kcal)	2.7
VITAMINS	
Vitamin A (mcg)	375 [a]
Vitamin D (mcg)	7.5 [b]
Vitamin K (mcg)	5
Vitamin E (mg)	3 [d]
Vitamin C (mg)	30
Thiamine (mg)	0.3
Riboflavin (mg)	0.4
Vitamin B_6 (mg)	0.3
Vitamin B_{12} (mcg)	0.3
Niacin (mg)	
(mg equivalents) [e]	5
Folate (mcg)	25
Pantothenic acid (mg)	2 [c]
Biotin (mcg)	10 [c]
MINERALS	
Calcium (mg)	400
Phosphorus (mg)	300
Magnesium (mg)	40
Iron (mg)	6
Iodine (mcg)	40
Zinc (mg)	5
Copper (mg)	0.4–0.6 [c]
Manganese (mg)	0.3–0.6 [c]
Sodium (mg)	120 [c]
Potassium (mg)	500 [c]
Chloride (mg)	180 [c]
Fluoride (mg)	0.1–0.5 [c]
Chromium (mcg)	10-40 [c]
Selenium (mcg)	10
Molybdenum (mcg)	15–30 [c]

[a] Retinol equivalents. One retinol equivalent equals 3.33 IU of vitamin A activity from retinol.

[b] Cholecalciferol. Ten mcg of cholecalciferol equals 400 IU of vitamin D.

[c] Estimated safe and adequate daily dietary intakes. Because there is less information on which to base allowances, some figures are provided as ranges of recommended intakes.

[d] T.E., alpha-tocopherol equivalents; 1 mg of δ-α-tocopherol equals 1α-T.E. The activity of α-tocopherol is 1.49 IU/mg.

[e] One niacin equivalent equals 1 mg of niacin or 60 mg of dietary tryptophan.

From Food and Nutrition Board, National Research Council, National Academy of Sciences, "Recommended Dietary Allowances," 10th ed., National Academy Press, Washington, D.C., 1989, p. 284.

Usual dilutions of unmodified cow milk and evaporated milk do not meet the standards (105). Iron deficiency and hyperphosphatemia are common complications in infants fed only cow milk. Furthermore, vitamin C supplementation is necessary in infants receiving only cow milk. The high protein and mineral content of cow milk increases the risk of hypernatremia and dehydration whenever diarrhea or other conditions increase the demand for water.

Nutritional requirements are best expressed as the amounts needed per 100 kcal of total food intake (Table 3), rather than amounts per kilogram of body weight. This system provides a convenient way to reflect the interaction of one nutrient with another, such as vitamin A and unsaturated fatty acids, and it can be applied to formulas of different caloric concentrations (24).

Protein The RDA for protein is 2.2 g/kg from birth to 6 months and 2.0 g/kg from 6 months to 1 year. Infant formulas must provide a minimum of 1.8 g/100 kcal of protein having a PER (protein efficiency ratio, derived from the weight gain per gram of protein fed) at least 100% that of casein (11). These recommendations apply primarily to formulas; human milk contains 1.5 g/100 kcal and is adequate for the full-term infant. If a formula has a PER less than 100% of casein, the amount of protein per 100 kcal should be increased to compensate for the lower PER. A formula that used a protein with a PER 75% that of casein would have to provide at least 2.4 g of protein per 100 kcal (1.8/0.75). Soy-protein infant formulas have a PER which is 70% of casein. No protein with a PER less than 70% that of casein can be used (105).

It is important that the protein source in formulas contain the amino acids isoleucine, leucine, lysine, methionine, phenylalanine, threonine, tryptophan, and valine. There is evidence that histidine also is necessary for the newborn (113). Both human and cow milk contain histidine in quantities exceeding estimated infant requirements of 26 mg/100 kcal and may be fed to newborns until the body begins to synthesize histidine (2–3 months after birth). Tyrosine and cystine, as well as histidine, may be needed in the first weeks of life for the preterm infant (113, 114).

Taurine is an amino acid found in abundant quantities in breast milk (115). This amino acid is not an energy source, nor is it used for protein synthesis. It is considered a conditionally essential nutrient. Conditional deficiency of taurine can result in adverse changes: retinal dysfunction; slow development of auditory brain stem-evoked response in preterm infants; and poor fat absorption in preterm infants and in children with cystic fibrosis. These conditions can be improved with taurine supplementation. Taurine provides a major nutritional role as a protector of cell membranes by attenuating toxic substances (e.g., oxidants, secondary bile acids, excess retinoids) and by acting as an osmoregulator (116). Taurine is now added to many infant formulas as a measure of prudence to provide the same margin of physiologic safety as found in human milk.

The protein in a formula may be derived from single or multiple sources and may be supplemented with L-amino acids or acceptable hydrolysates. Vegetable protein sources are acceptable. Hydrolysates are enzymatic breakdown products with reduced antigenicity. As measured by weight gain in rats, casein hydrolysates are 100% as efficient as casein (117).

Through electrodialysis or ion exchange, the amount of casein in cow milk may be altered to produce a whey-to-casein ratio resembling that of human milk (60:40, respectively). A new formula (Carnation Good Start H.A.) has been formulated with whey hydrolysate; therefore, this formula contains no casein.

Most commercial milk-based formulas use 2.3 g of protein per 100 kcal. Soy-protein formulas contain 2.7 g/100 kcal because of the lower PER of 70% of casein. The minimum quantity and quality of required protein (1.8 g/100 kcal) in commercial milk-based infant formulas promote growth and development equal to that of human milk (118, 119).

Levels of protein higher than 1.8 g/100 kcal in milk-based formulas do not confer any advantage when given to normal infants. LBW infants may have a higher protein requirement; however, too much protein may overwhelm the ability of the infant's kidney to excrete the nitrogenous waste. The FDA states that the maximum protein level should be 4.5 g/100 kcal (98).

Fat and Essential Fatty Acids Most commercial formulas have replaced butterfat with vegetable oil to obtain an easily digestible fat source. Vegetable oil digestibility is increased with a high proportion of unsaturated fatty acids and decreased with a large amount of long-chain fatty acids. Medium-chain fatty acids (8–10 carbons) that are unsaturated are absorbed most easily. Corn and soy oils are easier to digest than coconut oil, which has a relatively high number of long-chain saturated fatty acids. In some commercial formulas, about 85% of the fat is absorbed—the absorption rate of fat in human milk (120).

The FDA recommends a minimum of 3.3 g/100 kcal (30% of calories) and a maximum of 6.0 g/100 kcal of fat (93). A normal caloric distribution in an infant's diet derives 30–55% of the calories from dietary fat. Diets that supply more calories from fat may cause ketosis because ketone bodies are formed from excess free fatty acids (111). Fat is an efficient calorie source because of its high caloric density. It contains 9 kcal/g compared with 4 kcal/g for protein and carbohydrate. Fat in a diet increases palatability and enhances the absorption of lipid-soluble vitamins.

Fat also supplies the essential fatty acids not synthesized in the human body (linoleic and alpha-linoleic acids). The AAP recommends linoleic acid intakes of 300 mg/100 kcal or 2.7% of total calories (105). Linoleic acid and its derivatives, including arachidonic acid, enable optimum caloric intake use and proper skin composition (121). Linoleic acid represents the bulk of polyunsaturated fatty acids in infant formulas.

Carbohydrates Although there is no RDA for carbohydrates, an infant efficiently uses 35–65% of the total calories from a carbohydrate source (122). Most carbohydrate sources used in infant formulas are monosaccharides or disaccharides that are digested and absorbed more readily by the infant than polysaccharides (starch). Lactose is the major source of carbohydrates in milk-based formulas. It is hydrolyzed by acids and the enzyme lactase to glucose and galactose. Disaccharide hydrolysis in a newborn may be incomplete, and because lactase activity develops late in fetal life, infants born during the seventh or eighth month of gestation may be unable to hydrolyze the same amount of lactose that a full-term infant can generally metabolize. Preterm infants are especially prone to lactose intolerance (manifested by diarrhea, abdominal distention, and cramping) during the first weeks after birth (123).

Secondary lactase deficiency is a temporary reduction in intestinal lactase caused by gastroenteritis or malnutrition. Congenital lactase deficiency is a rare type of milk intolerance that results from an inborn error of metabolism (124). Low levels of lactase in the GI tract of these infants and in LBW infants can lead to an inability to metabolize the quantity of lactose found in breast milk or infant formulas. This is a temporary adverse reaction that most infants outgrow. Formulas with nutrient sources other than cow milk may be used when milk intolerance or hypersensitivities are suspected.

Other carbohydrates such as dextrins (tapioca), corn syrup solids, and sucrose are used in infant formulas when milk protein is to be avoided by allergic infants. Formulas that contain sucrose and corn syrup as carbohydrate sources have a sweeter taste than those that contain lactose.

Carbohydrates provide 40–50% of the calories in most infant formulas. If more than 50% of the calories are derived from carbohydrates, an infant's ability to hydrolyze disaccharides may be compromised; however, some special formulas (Pregestimil and Nutramigen) contain higher concentrations that are easily digestible because they are not high in dissaccharides. The increased passage of disaccharides in the feces creates an osmotic gradient in the colon that results in a loose, characteristically acidic, watery stool. The excess lactose in the ileocecal region is fermented by bacteria to produce carbon dioxide and lactic acid. The process irritates the colon and may cause diarrhea, resulting in dehydration and electrolyte imbalance. (See Chapter 13, *Antidiarrheal and Other Gastrointestinal Products.*)

Vitamins Vitamins are added to infant formulas to meet the following nutritional requirements established by the FDA (99).

Niacin Infant formulas should contain a minimum of 250 mcg of niacin per 100 kcal. One mg of niacin is derived from each 60 mg of dietary tryptophan, an amino acid precursor of niacin. The recommended protein level in formulas provides adequate tryptophan to supply the proper amount of niacin equivalents.

Pyridoxine The minimum recommendation for pyridoxine (vitamin B_6) is 35 mcg/100 kcal. Higher protein intake from certain formulas necessitates an increased amount of pyridoxine. At least 15 mcg of pyridoxine for each gram of protein is recommended.

Vitamin A The minimum recommendation for vitamin A is 250 IU/100 kcal. Most infant formulas contain about 300 IU/100 kcal.

Vitamin D A maximum of 100 IU/100 kcal of vitamin D (670 IU per liter of formula) is recommended. Most formulas contain 60 IU/100 kcal (400 IU/l) of vitamin D. The recommended higher levels of vitamin D more closely meet the requirements for LBW infants whose intake is low or whose absorption of fat is poor.

Vitamin K Milk-based formulas contain sufficient quantities of vitamin K to prevent deficiency. Furthermore, the bacterial flora generated by milk-based formulas in healthy infants contributes to an adequate supply of vitamin K. A level of 4 mcg/100 kcal of vitamin K in milk-based formulas is sufficient for normal infants. However, most milk-based formulas contain 8 mcg/100 kcal of vitamin K. Soy-protein and other milk-substitute formulas should contain a minimum of 8 mcg/100 kcal of vitamin K.

Vitamin E Vitamin E (tocopherol) is necessary to protect cell membranes from oxidative damage. Full-term infants require 0.7 IU/100 kcal of vitamin E and at least 1.0 IU of vitamin E per gram of linoleic acid. Tocopherol levels should be proportional to the oxidants (iron) and oxidizable substrate [polyunsaturated fatty acids (PUFA)] in the diet. Most infant formulas are supplemented to provide 0.8 IU/g of polyunsaturated fatty acids because cow milk is low in linoleic acid (contains only 20–25% as much as human milk) (125). About 2 IU/100 kcal (13 IU/l) of vitamin E is present in most infant formulas.

Preterm infants are born with disproportionately small body stores of vitamin E compared with those of full-term infants (126). Hemolytic anemia was reported in preterm infants who received formulas with high levels of polyunsaturated fatty acids supplemented with iron (127–130). The additional oxidant activity of iron (8 mg/kg or more) increases the risk for hemolytic anemia in preterm infants who have insufficient tocopherol levels.

To avoid hemolytic anemia in preterm infants, the ratio of vitamin E intake to polyunsaturated fatty acids (E/PUFA) should not be less than 0.4 (131) where E/PUFA is:

$$\frac{\text{Vitamin E per unit volume (IU of alpha-tocopherol)}}{\text{PUFA per unit volume (grams of linoleic and arachidonic acid)}}$$

Biotin, Choline, and Inositol The nutritional requirements for biotin, choline, and inositol are not known. The recommendation for biotin is a minimum of 1.5 mcg/100 kcal, which approximates that amount commonly used in milk-based formulas. Milk-based formulas provide choline in concentrations of 7 mg/100 kcal (or 45 mg of choline per liter). Inositol is present in most formulas in a concentration of 4 mg/100 kcal or 26 mg/l.

Electrolytes The levels of electrolytes and minerals in infant formulas should be near the minimal levels because maximal levels (based on cow milk) constitute a significant solute load. However, the amount of residue from cow milk can be excreted in isotonic urine (300 mOsm/l) by the normal healthy infant (132).

The amount of sodium, potassium, and chloride in infant formulas is based on the minimum levels found in human milk. The levels of sodium, potassium, and chloride in infant formulas should be 6–17, 14–34, and 11–29 mEq/l, respectively. These minimal levels can be expressed as sodium (20 mg/100 kcal), potassium (80 mg/100 kcal), and chloride (55 mg/100 kcal). These levels are sufficient to meet the growth needs of the infant and leave little residual for excretion in urine (98).

The ratio of sodium to potassium should not exceed 1.0:1, and the ratio of sodium plus potassium to chloride should be at least 1.5:1. These ratios in infant formulas are similar to those in human milk (sodium to potassium, 0.5:1; sodium plus potassium to chloride, 2.0:1).

Human milk provides about 1.0 mEq of sodium per kilogram per day. The amount of sodium in the diet of infants under 6 months of age was reduced from approximately 3 to 2 mEq/kg per day by the reduction or elimination of salt from strained and junior foods (133). This level of sodium intake has not been proven harmful. There is no evidence that intakes up to 9 mEq/kg per day predispose infants to subsequent hypertension (134).

The concentration of chloride should not be lower than 11 mEq/l. Maintenance of adequate chloride levels in infant formulations is necessary to prevent hypochloremic, hypokalemic alkalosis (133, 135).

Minerals The FDA has established the following minimum and maximum levels for minerals for normal full-term infants (98).

Calcium and Phosphorus The ratio of calcium to phosphorus should be no less than 1.0:1 and no more than 2.0:1. A ratio of calcium to phosphorus within this range ensures an alkaline ash diet similar to that of human milk. A high phosphate intake has been associated with hypocalcemic tetany (136, 137).

For preterm and LBW infants, additional calcium and phosphorus in special formulas are necessary for normal bone growth and mineralization (138). Formulas designed for full-term infants are deficient in calcium and phosphorus relative to the needs of the LBW or preterm infant.

Iron The FDA recommends that all formulas contain at least the lower level of iron found in human milk (0.5 mg/100 kcal or 1 mg/l) and that the iron be in a bioavailable form. Infants at risk for iron deficiency should be given formulas supplemented with 1 to 2 mg/100 kcal (approximately 6–12 mg/l) of iron. Most iron-supplemented formulas contain 12 or 13 mg/l.

Iron availability may be less in formulas with higher protein concentration; iron deficiency is more common in infants fed 2.4% protein (3.6 g/100 kcal) than in those fed 1.5% (2.3 g/100 kcal) in a milk formula (139).

Formulas for LBW infants contain 3 mg or less of iron per liter. Conservative levels of iron are used because iron supplementation in LBW infants up to 2 months of age has been associated with an increased risk of hemolytic anemia because of iron's interference with vitamin E metabolism. These formulas do not supply enough iron to meet the normal intrauterine accretion rate of iron. The decision to determine if or when iron supplementation is needed for infants fed LBW formulas should be made by the physician.

Zinc, Copper, and Manganese The minimum requirement for zinc by the infant is approximately 0.5 mg/100 kcal (3.2 mg of zinc per liter). Less zinc may be absorbed in soy-protein formulas because of the presence of phytate in soy protein (140). The minimum level for copper is 69 mcg/100 kcal. The requirement for manganese is unknown. The FDA recommends 5 mcg/100 kcal of manganese in the formula.

VITAMIN AND MINERAL SUPPLEMENTS

There is no evidence that vitamin and mineral supplementation is necessary for the full-term, formula-fed infant. Likewise, the normal, breast-fed infant of a well-nourished mother has not been shown conclusively to need any specific vitamin and mineral supplement (141). However, iron and vitamin D supplementation has been recommended for full-term, breast-fed infants (141).

Vitamin and mineral supplementation may be needed in preterm and LBW infants and in those whose mothers are inadequately nourished. These infants and those with other nutritional deficiencies, malabsorptive and other chronic diseases, rare vitamin dependency conditions, inborn errors of vitamin or mineral metabolism, or deficiencies related to the intake of drugs will need vitamin and mineral supplementation directed by a physician (141). Table 5 gives guidelines for supplementation.

Breast-Fed Infants

The antirachitic properties of the small amount of vitamin D in breast milk may be adequate for the normal, full-term infant of a well-nourished mother. Vitamin D is recommended as a supplement for breast-fed infants as a protective measure against rickets in case the mother's diet is deficient in vitamin D (142). However, rickets caused by vitamin D deficiency has been reported in relatively few breast-fed infants in the United States. In nearly every instance in these reports, the infant was dark skinned and had been protected from exposure to sunlight (143). The presence of fortified vitamin D foods in the diet of most mothers reduces the risk of diets deficient in vitamin D. If the mother's nourishment has been inadequate in vitamin D, supplements of 400 IU of vitamin D may be administered (144). Mothers should be encouraged to maintain a balanced diet and drink 5 to 6 glasses (8 oz per glass) of milk a day while breast-feeding to minimize vitamin and mineral deficiency (145).

Breast-fed preterm infants may demonstrate rickets (146, 147). This may be caused by the low phosphorus content (150 mg/l) of breast milk, in contrast to approximately 450–500 mg/l of phosphorus in milk-based and soy-protein infant formulas (144, 146). This condition is correctable with calcium, phosphate, and vitamin D supplementation in special preterm infant formulations.

Vitamin A deficiency rarely occurs in breast-fed infants; therefore, vitamin A may be omitted from supplements designed to provide vitamin D for infants.

Vitamin B_{12} deficiency has been reported in breast-fed infants of strict vegetarian mothers (148). This deficiency is relatively rare in the United States. A malnourished nursing mother and her infant should receive multivitamin supplements to prevent megaloblastic anemia.

TABLE 5 Guidelines for use of supplements in healthy infants

Infant	Multivitamin/ multimineral	Vitamin D	Vitamin E [a]	Folate	Iron [b]
TERM INFANTS					
Breast-fed	0	±	0	0	±
Formula-fed	0	0	0	0	0
PRETERM INFANTS					
Breast-fed [c]	+	+	±	±	+
Formula-fed [c]	+	+	±	±	+
OLDER INFANTS (>6 mo)					
Normal	0	0	0	0	±
High-risk [d]	+	0	0	0	±

Symbols indicate: +, a supplement is usually indicated; ±, it is possibly or sometimes indicated; 0, it is not usually indicated. Vitamin K for newborn infants and fluoride in areas where there is insufficient fluoride in the water are not shown.

[a] Vitamin E should be in a form that is well absorbed by small, preterm infants. If this form of vitamin E is present in formulas, it need not be given separately to formula-fed infants. Infants fed breast milk are less susceptible to vitamin E deficiency.

[b] Iron-fortified formula and/or infant cereal is a more convenient and reliable source of iron than a supplement.

[c] Multivitamin supplements (plus added folate) are needed primarily when calorie intake is below approximately 300 kcal a day or when the infant weighs 2.5 kg; vitamin D should be supplied at least until 6 months of age in breast-fed infants. Iron should be started by 2 months of age.

[d] Multivitamin–multimineral preparations including iron are preferred to use of iron alone.

Excerpted from *Pediatrics*, *66*, 1017 (1980).

Iron concentration in human milk averages about 0.3 mg/l (143). If an infant consumed a liter a day of human milk and absorbed 50% of the iron, the amount of iron absorbed would be 0.15 mg per day. This is less than the estimated requirement of absorbed iron of 0.6–0.7 mg per day (149). Iron deficiency is relatively common in children 12–36 months of age (150). An estimated prevalence of iron deficiency in this population is approximately 9% for all children and 20% for children below the poverty index ratio of the U.S. Department of Agriculture (151). Iron deficiency in children 12–36 months of age is probably caused by inadequate iron intake between birth and 1 year.

Breast-fed infants rarely develop iron deficiency anemia before 4–6 months of age because neonatal stores of iron are adequate. After 6 months of age, the neonatal stores may be depleted; consequently, in normal, breast-fed full-term infants, the addition of an iron supplement (2 mg/kg of ferrous sulfate) is desirable to supply adequate amounts of iron. An iron supplement is preferable to iron-fortified cereal. Cereal diluted with milk or formula provides about 7 mg of elemental iron per 100-g serving. A 4% absorption of iron from a 50-g serving of cereal yields only 0.14 mg or 20% of the requirement (143).

The most bioavailable iron preparations are chemically reactive and react in the presence of oxygen with polyunsaturated fatty acids in cereals. This reaction causes discoloration and oxidative rancidity (152). The bioavailability of the electrolyte iron powder used to fortify infant cereals has not been studied in human subjects. Because cereals contain potent inhibitors of iron absorption, cereal is a questionable source of iron (143).

Iron-fortified wet-packed cereal and fruit combinations marketed in jars offer no exposure of the iron sulfate to oxygen until the jar is opened; therefore, oxidative rancidity is not a problem. These products may be better sources of dietary iron supplementation than dry cereals (143). Products that require reconstitution of dehydrated flakes with water to produce instant baby foods appear to be nutritionally equivalent to the wet-packed foods (143).

The CON/AAP states that fluoride supplements can be initiated shortly after birth in breast-fed infants (138, 153, 154). This approach is based on the possibility that dental caries may be further reduced in breast-fed infants who consume little or no water. This issue is not significant when breast-feeding is maintained for only a few months. However, if an infant is breast-fed exclusively for more than 6 months, fluoride administration is warranted. Totally breast-fed infants in a nonfluoridated area should receive fluoride supplementation from birth; this regimen gives additional protection to the calcifying primary teeth with little risk of fluorosis in the permanent dentition (155, 156). In fluoridated areas where infants receive a diet supplemented by additional food and water, fluoride supplementation is not advised to avoid the risk of mild enamel fluorosis (151, 152). Table 6 contains the supplemental fluoride dosage schedule recommended by the CON/AAP.

Formula-Fed Full-Term Infants

Consumption of adequate amounts of an iron-fortified commercial milk-based formula by a full-term infant excludes the need for vitamin and mineral supplementation in the first 6 months of life (25). An iron-fortified formula is preferred because of the concern for adequate iron stores for growing infants. Studies have shown that infants fed iron-fortified formulas do not demonstrate a difference in stool consistency, fussiness, colic, or regurgitation compared to infants fed formulas not fortified with iron (157, 158).

Infants between 7 and 12 months of age who were fed formula and solid foods attained a more balanced intake of nutrients than infants fed cow milk and solid foods (159). The table foods fed to infants on cow milk were high in protein, sodium, and potassium and low in iron and linoleic acid. Thus, the overall diet of the infants fed cow milk and supplemental food had iron intakes of 52% of the RDA.

TABLE 6 Supplemental fluoride dosage schedule (mg per day)			
	Concentration of fluoride in drinking water (ppm) [a]		
Age	**<0.3**	**0.3–0.7**	**>0.7**
2 weeks–2 years	0.25	0	0
2–3 years	0.50	0.25	0
3–16 years [b]	1.00	0.50	0

[a] 2.2 mg sodium fluoride contains 1 mg of fluoride.

[b] The American Academy of Pediatrics recommends 16 as the termination age. The American Dental Association recommends 13 as the termination age.

Excerpted from *Am. J. Dis. Child.*, *134*, 866 (1980).

Vitamin and mineral supplements are not needed if an older infant (over 6 months of age) is receiving a diet of formula, mixed feedings, and increased amounts of table food. Cow milk, if used at this time, should be fortified with vitamin D. The diet should include an adequate source of vitamin C. A multivitamin with minerals may be needed in infants at special nutritional risk because of intercurrent illness or poverty.

If powdered or concentrated formula is used, fluoride supplements should be administered to infants only if the community water contains less than 0.3 ppm of fluoride. Ready-to-use formulas are manufactured with defluoridated water and contain less than 0.3 ppm of fluoride; therefore, recommendations for fluoride supplements for infants fed ready-to-use formulas are similar to those for breast-fed infants (154).

Preterm Infants

Preterm infants, either breast-fed or formula-fed, need vitamin and mineral supplementation. Their nutrient needs are proportionately greater than those of full-term infants because of their more rapid growth rate and because of decreased intestinal absorption (138, 160). Before these infants consume about 300 kcal/day or reach a body weight of 2.5 kg, a multivitamin supplement should be administered to provide the equivalent of the RDAs for full-term infants.

The multivitamin should include vitamin E in a form well absorbed by preterm infants, such as *d*-alpha-tocopheryl polyethylene glycol 1000 succinate (161). Because of conflicting data from clinical studies, it seems prudent to routinely monitor the supplementation of vitamin E for preterm infants and to maintain serum concentration of vitamin E between 1 and 3 mg/dl (162).

Folic acid deficiency has been reported in preterm infants (163). The instability of folic acid excludes its incorporation into liquid multivitamin and mineral preparations. Folate can be added to a multivitamin preparation in a concentration to provide a daily dose of 0.1 mg (U.S. RDA). The shelf life should be limited to 1 month, and the label should read "shake well" (147).

Iron supplementation should be withheld until the infant is several weeks old to minimize the possibility of hemolytic anemia in infants with insufficient vitamin E absorption. Iron is required at a dosage of 2 mg/kg per day starting by at least 2 months of age because neonatal iron stores may become depleted earlier than in full-term infants. Iron-fortified formulas supply sufficient iron to prevent iron deficiency in preterm infants (147).

Calcium, phosphorus, and vitamin D supplementation in preterm infant formulas is necessary to ensure adequate bone mineralization and thereby prevent osteopenia and rickets (164). The prevention of severe bone disease in preterm infants appears to depend on both high oral intakes of calcium and phosphorus and at least 500 IU of vitamin D per day (138). There is no evidence that administration of the active vitamin D metabolites, 25-dihydroxyvitamin D or 1,25-dihydroxy-vitamin D, to LBW or preterm infants is necessary (140). (See Chapter 17, *Nutritional Supplement, Mineral, and Vitamin Products.*)

TYPES AND USES OF INFANT FORMULAS

Commercial Formulas for Full-Term Infants

Although breast milk is the preferred feeding for full-term newborns, several studies indicate that growth rates of formula-fed infants are essentially similar to those of breast-fed infants (165–167). Infant formula is intended to replace or supplement breast milk when breast-feeding is not possible or is insufficient, or when mothers choose not to breast-feed.

Infant formulas are available in three types of formulations: liquid concentrate, liquid ready-to-feed, and powder. Ready-to-feed formula should be shaken before opening and does not need to be warmed before feeding to an infant. The liquid concentrate should be diluted with an equal amount of cooled, previously boiled water to supply 20 kcal per fluid ounce. The powder formulation requires adding 1 scoop (packed, level) to 2 fluid ounces of water to provide the appropriate caloric concentration of 20 kcal per fluid ounce.

Commercial formulas for full-term infants are basically milk-based or milk-based with added whey protein. These formulas must meet the minimum requirements for the various nutrients per 100 kcal as required by the FDA. Similac is an example of a milk-based formula. Enfamil, SMA, and Similac 60/40 are milk-based formulas with added whey protein.

Milk-Based Formulas

A milk-based formula is prepared from nonfat cow milk, vegetable oils, and added carbohydrate (lactose).

The added carbohydrate is necessary because the ratio of carbohydrates to protein in nonfat milk solids from cow milk is less than is desirable for infant formulas. Protein provides about 10% of calories, and fat furnishes 48–50% of calories (168). The most widely used vegetable oils are corn, coconut, safflower, and soy. Replacement of the butterfat allows better fat absorption and reduces the sour odor of vomitus from infants. Vitamins and minerals are added in accordance with the guidelines established by the FDA. Milk-based formulas are either iron fortified (1.8 mg/100 kcal) or low in iron (0.16 mg/100 kcal).

Milk-Based with Added Whey Protein

When whey is added in the proper amounts to nonfat cow milk, the ratio of whey proteins to casein can be made to approximate that of human milk. This ratio of 60% of protein from whey and 40% from casein differs considerably from cow milk, in which casein accounts for approximately 80% of the protein and whey for about 20% (169). Minerals can be removed from whey by electrodialysis or ion-exchange processes, and then minerals can be added to the formula to approximate the mineral content of human milk. Formulas containing partially demineralized whey proteins are not nutritionally superior to milk-based formulas for the normal infant. The high nutritional quality and relatively low renal solute load of these formulas are assets in the therapeutic management of ill infants (169).

Therapeutic Formulas

The use of therapeutic formulas is limited to disorders and conditions where the infant is being treated on an individual basis by medical specialists (Table 7). This type of limited use requires that nutrition specialists have flexibility in selecting sole-source nutrient formulations that meet the specific nutritional needs of the infant.

Soy-Protein Formulas

These formulas contain methionine-fortified isolated soy protein. Originally, soy flour was used as the source of protein, but these formulas produced loose, malodorous stools that stained diapers and frequently resulted in excoriation of the diaper area (170). Soy-isolate formulas are white, nearly odorless, and rarely cause loose or malodorous stools (170). Vegetable oils

TABLE 7 Indication for use of therapeutic infant formulas

Problem in infancy	Suggested formula	Rationale
Allergy to cow milk protein or soy protein	Protein hydrolysate (Nutramigen, Pregestimil, or Alimentum)	Protein sensitivity
Biliary atresia	Portagen	Impaired interluminal digestion and absorption of long-chain fats
Cardiac disease	SMA, Enfamil	Low electrolyte content
Celiac disease	Pregestimil, followed by soy formula, followed by cow milk formula	Advance to more complete formula as intestinal epithelium returns to normal
Constipation	Routine formula, increase sugar	Mild laxative effect
Cystic Fibrosis	Portagen	Impaired interluminal digestion and absorption of long-chain fats
Diarrhea—chronic nonspecific —intractable	Routine formula, Pregestimil, Alimentum	Appropriate distribution of calories; impaired digestion of intact protein, long-chain fats, and dissacharides
Failure to thrive (when intestinal damage is suspected)	Pregestimil, Alimentum	Advance to more complete formula as intestinal epithelium returns to normal
Gastroesophagal reflux	Routine formula	Thicken with 1 tbsp cereal per ounce of formula; small frequent feeds
Homocystinuria	Low Methoionine Diet Powder	Low content of methionine
Hepatitis—without failure —with failure	Routine formula Portagen	Impaired interluminal digestion and absorption of long-chain fats
Lactose intolerance	Soy-based formula	Impaired digestion and utilization of lactose
Maple syrup urine disease	MSUD Diet Powder	Low content of leucine, isoleucine, valine
Necrotizing enterocolitis (resection)	Pregestimil (when feeding is resumed)	Impaired digestion
Phenylketonuria	Lofenalac	Low content of phenylalanine
Renal insufficiency	Similac PM 60/40	Low phosphate content, low renal solute load

Modified from J. Guyboski and W. A. Walker, "Gastrointestinal Problems in the Infant," 2nd ed., W. B. Saunders, Philadelphia, Pa., 1983.

provide the fat content, and corn syrup solids and/or sucrose supply the carbohydrate in these formulas. Vitamin K is added to provide a level of 15 mcg/100 kcal. Other vitamins, taurine, and carnitine (necessary for optimal oxidation of fatty acids) are also added to soy-protein formulas. Carnitine supplementation to soy-protein formulas is necessary because of its low concentrations in foods of plant origin as compared to foods of animal origin (171).

About 15% of infants fed formulas receive soy-protein formulas, such as Isomil, Nursoy, Prosobee, and Soyalac (166). These formulas differ in amounts of ingredients, in the carbohydrate source, and in constitu-

ents for the fat source. For example, Isomil and Prosobee contain 105 mg/100 kcal and 94 mg/100 kcal of calcium, respectively. These differences in amount of ingredients are slight and do not constitute a significant variation among these formulas. The fat source in Soyalac is soy oil; Isomil contains soy oil and coconut oil; and Nursoy contains oleic oils (safflower) in addition to soy and coconut oils.

The carbohydrate source is an important factor in the use of these products. Isomil and Soyalac contain corn syrup solids and sucrose; Nursoy and I-Soyalac contain only sucrose; and ProSobee contains only corn syrup solids. Consequently, infants sensitive to corn and corn products who cannot tolerate a milk-based formula may benefit from the corn-free soy-protein formulas. Caution is advised, however, when the type of formulation is selected. The powder formulation of Nursoy contains corn syrup solids; the liquid concentrate and ready-to-feed formulations do not.

Soy-protein formulas are lactose free and, therefore, can be used in infants with primary lactase deficiency (e.g., galactosemia) or in secondary lactose intolerance resulting from enteric infection or other causes of mucosal damage (172–174). Resumption of a cow milk formula is generally possible 2 weeks after cessation of diarrhea.

RCF (Ross Carbohydrate Free) soy-protein formula does not contain a carbohydrate source. This infant formula may be used in the dietary management of infants unable to tolerate the type or amount of carbohydrates in milk or other infant formulas. A physician may select a carbohydrate source (sucrose, dextrose, or glucose polymers) that may be added before feeding. RCF is for use only under medical supervision.

Some infants with gastroenteritis develop intolerance to lactose and sucrose because of secondary lactase and sucrase deficiency. Isomil SF and ProSobee contain corn syrup solids (hydrolyzed corn starch, a glucose polymer) as the only carbohydrate source and can be used in this situation.

Food allergy may occur in infants because the immature digestive and metabolic processes may not be completely effective in converting dietary proteins into nonantigenic amino acids. The incidence of cow milk allergy in the first 2 years of life is estimated to be 0.4–7.5% of the infant population (175). The higher figure agrees with skin-testing data (176). An overall incidence of 0.5–1% was proposed and seems to be a median figure for infancy (177). The diagnosis of cow milk allergy is defined as symptomatology involving the respiratory tract, skin, or GI tract that disappears when cow milk is removed from the diet and reappears on two separate challenges when cow milk is given during a symptom-free period (175).

Soy-protein formulas are promoted for use in the management of infants who are allergic to milk or who are suspected of having milk allergy. However, the CON/AAP has recommended that protein-hydrolysate formulas rather than soy-protein formulas be used in infants with documented clinical allergy to cow milk and/or soy protein. (174). This recommendation is based on the concern that infants with severe manifestations of cow milk allergy, such as severe diarrhea, vomiting, laryngeal edema, wheezing, or urticaria, have intestinal mucosal damage sufficient enough to expose them to higher concentrations of foreign protein in soy-protein formulas. Such infants have demonstrated severe allergic manifestations when fed soy-protein formulas (178, 179).

In infants with a family history of atopy who have not shown clinical manifestations of allergy, a soy-protein formula may be used with caution (171). These infants should be monitored closely for allergy to soy protein.

The soy-protein source in these formulas provides an alternative for vegetarian families in which animal-protein formulas are not desired.

Soy-protein formula should not be used for the routine feeding of preterm and LBW infants and in the routine management of colic. Soy-protein formulas are also not recommended for infants with cystic fibrosis because of the presence of typsin inhibitors in the formula. This contributes to a risk of hypoproteinemia because infants on these formulas will lose substantial amounts of nitrogen through their stools (180).

Casein Hydrolysate-Based Formulas

Casein hydrolysate-based formulas are effective in the nutritional management of infants with a diversity of severe GI abnormalities where intolerance to enteral feeding and the malabsorption of standard forms of protein, fat, and carbohydrate are common. Indications for these formulas include severe or intractable diarrhea, severe food allergies, sensitivity to intact protein, transition from parenteral feeding to normal diet, disaccharidase deficiency, intestinal resection, malabsorption caused by dysfunction, steatorrhea from fat malabsorption, cystic fibrosis, protein-calorie malabsorption, and severe protein-calorie malnutrition.

Use of these formulas in infants for prophylaxis of allergy remains controversial. Many studies indicate that prolonged breast-feeding or extended use of hypoallergenic formulas and delayed introduction of solid foods help prevent allergic disease in infancy, but many other studies challenge these findings (181). To date, the effectiveness of dietary and environmental regimens in the prevention of allergic disease have not been conclusively proven by prospective studies. Infants with documented clinical allergic symptoms to cow milk may benefit from a protein hydrolysate formula because approximately 10% of these infants also react to soy protein (182).

Evidence from studies currently demonstrates that hydrolysate formulas are not needed in the routine management of colic. In selected instances, improvement occurs in infants with colic when cow milk or soy protein is eliminated, and a hydrolysate formula is introduced (183). However, in the vast majority of infants, symptoms of colic will persist. In cases where improvement is noted, it is difficult to definitively attribute this to a change in infant formula. The CON/AAP states that there is no evidence to support the use of hydrolysate formulas for the treatment of colic, sleeplessness, and irritability (183). These are common symptoms in infants but infrequently occur as a result of immune-mediated reaction to cow milk protein.

The extensively hydrolyzed casein protein makes these formulas less palatable. However, infants usually accept the feedings satisfactorily. If the formula should be rejected when first offered, it may be tried again after a few hours.

These products are designed to provide a sole source of nutrition for infants up to 4–6 months of age and provide a primary source of nutrition through 12 months of age when indicated. Extended use of hydrolysate formulas as a sole source of diet after 6 months of age should be monitored by physicians on a case-by-case basis (184).

Nutramigen, Pregestimil, Portagen, and Alimentum are infant formulas with enzymatic hydrolysates of casein as the protein source. Enzymatic hydrolysates of casein demonstrate nonantigenic polypeptides with <1,200 molecular weight (185); therefore, these hypoallergenic formulas can be fed to infants sensitive to intact proteins of milk or other foods. The casein hydrolysate formulas differ from other formulas in that alpha-amino nitrogen is supplied by enzymatically hydrolyzed, charcoal-treated casein rather than whole protein. These formulas are supplemented with three amino acids—L-cystine, L-tyrosine, and L-tryptophan—because of a reduction in these levels during charcoal treatment.

The carbohydrate sources in these formulas include one or more of the following: corn syrup solids, sucrose, modified corn starch, or modified tapioca starch. Nutramigen contains corn syrup solids and modified corn starch; Pregestimil, corn syrup solids and tapioca starch; Alimentum, sucrose and modified tapioca starch; and, Portagen, corn syrup solids and sucrose.

Glucose polymers in corn syrup solids or modified corn starch are particularly useful in infants with malabsorption disorders who are frequently intolerant to lactose, sucrose, and glucose. Glucose polymers are more easily digested and tolerated by infants whose capacity to handle lactose and sucrose may be impaired (186, 187). In addition, glucose polymers are a low osmolar form of carbohydrate and contribute very little to the total osmolar load in the diet. This is an advantage in infants with intestinal disorders who cannot tolerate the greater osmolar load of disaccharide or glucose-containing elemental diets.

The fat sources are MCTs and corn oil in Pregestimil and Portagen. Nutramigen contains only corn oil, and Alimentum contains safflower and soy oil (sources of linoleic acid) in addition to MCTs. MCTs do not require emulsification with bile and are more easily hydrolyzed than long-chain fats. The shorter chain fatty acids in MCTs are directly absorbed into the portal system. In addition, MCTs enhance the absorption of long-chain triglycerides. Formulas containing 40% of the fat as MCTs have been shown to relieve steatorrhea, promote weight gain, and improve calcium absorption in LBW infants (188–190).

Pregestimil Pregestimil has been proven effective in infants with massive bowel resection (short-gut syndrome), severe diarrhea, protein-calorie malnutrition, GI milk and soy-protein intolerance, transition from intravenous alimentation, GI immaturity, and cystic fibrosis. Pregestimil is also effective in the intractable diarrhea syndrome of infancy (IDSI). Pregestimil is not recommended for routine use in highly stressed LBW infants because of the increased risk of developing GI complications (184).

Nutramigen Nutramigen is effective for infants with severe diarrhea and GI disturbances, and in those allergic or intolerant to intact proteins of cow milk and other foods. In cases of galactosemia, a relatively rare disorder resulting from a deficiency of either galactose 1-phosphate uridyl transferase or galactokinase, it is necessary to eliminate dietary lactose, so that the body may convert glucose only to the amount of galactose it requires. Galactosemia is characterized in untreated infants by failure to thrive, liver disease, cataracts, and mental retardation. Infants with galactosemia can be fed formulas without lactose or sucrose: Nutramigen, Pregestimil, Alimentum, ProSobee.

Portagen Portagen contains MCTs as 87% of the fat source (compared with 40% MCTs in Pregestimil and 48% MCTs in Alimentum). Portagen also contains higher levels of vitamins, both lipid soluble vitamins (A, D, and E) and water-soluble vitamins (B_2, B_6, B_{12}, niacin). Higher levels of MCTs and vitamins in Portagen compensate for an impaired digestion of conventional food fat and absorption of the resulting long-chain fatty acids. Portagen has been effective in infants with pancreatic insufficiency (cystic fibrosis), bile acid deficiency, intestinal resection, and lymphatic anomalies. It can be used, according to physician recommendation, as a sole constituent of the diet or as a beverage to be consumed with each meal. Portagen should not be used in cases of abetalipoproteinemia (faulty chylomicron formation).

Alimentum The hydrolyzed casein in Alimentum is a blend of medium- and long-chain triglycerides. The addition of long-chain triglycerides (less extensively hydrolyzed peptide fraction) improves the palatability of the formulation but increases the allergenic potential in infants with cow milk allergy (191). Alimentum contains two carbohydrates (sucrose and modified tapioca starch) in lower concentrations than other hydrolysate formulas. These carbohydrates are digested and absorbed by separate mechanisms (principally, glucoamylase and sucrase-alpha-dextrinase). Noncompetitive digestive and absorptive mechanisms can produce a greater carbohydrate absorption than when either carbohydrate is fed alone (192). This infant formula is used in infants with protein sensitivity, pancreatic insufficiency (cystic fibrosis), and intractable diarrhea.

Whey Hydrolysate-Based Formulas

Casein hydrolysate has been used for many years for infants with defects in protein digestion and adverse reactions to intact cow milk protein. Recently, heat-treated whey proteins have been used as the protein source for an infant formula (Carnation Good Start H.A.) for similar purposes. Enzymatic hydrolysates of whey contain some peptides with >2,000 molecular weight, which increases the antigenicity of the product (181). In addition, the most prevalent allergic protein in cow milk is beta-lactoglobulin, the major protein found in the whey protein fraction (193, 194). Therefore, this type of formula should not be used in infants with documented allergy to cow milk protein. The effectiveness of whey-hydrolysate formula in infants with GI intolerance to cow milk, but who are not allergic, suggests that it may be an acceptable alternative to milk-based and soy-protein formulas. This product is promoted as having a pleasant taste, smell, and appearance, which may encourage better acceptance by mothers and infants than casein-hydrolysate formulas that have a noticeable difference in appearance and taste compared to milk-based and soy-protein formulas.

Low Sodium Formulas

Infants with congestive heart failure, hypertension, nephrosis, and acute nephritis often require a formula with an increased caloric concentration because they may tire in feeding before a volume with sufficient nutrients has been consumed. In addition, an excessive renal load must be avoided.

Lonalac contains a very low amount of sodium (approximately 1 mEq/l or 47 mg/100 kcal). Prepared from casein, coconut oil, lactose, minerals, and vitamins, it provides a caloric distribution similar to that of WCM. This formula can be used only for a short time before sodium must be supplemented. The formula presents a relatively high renal solute load (slightly less than that of WCM), and caution is required because of the limited liquid volume intake that is characteristic of the seriously ill heart patient.

The relatively low renal solute load and adequate caloric intake of whey-adjusted milk formulas (SMA, Similac 60/40, Enfamil) permit their use in long-term management of infants who require sodium restriction.

Of these formulas, SMA contains the lowest amount of sodium (15 mg/100 ml; equivalent to breast milk sodium levels).

Low Phenylalanine Formula

Phenylketonuria, an inborn error of amino acid metabolism, is due to an inability to convert phenylalanine to tyrosine in the body. Phenylalanine accumulation alters brain development and leads to mental retardation. Phenylalanine restriction is the only indication for Lofenalac. Lofenalac contains an enzyme hydrolysate of casein with various amino acids, including a trace of phenylalanine. The formula is supplemented with L-methionine, L-tyrosine, and L-histidine. Lofenalac provides approximately 18 mg of phenylalanine per 100 kcal and is inadequate as a sole source of this amino acid (195). Therefore, phenylalanine must be supplied in monitored quantities to achieve serum phenylalanine levels within acceptable limits (2–10 mg/dl) (196). Formulas that have a predominance of whey protein, which has less phenylalanine in casein, can be used as supplementary sources of phenylalanine.

Excessive phenylalanine restriction (blood levels below 2 mg/dl) has resulted in retarded bone growth, vacuolization of bone marrow cells, megaloblastic anemia, hypoglycemia, and death (197). Lofenalac, like other therapeutic formulas, should be used only as directed and as indicated.

Low Methionine Formula

Low Methionine Diet Powder formula is used for the dietary management of infants with homocystinuria. Homocystinuria develops from a lack of cystathionine synthase, an enzyme necessary for the normal conversion of methionine to cysteine. An excess accumulation of methionine and cysteine results in mental retardation, ectopia lentis, fine fair hair, malar flush, thromboembolic episodes, scoliosis, long extremities, and arachnodactyly. Low Methionine Diet Powder is a soy-protein formula that contains sufficient methionine (39 mg/100 kcal) to adequately meet the nutritional requirements for growth of infants with homocystinuria (198).

Low Leucine, Isoleucine, Valine Formula

MSUD Diet Powder is a branched-chain amino acid-free formula for the dietary management of maple syrup urine disease. Maple syrup urine disease (MSUD) is a familial, cerebral, degenerative disorder caused by disturbances in the metabolism of leucine, isoleucine, and valine. The characteristic odor of the urine, skin, and perspiration is present as early as the fifth day of life. Unless this disorder is detected and treated within

TABLE 8 Concentration and dilution of formula concentrates*

Desired caloric concentration (cal/oz)	Liquid formula concentrate (oz)	Water (oz)
10	1	3
15	1.5	2.5
20	1	1
24	3	2
26–27	3	1.5
28–29	5	2
30	3	1
32	2	0.5

*Currently marketed formula concentrates that require only the addition of water are 40 cal/oz.

From W. A. Walker and K. M. Hendricks, "Manual of Pediatric Nutrition," W. B. Saunders, Philadelphia, Pa., 1985, p. 74.

recommend the use of unsterilized equipment and hot tap water to prepare formula. The Committee recommends that some method of sterilization (preferably the terminal heating method), with emphasis on the need for 25 minutes of active boiling and the necessity for clean equipment, be used before feeding milk mixtures to infants (218).

The commercially sterilized liquid formulas and bacteriologically safe powdered formulas may be prepared more conveniently in single bottles. A day's supply of bottles may be sterilized in advance, adding the formula at feeding time. This practice eliminates the need for refrigerating bottled formula and warming bottles before a feeding.

The terminal heating method may allow bacterial growth during storage if instructions are not followed or if bottles are not thoroughly cleaned of milk film (219).

Feeding the Infant

The newborn infant may want to be fed at intervals of 2 to 3 hours. The schedule is permissible, but it does not allow the mother very much rest, and the infant may consume only small amounts (15 ml) of formula at a time. The baby should be encouraged to lengthen the interval to 4 hours as soon as possible. Most infants readily adopt a 4-hour schedule by the time they are 3–4 weeks old, but some prefer a shorter interval for several months (220).

Babies vary considerably in the amount of formula desired. The amount given should be consistent with the RDA for caloric intake (Table 4). Some pediatricians prescribe more formula than babies probably will accept, relying on each baby's own appetite to limit intake. This method works well if the mother does not urge or force the infant to take more than is desired at any one feeding. If an infant finishes a bottle and still seems hungry, another bottle should be offered.

Complaints about an infant's rejection of a formula may be resolved in some cases by examining the specific feeding problem. Spitting up is often caused by improper burping, feeding a large amount too quickly, laying the infant face down too soon after feeding, or having excess mucus in the nasopharynx. During feeding, the infant should be held in a well-supported position at a 45° angle, preferably with the head nestled in the curve of the arm. Infants should be burped after every 30–45 ml of formula by gently patting and rubbing the back interchangeably. After feeding, the infant should be positioned on the abdomen (on the right side) to prevent regurgitation and aspiration of formula. Many infants are chronic spitters of formula. If they are growing and gaining weight, there is no need to be greatly concerned.

TABLE 9 Concentration and dilution of powdered infant formulas[a]

Desired caloric concentration (cal/oz)	Powdered formula concentrate (tbsp)	Water (oz)
10	1	4
15	3	8
20	1	2
24	3	5
28	7	10
30	3	4
32	4	5

[a] Powdered infant formulas are 40 cal/tbsp (level, packed). Because the powder displaces the water and makes the volume larger and the formulas more dilute, for large volumes of formula, water should be added to the powder to equal the volume expected. For example, to make 32 oz of formula at 24 cal/oz, mix 19 tbsp with enough water (29 oz) to equal 32 oz.

[b] 1 tbsp = 1 scoop

From W. A. Walker and K. M. Hendricks, "Manual of Pediatric Nutrition," W. B. Saunders, Philadelphia, Pa., 1985, p. 74.

TABLE 10 Formula preparation

Terminal heating	Aseptic	Single-bottle*
1. Rinse the bottle and nipple with cool water immediately after the feeding. Wash the day's supply of bottles, nipples, and caps with hot, soapy water and rinse well.	1. Rinse the bottle and nipple with cool water immediately after the feeding. Wash the day's supply of bottles, nipples, and caps with hot, soapy water and rinse well.	1. Rinse the bottle and nipple with cool water immediately after the feeding. Wash the day's supply of bottles, nipples, and caps with hot, soapy water and rinse well.
2. Rinse the outside of the formula can and shake the contents well. Open the can with a clean can opener, mix the formula with water, or water-carbohydrate solution if prescribed, and pour the solution into bottles. Attach the nipples and cover them loosely with caps.	2. Boil the bottles, nipples, caps, can opener, and mixing utensils for 5 minutes in a deep pan with enough water to cover each item. Remove the items with tongs, and place the bottles on a clean towel or rack.	2. For formulas that require water, pour into each bottle the amount of water needed to prepare the feeding. Attach the nipples and cover them loosely with caps. Place the bottles on a rack in a deep pan containing ∼5–8 cm of water. Bring water to boil, cover, and allow it to boil gently for 25 minutes. Remove the pan from the stove, allow it to cool, and tighten the caps and bottles. The bottles may be left inside the pan until they are needed.
3. Place the bottles on a rack in a deep pan containing ∼5–8 cm of water. Heat water to boiling, and allow it to boil gently for 25 minutes while covered before removing from the stove.	3. While the equipment is being cleaned, boil water in a covered saucepan or teakettle for 5 minutes (slightly more water than the prescribed amount should be used to allow for evaporation).	3. For formulas that need no water, boil the bottles, nipples, caps, and can opener for 5 minutes. Put the nipples and caps on the bottles with aseptic care.
4. After the sides of the pan have cooled enough to be touched comfortably, remove the lid and the formula bottles. (Leaving the pan covered for this period is recommended to prevent formation of milk film on bottles and clogging of nipples.) Store in refrigerator until used.	4. Remove the boiled water from the stove, allow it to cool, and measure the required amount.	4. At feeding time, remove the cap and nipple aseptically. Add the appropriate amount of formula and replace the nipple. With the powdered formula, replace the cap and shake the bottle vigorously to mix.
5. Warm the bottle of formula to the desired temperature before feeding the infant.	5. Rinse, shake the can well, add the commercially processed formula or evaporated milk and carbohydrate mixture to the boiled water, and stir with a clean spoon. (If bottled milk or other unsterilized milk is used, it should be boiled with the water. Evaporated milk, carbohydrate modifiers, and commercially processed formulas usually are not boiled.)	5. Feed the infant while formula is at room temperature.
	6. Pour the formula into bottles, and attach the nipples and caps with aseptic care. Store them in the refrigerator. Formula should be used within 24 hours.	
	7. Warm the bottle of formula to the desired temperature before feeding the infant.	

*For supplementing the diet of breast-fed infant or when traveling.

Adapted from ''Handbook of Infant Formulas,'' 6th ed., J. B. Roerig, Division of Pfizer, New York, N.Y., 1969, pp. 86, 88, and H. N. Silver, *Pediatrics*, *20*, 997 (1957).

PRODUCT SELECTION GUIDELINES

Pharmacists should be able to discuss with parents the advantages and disadvantages of breast-feeding versus formula-feeding for a full-term infant. The limitations of breast-feeding should be recognized, such as the presence of certain drugs in breast milk and genetic disorders in infants. Mothers who cannot or do not wish to breast-feed should be reassured that normal growth and development in their infants is possible without breast-feeding.

In recommending the type of infant formula and its method of preparation, the pharmacist should consider the parents' ability to follow directions, their attitudes and preferences, and the sanitary conditions and refrigeration facilities available. Instruction in cleaning techniques may include step-by-step emphasis on the importance of sanitary conditions. For example, the top of the infant formula container should be cleaned thoroughly before opening, either by rinsing the top with hot tap water or by dipping it in boiling water for about 14 seconds before it is opened. Partially used formula cans should be kept covered, placed in the refrigerator, and stored no longer than 48 hours.

For many parents, cost may be a critical factor in the selection of an infant formula. The concentrated formula preparations are less expensive than the ready-to-feed products; the price of powdered preparations ranges between the other two formulations. Convenience is also a consideration. The powder and concentrated liquid formulas require more manipulative functions in preparation and more attention to aseptic technique. A formula should be well tolerated by the infant, convenient to prepare for the parents, and within the family budget.

SUMMARY

Pharmacists can monitor the response of infants to formula by questioning the parents. Detailed information obtained from discussions with parents about the type and severity of symptoms the infant may be experiencing and complaints by the parents may help the pharmacist make appropriate recommendations: change in feeding procedures, use of a different type of formula, or referral to a physician.

Questions concerning vitamin and mineral supplementation for infants taking formulas or breast milk must be answered accurately and completely. Informa-

tion presented in this chapter and Chapter 17, *Nutritional Supplement, Mineral, and Vitamin Products*, can be useful in making proper recommendations for iron, fluoride, and multivitamin supplementation. Pharmacists can encourage the use of iron-fortified infant formulas to conform with the CON/AAP recommendations. The use of an iron-fortified formula in young infants does not increase the incidence or severity of GI symptoms compared to infants not receiving iron-fortified formulas (153, 154). The parents should be advised that the stools of an infant receiving a formula or supplement containing iron may be darker. Prescribed fluoride supplementation should be based on the knowledge of the amount of fluoride in the water of the community and the type of feedings (breast milk, formula, or table food).

Pharmacists should keep current with the nutritional recommendations proposed by the FDA and the CON/AAP. A thorough understanding of the nutritional requirements of infant formulas can assist pharmacists in allaying the concerns of parents. Compliance with recall announcements for deficient infant formulas is necessary to prevent possible adverse reactions in infants.

REFERENCES

1 T. E. Cone, Jr., "200 Years of Feeding Infants in America," Ross Laboratories, Columbus, Ohio, 1976, p. 93.

2 H. J. Gerstenberger et al., *Am. J. Dis. Child.*, *10*, 249 (1915).

3 G. A. Martinez and F. W. Krieger, *Pediatrics*, *76*, 1004 (1985).

4 G. E. Hendershot, *Pediatrics*, *74* (suppl. no. 4, pt. 2), 591 (1984).

5 M. Mobassaleh et al., *Pediatrics*, *75* (suppl.), 160 (1985).

6 J. B. Watkins, *Pediatrics*, *75* (suppl.), 151 (1985).

7 M. Hamosh et al., *Pediatrics*, *75* (suppl.), 146 (1985).

8 E. E. Ziegler et al., "Proceedings of the International Symposium on Dietary Lipids and Postnatal Development," Milan, Italy, 1972.

9 E. Delachaume-Salem and H. Sarles, *Biol. Gastroenterol.*, *2*, 135 (1970).

10 B. Borgstrom et al, *Am. J. Dis. Child.*, *99*, 338 (1960).

11 K. E. Bergmann et al., in " Infant Nutrition," 2nd ed., S. J. Fomon, Ed., W. B. Saunders, Philadelphia, Pa., 1974, pp. 245–265.

12 C. M. Edelman, Jr., et al., *J. Clin. Invest.*, *39*, 1062 (1960).

13 L. I. Kleinman, in "Perinatal Physiology," U. Staue, Ed., Plenum Medical, New York, N.Y., 1978, pp. 589–616.

14 P. L. Piper, in "Nutrition in Infancy and Childhood," 4th ed., Times Mirror/Mosby College Publishing, St. Louis, Mo., 1989, pp. 86–119.

15 N. C. R. Raiha, *Pediatrics*, *75* (suppl.), 136 (1985).

16 G. E. Gaull et al., *Pediatrics*, *75* (suppl.), 142 (1985).

17 G. Carpenter, *Science*, *210*, 198 (1980).

18 G. Gaull et al., in "Membranes in Growth and Development," F. Hoffman et al., Eds., Alan R. Liss, New York, N.Y., 1982, p. 349.

19 R. G. Jensen et al., *Am. J. Clin. Nutr.*, *31*, 990 (1978).

20 U. M. Saarinen et al., *J. Pediatr.*, *91*, 36 (1977).

21 P. E. Johnson and G. W. Evans, *Am. J. Clin. Nutr.*, *31*, 416 (1978).

22 J. K. Welsh and J. T. May, *J. Pediatr.*, *94*, 1 (1979).

23 H. M. Seidel, in "*Pediatrics*," 2nd ed., M. Ziai, Ed., Little, Brown and Co., Boston, Mass., 1975, p. 209.

24 C. W. Woodruff, *J. Am. Med. Assoc.*, *240*, 657 (1978).

25 "Pediatric Nutrition Handbook," 2nd ed., G. B. Forbes and C. W. Woodruff, Eds., American Academy of *Pediatrics*, Elk Grove Village, Ill., 1979, pp. 1–421.

26 S. J. Fomon, in "Infant Nutrition," 2nd ed., W. B. Saunders, Philadelphia, Pa., 1974, p. 80.

27 S. J. Fomon, in "Infant Nutrition," 2nd ed., W. B. Saunders, Philadelphia, Pa., 1974, p. 81.

28 S. J. Fomon, in "Infant Nutrition," 2nd ed., W. B. Saunders, Philadelphia, Pa., 1974, p. 255.

29 C. W. Woodruff and J. L. Clark, *Am. J. Dis. Child*, *124*, 18 (1972).

30 C. W. Woodruff et al., *Am. J. Dis Child.*, *124*, 26 (1972).

31 J. F. Wilson et al., *J. Pediatr.*, *84*, 335 (1974).

32 C. P. Anyon and K. G. Clarkson, *N.Z. Med J.*, *74*, 24 (1971).

33 E. J. Eastman and W. A. Walker, *Pediatrics*, *60*, 477 (1977).

34 C. W. Woodruff, *Nutr. Rev.*, *34*, 33 (1976).

35 Committee on Nutrition, American Academy of Pediatrics, *Pediatrics*, *72*, 253 (1983).

36 M. G. Kovar et al., *Pediatrics*, *74* (suppl.), 615 (1984).

37 P. Froggatt et al., *Br. J. Prev. Soc. Med.*, *25*, 119 (1971).

38 J. W. Gerrard et al., *Acta Paediatr. Scand.*, *234* (suppl.), 1 (1973).

39 M. A. Valdes-Dapena, *Pediatrics*, *66*, 597 (1980).

40 G. L. France et al., *Am. J. Dis. Child.*, *134*, 147 (1980).

41 L. Gothefors et al., *Acta Paediatr. Scand.*, *64*, 807 (1975).

42 L. J. Mata and J. J. Urrutia, *Ann. N.Y. Acad. Sci.*, *176*, 93 (1971).

43 J. K. Welsh and J. T. May, *J. Pediatr.*, *94*, 1 (1979).

44 D. M. Fergusson et al., *Aust. Pediatr. J.*, *14*, 254 (1978).

45 D. M. Fergusson et al., *Aust. Pediatr. J.*, *17*, 191 (1981).

46 G. L. France et al., *Am. J. Dis. Child.*, *134*, 147 (1980).

47 M. R. Forman et al., *Am. J. Epidemiol.*, *119*, 335 (1984).

48 O. Schaefer and D. W. Spudy, *Can. J. Public Health*, *73*, 304 (1982).

49 C. R. Pullan et al., *Br. Med. J.*, *281*, 1034 (1980).

50 M. Downham et al., *Br. Med. J.*, *2*, 274 (1976).

51 C. J. Watkins et al., *J. Epidemiol. Commun. Health*, *33*, 180 (1979).

52 R. K. Chandra, *Acta Paediatr. Scand.*, *68*, 691 (1979).

53 A. S. Cunningham, *J. Pediatr.*, *95*, 685 (1979).

54 U. M. Saarinen, *Acta Paediatr. Scand.*, *71*, 567 (1982).

55 R. Paine and R. J. Coble, *Am. J. Dis. Child.*, *136*, 36 (1982).

56 J. A. Hildes and O. Schaefer, *J. Hum. Evolution*, *2*, 241 (1973).

57 F. J. W. Timmermans and S. Gerson, *Can. Med. Assoc. J.*, *122*, 545 (1980).

58 D. W. Hide and B. M. Guyer, *Arch. Dis. Child.*, *56*, 172 (1981).

59 H. Blair, *Arch. Dis. Child.*, *58*, 48 (1983).

60 D. M. Fergusson et al., *Arch. Dis. Child.*, *58*, 48 (1983).

61 B. Taylor et al., *J. Epidemiol. Commun. Health*, *37*, 95 (1983).

62 U. M. Saarinen et al., *Lancet*, *2*, 163 (1979).

63 M. S. Kramer and B. Moroz, *J. Pediatr.*, *98*, 546 (1981).

64 J. H. Himes, *J. Am. Diet. Assoc.*, *75*, 122 (1979).

65 U. M. Saarinen and M. A. Siimes, *Acta Paediatr. Scand.*, *68*, 245 (1979).

66 S. J. Fomon, *Am. J. Clin. Nutr.*, *46*, 171 (1987).

67 A. Stekel, in "Iron Nutrition in Infancy and Childhood," A. Stekel, Ed., Raven Press, New York, N.Y., 1984, pp. 1–10.

68 E. Hertrampf et al., *Pediatrics*, *78*, 640 (1986).

69 Committee on Nutrition, American Academy of Pediatrics, *Pediatrics*, *66*, 1015 (1980).

70 R. L. Poland et al., *Pediatr. Res.*, *14*, 1328 (1980).

71 R. L. Poland, *J. Pediatr.*, *99*, 86 (1981).

72 F. W. Rosa, *Am. J. Public Health*, *66*, 791 (1976).

73 G. M. Stirrat, *Obstet. Gynecol. Surv.*, *31*, 1 (1976).

74 J. J. Gellen, *J. Biosoc. Sci.*, *4* (suppl.), 149 (1979).

75 Committee on Nutrition, American Academy of Pediatrics, *Pediatrics*, *65*, 657 (1980).

76 J. G. Chopra, *Am. J. Clin. Nutr.*, *25*, 1202 (1972).

77 S. Koetsawang et al., *Fertil. Steril.*, *23*, 24 (1972).

78 G. H. Miller and L. R. Hughes, *Obstet. Gynecol.*, *35*, 44 (1970).

79 N. E. Borglin and L. E. Sandholm, *Fertil. Steril.*, *22*, 39 (1971).

80 A. K. Gupta et al., *Indian J. Med. Res.*, *62*, 964 (1974).

81 M. Karim et al., *Br. Med. J.*, *1*, 200 (1971).

82 J. Zanartu et al., *Obstet. Gynecol.*, *47*, 174 (1976).

83 V. S. Toddywalla et al., *Am. J. Obstet.*, *127*, 245 (1977).

84 B. Lonnerdal et al., *Am. J. Clin. Nutr.*, *33*, 816 (1980).

85 S. Nilsson et al., *Contraception*, *17*, 131 (1978).

86 S. Nilsson et al., *Am. J. Obstet. Gynecol.*, *132*, 653 (1978).

87 G. H. Miller and L. R. Hughes, *Obstet. Gynecol.*, *35*, 44 (1970).

88 H. C. Atkinson et al., *Clin. Pharmacokin.*, *14*, 217 (1988).

89 J. T. Wilson et al., *Clin. Pharmacokin.*, *5*, 1 (1980).

90 American Academy of Pediatrics, *Pediatrics*, *72*, 375 (1983).

91 L. Beely, *Clin. Obstet. Gynecol.*, *8*, 291 (1981).

92 J. T. Wilson in "Drugs in Breast Milk," ADIS Press, New York, N.Y., 1981.

93 R. J. Roberts in "Drug Therapy in Infants: Principles and Clinical Experience," W. B. Saunders, Philadelphia, Pa., 1984, pp. 346–372.

94   Committee on Drugs, American Academy of Pediatrics, *Pediatrics*, 72, 357 (1983).

95   P. O. Anderson, *Drug Intell. Clin. Pharm.*, 11, 208 (1977).

96   J. Riordan and M. Riordan, *Am. J. Nurs.*, 3, 323 (1984).

97   Committee on Nutrition, American Academy of Pediatrics, *Pediatrics*, 40, 916 (1967).

98   *Federal Register*, 50, 45106 (1985).

99   *Federal Register*, 47, 17016 (1982).

100   *Federal Register*, 50, 1833 (1985).

101   S. A. Anderson et al., in "A Background Paper on Infant Formulas," Life Sciences Research Office, Federation of American Societies for Experimental Biology, Bethesda, Md., 1980, pp. 1–33.

102   *Federal Register*, 44, 40343 (1979).

103   Infant Formula Council, Manual Registration No. 5574, Atlanta, Ga., 1973.

104   Food and Nutrition Board, National Research Council, National Academy of Sciences, "Recommended Dietary Allowances," 10th ed., National Academy Press, Washington, D.C., 1989, p. 33.

105   T. A. Anderson et al., *Lab. Clin. Med.*, 79, 31 (1972).

106   R. W. Krouskop et al., *Pediatr. Res.*, 8, 838 (1974).

107   T. V. Santulli et al., *Pediatrics*, 55, 376 (1975).

108   R. M. Tomarelli, *J. Pediatr.*, 88, 454 (1976).

109   C. L. Paxson et al., *Am. J. Dis. Child.*, 131, 139 (1977).

110   H. K. Silver, in "Current Pediatric Diagnosis and Treatment," 7th ed., C. H. Kempe et al., Eds., Lance Medical Publications, Los Altos, Calif., 1982, pp. 8–38.

111   S. J. Fomon, "Infant Nutrition," Medcom, New York, N.Y., 1972, p. 31.

112   Food and Nutrition Board, National Research Council, National Academy of Sciences, "Recommended Dietary Allowances," 9th ed., National Academy Press, Washington, D.C., 1980.

113   S. J. Fomon, in "Infant Nutrition," Medcom, New York, N.Y., 1972. p. 121.

114   G. Gaull et al., *Pediatr. Res.*, 6, 538 (1972).

115   D. K. Rassin et al., *Early Hum. Devel.*, 2, 1 (1978).

116   G. E. Gaull, *Pediatrics*, 83, 433 (1989).

117   S. J. Fomon, in "Infant Nutrition," 2nd ed., W. B. Saunders, Philadelphia, Pa., 1974, p. 59.

118   S. J. Fomon et al., *Acta Paediatr. Scand.*, 62, 33 (1973).

119   *Lancet*, 2, 1359 (1974).

120   "First After Mother's Milk," Wyeth Laboratories, Philadelphia, Pa., 1971, p. 6.

121   H. Schlenk, *Fed. Proc.*, 31, 1430 (1972).

122   K. M. Hambidge, *Pediatr. Clin. N. Amer.*, 24, 95 (1977).

123   S. J. Fomon, in "Infant Nutrition," Medcom, New York, N.Y., 1972, p. 194.

124   A. Holzel et al., *Lancet*, 1, 1126 (1959).

125   D. L. Phelps, *Pediatrics*, 63, 933 (1829).

126   M. Y. Dju et al., *Etudes Neonatates*, 1, 49 (1952).

127   H. Hassan et al., *Am. J. Clin. Nutr.*, 19, 147 (1966).

128   F. A. Oski and L. A. Barness, *J. Pediatr.*, 70, 211 (1967).

129   J. H. Ritchie et al., *N. Engl. J. Med.*, 279, 1185 (1968).

130   S. S. Lo et al., *Arch. Dis. Child.*, 48, 360 (1973).

131   M. W. Dicks-Bushnell and K. C. Davis, *Am. J. Clin. Nutr.*, 20, 262 (1967).

132   S. J. Fomon, in "Infant Nutrition," 2nd ed., W. B. Saunders, Philadelphia, Pa., 1974, p. 253.

133   S. Roy III and B. S. Arant, Jr., *N. Engl. J. Med.*, 301, 615 (1979).

134   "Sodium Intake by Infants in the United States," Committee on Nutrition, American Academy of Pediatrics, Evanston, Ill., 1979.

135   E. H. Garin et al., *J. Pediatr.*, 95, 985 (1979).

136   Committee on Nutrition, American Academy of Pediatrics, *Pediatrics*, 62, 826 (1978).

137   A. Mizrahi et al., *N. Engl. J. Med.*, 278, 1163 (1968).

138   Committee on Nutrition, American Academy of Pediatrics, *Pediatrics*, 75, 976 (1985).

139   P. R. Dallman, *J. Pediatr.*, 85, 742 (1974).

140   A. S. Prasad and D. Oberleas, *Lancet*, 1, 463 (1974).

141   Committee on Nutrition, American Academy of Pediatrics, *Pediatrics*, 66, 1015 (1980).

142   S. J. Fomon et al., *Pediatrics*, 63, 52 (1979).

143   S. J. Fomon, *Am. J. Clin. Nutr.*, 46, 171 (1987).

144   S. Bachrach et al., *Pediatrics*, 64, 871 (1979).

145   M. D. Jensen et al., in "Maternity Care: The Nurse and the Family," C. V. Mosby, St. Louis, Mo., 1977, p. 183.

146   J. C. Rowe et al., *N. Engl. J. Med.*, 300, 293 (1979).

147   P. O'Connor, *Clin. Pediatr.*, 16, 361 (1977).

148   M. C. Higginbottom et al., *N. Engl. J. Med.*, 299, 317 (1978).

149   A. Stekel, in "Iron Nutrition in Infancy and Childhood," A. Stekel, Ed., Raven Press, New York, N.Y., 1984, pp. 1–10.

150   G. M. Owen et al., *Pediatrics*, 53, 597, (1974).

151   S. M. Pilch and F. R. Senti, "Assessment of the Iron Nutritional Status of the U.S. Population Based on Data Collected in the National Health and Nutrition Examination Survey (Second, 1976–80)," Life Sciences Research Office, Federation of American Societies for Experimental Biology, Bethesda, Md., 1984, pp. 1–86.

152   S. J. Fomon, *J. Pediatr.*, 110, 660 (1987).

153   Committee on Nutrition, American Academy of Pediatrics, *Pediatrics*, 63, 150 (1979).

154   Committee on Nutrition, American Academy of Pediatrics, *Pediatrics*, 77, 758 (1986).

155   W. S. Driscoll and H. S. Horowitz, *Am. Dent. Assoc. J.*, 96, 1050 (1978).

156   W. S. Driscoll and H. S. Horowitz, *Am. J. Dis. Child.*, 133, 683 (1979).

157   F. A. Oski, *Pediatrics*, 66, 168 (1980).

158   S. E. Nelson et al., *Pediatrics*, 81, 360 (1988).

159   M. B. Montalto et al., *Pediatrics*, 75, 343 (1985).

160   Committee on Nutrition, American Academy of Pediatrics, *Pediatrics*, 60, 519 (1977).

161   S. Gross and D. K. Melhorn, *J. Pediatr.*, 85, 753 (1974).

162   H. M. Hittner et al., *N. Engl. J. Med.*, 305, 1365 (1981).

163   D. Stevens et al., *Pediatrics*, 64, 333 (1979).

164   J. J. Steichen et al., *J. Pediatr.*, 96, 526 (1980).

165   S. J. Fomon et al., *Acta Paediatr. Scand.*, 223 (suppl.), 1 (1971).

166   R. L. Jackson et al., *Pediatrics*, 33, 642 (1964).

167 L. J. Filer, Jr., "Abstracts of the Nutrition Foundation, Inc.," Food and Nutrition Liaison Committee, 1980.

168 S. J. Fomon and L. J. Filer, Jr., in "Infant Nutrition," 2nd ed., W. B. Saunders, Philadelphia, Pa., 1974, p. 383.

169 S. J. Fomon and L. J. Filer, Jr., in "Infant Nutrition," 2nd ed., W. B. Saunders, Philadelphia, Pa., 1974, p. 384.

170 S. J. Fomon and L. J. Filer, Jr., in "Infant Nutrition," 2nd ed., W. B. Saunders, Philadelphia, Pa., 1974, p. 387.

171 Committee on Nutrition, American Academy of Pediatrics, *Pediatrics, 72,* 359 (1983).

172 R. D. Leake et al., *Am. J. Dis. Child., 127,* 372 (1974).

173 M. Gabr et al., *Clin. Ther., 2,* 271 (1979).

174 B. T. Naidoo et al., *J. Int. Med. Res., 9,* 232 (1981).

175 J. W. Gerrard et al., *Acta Paediatr. Scand., 234* (suppl.), 1 (1973).

176 A. S. Goldman et al., *Pediatrics, 32,* 425 (1963).

177 S. Freier and B. Kletter, *Clin. Pediatr., 9,* 449 (1970).

178 G. K. Powell, *J. Pediatr., 93,* 553 (1978).

179 S. A. Bock, *J. Pediatr., 107,* 676 (1985).

180 P. A. di Sant'Agnese, in "Current Pediatric Therapy," S. S. Gellia and B. M. Kagan, Eds., W. B. Saunders, Philadelphia, Pa., 1973, p. 234.

181 Committee on Nutrition, American Academy of Pediatrics, *Pediatrics, 83,* 1068 (1989).

182 S. A. Bock, *Am. J. Dis. Child., 134,* 973 (1980).

183 L. Lothe et al., *Pediatrics, 70,* 7 (1982).

184 "Pediatric Products Handbook," Mead Johnson Nutritionals, Evansville, Ind., 1988, p. 19.

185 R. J. Knights, in "Nutrition for Special Needs in Infancy," F. Lifshitz, Ed., Marcel Dekker, Inc., New York, N.Y., 1985, pp. 105–115.

186 H. L. Greene et al., *J. Pediatr., 87,* 695 (1975).

187 J. O. Sherman et al., *J. Pediatr., 86,* 518 (1975).

188 B. F. Andrews and V. Lorch, *Pediatr. Res., 8,* 104 (1974).

189 P. Tantibhedyangkul and S. A. Haskim, *Pediatrics, 64,* 537 (1978).

190 P. Tantibhedyangkul and S. A. Haskim, *Pediatrics, 55,* 359 (1975).

191 L. Businco et al., *Pediatr. Res., 22,* 222 (1987).

192 B. Kerener et al., *Pediatr. Res., 17,* 191A (1983).

193 S. J. Taylor et al., in "Food Allergy," R. E. Chandra, Ed., Nutrition Research Education Foundation, Newfoundland, Canada, 1987, pp. 21–44.

194 S. L. Bahna and D. C. Heiner, in "Allergies to Milk," Grune and Stratton, Inc., New York, N.Y., 1980, pp. 11–22.

195 S. J. Fomon, in "Infant Nutrition," 2nd ed., W. B. Saunders, Philadelphia, Pa., 1974, p. 391–392.

196 "Pediatric Products Handbook," Mead Johnson Nutritionals, Evansville, Ind., 1988, p. 22.

197 "Amino Acid Metabolism and Generic Variation," W. I. Nyhan, Ed., McGraw-Hill, New York, N.Y., 1967, pp. 6–63.

198 "Pediatric Products Handbook," Mead Johnson Nutritionals, Evansville, Ind., 1988, p. 28.

199 "Pediatric Products Handbook," Mead Johnson Nutritionals, Evansville, Ind., 1988, p. 26.

200 G. B. Forbes, *Pediatr. Res., 12,* 434 (1978).

201 J. P. Shenai et al., *Pediatrics, 66,* 233 (1980).

202 S. J. Gross, *N. Engl. J. Med., 308,* 237 (1983).

203 D. P. Davis, *Arch. Dis. Child., 52,* 296 (1977).

204 P. R. Dallman, *J. Pediatr., 85,* 742 (1974).

205 B. D. Schmitt, in "Pediatric Telephone Advice," Little, Brown and Co., Boston, Mass., 1980, p. 46.

206 M. H. Klaus et al., *Pediatrics, 46,* 187 (1970).

207 L. S. Book et al., *J. Pediatr., 87,* 602 (1975).

208 H. I. Goldman and F. Deposito, *Am. J. Dis. Child., 111,* 430 (1966).

209 W. F. J. Cuthbertson, *Am. J. Clin. Nutr., 29,* 559 (1976).

210 C. D. May et al., *Am. J. Dis. Child., 80,* 191 (1950).

211 W. A. Cochrane et al., *Pediatrics, 28,* 771 (1961).

212 D. B. Coursin, *J. Am. Med. Assoc., 154,* 406 (1954).

213 J. D. Hydovita, *N. Engl. J. Med., 262,* 351 (1960).

214 P. B. Kulkarni et al., *J. Pediatr., 96,* 249 (1980).

215 R. F. Cifuentes et al., *J. Pediatr., 96,* 252 (1980).

216 Y. Tanaka et al., *J. Pediatr., 96,* 255 (1980).

217 H. K. Silver, *Pediatrics, 20,* 993 (1957).

218 Committee on the Fetus and the Newborn, American Academy of Pediatrics, *Pediatrics, 28,* 674 (1961).

219 C. C. Fischer and M. A. Whitman, *J. Pediatr., 55,* 116 (1959).

220 S. J. Fomon, in "Infant Nutrition," 2nd ed., W. B. Saunders, Philadelphia, Pa., 1974, p. 80.

INFANT FORMULA PRODUCT TABLE

	Ready-To-Feed (Iron Fortified) Isomil & Isomil SF (Ross)	Iron Fortified Soyalac (Loma Linda)	Iron Fortified ProSobee (Mead Johnson)	Iron Fortified Nursoy (Wyeth-Ayerst)	Iron Fortified SMA (Wyeth-Ayerst)	Iron Fortified Alimentum (Ross)
NUTRIENTS PER 100 CAL						
Protein, g	2.66	3.1	3	3.1	2.2	2.75
Fat, g	5.46	5.5	5.3	5.3	5.3	5.54
Carbohydrate, g	10.1	10	10	10.2	10.6	10.2
Water, g	133	128	134	133	134	133
Linoleic acid, mg	1300	2810	1000	500	500	1600
VITAMINS						
A, IU	300	312	310	300	300	300
D, IU	60	62	62	60	60	60
E, IU	3	2.3	3.1	1.4	1.4	3
K, mcg	15	7.8	15.6	15	8	15
Thiamine, mcg	60	78	78	100	100	60
Riboflavin, mcg	90	94	94	150	150	90
Pyridoxine, mcg	60	70	62	62.5	62.5	60
B_{12}, mcg	0.45	0.31	0.31	0.3	0.2	0.45
Niacin, mcg	1350	1250	1250	750	750	1350
Folic acid, mcg	15	23	15.6	7.5	7.5	15
Pantothenic acid, mcg	750	469	470	450	315	750
Biotin, mcg	4.5	9.4	7.8	5.5	2.2	4.5
C, mg	9	12	8.1	8.5	8.5	9
Choline, mg	8	16	7.8	13	15	8
Inositol, mg	5	16	4.7	4.1	—	5
MINERALS						
Ca, mg	105	94	94	90	63	105
P, mg	75	55	74	63	42	75
Mg, mg	7.5	12	10.9	10	7	7.5
Fe, mg	1.8	1.9	1.88	1.7	1.8	1.8
Zn, mg	0.75	0.78	0.78	0.8	0.8	0.75
Mn, mcg	30	156	25	30	15	30
Cu, mcg	75	78	94	70	70	75
I, mcg	15	7.8	10.2	9	9	15
Na, mg	44	44	36	30	22	44
K, mg	108	117	122	105	83	118
Cl, mg	62	65	83	55.5	55.5	80

[a] For babies over 6 months of age eating solid foods.

Iron Fortified Pregestimil (Mead Johnson)	Iron Fortified Nutramigen (Mead Johnson)	Ready-To-Feed (non-iron fortified)		Ready-To-Feed (iron fortified)		Iron-Fortified Good Start H.A. (Carnation)	Iron Fortified Good Nature[a] (Carnation)
		Similac (Ross)	Enfamil (Mead Johnson)	Similac (Ross)	Enfamil (Mead Johnson)		
2.8	2.8	2.22	2.2	2.22	2.2	2.4	3
4.1	3.9	5.37	5.6	5.37	5.6	5.1	3.9
13.4	13.4	10.7	10.3	10.7	10.3	11	13.2
127	134	133	134	133	134	135	134
1360	2000	1300	1100	1300	1100	450	700
310	310	300	310	300	310	300	250
62	62	60	62	60	62	60	65
2.3	3.1	3	3.1	3	3.1	1.2	0.8
15.6	15.6	8	8.6	8	8.6	8.2	8.1
78	78	100	78	100	78	60	80
94	94	150	156	150	156	135	96
62	62	60	62	60	62	75	66
0.31	0.31	0.25	0.23	0.25	0.23	0.22	0.32
1250	1250	1050	1250	1050	1250	750	1280
15.6	15.6	15	15.6	15	15.6	9	16
470	470	450	470	450	470	450	480
7.8	7.8	4.4	2.3	4.4	2.3	2.2	1.5
8.1	8.1	9	8.1	9	8.1	8	8
13.3	13.3	16	15.6	16	15.6	12	—
4.7	4.7	4.7	4.7	4.7	4.7	6.1	—
94	94	75	69	75	69	64	135
62	62	58	47	58	47	36	90
10.9	10.9	6	7.8	6	7.8	6.7	8.4
1.88	1.88	0.22	0.16	1.8	0.16	1.5	1.9
0.62	0.78	0.75	0.78	0.75	0.78	0.75	0.63
31	31	5	15.6	5	15.6	7	7
94	94	90	94	90	94	80	76
7	7	15	10.2	15	10.2	8	5.7
47	47	28	27	28	27	24	39
109	109	108	108	108	108	98	135
86	86	66	62	66	62	59	90

Glenn D. Appelt

19

WEIGHT CONTROL PRODUCTS

*Q*uestions to ask in patient/consumer counseling

What are your age, height, and weight?

How long have you had a weight problem?

How much overweight do you think you are?

Is there a family history of obesity? Does either of your parents have a weight problem?

Do you tend to eat excessively when you are anxious, nervous, or tired?

Have you consulted a physician about the problem?

Are you following a diet?

What diet preparations have you used previously? Were they effective?

What efforts have you made to lose weight? For example, do you belong to a self-help group, such as Weight Watchers?

Do you have a regular exercise program? Does your physician recommend that you exercise?

Are you being treated for any chronic disease, such as hypertension, diabetes, thyroid condition, or heart disease?

What medications are you currently taking?

Obesity is the pathologic accumulation of fat exceeding that needed for optimal body functioning (1). From a practical viewpoint, obesity may be defined as the physical state in which body weight, in relation to height, exceeds the ideal weight by 20%, according to Metropolitan Life Insurance data (Table 1) (2). Although the term "obese" often is associated with "overweight," the terms are not interchangeable. Athletes, for example, may be overweight but not obese. Measurement of skinfold thickness has been suggested as a practical means of determining the extent of obesity (1). Initially, the triceps skinfold, as measured by calipers, was reported to be the most representative of body fat (3). However, an expanded measuring system has been advocated, using four sites: biceps, triceps, subcapsular, and supraileac (4, 5). Attempts have been made to measure subcutaneous fat thickness by X-rays (6), but this technique is less convenient than skinfold measurement with little compensating advantage. Ultrasound measures have been employed to estimate body fat (7), although circumference measurements using calibrated fiberglass tape may provide a better estimation of body fat (8). The measurement of fatness by Quetelet's rule has been described and analyzed (9, 10). This body mass index is given by $QI = W/H^2$, where W is body weight in kilograms and H is height in meters.

Body circumferences have also been used to estimate body fat (11, 12), and the waist-to-thigh ratio has been reported to be an appropriate index for upper and central body fat distribution, especially in women

(13). The fat distribution after puberty is characteristically different in males and females. Women tend to store fat in the breasts, hips, and thighs (gynecoid distribution), whereas men tend to accumulate fat in the abdomen (android distribution). However, some women have a relatively central (or android) fat distribution, while some men exhibit a predominantly peripheral (or gynecoid) fat distribution. An android fat distribution may be more strongly associated with atherosclerosis, diabetes mellitus, and gouty arthritis than a similar amount of fat in a gynecoid distribution (9). Current interest extends to determining the proportion of abdominal fat that is subcutaneous or within the peritoneal cavity (14, 15) because growing evidence indicates that the metabolic complications of obesity may be related to the amount of intra-abdominal fat rather than subcutaneous fat located in the abdominal wall. Thus, it appears that the distribution of fat, rather than the total amount of fat, is an important factor in the metabolic effects of obesity.

Daily caloric allowances for persons with moderate physical activity may vary with age and sex (16). Values for average males (weight, 70 kg or 154 lb; height, 1.78 m or 5′10″) in a temperate climate range from 3,200 cal at 25 years of age to 2,550 cal at 65 years of age. Corresponding figures for average females (weight, 58 kg or 128 lb; height, 1.63 m or 5′4″) are 2,300 and 1,800 cal. The values for women increase slightly during pregnancy (300 cal) and significantly during lactation (1,000 cal).

It takes 3,500 excess calories to result in 0.454 kg (1 lb) of body fat. Most obesity cases involve overeating, particularly of carbohydrates or fats. The calories ingested beyond those necessary for normal energy requirements usually are deposited and stored as fat. Because the lack of food is rarely a problem in the United States, Americans must decide how much and what type of food to consume. Apparently, many make unwise choices, because obesity is a common American affliction. Obesity is estimated to occur in 24–45% of Americans over 30 years of age (17, 18). In children, the incidence is reported to be from 2 to 15% (17).

TABLE 1	Desirable weights for men and women, according to height and frame, ages 25 and over		
	Weight in pounds (in indoor clothing)		
Height (in shoes)*	**Small frame**	**Medium frame**	**Large frame**
MEN			
5′ 2″	112–120	118–129	126–141
3″	115–123	121–133	129–144
4″	118–126	124–136	132–148
5″	121–129	127–139	135–152
6″	124–133	130–143	138–156
7″	128–137	134–147	142–161
8″	132–141	138–152	147–166
9″	136–145	142–156	151–170
10″	140–150	146–160	155–174
11″	144–154	150–165	159–179
6′ 0″	148–158	154–170	164–184
1″	152–162	158–175	168–189
2″	156–167	162–180	173–194
3″	160–171	167–185	178–199
4″	164–175	172–190	182–204
WOMEN			
4′10″	92– 98	96–107	104–119
11″	94–101	98–110	106–122
5′ 0″	96–104	101–113	109–125
1″	99–107	104–116	112–128
2″	102–110	107–119	115–131
3″	105–113	110–122	118–134
4″	108–116	113–126	121–138
5″	111–119	116–130	125–142
6″	114–123	120–135	129–146
7″	118–127	124–139	133–150
8″	122–131	128–143	137–154
9″	126–135	132–147	141–158
10″	130–140	136–151	145–163
11″	134–144	140–155	149–168
6′ 0″	138–148	144–159	153–173

*1-inch heels for men and 2-inch heels for women.

Prepared by and reprinted with permission from the Metropolitan Life Insurance Company. Derived primarily from data of the *Build and Blood Pressure Study*, Society of Actuaries, 1959.

CLINICAL CONSIDERATIONS

Obesity is a subject of intense study. Many factors enter into metabolic equilibrium. Appetite control is only part of the answer. Psychologic components may contribute to or cause overeating, leading to obesity. Often self-therapy groups may help in treating the cause; the use of pharmacologic agents tends to treat only the symptoms. In addition, caloric expenditure by physical activity could promote the maintenance of a nonobese state in the motivated individual. However, it must be emphasized that excessive eating (caloric intake) is the major cause of obesity.

Etiology of Obesity

The question of why individuals ingest more calories than they expend is complex. The answer may be related to physiologic, genetic, environmental, or psychologic factors. Endocrine disorders, such as hypothyroidism or Cushing's syndrome, apparently are rarely involved in obesity. Obesity may result from an anatomical or biochemical lesion in the brain's feeding centers, although this hypothesis has not been proven in humans (19). Another theory suggests that the obese person has a deficiency of mitochondrial alpha-glycerol phosphate dehydrogenase, an enzyme responsible for alpha-glycerophosphate oxidation. This deficiency results in an increased availability of this substrate for triglyceride synthesis (20). One hypothesis suggests that prostaglandins are involved in the development of obesity through an effect on lipogenesis (21). Overproduction of prostaglandins in adipose cells may result in an increase in fatty tissue.

Some researchers believe that thin and obese people differ in the degree of thermogenesis after food ingestion (22). Overeating in nonobese subjects causes increased heat production, which tends to dissipate the excess calories. In obese subjects, the dissipation of thermal energy is less pronounced, resulting in fat storage. Although animal models of obesity have been shown to have a defective thermogenic component (23, 24), the evidence for this metabolic defect in human obesity is largely circumstantial (25). Certain studies, however, indicate that human subjects of the same height, weight, sex, and occupation maintain weight on a twofold range of energy intake (26, 27). Additionally, some individuals gain fat more easily than lean counterparts (28, 29). A subnormal thermogenic response to food has been reported in the obese (30–34) and in the postobese (35, 36). Although these studies may be criticized on the basis that reductions in diet-induced thermogenesis (DIT) may not be a cause but rather a result of the obesity and/or metabolic adaptation to a low caloric intake, the concept of a defective DIT in the etiology of obesity remains provocative. The thermogenesis theory was expanded to include a specialized form of fat tissue (brown fat), which participates in thermogenesis. The exact role of brown fat is unclear, but it appears to favor increased triglyceride hydrolysis (37).

Animal studies have indicated that sympathetic denervation of brown fat results in an increase in body fat in lean animals (37). Additionally, an increase in norepinephrine turnover in brown fat during elevated DIT (38), as well as the ability of norepinephrine to stimulate activity of brown adipose tissue (39), further implicates the sympathetic nervous system in obesity. Several reports present evidence that in humans the thermogenic response to food plays an important role in the relationship of the sympathetic nervous system to brown fat (35, 40–46).

A biochemical basis for obesity involving sodium–potassium adenosine triphosphatase (ATPase) has been suggested (47–50). Red blood cells in obese people were noted to have lower levels of sodium–potassium ATPase compared with individuals of normal weight. This enzyme facilitates the sodium–potassium pump process in body cells, which could result in caloric expenditure (47). In other words, obese individuals with reduced sodium–potassium ATPase activity are more likely to add fat because they burn fewer calories than nonobese individuals. Some investigators have disputed the relationship between obesity and sodium–potassium ATPase activity (51, 52), and other researchers have provided evidence for the genetic determination of obesity (53, 54).

The correlation of a primitive "hibernation response" with human obesity has been proposed (55). Adaptive reactions preparing the body for an impending shortage may be predominant in the obese individual. Although humans do not hibernate, an "endomorphic system," representing a relic of the human evolutionary past, may be operant and initiate the overeating typical of the obese person. It is suggested that this "hunger reaction" may be initiated by the beta-endorphins.

One belief holds that obese people sleep more than thin people. The connection that exists between metabolism and sleep may be related to obesity (56). Obesity has been correlated with the frequency of an ultraradian brain rhythm (non-REM and REM sleep). This observation lends credence to the proposal that the amount of sleep decreases in obese people when they lose weight (57). It has been observed that there is an increase in the amount of sleep time when anorectic patients gain weight (58).

Another hypothesis suggests that excess fat cells during infancy may predispose the individual to obesity later in life (59). Obese patients not only have larger than normal fat cells but also have an increased number of these cells. Apparently, as people lose weight on a low-calorie diet, the size of each fat cell decreases, but the total number of fat cells remains the same; when people return to increased weight levels, the fat cells regain their original size. Obesity in children may result from the addition of new fat cells; "adult onset obesity" may represent an expansion of fat cells already present (2). Previous experiments suggest that the earlier the onset of obesity, the greater the number of fat cells (60). After the age of 20, obesity is caused almost exclusively by the expansion of existent cells. Accordingly, an overweight child or adolescent may be more susceptible to obesity as an adult.

A child who has one obese parent has a 40% chance of being obese; if both parents are obese, the chance of obesity increases to 80% (61). These data suggest a direct genetic component, and although it has not been proven in human obesity, animal studies indicate this relationship (62). In experimental animals, genetic transmission of obesity is associated with modified organ size and composition (63, 64). Human data suggest fundamental relationships between body build and obesity (65, 66). Studies revealed that obese women differed from nonobese women in morphologic characteristics other than the degree of adiposity. Obese women were more endomorphic than nonobese women. Abdomen mass overshadowed thoracic bulk, all regions were notable for their softness and roundness, and the hands and feet were relatively small.

Obesity may result from environmental influence, such as the widespread advertising of food products. Occupational, economic, and sociocultural factors also may be considered in the broad environmental sense. It now appears that socioeconomic status and related social factors are important in obesity development. Obesity is seven times more common among women of low socioeconomic groups than among those of higher status (67). The mental health indices of the obese subjects in the low socioeconomic group reflected "immaturity," "rigidity," and "suspiciousness" in comparison with those individuals in the same group with normal weight. A defect in impulse control may be suggested by the "immaturity" rating. In another study, obesity again was found to be more prevalent in young females of low socioeconomic status than in those of a higher socioeconomic status (68). Another study confirmed the greater incidence of obesity among women of low socioeconomic status and found a similar but less marked trend in men. The prevalence of obesity in lower socioeconomic classes is first noted in early adulthood; also, children from manual labor backgrounds are more likely to become obese young adults when compared with their contemporaries from other work backgrounds (69). In addition, suggestive relationships between ethnic and religious factors and obesity were found for both sexes (79).

Obesity has a psychogenic component in 90% of the cases (71). Although the psychologic aspect of caloric excess usually is exemplified by compulsive overeating replacing other gratifications, other factors are also involved. Obesity may be related to physical activity and emotions (72). Decreased physical activity often coexists with mental depression and may play a role in the development and maintenance of obesity. This theory involves the aspect of caloric expenditure rather than caloric ingestion and stresses the function of caloric disequilibrium in obesity. Therefore, depression may not be an incidental occurrence in obese people but rather one of the main reasons for the obesity (72).

Another psychologic aberration in obese patients is the disturbance in body image, in which the body is viewed as "grotesque and loathsome" (73).

Appetite Control

The hypothalamus apparently contains centers that are involved in the food ingestion process. Studies in rats show a "satiety center" and an "appetite center" located in the hypothalamic region (74). Destroying the satiety center leads to marked overeating with subsequent obesity; conversely, obliterating the appetite center results in emaciation. These results indicate that there may be a feedback inhibition of the appetite center by impulses from the satiety center after food is ingested. The glucostatic hypothesis of appetite regulation states that hunger is related to the degree that glucose is used by cells called glucostats (75). When glucose utilization by glucostats in the satiety center is low, the inhibitory effect on the appetite center is reduced, favoring eating behavior. Conversely, when glucose utilization is high, the appetite center is inhibited, and the desire for food intake is reduced.

The hypothalamus contains high concentrations of noradrenergic terminals (76). A discrete fiber system that supplies the hypothalamus with most of its norepinephrine-secreting terminals is called the ventral noradrenergic bundle. Destroying the noradrenergic terminals in the hypothalamus or damaging the ventral noradrenergic bundle results in obesity in animals (77). Food-induced enhancement of sympathetic activity is modulated by the ventral noradrenergic bundle; in animals with lesions of this region, food intake increased significantly (78). It has been suggested that the ventral noradrenergic bundle normally mediates satiety and that it may serve as a substrate for amphetamine-induced appetite suppression (79).

The interpretation of visual and chemical food-related stimuli occurs in the cerebral cortex, and acceptance or rejection of the sight, aroma, or taste of foods involves this area of the central nervous system (CNS). An obese person may respond differently from people of normal weight to the appearance, taste, and sight of food (80).

Endogenous opioids increase food intake in animals (81–83), and naloxone (an opioid antagonist) decreases food intake in animals (84) and in obese humans (85). Opiate receptors, which exist in the central taste pathways (86), are believed to modulate human taste (87). Thus, an emerging hypothesis suggests that an endogenous opioid system is involved in human gustatory perceptions. Research involving the trigeminal nerve, a pathway relaying sensory input from the oral cavity to the hypothalamus, indicates this system's possible role in food intake. The trigeminal circuit is a system of oral touch, and the excessive nibbling common to obese individuals may be caused by their greater sensitivity to this stimulus (88).

Role of Obesity in Other Conditions

Studies have shown a significant association between early mortality and obesity. Cardiovascular and cerebrovascular diseases are associated with obesity and account for many early deaths (89–91). There is evidence that sustained hypertension is more common in overweight people, although the correlation between blood pressure and adiposity is not well established (92). Therefore, persons at high risk for hypertension, such as those with a family history of youthful obesity, should consider reducing their salt intake (93). The pharmacist should also recommend salt-intake reduction to persons who cannot control their obesity by other reasonable means. Although reduced sodium intake may reduce weight through water loss, providing some psychologic benefits, it should be stressed that this type of weight loss has no effect on fat cells.

The relationship between obesity and diabetes mellitus is well documented (89). An early study revealed that 85% of patients over 40 years of age who developed diabetes mellitus were overweight (94). Glucose intolerance commonly occurs with obesity, and relative insulin resistance is noted in obese subjects (92, 95). Obesity that persists over extremely long periods of time is associated with partial exhaustion of the beta cells with resultant hypoinsulinemia (96). In contrast, the hyperinsulinemia that occurs in obesity is related to increased body fat (97). Weight reduction results in improved glucose tolerance in the obese diabetic and reduced hyperinsulinemia in both nondiabetic and diabetic obese persons (98, 99). The severity of diabetes mellitus and the need for insulin or oral hypoglycemic agents often may be decreased by weight reduction. (See Chapter 16, *Diabetes Care Products*.)

In postmenopausal women, obesity is positively related to the risk of both breast and endometrial cancer. Obesity is associated with increased estrogen production secondary to peripheral aromatization. In postmenopausal women, this effect is proportionately more significant because the ovaries no longer contribute to production of estrogen (100). The peripheral aromatization of androstenedione (a major adrenal hormone) to estrone via the aromatase reaction in adipose tissue is the principal source of estrogen in postmenopausal women (101); an increased rate of this reaction has been reported in obese women (102, 103).

In addition to the correlations of obesity with these disease states, obese individuals have larger and more cellular organs (heart and liver) (104). Obesity may also be related to cholesterol gallstone formation because the level of this compound is characteristically elevated in obesity (105).

Hyperostosis of the spine (formation of bony bridges between the vertebrae) has been associated with hyperglycemia and obesity, although these factors are at least partly independent of each other (106). In addition, excessive obesity may contribute to respiratory stress. Obesity alters pulmonary function resulting in plethora, reduced lung volume, hypercapnia, and pulmonary hypertension (107). Charles Dickens describes Joe, the fat boy in *The Pickwick Papers*, as obese and somnolent. The description may be the first account of this condition in the literature; the "pickwickian syndrome" describes a person who is obese, exhibits narcoleptic behavior, and has an excessive appetite (108).

Certain skin disorders including candidiasis, tinea infections, furunculosis, pruritus vulvae, and trophic ulcerations occur frequently in obese individuals (109). These conditions have been associated with diabetes mellitus, which may explain the high incidence in obese persons. It should be noted, however, that scabies and psychosomatic skin disorders also occur in significant numbers of the obese. These conditions are not directly related to the diabetic state.

Although obesity generally is caused by overeating, it may mask malnutrition. Often the obese individual overconsumes carbohydrates at the expense of omitting other nutrients such as protein, vitamins, and minerals from the diet (110).

Symptoms of Obesity

Common complaints regarding obesity are often cosmetic, involving a desire to "look slim." However, remarks such as "I can't tie my shoes without getting out of breath" indicate actual physical discomfort. The obese individual may also complain of persistent backache and varicose veins.

Because obesity may be caused by inactivity due to mental depression, persons who remain obese after prolonged self-medication with nonprescription anorexigenic products should be referred to a physician (68). A psychogenic component involving inactivity due to depression or a compulsive anxiety reaction related to repeated "snacking" may be involved in such cases. The pharmacist should emphasize that weight loss will not occur unless caloric imbalance is corrected. Chronic use of nonprescription products to correct obesity may indicate a more severe underlying problem.

TREATMENT

Drug treatment of obesity is of limited value because the only satisfactory means of long-term weight control is caloric reduction and physical activity (111).

Amphetamines have been prescribed for obesity. Unfortunately, tolerance develops to the amphetamine's appetite suppressant activity, making long-term use undesirable. In addition, subtle or profound depression secondary to withdrawal from the effects of amphetamines can further complicate the effectiveness of other weight control measures. Because overeating seems to be controlled primarily by psychologic behavior factors, overeating will occur as soon as the anorexigenic effects disappear. Amphetamines and other related agents have the potential for abuse and dependence; their value is limited to short-term use (a few weeks) in obesity control as an adjunct to a controlled diet. Amphetamines should be used only when alternative therapy has been ineffective. Amphetamines and related prescription products apparently suppress appetite by stimulating the satiety center in the hypothalamic ventromedial nucleus. This process may occur indirectly on the frontal lobes of the cortex (112–113).

Another theory of appetite suppression is that anorexiants act primarily by lowering the body set point and only secondarily by suppressing appetite (114, 115). This theory is supported by the rapid regaining of body weight after cessation of appetite suppressants, such as amphetamines, in contrast to the relative stability of weight loss achieved without medication (116).

Human Chorionic Gonadotropin

Human chorionic gonadotropin (hCG) has been used by some clinicians in treating obesity. Several controlled clinical studies have indicated that hCG is no more effective than a placebo injection in weight reduction (117–123). One investigation supports the effectiveness of hCG (124); however, this study had a high dropout rate and uncertain control subjects (125). There appears to be no rationale in claims that hCG contributes to weight reduction regimens by influencing fat distribution, inducing a sense of well-being, or preventing hunger and fatigue in persons on a reducing diet. The Food and Drug Administration (FDA) has required the following addition to the indications in all hCG labeling (125):

> HCG has not been demonstrated to be effective adjunctive therapy in the treatment of obesity. There is no substantial evidence that it increases weight loss beyond that resulting from caloric restriction, that it causes a more attractive or "normal" distribution of fat or that it decreases the hunger and discomfort associated with calorie-restricted diets.

Phenylpropanolamine

Phenylpropanolamine, a sympathomimetic agent related chemically and pharmacologically to ephedrine and amphetamine, acts as an indirect sympathomimetic, exerting more prominent peripheral adrenergic effects compared with weak central stimulant actions (126). In the past, controversy has existed as to phenylpropanolamine's effectiveness as an anorexigenic agent (127). Early animal studies indicated its usefulness in diminishing food intake in animals (128, 129), and a qualitative difference between the anorexigenic activities of phenylpropanolamine and amphetamines was reported (130). The weight-reducing action of phenylpropanolamine may reflect a combined effect on both food intake and brown adipose tissue (BAT) thermogenesis (131). Later clinical studies indicated a possible appetite-suppressant activity. Results from one double-blind study indicated that phenylpropanolamine (25 mg), taken 30 minutes before lunch, reduced intake of a liquid diet (130). In another double-blind study, subjects who received the same dosage reported a significant reduction in their consumption of dinner and snacks (131). A double-blind clinical evaluation of a phenylpropanolamine–caffeine–vitamin combination compared with a placebo and diet showed a significantly greater weight loss over a 4-week period in patients on a 1,200-cal diet who received the same combination product (132). A 6-week double-blind study involving obese patients compared 37.5 mg of phenylpropanolamine and 140 mg of caffeine in a "sustained-action capsule" with placebo. Patients taking the phenylpropanolamine and caffeine combination lost an average of 4.64 pounds compared to 2.07 pounds for the placebo group (133).

In another study of healthy adults 18–60 years of age, 35 mg of phenylpropanolamine and 140 mg of caffeine in one capsule taken twice daily produced a weight loss of at least 6 pounds in 50% of the subjects (134); in the placebo group only 22% of the patients lost this much weight. In a physician-managed weight-reduction program that included behavior modification, mild caloric restriction, and exercise, phenylpropanolamine or placebo was added (135); this double-blind, 14-week clinical trial of 160 women demonstrated that subjects taking phenylpropanolamine lost significantly more weight (6.1 kg) than the placebo group (4.3 kg).

All authorities, however, do not agree on the effectiveness of phenylpropanolamine as an anorexigenic agent. The *AMA Drug Evaluations* states that weight control products containing phenylpropanolamine are "only minimally effective" (136). A basic pharmacology textbook states that the drug is ineffective as an appetite suppressant (137). However, a recent pharmacology text (138) cites reports of small but consistent weight loss, which accounts for the acceptance of phenylpropanolamine as an anorexigenic agent.

In 1982, the FDA advisory review panel on OTC miscellaneous internal drug products found phenylpropanolamine to be generally safe and effective for short-term weight control (139). The FDA permits a phenylpropanolamine dose of 37.5 mg in immediate-release products and 75 mg in sustained-release products. The maximum daily dosage is set at 75 mg (139).

Side effects may occur with phenylpropanolamine, especially if the recommended dosage is exceeded. Nervousness, restlessness, insomnia, headache, nausea, and excessive increase in blood pressure are some of phenylpropanolamine's adverse effects (126). Cardiovascular adverse reactions, including hypertensive episodes and stroke, have been reported following overdosage and recommended dosage of products containing phenylpropanolamine alone or in combination with other drugs (140–157). An extensive review article relating to nonprescription sympathomimetic agents and hypertension includes a comprehensive treatment of phenylpropanolamine (158). Intracerebral hemorrhage and cerebral vasculitis have been associated with prolonged use and overdose of phenylpropanolamine (159). Several other reports relate phenylpropanolamine to intracerebral hemorrhage (160–165); hypertension has been cited as the most likely cause of phenylpropanolamine-associated intracranial hemorrhage (166), especially in the basal ganglia (159). Vascular etiology involving multiple focal areas of arterial narrowing and segmental vascular injury has been implicated in lobar subcortical and subarachnoid hemorrhages (159). Cardiac arrhythmias, myocardial infarct, and atrioventricular blockage have also been attributed to phenylpropanolamine (167–171). Acute renal failure, sometimes associated with rhabdomyolysis, has been reported after phenylpropanolamine ingestion (172–175).

Hypertensive reactions in previously normotensive individuals have been reported with single oral doses of 85 mg of phenylpropanolamine in the immediate-release form (176, 177). In another instance, the same dosage form of phenylpropanolamine, taken with indomethacin, induced a severe hypertensive episode (178, 179). A double-blind study in young normotensive adults revealed that significant elevations in blood pressure may occur after a single dose of phenylpropanolamine (180). There is evidence that the immediate-release product in these studies was a different isomer, (+) norpseudoephedrine, rather than the racemic form, (±) norephedrine, which is available in the United States (181). It has been suggested that hypertensive effects are more likely to occur when phenylpropanolamine is in the immediate-release form rather than in a sustained-release preparation (182).

In contrast, controlled clinical studies have demonstrated an absence of significant side effects or hypertensive activity with phenylpropanolamine in obese patients (183) and in healthy nonobese subjects (184, 185). A recent study of obese normotensive patients (186) demonstrated the absence of significant pressor effects with a 75-mg phenylpropanolamine sustained-release form, even when combined with caffeine. Other reports (187–189) document the absence of pressor effects with phenylpropanolamine in recommended nonprescription dosages. Finally, in a pilot study, the safety and efficacy of phenylpropanolamine in therapeutic dosages were noted in adult patients with stable, controlled hypertension (190). These clinical evaluations indicate that recommended therapeutic dosages of phenylpropanolamine do not produce any significant cardiovascular adverse effects.

CNS stimulation as evidenced by convulsive seizures has been noted (191). Psychotic reactions have been described with 50 mg of phenylpropanolamine (in combination with isopropamide and phenyltoloxamine) (192). Mental disturbances have been described in considerable detail, and it is evident that the possibility of psychotic episodes exists (193, 194). "Amphetamine-like reactions" to phenylpropanolamine have been reported. Seven cases were reported from emergency room records over a 6-month period. All adverse effects occurred within 1 to 2 hours after ingestion of a single dose of either phenylpropanolamine alone or phenylpropanolamine in combination with caffeine. These effects included respiratory stimulation, tremor, restlessness, increased motor activity, agitation, and hallucinations (195). Psychiatric side effects attributed to phenylpropanolamine are noted in a review article (196). CNS disturbances—including paranoia, hallucinations, mania, and seizures—have been described following ingestion of phenylpropanolamine, often in combination with other drugs (197–201). "Legal" stimulants ("look-alikes" or "pseudo-speed") containing phenylpropanolamine, usually in combination with ephedrine and caffeine, have been associated with fatal cerebral hemorrhage and other severe adverse effects (202–204). The phenylpropanolamine, ephedrine, and caffeine product was declared an unapproved new drug by the FDA in 1982 and can no longer be marketed as a nonprescription preparation (205). Furthermore, in 1983 the FDA declared that the phenylpropanolamine and caffeine combinations found in several weight control products were "new drugs" requiring approved New Drug Applications (NDAs) before they could be marketed. Consequently, the combination phenylpropanolamine–caffeine products were removed from the market (206). Pharmacists can warn patients of the possible CNS effects of phenylpropanolamine. According to some clinicians, phenylpropanolamine "poses a danger to the public" and should be regarded as a drug with potential for abuse (207). However, a recent large-scale (837 healthy volunteers) double-blind, placebo-controlled study provides evidence that phenylpropanolamine in therapeutic dosages does not produce the euphoriant or "stimulant" subjective effects that characterize drugs of abuse (208).

Although the FDA advisory review panel on OTC cold, allergy, bronchodilator, and antiasthmatic drug products did not review anorexiants as such, it concluded that the incidence of side effects with phenylpropanolamine is low at oral therapeutic doses (209). Additionally, an analysis of 70 cases of accidental or deliberate overdosage with phenylpropanolamine or phenylpropanolamine with caffeine revealed that symptoms such as nausea or vomiting, nervousness, headache, tachycardia, or dizziness occurred in adults only if the dose ingested greatly exceeded the recommended therapeutic dosage (210). These authors further stated, "The lack of serious side effects in either the cases with only phenylpropanolamine or combinations of phenylpropanolamine with caffeine raises questions about the serious reactions noted in earlier published reports" (210).

Because phenylpropanolamine is an adrenergic substance, it may elevate blood glucose levels and produce cardiac stimulation. For these reasons, the labels on products containing phenylpropanolamine warn that individuals with diabetes mellitus, heart disease, hypertension, or thyroid disease should seek medical advice before taking this drug.

Phenylpropanolamine has been implicated in "drug–drug" interactions with monoamine oxidase inhibitors (211–214); indeed, phenylpropanolamine has been reported to have monoamine oxidase inhibitory activity (215). Severe hypertensive episodes may be more likely when preparations containing phenylpropanolamine in an immediate-release form, rather than in a sustained-release form, are ingested by patients already taking monoamine oxidase inhibitors (212, 213).

One report described a subject who had various adverse effects when phenylpropanolamine was ingested concurrently with aspirin and acetaminophen over a 3-week period. These adverse effects included nausea, vomiting, headaches, weakness, malaise, and severe muscle tenderness. Subsequently, brown-colored urine was noted, and a percutaneous renal biopsy revealed acute interstitial nephritis (216). A case of fatal ventricular arrhythmia induced by thioridazine was thought to be initiated by phenylpropanolamine administration (217). Severe hypertension has been reported when phenylpropanolamine was taken with methyldopa

or oxyprenolol (a beta-blocker similar to propranolol, which is an Investigational New Drug (IND) in the United States) (218). Phenylpropanolamine-induced hypertension has been treated with nifedipine (219) and propranolol (220). There is one report of a positive phentolamine test for pheochromocytoma in hypertension induced by phenylpropanolamine (221), and a pseudopheochromocytoma syndrome has been described following phenylpropanolamine use (222). One case report cites catatonia associated with phenylpropanolamine overdose and fluphenazine treatment (223).

The reports of adverse reactions with phenylpropanolamine and phenylpropanolamine-containing combinations should be interpreted within the total context. Many of these reports involve only one case or report multiple drug ingestion and are, in a sense, anecdotal in nature. Factors such as hypersensitivity, dosage and dosage forms ingested, concurrent pathology, and the presence of other drugs must be delineated before frank accusation of phenylpropanolamine as the "culprit drug" is warranted (224–231). The toxicity of phenylpropanolamine should not be evaluated on the basis of combination products or without detailed information on dosage ingested, analysis for presence of phenylpropanolamine, preexisting disease, patient drug history, and/or the possibility of multiple drug ingestion (227).

Reviews of phenylpropanolamine use in short-term weight control reflect the present status of this drug as a nonprescription weight control product (232, 233). Additionally, two comprehensive books are devoted entirely to phenylpropanolamine (234, 235).

Benzocaine

Benzocaine was first incorporated into a weight-control preparation in 1958 (236). A preparation containing benzocaine and methylcellulose in chewing gum wafers was tried for 10 weeks in 50 patients who were 5.5–46 kg overweight. The patients were instructed to chew one or two wafers, followed by a glass of water, just before meals. In addition, they were placed on low-calorie diets and were directed to chew the gum every 4 hours if there was a strong desire to eat. Results showed that 90% of the subjects lost weight. However, the study did not use a placebo control group, and the weight loss could have been caused by benzocaine, methylcellulose, or the diet alone. The benzocaine dosage was small, and any marked degree of numbness in the oral cavity was questionable. It is conceivable that subtle effects on taste sensitivity or taste modification may occur, and perceived analgesia or numbness is not necessary for possible appetite suppressant activity. Obese persons may be more sensitive to taste stimuli (88).

Constant snacking is characteristic of the "oral syndrome" in many obese persons. A nontraditional appetite-control plan using benzocaine, glucose, caffeine, and vitamins in a hard candy form was tried (237). The subjects ingested the candies when they wanted a snack and before and after meals. The purpose of this approach was to keep the patients orally active and at the same time elevate their blood glucose levels. The influence of benzocaine was considered to be an essential component of the significant weight reduction in the study group.

Capsules or tablets containing benzocaine are designed to be swallowed, and hence the drug does not come into contact with the oral cavity. Any appetite suppression would depend on an effect on the gastrointestinal (GI) mucosa. However, no conclusive clinical data support such an activity. The FDA advisory review panel on OTC miscellaneous internal drug products classified benzocaine as generally effective for short-term weight control (139). This panel also determined that a dose of 3–15 mg for use in gum, lozenges, or candy just prior to food consumption was generally safe and effective for weight control (139).

Although they are rare, cyanotic reactions have been reported following benzocaine administration (238). Methemoglobinemia in infants also has been reported (239–243). These reactions refer primarily to infants and therefore are not specifically relevant to the drug's use in the noninfant obese population. It is important, however, to be aware of potential benzocaine toxicity because benzocaine-induced methemoglobinemia has been recently reported in an adult (244). In addition, a fatal anaphylactic reaction occurred in an adult a few minutes after the ingestion of a throat lozenge containing benzocaine (245). Obese persons taking preparations containing benzocaine over long periods may expose themselves to the consequences of drug-induced hypersensitivity.

Bulk Producers

Typical examples of bulk producers are methylcellulose, carboxymethyl cellulose, psyllium hydrophilic mucilloid, agar, and karaya gum. Bulk-producing laxatives are a common source of these agents. It has been suggested that the bulk-producing activity produces a sense of fullness, reducing the desire to eat. The efficacy of the bulk-forming agents as appetite suppressants in controlling obesity has not been established (246). A radiographic study shows that a methylcellulose mass is almost entirely eliminated from the stomach in 30 minutes. In addition, intestinal peristalsis is actually accelerated by methylcellulose, as evidenced by the fact that most of the methylcellulose mass reaches the ileum in only 30 minutes (247). Therefore, neither bulk production by methylcellulose nor an increase in the rate of gastric transport offers a mechanism to produce satiety. No experimental evidence exists to support an appetite-suppressant claim. However, bulk-producing substances have been approved for dietary use by the FDA (248).

It is assumed that the benefit of bulk producers in obesity control is related to caloric intake reduction, irrespective of the ingestion of the bulk producer. Bulk producers probably are no more effective than a low-calorie, high-residue diet in a weight-reduction program. Moreover, their laxative effect may not always be desirable. Because of the danger of esophageal obstruction with methylcellulose wafers, generous amounts of fluid should accompany ingestion of bulk producers (199). Agents with anticholinergic properties reduce bowel motility. Concurrent use of these agents with bulk producers may be hazardous because they may produce intestinal obstruction. (See Chapter 15, *Laxative Products*.)

Other Products

Vitamins and minerals are present in some nonprescription weight-control products. If a dieting patient is not receiving adequate quantities of vitamins and minerals in the diet regimen chosen, then the addition is warranted. However, in a well-balanced, low-calorie diet, recommended daily allowances for vitamins and minerals are present. (See Chapter 17, *Nutritional Supplement, Mineral, and Vitamin Products*.)

Alginic acid, sodium bicarbonate, and carboxymethyl cellulose are found in some nonprescription products. The carbon dioxide evolved from the sodium bicarbonate combines with the alginic acid, and a foamy methylcellulose mass is formed (246). This bulk is purported to relieve the feeling of "emptiness" in the stomach. The alleged properties of grapefruit extract in accelerating fat metabolism have not been substantiated.

Dietary aids such as carbohydrate candy-type foods and low-calorie nutritionally balanced liquids are not considered drugs but are available as adjuncts in a weight-reduction program. In addition, synthetic sweeteners such as saccharin may be valuable in reducing excessive sugar consumption and thus lowering caloric intake.

Glucose

Preparations containing glucose and vitamins are claimed to elevate blood glucose levels when taken before meals or at snack time, so that the satiety center exerts an inhibitory influence on the appetite center. This assertion, however, is questionable. A clinical study reported that a glucose load (50 g) taken 20 minutes before lunch suppressed caloric intake relative to control load at lunch ($p < 0.01$) (249). Reactions to a glucose load's oral qualities may constitute the principal factor in the first 20 minutes rather than GI or postabsorptive effect on satiety. However, the efficacy of glucose in long-term weight-control programs has not been established.

Low-Calorie Balanced Foods

The "canned diet" products are considered substitutes for the usual diet. One product typical of this group supplies 70 g of protein per day, an amount the manufacturer states "is the recommended daily dietary allowance of protein for normal adults." It also contains 20 g of fat and 110 g of carbohydrate in a daily ration for a total daily calorie intake of 900 calories. Powder, granule, and liquid forms are available; these products are also formulated as cookies and soups.

These dietary foods are low in sodium. Weight loss in the first 2 weeks is probably caused, in part, by water loss from the tissues. It is questionable whether a weight loss over a short period is significant with regard to the effective long-term treatment of obesity.

The pharmacist should be aware that products that substitute 900 cal per day for the usual diet are usually effective in reducing weight. Moreover, it appears that any diet of 900 cal that supplies adequate protein and lowers carbohydrate and fat intake should enable an obese patient to lose weight.

Artificial Sweeteners

Sucrose overuse is common. A sucrose substitute, saccharin, provides no calories and may allow significant calorie reduction in certain patients. Saccharin is about 400 times more potent than sucrose as a sweetener. It produces a bitter taste in some individuals, and it is not heat stable; nevertheless, it is the most popular artificial sweetener, especially since the prohibition of nonregulated use of cyclamates. Saccharin may have considerable importance in reducing caloric intake in some individuals. For instance, if saccharin is used to sweeten a cup of coffee instead of one heaping teaspoonful of sugar, 33 calories are removed from the diet.

In 1972, bladder tumors were discovered in rats fed saccharin in utero and throughout life. The FDA then removed saccharin from the list of food additives generally recognized as safe. Saccharin is currently permitted in products labeled specifically as diet foods or beverages. It may accumulate in fetal tissues and therefore should not be used during pregnancy (250). As of June 1, 1978, pharmacies carrying saccharin-containing products are required to display posters containing the following warning statement (251):

> **SACCHARIN NOTICE** This store sells food including diet beverages that contain saccharin. You will find saccharin listed in the ingredient statement on most foods which contain it. All foods that contain saccharin will soon bear the following warning: Use of this product may be hazardous to your health. This product contains saccharin, which has been determined to cause cancer in laboratory animals. This store is required by law to display this notice prominently.

Human epidemiologic studies have not revealed a clearcut relationship between saccharin consumption and urinary bladder carcinoma (252). One study reported a positive relationship (253) but it has been criticized for deficiencies in design and analysis (254).

Aspartame is a synthetic dipeptide about 180 times as sweet as sugar. The FDA has determined that aspartame has been shown to be safe as a food additive. Products containing aspartame are required to carry the warning: "Phenylketonurics: Contains Phenylalanine." Because phenylalanine is contained in aspartame, individuals with phenylketonuria or patients who should avoid protein foods must be alerted to this fact. In addition, directions not to use aspartame in cooking or baking (the compound loses its sweetness) are required on "table products" of aspartame (255).

Acesulfam, a newly available artificial sweetener, is a chemical relative of saccharin (256). Approximately 200 times sweeter than sucrose, acesulfam has been approved by the FDA for use in certain food products, including chewing gum, dry beverage mixes, instant tea and coffee, puddings, gelatins, and nondairy creamers.

Fructose, sorbitol, and xylitol may be employed as alternates to saccharin. These sweeteners contain calories and should not be viewed as being a "sugar-free" diet item. Fructose and xylitol are sweeter than sucrose, and xylitol is less calorigenic and more expensive (257). Apparently, neither sorbitol nor xylitol causes tooth decay, and some products containing xylitol have a more pleasant taste (258). However, some evidence implicates xylitol in the development of urinary tract abnormalities, kidney stones, and tumors in laboratory animals (259). Further tests are under way to evaluate this possibility. The ingestion of sufficient amounts of dietetic candies containing sorbitol may result in an osmotic catharsis in small children (260).

Several naturally occurring compounds show promise as substitutes for sucrose (261). Monellin, thaumatin, and miraculin are proteins from plant sources, which are currently being investigated as possible sucrose substitutes.

Dosage Forms

Nonprescription products for obesity control are available as liquids, powders, granules, tablets, capsules, sustained-release capsules, wafers, cookies, soups, chewing gum, and candy preparations. If candy cubes, wafers, or chewing gum is substituted for high-calorie desserts or "snacks," the candy-like nature of the dosage form may offer patients a psychologic aid that is not found when a standard tablet or capsule is used. Ingesting large quantities of diet candy would, of course, contribute significantly to caloric intake.

Adjunctive Therapy

The only real therapy for most cases of obesity is diet alone or in conjunction with other therapeutic measures. The pharmacist should make sure that patients who are dieting are under a physician's supervision. Patients who are having difficulty in losing weight may find reinforcement in self-help groups and behavior modification.

Diet

High-protein, low-carbohydrate diets of 800–1,000 cal a day are used frequently in weight-reduction programs. Total fasting or semistarvation sometimes is proposed as a means of weight reduction in grossly obese persons (262, 263). Starvation, either total or partial, depletes the body of lean tissue and essential electrolytes in addition to fat (264). The ketosis and ketoacidosis resulting from a fasting state reflect a metabolic alteration. If total fasting is used to treat obesity, hospitalization is recommended to deal effectively with mood changes or alterations in physiologic functions such as cardiac arrhythmias (265). "Crash" diets involving 500 cal a day for 4–8 weeks have been implicated in the loss of scalp hair (266). This effect apparently reflects the trauma attributed to semistarvation.

Low-carbohydrate diets have been advocated on the basis that individuals may eat as much as they desire as long as no carbohydrates are ingested. Fat from food may be deposited as fat in the body, and proteins may be converted to fat. The excess fat metabolized may result in an increased production of ketones to the degree that ketosis, acidosis, and dehydration may occur. Some diets recommend inclusion of large quantities of fat in the diet (1, 267). Although a high-fat diet may suppress fat synthesis it doesn't prevent fat deposition. An additional problem encountered in these diets is the elevation of blood cholesterol.

A carbohydrate-free, high-fat diet does cause an immediate weight reduction due to water loss (dehydration), but it does not affect adiposity. The "drinking man's diet" adds alcohol to this regimen, which tends to add more calories and the increased liability of fat deposition. A high-meat (protein and fat), no-carbohydrate diet presents an extra burden to the kidney because of the resultant increased urea load. In addition, an increase in the uric acid levels in this diet may precipitate gouty arthritis in susceptible persons. A low-protein, low-fat "rice" diet was advocated several years ago. This unbalanced diet could lead to ill health (267).

A diet containing kelp, vinegar, lecithin, and vitamin B_6 has been proposed. Excess kelp, which contains high amounts of iodine, may decrease thyroid function by negative feedback mechanisms. The other ingredients in this diet do not have any established value in weight reduction. The weight loss in this diet is due to the low caloric intake, rather than the use of these specific additives.

The extent of injuries and deaths caused by the use of extremely low-calorie protein diets is unclear. However, it is apparent that studies oriented toward geographic incidence, concurrent pathology, age, and other factors need careful scrutiny. The complaints reported to the FDA frequently include nausea, vomiting, diarrhea (liquid preparations), constipation (dry preparations), faintness, muscle cramps, weakness or fatigue, irritability, cold intolerance, decreased libido, amenorrhea, hair loss, dry skin, cardiac arrhythmias, recurrence of gout, dehydration, and hypokalemia (268).

The possibility of "drug–food" interactions with low-calorie protein diets exists. Patients taking prescription medicines such as diuretics, antihypertensives, hypoglycemic agents, insulin, adrenergics, high doses of corticosteroids, thyroid preparations other than those used in replacement therapy, and lithium should not use the liquid protein diet.

The pharmacist should warn the patient not to undertake this type of diet approach without proper medical supervision. The patient's age also should be taken into consideration because elderly obese persons may be more susceptible to cardiovascular stress and gout.

A balanced diet containing no less than 12–14% protein, no more than 30% fat (unsaturated preferred), and the remainder carbohydrate (low sucrose) is preferable to potentially dangerous unbalanced diets of questionable value (1).

Group Therapy

Group therapy and behavior modification are effective in treating obesity. Groups such as TOPS (Take Off Pounds Sensibly) and Weight Watchers have been successful in the treatment of obesity (269). The group pressure resulting from praise or criticism apparently is an effective deterrent to overeating for many persons. Behavior modification that considers eating as a "pure" activity (not combined with any other activity), as well as eating more slowly, may be beneficial. In addition, keeping a diet diary and using a "unit dose" concept for food may prove helpful in a weight-reduction program. Psychotherapeutic approaches also show promise in obesity control (270).

Surgical Intervention

In refractory cases of gross obesity, intestinal bypass operations have been performed (271). This procedure is probably the most hazardous measure used to treat extreme obesity and has led to alternative, perhaps safer, procedures such as gastric partitioning to control morbid obesity (272).

SUMMARY

The effectiveness of a weight-reduction program depends largely on the patient's education and the acceptance of a regimen necessary to achieve long-term weight control. A patient should recognize the many facets of a successful weight-reduction program, including motivation, physical activity, reduced caloric intake, and possibly a pharmacologic "crutch" such as a nonprescription product. The role of the pharmacist is to supply pertinent and accurate information regarding these matters.

PRODUCT SELECTION GUIDELINES

In recommending a nonprescription product for weight control, the pharmacist should stress the importance of a diet plan and/or exercise program. Weight cannot be reduced without a concerted effort to change one's eating and exercise habits and to maintain the new habits. In light of the pharmacist's role in total health care, emphasis should be placed on alternate means of obesity control. The pharmacist should inquire about previous diet control regimens the patient has attempted so that other nonprescription diet management programs may be recommended. The pharmacist may also participate in monitoring the patient's weight-reduction efforts.

As a health care professional, the pharmacist should emphasize the importance of a rational, low-calorie, balanced diet and proper exercise to correct caloric imbalance, as well as the importance of individual effort in maintaining a diet management program. The patient may be referred to a reinforcing group.

The patient should appreciate the caloric value of various food types. A nonprescription obesity control product should be considered only as an adjunct to a planned weight reduction program. Vitamins sometimes are added to such products on the assumption that dieting individuals may not have an adequate vitamin intake. This practice may be justified in individual cases but cannot be applied to all patients.

REFERENCES

1 R. S. Goodhart and M. E. Shils, "Modern Nutrition in Health and Disease," Lea and Febiger, Philadelphia, Pa., 1980, pp. 721, 736.

2 A. Angel, *Can. Med. Assoc. J.*, *110*, 540 (1974).

3 C. C. Seltzer et al., *Pediatrics*, *36*, 212 (1965).

4 J. V. G. A. Durnin and M. M. Rahaman, *Br. J. Nutr.*, *21*, 681 (1967).

5 J. Womersly and J. V. G. A. Durnin, *Br. J. Nutr.*, *38*, 271 (1977).

6 J. M. Tanner, "Human Body Composition," J. Brozek, Ed., Pergamon Press, Oxford, Eng., 1965, pp. 211–236.

7 T. Weits et al., *Int. J. Obesity*, *10*, 161 (1986).

8 M. T. Fanelli et al., *Int. J. Obesity*, *12*, 125 (1988).

9 J. S. Garrow, in "Obesity and Related Diseases," J. S. Garrow, Ed., Churchill Livingstone, London, Eng., 1988, pp. 39–49.

10 J. S. Garrow and J. Webster, *Int. J. Obesity*, *9*, 147 (1985).

11 M. Ashwell et al., *Int. J. Obesity*, *6*, 143 (1982).

12 A. J. Hartz et al., *Am. J. Epidemiol.*, *119*, 71 (1984).

13 W. H. Mueller et al., *Int. J. Obesity*, *11*, 309 (1987).

14 M. Ashwell et al., *Br. Med. J.*, *290*, 1692 (1985).

15 H. Kvist et al., *Int. J. Obesity*, *10*, 53 (1986).

16 M. G. Wohl, "Modern Nutrition in Health and Disease," Lea and Febiger, Philadelphia, Pa. 1960, p. 532.

17 U.S. Public Health Service, "Obesity and Health: A Sourcebook of Current Information for Professional Health Personnel," Pub. No. 1485, Washington, D.C., 1966.

18 M. G. Wagner, *J. Am. Diet. Assoc.*, *57*, 311 (1970).

19 J. Mayer, *Annu. Rev. Med.*, *14*, 111 (1963).

20 D. J. Galton, *Br. Med. J.*, *2*, 1498 (1966).

21 P. B. Curtis-Prior, *Lancet*, *1*, 897 (1975).

22 D. S. Miller et al., *Am. J. Clin. Nutr.*, *20*, 1223 (1967).

23 G. A. Bray and D. A. York, *Physiol. Rev.*, *59*, 719 (1979).

24 D. S. Miller, in "Animal Models of Obesity," M. F. W. Festing, Ed., Macmillan, London, Eng., 1979, pp. 131–140.

25 E. Jequier, *Clin. Physiol.*, *3*, 1 (1983).

26 D. S. Miller, *Proc. Nutr. Soc.*, *41*, 193 (1982).

27 G. A. Rose and R. T. Williams, *Br. J. Nutr.*, *15*, 1 (1961).

28 D. S. Miller, in "Obesity in Perspective," G. A. Bray, Ed., U.S. Govt. Printing Office, Washington, D.C., 1973, pp. 137–143.

29 E. A. H. Sims et al., *Rec. Prog. Horm. Res.*, *29*, 457 (1973).

30 A. Golay et al., *Diabetes*, *31*, 1023 (1982).

31 M. L. Kaplan and G. A. Leveille, *Am. J. Clin. Nutr.*, *29*, 1108 (1976).

32 P. Pittet et al., *Br. J. Nutr.*, *35*, 281 (1976).

33 R. S. Schwartz et al., *Metabolism*, *32*, 114 (1983).

34 P. S. Shetty et al., *Clin. Sci.*, *60*, 519 (1981).

35 T. Bessard et al., *Am. J. Clin. Nutr.*, *38*, 680 (1983).

36 A. G. Dulloo and D. S. Miller, *Int. J. Obesity*, *10*, 467 (1986).

37 R. E. Smith and B. A. Horowitz, *Physiol. Rev.*, *49*, 330 (1969).

38 A. G. Dulloo and D. S. Miller, *Can. J. Physiol. Pharmacol.*, *62*, 235 (1984).

39 L. Landsberg et al., *Am. J. Physiol.*, *247*, E181 (1984).

40 A. G. Swick et al., *Int. J. Obesity*, *10*, 241 (1986).

41 J. Bazelmans et al., *Metabolism*, *34*, 154 (1985).

42 K. O'Dea et al., *Metabolism*, *31*, 896 (1982).

43 W. P. T. James et al., in "Animal Models of Obesity," M. F. W. Festing, Ed., Macmillan, London, Eng., 1979, pp. 221–235.

44 Y. Schutz et al., *Am. J. Clin. Nutr.*, *40*, 542 (1984).

45 M. E. J. Lean et al., *Int. J. Obesity*, *10*, 219 (1986).

46 R. S. Schwartz et al., *Int. J. Obesity*, *11*, 141 (1987).

47 M. DeLuise et al., *N. Engl. J. Med.*, *303*, 1017 (1980).

48 M. DeLuise and J. Flier, *J. Clin. Invest.*, *69*, 38 (1982).

49 M. DeLuise et al., *Metabolism*, *31*, 1153 (1982).

50 I. Klimes et al., *J. Clin. Endocrinol. Metab.*, *54*, 721 (1982).

51 B. M. Simat et al., *J. Clin. Endocrinol. Metab.*, *56*, 925 (1983).

52 L. F. Martin et al., *J. Surg. Res.*, *34*, 473 (1983).

53 E. Beutler et al., *N. Engl. J. Med.*, *309*, 756 (1983).

54 A. G. Mazelis et al., *Int. J. Obesity*, *11*, 561 (1987).

55 D. Margules, *Psychology Today*, Oct., 136 (1979).

56 K. Adams, *Br. Med. J.*, *2*, 234 (1977).

57 A. H. Crisp et al., *Psychother. Psychosom.*, *22*, 159 (1973).

58 J. H. Lacey et al., *Br. Med. J.*, *4*, 556 (1975).

59 J. Hirsch and J. I. Knittle, *Fed. Proc.*, *29*, 1516 (1970).

60 L. B. Salans et al., *J. Clin. Invest.*, *52*, 929 (1973).

61 S. R. Williams, "Nutrition and Diet Therapy," C. V. Mosby, St. Louis, Mo., 1967, p. 477.

62 J. Mayer, *Bull. N.Y. Acad. Med.*, *36*, 323 (1960).

63 K. J. Carpenter and J. Mayer, *Am. J. Physiol.*, *193*, 449 (1958).

64 N. B. Marshall et al., *Am. J. Physiol.*, *189*, 342 (1957).

65 C. C. Seltzer and J. Mayer, *J. Am. Med. Assoc.*, *189*, 677 (1964).

66 C. C. Seltzer and J. Mayer, *J. Am. Diet. Assoc.*, *55*, 454 (1969).

67 M. E. Moore et al., *J. Am. Med. Assoc.*, *181*, 962 (1962).

68 A. Stunkard et al., *J. Am. Med. Assoc.*, *221*, 579 (1972).

69 C. Power and C. Moynihan, *Int. J. Obesity*, *12*, 445 (1988).

70 P. B. Goldblatt et al., *J. Am. Med. Assoc.*, *192*, 1039 (1965).

71 "Drugs of Choice 1980–81," W. Modell, Ed., C. V. Mosby, St. Louis, Mo., 1980, p. 296.

72 A. Stunkard, *Psychosom. Med.*, *20*, 366 (1958).

73 A. Stunkard and M. Mendelson, *J. Am. Diet. Assoc.*, *38*, 328 (1961).

74 A. W. Hetherington and S. W. Ransom, *Am. J. Physiol.*, *136*, 609 (1942).

75 J. Mayer, *Ann. N.Y. Acad. Sci.*, *63*, 15 (1955).

76 V. Vngorstedt, *Acta Physion. Scand. Suppl.*, *365*, 1 (1971).

77 J. E. Ahlskog and B. G. Hoebel, *Science*, *182*, 166 (1973).

78 T. Sakaguchi et al., *Int. J. Obesity*, *12*, 285 (1988).

79 R. M. Gold, *Science*, *182*, 488 (1973).

80 B. G. Hoebel, *Annu. Rev. Physiol.*, *33*, 533 (1971).

81 J. E. Jalowiec et al., *Pharmacol. Biochem. Behav.*, *15*, 477 (1981).

82 R. Kumar et al., *Br. J. Pharmacol.*, *42*, 473 (1971).

83 D. J. Sanger and P. S. McCarthy, *Psychopharmacology*, *74*, 217 (1981).

84 W. C. Lynch and L. Libby, *Life Sci.*, *33*, 1909 (1983).

85 R. L. Atkinson, *J. Clin. Endocrin. Metab.*, *55*, 196 (1982).

86 M. Herkenham and C. B. Pert, *J. Neurosci.*, *3*, 1129 (1982).

87 J. M. Komorowski and A. Komorowska, *Int. J. Obesity*, *10*, 83 (1986).

88 H. P. Ziegler, *Psychol. Today*, Aug., 62 (1975).

89 H. H. Marks, *Metabolism*, *6*, 417 (1957).

90 S. I. Wilens, *Arch. Intern. Med.*, *79*, 120 (1947).

91 S. Heyden et al., *Arch. Intern. Med.*, *128*, 956 (1971).

92 G. V. Mann, *N. Engl. J. Med.*, *291*, 226 (1974).

93 J. Stamler, "The Hypertension Handbook," Merck Sharp & Dohme, West Point, Pa., 1974, p. 15.

94 G. F. Baker, "Clinic and Metropolitan Life Insurance Co.: Diabetes in the 1940's," New York Metropolitan Life Insurance Co. Press, 1940.

95 S. M. Genuth, *Ann. Intern. Med.*, *79*, 812 (1973).

96 F. P. Felber et al., *Int. J. Obesity*, *12*, 377 (1988).

97 A. Z. El-Khodary et al., *Metabolism*, *21*, 641 (1972).

98 J. H. Karam et al., *Lancet*, *1*, 286 (1965).

99 R. S. Yalow et al., *Ann. N.Y. Acad. Sci.*, *131*, 357 (1965).

100 R. J. Hershcopf and H. L. Broadlow, *Am. J. Clin. Nutr.*, *45*, 283 (1987).

101 J. M. Grodin et al., *J. Clin. Endocrinol. Metabl.*, *36*, 207 (1973).

102 C. D. Edman et al., *Am. J. Obstet. Gynecol.*, *130*, 439 (1978).

103 P. C. McDonald et al., *Am. J. Obstet. Gynecol.*, *130*, 448 (1978).

104 "The Merck Manual," 15th ed., Merck and Co., Inc., Rahway, N.J., 1987, p. 652.

105 "Muir's Textbook of Pathology," 9th ed., D. F. Cappell and J. R. Anderson, Eds., Edward Arnold Ltd., London, England, 1971, p. 587.

106 H. Julkunen et al., *Ann. Rheum. Dis.*, *30*, 605 (1971).

107 R. H. L. Wilson and N. L. Wilson, *J. Am. Diet. Assoc.*, *55*, 465 (1969).

108 C. S. Burwell et al., *Am. J. Med.*, *21*, 811 (1956).

109 A. M. Mousa et al., *Public Health Assoc.*, *52*, 65 (1977).

110 J. Woodsworth, "Diet Revolution," St. Martin's Press, New York, N.Y., 1977, p. 66.

111 *FDA Drug Bulletin* (December 1972).

112 S. Cole, *Psychol. Bull.*, *79*, 13 (1973).

113 W. C. Bowman et al., "Textbook of Pharmacology," Blackwell, Oxford, England, 1968, p. 332.

114 A. J. Stunkard, *Life Sci.*, *30*, 2043 (1982).

115 A. J. Stunkard, in "Anorectic Agents: Mechanisms of Action and Tolerance," S. Garattini and R. Somani, Eds., Raven Press, New York, N.Y., 1981, pp. 191–210.

116 L. W. Craighead et al., *Arch. Gen. Psychiatry*, *38*, 763 (1981).

117 L. S. Craig et al., *Am. J. Clin. Nutr.*, *12*, 230 (1963).

118 S. Carne, *Lancet*, *2*, 1282 (1961).

119 E. Sohar, *Am. J. Clin. Nutr.*, 7, 514 (1959).

120 B. W. Frank, *Am. J. Clin. Nutr.*, *14*, 133 (1964).

121 J. M. Harris and E. Warsaw, *J. Am. Ger. Soc.*, *12*, 987 (1964).

122 B. Hastrup et al., *Acta Med. Scand.*, *168 (fasc. 1)*, 25 (1960).

123 P. Lebon, *J. Am. Ger. Soc.*, *14 (2)*, 116 (1966).

124 W. L. Asher and H. W. Harper, *Am. J. Clin. Nutr.*, *26*, 211 (1973).

125 *FDA Drug Bulletin*, *5* (April–June, 1975).

126 L. D. Chait et al., *Psychopharmacology*, *96*, 212 (1988).

127 H. I. Silverman, *Am. J. Pharm.*, *135*, 45 (1963).

128 M. L. Tainter, *N. Nutr.*, *27*, 89 (1944).

129 A. Epstein, *Comp. Physiol. Psychol.*, *52*, 37 (1959).

130 P. J. Wellman and R. Crockroft, *Pharmacol. Biochem. Behav.*, *32*, 147 (1989).

131 P. J. Wellman and T. L. Sellers, *Pharmacol. Biochem. Behav.*, *24 (3)*, 605 (1986).

132 S. I. Griboff et al., *Curr. Ther. Res.*, *17*, 535 (1975).

133 S. Altschuler et al., *Int. J. Obes.*, *6*, 549 (1982).

134 M. Sebok, *Curr. Ther. Res. Clin. Exp.*, *37*, 701 (1985).

135 M. Weintraub et al., *Clin. Pharmacol. Ther.*, *39 (5)*, 501 (1986).

136 "AMA Drug Evaluations," 4th ed., American Medical Association, Chicago, Ill., 1980, p. 937.

137 A. Goth, "Medical Pharmacology," 7th ed., C. V. Mosby, St. Louis, Mo., 1974, p. 110.

138 G. D. Appelt and J. M. Appelt, in "Therapeutic Pharmacology," Lea & Febiger, Philadelphia, Pa., 1988, p. 133.

139 *Federal Register*, *47*, 8466 (1982).

140 P. R. Salmon, *Br. Med. J.*, *1*, 193 (1965).

141 S. R. Shapiro, *N. Engl. J. Med.*, *280*, 1363 (1969).

142 R. B. Peterson and L. A. Vasquez, *J. Am. Med. Assoc.*, *223*, 324 (1973).

143 S. Ostern and W. H. Dodson, *J. Am. Med. Assoc.*, *194*, 472 (1965).

144 P. H. Livingston, *J. Am. Med. Assoc.*, *196*, 1159 (1966).

145 J. McEwen, *Med. J. Aust.*, *2*, 71 (1983).

146 J. T. Higgins et al., *AJDC*, *139*, 331 (1985).

147 B. Mesnard and D. R. Ginn, *South. Med. J.*, *77*, 9 (1984).

148 R. B. Peterson and L. A. Vasquez, *J. Am. Med. Assoc.*, *223*, 324 (1973).

149 D. L. Howrie and J. H. Wolfson, *J. Pediatrics*, *102*, 143 (1983).

150 P. Pentel and F. Mikell, *Lancet*, *2*, 274 (1982).

151 J. King, *Med. J. Aust.*, *2*, 258 (1979).

152 C. F. Elliot and J. C. Whyte, *Med. J. Aust.*, *1*, 175 (1981).

153 J. McEwen, *Med. J. Aust.*, *2*, 71 (1983).

154 D. A. Johnson et al., *Lancet*, *2*, 970 (1983).

155 I. Biaggioni et al., *J. Am. Med. Assoc.*, *258*, 236 (1987).

156 P. Pentel et al., *Int. J. Obesity*, *9*, 115 (1985a).

157 C. R. Lake et al., *Am. J. Med.*, *85 (3)*, 339 (1988).

158 S. S. Chua and S. I. Benrimoj, *Med. Toxicol. Adverse Drug Exp.*, *3 (5)*, 387 (1988).

159 P. Maertens et al., *South Med. J.*, *80*, 1584 (1987).

160 D. G. Kitka et al., *Stroke*, *16*, 510 (1985).

161 R. Glick et al., *Neurosurgery*, *20 (6)*, 969 (1987).

162 L. M. Maher et al., *Neurology*, *37 (10)*, 1686 (1987).

163 C. S. Kase et al., *Neurology*, *37 (3)*, 399 (1987).

164 J. R. McDowell and H. J. Le Blanc, *West. J. Med.*, *142 (5)*, 688 (1985).

165 A. J. Stoessl et al., *Stroke*, *16*, 734 (1985).

166 R. J. Fallis and M. Fisher, *Neurology*, *35*, 405 (1985).

167 J. E. Clark and W. A. Simon, *Drug Intell. Clin. Pharm.* *17*, 737 (1983).

168 P. Pentel et al., *Br. Heart J.*, *47*, 51 (1982).

169 K. M. Weesner et al., *Clin. Pediatrics*, *21*, 700 (1982).

170 O. F. Woo et al., *J. Am. Med. Assoc.*, *253 (18)*, 2646 (1985).

171 B. T. Burton et al., *J. Emerg. Med.*, *2 (6)*, 415 (1985).

172 W. M. Bennett, *Lancet*, *2*, 42 (1979).

173 R. D. Swenson et al., *J. Am. Med. Assoc.*, *248*, 1216 (1982).

174 K. W. Rumf et al., *J. Am. Med. Assoc.*, *280*, 2112 (1983).

175 W. B. Duffy et al., *South. Med. J.*, *74*, 1548 (1981).

176 D. B. Frewin et al., *Med. J. Aust.*, *2*, 479 (1979).

177 J. D. Horowitz et al., *Med. J. Aust.*, *1*, 175 (1979).

178 K. Y. Lee et al., *Lancet*, *1*, 1110 (1979).

179 K. Y. Lee et al., *Med. J. Aust.*, *1*, 525 (1979).

180 J. D. Horowitz et al., *Lancet*, *1*, 60 (1980).

181 J. P. Morgan, in "Phenylpropanolamine," J. P. Morgan, Ed., Burgess, Fort Lee, N.J., 1986, pp. 13–25.

182 M. F. Cuthbert, *Lancet*, *1*, 367 (1980).

183 R. E. Noble, *Lancet*, *1*, 1419 (1982).

184 H. I. Silverman et al., *Curr. Ther. Res.*, *28*, 185 (1980).

185 M. B. Saltzman et al., *Drug Intell. Clin. Pharm.*, *17*, 746 (1983).

186 R. Noble, *Drug Intell. Clin. Pharm.*, *22*, 296 (1988).

187 R. P. Goodman et al., *Clin. Pharmacol. Ther.*, *40 (2)*, 144 (1986).

188 I. Liebson et al., *J. Clin. Pharmacol.*, *27*, 685 (1987).

189 G. L. Burton et al., *J. Am. Med. Assoc.*, *261 (22)*, 3267 (1989).

190 M. H. Bradley and J. Raines, *Curr. Ther. Res.*, *46 (1)*, 74 (1989).

191 P. D. Deocampo, *Med. Soc. N.J.*, *76*, 591 (1979).

192 F. J. Kane and B. Q. Green, *Am. J. Psychiat.*, *123*, 484 (1966).

193 G. Norvenius et al., *Lancet*, *2*, 1367 (1979).

194 B. C. Scavullo and B. Dimenti, *J. Am. Coll. Toxicol.*, *5 (6)*, 577 (1986).

195 A. J. Dietz, *J. Am. Med. Assoc.*, *245*, 601 (1981).

196 C. R. Lake et al., *Pharmacopsychiatry*, *21 (4)*, 171 (1988).

197 J. R. Cornelius et al., *Am. J. Psychiatry*, *141*, 120 (1984).

198 C. B. Schaeffer and M. W. Pauli, *Am. J. Psychiatry*, *137*, 1256 (1980).

199 M. B. Achor and I. Extein, *Am. J. Psychiatry*, *138*, 392 (1981).

200 B. H. Rumack et al., *Clin. Toxicol.*, *7*, 533 (1974).

201 J. F. Bale et al., *AJDC*, *138*, 683 (1984).

202 E. Bernstein and B. M. Diskant, *Ann. Emerg. Med.*, *11*, 311 (1982).

203 S. M. Mueller, *N. Engl. J. Med.*, *310*, 395 (1983).

204 S. M. Mueller, *Neurology*, *33*, 650 (1983).

205 *Federal Register*, *47*, 35344 (1982).

206 *Apharmacy Weekly*, *22*, 187 (1983).

207 A. Blum, Editorial, *J. Am. Med. Assoc.*, *245*, 1347 (1981).

208 J. P. Morgan et al., *J. Clin. Psychopharmacol.*, *9 (1)*, 33 (1989).

209 "Summary Minutes of the FDA OTC Panel on Cold, Cough, Allergy, Bronchodilator, and Antiasthmatic Drug Products," Washington, D.C., June 19–20, 1973.

210 B. R. Ekins and D. G. Spoerke, *Vet. Hum. Toxicol.*, *25*, 81 (1983).

211 C. M. Tonks and A. T. Lloyd, *Br. Med. J.*, *1*, 589 (1965).

212 A. M. S. Mason and R. M. Buckle, *Br. Med. J.*, *1*, 875 (1969).

213 M. F. Cuthbert et al., *Br. Med. J.*, *1*, 404 (1969).

214 S. Smookler and A. J. Bermodez, *Ann. Emerg. Med.*, *11*, 482 (1982).

215 P. H. Yu, *Res. Commun. Chem. Pathol. Pharmacol.*, *51 (2)*, 163 (1986).

216 W. M. Bennett, *Lancet*, 2, 42 (1979).

217 G. Choulnard et al., *Can. Med. Assoc. J.*, *119*, 729 (1978).

218 E. H. McLaren, *Br. Med. J.*, *2*, 283 (1976).

219 R. G. Gibson et al., *Am. Heart J.*, *113* (no. 2 pt. 1), 406 (1987).

220 P. R. Pentel et al., *Clin. Pharmacol. Ther.*, *37 (5)*, 488 (1985).

221 F. C. Duvernoy, *N. Engl. J. Med.*, *280*, 877 (1969).

222 J. S. Hyans et al., *J. Am. Med. Assoc.*, *253 (11)*, 1609 (1985).

223 S. Castellani, *J. Clin. Psychiatry*, *46 (7)*, 288 (1985).

224 M. B. Saltzman, *Lancet*, *1*, 1242 (1982).

225 H. I. Silverman and G. P. Lewis, *J. Am. Med. Assoc.*, *247*, 460 (1982).

226 W. C. Waggoner, *Lancet*, 2, 1503 (1983).

227 G. D. Appelt, *J. Clin. Psychopharmacol.*, *3*, 332 (1983).

228 G. A. Blewett and E. B. Siegel, *J. Am. Med. Assoc.*, *249*, 3017 (1983).

229 G. D. Appelt, *Am. J. Dis. Child.*, *139*, 651 (1985).

230 M. B. Saltzman, *Neurology*, *34*, 561 (1984).

231 W. C. Waggoner, *Drug Intell. Clin. Pharm.*, *18*, 823 (1984).

232 G. D. Appelt, *Colo. J. Pharm.*, *24*, 35 (1981).

233 H. I. Silverman, *N.Y. State Pharmacist-Century II*, *58*, 26 (1984).

234 "Phenylpropanolamine: Risks, Benefits, and Controversies," Clinical Pharmacology and Therapeutic Series, Vol. 5, J. P. Morgan et al., Eds., Praeger, New York, N.Y., 1985.

235 L. Lasagna, "Phenylpropanolamine: A Review," Wiley, New York, N.Y., 1988.

236 M. Plotz, *Med. Times*, *86*, 860 (1958).

237 C. W. McLure and C. A. Brusch, *J. Am. Med. Women's Assoc.*, *28*, 239 (1973).

238 B. M. Bernstein, *Rev. Gastroenterol.*, *17*, 123 (1950).

239 H. deC. Peterson, *N. Engl. J. Med.*, *263*, 454 (1960).

240 N. Goluboff and D. J. MacFadyen, *J. Pediatr.*, *47*, 22 (1955).

241 J. A. Wolff, *Pediatrics*, *20*, 915 (1957).

242 N. Goluboff, *Pediatrics*, *21*, 340 (1958).

243 P. Bachmann et al., *J. Toxicol. Clin. Exp.*, *6 (2)*, 123 (1986).

244 S. T. Anderson et al., *Anesth. Anal.*, *67 (11)*, 1099 (1988).

245 D. J. Hesch, *J. Am. Med. Assoc.*, *172*, 62 (1960).

246 "The Pharmacological Basis of Therapeutics," 6th ed., A. G. Gilman et al., Eds., Macmillan, New York, N.Y., 1980, p. 1004, 995.

247 E. J. Drenick, *J. Am. Med. Assoc.*, *234*, 271 (1975).

248 D. C. Fletcher, *J. Am. Med. Assoc.*, *230*, 901 (1974).

249 D. A. Booth et al., *Nature*, *228*, 1104 (1970).

250 *Med. Lett. Drugs Ther.*, *17*, 61 (1975).

251 *Federal Register*, *43*, 8793 (1978).

252 R. K. Kalkhoff and M. E. Levin, *Diabetes Care*, *1*, 211 (1978).

253 G. R. Howe et al., *Lancet*, 2, 578 (1977).

254 Editorial, *Lancet*, 2, 592 (1977).

255 *Federal Register*, *46 (142)*, 38284 (1981).

256 E. Brady, *Pharm. West*, *100 (9)*, 18 (1988).

257 J. D. Brunzell, *Diabetes Care*, *1*, 223 (1978).

258 W. H. Bowen, *Pharm. Times*, *43*, 25 (January 1977).

259 *Apharmacy Weekly*, *16*, 49 (1977).

260 J. R. Gryboski, *N. Engl. J. Med.*, *275*, 718 (1966).

261 G. D. Appelt, *Colo. J. Pharm.*, *22*, 50 (1979).

262 W. L. Bloom, *Metabolism*, *8*, 214 (1959).

263 S. M. Genut et al., *J. Am. Med. Assoc.*, *230*, 987 (1974).

264 R. E. Bolinger et al., *Arch. Intern. Med.*, *118*, 3 (1966).

265 I. C. Gilliand, *Postgrad. Med. J.*, *44*, 58 (1968).

266 R. B. Odum and D. K. Goette, *J. Am. Med. Assoc.*, *235*, 476 (1976).

267 F. Netter, "Fad Diets Can Be Deadly," Exposition Press, Hicksville, N.Y., 1975, pp. 98–103.

268 *FDA Drug Bull.* (Jan./Feb. 1978).

269 A. Stunkard et al., *Arch. Intern. Med.*, *125*, 1067 (1970).

270 A. Stunkard, *Arch. Gen. Psychiatry*, *26*, 391 (1972).

271 H. F. Conn, "Current Therapy," W. B. Saunders, Philadelphia, Pa., 1975, p. 406.

272 W. G. Pace, *Ann. Surg.*, *190*, 392–400 (1979).

APPETITE SUPPRESSANT PRODUCT TABLE

Product (Manufacturer)	Phenylpropanolamine Hydrochloride	Bulk Producer	Other Ingredients
Acutrim 16 Hour Steady Control Tablets (Ciba Consumer)	75 mg	hydroxypropyl methylcellulose	cellulose acetate stearic acid
Acutrim Late Day Tablets (Ciba Consumer)	75 mg	hydroxypropyl methylcellulose	cellulose acetate FD&C yellow #6 isopropyl alcohol propylene glycol riboflavin stearic acid titanium dioxide
Acutrim II Maximum Strength Tablets (Ciba Consumer)	75 mg	hydroxypropyl methylcellulose	cellulose acetate FD&C yellow #10 FD&C blue #1 FD&C yellow #6 povidone propylene glycol stearic acid titanium dioxide
Appedrine Tablets (Thompson Medical)	25 mg		vitamin A, 1,667 IU vitamin D, 133 IU thiamine, 1 mg riboflavin, 1 mg pyridoxine hydrochloride, 0.33 mg vitamin E, 10 IU folic acid, 0.13 mg vitamin B_1, 0.5 mg vitamin B_2, 0.56 mg vitamin B_6, 0.66 mg vitamin B_{12}, 2 mcg iodine, 50 mcg iron, 4 mg copper, 0.66 mg zinc, 5 mg cyanocobalamin, 0.33 mcg ascorbic acid, 20 mg niacinamide, 7 mg calcium pantothenate, 3.33 mg
Control (Thompson Medical)	75 mg		
Dex-A-Diet Extended Release (O'Connor)	75 mg		
Dex-A-Diet, Maximum Strength (O'Connor)	75 mg		
Dex-A-Diet with Vitamin C Capsules, Timed Release (O'Connor)	75 mg		ascorbic acid, 200 mg
Dexatrim Capsules (Thompson Medical)	50 mg		
Dexatrim, Maximum Strength (Thompson Medical)	75 mg		
Dexatrim Plus Vitamin C, Maximum Strength Capsules, Timed Release (Thompson Medical)	75 mg		ascorbic acid, 180 mg
Dexatrim Pre-Meal (Thompson Medical)	25 mg		

APPETITE SUPPRESSANT PRODUCT TABLE, continued

Product (Manufacturer)	Phenylpropanolamine Hydrochloride	Bulk Producer	Other Ingredients
Dexatrim Tablets, Caffeine Free Maximum Strength (Thompson Medical)	75 mg		
Diet Ayds (DEP)			benzocaine, 6 mg
Diet-Trim Tablets (Pharmex)	NS[a]	carboxymethyl-cellulose	benzocaine
Dieutrim T.D. (Legere)	75 mg	sodium carboxy-methylcellulose, 75 mg	benzocaine, 9 mg
Grapefruit Diet Plan with Diadax (O'Connor)	30 mg		grapefruit extract
Grapefruit Diet Plan with Diadax, Extra Strength (O'Connor)	75 mg		grapefruit extract
Grapefruit Diet Plan with Diadax, Extra Strength Vitamin Fortified Continuous Action Capsules (O'Connor)	75 mg		natural grapefruit extract, 100 mg ascorbic acid, 60 mg vitamin E, 30 IU
Phenoxine (Lannett)	25 mg		
Prolamine Capsules (Thompson Medical)	37.5 mg		caffeine, 140 mg
Super Odrinex (Fox)	25 mg		
Thinz Back-To-Nature (Alva Amco)	75 mg		caffeine lecithin kelp cider vinegar riboflavin pyridoxine
Thinz Before Meals (Alva Amco)	25 mg		dicalcium phosphate ascorbic acid ferrous sulfate potassium iodide thiamine hydrochloride
Thinz Drops (Alva Amco)	25 mg/5 drops		fructose pyridoxine potassium
Thinz-Span (Alva Amco)	75 mg		caffeine riboflavin ascorbic acid iron thiamine hydrochloride alpha tocopherol iodine
Unitrol (Republic Drug)	75 mg		

[a] Quantity not specified.

WEIGHT CONTROL PRODUCT TABLE

Product (Manufacturer)	Dosage Form	Calories Supplied	Essential Composition
BULK PRODUCERS			
Diet-Aid (Rexall)	tablet	NS[a]	alginic acid, 200 mg sodium carboxymethylcellulose, 100 mg sodium bicarbonate, 70 mg
Metamucil (Procter & Gamble)	powder	14/tsp	psyllium hydrophilic mucilloid, 3.4 g carbohydrate (sucrose), 3.5 g sodium, 1 mg potassium, 31 mg
Metamucil, Instant Mix (Procter & Gamble)	powder in single dose packets	4/packet < 1/packet (orange flavor)	psyllium hydrophilic mucilloid, 3.4 g citric acid sodium, 1 mg potassium, 290 mg aspartame sodium bicarbonate
Metamucil Orange Flavor (Procter & Gamble)	powder	30/tbsp	psyllium hydrophilic mucilloid, 3.4 g carbohydrate (sucrose), 7.1 g citric acid sodium, 1 mg potassium, 31 mg
Pretts (MiLance)	tablet	4.5	alginic acid, 200 mg sodium carboxymethylcellulose, 100 mg sodium bicarbonate, 70 mg
ARTIFICIAL SWEETENERS			
Equal (Searle)	packets	4/g	aspartame
Necta Sweet (Goody's)	tablet	0	¼ grain-sodium saccharin, 12.3 mg ½ grain-sodium saccharin, 24.6 mg 1 grain-sodium saccharin, 49.2 mg (contains sodium bicarbonate)
Sweeta (Squibb)	liquid tablet	0	saccharin sodium, 7 mg/drop 15 mg/tablet
LOW-CALORIE FOODS			
Dietene (Doyle)	powder	190/packet	nonfat dry milk cocoa carrageenan artificial flavor lecithin polysorbate 80 malt vitamins sucrose calcium caseinate minerals sodium, 5.2 mEq/packet
Slender (Carnation)	bar liquid powder to be mixed with milk	275/2 bar serving 225/can 170 mixed with 6 oz. skim milk 225 mixed with 6 oz. whole milk	nonfat dry milk sucrose vegetable oil (in liquid and bar version) artificial flavors vitamins minerals

[a] Quantity not specified.

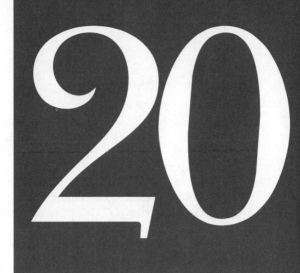

OPHTHALMIC PRODUCTS

Dick R. Gourley

Questions to ask in patient/consumer counseling

Is your vision blurred? Are your eyes painful as opposed to itching or stinging?

How long have these symptoms been present? What were you doing when you noticed them? Have you had a similar problem before?

Have you recently used a nonprescription eye product? Which one(s) did you use? For what symptoms?

Have you recently been in an accident or injured your head in any way?

Have you been working outside or in an environment that would cause your eyes to water or burn?

What is the nature of your work?

Have your eyes been exposed recently to irritants such as smog, chemicals, or sun glare? Have you recently used any pesticides or fertilizers?

Do you have any other eye problems (double vision, discharge, or twitch)?

Do you have a new pet?

Do you have a chronic disease such as diabetes, glaucoma, or hypertension?

Are you taking any prescription or nonprescription medications?

Do you wear contact lenses? Are they hard or soft lenses? What contact lens products do you use?

Do you have any allergies?

Have you recently had a head cold or sinus problem?

Do you use eye cosmetics? Do you use hair spray or spray deodorants?

Have you changed eye makeup brands or used a friend's eye makeup?

Pharmacists are often called upon to counsel patients experiencing ocular discomfort. In deciding between physician referral and self-medication, the pharmacist should have a thorough understanding of common eye problems. Minor symptoms may signal the beginning of a more serious problem that requires evaluation and treatment by a physician.

Nonprescription ophthalmic products are basically safe and effective only to relieve minor symptoms such as stinging, itching, tearing, "tired eyes," or "eye strain." These problems are usually self-limiting. Self-medication should be discouraged for people experiencing pain or blurred vision. These persons should be referred to a physician. A constraint with the use of nonprescription ophthalmic products is that conditions for which these products are useful generally require a hit-or-miss type of self-diagnosis. If the patient makes the wrong self-diagnosis, inappropriate therapy may exacerbate symptoms and possibly worsen the problem. Moreover, the active ingredients or preservatives in nonprescription products may cause allergic reactions. The Food and Drug Administration (FDA) advisory panel has issued some changes in its monograph on over-the-counter (OTC) ophthalmic drug products (1). The disorders and symptoms for which self-medication is indicated and may be effective or for which physician referral is indicated, as recommended by the FDA advisory review, are listed below.

Ocular disorders amenable to treatment with nonprescription products (1):

- Tear insufficiency—keratoconjunctivitis sicca (KCS) or dry-eye syndrome (medical diagnosis is indicated even if treatment is with nonprescription drugs);

- Corneal edema (medical diagnosis is indicated even if treatment is with nonprescription drugs);

- Inflammation and irritation of the eye—presence of loose foreign material in the eye, irritation from airborne pollutants and chlorinated water, and allergic conjunctivitis.

Ocular disorders for which self-medication may be effective (2):

- Hordeolum (stye);

- Blepharitis;

- Conjunctivitis.

Ocular disorders for which physician referral is indicated (2):

- Embedded foreign body;

- Uveitis;

- Glaucoma;

- Flash burns;

- Tear duct infections;

- Corneal ulcers.

EYE ANATOMY AND PHYSIOLOGY

The eye is divided into three general areas: the eyelids, the external eye, and the internal eye (Figure 1).

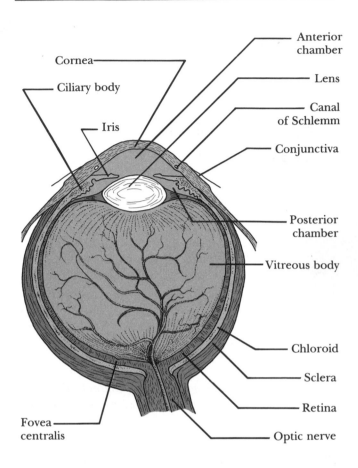

FIGURE 1 Horizontal cross-section showing the anatomy of the eyeball.

Eyelids

The eyelids are movable folds of tissue that protect the eye and distribute tears over the surface of the globe. The eyelids are covered anteriorly (externally) with skin, and lined posteriorly (internally) with conjunctiva, a thin transparent mucous membrane terminating at the corneal–scleral junction. Four types of glands are present in the lids: the meibomian glands, the glands of Zeis, Moll's glands, and the accessory lacrimal glands of Kraus and Wolfring. The meibomian glands are long sebaceous glands that secrete an oily substance that helps maintain the integrity of the tear film by preventing rapid evaporation. The glands of Zeis are smaller modified sebaceous glands associated with eyelash follicles; Moll's glands are modified sweat glands. The accessory lacrimal glands of Kraus and Wolfring supply most of the needed moisture to the conjunctival sac and cornea.

External Eye

The external eye consists of the lacrimal apparatus and the cul-de-sac that contains the lacrimal fluid. In the normal human eye, tears are constantly produced and removed, maintaining a resident volume of 7 mcl (3). The lacrimal fluid keeps the cornea and conjunctiva moist, protects the eye, clears away foreign materials from the eye (maintains a smooth optical surface), and inhibits the growth of microorganisms. Once formed, tears are conveyed across the corneal surface by the movement of the eyelids, finally collecting in the lower cul-de-sac for eventual drainage through the nasolacrimal duct into the nose.

Lid movement influences the drainage rate and thus physical movement of topically instilled drugs (3). The drainage apparatus begins at the punctum and ends in the nose. The passageway is a highly vascularized mucous membrane and consequently offers an extremely facile route for systemic absorption of topically instilled drugs, giving rise to the potential for systemic side effects (4–6).

Tear turnover in the precorneal area is rapid [16% per minute in humans (3)]. Any additional instilled fluid also drains away rapidly, with a rate constant proportional to the volume instilled (5). This process usually accounts for the loss of more than 90% of an instilled dose (7, 8); as a result, maintaining a high drug concentration for a prolonged period in the precorneal area is difficult.

Internal Eye

The eyeball (or globe) may be considered as a three-layered sac divided into three compartments filled with fluid. The three layers of the eye are an outer fibrous layer, consisting of the sclera (white of the eye) and the cornea; the middle vascular layer (uveal tract), consisting of the iris, ciliary body, and choroid; and the inner photoreceptor layer, consisting of the pigmented epithelium and retina. The three compartments are the anterior chamber, the space between the iris and the cornea; the posterior chamber, the space between the iris and the lens; and the vitreous cavity, the space posterior to the lens. Blood circulates through the conjunctiva, sclera, uveal tract, and other parts of the eye. Aqueous humor is found in both the anterior and posterior chambers of the eye; vitreous humor is found in the vitreous cavity.

The sclera makes up about 85% of the globe surface. Anteriorly, it joins with the cornea. The cornea is a smooth, nearly circular, layered structure averaging 1 mm thick in adults. The cornea consists of five distinct layers including the epithelium, Bowman's layer, the stroma, Descemet's membrane, and the endothelium. The corneal epithelium is lipophilic and will allow the passage of fat-soluble substances. Disruption of the corneal epithelium may alter the transport of topically applied drugs. The corneal stroma is hydrophilic and allows passage of water-soluble substances. The penetration of topically applied drugs through the cornea depends on phase solubility. The endothelium and, to a lesser degree, the epithelium provide a barrier to excessive corneal hydration. The cornea is also optically clear, thus allowing passage of light. Damage to either endothelium or epithelium tissue may lead to corneal edema and decreased transparency.

The iris, a thin, circular disk in front of the lens, regulates the amount of light reaching the retina by using two muscles, the sphincter pupillae and the dilator pupillae. Surrounding the globe just posterior to the limbus, where the cornea and sclera join, is the ciliary muscle. The ciliary body is composed of the ciliary muscles and the ciliary epithelium. The ciliary muscle changes the shape of the lens, enabling the eye to focus on near objects (accommodation). The ciliary epithelium is important in the production of aqueous humor. The choroid, which is mainly composed of blood vessels, supplies blood to the retinal pigment epithelium and the external layers of the retina (rods, cones, and inner nuclear layer). The internal layers of the retina are supplied by the central retinal artery.

The anterior chamber, the space between the iris and the cornea, is encircled by the trabecular meshwork, the outflow channel for aqueous humor via the canal of Schlemm. The canal of Schlemm is a circular modified venous structure in the anterior chamber angle. The meshwork consists of multiple perforated sheets (9–11). The aqueous humor is actively secreted by the ciliary epithelium of the ciliary body and flows from the posterior chamber through the pupillary opening into the anterior chamber.

The aqueous humor fills the anterior and posterior chambers. Its main functions are maintenance of the intraocular pressure and nourishment of the avascular lens and cornea. The aqueous humor turnover rate is 1–1.4% per minute, or about 2.75 mcl per minute, of which about 80% exits via the canal of Schlemm (12–14). The bulk flow of aqueous humor is a primary means of drug removal in the internal eye (15).

The lens is a biconvex structure located in the posterior chamber behind the iris. Its function is to focus light rays on the retina. Behind the lens is the vitreous cavity. Light passing through the cornea and lens converges in this space. The vitreous humor is a transparent jelly-like substance that fills the vitreous cavity, supports the structures within the eye, and helps maintain the transparency of the eye because it is impervious to cells and debris.

TABLE 2 Differentiation of the common types of conjunctivitis

Clinical findings and cytology	Viral	Bacterial	Chlamydial	Atopic (allergic)
Itching	Minimal	Minimal	Minimal	Severe
Hyperemia	Generalized	Generalized	Generalized	Generalized
Tearing	Profuse	Moderate	Moderate	Moderate
Exudation	Minimal	Profuse	Profuse	Minimal
Preauricular adenopathy	Common	Uncommon	Common only in inclusion conjunctivitis	None
In stained scrapings and exudates	Monocytes	Bacteria, PMNs*	PMNs*, plasma cells, inclusion bodies	Eosinophils
Associated sore throat and fever	Occasionally	Occasionally	Never	Never

*PMNs = polymorphonucleocytes.

Reprinted with permission from D. Vaughn et al., "General Ophthalmology," 12th ed., Appleton and Lange, San Mateo, Calif., and Norwalk, Conn., 1989, p. 76.

junctiva should be referred to an ophthalmologist for critical assessment of possible trauma to the globe or conjunctiva.

Conjunctival irritation due to foreign bodies, chemical irritants, or allergies generally is treated by removing the cause and administering nonprescription decongestants. A clue to chemical conjunctivitis, caused by airborne irritants such as smoke, smog, or garden sprays, is that both eyes are involved. Allergic conjunctivitis usually occurs on warm, windy days in the spring and during hay fever season. Typical symptoms, such as swelling, congestion, stinging, watering, and itching, affect both eyes.

Bacterial conjunctivitis usually is self-limiting and does not impair vision. If the patient awakens with the eyelids stuck together by dried exudate or if there is discharge or signs of swelling of the preauricular lymph node, the etiology is probably bacterial. In such cases, nonprescription ophthalmic products have only limited efficacy (19). Referral to a physician is needed because recovery may be hastened with an appropriate prescription drug, such as a sulfonamide or another antibiotic-containing ophthalmic product. Without treatment, most bacterial conjunctivitis lasts 10–14 days, although infections caused by species of *Staphylococcus* and *Moraxella* may become chronic. The more common forms of bacterial conjunctivitis (staphylococcal or diplococcal) are characterized by a purulent discharge. Corneal infections may exhibit symptoms similar to those of bacterial conjunctivitis. These infections are more serious and may rapidly obliterate vision. An accurate diagnosis is important. Pinkeye, a moderately contagious bacterial infection of the conjunctiva caused by species of *Hemophilus* in warm climates and species of *Pneumococci* in temperate climates, is characterized by an acute onset of conjunctival hyperemia and a moderate amount of mucopurulent discharge. If there is pain or photophobia, the cornea may be affected (20).

Viral conjunctivitis may resemble chemically induced conjunctivitis; symptoms may include red, perhaps swollen, watery, itching eyes and swollen preauricular lymph nodes. Unlike chemical irritations, however, viral conjunctivitis often is accompanied by systemic symptoms. In Newcastle disease conjunctivitis (a rare disorder that occurs in poultry workers, veterinarians, or laboratory helpers working with live virus), the patient may develop an influenza-like syndrome with symptoms including mild fever, headache, and arthralgia (19, 20). By careful patient questioning, the pharmacist may discover that the patient also has influenza. The reddened eyes in such cases suggest viral conjunctivitis, which is not amenable to specific drug therapy.

Lacrimal Disorders

The therapy of dacryoadenitis (inflammation of the lacrimal gland) is determined by etiology. Assessment should be made by a physician.

Decreased tear production may be associated with aging, physical trauma, and infection (trachoma), or may be induced by antihistamines or anticholinergic drug products. Symptoms are burning and constant foreign body sensation, and reddened and dry eyes.

Treatment is tear replacement with artificial tear products. These nonprescription products are very similar; however, a patient may be sensitive to a certain product because of the components in the formulation such as the vehicle, buffering agents, preservatives, or the pH of the product. If sensitive to a certain product, the patient should try a different product.

Continued self-medication of a dry-eye syndrome without professional diagnosis may exacerbate the underlying condition by delaying medical treatment. The FDA advisory review panel on OTC ophthalmic drug products concluded that "directions suggesting long-term use [of artificial tear products] should be limited to professional labeling and should not be a part of the OTC labeling. While these products are intended to serve as tear substitutes and are used on an ongoing basis, safeguards against the [long-term] unsupervised use of tear substitute preparations for long periods must be established through proper labeling, warning that professional consultation should be sought if symptoms persist for more than 72 hours" (21).

Some allergic reactions may cause excessive tearing, itching, and watery eyes. Cold water compresses and cool, clean air are beneficial for symptomatic relief, as are nonprescription vasoconstrictors. If, as in hay fever, the causative agent cannot be removed, oral antihistamines may be useful.

Internal Eye Conditions

Internal eye disorders may have far greater consequences than conditions of the external eye. Early diagnosis may help prevent partial or total loss of vision. The pharmacist should emphasize the importance of physician referral.

Glaucoma

Glaucoma is characterized by increased intraocular pressure, causing degeneration of the optic disk and defects in the visual field (19, 22, 23). It may be classified as either primary (including open-angle, narrow-angle, or hypersecretion glaucoma), congenital, or secondary. The most common form is primary open-angle glaucoma. Initial treatment of open-angle and secondary glaucoma may be medical; narrow-angle and congenital glaucoma treatment is generally surgical. Most chronic open-angle glaucoma will eventually require surgical intervention (24).

Primary open-angle glaucoma occurs as a result of decreased outflow (drainage) of aqueous humor from the anterior chamber of the eye. In patients with this disorder, the chamber angles appear normal. The decreased outflow is most likely caused by degenerative changes in the trabecular meshwork and canal of Schlemm. Open-angle glaucoma causes no early symptoms, and some loss of vision usually occurs late in the progress of the disease. Both eyes are nearly always involved, although one eye may be more severely affected (22). There is no pain with open-angle glaucoma.

Secondary glaucoma also occurs as a result of decreased outflow. Foreign bodies or tumors obstructing the trabecular meshwork, ocular inflammation, ocular trauma, hemorrhage, and topical corticosteroid therapy are causes of secondary glaucoma.

Narrow-angle glaucoma (angle-closure or acute glaucoma) is characterized by a sudden onset of blurred vision followed by excruciating pain that may be accompanied by nausea and vomiting. It occurs with sudden increase in intraocular tension due to a block of the anterior chamber angle by the root of the iris, which cuts off all aqueous outflow. The chamber angle is anatomically closed. Any abnormal dilation of the pupil (for example, from mydriatics) or swelling of the iris or lens may produce this obstruction. Narrow-angle glaucoma can be very dangerous and requires immediate referral to a physician or emergency room (23).

Cataracts

Approximately 15% of the individuals in the United States who are considered legally blind have cataracts as an underlying cause. A cataract is an opacity of the crystalline lens. At present, drug therapy is not a treatment for cataracts but only an aid for certain symptoms. However, the pharmacist may be questioned by patients concerned with cataracts. Many patients are under the misconception that medications are available without a prescription for treatment of cataracts. No medications, glasses, diet, or exercise will reduce the effect of a cataract once it is formed. The only way to improve the vision in an eye with a cataract is to surgically remove the opacity. Laser surgery has greatly improved this procedure (25).

Uveitis

Uveitis is a general term for inflammatory disorders of the uveal tract. Causes include infection, trauma, abnormalities such as cataracts, and systemic inflammatory disease. One or all three portions of the uveal tract may be involved simultaneously. Anterior uveitis refers to an inflammation of the iris (iritis) and/or the ciliary body (iridocyclitis); posterior uveitis refers to an inflammation of the choroid (choroiditis) and/or the retina (chorioretinitis) (19).

TREATMENT

Internal eye conditions are not amenable to treatment by nonprescription products. They must be diagnosed and treated by a physician. Most nonprescription ophthalmic products are promoted for relief of noninfectious conjunctivitis. If an irritant has not been sprayed or instilled directly into the eye and if the cornea is not abraded, nonprescription decongestants or artificial tears are useful in relieving the discomfort. It may be advisable to discontinue topical application of cosmetics while using a nonprescription decongestant. Nonprescription decongestants should not be used with other topical ophthalmic drugs because the pharmacokinetic characteristics of the drugs may be changed.

The following list gives specific recommendations for treatment of conditions that may be amenable to self-medication (2).

■ Tear insufficiency—KCS (dry-eye syndrome) may be treated with artificial tear products. The products with the more viscous vehicles, such as methylcellulose or polyvinyl alcohol, provide a longer contact time. Tear replacement is the first treatment; if this is not successful, other therapeutic measures such as ocular inserts or soft contact lens therapy are used. Selection of an ocular lubricant product will depend on patient acceptance as well as product quality (26). The various formulations of these products may result in sensitivity of patients to certain specific products. In this case, products with a different formulation should be suggested. Patients should be advised to consult a physician if these measures do not provide satisfactory relief.

■ Corneal edema—If corneal edema is not a result of recognized causes, such as elevated intraocular pressure, endothelial damage, or epithelial damage, self-medication may be helpful. Hypertonic solutions such as sodium chloride 5% (drops or ointment) may provide a sufficient dehydrating effect. The ocular decongestants may also be beneficial. If the condition persists for more than 24 hours, the patient should be referred to a physician.

■ Inflammation and irritation—Presence of loose foreign material in the eye such as dust or lint may be removed by flushing the eye with water or using an eyewash (Collyrium). The use of a medicated product is usually not necessary. Irritation from airborne pollutants and/or chlorinated water is amenable to treatment with nonprescription products. Ocular decongestants used after swimming will give relief, and in some cases use of artificial tear products may be helpful. Allergic conjunctivitis may be treated with ocular decongestants to give symptomatic re-

lief. If the symptoms do not resolve within 3 days, the patient should be referred to a physician.

■ Hordeola—External or internal hordeola (stye) may be resolved by use of hot compresses applied for 10 minutes, 3 or 4 times daily. Sometimes treatment will require application of antibiotic or ophthalmic solutions for several days. Minor styes may be resolved if they are treated early with hot compresses.

Eye patches are used in occlusion therapy of amblyopia, thereby forcing the patient to depend on the amblyopic eye for vision. Treatment of certain ocular conditions in young children includes eye patches applied for 1 or 2 days after treatment of corneal abrasion, removal of a foreign body, or an ultraviolet sunlamp burn. Eye patches should not be used unless they are recommended by a physician. In some cases (young children), eye patches may induce strabismus or amblyopia (26).

Ophthalmologists and optometrists (where state law permits) occasionally use steroids to treat allergic conjunctivitis. Pharmacists should watch for evidence of chronic steroid use (repeated requests for prescription renewal) because long-term use may cause glaucoma and/or cataracts and exacerbate herpetic corneal ulcers.

Patients experiencing pain or blurred vision should be referred to a physician. The pharmacist may suggest oral analgesics as an interim measure to relieve the pain until a physician can be contacted. (See Chapter 5, *Internal Analgesic Products*.)

Pharmaceutical Agents

The use of pharmaceutical (inactive) and medicinal (active) agents has been classified by the FDA as "monograph conditions" and "nonmonograph conditions." Monograph conditions refer to those conditions that are generally recognized as safe and effective and are not misbranded (old Category I), whereas nonmonograph conditions refer to those conditions that are not generally recognized as safe and effective and are misbranded, or available data are insufficient to classify as safe and effective and further testing is required (old Category II and Category III, respectively).

In general, nonprescription and prescription ophthalmic products must be initially sterile and must have bacteriostatic additives to maintain sterility. Bacteriostatic agents are not required for unit dose containers. These agents should be buffered, optically clear, and free from particles, filaments, and fibers. In addition, they must not contain any extraneous excipients such as coloring agents or fragrance, and they should approximate the tonicity and pH of tears as nearly as possible.

Although not a legal (i.e., FDA) requirement, good pharmaceutical practice suggests that all ophthalmic products should have an expiration date and should be used or discarded within 3 months from the date of opening. Another hazard associated with ophthalmic solutions is the introduction of drug crystals into the eye as a result of drug crystallization on the lip of the bottle or the dropper tip. However, microbial contamination is a more serious problem. Consequently, the patient should be warned not to touch the tip of the dispenser and to keep the container tightly closed when not in use. All ophthalmic solutions that are cloudy or discolored or that contain foreign particles should be discarded.

Nontherapeutic substances in nonprescription ophthalmic preparations include antioxidants, stabilizers, buffers, wetting or clarifying agents, antimicrobial preservatives, tonicity adjusters, vehicles for ointments, and viscosity-increasing agents. Because the eye is a sensitive organ, the FDA advisory review panel on OTC ophthalmic drug products reviewed inactive as well as active compounds. It noted that some agents traditionally considered inactive as formulation aids could be active in certain situations, such as agents used as emollients and demulcents. The panel ruled that labeling claims of this activity in the product necessitated classification of that agent as an active ingredient; if no claim was made for that activity, the agent was considered to be inactive (27).

The FDA panel determined that the ingredients listed in Table 3 meet the monograph condition for their respective ophthalmic drug class (1).

Antioxidants and Stabilizers

Edetic acid (sodium salt), sodium bisulfite (0.1%), sodium metabisulfite (0.1%), sodium thiosulfate (0.2%), and thiourea (0.1%) were classified as acceptable for use in ophthalmic solutions by the FDA advisory review panel on OTC ophthalmic drug products. Chemically, edetic acid chelates metal ions that would otherwise be free to catalyze redox reactions; the other four agents exercise their effectiveness by being oxidized preferentially instead of the active therapeutic component.

Buffers

Agents used as buffer components in nonprescription ophthalmic solutions include acetic acid, boric acid, hydrochloric acid, phosphoric acid, potassium bicarbonate, potassium borate and tetraborate, potassium carbonate, potassium citrate, the potassium phosphates (mono-, di-, and tribasic), sodium acetate, sodium bicarbonate, sodium biphosphate, sodium borate, sodium carbonate, sodium citrate, sodium hydroxide, and sodium phosphate. All are accepted by the FDA, although choice of a specific buffer depends on the drug used in the product being formulated.

Tears have a pH of 7.4; consequently, tear substitutes and all ophthalmic products should approximate this level. The acceptable pH range for ophthalmic products is 6.0–8.0 (28); products outside this range may be irritating. In an animal study, products outside the range of 4.0–10.0 with a strong buffer capacity caused corneal damage (29). The eye is able to tolerate products outside the acceptable range if the buffering capacity is low because the tears can overcome the buffer and return the eye to the physiologic level. This enables drug products to be formulated with a low pH for stability purposes and still allow the product to be relatively nonirritating. The buffer system contributes to the tonicity of the ophthalmic product. The tonicity of the entire formulation should approximate 0.9% sodium chloride solution to be isotonic with lacrimal fluid.

Wetting or Clarifying Agents

Polysorbate 80 (1.0%), polysorbate 20 (1.0%), poloxamer 282 (Pluronic L-92) (0.25%), and tyloxapol (Triton WR-1339) (0.25%) reduce surface tension, and thereby allow the solution to better wet the eye. However, they may decrease phenylmercuric nitrate antibacterial activity. Tyloxapol is used for in situ cleaning of artificial eyes.

Preservatives

Preservatives prevent growth of or destroy microorganisms accidentally introduced into the container after opening. The pharmacist should discuss proper instillation technique with the patient to lessen the opportunity for contamination.

The use of several preservatives has been classified by the FDA as monograph conditions. Benzalkonium chloride and benzethonium chloride are accepted as preservatives, although claims of effectiveness as cleaning agents or antibacterials have not been satisfactorily substantiated. When concentrations of benzalkonium chloride higher than 0.013% (0.017, 0.033, and 0.10%) were applied experimentally to rabbit eyes, corneal damage was reported. Benzalkonium chloride may be present in nonprescription products as a 0.013% concentration alone or in combination with edetic acid or an edetate salt. This concentration may be used safely within the eye. Benzalkonium chloride (0.02%) is available for instillation into the cul-de-sac to clean artificial eyes in situ. It is incompatible with nitrates and salicylates; however, very few ophthalmic products contain nitrates or salicylates. This product is not for use in the normal intact eye.

TABLE 3   Agents in ophthalmic drug products meeting FDA's monograph condition

Ophthalmic drug class	Ingredient	Ophthalmic drug class	Ingredient
Astringent	Zinc sulfate (0.25%)	Emollient (continued)	Light mineral oil (up to 50% in combination with one or more emollient agents included in the monograph)
Demulcent	Carboxymethylcellulose sodium (0.2–2.5%)		Mineral oil (up to 50% in combination with one or more emollient agents included in the monograph)
	Dextran 70 (0.1% when used with another polymeric demulcent agent included in the monograph)		Paraffin (up to 5% in combination with one or more emollient agents included in the monograph)
	Gelatin (0.01%)		Petrolatum (up to 100%)
	Glycerin (0.2–1%)		White ointment (up to 100%)
	Hydroxyethyl cellulose (0.2–2.5%)		White petrolatum (up to 100%)
	Hydroxypropyl methylcellulose (0.2–2.5%)		White wax (up to 5% in combination with one or more emollient agents included in the monograph)
	Methylcellulose (0.2–2.5%)		Yellow wax (up to 5% in combination with one or more emollient agents included in the monograph)
	Polyethylene gylcol 300 (0.2–1%)		
	Polyethylene glycol 400 (0.2–1%)		
	Polysorbate 80 (0.2–1%)	Eyewash	Water, tonicity agent(s), pH and buffering agent(s), and a preservative
	Polyvinyl alcohol (0.1–4%)		
	Povidone (0.1–2%)	Hypertonicity agent	Sodium chloride (2–5%)
	Propylene glycol (0.2–1%)	Vasoconstrictor	Ephedrine hydrochloride (0.123%)
Emollient	Anhydrous lanolin (1–10% in combination with one or more oleaginous emollient agents included in the monograph)		Naphazoline hydrochloride (0.01–0.03%)
			Phenylephrine hydrochloride (0.08–0.2%)
	Lanolin (1–10% in combination with one or more oleaginous emollient agents included in the monograph)		Tetrahydrozoline hydrochloride (0.01–0.05%)

From *Federal Register, 21*, 7089 (1988).

Benzethonium chloride in concentrations up to 0.01% may be present in products intended for instillation into the human eye. Products that are not intended for instillation directly in the eye may contain benzethonium chloride in a maximum concentration of 0.02%. Benzethonium chloride is also incompatible with nitrates and salicylates.

Chlorobutanol is another commonly used preservative. This agent hydrolyzes above a pH of 5 or 6 and

also permeates plastic. Hence, it may be partially or completely lost from a solution that is stored in a plastic container (with a comparable loss of effectiveness), depending on the container's wall thickness and the storage temperature.

Edetic acid is not effective alone as a preservative but enhances the action of benzalkonium chloride, thimerosal, and other agents. It is a weak primary sensitizer, and products containing this agent have been implicated in allergic reactions (30).

The mercurial preservatives (phenylmercuric acetate, phenylmercuric nitrate, and thimerosal) are moderately effective bacteriostats. However, they have a slow kill rate and may induce allergic reactions. Thimerosal may be a contact allergen because of the thio or mercuric radical. Thimerosal is used as an antiseptic in ophthalmic ointments used for conjunctivitis and corneal ulcers and to prevent infection following removal of foreign bodies. However, the FDA advisory review panel has not assessed the effectiveness of the compound as an antiseptic in the concentrations employed.

The advisory review panel is investigating several other agents, but there is insufficient evidence concerning their safety and efficacy. The use of cetylpyridinium chloride is classified as suitable for nonmonograph conditions because of its extensive binding capabilities.

Chlorhexidine hydrochloride and gluconate are not used routinely in the United States in ophthalmic products that are instilled into the eye. However, they are used in contact lens products that are not instilled. Parabens (methyl and propyl p-hydroxybenzoate) are efficient only at the limit of solubility, and they are irritating at that concentration. In addition, they are known sensitizers and a source of carbon for *Pseudomonas aeruginosa*. (See Chapter 21, *Contact Lenses and Lens Care Products*.)

Sodium propionate is a fungistat of questionable use in ophthalmics. Sodium benzoate and sorbic acid, alone or in combination with other agents, have not been shown to be safe and effective preservatives for ophthalmic use even though they have been used by the food, drug, and cosmetic industries for years. Other preservatives such as polyquaternium-1 (Polyquad) and polyaminopropyl biguanide (Dymed) have recently been introduced by various ophthalmic manufacturers (30).

Tonicity Adjusters

Products of 0.9 ± 0.2% sodium chloride equivalence may be considered isotonic and comparable to natural tears in tonicity. The eye tolerates 0.6–1.8% sodium chloride equivalence without damage (28–31). In addition to the danger of ocular damage, solutions at nonphysiologic tonicity may elicit excessive blinking or tearing. This severely hampers the products' bioavailability because of early washout by eye fluids (15). Agents used to adjust tonicity in ophthalmic preparations are dextrose, glycerin (1%), potassium chloride, propylene glycol (1%), and sodium chloride, in addition to those agents used as buffers.

Viscosity-Increasing Agents

Viscosity inducers may be used for their wetting, adhesive, and/or lubricating properties, specifically in dry-eye treatment (artificial tears). Increased viscosity moderately increases the bioavailability of therapeutic agents by increasing retention time (8, 33). Many of the polymers may influence interfacial tension, lowering surface tensions of saline from 72.2 dynes/cm to about 50 dynes/cm (42–66 dynes/cm) when present in a 1% concentration. They aid in wetting the eye by decreasing the contact angle of the solutions and therefore increasing the liquid's tendency to spread (32). They are virtually nontoxic in the concentrations used in ophthalmic products. Many of the polymers are film formers and may build up on contact lenses. The following agents are acceptable for use to increase viscosity in ophthalmic products:

- Cellulose derivatives—carboxymethyl cellulose sodium, hydroxyethylcellulose, hydroxypropyl methylcellulose, methylcellulose;

- Dextran 70;

- Gelatin (0.01%);

- Liquid polyols—glycerin, polyethylene glycol 300, polysorbate 80, propylene glycol, polyvinyl alcohol 2%, povidone.

There is insufficient evidence on acetylated polyvinyl alcohol, and it has been classified as nonmonograph conditions.

There are differences among artificial tear products, including their effect on tear breakup time (30). In general, products containing viscosity agents are retained about twice as long as saline solution (several minutes). The retention time depends on the viscosity and the drainage rate, and not entirely on the concentration of the polymer (33). Methylcellulose solutions, as formulated, are more viscous than polyvinyl alcohol solutions and tend to form crusts on the eyelids, which may be annoying to some patients. However, the methylcellulose solutions are retained longer than the polyvinyl alcohol solutions because of their higher viscosity for a given concentration. Products containing polyethylene glycol polymers are claimed to possess a mucomimetic property similar to gelatin and bovine mucin. Wetting of the corneal surface is facilitated in the presence of these substances (33).

Patients should be advised not to use alkaline borate products concomitantly with products containing polyvinyl alcohol because gummy deposits may result.

Vehicles in Ophthalmic Ointments

Many types of vehicles (petrolatum, vegetable oils, white and yellow waxes, mineral oils, lanolin, and lanolin substitutes such as polyethylene glycols) are used in ophthalmic ointments. Some of these substances are used as adjuncts to modify the product's consistency. These agents are considered to be safe and effective for lubricating the eye or providing an emollient effect, or as drug delivery systems. Consideration must be given to the preservatives necessary to maintain sterility because the significant increase in retention time could result in corneal damage by these agents.

Medicinal Agents

Therapeutic agents contained in nonprescription ophthalmic products include antipruritics, anti-infectives, astringents, and decongestants/vasoconstrictors. Few of these drugs have been proven effective. Many are contraindicated in specific conditions.

Antipruritics

Antipyrine (0.1–0.4%), camphor, and menthol are present in some nonprescription ophthalmic medications because of their mild local analgesic and cooling effect. Such products are considered generally unsafe because the local analgesia produced may mask the presence of foreign bodies, leading to severe corneal abrasions.

Anti-infectives

There is no acceptable nonprescription ophthalmic anti-infective available for treatment of minor external eye infections. Boric acid is weakly effective at best and at worst may be dangerous because systemic absorption may result in boron toxicity. Silver protein products are effective but lack patient acceptability because of their staining properties. Yellow mercuric oxide has been marketed in the past, and there is recent evidence to support its efficacy in the treatment of blepharitis (34). The FDA categorizes the use of these products for monograph conditions.

The FDA advisory review panel has reviewed sulfacetamide 10% (available only on prescription) for deregulation to nonprescription standing to treat surface infections of eyelids and conjunctiva. Evaluation of the data suggest that it would not be safe for nonprescription use because of its irritating and allergic potential. In addition, indiscriminate use could lead to overgrowth of resistant strains of organisms (35).

Astringents

Astringents are applied locally to precipitate proteins and reduce local edema and inflammation. These agents help to clear mucus from the outer surface of the eye and are used for the temporary relief of minor eye irritations. In high concentrations, many astringents are irritating or caustic; therefore, they must be formulated in concentrations low enough to be nonirritating. Barberine, hydrastine, peppermint oil, rose geranium oil, and infusion of rose petals were promoted as astringents in ophthalmic products. These products were judged unacceptable by the FDA advisory review panel because there was no substantive evidence of safety and effectiveness (36).

The only astringent recommended by the FDA advisory review panel for use in OTC ophthalmic products is zinc sulfate (0.25%) used together with a preservative, buffer, and tonicity adjusters. The dosage for adults and children is 1 to 2 drops of a 0.25% solution instilled in the affected eye up to 4 times a day. Zinc salts have no decongestant action; however, they may be used in combination with a single vasoconstrictor. By themselves, they are mild vasodilators in the concentrations used. Zinc sulfate is indicated for temporary relief from minor eye irritations.

Demulcents

Demulcents are usually water-soluble polymers that are applied topically to the eye to protect and lubricate mucous membrane surfaces and relieve dryness and irritation that may be caused by exposure to wind and sun.

The water-soluble polymers used in this capacity also have viscosity-increasing properties and have been discussed in the section on viscosity-increasing agents. Formulations may contain up to three demulcents, a preservative, buffers, and tonicity adjusters. See Table 3 for a list of these agents.

Decongestants/Vasoconstrictors

Vasoconstrictors are effective in the symptomatic treatment of allergic conjunctivitis and offer temporary relief of redness of the eye caused by minor eye irritations. Reddened eyes usually are rapidly whitened by vasoconstrictors that limit the local vascular response by constricting the blood vessels. The vasoconstrictors, which are all sympathomimetic amines, not only affect the vascular receptors but also may stimulate alpha-adrenergic receptors on the dilator pupillae causing pupillary dilation.

These agents generally are contraindicated in known narrow-angle glaucoma patients. They are designed specifically for short-term, primarily cosmetic use and should not be used on a regular basis. They are potentially hazardous in that they may mask symptoms of a serious problem, thereby delaying necessary medical treatment.

If an ophthalmic decongestant is used when there is disease of the globe interior, no relief can be expected, and complications from the lack of primary treatment may occur. Furthermore, bacterial or other infections also may be masked by the use of symptomatic treatment. If an ocular condition persists for more than 72 hours, the patient should be referred to a physician. Drugs used as decongestants/vasoconstrictors are ephedrine hydrochloride (0.123%), naphazoline hydrochloride (0.01 to 0.03%), phenylephrine (0.08 to 0.2%), oxymetazoline (0.025%), and tetrahydrozoline (0.01 to 0.05%) (1, 30, 37).

Ephedrine is similar to epinephrine in that it is short acting and produces rebound congestion. However, it is more stable than epinephrine.

The imidazoline derivatives, naphazoline, oxymetazoline, and tetrahydrozoline, are more stable and have a longer duration of action than epinephrine (2 to 3 hours). They are buffered to pH 6.2. Naphazoline is used in prescription ophthalmic solutions at a concentration of 0.1%; however, this high concentration is not considered safe for nonprescription use. Untoward effects occurring after use of imidazoline class drugs have been reported, particularly central nervous system (CNS) stimulation after accidental ingestion by children. Although rebound congestion was reported after prolonged intranasal use of naphazoline, it has not been reported after ophthalmic use.

Phenylephrine is the vasoconstrictor used most commonly in nonprescription ophthalmic products. Its effectiveness is variable because of its relative instability (30). Solutions usually are effective initially, but with continued use, oxidation may reduce the product's activity significantly although no evidence of discoloration is present. Furthermore, phenylephrine products in polyethylene containers may be less stable than those packaged in glass. Oxygen diffuses through the polyethylene and hastens oxidation of the amine unless an oxygen-resistant coating is put over the plastic bottle. Patients allergic to epinephrine may show cross-sensitivity to phenylephrine.

Rebound congestion may occur following the prolonged use of vasoconstrictors in the eye. The tissues become more congested and edematous as the vasoconstriction action of the drug subsides. The phenomenon causes a vicious cycle because it leads to more frequent use of the drug that causes it.

A typical formulation would contain a single vasoconstrictor (or a single vasoconstrictor and zinc sulfate as an astringent), preservatives, buffers, tonicity agents, stabilizers, and viscosity agents (38).

Emollients

Emollients are usually oleagenous materials applied locally to the eyelids to protect or soften tissues and prevent drying and cracking. An emollient is used as an eye lubricant to relieve dryness and irritation that may be caused by exposure to wind and sun. In this respect, an emollient is similar to a demulcent. These agents are also used as vehicles in ophthalmic ointments and are discussed in the section on ophthalmic ointment vehicles.

Formulations usually contain two or more emollients and a preservative. See Table 3 for a list of these agents.

Eye Washes

Eye washes contain no active ingredient and are intended for bathing or mechanically flushing the eye to remove loose foreign material, air pollutants, or chlorinated water.

Eye washes simply contain preservatives, buffers, and tonicity agents.

Hypertonic Agents

Symptomatic relief of corneal swelling may be produced by hypertonic solutions. The only acceptable hypertonic agent for nonprescription use is sodium chloride in a concentration of 2–5%. Sodium chloride is available for nonprescription use as a sterile solution or ointment. The dosage for adults and children is 1 to 2 drops of a 2–5% concentration instilled in the affected eyes every 3 or 4 hours or as directed by a physician. Pharmacists should warn the patient of transient stinging and burning. Although available for nonprescription use, such concentrated solutions should be used only under the advice of a physician.

A formulation contains sodium chloride (2–5%), preservatives, and viscosity agents (38).

Pharmacokinetic Considerations

Properties of the drug, its formulation, and the eye itself influence the pharmacokinetics of topical ophthalmic products. Pharmacists should consider these factors when recommending a nonprescription ophthalmic preparation.

The physical drug properties that probably have the most effect on transport of the drug into and through the eye are lipid solubility and water solubility (39). Protein-binding of drugs in the tear fluids may further reduce the amount of free drug available for absorption and thus adversely affect its bioavailability. Metabolism in the precorneal area and absorption by tissues other than the cornea also are potential drug loss mechanisms (39–42). Because the conjunctiva and nasolacrimal duct are highly vascularized, drugs may be absorbed into the bloodstream and lost from the target site (43). Moreover, because drugs in the eye are eliminated primarily by bulk flow, elimination may be either enhanced or retarded by a drug's pharmacologic effect. In a glaucomatous eye, the reduction of intraocular pressure brought about by increased outflow could lessen the duration of action of the drug (15).

The concentration, volume instilled, and contact time also are important variables that may affect a drug's ocular availability and effectiveness. High concentrations may cause irritation, which in turn causes tearing and thus flushing of the precorneal area, removing the drug from the absorption site (15). Because the nasolacrimal drainage rate also is a function of instilled volume, it is desirable to administer the smallest volume of product possible. In addition, patients instilling more than one medication into the eye should wait at least 3–5 minutes between drops. This procedure ensures that the first drop is not flushed away by the second drop or, conversely, the second drop is not diluted by the first. Both conditions would reduce bioavailability (5, 44).

The eye is a unique system relative to biopharmaceutics and pharmacokinetics. Several factors not dependent on the drug molecule itself greatly influence the activity of the applied drug. The absorption and elimination rate constants used to explain the kinetics of drug transport are a complication of the various processes going on in the whole system, dominated by an apparent parallel elimination in the precorneal area, distribution in the aqueous humor, and bulk flow from the aqueous humor (15).

PRODUCT SELECTION GUIDELINES

The following general guidelines should help the pharmacist in selecting a suitable nonprescription ophthalmic product:

- Nonprescription ophthalmic products should be used only in situations where vision is not threatened and should not be used for longer than 72 hours without medical referral, unless a stye is involved; nonprescription treatment of a stye may take 3 or 4 days before the stye subsides.

- Nonprescription ocular medications should not be recommended to patients who have demonstrated an allergy to any of the active ingredients, preservatives, or other agents in the product.

- Patients with narrow-angle glaucoma should not use sympathomimetic amines, and patients with open-angle glaucoma should use these drugs only on the advice of a physician.

- Patients already using a prescription ophthalmic product should use nonprescription ophthalmic products only after consulting with a pharmacist or a physician.

The pharmacist should instruct the patient on the proper use of ophthalmic products (45). Before administration, the hands should be washed and the product inspected for expiration date, contamination, discoloration, or other problems. The detection of contamination and discoloration may be difficult for the patient because of the use of plastic bottles. Therefore, the pharmacist should stress appropriate storage and administration techniques.

Ophthalmic drops should be administered to the patient with the head tilted back and up. The skin below the eye just above the cheekbone should be pulled down, and the fluid dropped into the lower conjunctival sac away from the tear ducts. To avoid contamination, the dropper tip should not touch the eye or lid. Suspension fluids should be shaken well before they are instilled.

To administer ophthalmic ointments, the patient should assume the same position. A thin line of ointment should be applied along the conjunctival surface of the lower lid. The patient should be instructed to close the eyes for a short period to allow the medication to be dispensed throughout the eye. Gently massaging the eye to distribute the ointment over the cornea is helpful. The tip of the ointment tube should not touch the eye, and the cap should be replaced immediately.

Eyecups should be discouraged as a method for administering ophthalmic solutions because they may harbor bacteria that cause infections. When an eyecup must be used, the pharmacist should caution the patient to rinse the cup well with clean water before and after each use.

SUMMARY

The eye is one of the most sensitive areas of the human body and may be subject to many types of disorders. Pharmacists often are the first health care professionals to be informed of a patient's ocular condition. The decision to recommend self-medication with a nonprescription product or physician referral rests with the pharmacist. Ocular problems lasting more than 72 hours should be referred to a physician. Usually nonprescription ophthalmic preparations relieve only symptoms; they do not treat the disorder. Self-medication by the patient is generally trial and error with the possibility of a wrong guess leading to exacerbation of symptoms. The pharmacist should exercise professional judgment when suggesting ophthalmic products for ocular disorders such as tear insufficiency, corneal edema, and minor inflammation and irritation of the eye including some minor external infections such as hordeolum, blepharitis, and conjunctivitis. Patients with ocular disorders such as an embedded foreign body, uveitis, glaucoma, flash burns, tear duct infections, and corneal ulcers should be referred to a physician. Symptoms of these conditions include pain, blurred vision, and mucopurulent discharge.

The Nonprescription Drug Manufacturers Association (formerly The Proprietary Association) has recently endorsed several resolutions of the U.S. Pharmacopeia, one of which mandates the labeling of inactive as well as active compounds that are present in a nonprescription drug product (46). If NDMA member companies follow this policy, it will be reasonably easy for the professional to assist the consumer in product selection.

REFERENCES

1   *Federal Register*, *53*, 7076–93 (1988).
2   *Federal Register*, *45*, 3006–12 (1980).
3   S. Mishima et al., *Invest. Ophthalmol.*, *5*, 264 (1966).
4   J. J. Greco and D. C. Kelman, *Ann. Ophthalmol.*, *5*, 57 (1973).
5   S. S. Chrai et al., *J. Pharm. Sci.*, *63*, 333 (1974).
6   E. Epstein, *Ann. J. Ophthalmol.*, *59*, 109 (1965).
7   L. Harris and M. Galin, *Arch. Ophthalmol.*, *84*, 105 (1970).
8   S. S. Chrai et al., *J. Pharm. Sci.*, *62*, 1112 (1973).
9   A. Bill and B. Svedbergh, *Acta Ophthalmol.*, *50*, 295 (1972).
10   D. G. Cole and R. C. Tripathi, *Exp. Eye Res.*, *12*, 25 (1971).
11   A. Bill, *Invest. Ophthalmol.*, *14*, 1 (1975).
12   P. Ellis and D. Smith, "Handbook of Ocular Therapeutics and Pharmacology," 5th ed., C. V. Mosby, St. Louis, Mo., 1977, pp. 83–85.
13   J. G. Daubs, *Am. J. Ophthalmol.*, *49*, 1005 (1972).
14   E. Weigelin et al., *Eye Ear Nose Throat Mon.*, *54*, 13 (1975).
15   M. C. Makoid and J. R. Robinson, *J. Pharm. Sci.*, *68*, 435 (1979).
16   L. A. Wilson et al., *Am. J. Ophthalmol.*, *79*, 596 (1975).
17   S. Aronson and E. Yamamoto, *Invest. Ophthalmol.*, *5*, 75 (1966).
18   B. D. Zuckerman, *Am. J. Ophthalmol.*, *62*, 672 (1966).
19   D. Vaughn et al., "General Ophthalmology," 12th ed., Appleton and Lange, San Mateo, Calif., 1989, pp. i, 74–98, 131–143, 190–205.
20   *Med. Lett. Drugs Ther.*, *18*, 70–72 (1976).
21   *Federal Register*, *45*, 30044 (1980).
22   T. H. Roy, "Practical Management of Eye Problems: Glaucoma, Strabismus, Visual Fields," Lea and Febiger, Philadelphia, Pa., 1975, pp. 9–17.
23   D. R. Gourley and C. McKenzie, in "Clinical Pharmacy and Therapeutics," E. T. Herfindal et al., Eds., Williams and Wilkins, Baltimore, Md., 1988, pp. 534–551.
24   A. M. Potts, *Am. J. Ophthalmol.*, *86*, 743 (1978).
25   D. R. Gourley and R. E. Records, *U.S. Pharmacist*, *5*, 7 (1980).
26   "Manual of Ocular Diagnosis and Therapy," D. Pavan-Langston, Ed., Little, Brown and Co., Boston, Mass., 1980, pp. 99–100.
27   *Federal Register*, *45*, 30023 (1980).
28   "Remington's Pharmaceutical Sciences," 17th ed., Mack Publishing, Eaton, Pa., 1985, pp. 1555–1557.
29   J. M. Conrad and J. R. Robinson, *J. Pharm. Sci.*, *66*, 219 (1977).
30   J. D. Barlett and S. D. Jaanus, "Clinical Ocular Pharmacology," 2nd ed., Butterworths, Boston, Mass., 1989, pp. 21–22.
31   J. E. Hoover, "Dispensing of Medications," 8th ed., Mack Publishing, Easton, Pa., 1976, p. 236.
32   M. A. Lemp and F. J. Holly, *Ann. Ophthalmol.*, *4*, 15 (1972).
33   T. F. Patton and J. R. Robinson, *J. Pharm. Sci.*, *64*, 1312 (1975).
34   P. R. Kastl et al., *Ann. Ophthalmol.*, *19*, 376–379 (1987).
35   *Federal Register*, *45*, 30028 (1980).
36   *Federal Register*, *45*, 30037 (1980).
37   *Federal Register*, *45*, 30033–35 (1980).
38   *Federal Register*, *45*, 29788 (1980).
39   K. D. Swan and N. G. Shite, *Ann. J. Ophthalmol.*, *25*, 1043 (1942).
40   S. Y. Butelho, *Sci. Am.*, *2112*, 78 (1964).
41   N. Ehlera, *Acta Ophthalmol.* (Suppl.), 81 (1965).
42   O. F. Erickson, *Am. J. Ophthalmol.*, *43*, 295 (1957).
43   T. F. Patton and J. R. Robinson, *J. Pharm. Sci.*, *65*, 1295 (1976).
44   C. Asseff et al., *Am. J. Ophthalmol.*, *75*, 212 (1973).
45   H. F. Wedemeyer et al., in "Handbook for Institutional Pharmacy Practice," T. R. Brown and M. C. Smith, Eds., Williams and Wilkins, Baltimore, Md., 2nd ed., 1986, pp. 355–357.
46   USP Quinquennial Meeting, Rockville, Md., March 1985.

ARTIFICIAL TEAR PRODUCT TABLE

Product (Manufacturer)	Viscosity Agent	Preservative	pH	Other Ingredients
Adsorbotear (Alcon)	hydroxyethylcellulose povidone, 1.67%	edetate disodium, 0.1% thimerosal, 0.004%	NS[a]	
Akwa Tears (Akorn)	polyvinyl alcohol	benzalkonium chloride, 0.01% edetate disodium	NS[a]	sodium chloride
Artificial Tears Solution (Rugby)	polyvinyl alcohol, 1.4%	edetate disodium chlorobutanol	NS[a]	
Celluvisc (Allergan)	carboxymethylcellulose sodium, 1%		NS[a]	calcium chloride potassium chloride sodium chloride sodium lactate
Comfort Tears (Barnes-Hind)	hydroxyethylcellulose polyvinyl alcohol	edetate disodium, 0.005% benzalkonium chloride, 0.02%	NS[a]	
Hypotears (Iolab)	polyvinyl alcohol, 1%	benzalkonium chloride, 0.01%	6.6	
I-Liqui Tears (Americal)	polyvinyl alcohol, 1% hydroxyethylcellulose, 0.5%	benzalkonium chloride, 0.01% edetate disodium	NS[a]	sodium chloride
Isopto Alkaline (Alcon)	hydroxypropyl methyl-cellulose, 1%	benzalkonium chloride, 0.01%	NS[a]	
Isopto Plain (Alcon)	hydroxypropyl methyl-cellulose, 0.5%	benzalkonium chloride 0.01%	NS[a]	
Isopto Tears (Alcon)	hydroxypropyl methyl-cellulose, 0.05%	benzalkonium chloride, 0.01%	NS[a]	
Just Tears (Blairex)	hydroxypropyl methylcellulose	benzalkonium chloride, 0.01% edetate disodium, 0.025%	NS[a]	sodium chloride potassium chloride sodium borate boric acid
Lacril (Allergan)	hydroxypropyl methyl-cellulose, 0.5% gelatin A, 0.01%	chlorobutanol, 0.5%	NS[a]	
Liquifilm Forte (Allergan)	polyvinyl alcohol, 3%	edetate disodium thimerosal, 0.002%	NS[a]	
Liquifilm Tears (Allergan)	polyvinyl alcohol, 1.4%	chlorobutanol, 0.5%	NS[a]	sodium chloride
Milroy Artificial Tears (Milroy)	methylcellulose	benzalkonium chloride, 0.002%	8.0-8.6	boric acid sodium borate
Moisture Drops (Bausch & Lomb)	hydroxypropyl methyl-cellulose, 0.5% dextran 40, 0.1%	edetate disodium benzalkonium chloride, 0.01%	NS[a]	sodium chloride potassium chloride sodium borate boric acid
Murine (Ross)	polyvinyl alcohol, 1.4% povidone, 0.6%	benzalkonium chloride edetate disodium	NS[a]	dextrose potassium chloride sodium bicarbonate sodium chloride sodium citrate sodium phosphate
Muro Tears (Bausch & Lomb)	hydroxypropyl methyl-cellulose dextran 40	benzalkonium chloride, 0.01% edetate disodium	NS[a]	boric acid sodium chloride

ARTIFICIAL TEAR PRODUCT TABLE, continued

Product (Manufacturer)	Viscosity Agent	Preservative	pH	Other Ingredients
Murocel (Bausch & Lomb)	methylcellulose, 1%		NS[a]	propylene glycol sodium chloride boric acid parabens
Refresh (Allergan)	polyvinyl alcohol, 1.4% povidone, 0.6%		NS[a]	sodium chloride
TearGard (Medtech)	hydroxyethylcellulose	edetate disodium, 0.1%	NS[a]	sorbic acid, 0.25%
Tearisol (Iolab)	hydroxypropyl methyl-cellulose, 0.5%	benzalkonium chloride, 0.01%	7.5	boric acid potassium chloride sodium carbonate
Tears Naturale (Alcon)	hydroxypropyl methyl-cellulose dextran 70	benzalkonium chloride, 0.01% edetate disodium, 0.05%	7.0	
Tears Naturale II (Alcon)	hydroxypropyl methyl-cellulose, 0.3% dextran 70, 0.1%	edetate disodium	NS[a]	potassium chloride sodium chloride polyquaternium-1, 0.001%
Tears Plus (Allergan)	polyvinyl alcohol, 1.4% povidone, 0.6%	chlorobutanol, 0.5%	NS[a]	
Tears Renewed (Akorn)	hydroxypropyl methylcellulose dextran 70	benzalkonium chloride, 0.01% edetate disodium, 0.05%	NS[a]	sodium chloride
Ultra Tears (Alcon)	hydroxypropyl methyl-cellulose, 1%	benzalkonium chloride, 0.01%	7.5	

[a] pH not stated.

OPHTHALMIC DECONGESTANT PRODUCT TABLE

Product (Manufacturer)	Viscosity Agent	Vasoconstrictor	Preservative	Buffer	pH	Other Ingredients
Adsorbonac (Alcon)	povidone		EDTA, 0.1% thimerosal, 0.004%		NS[a]	sodium chloride, 2%, 5%
AK-Nefrin (Akorn)	hydroxyethyl-cellulose, 0.5%	phenylephrine hydrochloride, 0.12%	benzalkonium chloride, 0.01% EDTA		NS[a]	sodium chloride
Allerest Eye Drops (Pharmacraft)		naphazoline hydrochloride, 0.012%			NS[a]	
Clear Eyes (Ross)		naphazoline hydrochloride, 0.012%	benzalkonium chloride EDTA	boric acid sodium borate	NS[a]	glycerin, 0.2%
Collyrium w/Tetra-hydrozoline (Wyeth-Ayerst)		tetrahydrozoline hydrochloride, 0.05%	benzalkonium chloride, 0.01% EDTA, 0.1%	boric acid sodium borate	NS[a]	glycerin, 1%
Comfort Eye Drops (Sola/Barnes-Hind)	hydroxyethyl-cellulose polyvinyl alcohol	naphazoline hydrochloride, 0.03%	benzalkonium chloride, 0.005% EDTA, 0.02%	mono- and dibasic sodium phosphate	NS[a]	sodium chloride
Degest 2 (Sola/Barnes-Hind)	hydroxyethyl-cellulose	naphazoline hydrochloride, 0.012%	benzalkonium chloride, 0.0067% EDTA, 0.02%	sodium citrate	NS[a]	
Eye-Zine (Ocumed)		tetrahydrozoline hydrochloride, 0.05%				
Isopto-Frin (Alcon)	hydroxypropyl methylcellu-lose, 0.5%	phenylephrine hydrochloride, 0.12%	benzalkonium chloride, 0.01%	sodium citrate sodium phosphate sodium biphosphate	7.3	
Mallazine Drops (Hauck)		tetrahydrozoline hydrochloride, 0.05%		sodium borate boric acid		sodium chloride
Murine Plus (Ross)		tetrahydrozoline hydrochloride, 0.05%	benzalkonium chloride, 0.01% EDTA, 0.1%		NS[a]	
Naphcon (Alcon)		naphazoline hydrochloride, 0.012%	benzalkonium chloride, 0.01%		NS[a]	
OcuClear (Schering)		oxymetazoline hydrochloride, 0.025%	benzalkonium chloride, 0.01% EDTA			
Ocu-Phrin (Ocumed)		phenylephrine hydrochloride, 0.12%			NS[a]	
Optigene III (Pfeiffer)	povidone	tetrahydrozoline hydrochloride, 0.05%	benzalkonium chloride, 0.004% EDTA, 0.1%		NS[a]	

OPHTHALMIC DECONGESTANT PRODUCT TABLE, continued

Product (Manufacturer)	Viscosity Agent	Vasoconstrictor	Preservative	Buffer	pH	Other Ingredients
Optised (Various manufacturers)		phenylephrine hydrochloride, 0.12%				zinc sulfate, 0.25%
Phenylzin (CooperVision)	hydroxypropyl methylcellulose	phenylephrine hydrochloride, 0.12%	benzalkonium chloride, 0.01% EDTA, 0.01%		NS[a]	sodium bisulfite zinc sulfate, 0.25%
Prefrin Liquifilm (Allergan)	polyvinyl alcohol, 1.4%	phenylephrine hydrochloride, 0.12%	benzalkonium chloride, 0.005%	mono- and dibasic sodium phosphate	NS[a]	
Relief (Allergan)	polyvinyl alcohol, 1.4%	phenylephrine hydrochloride, 0.12%		mono- and dibasic sodium phosphate	NS[a]	
Soothe (Alcon)	povidone	tetrahydrozoline hydrochloride, 0.05%	benzalkonium chloride, 0.004% EDTA, 0.1%		NS[a]	
Tetrahydrozoline Hydrochloride (Various manufacturers)		tetrahydrozoline hydrochloride, 0.05%				
20/20 Eye Drops (S.S.S.)		naphazoline hydrochloride, 0.012%	thimerosal, 0.005%	boric acid, 1.22% sodium carbonate, 0.004%	6	potassium chloride, 0.73% zinc sulfate, 0.06%
VasoClear (Iolab)	polyvinyl alcohol	naphazoline hydrochloride, 0.02%	benzalkonium chloride, 0.01% EDTA		NS[a]	PEG-8000
VasoClear A (Iolab)	polyvinyl alcohol, 0.25%	naphazoline hydrochloride, 0.02%	benzalkonium chloride, 0.005% EDTA			zinc sulfate, 0.25% PEG-8000
Visine (Leeming)		tetrahydrozoline hydrochloride, 0.05%	benzalkonium chloride, 0.01% EDTA, 0.1%	boric acid sodium borate	NS[a]	sodium chloride
Visine A.C. (Leeming)		tetrahydrozoline hydrochloride, 0.05%	benzalkonium chloride, 0.01% EDTA, 0.1%	boric acid sodium citrate	NS[a]	zinc sulfate, 0.25% sodium chloride
Visine Extra (Leeming)		tetrahydrozoline hydrochloride, 0.05%	benzalkonium chloride, 0.013% EDTA, 0.1%	boric acid sodium borate	NS[a]	PEG-400, 1% sodium chloride
Zincfrin (Alcon)		phenylephrine hydrochloride, 0.12%	benzalkonium chloride, 0.01%		NS[a]	zinc sulfate, 0.25%

[a] pH not specified.

EYE WASH PRODUCT TABLE

Product (Manufacturer)	Buffer	pH	Preservative	Other Ingredients
Blinx (Barnes-Hind)	sodium phosphate	NS[a]	benzalkonium chloride, 0.005%	
Collyrium Eye Lotion (Wyeth-Ayerst)	boric acid sodium borate	NS[a]	thimerosal, 0.0002%	
Collyrium for Fresh Eyes (Wyeth-Ayerst)	boric acid sodium borate	NS[a]	thimerosal, 0.002%	
Dacriose (Iolab)	sodium phosphate	NS[a]	benzalkonium chloride, 0.01% edetate disodium, 0.3%	potassium chloride sodium chloride
Enuclene[b] (Alcon)		NS[a]	benzalkonium chloride, 0.02%	tyloxapol, 0.25%
Eye-Stream (Alcon)	sodium acetate, 0.39% sodium citrate, 0.17%	NS[a]	benzalkonium chloride, 0.013%	calcium chloride, 0.048% magnesium chloride, 0.03% potassium chloride, 0.075% sodium chloride, 0.64% sodium hydroxide and/or hydrochloric acid
Eye Wash (Hauck)	boric acid, 1.2%	NS[a]	edetate disodium, 0.05% benzalkonium chloride, 0.01%	potassium chloride, 0.38% sodium carbonate anhydrous, 0.014%
Lauro Eye Wash (Otis Clapp)	sodium phosphate	7	edetate sodium benzalkonium chloride	sodium chloride
Lavoptik Eye Wash (Lavoptik)	sodium biphosphate, 0.4% sodium phosphate, 0.45%	NS[a]	benzalkonium chloride, 0.005%	sodium chloride, 0.49%
Op-thal-zin (Alcon)		7.5	benzalkonium chloride, 0.01%	zinc sulfate, 0.25%
Trisol Eye Wash (Buffington)	sodium phosphate	7	edetate sodium benzalkonium chloride	sodium chloride

[a] pH not stated.
[b] For artificial eyes.

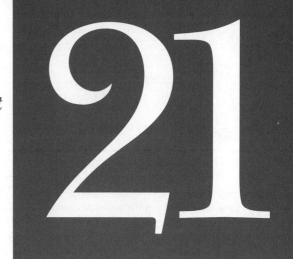

Thomas A. Gossel and J. Richard Wuest

CONTACT LENSES AND LENS CARE PRODUCTS

Q*uestions to ask in patient/consumer counseling*

What types of problems are you having with your lenses? Are they related to eye irritation or changes in vision?

———

Have you recently changed brands of any of your solutions?

———

What types of lenses do you wear? Hard, soft, or rigid gas permeable?

———

How long have you been wearing lenses? When did the problems start?

———

What nonprescription and prescription medications are you now taking?

———

Have you become pregnant or begun using oral contraceptives since you were fitted for lenses?

———

How many hours per day do you wear your lenses before problems start?

———

Do you remove your lenses during the day?

———

When did you last see your optometrist or ophthalmologist?

———

Do you have any allergies?

———

How often do you clean your storage container? Does it need to be replaced?

———

Hard Lens Wearers

Do you soak your lenses when not in use?

———

How long have you been using your present supply of lens solutions?

———

Do you use any lens solutions that are not manufactured strictly for use in the eyes or for contact lens care?

———

Do you wash your hands each time before putting in or taking out your lenses?

———

Are you ever exposed to dust, chemicals, excessive wind, or other environmental particles that could get into your eyes and cause problems?

———

How often do you replace solutions in your lens storage container?

———

How often do you clean your lenses?

———

Do you use enzyme tablets?

———

What products do you use? Do you use a combination-type solution?

———

Soft Lens Wearers

Do you clean your lenses before disinfection?

———

What method of disinfection do you use?

———

How often do you disinfect your lenses?

———

Do you use commercial saline solutions or do you mix your own? How often do you replace it?

———

Do you use any cosmetics or medications (nonprescription or prescription) that are applied to the eye area? How do you apply these products?

———

Editor's Note: This chapter is based in part on the chapter with a similar title that appeared in the 8th edition but was authored by James R. Boyd.

The first corneal plastic contact lens was introduced in the United States in 1939, but it was not until the advent of the contour-fitting principle in 1955 that lens use began to gain wide acceptance. "Contour-fitting" is the use of lenses with multiple inside radii rather than a single posterior curve; it soon became standard practice to tailor lenses for the individual cornea. These early lenses were so successful and popular that today nearly 20% of patients requiring corrective lenses choose contact lenses.

Annual sales of contact lens care products now exceed $400 million, and are growing faster than any other category of nonprescription items (1). It is estimated that by the year 2000 the number of persons wearing contact lenses will be the same as those who use eyeglasses (2). With the introduction of soft contact lenses in the 1970s, the greatly enhanced comfort of lenses led to a significant expansion of the contact lens market. Similarly, developments with rigid gas-permeable hard lenses provide the greater comfort of soft lenses and the enhanced optical qualities of hard lenses, which promises continued growth for this mode of vision correction. Extended wear lenses, toric lenses for astigmatism, tinted lenses, bifocal contacts, and disposable lenses greatly expand the potential patient population who will desire and benefit from contact lenses.

With increasing evidence of contact lens problems associated with improper cleaning and disinfecting practices, more emphasis has been placed on developing and marketing contact lens products that increase patient care, convenience, and compliance. For example, disposable soft contact lenses (Acuvue) and multipurpose cleaning, disinfecting, rinsing, and soaking solutions were recently introduced.

Of the 25 million Americans wearing contacts, nearly 90% use contact lenses to correct vision of the otherwise healthy eye. Although much of the motivation to wear contact lenses may be cosmetic, properly fitted contact lenses can provide significant vision advantages over spectacle lenses; contact lenses reduce size distortion and prismatic effects, and improve peripheral vision. Elimination of spectacle fogging, dirt accumulation, and frame distraction may also be a significant advantage to many users, and most contact lens wearers state that their contact lenses are more comfortable than eyeglasses.

However, it has been well established that corneal contact lenses, even when expertly fitted, produce some degree of alteration of ocular tissues and changes in the corneal metabolism. This alteration makes it imperative that both the user and the health professional understand the proper care, maintenance, and safe use of these products. Failure to use such methods can greatly increase the chance of corneal infection, corneal ulcers, and other ocular conditions that may result in permanent eye damage.

More than 150 nonprescription contact lens products are available. Selection of products depends on their compatibility with each other as well as with the specific lens device. Consumers are likely to be overwhelmed at the variety of products. Except for the lens fitter, pharmacists are the most qualified to counsel contact lens wearers (3). These considerations place a direct responsibility on the pharmacist to understand this area of professional practice and be an effective, up-to-date information consultant to the contact lens wearer (4, 5).

INDICATIONS FOR CONTACT LENS USAGE

One important consideration in contact lens usage is that the decision to wear lenses is sometimes based on therapeutic necessity (6–8). Keratoconus is a gradual protrusion of the central cornea, and satisfactory vision is usually unattainable with ordinary eyeglasses. This condition responds only to contact lenses or corneal transplantation (9, 10).

Aphakia results when the crystalline lens of the eye is removed because of an opacified lens or cataract (11). Aphakic individuals characteristically show improved quality of vision with cataract contact lenses compared with cataract spectacles. Extended wear contact lenses are particularly beneficial for such patients because their poor visual acuity makes it difficult to insert and remove lenses.

Visual aberrations caused by corneal scarring are also often better corrected by contact lenses (12). The close proximity of the lens actually transforms the corneal topography; eyeglasses simply correct refractive error by changing the direction of the incident light.

Other indications for the use of contact lenses include refractive errors such as myopia (nearsightedness), hyperopia (farsightedness), astigmatism, and presbyopia (old vision).

Presbyopia is a condition caused by aging, in which the crystalline lens cannot properly focus on near objects. Contact lenses have not been overly successful in this condition; because vision correction is needed for both near and far, two optical corrections are required in each bifocal contact lens.

The method for correcting presbyopia with spectacles is with use of bifocal or trifocal lenses (often called multifocal lenses). Monovision is one method of contact lens correction that has been successful in some cases; the dominant eye is fitted with a lens for far vision, and the other eye with a lens that corrects for close-up objects and reading. In most individuals, the eyes will adjust in a relatively short time; reading will be done with the nondominant eye, and everything else will be noted with the dominant eye.

Monovision eliminates the need for bifocal or trifocal spectacles and is much more acceptable than bifocal contact lenses. It serves most presbyopia patients well in everyday life.

Perhaps the main reason for choosing contact lenses among many wearers is the perceived improvement in personal appearance (13). Other strongly influencing factors favoring contact lens wear include: no obstruction of vision from eyeglass frames (14–16), greater clarity in the peripheral visual field, no fogging of lenses caused by sudden temperature changes, and more freedom of motion during vigorous activity. Although it has been demonstrated that there is no substantial difference in central visual acuity between contact lenses and eyeglasses, a number of factors contribute to a subjective perception of improvement by the contact lenses wearer (17). Increased sensitivity to light and improved quality of the retinal image often occur with contact lens wear (18, 19). With eyeglasses, the myopic individual sees a smaller than normal image and the hypermetropic individual sees a larger than normal image. With contact lenses, both myopic and hypermetropic individuals see objects in nearly their true sizes; for highly myopic persons, the image size increase with contact lenses is significant and decidedly beneficial.

Contraindications

Certainly, contact lenses are not for everyone. Some individuals who require vision correction cannot or should not wear contact lenses. Contraindications are often based on lifestyle as well as medical history.

Occupational conditions that may prohibit the wearing of contact lenses include exposure to dust and particulate matter, wind, glare, molten metals, irritant chemicals, tobacco smoke, and chemical fumes (20). Certain chemical fumes have been suggested to be particularly hazardous because of the potential concentration of irritants under a hard lens or inside a soft lens. The lens theoretically prolongs contact of such substances with the cornea and can lead to corneal toxicity. These theoretical occupational contraindications have not been proven, however; the contact lens wearer does not appear to be at significantly greater risk than an individual without contact lenses. In any situation in which occupational exposure to airborne contaminants is significant, workers should wear safety goggles—with or without contact lenses.

Corneal contact lenses should not be used for cosmetic reasons if a patient has active pathologic intraocular or corneal conditions, although they may be used in cases of open-angle glaucoma (9). Medical reasons that contraindicate contact lens wear include chronic conjunctivitis; blepharitis; recurrent viral, bacterial, or fungal infections; poor blink rate or incomplete blink; and insufficient or abnormal tear production. An obstructed nasolacrimal duct, anatomical or physiologic abnormalities, and various clinical conditions, such as ocular herpes simplex, also contraindicate contact lens use (21). Diabetics are often advised against extended wear contact lenses because of retarded healing processes and the tendency toward prolonged corneal abrasion with such use. This precaution is probably unnecessary for daily wear of lenses unless problems occur. Chronic common colds or allergic conditions such as hay fever and asthma may make lens wear extremely uncomfortable or impossible.

The successful wearing of contact lenses depends on adequate tear production. Because the cornea is avascular, tears provide oxygen and remove waste products in addition to providing lubrication and serving as a barrier to microorganisms. Insufficient tear production, a deficiency or excess of mucin, excessive lipid production, or excessively dry environments may preclude successful contact lens use.

Dry spots on the cornea, often found in postmenopausal women, prevent the successful use of lenses (22). These spots, possibly caused by the absence of the precorneal film, are often identified with lacrimal insufficiency caused by subclinical hypothyroidism and Sjogren's syndrome (a chronic systemic inflammatory disorder characterized by dryness of the mouth, eyes, and other mucous membranes).

Cautions

Contact lenses should be used with caution in patients with epilepsy, diabetes mellitus, high blood pressure, heart disease, or severe arthritis. The corneal topography may be altered by pregnancy or use of oral contraceptives (21, 22). Although the newer "low-dose" oral contraceptives cause fewer problems, the fluid-retaining properties of estrogen may lead to edema of the cornea and eyelids as well as decreased tear production. Patients taking oral contraceptives for at least 6 months prior to fitting of contact lenses generally do much better than those who begin use of oral contraceptives after regular contact lens use. Likewise, a lens wearer who stops using oral contraceptives may develop problems with lens fit because of topographical and other edematous changes in the cornea. Contact lenses should also be used with caution by elderly persons, because of possible lacrimal insufficiency, and by individuals with arthritis, which may restrict the movement and dexterity needed to insert lenses.

Diseases secondary to contact lens wear have been described (23). Lens wearers moving from a low to a high altitude may encounter hypoxia or metabolic deficiency, resulting in irritation and corneal abrasions (24).

Many systemic medications, such as diuretics, estrogens, oral contraceptives, antihistamines, anticholinergics, decongestants, and tricyclic antidepressants, affect the eyes and therefore may reduce lens tolerance (21, 22, 25). Microedema caused by hormonal therapy as well as premenstrual edema may also cause problems in the use of contact lenses (26). Orally administered antihistamines and decongestants may decrease tear production and cause mild keratitis, interfering with lens wear (27, 28).

During the adaptive period to rigid contact lenses, the eyelids may become hyperemic; this condition may lead to blepharitis, especially in the upper lid (29). Short pseudoblinks, often found in new wearers of hard lenses, may irritate the conjunctiva of the upper eyelid. Chin elevation and squinting may result from irritating lenses (29).

Cosmetics and Contact Lenses

Cosmetics must be chosen with care (30). Women should be advised to insert lenses before applying makeup, and to avoid touching the lens with eyeliner or mascara. Many eye cosmetics have an oily base and cause greasy smudges on the lenses that can be difficult to remove. Cosmetics with an aqueous base should be used because oil-based products may cause blurred vision and irritation if they are deposited on the lens. Powders may also be irritating if small particles become lodged under the lens. Mascara should be applied only to the very tips of the lashes. Hair sprays, in particular, must be used with caution. Irritation may occur if some of the spray particles are trapped in the tear layer beneath the lens, and some sprays may actually damage the lens. One way to avoid a problem is to insert the lenses, go to another room, cover the eyes with a cloth, apply hair spray, and then leave the area with the eyes still closed.

Nail polish, hand creams, and perfumes should be applied only after the lens has been inserted. Men frequently contaminate their lenses with hair preparations; they should take special care to clean their hands thoroughly before handling contact lenses. Soaps containing cold cream or deodorants should be avoided

because they can leave a film on the fingers after rinsing. This residue is readily transferred to a soft lens and can cause blurred vision.

LENS CHOICE: HARD, RIGID GAS-PERMEABLE, OR SOFT?

Contact lenses are often broadly classified into three distinct groups based on the chemical make-up and physical properties of the lens. Lenses that are relatively inflexible, do not appreciably absorb water, and retain their shape when removed from the eye are commonly called hard lenses. Lenses that are moderately to highly flexible, absorb a high percentage of water, and conform to the shape of a supporting surface are commonly called soft lenses. The third group is called rigid gas-permeable lenses; although rigid in shape, they are oxygen permeable. This improves comfort. Approximately 80% of lens wearers use soft lenses, 19% use rigid gas-permeable lenses, and only 1% now use hard lenses (31).

Lens wearers may have strongly preconceived notions about selection among the various lenses available. Advice from friends, relatives, or contact lens fitters who have had experiences with a particular type of lens, promotional claims through media advertising, and connotations associated with the words "hard" and "soft" with respect to a perception of comfort may influence a lens wearer's choice. However, it is important to note that the lens of choice, and the ultimate success of visual correction and comfort, may be influenced by a number of factors that vary from individual to individual. No single type of lens will be ideally suited to all people. Therefore, the lens selection decision should be determined primarily by a vision care specialist, based on the specific optical requirements of the eye and other important related variables.

Conventional Hard Lenses

Hard lenses are polymerized products of esters of acrylic acid or methacrylic acid (32). The most common plastic found in hard lenses is polymethlymethacrylate (PMMA), which is known commercially as Lucite or Plexiglas.

Contact lenses made of PMMA are hydrophobic (33). However, PMMA possesses many characteristics that make it ideal for an over-the-eye corrective lens:

- Lenses are very light because of a specific gravity of 1.18–1.20.

- The refractive index, 1.49–1.50, is similar to glass spectacle lenses.

- Lenses allow a light transmission of 90–92%.

- Lenses are not affected by weak alkalis or weak acids.

- The plastic does not cause sensitivity reactions when placed onto the cornea.

The "hardness" of these hard lenses is less than that of glass, however, and reasonable care must be exercised to avoid scratching and chipping.

Rigid Gas-Permeable Hard Lenses

The new generation of rigid lenses combines the optical qualities of PMMA and the oxygen permeability of soft lenses. Rigid gas-permeable hard lenses are available in several materials.

One type of rigid gas-permeable hard lenses is composed of silicone acrylates that combine PMMA and silicone in varying amounts. This material is relatively stable, and the lens allows 1–7% oxygen transmission, depending on lens thickness. A disadvantage of most silicone acrylates is a decrease in surface wettability when compared with PMMA. This occurs because of the relatively higher hydrophobicity of silicone.

Another type of rigid gas-permeable hard lens is made of cellulose acetate butyrate (CAB). CAB lenses will transmit up to 5% oxygen depending on their thickness; they possess the optical qualities of other hard lenses. However, CAB has several disadvantages, including its relative ease of surface scratching and its tendency to warp.

Polystyrene is another type of rigid gas permeable hard lens. The new generation of polystyrene lens is thought to be much more stable than its predecessors.

All three types of rigid gas-permeable hard lenses have been investigated for extended wear use. Some have been approved for 1–7 days extended wear.

Pure silicone contact lenses have been available for many years but have experienced limited market success and consumer popularity. These lenses can be made in both a hard resin and a flexible variety, and are by far the most permeable to oxygen of all contact lenses. However, pure silicone lenses are uncomfortable because of the extremely hydrophobic nature of the material.

Rigid gas-permeable lenses have been implicated in causing corneal ulcers—eruptions on the corneal surface. In some cases, these corneal ulcers can lead to

TABLE 1 Examples of rigid gas-permeable lenses

Trade name	Manufacturer	Lens material
Airlens	Wesley-Jessen	Airfocon (t-butyl styrene)
Boston II	Polymer Tech	Itafocon B
Boston IV	Polymer Tech	Itafocon A
Cooper Vision HGP	Cooper Vision	Itafocon A
FluoroPerm	Paragon	Paraflucon A
GP II	Barnes-Hind	Parafocon
Meso	Danker	Cellulose acetate butyrate
Optacryl	Optacryl	PMMA/Silicon
OxyFlow	Product Development	Pasifocon A/B
Paraperm	Paragon	Pasifocon A-C
Permaflex HGP	CooperVision	Itafocon B
Polycon	Sola	Silafocon
Rx-56	Rynco	Cellulose acetate butyrate
S.G.P.	Kontur	Telefocon A
Sofperm	Barnes-Hind	Synergicon
Sila Rx	Danker	Silicone
Silcon VFL	Conforma	Silicone

partial or complete blindness (34). Table 1 lists examples of rigid gas-permeable hard contact lenses currently available in the United States.

Soft Lenses

The main chemical difference between the hydrophobic, rigid hard lens and the hydrophilic soft lens is that the soft lens contains hydroxyl or hydroxyl and lactam groups that allow it to absorb and hold water. Table 2 lists some examples of daily wear soft lenses available in the United States. Nearly all lenses are composed of 2-hydroxyethylmethacrylate (HEMA) with small amounts of cross-linking agents that form a hydrophilic gel (hydrogel) network (35). The degree of cross-linking determines lens hydrophilicity. Greater cross-linking means fewer hydrophilic groups available for interaction with water, which in turn produces a less flexible, less hydrated lens than those originally available (31, 36).

TABLE 2 Examples of soft contact lenses for daily wear

Trade Name	Manufacturer	% Water/Saline
A O Soft	Ciba Vision	42.5
AL 47	Alden	35–47
Amsof	Channel	43
Aquasight	Channel	43
Ciba Soft	Ciba Vision	37.5
Cooperthin	Cooper Vision	38
Custom-Eyes	CTL	38
DuraSoft	Wesley-Jessen	30-55
Flexlens	Flexlens	45
Fre-Flex	Optech	55
Hydrasoft	Coast Vision	55
Hydrocurve II	Barnes-Hind	45.5
Hydromarc	Vistacon	43
Hydrosoft	National Contact Lens	43
Metrosoft II	Metro Optics	38
Mini/Zero	American Hydron	38
Omega D	Omega	43
Omega Soft	Omega	38.6
Optima 38	Bausch & Lomb	38.6
PDC Soft Lens	PDC	38
Soflens	Bausch & Lomb	38.6
Soft Mate	Barnes-Hind	45
Softact II	C. L. Corp.	38
Softcon	Ciba Vision	55
Softsite	Softsite	45
VT45	Visiontech	45

The water content of soft lenses varies from 30 to 80%. Increasing water content improves the oxygen permeability of a material, although oxygen transmissibility of a lens also depends on lens thickness. Lenses with a high water content must be thickened to offset fragility; therefore, the two factors often cancel each other where oxygen transmissibility is concerned. Increased oxygen permeability of soft contact lenses enables certain lenses to be "broken in" more quickly, and worn continuously. Table 3 lists examples of soft contact lenses approved for extended wear in the United States. Extended wear lenses were originally intended to be worn for weeks. However, because of problems with contamination and infection, they should not be worn for more than 7 days (37). Recent evidence strongly supports the removal of extended wear contact lenses overnight to reduce the risk of ulcerative keratitis (38, 39).

The water content of nonspecialty soft lenses has gradually decreased since they were introduced. The water content of a HEMA-type material can vary between 5 and 90%, but a theoretical "ideal" value might be 75–78%, which matches the hydration level of the corneal stroma.

Highly hydrated lenses are more comfortable, but they are also more fragile and therefore more susceptible to cuts and tears from fingernails during insertion and removal. Lowering the water content produces a more durable and longer lasting lens. In addition, reducing the percentage of water in a soft HEMA lens also reduces the thickness of the hydrated lens. This reduction improves the comfort level for lens wearers.

When a soft lens is placed on the cornea, its shape conforms to the corneal topography. Unlike a hard lens that resists flexure and therefore masks corneal astigmatism, the soft lens is severely limited in its ability to correct corneal astigmatism. Soft lenses can be fitted to eyes with an upper limit of astigmatism of about 1.00 diopters, a figure highly dependent on criticality and motivation of the patient. A diopter is a unit of refracting power used as a quantitative measure of the abnormal refraction of light at surfaces such as the cornea.

Toric soft lenses have been developed specifically to correct astigmatic visual conditions. Traditional soft lenses do not correct astigmatism because they conform to the corneal surface rather than retain their original shape, as do hard lenses. Toric soft lenses are fabricated with both spherical and cylindrical optical corrections and remain "on axis" because of design features such as weighting the bottom edge of the lens. Table 4 lists

TABLE 3 Examples of soft contact lenses for extended wear

Trade Name	Manufacturer	% Water/Saline
B & L 70	Bausch & Lomb	70
Ciba Thin	Ciba Vision	37.5
CSI	Sola	38.5
Custom Eyes	CTL	38.6
CW 79	Bausch & Lomb	79
DuraSoft	Wesley-Jessen	55–74
Genesis-4	Channel	70
Hydrocurve II	Barnes-Hind	55
Kontur 55	Kontur	55
Optima EW	Bausch & Lomb	38.6
Permaflex	CooperVision	43–74
Permalens	CooperVision	71
Q & E 70	Breger	70
Sofcon EW	Ciba Vision	55
Softlens 03/04	Bausch & Lomb	38.6
Softmate I-II	Barnes-Hind	45–55
Softsite	Softsite	45
Vistmarc	Vistacon	58
VT70	Visiontech	70–79
X-70/Zero	American Hydron	38–70

TABLE 4 Examples of toric and bifocal soft contact lenses

Trade Name	Manufacturer	% Water/ Saline
TORIC LENSES (for astigmatism)		
Accugel	Strieter	46.6
B & L Toric	Bausch & Lomb	45
Durasoft	Wesley-Jessen	38–55
FreFlex Toric	Optech	55
Hydrasoft Toric	Coast Vision	45
Hydrocurve II Toric	Barnes-Hind	55
Hydromarc Toric	Vistakon	43 & 55
Hydro-Toric	American Hydron	38
Kontur 55	Kontur	55
Metrosoft Toric	Metro Optics	38
Ocu-Flex 53	Ocu-Ease	53
Optima Toric	Bausch & Lomb	45
Torisoft	Ciba Vision	37.5
Zero T	American Hydron	38
BIFOCAL LENSES (for presbyopia)		
ALGES	University Optical	45
Bi-Soft	Ciba Vision	37.5
DuraSoft 2	Wesley-Jessen	38
Hydrocurve II	Barnes-Hind	45
Soflens	Bausch & Lomb	38.6
Softsite	Softsite	45
VT45 Cresent	Visiontech	45

examples of available toric soft lenses and bifocal lenses.

Soft lenses in the nonhydrated (dry) state are rigid and extremely brittle. They should never be handled in the dry state by the wearer. When hydrated, they expand as water is absorbed into the gel matrix (34). They are most comfortable when they are at least the diameter of the cornea, have thin edges, and undergo little movement on the eye, although adequate movement is necessary to ensure lubrication of the ocular surface under the lens. Many lens wearers find that they cannot tolerate lenses with a thickness above 0.4 mm because of lid discomfort. For those who cannot tolerate regular soft lenses, several ultrathin soft lenses are available with a thickness as low as 0.07 mm.

Table 5 provides a comparative summary of the characteristics that differentiate conventional hard lenses, soft lenses, and rigid gas-permeable hard lenses.

Advantages of Soft Lenses

Soft lenses provide certain advantages that make them more attractive to the lens wearer. They are easier to apply, and are considerably more comfortable than hard lenses. This effect is most apparent during the initial break-in period (40, 41). Photophobia is not likely to occur with soft lenses and glare is reduced significantly. As with hard lenses, however, flare around the periphery may be noticed at night, particularly in individuals who have large pupils (42). This flare is caused by refractive light entering the eye through the edge margin of the contact lens.

Soft lens wearers can change more easily from their lenses to eyeglasses after a period of wear. A common problem among hard lens wearers is "spectacle blur," or "contact blindness." Nonpathologic spectacle blur is simply a refractive change caused by the corneal curvature modifying effect of a hard lens. It may last for a short time or up to hours or days. The net result is unclear vision after the person has removed contact lenses and put on eyeglasses. The typical soft lens wearer does not usually experience spectacle blur.

Soft lenses are also less likely to dislodge or fall out as often as hard lenses (43). Therefore, soft lenses are better suited for occasional wear and sports, including contact sports. Soft lenses are less likely than hard lenses to trap dust particles, eyelashes, or other foreign material under the lens.

TABLE 5 Comparison of contact lens characteristics

	Conventional hard lenses	Soft contact lenses	Rigid gas-permeable hard lenses
LENS CHARACTERISTICS			
Rigidity	+++	0	+++
Durability	+++	+	++
Oxygen transmission	0	+	+++
Adsorbs chemicals	0	+++	0
OPTICAL QUALITY			
Visual acuity	+++	+	+++
Corrects astigmatism	Yes	Toric	Yes
Photophobia	+++	+	++
Spectacle blur	+++	–	++
CONVENIENCE			
Comfort	+	+++	++
Adaptation period	Weeks	Days	Days
Extended wear	No	Yes	Yes
Intermittent wear	No	Yes	No

Disadvantages of Soft Lenses

Although many people prefer the comfort of soft lenses, it has been shown that not all soft lens wearers can achieve excellent visual acuity (44, 45). The hydration of the lens may change either in or out of the eye (particularly with extreme temperatures and low relative humidity); this change can decrease the quality of the visual image (44). Because a soft lens conforms in large part to the corneal shape, it is difficult to predict the degree of vision improvement before actually placing the lens on the eye. Also, because soft lenses cannot be precisely tailored to the specific requirements of an individual cornea, the fitting process is less exact than with rigid lenses. As a result, the overall quality of vision with soft contact lenses does not usually equal that of a properly fitted pair of hard lenses. Fortunately, these differences are small and should not be a cause for concern to the average wearer. The major consequence of these differences is seen only when a lens wearer switches from hard to soft contact lenses (32, 33). In some cases, the decrease in vision quality is unacceptable to the established hard lens wearer.

Unlike hard lenses, soft lenses can absorb chemical compounds from topically administered ophthalmic products (46–50). Occular irritation may result, and the lens may be damaged (51). Drugs such as epinephrine can enter the hydrogel and discolor it because of colored oxidative breakdown products. Other drugs may bind to the matrix and cause oxidative breakdown of the plastic (52). Drugs such as sulfasalazine (yellow) and rifampin (red-orange) that are secreted into tear fluid may also discolor contact lenses. All manufacturers of soft lenses emphasize that with exception of a few specially formulated rewetting solutions, no solutions should be placed into the eye with the soft lens in place. If a drug solution is placed into the eye prior to lens insertion, the wearer must wait until the drug solution has cleared from the precorneal (conjunctival) pocket. For most drug solutions, about 5 minutes is adequate. In some instances, the ophthalmologist may prefer the lenses to be worn while a prescription medication is instilled in the eye so that the lens serves as a reservoir for the drug. If no instructions accompany an ophthalmic prescription for a soft lens wearer, a physician should be contacted. This is also true for any nonprescription ophthalmic product not specifically designed for use with contact lenses. When topical ophthalmic ointments are being used, the lenses should not be worn at all.

Unlike hard lenses, soft lenses cannot be marked to identify which is for the left and right eyes. In hard lenses, a small colored dot marker on one hard lens identifies it as the left or right. This marker, located at the outer periphery of the lens, is not perceived by the wearer when the lens is on the cornea. A soft lens wearer who is uncertain of the positional identity of the lenses may have to see a vision specialist for proper determination. Always removing and inserting lenses in the same order reduces the chance of a mix-up.

Soft lenses generally cost more than hard lenses (43). Although the initial cost of acquiring soft lenses has decreased with the increased number of new users, the overall cost is greater because of more frequent replacement requirements and increased use of lens cleaning and disinfection solutions. In addition to replacement necessitated by changes in the refractory requirements of the eye, soft lenses are less durable.

The care given to contact lenses varies considerably with each wearer. Inadequate care or neglect of hard lenses may lead to corneal problems and/or wearer discomfort, but the lens will still maintain its optical qualities. However, soft lenses rapidly degenerate to useless pieces of plastic if they are neglected. When used with a conscientious care and cleaning program, daily wear soft lenses can be expected to have an average life of 18–24 months compared with 2–3 years for a similarly used rigid gas-permeable lens (53).

Insertion of Soft Lenses

When inserting soft lenses, the wearer should carefully follow these steps:

- Wash the hands with noncosmetic soap and rinse thoroughly; dry the hands with a lint-free towel.

- Remove the lens for the right eye from its storage container. Rinse it with saline solution to dilute any preservatives left from disinfection.

- Place the lens on the top of a finger and examine to be sure it is not "inside-out."

- Examine the lens for cleanliness. If necessary, clean it and again rinse with saline.

- Insert the lens on the right eye.

- Repeat the process for the left eye.

Corneal Effects of Hard and Soft Lenses

Corneal Hypoxia and Edema

As with any other tissue, the cornea requires oxygen. Because it does not have a direct blood supply, nearly all of the cornea's oxygen must be transferred through tear fluid. This process means that an adequate supply of oxygen can be provided only if the cornea is continuously bathed with oxygenated tears (54–57). A contact lens interferes with normal corneal oxygen uptake because it restricts available oxygen from reaching the cornea. Additionally, because hard and many soft lenses are generally less permeable to oxygen than are the tears, it is crucial that lenses be fitted to maximize tear movement between the lens and the cornea (37).

Metabolic byproducts from the surface epithelium are flushed out from under contact lenses and oxygen brought in as tear fluid is pumped in and out from under contact lenses when they move toward and away from the cornea during blinking. Even when properly fitted, both rigid and soft lenses can produce a progressive hypoxia of the cornea while the lenses are in place (54–59), especially in persons who do not blink often enough.

One major effect of this hypoxia is edema of the corneal tissues (58, 60–62). It has been demonstrated that corneal thickness is increased to a greater extent by hard lenses (61–63). After approximately 16 hours of continuous wear, hard and, to lesser extent, soft lenses cause the glycogen content of the cornea to fall to a level that is accompanied by significant edema. If lenses are then removed for 6 hours, the glycogen levels return to approximately 93% of the normal value and about 98% in 8 hours. To prevent edema from reaching this extent, lenses should be removed for a 1-hour rest period after 7–9 hours of wear. The lenses may then be reinserted for up to 8 hours if necessary. Wearing rigid gas-permeable or soft lenses uninterrupted for 14–18 hours once or twice a week will not usually cause problems; continuing such a practice on a daily basis should be discouraged. Tolerance to contact lens wear does occur.

Corneal Abrasions

Corneal abrasions are surface defects in the epithelial layer of the cornea. Causes of these abrasions range from poorly fitted lenses or simple overwear to scratches caused by entrapment of foreign bodies such as dust, makeup, or eyelashes under the lens. The cornea is sensitive to pain upon abrasion, so that reflex lid closure (blepharospasm), lacrimation, and raising of the hands to the affected eye are immediate. Rubbing the eye, although almost reflexive, must be avoided because it can cause more extensive damage while the lens remains in the eye.

Fortunately, the pain associated with corneal abrasion is usually of greater magnitude than the damage that is present. The epithelium regenerates quickly so that most minor epithelial defects (22 mm in diameter or less) generally heal within 12–24 hours. The lens should be left out for 2 days to a week. The wearer may then proceed using a modified break-in schedule suggested by the vision specialist. More extensive abrasions require the attention of an ophthalmologist.

SIGNS AND SYMPTOMS OF LENS PROBLEMS

A "symptom" may be defined as a subjective patient complaint; a "sign" is an objective measurement of observation by a trained practitioner. Lens wearers may initially encounter various problems in adapting to lenses, particularly rigid gas-permeable lenses; even long-time wearers occasionally experience some type of difficulty. The following listing provides a perspective for counseling a lens wearer who seeks advice. Many of these problems arise from different causative factors, and the identification and resolution of a specific problem may require a trained vision specialist. Most of this information is particularly applicable to hard lens wear.

- Deep aching of eye—This pain persists even after the lens is removed and may be caused by poorly fitted lenses (too tight). The lens diameter must be increased.

- Blurred vision—This effect may be produced by improper refractive power; tear film buildup (cosmetics and surface scratches on the outer face of the lens enhance protein buildup); cosmetic film buildup (eye makeup and cosmetics can be transferred to the lens from the fingers); switched lenses; corneal edema; or oral contraceptive use.

- Excessive tearing—Tearing is a normal symptom when lens wear is first initiated; however, tearing may also be caused by poorly fitted lens (too tight causes poor tear circulation; too loose causes excessive contact with lids and reflex lacrimation), or chipped, rough edges on the lenses.

- Fogging—"Misty" or "smoky" vision can be caused by corneal edema; overwearing of contact lenses; coatings or deposits on lens surfaces; or poor wetting of lens while on the eye.

- Itching—This problem may be caused by allergic conjunctivitis and may be treated with short-term use of topical steroids.

- Lens falls out of eye—Poorly fitted lenses are probably the cause. However, hard lenses may occasionally slide off of the cornea or be blinked out of the eye even when properly fitted.

- Inability to wear lenses in morning—This may be caused by corneal edema or mild conjunctivitis.

- Pain after removal of lens—This effect is usually caused by corneal abrasion. The presence of the lens anesthetizes the cornea; sensation returns after 4–6 hours and pain develops. For this reason, the wearer may not directly link the cause to the lenses.

- Sudden pain in the eye—A foreign body or chipped lens may be the problem.
- Squinting—This effect is caused by excessive lens movement or a poorly fitted lens. The wearer squints to center optical portion of lens over the pupil.

CARE OF HARD AND RIGID LENSES

For the cornea to sustain normal metabolic balance and maintain proper refractory characteristics for optical clarity, it must have relatively constant exposure to the atmosphere during waking periods (55, 56). This exposure permits atmospheric oxygen to dissolve in the precorneal fluid and transfer to the cornea. This precorneal fluid also must constantly bathe the corneal surface; this process is aided by blinking. The presence of a hard contact lens impairs these normal processes. To minimize the stress on these processes, hard contact lens wear must be supported with concurrent use of lens care products. Such solutions aid the wearer by providing comfort and safety.

Cleaning Products

Normal tears are composed of secretions from many specialized glands lining the lacrimal apparatus, conjunctiva, and lids. Many components are somewhat hydrophobic and tend to adhere to the surface of a hard lens during normal daily wear. This residue, primarily proteinaceous debris and oils, acts as a growth medium for bacteria. If this material is not routinely removed by daily cleaning, it may harden to form coatings or tenacious deposits that create an irregular surface on the lens. This residue will eventually irritate the lids and corneal epithelium, and may progress to infection or other pathology. Decreased visual acuity and lens wear time are likely consequences of a cloudy lens or allergenic reactions.

Typical cleaning solutions contain nonionic or amphoteric surfactants that emulsify oils and aid in solubilizing other debris. Proteins and lipids are soluble in highly alkaline media, but a high pH can cause lens decomposition. Weak alkaline solutions may be helpful in dislodging deposits from the lens in conjunction with the surface tension lowering properties of the surfactants.

Lenses should be thoroughly rinsed after cleaning because residual cleaning agents may lead to ocular irritation. Lenses should never be wiped dry with tissue as this can cause surface scratches.

Contact lenses should be cleaned immediately after removal from the eye. Routine daily removal of accumulated deposits will do much to ensure a clear, comfortable lens. Many complaints of lens discomfort or unclear vision can be traced to inadequate or improper cleaning procedures.

There are four basic techniques for cleaning hard lenses.

Friction Rubbing

A contact lens cleaning solution or gel is applied to both surfaces of the lens. The lens is then rubbed between the thumb and forefinger or between the forefinger and palm of the opposite hand for about 20 seconds. Friction rubbing is the most common cleaning method (32) and it is effective, but it may result in scratched and warped lenses if rubbing is too vigorous.

Spray Cleaning

The lenses are placed into a perforated holder and held under a stream of running water from an ordinary faucet. The pressure of the water flow dislodges debris that has been loosened by overnight soaking in the storage case.

Hydraulic Cleaning

The lenses are placed into separate baskets in a plastic container that has a rotating cap. The cap, which is connected to the baskets in which the lenses are placed, is rotated for 20–30 seconds to provide a high level of turbulence. The unit is filled with a special cleaning solution to assist in removal of deposits.

Ultrasonic Cleaning

The lenses are placed in a water bath through which ultrasound waves are passed. These specialized cleaning units have not been shown to be superior in cleaning contact lenses, and their cost limits use to in-office cleaning by the practitioner.

Soaking Solutions

A soaking solution is used to store a hard contact lens whenever it is removed from the eye. The solution serves for maximum comfort and visual acuity. It also aids in the removal of deposits that accumulate on the lens during wear (64).

A rigid lens absorbs between 1 and 3% moisture by weight. Upon exposure to air, the lens dehydrates; the lens subsequently rehydrates when it comes in contact with a soaking solution or the lacrimal fluid (65). Placing a dehydrated lens into the eye, with or without a wetting solution, causes discomfort as the lens absorbs tears from the precorneal eye (66). In addition, a dehydrated lens is flatter than a hydrated lens; this factor causes problems with both comfort and visual acuity until the lens' moisture content stabilizes (67, 68).

During normal wear, rigid lenses absorb tear constituents, which results in an accumulation of deposits. If lenses are allowed to dry out during overnight storage, the deposits are more difficult to remove by normal cleaning methods. Thorough cleaning of lenses after removal and subsequent storage in a soaking solution reduce the likelihood of deposit.

To maintain sterility, storage solutions use essentially the same preservatives as wetting solutions. The main difference is that the concentration can be somewhat higher in a soaking solution because it is rinsed from the lens before insertion. However, preservative levels are carefully selected because higher levels do not necessarily give increased effectiveness and may lead to impaired wetting or corneal irritation because of the adsorption of preservatives onto the lens (69, 70).

Wetting Solutions

The functions of an ideal wetting solution are:

- To convert the hydrophobic lens surface to a hydrophilic surface by means of a uniform film that does not easily wash away (71–73);

- To increase comfort by providing a cushioning and lubricating effect between the corneal surface and the inner surface of the lens, and between the lens and the inner surface of the eyelid (72, 74);

- To establish a viscous coating on the lens to protect it from oily deposits on the fingers during insertion;

- To stabilize the lens on the fingertip to facilitate insertion, particularly for individuals with poor manual dexterity or unsteady hands (32).

The term "contact lens" is a misnomer because, when properly positioned, the lens does not actually contact the corneal surface. Rather, a hard lens should float freely on a layer of tears and rotate during blinking. For this to occur, tear fluids must "wet" the hydrophobic lens surface.

If the lens is thoroughly cleaned before insertion, the lacrimal fluid could adequately wet the lens. Indeed, the "wetting action" of popular wetting solutions is not significantly better than saline, and those whose tears are capable of wetting a lens almost immediately upon insertion often do not use these solutions prior to insertion on the eye.

The basic wetting solution is comprised of components from four main functional categories:

- Cushioning agents, such as viscosity-inducing additives (usually cellulose gum derivatives such as methylcellulose or hydroxypropyl methylcellulose);

- Wetting agents, such as polyvinyl alcohol or other surfactants;

- Preservatives, such as benzalkonium chloride, thimerosal, polyquaternium-1, sorbic acid and sorbates, and polyamino propyl biguanide;

- Buffering agents and salts to adjust pH and tonicity.

The cushioning effect of a wetting solution is caused by the presence of hydrophilic polymers that lubricate the interface between the lens and the surfaces of the cornea and eyelid. Cellulose gum derivatives are often used because they are effective lubricants. Although compounds such as methylcellulose possess a degree of surfactant activity, they do not promote uniform wetting of a rigid lens. For this reason, polyvinyl alcohol frequently is used in combination with these agents to decrease surface tension.

The concentration of the cushioning polymer in wetting solutions affects both the comfort of the lens in the eye and the quality of vision immediately following insertion. In some individuals, a concentration that is too low causes discomfort after only a short period of lens wear. In other wearers, a high polymer concentration results in blurred vision because of poor mixing of the viscous solution with tears. In addition, overspill of solution onto the lids and eyelashes causes crusting as the solution dries; this crusty residue can be a source of foreign material falling into the eye. Saliva should never be used to wet contact lenses because it can lead to infection by *Acanthamoeba*, *Pseudomonas aeruginosa*, or other pathogens (32).

Multifunctional Products

There has been a trend toward the use of combination solutions for the cleaning, soaking, and wetting of hard contact lenses. Initially, manufacturers recommended three different solutions, specially formulated, for these functions. Soon, solutions claiming to be effective for both wetting and soaking, or for soaking and cleaning, were introduced. Some manufacturers offer a single solution claimed to be effective for all three basic procedures.

The major problem with an all-purpose solution is that, to some extent, ingredients required in the formulation perform different and somewhat incompatible functions (32). For example, high concentrations of benzalkonium chloride are necessary to kill bacteria in soaking solutions; these same concentrations can cause ocular irritation when placed directly on the eye with a contact lens.

If lenses are stored overnight in a solution containing a high concentration of polymers for cushioning and wetting, the lenses may become "gummy" and cause discomfort. Likewise, if lenses are stored overnight in a cleaning solution containing an anionic surfactant, the detergent may eventually build up on the lens and cause irritation. Although there is a need for a single agent that will adequately perform all three basic functions, no such agent currently exists. The present all-purpose solutions should be considered compromises. They are marginally effective, but they cannot be expected to perform as well as separate solutions. Some persons will do quite well with an all-purpose solution, but others will undoubtedly do better with a multiple solution approach.

Rewetting Products

These solutions are intended to clean and rewet the contact lens while the lens is in place on the eye (75). They depend on the use of surfactants to loosen deposits; removal is assisted by the natural cleaning action of blinking. An agent used to promote this action is polyoxyl 40 stearate. Although these products function well to recondition the in situ lens, the cornea benefits more from actual removal, cleaning, and rewetting of the lens. Removal of the lens for even a brief time during the normal wear period allows the cornea to recover some of its depleted glycogen levels. The use of an in-the-eye rewetting solution, although expedient, does not provide this needed respite.

Miscellaneous Lens Care Products

Preinsertion Solutions

Preinsertion solutions are used to prepare lenses for insertion onto the cornea. These products are generally high viscosity polymer solutions that further

cushion placement of the lens on the cornea. They may be especially useful during the initial break-in period for individuals with particularly high corneal sensitivity. The high viscosity of these solutions may cause blurred vision for a little while after insertion, which some patients may find annoying.

Conditioners

Conditioners are recommended when tears do not supply a sufficient wetting action or cushioning effect. They are also used to clear the eye of potential debris-forming substances before lens insertion, and they can be applied to the eye as frequently as 3 or 4 times a day while the lens is being worn (75).

Other Products

Other ophthalmic products are available to the hard lens wearer for occasional use. Some, such as artificial tears and ocular decongestants, are not recommended for use with the lenses in place. Because of their emollient and lubricating effect, artificial tears can be used to soothe the eye. Ocular decongestants reduce mild conjunctival hyperemia associated with prolonged lens wear. Routine use of these products should be avoided. If symptoms requiring their use persist, a visit to a vision specialist is advised to determine the cause. (See Chapter 20, *Ophthalmic Products.*)

Formulation Considerations

The manufacturing and marketing of contact lenses are regulated by the ophthalmic devices division of the Food and Drug Administration (FDA). Even though contact lens solutions are not considered drug products, formulation considerations still apply. Formulation of a contact lens product must be guided by the knowledge that a contact lens solution may be used daily for months or even years. The potential for cumulative effects on ocular tissues or the lens is significant. Because these products are often used by inexperienced people after minimal counseling, all ingredients must be effective and provide a high margin of safety.

The basic considerations for a well-formulated contact lens solution include isotonicity with tears, pH, viscosity, stability, sterility, and provision for maintenance of sterility (bactericidal action). The pH range for comfort is not well defined because tear pH varies among individuals; normal tear pH is 7.4. It is best to have a weakly buffered solution that can readily adjust to any tear pH because highly buffered solutions can cause significant discomfort, even ocular damage, when instilled. However, as with therapeutic ophthalmic solutions, stability of the solution components takes precedence over comfort. For this reason, many contact lens solutions are formulated with pH values above or below 7.4, some as much as 3 pH units (76). However, these systems are weakly buffered and are well tolerated by the eye.

Routine daily use of any contact lens solution allows the potential for bacterial contamination. Depending on the individual's specific lens care procedures, a single container may last for a month or more. The solution must therefore contain a suitable bactericidal agent that is both effective over the long-term and nonirritating with daily use in the eye. Few preservatives fulfill these criteria (77, 78). The most commonly used agents are benzalkonium chloride, thimerosal, and sorbic acid products. These agents are not free from irritation potential, depending on concentration and patient sensitivity. Solutions from different manufacturers should not be mixed because a precipitate may result. For instance, a product containing alkaline borate buffers forms a gummy, gel-like precipitate on lenses if mixed with a wetting solution containing polyvinyl alcohol.

Contact lens solutions specifically formulated for hard lenses should *not* be used for soft lens care. Certain preservatives and agents in rigid lens solutions may bind to and adversely affect soft contact lenses. In addition, some otherwise compatible agents in hard lens solutions may be too concentrated for use with soft lenses. Contact lens wearers should use only lens care products that have been approved by the FDA for use with their specific contact lens material.

Soft contact lens solutions, on the other hand, may generally be used with hard lenses. However, efficacy of soft lens solutions for cleaning, wetting, or storing hard lenses may not be as great as solutions specifically formulated for hard lenses.

CARE OF SOFT LENSES

Wearers of hydrophilic contact lenses should be particularly cautious in exposing their lenses to chemicals. These chemicals, many of which penetrate and bind with the lens material, come from cosmetics, environmental pollutants, and nonprescription and prescription ophthalmic and systemic products (46, 47). Conventional hard lens solutions are contraindicated for use with soft lenses because absorption of the ingredients can damage lenses (49, 56, 79, 80). Because soft lenses contain a high percentage of water, they are most prone to bacterial contamination (81). Lens disinfection must be maintained to prevent ocular infection and damage to the lens material by bacteria and fungi (82). Actually, the term "sterility" is a misnomer because maintaining true sterility of a soft lens, especially while worn in the eye, is not possible. The term "disinfection" more accurately reflects the routine procedures used to eliminate bacterial contamination before it increases to harmful levels in the lens.

The basic regimen of care is more important for soft lenses than hard lenses in maintaining comfort and optical clarity and quality. Several types of cleaning and disinfectant products have been developed.

Cleaning Products

A troublesome aspect of soft lens wear is the accumulation of deposits on the lens (51, 83). The nature of these deposits is varied, but generally they consist of proteins and lipids from the wearer's lacrimal secretions. The rate at which these deposits accumulate depends on the lens and the tears. Deposits are a greater problem with the more highly hydrated lenses. However, some wearers experience little difficulty and wear soft lenses for long periods without significant buildup; others may show deposits in as little as 2 or 3 days. Whatever the cause or accumulation rate, the result is an uncomfortable lens of poor optical quality (84–86). Specific cleaning procedures have been developed to help the wearer maintain clear lenses for a prolonged period (87–91).

Surface-Active Cleaners

A common method of cleaning soft lenses involves use of surface-active materials and friction rubbing. Several drops of a cleaning product are placed onto the lens surface and the lens is gently rubbed between the thumb and forefinger. Another method is to place the lens in the palm of the hand and rub gently with a fingertip. With both methods, care must be used to avoid cutting the soft lens with a fingernail or scratching lens surfaces with grit or dirt not washed from the hands. Soft lens cleaning solutions generally contain a nonionic detergent, a wetting agent, a chelating agent, buffers, preservatives, and, in some cases, polymeric cleaning beads. Friction cleaning usually takes about 20–30 seconds, and then the cleaner must be thoroughly rinsed from the lens. Rinsing is an essential part of soft lens care; it should be carried out using a sterile isotonic buffered solution (32). Some products have a lower viscosity and may be easier to rinse off the lens.

Weekly (Enzymatic) Cleaners

The surface-active cleaners generally are quite effective in removing lipid deposits. They are less successful in removing tenacious protein debris. Weekly cleaners are an additional cleaning aid that can help to solve this problem. Lenses are soaked in an enzyme solution (papain, pancreatin, or subtilisin) for several hours or overnight. These enzymes hydrolyze polypeptide bonds of protein and dissolve the protein deposits. The lenses should then be cleaned to remove all traces of enzyme to prevent eye irritation. It is usually sufficient to use enzyme cleaning as a once-a-week supplement to daily cleaning with surface-active chemicals. Enzymatic regimens have been developed to be used simultaneously with thermal and chemical disinfection.

Disinfection of Soft Lenses

The FDA recommends "sterilization" of soft contact lenses before each reinsertion. Two methods are currently approved for use: thermal and chemical. Studies have shown that microorganisms do not actually enter the matrix of soft lenses (92, 93), but that surface contamination could lead to ocular infection (94, 95). Both disinfecting methods are reliable. The disinfecting step occurs after cleaning the lens. Chemical disinfection with hydrogen peroxide has increased in popularity over thermal and earlier chemical disinfectants.

Thermal Disinfection

The basic method of thermal (heat) disinfection involves placing the cleaned lenses into separate compartments of a storage case filled with saline. The case is then placed into a heating unit and the temperature increased to a specific level for a prescribed time (96). Originally, the lenses were disinfected by raising the temperature to the boiling point for about 20 minutes. Units that use a lower temperature (about 80°C or 176°F) for a longer time are now available. The FDA requirement is 80°C for at least 10 minutes. This process is as effective as boiling and prolongs lens life. The procedure is usually undertaken at night so that lenses are ready for wear in the morning.

Thermal disinfection has several advantages. It is preservative-free and therefore less likely to cause eye irritation. Additionally, thermal disinfection kills microbial contamination better than any other method. Thermal disinfection is the only contact lens disinfecting method known to be effective against cysts of *Acanthamoeba* and is generally more effective against chemically resistant microorganisms such as fungi and bacillus species. When requiring maximum kill, thermal disinfection is best. It kills organisms on and surrounding contact lens cases, further preventing potential lens contaminants from entering the lenses.

Although many wearers consider thermal disinfection to be the best, it does have several drawbacks. Some find the method cumbersome and less convenient than chemical disinfection. There is a high initial cost for thermal disinfection equipment for the user, although long-term costs of chemical disinfectant solutions may offset this. The user must take care to remove proteinaceous and other debris by cleaning lenses before thermal disinfection. Lens cases used with thermal units, and the units themselves, should be routinely inspected for damage, cracks, or leaks and replaced at the earliest sign of a problem.

Chemical Disinfection

Chemical disinfection may also be termed "cold" sterilization because heat is not used to kill microorganisms. The lenses are stored for a prescribed period of time in a solution containing bactericidal agents that are compatible with soft lens materials.

There are two basic forms of chemical disinfecting systems in the United States. First, antimicrobial preservatives of sufficient concentration in storage solutions primarily composed of saline were the original chemical disinfecting solutions. Initial disinfecting solutions contained chlorhexidine and thimerosal. Thimerosal induced sensitivity reactions in many patients. Several disinfecting solutions still contain chlorhexidine. Patients are less sensitive to chlorhexidine, and it appears to be better tolerated than thimerosal.

Several new disinfecting preservatives are marketed for soft contact lens solutions to avoid sensitivity reactions. These preservatives are sorbic acid, Polyquad, and Dymed, touted to be much less toxic or allergenic than their early antimicrobial predecessors. However, these agents may be less effective against fungi and protozoans.

The second chemical method uses hydrogen peroxide as the antimicrobial agent. Soft lenses are placed in purified hydrogen peroxide, and the liberation of oxygen from peroxide provides effective disinfection. Following disinfection, peroxide is neutralized to trace levels by catalytic action of platinum or peroxidase, or by soaking lenses in sodium thiosulfite solution. The soft lens wearer should ensure that the peroxide has been neutralized, because a peroxide-soaked lens placed on the eye will cause great pain, photophobia, redness, and, perhaps, corneal epithelial damage. Household hydrogen peroxide solutions should not be used to disinfect soft lenses because contaminants and other chemicals within such solutions may discolor the lenses.

Soft lens wearers may freely switch from thermal disinfection to chemical methods, but the switch from chemical to thermal may present problems. If lenses that have been subjected to a chemical disinfecting solution are not completely free from all traces of the chemicals, the lens can be damaged by heating. Prolonged soaking in several changes of saline is recommended to purge the lens before using a heating unit.

Saline Solutions

Because the hydrophilic soft contact lens absorbs water, it must be maintained in a constant state of hydration. Furthermore, the hydrated lens must be isotonic with tears because changes in tonicity can alter the conformation and optical properties of the lens. Isotonic normal saline is the basic solution used for rinsing, thermal disinfection, and storage of soft contact lenses.

Prepared saline is available in either preserved or preservative-free forms. Because thimerosal and chlorhexidine can cause sensitivity reactions or irritation in a substantial number of patients, sorbic acid-preserved products are therefore commonly promoted for "sensitive eyes" and appear to be acceptable to the majority of wearers. Salines preserved with Polyquad and Dymed are also promoted for patients who are sensitive to other preservatives.

If avoiding preservatives altogether is desired or essential, several preservative-free salines are available. Preservative-free buffered saline is available in unit-of-use containers, which should be used or discarded once opened. Unpreserved salines are available as aerosol sprays.

Some persons may choose to prepare their own preservative-free saline using salt tablets and USP purified water. The use of salt tablets is inexpensive compared with other forms of saline, but the clear superiority of commercial salines argues strongly against the use of salt tablets. The use of homemade saline from salt tablets and application of improper lens care are the greatest predisposing factors to acanthamoeba keratitis, a rare vision-threatening eye disease, and to many anterior eye infections contracted by hydrophilic lens wearers (34, 97–99). The FDA no longer condones the use of salt tablets, and neither should a concerned pharmacist.

Acanthamoeba, of which there are 15 species, is an opportunistic protozoan. Usually nonpathogenic, *Acanthamoeba* has been isolated from airborne dust, soils, surface water, tap water, and even distilled water. In unfavorable environments, the protozoan forms a very resistant cyst that can survive many antimicrobial agents, even though its vegetative form (trophozoite) may be susceptible. Viable cysts have been found in swimming pools and hot tubs that are adequately chlorinated to kill trophozoites.

Most victims of acanthamoeba keratitis have used nonsterile saline solution—made from salt tablets and distilled water—or have used tap water in the maintenance of their soft contact lenses. Because cysts are very resistant, *Acanthamoeba* often can survive attempts to antimicrobially eradicate them from the eye. Multiple antibiotic regimens have been applied; however, many cases of acanthamoeba keratitis have resulted in keratoplasty to save the eye. Although a rare eye disease, this form of keratitis is devastating. As diagnosis of the keratitis has become more definitive and awareness of the disease more acute, the apparent incidence of acanthamoeba keratitis has risen from 11 cases reported between 1973 and 1983, to 24 cases between mid-1985 and February 1986. Over 200 cases have been diagnosed through the first quarter of 1989. The uses of tap water and/or salt tablets with contact lenses is, therefore, to be discouraged.

Other Soft Lens Products

Accessory solutions for use with soft lenses have been formulated to permit cleaning, lubricating, and rewetting of the lens in the eye. These solutions typically contain a low concentration of a nonionic surfactant to promote cleaning and a polymer to lubricate the lens surface, along with buffering agents. They are particularly useful to patients with highly hydrated lenses, such as the extended-wear type (3). Exposure of lenses to wind and high temperature causes a degree of dehydration even with the lens in place in the eye (44). The resulting discomfort can sometimes be relieved by 1 or 2 drops of these solutions. To minimize contaminations, the tip of the applicator bottle should not touch the eye, eyelid, or any other surface.

CARE OF RIGID-GAS PERMEABLE LENSES

The diversity and variation in materials used in rigid gas-permeable lenses preclude generalizations about products and regimens used in their care. Lens wearers should be advised by their eye care professionals about the products and regimens recommended for their particular lenses. The labeling for contact lens products also indicates the lenses for which they are approved.

Conventional hard lens solutions are generally compatible with rigid gas-permeable lenses. Use of cleaning, soaking and disinfection, and wetting solutions is recommended.

Lenses containing silicone require a conditioning solution, essentially a specially formulated wetting solution, because of the hydrophobic nature of silicone.

The conditioner system enhances wettability of the lens, increases comfort, and disinfects the lens. Silicone acrylate lenses (acrylate) have an active surface that promotes binding of tear constituents. Cleaners designed for conventional rigid lenses may not be effective in removing the more tenacious deposits. Cleaning products designed for this type of lens are formulated with polymercuric beads that mechanically break the adhesive bonds that have formed between the lens and deposits. These cleaning products may cause hairline scratches in the lens, and, if not rinsed carefully, ocular irritation.

Products containing chlorhexidine gluconate should *not* be used with silicone or styrene lenses because this agent will make the lens surface more difficult to wet. Thermal disinfection should also not be used with these lenses, because it can warp them.

PRESERVATIVES USED IN CONTACT LENS SOLUTIONS

Benzalkonium Chloride

Benzalkonium chloride is a surface-active agent and germicide effective against a variety of Gram-positive and Gram-negative bacteria (100–102). In sufficient concentration, it is also effective against perhaps the most worrisome ocular pathogen, *P. aeruginosa.* Several properties of benzalkonium chloride require that care be exercised with respect to its concentration in a hard lens solution. Benzalkonium chloride is incompatible with soft contact lenses and must not be used with them.

High concentrations of benzalkonium chloride cause ocular damage, either directly by instillation into the eye or indirectly by adsorption onto the lens (103). The maximum tolerable concentration is reportedly about 0.03% (1:3,000), with solutions of 0.02% having been shown to be tolerated up to several times a day (104). However, most solutions for direct instillation into the eye contain concentrations well below this (0.004%).

Some persons using a solution preserved with benzalkonium chloride develop ocular irritation because of buildup of the surfactant on their lenses. Switching to a solution with a lower benzalkonium chloride concentra-

tion may alleviate this, but change to a solution with a completely different preservative or cleaning agent may be required.

Thimerosal

Thimerosal, or sodium ethylmercurithiosalicylate, was introduced as an alternative to benzalkonium chloride. It is effective against *P. aeruginosa,* but it is slow to act because it depends on sustained release of mercurial ions that penetrate the bacterial cell (105–107). It is incompatible with benzalkonium chloride. Like other mercurials, it may also cause sensitization in some individuals after repeated application. In general, thimerosal is not a significant problem except for soft contact lens use. Apparently, the concentration of the preservative carried to the eye via soft lenses causes a significant incidence of irritation. Like benzalkonium chloride, it acts by interfering with cell metabolism, glycolysis, and respiration. Most practitioners have discouraged the use of soft lens care products with thimerosal because of the high incidence of sensitivity in the population.

Phenylmercuric Nitrate

Phenylmercuric nitrate also is a mercurial preservative, similar in action to thimerosal. It is usually used in dilute concentration and is not precipitated in an acidic pH. When used alone, however, it is not very effective against *P. aeruginosa* (108, 109). Organic mercurials can be effective preservatives, but their usefulness in ophthalmic solutions is severely limited because of their slow action (107).

Sorbic Acid or Potassium Sorbate

Sorbic acid is becoming increasingly popular as a preservative. It is less irritating than mercurials. It is also the preservative ingredient often included in products labeled "thimerosal-free." It is reported to possibly increase age-associated yellowing of some lenses, particularly those containing a methacrylic acid (32).

Chlorhexidine

Chlorhexidine can irritate the eyes, and its degradation products may produce a yellow-to-green discoloration (83).

Sodium Edetate

Sodium edetate (tetrasodium ethylenediaminetetraacetate, or EDTA) is often used in lens solutions because it disrupts the integrity of bacterial cell walls. As such, it enhances the action of other preservatives (110). It also complexes with other substances, such as metallic ions, that might reduce benzalkonium chloride activity. By complexation, calcium deposits on lenses may be prevented. EDTA is often used in contact lens solutions that contain another chemical agent as their primary preservative. Solutions of EDTA cannot be claimed to be preservative-free, even if there is no other primary preservative.

PRODUCT SELECTION GUIDELINES

Hard Lens Products

The variety of lens care solutions available to hard lens wearers poses a puzzling selection problem. The availability of single- and multiple-function products within the same product line can further frustrate and confuse some wearers. This situation means that selection of contact lens products is an area where pharmacists can perform a much needed role as a consultant. Unfortunately, available information is not always sufficient to provide a complete foundation for patient consultation in all aspects of lens wear. Product labeling is often incomplete or limited to general information. Preservative concentration is usually listed adequately in terms of the specific agents and concentrations, but concentrations of cushioning and lubricating polymers are often absent. Furthermore, other ingredients are often listed simply as "cleaning agents" or "buffers," making alternate selections a random process for patients with sensitivities to these components. One factor that could be used in determining which products to recommend when no specific brand is requested is to select those with adequate labeling.

A very important factor for a hard lens wearer who is experiencing ocular irritation is how long the lenses are worn each day. The presence of a hard lens on the cornea reduces corneal sensitivity to the extent that the wearer may not be aware of overwear abrasion or edema until several hours after the lenses are removed. Often, many cases of burning, itching eyes can be solved by using short periods of lens removal (rest periods) for patients who must routinely wear their lenses for long hours during the day and evening.

Soft Lens Products

Although most soft lens care regimens are initially recommended by the prescriber, pharmacists can assist wearers who experience difficulty or express dissatisfaction. Many problems associated with soft lens wear arise from the way people handle their lenses. Unsatisfactory results with soft lens products may stem from improper procedures rather than an inadequate product (32, 111, 112). In one investigation, only 26% of contact lens wearers fully complied with care instructions. Noncompliance was directly correlated to the occurrence of signs and symptoms of potential wearing problems. Specific questions about the care and maintenance regimen used by a wearer can often bring these problems to light. Compatibility of lifestyle and lens care regimen is particularly essential for comfortable and trouble-free soft lens wear.

Rigid Gas-Permeable Lens Products

The appropriate lens care regimen for rigid gas-permeable lenses must be compatible with the particular lens. Lens wearers should be advised against substituting products for those specifically recommended by their eye care professional.

PATIENT COUNSELING

The following are general instructions for successful contact lens wear:

- The hands should be washed and thoroughly rinsed before contact lenses are touched.

- When handling lenses over a sink, the drain should be covered or closed to prevent loss of a lens.

- Contact lenses are individually fitted to correct the accommodation error of each eye. To avoid mixing up the lenses, it is helpful to always work with the same lens first (always insert or remove the right lens first and then the left). Hard lenses may be marked to avoid confusion.

- Oily cosmetics should be avoided while lenses are being worn. Bath oils or soaps with a bath oil or cream base may leave an oily film on the hands that will be transferred to the lenses. Therefore, special care should be used in cleaning the hands before touching lenses.

- Aerosol cosmetics, such as hair sprays or spray deodorants, damage the lens and should be applied before lens insertion, or with eyes closed until air is clear of spray particles.

- Lenses should not be inserted in red or irritated eyes. If the eyes become irritated while wearing lenses, they should be removed until irritation subsides. Should irritation or redness not subside, a lens practitioner should be contacted.

- Except for extended wear lenses, *contact lenses must not be worn while sleeping*. Damage to the eye may result.

- Lenses should not be worn while sitting under a hair dryer if excessive dryness of the eyes results. The same applies to overhead fans or air ducts at work or home.

- The eyes should be protected when lenses are worn outside on windy days because windblown soot and other particles may become trapped under the lens and scratch the cornea.

- Contact lenses do not preclude the use of eye protection in industry, for sports, or for any other occupation or hobby that has the potential for eye damage.

- Contact lens solution should never be reused.

- Contact lenses should always be stored in a proper lens case when not in use. This prevents lens loss and damage.

- Contact lens care instructions should be carefully followed.

- Soaking solutions in lens cases should be replaced after each use. Lenses should not be stored in tap water.

- Contact lenses should be cleaned only with agents specifically made for that purpose. Household cleaners will damage contact lenses.

- Each type of lens should be cared for only with products made specifically for that type of lens.

- Contact lens care products from different manufacturers may not be chemically compatible with each other and should not be mixed.

- Contact lens care products should be discarded if the labeled expiration date has passed.

- Contact lenses should not be worn in swimming pools (or hot tubs) unless special lenses for this purpose are being used, or the eyes are kept shut.

- To prevent contamination, dropper tips or the tips of lens care product containers should not be touched.

- Contact lenses and contact lens care products should be kept out of the reach of children.

- Saliva should never be used to wet contact lenses. This practice can result in eye infections.

The following special instructions will help ensure successful hard contact lens wear:

- The eyes should not be rubbed while lenses are in place. Rubbing could result in cuts or abrasions of the cornea.

- Contact lenses should not be rinsed with very hot or very cold water because temperature extremes may warp the lenses.

The following special instructions will help ensure successful soft contact lens wear:

- Soft contact lenses must be thoroughly cleaned before thermal disinfection.

- Chemical disinfectants must be completely rinsed off before placing the lens in the eye.

- Hydrogen peroxide disinfectants must be completely neutralized before placing the lens in the eye.

- Salt tablets or homemade saline solution should not be used with contact lenses.

- Enzyme cleaner tablets should be discarded if any discoloration has appeared.

- The many types of soft lenses each require a specific care regimen. Only care products recommended for the patient's type of soft lens should be used.

- Soft lenses must be handled with care because they are very fragile and can easily be torn.

- Soft contact lenses should be removed before instillation of any ophthalmic preparation that is not specifically intended for concurrent use with soft contact lenses. The wearer should wait at least 20–30 minutes before reinserting the lenses unless directed otherwise by an eye care specialist. Lenses should not be worn at all when a topical ophthalmic ointment is being used.

■ Soft contact lenses should not be worn in the presence of irritating fumes or chemicals.

■ Extended wear soft lenses should not be worn continuously for more than 7 days without complete cleaning and disinfection.

■ Disposable soft contact lenses should be used strictly in accordance with manufacturer's guidelines and under supervision of a lens specialist. Overextending the wear requirements of these lenses can result in eye infection or other adverse ocular consequences.

SUMMARY

The continued growth of contact lens use for both cosmetic and therapeutic reasons further increases the need for pharmacists to keep up to date with all aspects of lens products, lens materials, and care and maintenance programs. When maintaining a patient medication profile, pharmacists should note that the person is a contact lens wearer. Specific information regarding the patient's sensitivities to ingredients in lens care products should be included in the profile. Concurrent use of any systemic drug that could affect tear flow or discolor lenses should be considered when counseling a lens wearer about health care. Particular attention should be given to the possible effects of ophthalmic medications on contact lenses.

Because of the wide variety of lens care products, stock should be carefully selected to provide a complete care program for most wearers. Use of Plan-O-Grams will help to reduce inventory cost. When choosing a product line, pharmacists should consider stocking all products in the line to properly serve contact lens wearers. Conscientious and knowledgeable pharmacists can provide an important and needed service to the public.

REFERENCES

1 "Pharmacists' Handbook of Contact Lenses and Contact Lens Solutions," H. W. Hind and V. S. Zuccharo, Eds., Barnes–Hind, Sunnyvale, Calif., 1986, pp. 3–48.

2 J. L. Bagley, *Am. Drug. 192* (6), 70 (1985).

3 D. L. MacKeen, *Am. Pharm. NS26, 27* (1986).

4 J. R. Scholles, *Contact, 1,* 5 (1989).

5 J. J. Carlson, *For the Defense, 29,* 115 (1987).

6 J. N. Buxton and C. R. Locke, *Am. J. Ophthalmol., 72,* 532 (1971).

7 *Br. Med. J., 2,* 655 (1977).

8 A. R. Gasset and L. Lobo, *Ann. Ophthalmol., 8,* 843 (1977).

9 L. J. Girard, in "Corneal Contact Lenses," L. J. Girard, Ed., C. V. Mosby, St. Louis, Mo., 1972, pp. 107–120.

10 B. A. Weissman, in "Contact Lens Primer," Lea & Febiger, Philadelphia, Pa., 1984, pp. 49–55.

11 J. Hartstein, in "Questions and Answers on Contact Lens Practice," C. V. Mosby, St. Louis, Mo., 1973, pp. 60–67.

12 C. Thranberend, *Klin. Monatsbl. Augenhetlkd., 164,* 509 (1974).

13 R. L. Terry, *Contact Lens. Spectr., 4,* 58 (1989).

14 F. Dickenson, *Contacto, 11,* 12 (1967).

15 C. H. May, *Contacto, 4,* 41 (1960).

16 T. F. Gumpelmayer, *Am. J. Optom., 47,* 879 (1970).

17 J. A. Baldone, *Trans. Am. Acad. Ophthalmol. Otol., 78,* OP-406 (1974).

18 M. Millodot, *Arch. Ophthalmol., 82,* 461 (1969).

19 "Contact Lens Practice," R. B. Mandell, Ed., Charles C. Thomas, Springfield, Ill., 1974, pp. 83–116.

20 O. H. Dabezies et al., *Patient Care, 12,* 98 (1978).

21 L. J. Girard, in "Corneal and Scleral Contact Lenses," L. J. Girard, Ed., C. V. Mosby, St. Louis, Mo., 1967, pp. 40–48.

22 L. J. Girard, in "Corneal and Scleral Contact Lenses," L. J. Girard, Ed., C. V. Mosby, St. Louis, Mo., 1967, pp. 1–17.

23 M. Rubin, *Lancet, 1,* 138 (1976).

24 J. C. Casebeer, *Am. J. Ophthalmol., 76,* 165 (1973).

25 H. M. Rosenwasser, *Opt. J. Rev. Optom., 100,* 41 (1963).

26 K. Dalton, in "Contact Lenses, A Textbook for Practitioner and Student," 2nd ed., Vol. 1, J. Stone and A. J. Phillips, Eds., Butterworth's, Boston, Mass., 1980, pp. 179–180.

27 O. W. Cole, *Contacto, 15,* 5 (1971).

28 "Contact Lens Practice," R. B. Mandella, Ed., Charles C. Thomas, Springfield, Ill., 1974, pp. 108–109.

29 "Symposium on Contact Lenses," C. V. Mosby, St. Louis, Mo., 1973, pp. 1–12.

30 G. Mulrooney, *Can. J. Optom., 33,* 74 (1971).

31 M. B. Smith, *Contact, 1,* 14 (1988).

32 "The Pharmacist's Guide to Contact Lenses and Lens Care," G. Lowther et al., Eds., Ciba Vision, 1988, pp. 1–8.

33 O. H. Dabezies, in "Corneal and Scleral Contact Lenses," L. J. Girard, Ed., C. V. Mosby, St. Louis, Mo., 1967, pp. 347–361.

34 F. B. Hoefle, *Trans. Am. Acad. Ophthalmol. Otol., 78,* OP-386 (1974).

35 "Soft Contact Lens," A. R. Gasset and H. E. Kaufman, Eds., C. V. Mosby, St. Louis, Mo., 1972, pp. 233–239.

36 "Soft Contact Lens," A. R. Gasset and H. E. Kaufman, Eds., C. V. Mosby, St. Louis, Mo., 1972, pp. 175–183.

37 P. F. Bommarito, *You and Your Health, 2,* 8 (1986).

38 O. D. Schein et al., *N. Engl. J. Med., 321,* 773 (1989).

39 R. M. Kershner, *J. Am. Med. Assoc., 261,* 3549 (1989).

40 "Contact Lens Practice," R. B. Mandell, Ed., Charles C. Thomas, Springfield, Ill., 1974, pp. 437–454.

41 "Symposium on the Flexible Lens," J. L. Bitonte and R. H. Keates, Eds., C. V. Mosby, St. Louis, Mo., 1972, pp. 35–51.

42 "Soft Contact Lens," A. R. Gasset and H. E. Kaufman, Eds., C. V. Mosby, St. Louis, Mo., 1972, pp. 83–86.

43 J. R. Wuest and T. A. Gossel, *Ohio Pharm., 34,* 5 (1984).

44 "Contact Lens Practice," R. B. Mandell, Ed., Charles C. Thomas, Springfield, Ill., 1974, pp. 83–116.

45 R. L. Sutherland and W. N. Van Leeuwen, *Can. Med. Assoc. J., 107,* 49 (1972).

46 "Symposium on Contact Lenses," C. V. Mosby, St. Louis, Mo., 1973, pp. 174–180.

47 "Soft Contact Lens," A. R. Gasset and H. E. Kaufman, Eds., C. V. Mosby, St. Louis, Mo., 1972, pp. 199–209.

48 J. Z. Krezanoski, *J. Am. Optom. Assoc.*, *43*, 305 (1972).

49 W. R. Bailey, *Contact Lens Society Am.*, *6*, 33 (1972).

50 M. J. Sibley and G. Yung, *Am. J. Optom.*, *50*, 710 (1973).

51 S. Stenson, *J. Am. Med. Assoc.*, *257*, 2823 (1987).

52 J. Sugar, *Arch. Ophthalmol.*, *91*, 11 (1974).

53 *Br. Med. J.*, *3*, 254 (1972).

54 F. H. Adler, in "Physiology of the Eye," 4th ed., C. V. Mosby, St. Louis, Mo., 1965, pp. 48–49.

55 I. Fatt, *Contact Lens*, *14*, 3 (1972).

56 R. M. Hill and I. Fatt, *Am. J. Optom.*, *35*, 873 (1964).

57 J. F. Hill, *Optom. Weekly*, *64*, 943 (1973).

58 L. J. Girard, in "Corneal Contact Lenses," L. J. Girard, Ed., 2nd ed., C. V. Mosby, St. Louis, Mo., 1970, pp. 18–24.

59 R. M. Hill and I. Fatt, *Am. J. Optom.*, *41*, 678 (1964).

60 "Symposium on Contact Lenses," C. V. Mosby, St. Louis, Mo., 1973, pp. 65–81.

61 S. G. El Hage et al., *Am. J. Optom. Physiol. Optics*, *51*, 24 (1974).

62 D. R. Korb, *J. Am. Optom. Assoc.*, *44*, 246 (1973).

63 L. Krejel and H. Krejcova, *Br. J. Ophthalmol.*, *57*, 675 (1973).

64 "Soft Contact Lens," A. R. Gasset and H. E. Kaufman, Eds., C. V. Mosby, St. Louis, Mo., 1972, pp. 61–71.

65 J. C. Neil and J. J. Hanna, *Contacto*, *7*, 10 (1963).

66 C. E. Watkins, *Optom. World* (Oct. 1964).

67 R. A. Koetting, *Optom. Weekly* (Oct. 1963).

68 R. A. Koetting, *Optom. Weekly*, *57*, 52 (1966).

69 O. H. Dabezies, *Eye Ear Nose Throat Mon.*, *45*, 78 (Oct. 1966).

70 O. H. Dabezies and T. Naugle, *Eye Ear Nose Throat Mon.*, *50*, 378 (Oct. 1971).

71 I. J. Szekely, *S. Pharm. J.*, *52*, 17 (1960).

72 H. L. Gould, *Eye Ear Nose Throat Mon.*, *41*, 359 (1962).

73 *Contacto*, *3*, 262 (1959).

74 H. W. Hind and I. J. Szekely, *Contacto*, *3*, 66 (1959).

75 M. J. Sibley and D. E. Lauck, *Contact Lens J.*, *8*, 10 (1974).

76 H. L. Gould and R. Inglima, *Eye Ear Nose Throat Mon.*, *43*, 39 (1964).

77 D. A. Norton et al., *J. Pharm. Pharmacol.*, *26*, 841 (1974).

78 S. R. Kohn et al., *J. Pharm. Sci.*, *52*, 967 (1963).

79 R. E. Phares, *J. Am. Optom. Assoc.*, *43*, 308 (1972).

80 J. Z. Krezanoski, *Ophthal. Optician*, *12*, 1035 (1972).

81 "Symposium on the Flexible Lens," J. L. Bitonte and R. H. Keates, Eds., C. V. Mosby, St. Louis, Mo., 1972, pp. 205–212.

82 G. L. Cureton and N. C. Hall, *Am. J. Optom. Physiol. Optics*, *51*, 406 (1974).

83 R. C. Tripathi and B. J. Tripathi, *Ophthalmic Forum*, *2*, 80 (1984).

84 M. F. Refojo and F. J. Holly, *Contact Intraocular Lens Med. J.*, *3*, 23 (1977).

85 J. S. Cumming and H. Karageozian, *Contacto*, *19*, 8 (July 1975).

86 G. E. Lowther, *Am. J. Optom. Physiol. Optics*, *54*, 76 (1977).

87 J. Z. Krezanoski, *Contact Lens Soc. Am. J.*, *7*, 9 (1974).

88 J. A. Baldone, *Contact Lens Med. Bull.*, *4*, 9 (1971).

89 J. Z. Krezanoski, *Ont. Optician*, *5*, 9 (1974).

90 W. Sagan and K. N. Schwaderer, *J. Am. Optom. Assoc.*, *45*, 266 (1974).

91 M. S. Favero et al., *Science*, *173*, 836 (1971).

92 B. R. Matas et al., *Arch. Ophthalmol.*, *88*, 287 (1972).

93 "Symposium on the Flexible Lens," J. L. Bitonte and R. H. Keates, Eds., C. V. Mosby, St. Louis, Mo., 1972, pp. 222–234.

94 A. M. Charles, *J. Am. Optom. Assoc.*, *43*, 661 (1972).

95 A. J. Milauskas, *Am. Acad. Ophthal. Otolaryngol. Trans.*, *76*, 511 (1972).

96 J. C. Busschaert et al., *J. Am. Optom. Assoc.*, *45*, 700 (1974).

97 M. B. Moore et al., *Am. J. Ophthalmol.*, *100*, 396 (1985).

98 J. D. Auran et al., *Cornea*, *6*, 2 (1987).

99 R. G. Fiscella, *U.S. Pharmacist*, *14*, 75 (1989).

100 Z. Baker et al., *J. Exp. Med.*, *73*, 249 (1941).

101 C. G. Dunn, *Am. J. Surg.*, *41*, 268 (1938).

102 C. G. Dunn, *Proc. Soc. Exp. Biol. Med.*, *37*, 661 (1938).

103 K. C. Swan, *Am. J. Ophthalmol.*, *27*, 1118 (1944).

104 *Contacto*, *15*, 20 (1971).

105 D. P. Bixler, *Am. J. Ophthalmol.*, *62*, 324 (1966).

106 S. Riegelman, *Am. J. Ophthalmol.*, *64*, 485 (1967).

107 S. Riegelman et al., *J. Am. Pharm. Assoc. Sci. Ed.*, *45*, 93 (1956).

108 H. W. Hind and F. M. Goyan, *J. Am. Pharm. Assoc., Sci. Ed.*, *36*, 33 (1947).

109 P. P. Hopf, *Manuf. Chemist*, *24*, 444 (1953).

110 D. R. McGregor and P. R. Elliker, *Can. J. Microbiol.*, *4*, 499 (1958).

111 M. G. Harris, *Int. Contact Lens Clinic*, *15*, 143 (1988).

112 M. J. Collins and L. G. Carney, *Am. J. Optom. Physiol. Optics*, *63*, 952 (1986).

HARD LENS PRODUCT TABLE

Product (Manufacturer)	Suggested Use	Viscosity Agent	Preservative	Other Ingredients
Adapettes (Alcon)	rewetting	adsorbobase povidone	thimerosal, 0.004% EDTA, 0.1%	
Adapt (Alcon)	wetting rewetting	adsorbobase hydroxyethylcellulose	thimerosal, 0.004% EDTA, 0.1%	
Blink-N-Clean (Allergan)	cleaning wetting	polyoxyl 40 stearate polyethylene glycol 300	chlorobutanol, 0.5%	
Boston Cleaner (Polymer Tech)	cleaning			sodium chloride sulfate surfactant
Boston Reconditioning Drops (Polymer Tech)	cleaning soaking	polyvinyl alcohol hydroxyethylcellulose	EDTA chlorhexidine gluconate	
Clean-N-Soak (Allergan)	cleaning soaking		phenylmercuric nitrate, 0.004%	cleaning agent
Clens (Alcon)	cleaning		benzalkonium chloride, 0.02% EDTA, 0.1%	cleaning agents
Clerz (Wesley-Jessen)	rewetting lubricating	hydroxyethylcellulose	thimerosal, 0.001% sorbic acid EDTA, 0.1%	poloxamer 407
Clerz 2 (Wesley-Jessen)	rewetting	hydroxyethylcellulose	sorbic acid EDTA	poloxamer 407 sodium chloride potassium chloride sodium borate boric acid
Concentrated Cleaner (Bausch & Lomb)	cleaning			sodium chloride sulfate surfactant
Contique Cleaning Solution (Alcon)	cleaning		benzalkonium chloride, 0.02%	
Contique Clean-Tabs[a] (Alcon)	cleaning			cleaning agents
Contique Soak-Tabs[a] (Alcon)	soaking		thimerosal, 0.08% benzethonium chloride, 4%	
Contique Wetting Solution (Alcon)	wetting	hydroxypropyl methylcellulose	benzalkonium chloride, 0.004% EDTA, 0.025%	
de•Stat (Sherman)	cleaning soaking		benzalkonium chloride, 0.01% EDTA, 0.25%	surfactant
de•Stat 3 (Sherman)	cleaning soaking disinfecting		EDTA, 0.5%	octylphenoxy-polyethoxyethanol benzyl alcohol, 0.1%
d-film Gel (Wesley-Jessen)	cleaning		benzalkonium chloride, 0.025% EDTA, 0.25%	poloxamer 407
duo Flow (Wesley-Jessen)	cleaning soaking		benzalkonium chloride, 0.013% EDTA, 0.25%	poloxamer 188

HARD LENS PRODUCT TABLE, continued

Product (Manufacturer)	Suggested Use	Viscosity Agent	Preservative	Other Ingredients
EasyClean/GP (Allergan)	cleaning	cocoamphocarboxy-glycinate		sodium chloride sodium phosphate sodium lauryl sulfate hexylene glycol
Gas Permeable Wetting & Soaking (Sola/Barnes-Hind)	wetting disinfection storage	hydroxyethylcellulose polyvinyl alcohol povidone	chlorhexidine gluconate, 0.005% EDTA, 0.02%	surfactants propylene glycol sodium chloride
Gas Permeable Daily Cleaner (Sola/Barnes-Hind)	cleaning	hydroxyethylcellulose	potassium sorbate, 0.13% thimerosal, 0.004% EDTA, 2%	surfactant trisamino
Gas Permeable Protein Remover (Sola/Barnes-Hind)	cleaning		potassium sorbate, 0.13% EDTA, 0.1%	surfactants propylene glycol borate buffer
Gas Permeable Comfort Drops (Sola/Barnes-Hind)	wetting lubricating	hydroxyethylcellulose	potassium sorbate, 0.13% EDTA, 0.1%	surfactant sodium chloride
Gel Clean (Sola/Barnes-Hind)	cleaning		thimerosal, 0.004%	nonionic surfactant
hy-Flow (Wesley-Jessen)	wetting	polyvinyl alcohol hydroxyethylcellulose	benzalkonium chloride EDTA	
LC-65 (Allergan)	cleaning		thimerosal, 0.001% EDTA	cleaning agent
Lens Fresh Drops (Allergan)	rewetting lubricating	hydroxyethylcellulose	sorbic acid, 0.1% EDTA, 0.2%	sodium chloride boric acid sodium borate
Lens Lubricant (Bausch & Lomb)	rewetting lubricating	povidone	thimerosal, 0.004% EDTA, 0.1%	polyoxyethylene
Lensine Extra Strength Cleaner (Wesley-Jessen)	cleaning		benzalkonium chloride, 0.01% EDTA, 0.1%	cleaning agents
Lens-Mate (Alcon)	cleaning soaking wetting	polyvinyl alcohol hydroxypropyl methylcellulose	benzalkonium chloride, 0.01% EDTA, 0.1%	
Lens-Wet (Allergan)	wetting lubricating	polyvinyl alcohol	thimerosal, 0.002% EDTA, 0.01%	mono- and dibasic sodium phosphate sodium chloride
Liquifilm Tears (Allergan)	wetting	polyvinyl alcohol, 1.4%	chlorobutanol, 0.5%	sodium chloride hydrochloric acid or sodium hydroxide
Liquifilm Wetting Solution (Allergan)	wetting	hydroxypropyl methylcellulose polyvinyl alcohol	benzalkonium chloride, 0.004% EDTA	sodium chloride potassium chloride
MiraFlow Extra Strength (Ciba Vision)	cleaning			isopropyl alcohol, 20% poloxamer 407 amphoteric 10
Murine Sterile Lubricating & Rewetting (Ross)	rewetting lubricating	hydroxyethylcellulose	sorbic acid, 0.1% EDTA, 0.2%	sodium chloride boric acid sodium borate
Opti-Clean (Alcon)	cleaning		thimerosal, 0.004% EDTA, 0.1%	polymeric cleaning beads polysorbate 21

HARD LENS PRODUCT TABLE, continued

Product (Manufacturer)	Suggested Use	Viscosity Agent	Preservative	Other Ingredients
Opti-Clean II (Alcon)	cleaning	hydroxyethylcellulose	EDTA, 0.1%	cleaning agent polysorbate 21 polyquaternium-1, 0.01%
Ova-Nite (Milroy)	cleaning soaking		benzalkonium chloride, 0.02% EDTA, 0.25%	nonionic surfactants
ProFree/GP Weekly Enzymatic[a] (Allergan)	cleaning	papain	EDTA	sodium chloride sodium carbonate sodium borate
Resolve/GP Daily (Allergan)	cleaning	cocoamphocarboxy-glycinate		fatty acid amide sodium lauryl sulfate hexylene glycol alkyl ether sulfate surfactants
SilaClean (Professional Supplies)	cleaning		benzalkonium chloride EDTA	cleaning agent
SLC (Ocular)	cleaning		sorbic acid, 0.1% EDTA, 0.1%	cleaning agent
Soaclens (Alcon)	soaking wetting		thimerosal, 0.004% EDTA, 0.1%	buffers wetting agents
Soakare (Allergan)	soaking		benzalkonium chloride, 0.01% EDTA, 0.25%	sodium hydroxide
Soquette (Sola/Barnes-Hind)	soaking	polyvinyl alcohol	benzalkonium chloride, 0.01% EDTA, 0.2%	
Stay-Brite (Sherman)	cleaning		benzalkonium chloride, 0.01% EDTA, 0.25%	cleaning agent
Stay-Wet (Sherman)	wetting rewetting	polyvinyl alcohol hydroxyethylcellulose povidone	benzalkonium chloride, 0.01% EDTA, 0.025%	sodium chloride potassium chloride sodium carbonate
SWS (Ocular)	soaking wetting	polyvinyl alcohol hydroxyethylcellulose	benzalkonium chloride, 0.01% EDTA, 0.025%	sodium chloride potassium chloride
Titan (Sola/Barnes-Hind)	cleaning		benzalkonium chloride EDTA	nonionic cleaner buffers
Total All-in-One Contact Lens Solution (Allergan)	cleaning soaking wetting	polyvinyl alcohol	benzalkonium chloride EDTA	
Visalens Soaking/Cleaning (Leeming)	cleaning soaking		benzalkonium chloride, 0.02% EDTA, 0.1%	cleaning agents sodium borate boric acid sodium chloride
Visalens Wetting Solution (Leeming)	wetting	polyvinyl alcohol hydroxypropyl methylcellulose	benzalkonium chloride, 0.01% EDTA, 0.1%	sodium chloride sodium hydroxide
Wet-Cote (Milroy)	wetting	polyvinyl alcohol hydroxyethylcellulose	benzalkonium chloride, 0.01% EDTA, 0.25%	sodium chloride potassium chloride
Wet-N-Soak (Allergan)	soaking wetting	polyvinyl alcohol	benzalkonium chloride, 0.004% EDTA, 0.004%	

HARD LENS PRODUCT TABLE, continued

Product (Manufacturer)	Suggested Use	Viscosity Agent	Preservative	Other Ingredients
Wet-N-Soak Plus Wetting and Soaking (Allergan)	wetting soaking	polyvinyl alcohol	benzalkonium chloride, 0.003% EDTA	
Wetting and Soaking Solution (Sola/Barnes-Hind)	soaking wetting	polyvinyl alcohol povidone hydroxyethylcellulose	benzalkonium chloride, 0.005% EDTA, 0.1%	
Wetting Solution (Sola/Barnes-Hind)	wetting	polyvinyl alcohol	benzalkonium chloride, 0.004% EDTA, 0.02%	

^a Tablet must be dissolved in water.

SOFT LENS PRODUCT TABLE

Product (Manufacturer)	Suggested Use	Viscosity Agent	Preservative	Other Ingredients
Adapettes For Sensitive Eyes (Alcon)	lubricating rewetting	povidone	thimerosal, 0.004% EDTA, 0.1%	polymers
Allergan Hydrocare Cleaning & Disinfecting Solution (Allergan)	chemical disinfection		thimerosal, 0.002% hydrochloric acid tris (2-hydroxyethyl) tallow ammonium chloride, 0.013% bis (2-hydroxyethyl) tallow ammonium chloride	polysorbate 80 sodium bicarbonate propylene glycol sodium phosphate soluble polyhema
Allergan Hydrocare Preserved Saline Solution (Allergan)	rinsing thermal disinfection storing		thimerosal, 0.001% EDTA, 0.01%	sodium hexametaphosphate sodium chloride boric acid sodium borate sodium hydroxide
Allergan Enzymatic Contact Lens Cleaner Tablets (Allergan)	weekly protein cleaner		EDTA	sodium chloride papain sodium carbonate sodium borate
Allergan Sorbi-Care Saline Solution (Allergan)	rinsing thermal disinfection storing		sorbic acid, 0.1%	sodium chloride sodium borate boric acid sodium hexametaphosphate
Amcon 250[a] (Amcon)	salt tablets for saline			sodium chloride, 250 mg
Aosept (Ciba Vision)	rinsing chemical disinfection storing			hydrogen peroxide, 3% sodium chloride, 0.85% sodium stannate sodium nitrate phosphate buffer
Boil n Soak (Alcon)	rinsing thermal disinfection storing		thimerosal, 0.001% EDTA, 0.1%	boric acid sodium borate sodium chloride, 0.7%
Blairex Sterile Saline Solution (Blairex)	rinsing thermal disinfection storage			sodium chloride, 0.9% boric acid sodium borate
Ciba Vision Saline (Ciba Vision)	rinsing thermal disinfection storing			sodium chloride boric acid
Ciba Vision Cleaner (Ciba Vision)	cleaning	cocoamphocarboxyglycinate	sorbic acid, 0.1% EDTA, 0.2%	sodium lauryl sulfate hexylene glycol
Clerz (Wesley-Jessen)	rewetting lubricating	hydroxyethylcellulose	thimerosal, 0.001% EDTA, 0.1%	sodium borate poloxamer 407 sorbic acid
Clerz 2 (Wesley-Jessen)	rewetting lubricating	hydroxyethylcellulose	sorbic acid EDTA	sodium chloride potassium chloride sodium borate poloxamer 407 boric acid

SOFT LENS PRODUCT TABLE, continued

Product (Manufacturer)	Suggested Use	Viscosity Agent	Preservative	Other Ingredients
Comfort Tears (Sola/Barnes-Hind)	rewetting lubricating	hydroxyethylcellulose	benzalkonium chloride, 0.005% EDTA, 0.02%	
Daily Cleaner (Bausch & Lomb)	cleaning	hydroxyethylcellulose polyvinyl alcohol	thimerosal, 0.004% EDTA, 0.2%	tyloxapol sodium phosphate sodium chloride
Disinfecting Solution (Bausch & Lomb)	rinsing chemical disinfection storing		thimerosal, 0.001% chlorhexidine gluconate, 0.005% EDTA, 0.1%	sodium chloride sodium borate boric acid
DURAcare (Blairex)	cleaning		thimerosal, 0.004% EDTA, 0.001%	nonionic detergents
DURAcare II (Blairex)	cleaning		sorbic acid, 0.1% EDTA, 0.25%	block copolymers of ethylene and propylene oxide octylphenoxy polyethoxyethanol
Easy Eyes 250 mg [a] (Eaton Medicals)	salt tablets for saline			sodium chloride, 250 mg
Extenzyme Protein Cleaner (Allergan)	weekly protein cleaner		EDTA	stabilized papain sodium chloride sodium carbonate sodium borate
Flex-Care (Alcon)	rinsing chemical disinfection		thimerosal, 0.001% chlorhexidine gluconate, 0.005% EDTA, 0.1%	sodium chloride sodium borate boric acid
Hypo-Clear (Bausch & Lomb)	rinsing thermal disinfection storing			sodium chloride, 0.9%
LC-65 (Allergan)	cleaning		thimerosal, 0.001% EDTA	cleaning agent
Lens Clear (Allergan)	cleaning	cocoamphocarboxyglycinate	sorbic acid, 0.1% EDTA, 0.2%	sodium lauryl sulfate hexylene glycol
Lens Drops (Ciba Vision)	rewetting lubricating		sorbic acid, 0.15% EDTA, 0.2%	sodium chloride borate buffer carbamide poloxamer 407
Lens Fresh (Allergan)	rewetting lubricating	hydroxyethylcellulose	sorbic acid, 0.1% EDTA, 0.2%	sodium chloride boric acid sodium borate
Lens Lubricant (Bausch & Lomb)	rewetting lubricating	povidone	thimerosal, 0.004% EDTA, 0.1%	polyoxyethylene
Lens Plus Daily (Allergan)	cleaner	cocoamphocarboxyglycinate	EDTA	sodium lauryl sulfate hexylene glycol sodium chloride sodium phosphate
Lens Plus Oxysept-1 (Allergan)	disinfection			hydrogen peroxide, 3% sodium stannate sodium nitrate phosphate buffers

SOFT LENS PRODUCT TABLE, continued

Product (Manufacturer)	Suggested Use	Viscosity Agent	Preservative	Other Ingredients
Lens Plus Oxysept-2 (Allergan)	rinsing/ neutralizing		EDTA	catalase sodium chloride mono- and dibasic sodium phosphates
Lens Plus Rewetting Drops (Allergan)	rewetting			sodium chloride boric acid
Lens Plus Sterile Saline Solution (Allergan)	rinsing thermal disinfection storing			sodium chloride boric acid
Lensrins (Allergan)	rinsing thermal disinfection		thimerosal, 0.001% EDTA, 0.1%	sodium chloride sodium phosphate buffers sodium hydroxide and/or hydrochloric acid
Lensept (Ciba Vision)	rinsing chemical disinfection neutralizing storing		sorbic acid (rinse & neutralizer) EDTA (rinse & neutralizer)	rinse & neutralizer: sodium chloride sodium borate decahydrate boric acid bovine catalase disinfecting solution: hydrogen peroxide, 3% sodium stannate sodium nitrate phosphate buffer
Lens-Wet (Allergan)	rewetting lubricating	polyvinyl alcohol	thimerosal, 0.002% EDTA, 0.01%	dibasic sodium phosphate monobasic sodium phosphate monohydrate sodium chloride
Marlin Salt System II (Marlin)	salt tablets for saline			sodium chloride, 250 mg
MiraFlow Extra Strength (Ciba Vision)	cleaning			isopropyl alcohol, 20% poloxamer 407 amphoteric 10
MiraSept System (Wesley-Jessen)	rinsing chemical disinfection neutralizing storing		sorbic acid (rinse & neutralizer) EDTA (rinse & neutralizer)	rinse & neutralizer: boric acid sodium borate sodium pyruvate disinfecting solution: hydrogen peroxide, 3% sodium stannate sodium nitrate
Murine Contact Lens (Ross)	cleaning	hydroxypropyl methylcellulose	sorbic acid, 0.25% EDTA, 0.5%	poloxamine sodium chloride borate buffer
Murine Preserved All-Purpose Saline Solution (Ross)	rinsing thermal disinfection storing		sorbic acid, 0.1% EDTA, 0.1%	sodium chloride
Murine Sterile (Ross)	rewetting lubricating	hydroxyethylcellulose	sorbic acid, 0.1% EDTA, 0.2%	sodium chloride boric acid sodium borate
Opti-Clean (Alcon)	cleaning		thimerosal, 0.004% EDTA, 0.1%	tween 21

SOFT LENS PRODUCT TABLE, continued

Product (Manufacturer)	Suggested Use	Viscosity Agent	Preservative	Other Ingredients
Opti-Clean II (Alcon)	cleaning	hydroxyethylcellulose	EDTA, 0.1%	polysorbate 21 polyquaternium-1, 0.01% cleaning agent
Opti-Free (Alcon)	rinsing chemical disinfection storing		EDTA, 0.05%	citrate buffer sodium chloride polyquaternium-1, 0.001%
Opti-Soft (Alcon)	rinsing thermal disinfection storing		EDTA, 0.1%	sodium chloride borate buffer polyquaternium-1, 0.001%
Opti-Tears (Alcon)	rewetting lubricating	hydroxypropyl methylcellulose	EDTA, 0.1%	dextran sodium chloride potassium chloride polyquaternium-1, 0.01%
Opti-Zyme Enzymatic[a] (Alcon)	weekly protein cleaner			pancreatin
Pliagel (Wesley-Jessen)	cleaning		sorbic acid, 0.25% EDTA, 0.5%	poloxamer 407 sodium chloride potassium chloride
Preflex for Sensitive Eyes (Alcon)	cleaning	hydroxyethylcellulose polyvinyl alcohol	thimerosal, 0.004% EDTA, 0.2%	sodium chloride sodium phosphate tyloxapol
Preserved Saline Solution (Bausch & Lomb)	rinsing thermal disinfection storing		thimerosal, 0.001% EDTA	boric acid sodium chloride
Pure Sept (Ross)	rinsing storage chemical disinfection		sorbic acid, 0.1% (rinse & neutralizer) EDTA, 0.1% (rinse & neutralizer)	rinse & neutralizer: borate buffer sodium chloride disinfecting solution: hydrogen peroxide, 3% sodium stannate sodium nitrate phosphate buffer
Purisol 4 (Amcon)	rinsing storing			sodium chloride boric acid sodium borate
Quick-Sept System (Bausch & Lomb)	rinsing storing chemical disinfection		sorbic acid (cleaning & storing) EDTA (cleaning & storing)	cleaning: sodium chloride borate buffer surfactant disinfecting solution: hydrogen peroxide, 3% sodium stannate sodium nitrate phosphate buffer storing: sodium chloride borate buffer
ReNu Effervescent Enzymatic[a] (Bausch & Lomb)	weekly protein cleaner			subtilisin PEG sodium carbonate sodium chloride tartaric acid

SOFT LENS PRODUCT TABLE, continued

Product (Manufacturer)	Suggested Use	Viscosity Agent	Preservative	Other Ingredients
ReNu Multi-Action (Bausch & Lomb)	rinsing chemical disinfection storing		EDTA	sodium chloride sodium borate boric acid poloxamine polyaminopropyl biguanide, 0.00005%
ReNu Saline (Bausch & Lomb)	rinsing thermal disinfection storing		EDTA	sodium chloride boric acid polyaminopropyl biguanide, 0.00003%
Sensitive Eyes Daily (Bausch & Lomb)	cleaning	hydroxypropyl methylcellulose	sorbic acid, 0.25% EDTA, 0.5%	sodium chloride borate buffer surfactant
Sensitive Eyes Drops (Bausch & Lomb)	rewetting		sorbic acid, 0.1% EDTA	borate buffer
Sensitive Eyes Saline/ Cleaning Solution (Bausch & Lomb)	cleaning		sorbic acid EDTA	sodium chloride borate buffer surfactant
Sensitive Eyes Saline Solution (Bausch & Lomb)	rinsing thermal disinfection storing		sorbic acid, 0.1% EDTA	sodium chloride borate buffer
Sof/Pro-Clean (Sherman)	cleaning		thimerosal, 0.004% EDTA, 0.1%	salts detergents
Sof/Pro-Clean (s.a.) (Sherman)	cleaning		sorbic acid, 0.1% sodium bisulfite, 0.1% EDTA, 0.25%	salt buffers ethylene and propylene oxide copolymers octylphenoxy polyethoxyethanol imidazoline lauryl sulfate
Soft Mate Comfort Drops (Sola/Barnes-Hind)	cleaning rewetting lubricating	hydroxyethylcellulose	thimerosal, 0.004% EDTA, 0.1%	borate buffer octylphenoxyethanols
Soft Mate Comfort Drops For Sensitive Eyes (Sola/Barnes-Hind)	rewetting lubricating		EDTA, 0.1%	borate buffer potassium sorbate, 0.13%
Soft Mate Consept-1 (Sola/Barnes-Hind)	cleaning disinfection			hydrogen peroxide, 3% polyoxyl 40 stearate sodium stannate sodium nitrate phosphate buffer
Soft Mate Consept-2 (Sola/Barnes-Hind)	rinsing neutralizing			sodium thiosulfate, 0.5% sodium chloride borate buffer
Soft Mate Daily Cleaning Solution (Sola/Barnes-Hind)	cleaning	hydroxyethylcellulose	thimerosal, 0.004% EDTA, 0.2%	sodium chloride
Soft Mate Daily Cleaning For Sensitive Eyes (Sola/Barnes-Hind)	cleaning	hydroxyethylcellulose	potassium sorbate, 0.13% EDTA, 0.2%	sodium chloride octylphenoxyethanol
Soft Mate Hands Off Daily Cleaner (Sola/Barnes-Hind)	cleaning	hydroxyethylcellulose	potassium sorbate, 0.13% EDTA, 0.20%	sodium chloride octylphenoxyethanol

SOFT LENS PRODUCT TABLE, continued

Product (Manufacturer)	Suggested Use	Viscosity Agent	Preservative	Other Ingredients
Soft Mate Disinfecting Solution (Sola/Barnes-Hind)	rinsing chemical disinfection storing	povidone	chlorhexidine gluconate, 0.005% EDTA, 0.1%	octylphenoxyethanols sodium chloride
Soft Mate Enzyme Plus (Sola/Barnes-Hind)	cleaner			subtilisin surfactant
Soft Mate Lens Drops (Sola/Barnes-Hind)	rewetting lubricating		potassium sorbate, 0.13% EDTA, 0.025%	sodium chloride
Soft Mate Protein Remover Solution (Sola/Barnes-Hind)	cleaner			surfactants borate buffer
Soft Mate ps Comfort Drops (Sola/Barnes-Hind)	cleaning rewetting lubricating	hydroxyethylcellulose	potassium sorbate, 0.13% EDTA, 0.10%	octylphenoxyethanol sodium chloride borate buffer
Soft Mate ps Daily Cleaning Solution (Sola/Barnes-Hind)	cleaning	hydroxyethylcellulose	potassium sorbate, 0.13% EDTA, 0.20%	sodium chloride borate buffer
Soft Mate ps Saline Solution (Sola/Barnes-Hind)	rinsing thermal disinfection storing		potassium sorbate, 0.13% EDTA, 0.025%	sodium chloride borate buffer
Soft Mate Saline For Sensitive Eyes (Sola/Barnes-Hind)	rinsing storing thermal disinfection		potassium sorbate, 0.13% EDTA, 0.025%	sodium chloride
Soft Mate Saline Preservative-Free (Sola/Barnes-Hind)	rinsing thermal disinfection storing			sodium chloride borate buffer
Soft Mate Saline Solution (Sola/Barnes-Hind)	rinsing thermal disinfection storing		thimerosal, 0.001% EDTA, 0.01%	sodium chloride borate buffer
Soft Mate Saline Spray (Sola/Barnes-Hind)	rinsing thermal disinfection storing			sodium chloride borate buffer
Soft Mate Weekly Cleaning Solution (Sola/Barnes-Hind)	cleaning		thimerosal, 0.001% EDTA, 0.1%	sodium chloride
Soft Rinse 135[a] (Professional Supplies)	salt tablets for saline			sodium chloride, 135 mg
Soft Rinse 250[a] (Professional Supplies)	salt tablets for saline			sodium chloride, 250 mg
Sterile Lens Lubricant (Blairex)	rewetting lubricating	hydroxypropyl methylcellulose	sorbic acid, 0.25% EDTA, 0.1%	borate buffer sodium chloride glycerin
Sterile Saline (Bausch & Lomb)	rinsing thermal disinfection storing		EDTA	sodium chloride borate buffer
Ultrazyme Enzymatic (Allergan)	weekly protein cleaner			subtilisin A effervescing agents buffers

SOFT LENS PRODUCT TABLE, continued

Product (Manufacturer)	Suggested Use	Viscosity Agent	Preservative	Other Ingredients
Unisol (Wesley-Jessen)	rinsing storing thermal disinfection			sodium chloride sodium borate boric acid
Unisol 4 (Wesley-Jessen)	rinsing storing thermal disinfection			sodium chloride sodium borate boric acid

^a Tablet must be dissolved in water.

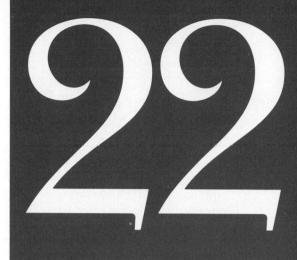

Keith O. Miller

OTIC PRODUCTS

*Q*uestions to ask in patient/consumer counseling

Earache

Do you have an earache?
———

Is the pain sharp and localized or dull and generalized?
———

How long have you had the earache?
———

Is it a constant pain or is it made worse by chewing or by pulling on the ear?
———

Do you have a cold or the flu?
———

Do you have a fever?
———

Have you been swimming in the past few days?
———

Have you attempted to clear your ears recently to remove ear wax? If so, what method did you use?
———

Are your ear canals either dry and flaky or wet and sticky?
———

Have you had similar symptoms in the past?
———

What have you already done to treat your earache?
———

Do you wear dentures or have any dental problems?
———

What is your occupation?
———

Hearing Loss

How long have you noticed that your hearing is not as good as it used to be?
———

What is your occupation?
———

Do you have a cold or the flu?
———

Have you been swimming in the past few days?
———

Are your eardrums intact?
———

Have you been traveling in an airplane recently or been in any places where the air pressure has changed suddenly (fast elevators)?
———

Are you taking any prescription medications, even for other medical problems?
———

Tinnitus

Are the sounds continuous or intermittent?
———

Are you taking aspirin or any medications that your physician has prescribed or that you have purchased without a prescription?
———

Discharge

Could you describe the appearance and amount of the discharge?
———

Was your ear itchy before the discharge appeared?
———

Did you have any pain after the discharge appeared?
———

Did you have pain before the discharge started?
———

Have you taken aspirin or tried to rinse out the ear?
———

Do you have diabetes or any other medical problems?
———

Do you have a problem with dandruff?
———

Ear disorders are very common and in most cases cause discomfort. Patients usually complain of "earache," "impacted ear," "running ear," "cold in the ear," or a combination of these symptoms. Before recommending any nonprescription product to persons with ear disorders, the pharmacist should have a clear picture of the symptoms of ear disorders and their corresponding pathophysiology. This information will help the pharmacist understand the recommended treatment plans and permit an accurate evaluation of the problem.

Ear disorders may be caused by a disease of the auricle, external auditory meatus (external ear canal), or middle ear or by a disease in another area of the head or neck. A traumatic or pathologic condition of the tongue, mandibles, oropharynx, tonsils, or paranasal sinuses may cause referred pain to the ear and may appear to the patient as an "earache." These conditions often are caused by some underlying disease process that requires accurate diagnosis and treatment by a physician. Therefore, self-medication may be unwise.

Home remedies and nonprescription drugs usually are restricted to self-limiting disorders related only to the external ear. Self-medication should be reserved for minor conditions. In addition, it may be used effectively for prophylaxis to aid the normal body defenses and to improve the integrity of the skin lining the auricle and external auditory canal.

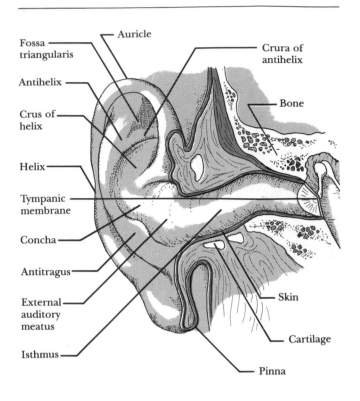

FIGURE 1   Anatomy of the auricle and external ear.

EAR ANATOMY AND PHYSIOLOGY

The external ear is composed of the auricle (pinna) and the external auditory meatus (Figure 1). The auricle is the external appendage of cartilage (elastic type) covered by a thin layer of normal skin that is highly vascularized except for the lobule, which is mainly fatty tissue. The auricle is a flattened, irregular oval structure that is considered an extension of the cartilaginous ear canal. A thin tissue layer called the perichondrium covers both the cartilaginous auricle and the outer cartilaginous half of the external auditory canal (1). The periosteum, a specialized connective tissue, covers the inner bony half of the external auditory canal. The skin covering the ear is thinner than skin elsewhere in the body because it lacks a protective layer of fat and has essentially only a layer of blood vessels. The auricular skin is more subject to frostbite than any other part of the body (2).

The external auditory meatus is tubular, forming a channel for sound waves to pass to the tympanic membrane (eardrum) and protecting the membrane from injury. In adults, the external auditory canal is about 24 mm long and has a volume of about 0.85 ml (17 drops) (2, 3). Both the auricle and the external auditory canal show much individual variation in size and shape. The auditory meatus is the only epidermal-lined cul-de-sac in the body.

The channel narrows about 7 mm from the tympanic membrane; this area is called the isthmus (2). Proximal to the isthmus, the canal floor dips downward to the junction of the annular ring of the tympanic membrane to the canal wall, forming a depression termed the "tympanic recess." Excess water and fluids in the tympanic recess may cause a feeling of fullness in the ear. Fluid removal is accomplished by having the patient tilt the head on the side with the affected ear down. This position permits the excess fluid to drain out of the ear by gravity. To permit direct visual examination of the tympanic membrane, it may be necessary to straighten the canal by applying upward and backward traction on the auricle.

The auricular skin is continuous and lines the entire auditory meatus and the outer covering of the tympanic membrane (4). The skin covering the cartilaginous portion is thicker than the skin covering the bony portion. The skin of the cartilaginous part of the canal contains hair follicles, large sebaceous glands, which open either to the skin surface or into the hair follicle lumen, and ceruminous glands (3). There are 1,000–2,000 ceruminous glands in the average ear, although older people may have fewer (3). The hairs appear to fulfill a protective function, evidenced by their ability to trap foreign bodies in their waxy network. No hair follicles or glands (sebaceous and ceruminous) are found in the inner half of the external auditory canal.

Cerumen (earwax) is derived from the watery secretions of the apocrine glands and the oily secretions of the sebaceous glands (3). The apocrine glands mature and become functional at puberty. Collectively these glands are referred to as ceruminous glands. These glands are abundant in the skin of the cartilaginous portion of the canal but are absent from the skin of the bony portion of the canal. This colorless, watery, fluid secretion is composed of polypeptides, lipids, fatty acids, amino acids, and electrolytes (3, 5). Cerumen turns brown when it mixes with desquamated epithelial cells and dust particles. The cerumen lubricates the skin and traps foreign material entering the external auditory canal, providing a protective barrier (2, 4, 6). Under normal conditions, the cerumen forms small, round droplets and dries into a semisolid. It then is expelled unnoticed by epithelial migration. This migration is the movement of epithelial cells across the surface of the tympanic membrane and the epithelial lining of the external auditory meatus to the outside during the process of mastication and talking (2, 7). The skin of the normal external auditory meatus is acidic with a pH between 5.0 and 7.2 (3). This "acid mantle" provides protection against opportunistic bacteria and fungi (4).

The tympanic membrane is pearl-gray, egg shaped, semitransparent, and about 0.1 mm thick and 8–9 mm wide (the narrow portion is at the bottom) (3). Its outer epithelial layer is continuous with the epidermis of the external auditory canal; the middle layer is tough, fibrous tissue; and the innermost layer is a mucous membrane continuous with the tympanic cavity lining (7). In adults, the membrane forms an approximately 45° angle with the external meatus floor, and is almost horizontal in infants (3). It provides protection to the middle ear from external foreign material and also aids in transmitting airborne sound waves into the middle ear. Anatomically, the tympanic membrane is part of the external auditory canal because it is attached to the canal's medial terminal end (Figure 1); however, functionally, it is considered part of the middle ear (tympanic cavity) (3).

ETIOLOGY OF EAR CONDITIONS

Predisposing factors often lead to the breakdown of natural barriers of the normal ear canal; hairs in the outer half of the meatus, the size of the ear canal and its isthmus, and cerumen collectively prevent the introduction of foreign material that may cause injury or infection. The integrity of the skin layers and the acid pH of the canal provide natural protection against infection.

An inherited narrowed ear canal, a malformation of the mandible, and/or excess hair growth in the canal may impair the normal cleansing process and decrease the efficiency of the epithelial migration. Hyperactive ceruminous glands may cause excessive wax production to accumulate and become impacted. Black people have shorter and straighter ear canals, and external otitis occurs less frequently in blacks than in nonblacks (8).

Certain conditions and activities contribute to the breakdown of natural barriers of the normal ear canal. Warm humid climates, with intense heat and humidity, accompanied by sweating, and exposure to water (swimming and bathing) during the summer months have been implicated. The increased exposure to moisture may result in tissue maceration that breaks down the protective barrier of the skin and alters the pH of the skin. These collectively predispose the ear canal to infection (4). There is a positive correlation between the amount of water exposure in the ear canal and the incidence of external otitis (8).

The etiology of ear disorders may be due to a variety of trauma-induced causes. Improperly cleaned or poorly fitted ear plugs may cause trauma and/or maceration of the skin in the ear canal. They also may be sensitizing. Poorly fitted hearing aids may be another source of trauma-induced injury.

Patients commonly use an instrument, a cotton applicator, or other device to clean their ears; such use is likely to push the earwax deeper in the ear canal and cause it to become tightly impacted, increasing the difficulty of subsequent removal. Its subsequent removal or modification of protection by the cerumen may increase the predisposition for bacterial or fungal infection in the ear canal. This cleaning process often causes trauma to the skin covering the ear canal and further predisposes the ear to infection. Mechanical cleaning of the ear decreases the ear's normal natural cleaning process. The normal healthy ear cleans itself, thus negating any need for cleaning with mechanical devices or instruments.

After the protective layer of the skin of the ear canal has been compromised, a preinflammatory stage occurs; the patient most likely will involuntarily scratch the ear or rub the auricle in response to an itch (9). These involuntary maneuvers further abrade the skin,

TABLE 1 Symptoms of otic disorders

	Boil	Otomycosis	Bacterial external otitis	Nonsuppurative otitis media	Impacted cerumen	Suppurative otitis media
Pain*	Often	Possibly	Often	Rarely	Rarely	Usually
Hearing deficit	Rarely	Possibly	Possibly	Possibly	Often	Usually
Purulent discharge	Rarely	Rarely	Often	Rarely	Rarely	Occasionally and indicative of perforation
Bilateral symptoms	Rarely	Rarely	Possibly	Often	Rarely	Occasionally
Appropriateness of self-medication	Auricle only	Never	Never	Never	Never	Never

*Pain is increased with chewing, traction on the auricle, and medical pressure on the tragus except in otitis media, where it is knifelike and steady.

causing deep fissures in the epidermis of the cartilaginous portion of the ear canal. An inflammatory reaction follows this fissure formation, causing edema, pain, swelling, and redness of the affected areas. This area becomes a good culture medium for bacteria or fungi, making subsequent infection likely.

Neurodermatitis sometimes occurs in middle-aged patients and is a cause of involuntary rubbing, scratching, or cleaning the ear canal in response to a vague itch or a feeling of fullness (4, 10). Overproduction of cerumen may produce similar symptoms. In some people experiencing high emotional stress and/or excessive temperatures, the ceruminous glands may respond excessively, and the acid environment of the ear canal skin may beome compromised.

COMMON PROBLEMS OF THE EAR

Many disorders of the ear are minor and easily resolved. However, the pharmacist should keep in mind that the pain associated with even minor disorders can be significant. Some untreated ear problems can result in hearing loss. The pharmacist can assist the patient by helping evaluate the disorder (Table 1), by discussing the proper course of action (self-treatment or referral

to a physician), and by recommending an efficacious nonprescription product, if appropriate.

Disorders of the Auricle

The disorders associated with the auricle, the part of the ear not within the head, are generally minor and involve lacerations, boils, and dermatitis. These conditions are generally self-limiting. Table 2 gives examples of some common physical findings related to disorders of the external ear.

Trauma

Lacerations, including scrapes and cuts, involving only the auricle skin usually heal spontaneously. A wound that does not heal normally should be checked by a physician. Deep wounds that may involve injury to the cartilage also require examination by a physician. Injury to the auricle that does not perforate the subperichondrium may cause subcutaneous bleeding and produce a hematoma. A hematoma requires aspiration or incision by a physician because the red-blue swelling may obliterate normal auricular contours and frequently results in inflammation and in perichondritis or "cauliflower ear." The swelling can also cause local pruritus and pain upon touch.

Boils

Boils (furuncles) are usually localized infections of the hair follicles. The etiology is uncertain. Fatigue and emotional stress appear to predispose individuals to furuncles. Anemia and diabetes mellitus as well as malnutrition have been found to be predisposing factors in some populations. In a high percentage of cases in young adults, no specific causative or predisposing factor has been established. Poor body hygiene is generally contributory to boils (11).

Boils often involve the anterior external auditory meatus. They usually begin as a red papule and may progress into a round or conical superficial pustule with a core of pus and erythema around the base. The lesion gradually enlarges, becomes firm, then softens and opens spontaneously (after a few days to as long as 2 weeks), discharging the purulent contents. Because the skin is very taut, even minimal swelling may cause severe pain.

Boils are usually self-limiting; however, they may be severe, autoinoculable, and multiple. Deeper lesions may lead to perichondritis (inflammation of the connective tissue). The etiologic organism of a boil is usually *Staphylococcus aureus* (2, 9).

Small boils may be treated by good hygiene combined with topical compresses. Hot compresses of saline solution may be applied to the auricle and the side of the face. Cases in which boils do not respond rapidly to topical dressings should be referred to a physician. In addition, patients with recurring boils should be referred to a physician for evaluation and possible systemic antibiotic therapy.

Perichondritis

Perichondritis is an inflammation involving the perichondrium (the fibrous connective tissue surrounding the auricular cartilage) usually following a poorly treated or untreated burn, injury, hematoma, or local infection.

The onset of perichondritis is characterized by a sensation of heat and stiffness of the auricle with pronounced pain. As the condition progresses, an exudate forms and the auricle becomes dark red and swollen. The entire auricle becomes shiny and red with uniform thickening caused by edema and inflammation. The lesions usually are confined to the cartilaginous tissue of the auricle and external canal. Constitutional disturbances may include generalized fever and malaise.

Perichondritis frequently results in severe auricular deformity, and atresia (a pathologic closure) of the external auditory canal may occur. A patient suspected of having perichondritis should be seen by a physician.

TABLE 2 Interpretation of physical findings of the external ear

Physical findings	Probable appearance	Physiologic basis	Example
Enlarged lymph node	Swollen, tender to touch, pre- and postauricular	Inflammation of lymph node; spread of infection outside the ear	Mastoiditis, otitis media
Tophus	Hard, pale node on helix, chalklike dust upon rupture	Urate crystals	Gout
Sebaceous cyst	Swollen, erythematous postauricle lesion in the skin of the ear	Inflammation of sweat gland	Skin infection
Cerumen	Red-orange pastelike discharge	Normal secretion of wax	Normal finding
Blood	Red-blue discharge	Ruptured blood vessel	External otitis
Serous fluid	Clear discharge	Blocked eustachian tube	Chronic (purulent) otitis media
Pus	Yellowish discharge	Acute inflammation	Acute suppurative otitis media

Adapted with permission from R. Leon Longe and Jon C. Calvert, *Drug Intell. Clin. Pharm., 11*, 660 (1977).

Dermatitis of the Ear

An inflammatory condition of the skin may result from an abrasion of the auricle and, if untreated, may develop into an infection of these skin layers. Inflammatory conditions such as seborrhea, psoriasis, and contact dermatitis (poison ivy and poison oak) also may affect the skin of the auricle and the external ear canal. Contact dermatitis also may be caused by an allergic response to jewelry, cosmetics, detergents, or topical drug applications (dermatitis medicamentosa) (7, 12). The lesions may spread to the auditory canal, neck, and facial areas (9). Allergens most common to the ear include antihistamines and the antibiotics gentamicin, neomycin, and polymyxin B (12, 13). Triethanolamine oleopeptide is known to irritate and inflame the skin of the ear canal (2).

Symptoms of dermatitis of the ear usually include itching and local redness followed by vesication, weeping, and erythema. The lesions form scales and yellow crusts on the skin (7, 10). They may spread to adjacent unaffected areas, and excessive scratching may cause them to become infected. Topical drugs should be used cautiously with dermatitis because of their potential allergenicity, which could exacerbate the condition. Seborrheic dermatitis of the ear is usually associated with dandruff. Treatment with dandruff-control shampoos is recommended (9). Cases that are difficult to control should be referred to a physician.

Itching or Pruritus of the Ear

An itchy ear canal is a common symptom and may mask the preinflammatory stages of acute external otitis. Itching can also occur without visible lesions of the ear. Inadequate or abnormal cerumen may be annoying to the patient and may be associated with dermatologic disorders such as seborrheic dermatitis. Symptoms include scaling, itching, and cracking of the ear canal (2). Patients with chronic external otitis experience itching caused by dry ears that may lack sufficient cerumen. Itching rather than pain is the chief complaint of persons with chronic external otitis (2). Itching may also be caused by eczema of the skin around the ears, infections, allergic seborrheic dermatitis, psoriasis, contact dermatitis, or neurodermatitis (4, 14).

Itching commonly begins as an annoying itch–scratch cycle that results in trauma, infection, epidermal barrier destruction, and inflammation of the affected areas following repeated scratching. Ear scratching has been known to be a nervous habit that may be addictive (9). Careful observation to determine the cause of itching often is helpful prior to any attempt to afford symptomatic relief.

Aural Drainage

Any patient with a discharge or drainage from the ear should be referred to a physician for proper diagnosis and treatment. The drainage or discharge may be blood, watery fluid (serum), or purulent or mucoid material. Head trauma may cause leakage of cerebrospinal fluid into the ear, or an infection of the external ear canal may produce a watery discharge. A ruptured tympanic membrane usually produces a serosanguineous fluid. Any trauma to the ear canal may cause bleeding and, if infected, the ear may exude a purulent fluid from which the causative organisms may be cultured and appropriate antibiotics chosen.

In 1982, the Food and Drug Administration (FDA) advisory review panel on topical over-the-counter (OTC) otic drug products, recommended that self-medication is inappropriate and not safe whenever drainage, pain, or dizziness is present; whenever an infection is suspected; in the presence of known injury or perforation (hole) in the eardrum; or within 6 weeks following surgery (15). This has been confirmed in a recent FDA final monograph establishing criteria for OTC products for the ear (16).

Disorders of the External Auditory Canal

Boils

Boils of the external auditory canal are pathologically similar to those of the auricle and external auditory meatus. Symptoms include pain at the infected site, which is usually exacerbated by mastication. The auditory meatus may be partly occluded by swelling, but hearing is impaired only if the opening is completely occluded. Edema and pain over the mastoid bone directly behind the auricle may occur. Traction of the auricle or the tragus is very painful. Patients with boils in the external auditory canal should be referred to a physician because unresolved conditions may lead to a generalized infection of the external auditory canal.

Otomycosis

Otomycosis, external fungal infection of the ear, is more common in warmer, tropical climates than in mild, temperate zones. Species of *Aspergillus* and *Candida* are the most common causative agents (4, 9, 16). *Aspergillus niger* produces a black exudate along the canal (2). Antibiotic treatment of a bacterial ear infection, with resultant suppression of normal bacterial flora along with diabetes mellitis, may predispose an individual to a mycotic external ear infection (9).

A superficial mycotic infection of the external auditory meatus is characterized by pruritus with a feeling of fullness and pressure in the ear. Intense itching is the primary complaint of persons with otomycosis (2). Pain may be present, increasing with mastication and traction on the pinna and the tragus. The fungus forms an accumulation of epithelial debris, exudate, and cerumen and, in the acute state, may obstruct the external auditory meatus. Hearing may be impaired.

Depending on the nature of the fungus, the color of the mass may vary. The skin lining the external auditory canal and the tympanic membrane becomes beefy-red and scaly and may be eroded or ulcerated (3). A scant, colorless mucoid discharge is common. Otomycosis is particularly serious in diabetic patients because of the microangiopathy and associated cutaneous manifestations common to diabetes mellitus (4). Mycotic ear infections must be treated by a physician. (See Chapter 16, *Diabetes Care Products*.)

Keratosis Obturans

This condition is rare and its etiology is unclear (4). Wax accumulates in the deeper parts of the external auditory canal and, with adjacent epithelial cells that contain cholesterol, forms an obstruction that exerts pressure on the surrounding tissue. It may result in erosion of the epithelial tissues surrounding it, forming a potential entrance for bacteria (1). The infection may form abscesses in the subcutaneous tissue or mastoid bone.

Pain in the ear and decreased hearing are common symptoms. A discharge and tinnitus (ringing in the ear) also may occur. Mechanical removal of the obstruction is necessary but often difficult. Removal should be performed by a physician. Patients should not attempt to remove the obstruction themselves.

Foreign Objects in the Ear

Young children often insert into the ear canal small items such as candy, pretzel sticks, pencil erasers, toy stuffing, beans, peas, marbles, pebbles, beads, or metal nuts unscrewed from toys (17). If an object becomes lodged in the ear canal, it may cause significant hearing loss. Vegetable seeds, such as dried beans or dried peas, lodged in the external auditory meatus swell when moistened during bathing or swimming and become wedged in the bony portion of the canal, causing severe pain. Furthermore, if an obstruction of the external auditory meatus is not removed promptly, acute bacterial otitis may result. Insects may enter the meatus and cause distress by beating their wings and crawling. Olive oil (sweet oil) drops may be used to suffocate the insect and stop the movement.

Foreign objects lodged in the ear canal may not cause symptoms and may be found only during a routine physical examination. Usually an object in the ear canal will cause a hearing deficiency, pain, or pressure in the ear during mastication. An exudate may form because of secondary bacterial infection. Mechanical removal should be done only by a physician because unskilled attempts at removal often damage the skin surrounding the external auditory meatus.

Impacted Cerumen

The accumulation of cerumen in the external auditory meatus may be caused by any of three factors: overactive ceruminous glands, an abnormally shaped external auditory meatus, or abnormal cerumen secreted by the ceruminous glands. Overactive ceruminous glands cause cerumen to accumulate in the external auditory canal. A tortuous or small canal or abnormal narrowing of the canal may not permit normal migration of the cerumen to the outside. Abnormal cerumen may be drier or softer than normal cerumen and may interfere with the normal epithelial migration process. People who get water in their ears while swimming or showering sometimes will experience the sudden loss of hearing in one ear. This may be caused by the increased bulk of the earwax or by water trapped behind the wax (2). Cerumen often is packed deeper into the external auditory meatus by repeated attempts to remove it. Ordinarily there is no pain unless the ear is secondarily infected (2). There usually is no cerumen in the inner half of the meatus unless it has been pushed there. In elderly persons, cerumen is frequently admixed with long hairs in the meatus, preventing normal expulsion and forming a matted obstruction in the ear.

External Otitis

External otitis (inflammation of the skin lining the external auditory canal often due to infection) is one of the most common diseases of the ear. It is very painful and annoying. The external auditory canal is considered a blind canal lined with skin. It is a dark, warm cul-de-sac that is well suited for collecting moisture. Prolonged exposure to moisture tends to disrupt the continuity of the epithelial cells, causing skin maceration and fissures, that provide a fertile environment for bacterial growth. Additionally, this prolonged exposure to moisture tends to raise the skin pH above the normal range of 5–7 (17), which improves the growth environment for bacteria. Factors contributing to susceptibility to external otitis are race, age, climate, and occupation (9). The most common causative organisms of external otitis include species of *Pseudomonas*, *Staphylococcus*, *Bacillus*, and *Proteus*. Fungi may be the causative organisms in some cases (9).

There is very little subcutaneous tissue between the skin tightly bound to the perichondrium on the cartilaginous portion and the periosteum on the bony portion of the external auditory canal. Consequently, there is disparity between the size of the visible swelling and the amount of pain associated with the condition. The lack of space available for expansion increases skin tension. Inflammation causing edema provokes severe pain in the inflamed skin that is out of proportion to visible swelling. As the inflammation increases, pain may be increased significantly during mastication. Symptoms often develop following attempts to clean the ear of foreign debris (with cotton swabs, hairpins, matchsticks, pencils, fingers, or other objects) or to scratch the ear to relieve itching. This may traumatize and damage the horny skin layer, forming an opening that allows invasion of organisms.

A normal, healthy external auditory canal is impervious to pathologic organisms. Generally, individuals must be susceptible to bacterial infections, and the skin integrity must be interrupted before an organism can produce an infection.

Another type of trauma-induced external otitis is called "swimmer's ear," or desquamative external otitis (9). Excessive moisture in the external auditory meatus may cause water to accumulate in the tympanic recess, resulting in tissue maceration because of water absorption into the stratum corneum. This excessive moisture accumulation may be important in predisposing the ear canal to infection. After bathing or swimming, patients frequently attempt to clear the ear canal of water with objects that cause abrasions or lacerations of the skin lining. Also, cerumen accumulated in the external auditory meatus absorbs water and expands. The trapped water provides a medium for infection (3). Within a few hours to 1 day following exposure to excess water, symptoms of itching, pain, and possible draining from the ear with partial occlusion occur.

Often the patient first complains of an itching feeling. Then within a few hours or up to 24 hours later, the complaints are followed by a feeling of wetness of the ear canal and discomfort leading to pain. The amount of wetness may vary from minimal to frank otorrhea (discharge). The discharge is usually cream colored or yellow. Any secondary hearing loss may be caused by epithelial debris mixed with purulent discharge causing blockage (14).

A bacterial infection of the external auditory canal leads to inflammation and epidermal destruction of the tympanic membrane (4). The infection may progress through the fibrous layer of the tympanic membrane and cause perforation and spreading of the infection into the middle ear, resulting in intense pain and discomfort. External otitis caused by infection, like otomycosis, is particularly difficult to control in individuals who have diabetes (4, 18).

Symptoms of acute external otitis are related to the severity of the pathologic conditions. There usually is mild or moderate pain that becomes pronounced by pulling upward on the auricle or by pressing on the tragus. There may be a discharge. Hearing loss may occur if the ear canal is obstructed by swelling and edema, debris, or a cerumen plug.

Chronic external otitis usually is caused by the persistence of predisposing factors. The most common symptom is itching, which prompts patients to attempt to scratch the ear canal to reduce or relieve the itching. This scratching can break the skin (10).

In allergic external otitis and dermatitis of the external auditory canal caused by seborrhea, a common symptom is itching, burning, or stinging of the lesions. Often the complaints seem excessive compared with the visible signs.

Chronic cases and those cases with symptoms of severe pain, lymphadenopathy, discharge, possible hearing loss, and fever should be referred to a physician (3). Tender nodes may be felt anterior to the tragus, behind the ear, or in the upper neck just below the pinna. (Figure 3 in Chapter 23, *Oral Health Products* shows the major lymph node areas of the neck.) Minor cases of chronic and allergic external otitis, especially swimmer's ear, often may be treated adequately with nonprescription products. All progressive symptoms of disease processes pertaining to the external ear canal or auricle should be treated only under a physician's supervision.

Malignant external otitis is the most progressive form of otitis. It occurs most frequently in elderly patients and patients with chronic lymphocytic leukemia, granulocytopenia, or poorly controlled diabetes mellitus (19, 20). In these patients, the ear becomes inflamed, and spreading proceeds to the temporal bone area. The common complaint is severe persistent pain and swelling. Clinical response to conventional therapy is not consistent. Clinical findings include persistent aural drainage, severe tenderness, and swelling in the region of the ear and mastoid bone. The tragus is always tender to touch and the auricle tender to traction.

Disorders of the Middle Ear

Disorders involving the middle ear should not be treated with nonprescription otic products. However, a brief overview of the common conditions involving the middle ear will aid the pharmacist in evaluating symptoms. Although some symptoms of middle ear disorders are the same as those of external ear disorders, others are not (Table 3). All bacterial infections of the middle

TABLE 3 Some abnormal physical findings of the middle ear

Physical findings	Probable appearance	Interpretation
Perforation	Dark, thin, oval discoloration	Rupture of the eardrum
Acute purulent otitis media	Yellowish pus behind eardrum; bulging, hyperemic membrane; light reflex absent	Acute infection of the middle ear
Chronic serous otitis media	Amber-like fluid behind eardrum; observable fluid level with air bubbles; retraction of handle of malleus	Blockage of eustachian tube

Reprinted with permission from R. Leon Longe and Jon C. Calvert, *Drug Intell. Clin. Pharm. 11*, 661 (1977).

ear should be promptly evaluated and treated by a physician. The usual treatment is systemic antibiotics.

Otitis Media

Otitis media is an inflammatory condition of the middle ear that occurs most often during childhood. Conditions that interfere with the eustachian tube function, such as upper respiratory tract infection, allergy, adenoid lymphadenopathy, and cleft palate, predispose individuals to otitis media (4). Blockage of the eustachian tube allows the oxygen in the middle ear cleft to be absorbed. This leaves a relative negative pressure or vacuum that results in a transudation (movement) of fluid into the middle ear cleft. Generally, symptoms of eustachian tube blockage are mild intermittent pain, mild hearing loss, and fullness in the ear. The tympanic membrane is retracted; if infection is absent, its color is pearlish gray. Inflation of the eustachian tube by Valsalva's maneuver (blowing against pressure) or by swallowing may assist the transport of air up the eustachian tube. The tube should not be inflated when the nasopharynx is infected because of the danger of spreading the infection into the middle ear.

Chronic middle ear infections are often treated with a myringotomy and placement of drainage tubes in order to relieve the pain and equalize the air pressure (2). Nose blowing and sneezing against occluded nostrils may worsen the condition and therefore should be avoided (21, 22). If the serous fluid in the middle ear

cavity remains sterile, the condition is termed serous otitis media and is most often of viral origin; if infected, it is termed purulent otitis media and is most often of bacterial origin.

Children often experience repeated episodes of eustachian tube obstruction caused by masses of adenoids that become edematous and block the eustachian tube openings, resulting in otitis media. Adenoidectomy usually prevents future occurrence. In adults, recurrent otitis media may be caused by nasopharyngeal tumors.

The most common symptoms in the acute phase of purulent otitis media are pain, hearing loss, fever as high as 104° F (40° C), and malaise (23). As noted by one author, "the strategic location of the middle cleft and mastoid cells separated from the sigmoid sinus and meninges by a mere thin shell makes every infection of the middle ear capable of intracranial infection" (4). Severity of symptoms increases as the condition worsens. Pain arises from the pressure of the fluids in the middle ear. This causes an outward tension on the tympanic membrane, which is innervated by sensory nerves. The rapid production of fluid and tension in a short period is responsible for the acute pain described as sharp, knifelike, and steady. The pain usually does not increase with mastication or when traction is applied to the auricle or tragus. Excessive nose blowing, especially against occluded nostrils, may force additional purulent mucus into the eustachian tube, perpetuating the condition.

If patients are not treated promptly, the pressure inside the middle ear may increase, leading to distention and bulging of the tympanic membrane. As bulging increases, so does necrosis, leading to perforation and escape of the purulent material from the middle ear. The mucopurulent discharge may cause a secondary bacterial external otitis infection. The appearance of a discharge is usually accompanied by a lessening of pain due to the decreased tension on the tympanic membrane. The initial discharge may be bloodstained, followed by a foul-smelling, purulent, serous fluid (7). The tympanic membrane usually loses its pearl-gray luster and appears yellow to orange-pink to rusty purple, representing a spectrum of increasing severity. Ear drops do not assist in the resolution of acute otitis media while the tympanic membrane is intact. The use of nonprescription otic drugs for the treatment of any form of otitis media is not recommended.

Symptoms of serous otitis media include a sensation of fullness in the ear accompanied by hearing loss (24). The condition worsens as the fluid accumulates and fills the middle ear cleft. The sensation of fullness is associated with voice resonance, a congested feeling in the ears, a hollow sound, or a popping or cracking noise in the ears especially during swallowing or yawning. These symptoms usually are not present in external otitis.

Chronic Otitis Media

In chronic serous otitis media, the fluid in the middle ear may be thin and serous or thick and viscous ("glue ear") (4). Chronic serous otitis media occurs most often in small children. It may be caused by inadequate treatment of previous episodes of otitis media or by recurrent upper respiratory tract infections associated with eustachian tube dysfunction (24).

The most common symptom is impaired hearing, but the onset is often insidious; children may have no acute symptoms (24). Frequently parents accuse the child of being inattentive and disobedient. Pain is usually absent. The diagnosis is performed by visual inspection of the tympanic membrane. The tympanic membrane appears yellow or orange and lusterless, and its flexibility is lost. It is not perforated but often appears to be retracted. Often, long-standing fluid becomes more and more viscous, thus the term glue ear.

Treatment may involve evacuation of the fluid by aspiration through an incision in the tympanic membrane (myringotomy) and implantation of a temporary, pressure-equalizing tube (24). This procedure usually is performed bilaterally and is useful in patients who do not have hypertrophied adenoids and when an adenoidectomy is not indicated. The tubes allow equalization of pressure between the middle ear space, thereby compensating for eustachian tube dysfunction (2). It is common for children under 10 years of age to wear the tubes for 6–12 months. Usually during this time, the tubes are extruded spontaneously; repeated implantation of the pressure-equalizing tubes is generally unnecessary.

The tubes are especially helpful during acute or persistently frequent episodes of eustachian tube obstruction (a common complication of acute serous otitis media or barotrauma). They permit normal atmospheric environmental changes in the middle ear cavity and allow for changes in air pressures that are not dependent on the eustachian tube. The mucosal and epithelial linings then return to normal function.

Chronic purulent otitis media is usually secondary to a persistent tympanic membrane perforation. With exacerbation of the condition, the patient may exhibit the symptoms of acute purulent otitis media with mucopurulent discharge.

Tympanic Membrane Perforation

The most common causes of traumatic perforation of the tympanic membrane are water sports, such as diving or water-skiing (7). Any corrosive agent introduced into the ear canal may produce tympanic membrane perforation. Other causes of perforation include blows to the head with a cupped hand, foreign objects entering the ear canal with excessive force, and forceful irrigation of the ear canal. At the moment of injury, the pain is severe, but it decreases rapidly. Hearing acuity usually diminishes. An untreated injury may lead to otitis media. Other complications may include tinnitus, nausea, and vertigo, and may progress to mastoiditis. Any patient suspected of having an acute perforated tympanic membrane should be referred to a physician for examination.

Barotrauma (Acute Aero-otitis Media)

Barotrauma occurs during quick descent from high altitude (10, 24). The middle ear fails to ventilate, resulting in a negative pressure in the middle ear. This negative pressure causes a suction and forces the tympanic membrane to retract, causing pain. In addition, edema is formed, with transudation and hemorrhage into the middle ear space. Barotrauma may also occur in individuals who fly with an upper respiratory tract infection or any condition associated with impaired eustachian tube ventilation.

Upon examination, the tympanic membrane appears inflamed and retracted and is similar to that seen with acute otitis media, confusing the differential diagnosis.

Pretreatment with antihistamines and/or decongestants may help to avoid serious symptoms during air travel for patients susceptible to barotrauma. Treatment of acute episodes consists of oral decongestants, antihistamines, and autoinflation of the eustachian tube (Valsalva's maneuver) (4, 24). Blowing against pressure or swallowing may also inflate the eustachian tubes.

Hearing Disorders

Obstructive Hearing Loss

Accumulated cerumen is a common cause of hearing loss, especially in persons with overactive cerumen glands. The accumulated cerumen causes an obstruction and produces a feeling of fullness or diminished hearing. A hearing impairment may occur when the cerumen occludes the canal, impairing the transmission of sound waves to the tympanic membrane. Impacted cerumen can be removed only by direct manipulation; the procedure should not be attempted by the patient or untrained persons. After the patient swims or bathes, water can be trapped in the ear canal. The trapped water is absorbed by cerumen that occludes the canal, causing a sudden hearing deficit. As discussed previously in the section on external otitis, a temporary hearing impairment may result from excessive edema, which with accumulated cerumen and debris, may occlude the canal.

Tinnitus

Tinnitus may be associated with hearing loss, exposure to high noise levels, or acoustic trauma, or may be a symptom of a systemic disease or a drug toxicity (22). Disequilibrium (vertigo) may be of otic origin. It may be due to drug toxicity, intracranial or neurologic diseases, infection, hyperventilation, or severe ceruminal impaction (25). Tinnitus is defined as a noise or ringing in the ear. It is usually subjective and audible only to the patient. It is usually a sign of a hearing disorder and may be the first and only symptom (2). Tinnitus can be very annoying and may be constant or intermittent. It is described as sounding like steam escaping from a small pipe, ringing, roaring, pulsating, chirping (crickets), or humming (26). The intensity of the disturbance varies from patient to patient, and patients' reactions may vary from minor distraction to severe mental depression. Tinnitus can arise from a variety of causes often involving the inner ear. It may be the result of blockage of the ear canal, or the eustachian tube and middle ear cavity, which is easily corrected following proper diagnosis.

Serous otitis media, external otitis, acute otitis media, and chronic otitis media seldom produce tinnitus as the sole or predominant complaint. Most patients have sensory insult from loud noise exposure, ototoxicity, head trauma, Meniere's disease, or acoustic neurinoma (24).

Patients with tinnitus caused by such drugs as salicylates (arthritis patients), quinidine (heart patients), and quinine (malaria patients or patients with leg cramps) usually will notice a decrease in the intensity of the tinnitus following discontinuation of the offending medication. Any patient who experiences any symptom of tinnitus should receive a medical examination and evaluation. Nonprescription ear drops are not effective and are not recommended for the treatment of tinnitus.

ASSESSMENT

To choose appropriately between self-treatment and physician referral, the pharmacist must be able to assess the nature and severity of the patient's otic condition by evaluating the signs and symptoms (Table 1). The most common complaints may include one or more of the following: localized pain, itchiness in the ear canal, a feeling of fullness, hearing loss, lymphadenopathy, fever, and malaise.

Ear Pain

Pain in the ear, commonly expressed by the patient as an earache, may be caused by a variety of disorders. Careful inspection with proper instrumentation by trained personnel often is necessary to determine the etiology of the pain. External otitis, foreign material (cerumen) packed against the tympanic membrane, and acute otitis media with its possible complications (mastoiditis or abscess) are all common causes of ear pain. Some pain is referred to the ear from the sinuses, nasopharynx, tongue, hypopharynx, larynx, or temporomandibular joint. Loose-fitting dentures may also induce frank ear pain. In all such cases, proper diagnosis and determination of pain source should be advised rather than self-medication.

Applied pressure on the pinna or the tragus increases pain in external otitis (27). Patients with otitis media rarely report increased pain with pressure on the pinna or tragus. Mastication may cause increased pain in patients with either external otitis or otitis media. This is an important consideration in diagnosis.

Boils

The signs and symptoms of a boil in the ear canal include a localized, burning pain that increases when the patient chews, when traction is applied to the auricle, and when the tragus is pressed medially. A red, inflamed, raised lesion can be seen along the ear canal. The skin around the affected area is intact and not broken, provided the patient has not attempted to scratch it. The patient's subjective hearing is usually intact. If lymphadenopathy, fever, malaise, or severe pain is present, the patient should be referred to a physician for treatment.

Foreign Objects

The signs and symptoms of a foreign object in the ear usually include a feeling of fullness with hearing loss from the affected ear. Pain may be present and increased by chewing, traction on the auricle, and pressure applied medially on the tragus. Lymphadenopathy, fever, or malaise does not occur acutely but may develop later with a foul-smelling discharge from the affected ear. Collectively, these characteristics indicate a secondary infection. All patients with foreign objects in ear, with or without secondary infection, should be seen and treated by a physician.

External Otitis

The only conclusive means by which bacterial or fungal external otitis may be ruled out is by microbiologic culture. However, a culture is not always practical or necessary. Pain and swelling localized in the ear canal are usually the motivating symptoms that cause the patient to seek professional help (Table 4). A bacterial infection may be characterized by increased pain with chewing, traction applied on the auricle, and pressure applied medially on the tragus. Lymphadenopathy, a feeling of fullness, and fever and associated malaise may be additional characteristics. Otoscopic examination is painful and reveals a swollen inflamed ear canal and an inflamed tympanic membrane. A purulent, foul-smelling discharge may block visual inspection of the tympanic membrane. Any foul-smelling mucopurulent discharge indicates a bacterial infection. Patients with external otitis should be referred to a physician for thorough cleansing and inspection of the ear canal.

TABLE 4 Differential diagnosis of acute external otitis and acute otitis media

	Acute external otitis	Acute otitis media
Season	Summer	Winter
Movement of tragus painful	Yes	No
Ear canal	Swollen	Normal
Eardrum	Normal (or red)	Perforated or bulging
Discharge	Yes	Yes, but through a perforation
Nodes	Frequent	Less frequent
Fever	Yes	Yes
Hearing	Normal or decreased	Always decreased

Adapted with permission from D. DeWeese et al., "Otolaryngology—Head and Neck Surgery," 7th ed., C. V. Mosby, 1988, p. 398.

Hearing Loss

Hearing loss is a subjective complaint unless diagnosed and evaluated by an audiologist. Acute hearing loss without pain may be caused by impacted cerumen, which may be observed during direct visualization of the ear canal. Impacted cerumen in the ear canal obstructs the tympanic membrane and prevents its visualization.

Patients with impacted cerumen without secondary complications may be treated safely with nonprescription cerumen-softening agents. Patients with hearing loss without pain, and whose tympanic membrane is visible and not obstructed, should be evaluated and treated by a physician. A perforated tympanic membrane results in decreased hearing. Usually the patient has experienced a sharp pain of short duration at the time of injury. Treatment for a perforated tympanic membrane includes repair and medical therapy to prevent infection in the middle ear.

Otomycosis

Patients with otomycosis usually complain of itching and a feeling of fullness in the affected ear. A color-

less discharge may or may not be present. Pain usually is not present but may occur in severe cases. The pain increases with chewing, traction on the auricle, and pressure applied medially on the tragus. Constitutional disturbances usually occur only in severe cases, which often are due to secondary bacterial infections with obstruction of the ear canal causing a hearing loss.

Otitis Media

The only conclusive means of diagnosing otitis media is a complete physical examination, using a pneumatic otoscope, and a complete patient history. In most cases, otitis media is caused by eustachian tube dysfunction. It is found most commonly in children. Patients may be asymptomatic or may complain of occasional fullness and "cracking" or a "hollow sound" in the ears. The effect is usually bilateral. Otoscopic findings are specific and may demonstrate typical changes in tympanic membrane mobility consistent with the symptoms and degree of severity of the disorder.

A complication of prolonged serous otitis media is caused by bacteria and viruses extending along the eustachian tube causing suppurative otitis media. Pneumatic otoscopic findings are specific and demonstrate a bulging, poorly resilient tympanic membrane. Deformity of the tympanic membrane is caused by the pus and exudate that accumulate behind the tympanic membrane. The patient usually experiences pain that is dull and throbbing at first and then rapidly becomes sharp, knifelike, and agonizing. These symptoms usually follow an upper respiratory tract infection. Constitutional symptoms include chills, fever, and malaise. A purulent discharge occurs only after tympanic membrane perforation, at which time the patient experiences sudden relief from pain. A bloody, purulent, foul-smelling drainage flows from the ear. Following drainage, temperature rapidly returns to normal.

Patients with any of these symptoms should be treated by a physician because middle ear disorders are often associated with an underlying cause and require thorough diagnostic evaluation and treatment.

TREATMENT

Normally, the skin lining the external auditory meatus provides adequate protection against bacterial or fungal infection; cerumen lubricates the skin to maintain its integrity. The hair helps shield the meatus from dust and debris. Cerumen provides a continuing, self-cleaning process that removes particulate matter and debris from the external auditory meatus. An infection of the auricle or external auditory meatus is a skin infection and should be treated as such.

Progressive symptoms of otic disease should be evaluated and treated only under a physician's supervision. Cerumen-softening and cerumenolytic agents only soften and loosen cerumen to enable its easy removal by a physician. These agents do not readily remove cerumen. Effective mechanical removal by irrigation or instrumentation should be reserved for the physician. Surgical intervention may be necessary for deep cuts, bruises, or abrasions of the ear. Severe infections often require both systemic and local antibiotics.

Self-treatment of boils may be instituted by applying heat followed by a bland ointment to the affected area. A soft cotton applicator is useful for application over and around the boil. An antibiotic ointment may be used in the absence of known or suspected sensitivity. The lesion usually is self-limiting and clears after several days of frequent applications of heat and ointment. Resistant lesions require incision and drainage by a physician.

Treatment of external otitis typically includes antibiotic and hydrocortisone drops applied in the ear canal. When cellulitus and lymphadenopathy are present,

oral antibiotics are effective. Trauma to the ear should be avoided. The ear canals should be kept clean and dry at all times. After the patient swims or bathes, the ear canals may be filled for 1 or 2 minutes with alcohol, glycerin, propylene glycol, or water acidified to a pH of 4–5 to help restore the normal acidic pH to the ear canal (4). A 5% aluminum acetate solution (Burow's solution) may be used as an astringent to obtain rapid resolution of eczematous or weeping skin (2).

Patients who have repeated episodes of external ear infections should be advised to use an acidifying agent and/or alcoholic solution when exposed to high humidity (e.g., while swimming).

Soaking with warm water, saline, or Burow's solution is often useful in the treatment of crusting and edema involving the auricle and surrounding tissue (20).

Cleansing the ear with a soft rubber bulb ear syringe may be uncomfortable, but should never be painful. If frank pain does occur, irrigation must be stopped at once. Severe knifelike pain occurs if the tympanic membrane is ruptured and may be followed by intense vertigo. The irrigation solution should always be at room temperature. If the solution is too hot or too cold, the patient may experience vertigo (28, 29). Many times cleansing with saline or water at body temperature helps to clear debris from the ear canal.

External otitis should always be treated promptly for a satisfactory outcome. If not treated properly, spreading to the mastoid bone or to the middle ear cavity is likely. Severe cases may result in permanent hearing loss.

Minor symptoms of otomycosis (rare) may be treated prophylactically with alcohol, propylene glycol, glycerin, or water that has been acidified. Aluminum acetate solution also may be used for its astringent effect. These ingredients have been demonstrated to be safe and effective for maintaining a clean, dry ear canal and promoting aural hygiene (4). The choice of the product depends on availability. Patients with severe otomycosis and impacted mycotic debris should have their ear canals cleaned and treated by a physician.

Primary Nonprescription Pharmacologic Agents

Nonprescription products used for palliative treatment of auricular ear disorders should include selective products useful for the treatment of skin disorders.

When applied to the skin, salicylic acid acts as a mild irritant; continuous application may cause dermatitis (30). The use of salicylic acid in topical preparations applied to the ear canal is considered inadvisable unless recommended by a physician.

Antibiotic ointments, such as neomycin and bacitracin ointments, alone or in combination with polymyxin B sulfate, are adequate for treating minor lesions of the auricle. They should be used only in the absence of known or suspected sensitivity. Antibiotics do not readily penetrate abscesses; therefore, incision and drainage may be required.

Acetic Acid Solutions

Weak acetic acid solutions are used to treat mild forms of external otitis and swimmer's ear. Acetic acid solution in the form of household vinegar has been used successfully for many years to treat external otitis (31). The use of acetic acid for the treatment of ear disorders was first described in an Assyrian medical textbook, which was translated by Thompson (32). Acetic acid has bactericidal and fungicidal properties if properly used. An environmental pH of 7.2–7.6 appears to be optimal for bacterial growth, as indicated by a study of 42 otitis cases in which pus cells and bacteria were observed in a pH range of 6.5–7.2 (33). The recommended treatment of 4 drops placed into the ear canal 4 times daily provides an environmental pH of <3 (33). Recommended prophylaxis is 4 drops placed into the ear canal after swimming, showering, bathing, or washing hair. Concentrations of 2 to 3% provide effective and dependable treatment for mild forms of otitis by lowering the pH of the ear canal; however, solutions of less than 1% lack bactericidal properties (34).

A suitable concentration of acetic acid can be made easily and inexpensively in the pharmacy from white distilled household vinegar, which is usually 5% acetic acid. A 50:50 mixture of distilled household vinegar with either water, propylene glycol, glycerin, or rubbing alcohol (70% isopropyl alcohol or 70% ethyl alcohol) will provide a 2.5% solution (35). Because propylene glycol is viscous, mixing it with vinegar will increase the contact time of acetic acid on the epithelium. Anydrous glycerin alone or mixed with vinegar will help to remove water from the ear. Alcohol alone or mixed with vinegar has local anti-infective properties and provides a drying effect (7, 28, 36). Decreasing the alcohol concentration may lessen the burning sensation and also decrease the drying effect, whereas increasing the alcohol concentration will increase the drying effect. Instilling acidified alcohol into the ear after swimming, showering, bathing, or washing hair has been shown to prevent the growth of bacteria, including species of *Pseudomonas* (6, 35). However, patients should be cautioned that denaturants in 70% rubbing alcohol formulations may cause sensitization.

The FDA advisory review panel on OTC topical otic products has concluded that acetic acid is safe for use in the ear but that data are inadequate to demonstrate effectiveness (37).

Aluminum Acetate Solution (Burow's Solution)

External otitis or local itching of the external ear caused by external ear dermatitis may be treated with an astringent such as 1:20 or 1:40 aluminum acetate solution (3, 35, 38, 39). One tablet or packet dissolved in 500 ml of water yields a concentration of 1:40. Aluminum acetate solution is used widely for conditions involving the external ear. Its major value is its acidity, which restores the normal antibacterial pH of the ear canal. Applied locally as protein precipitants, astringents dry the affected area by reducing the secretory function of the skin glands (39). Contraction and wrinkling of the affected tissue may be seen; astringents also toughen the skin to assist the prevention of reinfection. When applied properly, this preparation is useful for treating bacterial infections as well as otomycosis.

Aluminum acetate solution is often useful for resolving the edema and crusting associated with acute moist ear canals. Special cleansing is sometimes necessary because of the abundant desquamative debris that forms (7).

A wet compress may also be used with a gauze dressing on the auricle (3, 20). Drops may be instilled into the meatus. Usually the dosage is 4–6 drops every 4–6 hours until the itching or burning subsides. The drops also may be used prophylactically against swimmer's ear to help clean and dry the ear canal after swimming or bathing. Aluminum acetate solution is suitable for children and adults. Used properly, it is nonsensitizing and well tolerated (30). Adverse reactions are rare.

Antipyrine

The FDA advisory review panel on OTC topical analgesic, antirheumatic, otic, burn, and sunburn treatment drug products concluded that antipyrine is neither safe nor effective for nonprescription use as a topical otic analgesic and anesthetic and should be used only under the advice and supervision of a physician (40). The clinical effectiveness and safety of antipyrine in treating otic disorders have not been substantiated. (See Chapter 32, *External Analgesic Products*.)

Benzocaine

The utility of benzocaine or other local anesthetics for local analgesia in the ear canal is not clear. The FDA advisory review panel concluded that benzocaine is neither safe nor effective for nonprescription use as a topical analgesic and suggested that benzocaine is ineffective topically as an analgesic and/or anesthetic on the tissue of the tympanic membrane and ear canal (15, 40). Hypersensitivity to benzocaine is considered a general contraindication to its topical use in the ear or applied elsewhere to the skin.

The topical application of any local anesthetic may produce the same untoward effects as those following parenteral administration. Reactions or complications are usually avoided by applying the minimal effective dose. Special caution should be exercised in patients with known drug sensitivity and in those with severe trauma or sepsis of the areas of application.

Boric Acid

Boric acid is an ingredient in several ear preparations. It is a weak, local anti-infective and is nonirritating to intact skin in a dilute solution of 1–5%. Supersaturated alcoholic boric acid solutions have improved the antibacterial action over alcohol itself (either 99% isopropyl or 70% ethyl alcohol). The addition of acetic acid or boric acid will increase the acidity of the preparation, which when applied topically will increase the acidity of the skin (6, 35). Because of its toxicity, boric acid should be used with caution, particularly in children and on open wounds where the potential for systemic absorption is high (39).

Camphor

Camphor is used in eardrops and earwax softeners as a weak antiseptic and a mild anesthetic intended to suppress itching. However, its effectiveness in the concentrations used has not been substantiated.

Carbamide Peroxide

The antibacterial properties of carbamide peroxide (urea hydrogen peroxide) are due to its release of nascent oxygen; its main value is to clean wounds. The effervescence caused by the oxygen release mechanically removes debris from inaccessible regions. In otic preparations, the effervescence disintegrates wax accumulations. Carbamide (urea) helps debride the tissue. These actions soften the residue in the ear, and removal of the liquefied cerumen may be assisted by warm water irrigation.

The FDA advisory review panel on OTC topical otic products has concluded that carbamide peroxide 6.5% formulated in an anhydrous glycerin vehicle is safe and effective for occasional nonprescription use as an aid to soften, loosen, and remove excessive earwax (16). The panel recommends usage twice a day for up to 4 days if needed, or as directed by a physician. Five drops of the solution should be instilled into the affected ear and allowed to remain at least 15 minutes, either by tilting the head (affected ear up) or by insert-

ing a small amount of cotton into the canal opening. The applicator tip should not enter the canal. Wax remaining after treatment may be removed by gently flushing the ear with warm water, using a soft rubber bulb ear syringe. The process may be repeated a second time, if necessary. It is not recommended for children under 12 years of age. Failure to obtain relief after 4 days of treatment could indicate a more serious condition for which a physician should be consulted.

Carbamide peroxide should not be used in the presence of ear drainage, pain, or dizziness. It should not be used in the presence of known injury or perforation (hole) of the eardrum or within 6 weeks following ear surgery except with physician supervision.

This treatment should be discontinued whenever irritation or rash appears. It is not recommended for treating pain of raw inflamed tissue, swimmer's ear, or itching of the ear canal.

Chloroform

Chloroform is an irritant and preservative used in some eardrops. It is volatile and evaporates on exposure to the air. Its effectiveness for treating ear disorders has not been substantiated.

Glycerin

Glycerin may be used as a solvent or an emollient, and also as a humectant because of its hydroscopic properties. Glycerin is widely used as a solvent and a vehicle in many otic preparations (prescription and nonprescription). It is safe and nonsensitizing when applied to open wounds or abraded skin.

The FDA advisory review panel on OTC topical otic drug products has concluded that glycerin is considered safe for use in the ear but that data are inadequate to demonstrate effectiveness (16). Dehydrated glycerin contains no less than 98.5% glycerin. Glycerin USP contains no less than 95% glycerin (it may contain a maximum of 5% water) (41, 42). Anhydrous glycerin may be prepared by heating glycerin USP at 150°C for 2 hours to drive off the moisture (16). Because of glycerin's hygroscopic properties, patients should be advised not to rinse the applicator, as this will dilute the glycerin and reduce its effectiveness.

Ichthammol

Ichthammol is a weak antiseptic and irritant with demulcent and emollient properties. Its primary contribution is as an emollient, not as an antiseptic. Ichthammol ointment (10%) is used for treating local inflammation associated with minor boils or abscesses. It may be employed with glycerin in external otitis and cellulitis. Evidence to support effectiveness and efficacy is not available (11).

Menthol

Menthol, which is included in some earwax softeners, is an antipruritic and counterirritant when applied locally. Menthol's clinical effectiveness in treating ear disorders has not been substantiated.

Olive Oil (Sweet Oil)

Olive oil, a fixed oil containing mixed glycerides of oleic acid (about 83%), is used as an emollient and topical lubricant (42). It is often instilled into the ear canal to alleviate itching and burning. It is also helpful for softening ear wax (18). If an insect becomes trapped in the ear canal, olive oil can be used to smother the insect and stop its crawling.

Phenol in Glycerin

Phenol in glycerin (5–10%) was formerly prescribed to treat pain caused by ear disorders (43). Its use is not recommended because of inherent dangers of necrosis and perforation of the tympanic membrane (11, 44). Phenol is a potent but toxic bactericide. It is absorbed by the skin and has caused severe toxic effects and death when used in excess (11).

Propylene Glycol

Propylene glycol is a solvent that has preservative properties and is a useful humectant. Used in both prescription and nonprescription otic preparations, propylene glycol is a clear, colorless, nonirritating, viscous liquid. Its viscosity provides increased contact time to the tissues of the external auditory meatus. Adding acetic acid to propylene glycol increases the solution's acidity, enhancing its anti-infective properties (45). If used over a long period of time, propylene glycol has been known to cause allergic reactions or dermatitis (2, 13).

Thymol

Thymol, a phenol obtained from thyme oil, has a more agreeable odor than phenol. It has antibacterial and antifungal properties in a concentration of 1% (31). In the presence of large amounts of proteins, its antibacterial activity is greatly reduced. It has been used traditionally in topical preparations partly because of its deodorant properties. Thymol in 95% ethyl alcohol has been used for the treatment of resistant fungal infections of the ear. Contact time is increased by the use of a cotton wick placed in the ear (2). The clinical effective-

ness of thymol for treating ear disorders has not been well studied and therefore is not substantiated.

Other Cerumen-Softening Products

Other products used to soften earwax include light mineral oil, a mixture of warm water and 3% hydrogen peroxide in a ratio of 1:1, and a 3% hypertonic sodium chloride solution (28). The use of undiluted 3% hydrogen peroxide and the indiscriminate use of aqueous hydrogen peroxide (1:1) instilled in the ear canal are unwise because they may cause maceration of the skin and predispose it to infection (9). Cerumen-softening agents only soften the hardened, impacted cerumen. They do not and should never be expected to both soften and remove cerumen. Patients can be instructed to use the cerumen-softening agents for up to 3 days, after which time the cerumen should be softened enough to be easily removed (2). The impacted cerumen should be removed only by a physician through irrigation or mechanical means.

Removal of the cerumen, desquamated debris, and dried secretions often is best accomplished by suction or use of a small cotton-tipped applicator. (This method should be performed only by trained personnel.) Gentle irrigation with an ear syringe or a forced water spray should be performed only if the tympanic membrane is known to be intact. Ordinary tap water may be used, but it must be at body temperature or vertigo will develop from vestibular stimulation (2). Direct visualization of the ear canal is important for the patient's safety. In patients who have difficulty with hard, impacted cerumen, the occasional instillation of olive oil, mineral oil, glycerin, diluted hydrogen peroxide solution, or propylene glycol in the ear may soften the cerumen and promote the normal process of removal.

The patient may irrigate the ear canal with warm water, normal saline, a mixture of 20–30% alcohol and water, or aluminum acetate solution to help prevent cerumen buildup (35). If the tympanic membrane is perforated or if it is not known whether the tympanic membrane is intact, these cerumen-softening products should be used only under a physician's supervision.

In mild cases of external otitis, topical treatment is all that is necessary (2). Following careful cleansing, a bland soothing liquid placed in the ear canal is suitable. An important feature of any otic solution is that the pH is acidic, because most bacteria or fungi do not thrive in acidic environments (2). This treatment is preferred except in diabetic patients and in unusually severe cases of external otitis. In severe cases, these solutions may be used to irrigate the debris from the ear canal to improve the effectiveness of topical antibacterial otic drops (4). Dilute alcohol 10–20% is less irritating for the patient with acute ear pain. However, as inflammation diminishes, 70% acidified alcohol may be used to keep the ear canal clean and dry. Patients may be advised to use an alcohol solution in the ear any time water enters the ear canal (7). Patients should also be advised that future episodes may be avoided by keeping the ears dry with routine use of dilute acidified alcohol at least 3 times weekly, especially after swimming. Patients should also be advised against scratching the ear canal with cotton applicators (7). Patients with a known tympanic membrane perforation should not use otic preparations without their physicians' consent.

All nonprescription otic preparations may be contraindicated because of local irritation and hypersensitivity caused by the ingredients. Patients should be advised that if a rash, local redness, or other noticeable adverse symptoms occur, the medication should be discontinued.

PRODUCT SELECTION GUIDELINES

Patient Considerations

The pharmacist's evaluation of the patient's present health status must be based on information in the medical and drug history, including current symptoms. This information should include the presence of chronic diseases that may impair healing, such as diabetes mellitus (patients using insulin or oral hypoglycemics), or conditions that may influence the patient's response to self-medication.

Other considerations include deformities or ear scars. An earache caused by otitis media, secondary to an upper respiratory tract infection, should be ruled out before the pharmacist suggests self-treatment of an external ear disorder. A history of pressure in or referred pain to the ear may be caused by a pathologic condition in the area around the ear. Recent injury or trauma to the head or neck regions may also cause referred pain to the ear. Adults with recurrent otitis who respond poorly to treatment should be examined by a physician to exclude nasopharyngioma.

Management of ear disorders often may be difficult because of underlying diseases or predisposing factors. The skin of patients with diabetes mellitus is more prone to infection (bacterial and fungal), especially when the diabetes is uncontrolled. Infections in diabetics tend to resolve more slowly and to recur more frequently. The increased predisposition to infection of the ear canal may be related to impairment of the skin's integrity, increased glucose concentrations, and abnormalities in immunologic responses. Ear infections, especially external otitis, are difficult to treat in diabetic patients. Rigid control of diabetes cannot be overemphasized for favorable outcome of treatment. (See Chapter 16, *Diabetes Care Products*.)

The pharmacist should ask specific questions regarding the patient's medical history, such as whether the patient has experienced similar symptoms previously and, if so, when and how they were treated. The pharmacist should ask the patient to describe the symptoms. The patient's medical history should reveal underlying disease states and predisposing factors, including allergies, that may influence the response to self-medication.

The pharmacist first should consider whether the patient can be appropriately treated with nonprescription drugs. Health professionals (pharmacists and nurses) properly trained to visualize the tympanic membrane and ear canal with a suitable otoscope and those properly instructed in aural hygiene may, in most cases, perform irrigation safely with an ear syringe or a forced water spray. Pharmacists may assess the severity of the otic disorder and either provide appropriate nonprescription medication with instructions or refer the patient to a physician. Appropriately selected nonprescription drug products can be relied upon to provide a suitable therapeutic response. Proper selection and instruction by the pharmacist require a clear knowledge of the symptoms and pathophysiology of the illness. Referral to medical treatment by a physician requires an ability to recognize the severity of the illness or the potential or actual complications associated with the condition. The patient should always be referred to a physician if any of the following symptoms exist: severe pain, lymphadenopathy, discharge from the ear, possible hearing deficit, or fever.

Patient Consultation

Many physicians feel that cleansing procedures and self-medication for treating ear disorders should not be delegated to the patient, or to anyone who is not properly trained. Patients must be evaluated for their ability to understand the hazards of inappropriate self-medication. The pharmacist with proper instruction in aural visualization and irrigation procedures can usually make these judgments.

The use of nonprescription drugs for the ear should be supervised as are other drug products dispensed by the pharmacist (46). The proper use of medicine droppers for administering eardrops into the ear and ear syringes for irrigating the ear should be fully understood by the patient. Eardrops should be warmed to body temperature by holding the medication container in the palm of the hand or in a vessel of warm water for a few minutes before administration. Eardrops heated to hot temperatures should never be applied to the ear canal. Hot eardrops are potentially dangerous and are likely to damage the ear. Also, excessive heat may damage the ingredients in the eardrop container.

Eardrops may be applied as frequently as 4 drops 4 times daily. The involved ear should be tilted up for at least 2 minutes following the placement of the eardrops to permit effective contact of the medication (2).

A cotton wick may be inserted gently to help the medication maintain contact with the skin in the ear canal. Cotton wicks, however, usually require insertion with appropriate instruments and should be used only by trained personnel. Pulling the auricle back may allow the medication to reach a greater depth in the ear canal. If irrigation of the ear canal is necessary, it should be performed only by trained persons using either an ear syringe or a forced water spray, such as a Water Pik; the direction of the water column should be superior against the canal wall and the tympanic membrane, because most debris and foreign material will gather along the inferior portion of the canal (2). In addition, patients should be advised to consult a physician if symptoms persist or increase in severity within a few days following the initiation of self-medication. Symptoms usually begin to subside within 1–2 days if self-medication is appropriate. If symptoms persist or if an adverse reaction to the medication occurs, the patient should be referred to a physician immediately.

SUMMARY

Otic disorders affect both young and old people, and their visible signs are not always proportional to the amount of pain suffered. Nonprescription products are available for treatment of disorders of both the auricle and the external auditory canal. Disorders involving the middle ear should not be treated with nonprescription products.

By assessing the complaint and reviewing the patient's history, the pharmacist should be able to judge whether symptoms may be self-treated or if referral to a physician is indicated. Health professionals trained in otic procedures may examine the tympanic membrane

with an otoscope and irrigate the ear canal gently with a syringe or a forced water spray. This procedure should be performed only if the tympanic membrane is known to be intact and there are no underlying disorders.

Objects such as hairpins, pencils, matchsticks, cotton swabs, or other sharp instruments should never touch the external auditory canal, and objects smaller than a finger draped with a clean washcloth should never enter the external auditory canal. Patients should be advised never to place objects in the ear canal. Good personal hygiene, especially of facial and neck areas, should be maintained. Dandruff and dirty hair may be controlled with appropriate shampoos and washing. A skin infection must not be neglected because it may be transferred very easily to uninfected areas.

Most nonprescription otic products have been shown to be safe and effective, and the choice of a specific product generally depends on availability and patient preference. The pharmacist should advise the patient to consult a physician if symptoms do not subside within 1 or 2 days after treatment is initiated or if adverse reactions occur.

REFERENCES

1 I. Hall and B. Colman, "Diseases of the Nose, Throat and Ear," 10th ed., Williams and Wilkins, Baltimore, Md., 1973, pp. 278, 315, 324.

2 D. DeWeese et al., "Otolaryngology—Head and Neck Surgery," 7th ed., C. V. Mosby, St. Louis, Mo., 1988, pp. 347, 349, 351, 395–397, 399, 401, 402, 409, 413, 423, 479.

3 I. Friedman, "Pathology of the Ear," Blackwell Scientific Publications, London, England, 1974, pp. 10, 14, 15, 27.

4 M. M. Paparella and D. A. Shumick, "Otolaryngology," Vol. 2, W. B. Saunders, Philadelphia, Pa., 1980, pp. 31, 1345–1349, 1393, 1412, 1413, 1419, 1445.

5 S. Riegelman and D. L. Sorby, in "Dispensing of Medication," 7th ed., E. W. Martin, Ed., Mack, Easton, Pa., 1971, p. 908.

6 G. L. Adams et al., "Fundamentals of Otolaryngology," 5th ed., W. B. Saunders, Philadelphia, Pa., 1978, pp. 181, 184.

7 "Diseases of Nose, Throat, Ear, Head, and Neck," 13th ed., J. J. Ballenger et al., Eds., Lea and Febiger, Philadelphia, Pa., 1985, pp. 881, 1092, 1093, 1096, 1123, 1130.

8 *Federal Register*, *42*, p. 63559 (1977).

9 S. R. Mawson and H. Ludman, "Diseases of the Ear," 4th ed., Yearbook Medical, Chicago, Ill., 1979, pp. 252, 257, 261, 267.

10 B. H. Senturia et al., "Diseases of the External Ear, An Otologic-Dermatology Manual," 2nd ed., Grune and Stratton, New York, N.Y., 1980, pp. 79, 80.

11 A. Rook et al., "Textbook of Dermatology," Blackwell Scientific Publications, London, England, 1979, pp. 443, 553.

12 J. Rutka and P. Alberti, "Toxic and Drug Induced Disorders in Otolaryngology," The Otolaryngologic Clinics of North America, 1984, pp. 761–774.

13 J. Booth, in "Scott-Brown's Otolaryngology," 5th ed., A. Kerr, Ed., Butterworth's & Co. Ltd., London, England, 1987, pp. 55, 56, 164.

14 C. S. Karmody, "Textbook of Otolaryngology." Lea & Febiger, Philadelphia, Pa., 1983, p. 56.

15 *Federal Register*, 47, 30014, 30018, (1982).

16 *Federal Register, 51*, 28656–661 (1986).

17 J. Bordely et al., "Ear, Nose, and Throat Disorders in Children," Raven Press, New York, N.Y., 1986, pp. 56, 57, 61, 89.

18 A. Cohn, *Arch. Otolaryngol.*, *99*, 138 (1974).

19 J. G. Corcoran and S. G. Atline, "Infectious Diseases in the Geriatric Patient: Symposium on Geriatric Otolaryngology," Otolaryngologic Clinics of North America, 1983, p. 425.

20 F. E. Lucente, in "Otolaryngology—Diseases of the Ear and Hearing," G. M. English, Ed., Vol. 1, Harper & Row, Philadelphia, Pa., 1983, p. 1–12.

21 J. Bossi and J. Jackman, *Drug Intell. Clin. Pharm.*, *11*, 665 (1977).

22 G. D. L. Smyth, "Chronic Otitis Media in Otolaryngology," Vol. 1, G. M. English, Ed., Harper & Row, Philadelphia, Pa., 1976, p. 2.

23 D. Elliott et al., *Patient Care*, *5*, 20 (1971).

24 K. J. Lee, "Differential Diagnosis, Otolaryngology," Arco, New York, N.Y., 1978, pp. 91, 94, 115.

25 R. P. Wood and F. L. Northern, "Manual of Otolaryngology," Williams and Wilkins, Baltimore, Md., 1979, pp. 39, 42.

26 L. J. Bradford and W. G. Hardy, "Hearing and Hearing Impairment," Grune and Stratton, New York, N.Y., 1979, pp. 106–107.

27 D. Wright and F. Alexander, *Arch. Otolaryngol.*, *99*, 16–18 (1974).

28 K. J. Lee, Ed., "Essential Otolaryngology: Head & Neck Surgery," 32nd ed., Medical Examination Publishing Co., Inc., New Hyde Park, N.Y., 1983, p. 164.

29 K. G. Marshall and E. L. Attia, "Disorders of the Ear," John Wright PSG, Littleton, Mass., 1983, p. 25.

30 A. Wade and J. E. Reynolds, "Martindale, The Extra Pharmacopoeia," 27th ed., Pharmaceutical Press, London, Eng., 1979, pp. 212, 272.

31 I. Ochs, *Arch. Otolaryngol.*, *52*, 935–937 (1950).

32 R. Thompson, *J. Roy. Asiatic Soc.*, (1931).

33 F. Goffin, *N. Eng. J. Med.*, *268*, 287–289 (1963).

34 E. Jones and P. McIain, *Laryngoscope, 71*, 928–935 (1961).

35 "AMA Drug Evaluations," 5th ed., American Medical Association, Chicago, Ill., 1983, pp. 543, 1392.

36 D. Wright and M. Dinen, *Arch. Otolaryngol.*, *95*, 245 (1972).

37 *Federal Register, 51*, 27369, 27372 (1986).

38 "Drugs of Choice," W. Modell, Ed., C. V. Mosby, St. Louis, Mo., 1984, p. 743.

39 "Remington's Pharmaceutical Sciences," 16th ed., Mack, Easton, Pa., 1985, pp. 777, 788.

40 *Federal Register, 42*, 63564 (1977).

41 "The United States Pharmacopoeia," 21st ed., Mack, Easton, Pa., 1985, p. 464.

42 "The United States Dispensatory," 27th ed., A. Osol and R. Pratt, Eds., J. B. Lippincott, Philadelphia, Pa., 1973, pp. 199, 804.

43 M. S. Ersner, in "Diseases of the Nose, Throat and Ear," 1st ed., C. Jackson and C. L. Jackson, Eds., W. B. Saunders, Philadelphia, Pa., 1945, p. 266.

44 L. R. Boies, "Fundamentals of Otolaryngology," W. B. Saunders, Philadelphia, Pa., 1950, pp. 66, 67.

45 *Medical Notes of External Otitis*, Burroughs Wellcome Co., 1972.

46 "Self-Medication," J. A. D. Anderson, Ed., University Park Press, Baltimore, Md., 1979, pp. 49, 68.

OTIC PRODUCT TABLE

Product (Manufacturer)	Ingredients
Aqua-Otic-B (Ortega)	aluminum acetate; boric acid, 1%; acetic acid, 1%; propylene glycol; benzyl alcohol, 0.5%
Aurinol Ear Drops (Various Manufacturers)	chloroxylenol; acetic acid; benzalkonium chloride; glycerin
Aurocaine Ear Drops (Republic)	carbamide; glycerin; propylene glycol; chlorobutanol, 0.5%
Aurocaine 2 (Republic)	boric acid, 2.75%; isopropyl alcohol
Auro-Dri (Commerce)	boric acid, 2.75%; isopropyl alcohol
Auro Ear Drops (Commerce)	carbamide peroxide, 6.5%
Benzodyne (Kay Pharm)	chloroxylenol; acetic acid; benzalkonium chloride; glycerin
Debrox Drops (Marion)	carbamide peroxide, 6.5%; glycerin; propylene glycol
Dents Ear Wax Drops (C.S. Dent)	glycerin, 96%
Dri/Ear Drops (Pfeiffer)	boric acid, 2.75%; isopropyl alcohol
Ear-Dry (Scherer)	boric acid, 2.75%; isopropyl alcohol
Earsol (Parnell)	alcohol, 44%; propylene glycol; benzylbenzoate; fragrance
E.R.O. (Scherer)	carbamide peroxide, 6.5%; anhydrous glycerin
Halogen Ear Drops (Halsey)	chloroxylenol; acetic acid; benzalkonium chloride; glycerin
Mollifene Ear Drops (Pfeiffer)	glycerin; camphor; cajuput oil; eucalyptus oil; thyme oil
Murine Ear Wax Removal System and Ear Drops (Ross)	carbamide peroxide, 6.5%; alcohol, 6.3%; glycerin; polysorbate 20
Otix Ear Drops (DeWitt)	carbamide peroxide, 6.5%; anhydrous glycerin
Swim-Ear (Fougera)	isopropyl alcohol, 95%; anhydrous glycerin, 5%

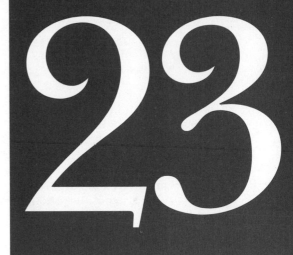

Karen A. Baker

ORAL HEALTH PRODUCTS

Questions to ask in patient/consumer counseling

How long have you had this dental problem? Have you seen a dentist about the problem? When?

Is the problem painful or severe? Is the pain continuous, dull, and/or deep? Is it triggered by hot or cold substances or by chewing?

Are there any prior events such as trauma associated with the pain?

Are there any other symptoms associated with the pain? Do you have a cold or sinus or ear infection?

Are your teeth loose? Do your gums bleed when you brush your teeth?

Does the condition produce continuous bad breath?

How do you clean your teeth or dentures? How often? Do you use dental floss?

How often do you see your dentist? Do you use supplemental fluoride in any form? Is your water fluoridated?

Do you wear dentures? Are your dentures loose? Do they cause sore spots?

Is the sore visible, and is there a pus discharge? Do you have a fever? Is the sore white in color?

Do you suffer from any chronic medical illnesses such as diabetes mellitus, rheumatic heart condition, asthma, epilepsy, or high blood pressure? Do you have a pacemaker?

What medications are you taking?

Do you have any allergies to foods or medications? What are they?

In 1976, the Department of Health, Education, and Welfare's Committee on Nutrition indicated that dental caries was the most prevalent disease of all age groups beyond infancy (1). However, a more recent National Dental Caries Survey by the National Institute for Dental Research (NIDR) indicated a 32% decline in caries rate among children 5–17 years of age over the period 1970–1980 (2). As adults are retaining greater numbers of teeth later in life, caries affecting the exposed root surfaces is becoming an increasingly important oral health problem (3). Periodontal disease has long been considered the major adult oral disease and is the principal reason for loss of teeth in persons over 35 years of age (4). Most U.S. regional surveys indicate that 41–75% of Americans have varying degrees of periodontal disease (5–7). Nationwide, approximately 70% of tooth loss can be attributed to periodontal disease; the remaining 30% is caused by caries, direct trauma, and orthodontic extraction. It has been estimated by the National Center for Health Statistics that more than 22.6 million people in the United States are edentulous (without natural dentition) (8). In addition, approximately $2.2 billion are spent annually on oral hygiene products in the United States (9). It becomes clear from these statistics that dental disease is one of the most

Editor's Note: This chapter is based in part on the chapter by the same title that appeared in the 8th edition but was authored by Karen A. Baker and Dennis K. Helling.

frequently encountered health care problems in the United States, and many health care dollars are spent on prevention as well as treatment of dental disease.

The American Dental Association (ADA) considers the pharmacist to be an integral team member in the prevention and treatment of dental disease (10). Pharmacists routinely consult with individuals on the use of oral health products and, when appropriate, refer patients for dental supervision (11).

This chapter provides pharmacists with basic information concerning common dental problems, patient counseling, when to make referrals to dentists, and when to recommend nonprescription dental hygiene and treatment products. Specific dental problems to be discussed include caries, periodontal disease, oral and perioral ulcers, damaged or misfitting prostheses and teeth, and other common oral disorders.

DENTAL ANATOMY AND PHYSIOLOGY

The teeth and supporting structures are necessary for normal mastication and articulation and for esthetic appearance. Normally, people are provided with two sets of teeth—the primary or deciduous dentition, followed by the permanent dentition. The primary dentition first appears at approximately 6 months of age with the eruption of the mandibular (lower jaw) central incisor and is usually complete with the eruption of the upper second molars by approximately 24 months (Figure 1). There are 20 deciduous teeth, 10 in each arch. Generally, the permanent dentition initially appears with the eruption of the mandibular first molar behind the deciduous second molar at approximately 6 years and continues in a regular pattern replacing shedding deciduous teeth. The last permanent teeth to erupt into the oral cavity are the third molars (wisdom teeth), which appear between 17 and 21 years of age.

Anatomically, the teeth are grossly viewed as having two parts, the crown and the roots (Figure 2). The roots are normally below the gingival (gum) line or margin and are essential for support and attachment of the tooth with the surrounding tissues. The crown is above the gingival margin and is the part of the tooth responsible for mastication. The teeth are comprised of four basic components: the enamel, the dentin, the cementum, and the pulp.

Enamel is comprised of very hard, crystalline calcium salts (hydroxyapatite) and covers the crown of the tooth to the cementoenamel junction. Enamel protects the underlying tooth structure and serves as the surface material of the crown that withstands the wear of mastication. Dentin lies beneath the enamel and comprises

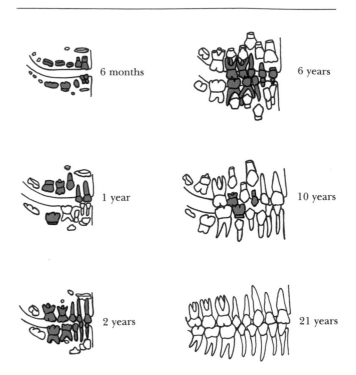

FIGURE 1   Stages of formation and eruption of deciduous and permanent dentition.

the largest part of the tooth structure. Dentin is softer than enamel. Its tubules enable transport of nutrients from the dental pulp. The dentin protects the dental pulp from mechanical, thermal, and chemical irritation.

The pulp occupies the pulp chamber and is continuous with the tissues surrounding the tooth by means of the apical foramen, an opening at the apex of the root. The pulp consists of mostly vascular and neural tissues. The only type of nerve endings in the pulp are free nerve endings; any type of stimulus to the pulp is interpreted as pain.

The bonelike cementum is softer than dentin and covers the root of the tooth, extending apically from the cementoenamel junction. The major function of cementum is to provide attachment of the tooth with the periodontal ligament via periodontal fibers. The cementum is considered to be one of the four major components of the periodontium or supporting tooth structures.

The periodontium includes the cementum, periodontal ligament, the encompassing alveolar bone, and the gingiva. The periodontal ligament is connective tissue and provides attachment of the tooth to surrounding alveolar bone and gingival tissue. The four functions of the periodontal ligament are supportive, formative, sensory, and nutritive.

The alveolar bone forms the sockets of the teeth. Alveolar bone is thin and spongy and attaches to the principal fibers of the periodontal ligament.

Gingiva (gum tissue) is the soft tissue surrounding the teeth and is firmly attached to the underlying alveolar bone. It is normally pink and is keratinized. The gingiva is attached to the cementum by the gingival group of periodontal ligament fibers.

Dentistry is concerned not only with the dentition and surrounding supportive tissues, but also with the other oral and extraoral tissues involved in pathologic processes of the head and neck. A thorough dental exam often includes examination of all intraoral tissue including the pharynx, tongue, hard and soft palates, floor of the mouth, vestibule (between the alveolar ridge and cheek), buccal (cheek) tissue, and salivary glands. Oral cancer screening is an important part of a general dental examination.

The mucosa covering the pharyngeal region, soft palate, floor of the mouth, vestibule, and cheeks is normally more pinkish-red than the gingiva. The outer surface of the mucosa is stratified squamous epithelium but does not have a keratinized stratum corneum outer layer as does the gingiva, which accounts for the difference in color.

The tongue is important in the functions of mastication, swallowing, taste, and articulation of speech. The dorsal or upper surface of the tongue is usually irregular and rough in appearance. Taste buds are usually small, oval-shaped organs of flat epithelial cells surrounding a small opening (taste pore). Taste buds are in fungiform papillae, on the surface of and surrounding circumvallate papillae at various locations of the tongue. The epithelium covering the tongue is keratinized, especially at the crests of the filiform papillae.

The major salivary glands are the parotid, submandibular, and sublingual salivary glands. They are responsible for secretion of saliva, which is an alkaline, slightly viscous, clear secretion containing enzymes (lysozymes and ptyalin), serum albumin, epithelial mucin (a mucopolysaccharide), immune globulin, leukocytes, and minerals. Normal salivary gland function promotes good oral health in a number of ways. Saliva components clear carbohydrates and microorganisms from the oral cavity. Saliva also reduces the amount of acid formed by carbohydrate fermentation and buffers the pH fall caused by acid production. Many other effects have been postulated.

The dental practitioner is also trained to examine perioral and extraoral tissues, such as the lips, the angles of the mouth, the symmetry of the head and neck, and the lymph nodes of the region (Figure 3).

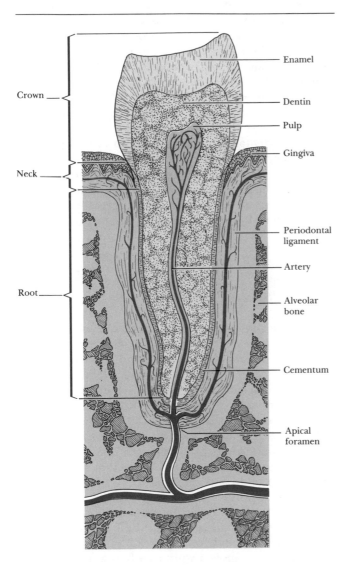

FIGURE 2   Anatomy of the tooth.

Crown

Neck

Root

Enamel

Dentin

Pulp

Gingiva

Periodontal ligament

Artery

Alveolar bone

Cementum

Apical foramen

ETIOLOGY AND PATHOPHYSIOLOGY OF COMMON ORAL PROBLEMS

Dental Caries

Dental caries is now understood to be a multifactorial disease related to oral bacteria, diet, and host resistance (12). Dental caries formation requires growth and implantation of cariogenic microorganisms (*Streptococcus mutans, Streptococcus sanguis, Lactobacillus casei*, and *Actinomyces viscosus*) on exposed surfaces. If oral hygiene is neglected, dental plaque containing these organisms remains on the tooth surfaces, allowing the carious process to proceed.

Diet and other personal habits constitute other factors in caries development. Foods with a high concentration of refined sugar (sucrose) are strongly cariogenic. Sucrose is converted by bacterial plaque into volatile acids (lactic, pyruvic, acetic, propionic, and butyric acids), which attack, dissolve, and solubilize the calcium salts found in tooth structure (13). Unfortunately, sugar-containing foods are highly popular with the young age group in which the greatest susceptibility to caries occurs. Saccharin, a potent noncariogenic sugar substitute, is still widely used despite animal studies showing dose-dependent carcinogenicity. Oral hygiene products such as mouthwashes and dentifrices contain such low concentrations of saccharin that ingestion from such products poses no hazard (14). The Food and Drug Administration (FDA) limit on saccharin is 1 g per day for adults; ingestion of both mouthwash and dentifrice would result in a total saccharin exposure of only 20–40 mg per day (14). Other noncariogenic sugar substitutes such as aspartame, sorbitol, and xylitol are currently used to sweeten a wide variety of products (15). The chewing of gum increases salivary flow, which apparently produces a beneficial buffering effect against acids in the oral cavity. Moreover, some clinical trials have demonstrated that xylitol-containing chewing gum is cariostatic (16).

Excessive sugar intake is not the only source of dental caries. Other types of fermentable carbohydrates, such as fructose (found in fruit) and lactose (found in milk), also are cariogenic but to a far lesser extent than sucrose (17). Also, except during pregnancy and childhood, ingesting dairy products or other calcium-rich foods has little or no effect on prevention of caries in fully developed teeth although positive plaque pH effects may be seen.

The pathophysiology of dental caries is basically one of demineralization caused by organic acids, such as lactic acid, produced (usually anaerobically) by microorganisms resident in dental plaque. This demineralization is actually chronic in nature with a carious lesion starting slowly on the enamel surface and initially exhibiting no clinical symptoms. Early dental caries appears as a faint white opacity or chalky area. The lesion becomes bluish-white as the enamel is penetrated and eventually brown or yellow as excavation proceeds. Once the demineralization progresses through the enamel to the softer dentin, the destruction is much more rapid and becomes clinically evident as a carious lesion. At this point, the patient can become aware of the process by visualization or by symptoms of sensitivity (toothache) to stimuli such as heat, cold, or percussion. If untreated, the carious lesion can result in damage to the dental pulp itself (with continuous pain as a common symptom) and eventually necrosis of the vital pulp tissue. Because an opening exists between the pulp and surrounding supporting tissues via the apical foramen, the infectious process can progress apically and result in bone loss, abscesses, cellulitis, or osteomyelitis.

Plaque and Calculus

The accumulation of dental plaque is very much associated with dental caries and periodontal disease. Plaque is thought to start with the formation of acquired pellicle on a clean tooth surface. Pellicle appears to be a thin, acellular, glycoprotein–mucoprotein coating that adheres to the enamel within minutes after cleaning a tooth. Its source is thought to be saliva. The pellicle seems to serve as an attachment for cariogenic bacteria that produce, along with acids, long-chain polymers such as dextrans and levans that adhere to the pellicle and tooth surface. This sticky adherent mass is called dental plaque.

After meals, food residue may be incorporated into plaque by bacterial degradation. Left undisturbed, the plaque thickens and bacteria proliferate (18). Dental plaque, if not removed within 24 hours, begins to calcify by calcium salt precipitation from the saliva and forms calculus, or "tartar." This hardened, adherent deposit is removable only by professional dental cleaning (18). Plaque is commonly recognized as the source

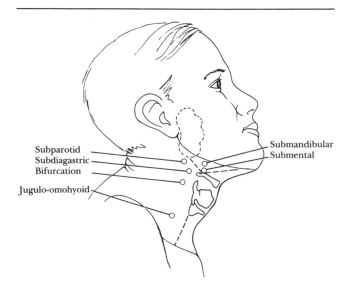

Subparotid
Subdiagastric
Bifurcation

Jugulo-omohyoid

Submandibular
Submental

FIGURE 3   Major lymph node areas of the neck.

of microbes that cause caries and periodontitis; thus plaque buildup is related to incidence of oral disease. Calculus is now generally considered to be a substrate on which plaque can develop and is not regarded as the primary causative oral accumulation in periodontal disease (18). However, most periodontists agree that supragingival and subgingival calculus can promote the progression of periodontal disease in several ways. Calculus can promote the retention of new bacterial plaque accumulation and can interfere with local self-cleaning processes and patient plaque removal. Subgingival calculus can increase the rate of epithelial junction displacement and extend the bone destruction beyond that resulting from plaque alone. Therefore, thorough removal of subgingival calculus is an important step in periodontal therapy. The reduction of supragingival calculus formation has not been shown to reduce gingivitis, but is at the very least cosmetically beneficial.

The best way to promote dental health is to remove plaque buildup by mechanical means, mainly by brushing and flossing regularly. Chewing gum or eating fibrous foods, such as celery or carrots, does not prevent plaque accumulation or aid in its removal (19). Newly developed agents for the chemical management of plaque and calculus can enhance mechanical removal in selected patients.

Fractured Dentition, Restorations, and Dentures

Fractures of the natural dentition are correctable only by a dentist. Besides being esthetically unappealing (especially if it involves an anterior tooth), fractured teeth can result in pulp exposure, irritation to adjacent soft tissues, pain, malocclusion, rapid carious breakdown, compromised mastication, or infection. Minor chips in the tooth's crown may be adequately repaired with restorative materials and techniques. However, a large fracture may require endodontic treatment (root canal therapy), extensive restorative procedures, or extraction of the tooth.

Fractured or Misfitting Restorations and Dentures

Loose, displaced, or broken dental restorations (fillings) and nonremovable prostheses (crowns and bridges) can be evaluated and treated adequately only by a dentist. Fillings, crowns, and bridges that need repair may result in loss of normal function, tooth breakdown, or malocclusion.

Loose, misfitting, or broken removable dental prostheses (partial or full dentures) may also cause serious consequences. Ill-fitting or broken dentures can contribute to accelerated bone loss, ulceration, irritation, tumorous growths, and compromised oral function. Refitting, relining, or repairing dentures to ensure their proper functioning requires professional dental treatment.

Periodontal Disease

Gingivitis and periodontitis have been classified many ways (20). Only the more common forms of chronic gingivitis and periodontitis are discussed.

Chronic Gingivitis

Chronic gingivitis (inflammation of the gingiva) left untreated can be a common precursor to the more advanced inflammatory condition of chronic destructive periodontal disease or periodontitis. Periodontitis is the inflammation and destruction of the periodontium. The etiology of chronic gingivitis is thought to be associated with the presence of microorganisms in the plaque in the gingival sulcus (space between the gingiva and tooth). These organisms are capable of producing harmful products such as acids, toxins, and enzymes that damage cellular and intercellular tissue. Dilatation of gingival capillaries, proliferation of capillaries, and increased blood flow with resultant erythema (redness) of the gingiva are found in early stages of chronic gingivitis. (See *Plate 1–2*.) In time, the capillaries become engorged, venous return is slowed, and localized anoxemia gives a bluish hue to areas of the reddened gingiva. The gingiva may also increase in size, appear swollen, and change shape as a result of the inflammation. The presence of red cells in extravascular tissue and the breakdown of hemoglobin also deepen the color of the gingival tissue. The gingiva generally bleeds readily when probed or during toothbrushing. The progression of these events is usually slow and often painless to the patient.

Chronic gingivitis may be localized to one or several teeth or it may be generalized, meaning the gingiva around all of the teeth is involved. The inflammation may involve just the marginal gingiva (the border of the gingiva surrounding the neck of the tooth) or may be more diffuse and involve all of the gingival tissue surrounding the tooth. Changes in gingival color, size, shape, and ease of gingival bleeding are common indications of chronic gingivitis that the patient as well as the pharmacist can recognize.

Gingival Disease in Pregnancy

Gingival disease in pregnancy, or pregnancy gingivitis, is caused by local factors, as is gingivitis in nongravid patients. Pregnancy causes a modification in the host's response to dental plaque. Several studies have shown that the incidence and severity of gingival redness, swelling, bleeding, and exudation increase from the second month of gestation to the eighth month and then decrease (21, 22). Perhaps high progesterone levels during pregnancy increase capillary permeability and gingival swelling (23). Metabolic alterations and changes in immune response during pregnancy may also contribute to pregnancy gingivitis. Pregnancy gingivitis can be resolved by careful attention to plaque control, which emphasizes the fact that the hormonal changes simply modify the tissue response to bacterial substances (24). The severity of the gingivitis will decrease postpartum, returning to prepregnancy levels after approximately 1 year.

Acute Necrotizing Ulcerative Gingivitis

Acute necrotizing ulcerative gingivitis (ANUG), also referred to as "Vincent's stomatitis" and "trench mouth," is characterized by necrosis and ulceration of the gingival surface with underlying inflammation. The disease most commonly starts in the gingiva between teeth and displays "punched out" papillae (the raised interproximal gingiva). Spirochete and fusiform bacteria proliferate and invade the gingiva (25). The interdental and marginal gingiva exhibit a necrotic and grayish slough, while the adjacent gingiva usually exhibits marked erythema. The disease may involve a single tooth or group of teeth, or the entire oral cavity. Accompanying symptoms often include severe pain, bleeding gingival tissue, halitosis, foul taste, and increased salivation. Lymphadenopathy, fever, and malaise less frequently accompany the disease.

ANUG is seen most frequently in the United States in teenagers and young adults (26, 27). Predisposing factors associated with the disease include anxiety and emotional stress, smoking, malnutrition, and poor oral hygiene (26). The association between the disease and these predisposing factors is not clear. Contrary to some articles in the literature, acute necrotizing ulcerative gingivitis has not been demonstrated to be communicable (26, 27). The precise cause of ANUG is not known; however, the ulcerative stage of the disease seems to be associated with overgrowth of spirochete and fusiform organisms (26, 27). Although ANUG has been reported to go into remission spontaneously without treatment, it can result in progressive tissue destruction, septicemia, and serious systemic sequelae (27). Treatment consists of local debridement and elimination of predisposing factors. Patients with widespread lesions or regional lymph node enlargement have been successfully treated with penicillin VK or metronidazole (28).

Periodontitis

Periodontitis and gingivitis, the two most common periodontal diseases, can be distinguished in the following way. As previously discussed, gingivitis is inflammation of the gingiva without loss or migration of epithelial attachment to the tooth. Periodontitis occurs when the periodontal ligament attachment and alveolar bone support of the tooth have been lost (29). This process involves the apical migration of the epithelial attachment from the enamel to the root surface. (See *Plate 1–3.*)

The American Academy of Periodontology (AAP) has developed a periodontal disease classification system; the most common forms of periodontitis are (29):

A. Periodontitis in adults
   1. AAP Classification I, II, III, IV
   2. Epidemilogic: moderately and rapidly progressing periodontitis
   3. Clinical based on treatment: refractory and recurrent

B. Periodontitis in juveniles
   1. Localized juvenile periodontitis
   2. Generalized juvenile periodontitis

The AAP describes adult periodontitis type I as gingivitis characterized by changes in color, form, position, surface appearance, and the presence of bleeding and/or exudate. Type II is slight periodontitis characterized by progression of gingival inflammation into deeper tissues and the alveolar bony crest with slight bone loss. The periodontal pocket is 3–4 mm deep and there is slight loss of connective attachment and alveolar bone. Type III is moderate periodontitis characterized by noticeable loss of bony support and possible increased tooth mobility. Type IV is advanced periodontitis characterized by major loss of alveolar bone support usually accompanied by increased tooth mobility (29, 30).

Adult periodontitis, especially slight or moderate, is very common (29). Most adults with periodontitis have moderately progressing disease, and perhaps 10% have rapidly progressing disease. As shown in the AAP classification system, diagnosis of adult periodontal disease can be based on response to therapy (29). Recurrent periodontitis is destruction of the attachment apparatus occurring in a patient who has been successfully treated in the past. It often results from inadequate maintenance therapy and is relatively common. It appears to occur in localized areas but may be generalized in immunodeficient patients. Refractory periodontitis does not respond even to well-performed, completed therapy (29).

Periodontitis in juveniles is relatively rare; localized juvenile periodontitis (LJP) affects less than 1% of teenagers and young adults. LJP occurs most often in teenagers and young adults with an overall prevalence of 0.1% in this age group (29). LJP is characterized by pocket formation, attachment loss, and alveolar bone loss affecting mainly the first molars and incisors. Occasionally, premolars and second molars are involved. These patients rarely display gingivitis and have little or no plaque or calculus. LJP displays a marked familial tendency and is associated with a particular type of bacteria. Generalized juvenile periodontitis (GJP) affects a slightly older age group and is much less prevalent than LJP. Severe gingival inflammation with extensive plaque and calculus deposits distinguish GJP from LJP.

In order to diagnose, treat, and monitor periodontal disease, the dentist should include a periodontal component in the oral examination of all patients. The periodontal exam includes an assessment of the gingiva and attachment apparatus and examination of the entire periodontium with charting of all teeth in the dental record. The gingiva should be assessed visually and by gingival bleeding measures. Periodontal probing depths measured in millimeters should be performed to measure pocket depth and attachment levels. Tooth mobility measurements and a radiographic survey of alveolar bone levels should also be included (30). Patients have a good prognosis if an initial comprehensive course of therapy is successful. Unfortunately, alveolar bone loss is irreversible. Prospects for disease control are not good if plaque and calculus control is poor or if resolution of inflammation is inadequate despite comprehensive treatment (30).

Common Oral Lesions

Canker Sores

Canker sores, also referred to as recurrent aphthous ulcers (RAU) or recurrent aphthous stomatitis (RAS), affect approximately 20–50% of Americans (31). The cause of aphthous ulcers is unknown; however, evidence suggests that the ulcers may result from a hypersensitivity to antigenic components of pleomorphic *Streptococcus sanguis* (32–36). Evidence also suggests that cell-mediated immunity may play a role in causing aphthous ulcers. Lymphocytes from patients with aphthous lesions are cytotoxic to mucosal epithelial cells in vitro (36–38). There appears to be a familial factor in aphthous ulcers. Offspring of parents with a

history of aphthous ulcers are more likely to suffer from aphthous ulcers themselves (36). Recent studies seem to indicate that aphthous ulcers are caused by a dysfunction of the immune system that is initiated by minor trauma (39).

Aphthous lesions can appear on any nonkeratinized mucosal surface in the mouth, such as the lips, buccal mucosa, tongue, floor of the mouth, or soft palate (40). Rarely, lesions affect keratinized tissue such as gingiva. Patients may experience a burning or itching sensation preceding the actual appearance of an aphthous lesion. Patients may experience a single lesion or as many as 30 or more. Most aphthous lesions persist for 10–14 days and heal without scarring (35).

Canker sores usually range from 3 to 5 mm in diameter; however, several lesions may coalesce to form larger, irregularly shaped lesions. Individual aphthous lesions are usually round or oval in shape and are either flat or crater-like in appearance. (See *Plate 1–4*.) The color is usually gray to grayish-yellow with an erythematous halo of inflamed tissue surrounding the ulcer. The lesions can be very painful and may inhibit normal eating, drinking, talking, and routine home oral care. Although many patients have recurrent episodes of oral lesions with periods of remission (no lesions), some patients may chronically experience one or more lesions in the mouth for very long periods. There usually is no fever or lymphadenopathy accompanying aphthous lesions although these symptoms arise if the ulcerations become secondarily infected.

Cold Sores

Cold sores or fever blisters are caused most often by the herpes simplex type 1 virus and are referred to as herpes simplex labialis because they most commonly occur on the lip or areas bordering the lip. They are recurrent, often arising in the same location repeatedly. The lesions are painful and cosmetically objectionable. Patients who suffer from herpes labialis have previously been primarily infected with herpesvirus (36, 40). Patients may or may not relate a history of primary herpetic stomatitis. Most primary oral infections of herpes seem to be subclinical and, therefore, most patients are unaware of the previous primary exposure (40). The primary infection, historically, has been reported most frequently in childhood; however, it is now estimated that 15% of adults experience the primary infection (36). After the primary infection, the virus apparently remains in host cells. These "resident" viruses are thought to be responsible for recurrent herpes labialis.

Cold sores often are preceded by a prodrome, when the patient notices burning, itching, or numbness in the area of the forthcoming lesion. The lesion first becomes visible as small red papules of fluid-containing vesicles 1–3 mm in diameter. Often many lesions coalesce to form a larger area of involvement. An erythematous border around the vesicles may or may not be present. A mature lesion often has a crust over the top of many coalesced, burst vesicles. The base of the lesion is erythematous. The presence of pustules or pus under the crust of a cold sore may indicate a possible secondary bacterial infection. Cold sores are self-limiting and heal without scarring, usually within 10–14 days. The recurrence rate and extent of lesions vary greatly from patient to patient. Some patients may experience several large lesions every few weeks; other patients may have only a single small lesion perhaps once a year. Patients often will associate predisposing factors such as sun or wind exposure, fever, systemic disease (colds and flu), or trauma with the onset of cold sores.

Herpesvirus type 1 is contagious and thought to be transmissible by direct contact because the virus does not live outside the host environment (41). Saliva, stratum corneum cells, fluid from herpes vesicles, and mucosal secretions may serve to transmit the virus from patient to patient (36, 41). Herpes simplex type 2 virus, which is the cause of genital lesions, has been demonstrated in herpes lesions of the lip (42).

Common Oral Infections

Dentopyogenic Infections

Dentopyogenic infections are pus-producing infections that are associated with a tooth or its supporting structures (gingiva, periodontal ligament, cementum, and alveolar bone) (43). The symptoms of these infections vary greatly, from mildly symptomatic to fever, malaise, swelling, erythema, warmth at the infection site, and septic shock. The symptoms and severity of these infections are determined by several factors. The anatomic features of the infection site, local and systemic host resistance, virulence of the causative organisms, and time between onset of infection and treatment all play a part in the clinical presentation. Dentopyogenic infections range in severity from small, well-localized abscesses with no systemic signs of infection to a diffuse, rapidly spreading cellulitis or osteomyelitis with a high morbidity and mortality. Patients with severe symptoms associated with dentopyogenic infections usually seek dental attention as soon as possible; however, persons with minimal symptoms may unwisely delay dental treatment and try self-treatment.

There are four common dental abscesses: periapical abscess, periodontal abscess, pericoronal abscess, and subperiosteal abscess. A periapical abscess, located around the apex of a tooth root, originates from a necrotic, infected dental pulp and gains access to the periapical area by the apical foramen. The two most common causes of dental pulp infection and necrosis with a subsequent periapical abscess are dental caries that expose the pulp to oral bacteria and trauma that causes a decrease or stoppage of blood flow to and from the pulp.

A periodontal abscess is usually a result of periodontitis. Periodontitis leads to destruction of supporting tooth structures and the subsequent formation of deep periodontal pockets. The bacteria associated with periodontitis move toward the apex of the tooth within the deepening pocket. The accumulated bacteria within this pocket form an abscess in surrounding tissue if host resistance decreases or if the bacteria are forced into the surrounding tissue from occlusion of the pocket or trauma.

Pericoronal abscesses are most frequently associated with mandibular third molars (lower wisdom teeth). Mandibular third molars in the process of erupting or those that do not fully erupt often have gingiva covering a portion of the crown. This gingival tissue can be traumatized by the opposing upper third molar when the patient bites down. Food, bacteria, and debris also collect beneath this flap of gingiva resulting in an abscess in the tissue surrounding the lower molar.

A subperiosteal abscess is a bone abscess located beneath the thin connective tissue covering (periosteum) of the bone surrounding or underlying a tooth socket. These infections are most common after extraction of a tooth.

Dentopyogenic abscesses are usually mixed bacterial infections containing more than one species of microorganisms (43–45). Hundreds of different organisms have been isolated from oral abscesses. The most frequently isolated organisms have been facultative Gram-positive cocci (the viridans group of *Streptococcus* and others) and anaerobic Gram-negative rods (including species of *Bacteroides*) (43–45).

These oral abscesses, even if well-localized and seemingly not serious, may progress to more severe acute or chronic infections. They usually require dental surgical intervention with or without antibiotic therapy (46).

Candidiasis

Candida is a true fungus and is found as normal flora in the GI tract and oral cavity in 60% of healthy adult patients (47, 48). *Candida albicans* is by far the most common opportunistic pathogen associated with oral infections. There are three morphologic forms: the yeast cell, hypha, and mycelium. The mycelial form is the pathologic form found in oral candidiasis.

Symptomatically, oral candidiasis appears commonly in one of four forms: acute pseudomembranous candidiasis, acute atrophic candidiasis, chronic hyperplastic candidiasis, or chronic atrophic candidiasis (49). The acute pseudomembranous form is often referred to as "thrush" and is characterized by white plaques with a "milk curd" appearance that are attached to the oral mucosa. These plaques usually can be detached easily, displaying erythematous, bleeding, sore areas beneath them. (See *Plate 1–5.*) Thrush is most common in infants, pregnant women, and debilitated patients.

Acute atrophic candidiasis, sometimes referred to as "antibiotic tongue" or "antibiotic sore mouth," is characterized by erythematous, painful, sometimes bleeding areas of the mouth. The entire upper surface of the tongue or the entire oral cavity may be involved. This form is thought to be similar to thrush but without the white plaques. Broad-spectrum antibiotic therapy is the most common predisposing factor.

Chronic hyperplastic candidiasis most commonly appears as firm, well-attached, persistent, white plaques on the cheeks, tongue, palate, or lips. Unlike the plaques of thrush, these plaques cannot be detached, are resistant to treatment, and are usually painless. This form of oral candidiasis is sometimes referred to as "Candida leukoplakia" or "speckled leukoplakia" (49).

Chronic atrophic candidiasis, sometimes referred to as "denture stomatitis" or "denture sore mouth," is commonly found in patients with full or partial dentures (49). Symptomatically, this form is characterized by generalized inflammation of the denture-bearing area. The tissue may be erythematous and edematous with soreness or a burning sensation, or the tissue may be granular in appearance (49). Inflammation secondary to the trauma of ill-fitting dentures is usually localized to the specific area of trauma; inflammation secondary to *Candida* is generalized to the entire denture-bearing tissue area. It appears that the candidal organisms adhere to the denture material or reside in pores of the denture material (50–52). Failure to remove the denture at bedtime and to clean the denture regularly worsens this condition. Angular cheilitis (inflammation of the corners of the mouth) is commonly associated with chronic atrophic candidiasis and other forms of oral candidiasis (49). Cultures of these angular cheilitis lesions frequently are positive for *Candida albicans* and *Staphylococcus aureus* (49, 53).

Candidiasis is often called "the disease of the diseased" because it appears in debilitated patients and patients taking a variety of drugs. Associated predisposing factors include:

- Physiologic factors—early infancy, pregnancy, and old age;

- Endocrine disorders—diabetes mellitus, hypothyroidism, hypoparathyroidism, and hypoadrenalism;

- Malnutrition and malabsorption syndromes—iron-deficiency anemia, pernicious anemia, postgastrectomy, and alcoholism;

- Malignant diseases—leukemias, agranulocytopenia, and granulocytopenia;

- Drugs causing depression of defense mechanism—immunosuppressives, corticosteroids, cytotoxics, and radiation therapy;

- Drugs commonly causing xerostomia—anticholinergics, antidepressants, antipsychotics, antihypertensives, and antihistamines;

- Other changes in host environment—trauma, chemical damage, postoperative states, radiation therapy, and antibiotics and anti-infectives.

Halitosis

Halitosis, also called fetor oris, is an offensive odor emanating from the oral cavity. Unlike caries, periodontal disease, ANUG, and the other oral pathology discussed in this section, halitosis is a symptom of a disease process or problem (54). Foul breath can be a useful diagnosis aid, as in the case of ANUG. Halitosis has many causes; it should be determined if the source is oral or nonoral. Common oral causes of halitosis include odoriferous food particles, debris, plaque-coated tongue, and periodontal disease. These can be the result of poor oral or denture hygiene, ANUG, caries, postsurgical states, extraction wounds, purulent infections, chronic periodontitis, and smoking. Common nonoral sources of halitosis include pulmonary disease such as purulent lung infections, tuberculosis, bronchiectasis, sinusitis, tonsillitis, and rhinitis. Other common nonoral causes of halitosis include the elimination of chemical substances from the blood through the lungs upon exhalation. Examples include alcoholic breath, acetone breath in severely hyperglycemic diabetics, and foul breath from dimethyl sulfoxide use.

Oral Cancer

Oral cancer is of major concern even though it occurs less frequently than periodontitis, caries, aphthous ulcers, and other oral problems. Because of the serious consequences of oral cancer, it must always be considered in the differential diagnosis of persistent oral lesions. By far, the most common form of oral cancer is squamous cell carcinoma. Most oropharyngeal squamous cell carcinomas occur in males over 50 years of age, although the incidence in females has increased in recent years (55). Clinically, oral carcinomas can appear as red or white lesions, ulcerations, or tumors. As with other carcinomas, the cause of oral and perioral carcinomas is unknown. However, tobacco use, both combustible and smokeless, and chronic alcohol consumption appear to be risk factors (56, 57). The role of alcohol consumption in the etiology of oral cancer is complicated by concurrent cigarette smoking, but high rates of alcohol consumption, hepatic cirrhosis, and oral cancer appear to be related (58). Other possible risk factors in oral cancer include iron deficiency, chronic candidiasis, herpes simplex virus, syphilis, and poor oral hygiene (58).

PATIENT ASSESSMENT

Pharmacists should be able to recognize common oral problems and give appropriate guidance to patients. An effort to determine the severity or potential severity of oral complaints must be made when helping and advising patients. To assess an oral problem and aid in proper treatment, the pharmacist can use visual observation and the patient's verbal history to evaluate signs and symptoms. The pharmacist should gather as much useful information as possible from the patient concerning the oral problem before counseling.

Pain is one symptom that can accompany all common oral problems. Questioning the patient about pain and associating it with other symptoms helps the pharmacist better understand the problem. Tooth pain triggered or worsened by heat, cold, or percussion is often indicative of a pulpal response to deep carious lesions or a cracked or broken tooth. Continuous tooth pain may indicate pulpal infection and necrosis, an abscess, or serious periodontal disease. Continuous soreness or pain that is associated with soft tissues of the mouth and is more severe upon eating or drinking, is a common complaint with canker sores and acute atrophic candidiasis. Pain along the gingival ridge under the denture indicates the common problems of ill-fitting dentures or denture stomatitis candidiasis. These different features of pain indicate different underlying problems.

Visual signs are helpful in evaluating a patient's oral complaint. The color, shape, and location of various anomalies help in assessing the oral problem. Some examples of color changes include the white plaques of candidiasis, the erythema associated with the margins of canker and cold sores, and the gingival erythema associated with periodontitis. The irregular shape of coalesced cold sore vesicles, the swelling and asymmetrical shape of a patient's face caused by an oral abscess, and the large defect left by a dislodged dental restoration can aid in evaluating an oral problem. Recurrent oral sores on nonkeratinized oral mucosa (such as canker sores), recurrent vesicular sores on the skin bordering the lip (cold sores), and inflammation under seldom-cleaned dentures (denture stomatitis) are examples of lesion locations that can help define oral problems.

Patients' oral hygiene habits and frequency of dental care should be evaluated. If patients admit to poor oral hygiene and infrequent dental care, this can greatly increase the likelihood of dental caries, periodontal disease, misfitting dentures, broken dentures, infection, and other oral problems. Bleeding gingiva, the presence of plaque and calculus on teeth, and loose teeth are sometimes noticed by patients during brushing and flossing and should be investigated. Halitosis commonly results from poor oral hygiene, ANUG, and dentopyogenic infections, and it merits inquiry.

Other signs and symptoms such as fever, purulent matter (pus), malaise, xerostomia (dry mouth), and changes in taste help identify an oral problem and determine its severity.

An important area of inquiry and evaluation by the pharmacist is the patient's medical and drug history. If available, the patient's medication profile should be reviewed. The pharmacist should ask about past or current medical conditions or disease states, such as rheumatic heart disease, diabetes mellitus, prosthetic joints, and hematologic disorders. The pharmacist should also inquire about any medications the patient has recently taken or is currently taking. This history should include prescription, nonprescription, and illicit or "recreational" drug use. The medical and drug history may suggest to the pharmacist potentially serious dental or medical complications such as endocarditis secondary to an oral abscess in a patient with rheumatic heart disease. These historical data also alert the pharmacist to predisposing factors of suspected oral conditions. Examples include a patient with signs and symptoms of oral candidiasis taking an antihistamine that dries the mouth, an orally inhaled steroid that decreases the immune response in the mouth, or a broad-spectrum antibiotic that results in superinfection.

PRODUCT SELECTION GUIDELINES

Plaque Removal Products

Toothbrushes

Toothbrushes are the most effective nonprescription product available to remove dental plaque and maintain good oral hygiene (59). There are no specific recommendations as to which is the best type of toothbrush to use. Dentists recommend toothbrushes based on the patient's manual dexterity, oral anatomy, and periodontal health. In general, soft, rounded, nylon bristle brushes are preferred by many dentists and dental hygienists. Clinical trials have shown soft bristles to be more effective than harder bristles in plaque removal below the gingival margin and on proximal tooth surfaces. Investigators have found that short strokes with rounded, soft bristles significantly decreased cervical abrasion and gingival injury compared to longer strokes with a harder toothbrush. The most common adverse effects caused by toothbrushing are cervical abrasion on the buccal surface of the first premolars, irritation of the anterior gingival margins, and gingival recession with associated hypersensitivity (60).

The proper frequency of brushing and method of brushing have not been established and may vary from patient to patient. Thoroughness of brushing without trauma is more important than the method of brushing (61). The proper method and frequency of brushing are best taught to each individual patient by the dentist or dental hygienist after evaluating the patient. In general, patients should brush thoroughly at least once a day, and preferably, twice daily, taking time to clean commonly neglected areas such as interdental surfaces, areas behind the back molars, and all sulcular areas (62). Gentle brushing of the upper surface of the tongue is often recommended because it too accumulates plaque. Toothbrushing alone has not been shown to remove plaque adequately from interproximal surfaces of the teeth (61). Toothbrushing will not remove dental calculus (61). Calculus removal must be done by dentists or dental hygienists.

How often should the patient buy a new toothbrush? Ideally, patients should alternate two toothbrushes to allow each to dry completely, thereby decreasing bristle wear and matting. A unique study related the state of toothbrush wear to its effectiveness in removing plaque (63). Brush wear greatly inhibits plaque removal in the difficult-to-reach areas of the mouth compared to easily accessible areas, and it is apparent that matting, rather than tapering, of bristles is the primary cause of decreased plaque removal. Therefore, patients should be told to replace toothbrushes at the first sign of bristle matting rather than after a set period of use. The ADA Council on Dental Materials, Instruments, and Equipment (CDMIE) has recognized the following toothbrushes as safe and effective: Aim, Disney, and Pepsodent (Chesebrough–Pond's); Arco (Arco International); Butler (John O. Butler Company); Improve (Prevent Care Products); Lactona (Lactona); McDonald (Harry Panzer International); Milor and Milor Angle Plus (Milor Corporation); Oral–B (Oral–B Laboratories); Prevent, Reach, and Reach Gentle (Johnson & Johnson); and Py-Co-Pay

Softex, Py-Co-Twin, Sensodyne Gentle, and Sensodyne Search (Block Drug Company).

Electric Toothbrushes Standard electric toothbrushes mimic the horizontal or vertical motions of hand brushing and have not been proven superior to properly manipulated manual toothbrushes (64, 65). However, electric toothbrushes may benefit patients lacking manual dexterity, patients who require someone else to clean their teeth, some patients with orthodontic appliances, and patients motivated by the novelty of a powered toothbrush (66). Electric toothbrushes are available from numerous manufacturers and use many brush-head motions to clean. Best results can be obtained, in general, if a patient uses a brush carrying the ADA seal of acceptance and follows the specific directions of a dentist or dental hygienist. The conventional electric toothbrushes accepted by the ADA include: Broxodent (Squibb), Braun Appliances (Braun), Sunbeam automatic toothbrush (Northern Electric), and Waterpik automatic toothbrush (Teledyne Water Pik).

New types of rotary plaque-removal devices have recently been marketed and evaluated. Dentifrices will clog these machines and cannot be used. The Rota-Dent by Pro-Dentec comes with three brush heads shaped like interproximal brushes and rotates in a fashion similar to instruments used during a professional prophylaxis (67). Clinical trials comparing the Rota-Dent to conventional manual plaque-removal devices show the Rota-Dent to be generally superior to manual toothbrushes in removing plaque (68, 69) and equivalent to manual toothbrushing in combination with flossing and use of toothpicks (70).

The Interplak by Dental Research Corporation has a brush head with two rows of bristles, each tuft linked to a maze of rack and pinion gearing. Each tuft spins independently at 4,200 rpm. For most patients, the Interplak, if used properly, is more effective than manual brushing in eliminating plaque (71). Patients with orthodontic bands may also find this device beneficial. Rotary oral hygiene devices may be helpful for patients who cannot accomplish effective plaque removal by manual brushing and flossing. Patients should be counseled to use a fluoride rinse because they cannot use a fluoride dentifrice with these devices. Both Rota-Dent and Interplak have been recognized by the Council on Dental Therapeutics (CDT) as safe and effective.

Pediatric Toothbrushes As with adult toothbrushes, no specific size or shape of toothbrush is uniformly recommended for children. In general, the size of the child's toothbrush is smaller than an adult toothbrush and should be individualized according to the size of the child's mouth. Children can usually remove plaque more easily with a brush having shorter and narrower bristles than those available in most adult toothbrushes. No matter what type of toothbrush is used, children are usually unable to brush by themselves until they are 4 or 5 years old. Most children require some supervision until 8 years of age.

Oral Irrigating Devices

Oral irrigators work by directing a high-pressure steady or pulsating stream of water through a nozzle to the tooth surfaces. Oral irrigators cannot be viewed as substitutes for the toothbrush, floss, or other plaque-removing devices. At best, they can be considered adjuncts in maintaining oral hygiene (72). Studies have shown that oral irrigators are able to remove only a minimal amount of plaque from tooth surfaces (72, 73). The ADA views these devices as potentially useful for "removing loose debris from those areas that cannot be cleaned with the toothbrush such as around orthodontic bands, fixed bridges, and periodontal pockets" (72). Some periodontal groups, however, have stated that "there is no scientific justification for recommending them as an aid in oral hygiene"; in view of the risks of bacteremia and traumatic lesions, the drawbacks may outweigh the device's value (73). Oral irrigation devices have been reported to cause bacteremia and may be considered contraindicated in patients predisposed to bacterial endocarditis. Patients with significant periodontal disease should use these devices only under the supervision of a dentist (72). Oral irrigators have been valuable as vehicles for administering chemotherapeutic agents that inhibit microbial growth in inaccessible regions of the mouth (74).

Two types of oral irrigation devices are available—pulsating (intermittent low- and high-water pressure) and steady stream (constant water pressure). Neither type has shown superior ability to remove debris or plaque. In general, steady-stream types are less expensive than pulsating models. The ADA has evaluated and given its seal of acceptance to several brands of irrigating devices including Dento Spray (Texell Products), Gum Machine (Gum Machine Company), Propulse 7618 (Propulse), and Sunbeam Models 6271, 6272, and 6280 (Northern Electric). The Waterpik by Teledyne Water Pik has been accepted in the "powered oral hygiene device" category instead of the oral irrigating device category even though plaque-removal efficacies appear to be similar.

Oral irrigators should be operated with warm or tepid water within recommended water pressure levels. Operating these devices parallel to the long axis of the teeth may cause soft tissue trauma or impaction of food within a periodontal pocket.

Dental Floss

Dental flossing is the most widely recommended method of cleansing proximal tooth surfaces (61). Floss is available as a multifilament nylon yarn that is waxed or unwaxed, and thick or thin. Because no particular product has been proven superior, patient factors such as tightness of tooth contacts, tooth roughness, and manual dexterity should be considered when selecting a product (61). Recent studies show no difference between waxed and unwaxed floss in terms of plaque removal and prevention of gingivitis (75, 76). Concern about a residual wax film on tooth surfaces is unfounded (77). Supervised brushing and flossing have been shown to decrease plaque and gingival inflammation (72). Flossing, however, has not been conclusively shown to achieve a reduction in dental caries (72).

Proper flossing requires some finger dexterity and a few practice sessions. Patients should be instructed to use 18 inches of floss and wrap most of it around a middle finger. The remaining floss should be wound around the same finger of the opposite hand. About an inch of floss should be held between the thumbs and forefingers. The patient should use a gentle, sawing motion to guide the floss between teeth. When the floss reaches the gumline, it should be curved into a C-shape against one tooth and gently slid into the space between the gum and tooth until there is resistance. The patient should hold the floss tightly against the tooth and gently scrape the side of the tooth while moving the floss away from the gums. Next, the patient should curve the floss around the adjoining tooth and repeat the procedure. Waxed floss may pass interproximally between tight-fitting teeth easier than unwaxed floss and without shredding. If contacts at the crowns of teeth are too tight to force floss interdentally, then floss threaders can often be used to pass floss between teeth and around fixed bridges. Floss threaders are usually thin plastic loops or soft plastic, needle-like appliances and should be used cautiously so as not to traumatize the gingiva physically. One manufacturer offers special precut floss with a stiff "floss threader" at the end of the floss (Oral-B Super Floss). Floss holders are recommended for patients lacking manual dexterity and for nursing personnel assisting handicapped or hospitalized patients. A floss holder should have one or two forks rigid enough to keep floss taut, and a mounting mechanism that allows quick rethreading of floss (61).

The CDMIE has recognized the following brands of dental floss as safe and effective: Butler, Dr. Flosser by Flossrite, Johnson & Johnson, and Oral-B.

Specialty Aids

Cleaning devices that adapt to irregular tooth surfaces better than dental floss are recommended for interproximal cleaning of teeth with large interdental spaces, such as those found in patients with periodontal disease (61). Specialty brushes and aids are available to remove plaque from difficult-to-clean areas and dentures. The most common types are tapered wooden toothpicks that are round or triangular (Stim-U-Dent, Perio-Aid), miniature bottle brushes (Py-Co-Prox, Proxabrush), rubber stimulator tips, denture brushes, and denture clasp brushes. A recent study demonstrated no difference in plaque-removal efficacy when comparing dental floss, an interdental brush, and a rubber stimulator tip (78). All three devices improved plaque removal in patients who brushed normally.

The CDMIE has recognized the following oral hygiene aids as safe and effective: Proxabrush and Stimulator (John O. Butler Company), Sakool Tongue Cleaner (Sakool Company), Stim-U-Dent (Johnson & Johnson), Oral-B Interdental Brushes (Oral-B Laboratories), Orapik (Dental Concepts), and Silverak Tongue Cleaner (Gautamas).

Dentifrices

Dentifrices are products that are used with a toothbrush for cleaning accessible tooth surfaces. Dentifrices are available in three forms—powders, pastes, or gels. The gels and pastes commonly contain a surfactant, a humectant, suspending agents, flavoring agents, an abrasive, and sometimes fluoride. The powders commonly contain an abrasive and flavoring and sometimes a surfactant. Dentifrices enhance the removal of stain and dental plaque by the toothbrush (79). The beneficial effects of dentifrice use include decreased incidence of dental caries and gum disease, reduced mouth odors, and enhanced personal appearance (79).

Abrasives are generally considered to be the component in dentifrices responsible for physically removing plaque and debris. The ideal abrasive would maximally aid in cleaning and minimally abrade and damage tooth surfaces. Unfortunately, because of the variance in patient brushing techniques and oral conditions, the ideal dentifrice abrasive does not exist. Abrasives in dentifrices have not been shown to damage dental enamel appreciably (80). However, exposed root surfaces (cementum) and dentin can be damaged by toothbrushes and abrasives and may lead to tooth hypersensitivity (80). Although 15% of the population 20–24 years of age have such surfaces, 58% of those 50–59 years of age have exposed surfaces that could be severely abraded. A number indicating relative abrasivity is included in the Toothpaste Product Table and is based on a radioactive dentin abrasion (RDA) assay (81). Abrasivity increases as the numbers increase. Based on current data regarding dentifrice abrasivity, the following points are clear:

- An RDA range of 50–200 is adequate to ensure safe removal of stained pellicle.

- Under normal use, nonabrasive dentifrice will not effectively remove stained pellicle.

- The lowest effect value for dentifrice abrasivity has not been definitively established (80).

Dentifrice abrasives are pharmacologically inactive and insoluble compounds. Common abrasives include silicates, dicalcium phosphate, sodium metaphosphate, calcium pyrophosphate, calcium orthophosphate, calcium carbonate, magnesium carbonate, and aluminum oxides (80). Dentifrices vary greatly in abrasiveness (80, 81). In general, patients might best be advised to use the least abrasive dentifrice, which provides effective pellicle removal, unless they are advised otherwise by their dentist. Certainly, patients with periodontal disease and exposed root surfaces should use a low-abrasive dentifrice.

Surfactants are incorporated into most dentifrices to aid in removing debris by their detergent action and because the "foaming" they cause is desirable to most patients. The most common surfactants are sodium lauryl sulfate and sodium *N*-lauroyl sarcosinate (82, 83). There is no evidence that surfactants in dentifrices possess anticaries activity or reduce periodontal disease, and they are considered inactive ingredients by the FDA (84).

Humectants and suspending agents are used in paste and gel dentifrices. The humectants prevent the preparation from drying out and usually include sorbitol, glycerin, and propylene glycol (83). The suspending agents suspend and stabilize the various ingredients and often thicken the preparation. Common suspending agents include methylcellulose, carboxymethyl cellulose, Veegum, bentonite, tragacanth, karaya gum, and sodium alginate (83).

Flavoring and sweetening agents are incorporated in these preparations to make them more appealing. Most dentifrices contain saccharin, sodium saccharin, or sorbitol as sweeteners. Flavoring agents include a host of essential oils and other flavorings (83).

Fluoride Dentifrices Fluoride dentifrices are accepted by the ADA as being safe and effective agents in caries prevention. Sodium monofluorophosphate (NaMFP) 0.76% or 0.80% has been the most common fluoride compound and has been associated with caries reductions ranging from 17 to 42% when compared to nonfluoride dentifrices (85). Recently, the number of accepted sodium fluoride dentifrices has increased; the number of approved NaF and NaMFP dentifrices are now equal. Most accepted dentifrices contain 0.24% sodium fluoride (NaF) and have produced caries reductions ranging from 13 to 41% (85–87). One of these dentifrices, Gleem, has submitted all the necessary caries data to the ADA but the manufacturer chooses not to display the seal of acceptance. Included in the ADA-accepted dentifrices are the standard 1,000 ppm and 1,100 ppm fluoride ion concentrations as well as a new 1,500 ppm fluoride ion product. This extra-strength MFP product is clinically and statistically superior to its regular-strength MFP counterpart (88). However, because of concerns about excessive fluoride ingestion in children, the CDT has required that the following directions appear on the Extra-strength Aim carton:

- Not for use by children under 2 years of age;

- Children 6 years of age or younger should be supervised while using the dentifrice;

- Brush teeth thoroughly at least once daily (88).

In a recent review of clinical studies of high-potency fluoride dentifrices (89), the author concluded the following with regard to caries efficacy:

- High-potency 1,500-ppm NaMFP dentifrice is superior to 1,100-ppm NaMFP dentifrice.

- High-potency 2,000–2,500-ppm NaMFP dentifrice is superior to 1,100-ppm NaMFP dentifrice.

- High-potency 2,800-ppm NaMFP dentifrice is superior to 1,100-ppm NaF dentifrice.

- There is insufficient evidence to claim that 2,000–2,500-ppm NaMFP dentifrice is superior to 1,500-ppm NaMFP dentifrice.

- The combination of NaF and NaMFP in a dentifrice does not enhance the cariostatic benefits of the dentifrice compared to each compound used alone in equal total fluoride concentrations.

- Additional evidence is needed to confirm the claim that a high-potency mixed fluoride dentifrice with 1,450–2,500-ppm fluoride (NaF + NaMFP) is superior to a single or mixed fluoride dentifrice in conventional concentrations.

Little is known about the anticaries benefit of fluoridated dentifrices in adult populations. However, it appears that use of an 1,100-ppm NaF dentifrice can have a beneficial effect on both coronal and root surface caries in an older population (90).

Fluorides are anticariogenic because they replace the hydroxyl ion in hydroxyapatite with fluoride ion to form fluorapatite. Fluorapatite in the outer surface of dental enamel is harder and more resistant to acids than hydroxyapatite and, therefore, the enamel is less susceptible to carious breakdown (91). In addition to the formation of fluorapatite, topical fluoride preparations also have been shown to have an antibacterial and anti-enzyme effect on plaque bacteria resulting in decreased acid production (91–93). Fluoride-containing dentifrices are thought to be of greatest benefit when used by children in areas with a nonfluoridated water supply; however, they can help reduce caries incidence even in patients residing in communities with a fluoridated water supply (85). Fluoride-containing dentifrices do not cause dental fluorosis unless excessive amounts are chronically ingested. (See *Plate 2–6*.)

Antiplaque Dentifrices Several dentifrice manufacturers make claims of antiplaque effectiveness. However, no dentifrice is currently accepted by the ADA as efficacious in this regard. Certain fluoride dentifrices for which antiplaque claims are made bear the ADA seal of approval for anticaries effect. To gain the ADA seal for plaque and gingivitis control, the product must fulfill very stringent guidelines outlined by the ADA (94). Criteria regarding study design, study duration, microbiological assessments, and effects on plaque and gingivitis are described. Only those chemotherapeutic products that fulfill these criteria in the data submitted to the CDT will receive the ADA seal of acceptance in the antiplaque/antigingivitis therapeutic category. Only one nonprescription product (Listerine mouthwash) has fulfilled these criteria, and it will be discussed in the mouthwash section of the chapter. The antiplaque ingredients of these dentifrices include micronized silica abrasives, sodium bicarbonate, and a variety of other ingredients (81).

Anticalculus Dentifrices A number of fluoride dentifrices containing anticalculus compounds are currently marketed. Several of these products carry the ADA seal of acceptance for anticaries efficacy but the anticalculus claims have not been evaluated by the ADA. The ADA regards inhibition of supragingival calculus as a nontherapeutic use and therefore does not evaluate the anticalculus claims. The ingredients that prevent new calculus formation are zinc chloride, zinc citrate, and 3.3% pyrophosphate. Placebo-controlled clinical trials testing these dentifrices separately have produced a range of 20–50% for calculus reduction (95, 96). Patients who are heavy calculus formers should consider using these products instead of a plain fluoride dentifrice. There is some preliminary evidence that some anticalculus compounds may enhance dentinal sensitivity by preventing tooth surface remineralization (97). Until more is known about this effect, patients with sensitive teeth should avoid anticalculus products.

Cosmetic Dentifrices Cosmetic dentifrices make no therapeutic claims and are usually chosen by patients because of taste or "whitening ability." Dentifrices claiming to remove tough tobacco stains are sometimes more abrasive than other formulations and could be hazardous in patients with exposed root surfaces. A new cosmetic dentifrice called Epi-Smile is purported to whiten teeth by a pellicle dissolution action of calcium peroxide. This product is no more abrasive than regular fluoride toothpaste, but claims of superior whitening ability have not yet been substantiated in the literature. Popular gel dentifrices are flavored more like mouthwashes and disperse rapidly in the oral cavity. Manufacturers of gel dentifrices have advertised that children brush longer and more thoroughly because of the gel's consistency, translucent appearance, dispersibility, and flavor. A recent study documented the brushing times and patterns of two groups of children (10–16 years of age) who used either a translucent gel or a conventional paste for 1 month (98). There was no difference in duration or pattern of brushing between the paste and the gel, and average brushing time was 1 minute.

Desensitizing Dentifrices Dentifrices for hypersensitive teeth should be used regularly only if the patient's dentist recommends them (99). Because the most common cause of tooth sensitivity is exposed dentin, a desensitizing dentifrice must inhibit sensitization while being nonabrasive. Many agents have been used to treat dentinal hypersensitivity but only 5% potassium nitrate (Denquel, Promise, and Mint Sensodyne), 10% strontium chloride hexanitrate products (Sensodyne), and dibasic sodium citrate 2% in pluronic gel (Protect) have been accepted by the ADA (99). All of these agents probably alter the function of dentinal tubules but their exact mechanism is not known (99). In one clinical trial, subjects brushed twice daily for 1 month with either Denquel, Sensodyne, Protect, or Thermodent (100). Sensitivity was assessed by electrical and cold-air stimulus and by the patient's subjective assessment. Denquel showed significantly greater reductions in sensitivity than did any other dentifrice. Sensodyne was ranked next, and the other two dentifrices were rated as no more effective than placebos. However, other trials have shown all agents to be useful for dentinal sensitivity. These dentifrices should be used until the sensitivity subsides; the patient should then switch to a low-abrasion dentifrice. The desensitizers do not currently contain fluoride, so patients should be advised to use fluoride rinses during therapy (99).

Miscellaneous Hygiene Products

Disclosing Agents

Disclosing agents are used as aids in visualizing dental plaque. They are used both at home by the pa-

tient and in the dental office. By staining the dental plaque and making it more easily visible, patients can better evaluate their oral hygiene efforts and detect areas of needed improvement. (See *Plate 2–7.*) In this way, it is hoped that the patient will be motivated to improve oral hygiene.

Disclosing agents are available for home use as either a solution or chewable tablet. They are intended for occasional use as an indicator and not for continuous long-term use. Disclosing products should be expectorated completely (not swallowed), the mouth should be rinsed with water, and the water expectorated. Solutions are often preferred because they can easily be applied with a cotton-tipped applicator to a handicapped patient's dentition by another person and they can be diluted with water. In addition, solutions are often more acceptable than the tablets in small children. The FDA has found D&C Red No. 28 and FD&C Green No. 3 safe when used at approved dosages and expectorated. Most nonprescription disclosing products contain D&C Red No. 28 as a single agent because it has the advantage of staining red (matching oral soft tissues) and not markedly staining hard tissues. However, D&C Red No. 28 does have the disadvantage of not differentiating plaque well at the gingival margin (101). A mixture of D&C Red No. 28 and FD&C Green No. 3 has shown the ability to color differentiate between thick and thin plaque (101). This mixture has the advantage of demonstrating areas of rapidly accumulating plaque or areas that the patient neglects during oral hygiene. Fluorescein dye also has been recommended as a dental plaque disclosing agent (101). It is readily taken up by plaque, is basically colorless in normal light, and fluoresces with a strong yellow color under 4,800 Å (ultraviolet light). Fluorescein has the disadvantages of being costly (especially when an ultraviolet light source is required) and has the potential to cause tissue damage secondary to ultraviolet light overexposure.

Artificial Saliva Products

Artificial salivas are preparations designed to mimic natural saliva both chemically and physically. They do not stimulate natural salivary gland production and must be considered as replacement therapy, not as a cure for xerostomia (dry mouth). Patients complaining of xerostomia may have permanent salivary gland atrophy caused by head and neck radiation, Sjogren's syndrome, or advanced age (102). Temporary xerostomia is often drug-induced, and normal saliva flow returns after discontinuing therapy. Common adverse effects of chronic xerostomia include the following: reduced denture wearing time; stomatitis and burning tongue; difficulty swallowing and speaking; disturbed sleep patterns; rampant caries; and periodontal disease. Treatment should be directed toward the control of dental decay and the relief of soft tissue distress. The commercially available artificial salivas relieve this soft tissue discomfort and are more effective and longer lasting than simple rinses and lozenges.

Artificial saliva closely resembles natural saliva with regard to the following factors:

- Viscosity (carboxymethycellulose and glycerin are used to mimic natural saliva viscosity);

- Mineral content (All products contain calcium and phosphate ions, and three also contain fluoride. With normal use no product has demonstrated the ability to remineralize enamel. Therefore, the ADA does not recognize any such claims made by the manufacturers.);

- Preservatives (all products except Salivart contain preservatives such as methyl- or propylparaben. Certain patients may have hypersensitivity reactions.);

- Palatability (the most common flavorings are mint, sorbitol, and xylitol).

In xerostomic patients, the oral flora's ability to ferment sorbitol may be enhanced, thereby increasing caries rate (103). The xerostomic patient with a history of caries susceptibility should use a professionally designed topical fluoride program in addition to artificial saliva products. The ADA-approved artificial salivas are Moi-Stir and Moi-Stir Oral Swabsticks (Kingswood Laboratories), Orex (Young Dental Manufacturing Company), Salivart (Westport Pharmaceuticals), Saliva Substitute (Roxane Laboratories), and Xero-Lube (Scherer Laboratories).

Mouthwashes

Mouthwashes are solutions that often contain breath-sweetening, astringent, demulcent, detergent, or germicidal agents used for freshening and cleaning the oral cavity by gargling (104). They may be cosmetic or may contain a therapeutically effective agent.

Cosmetic Mouthwashes These mouthwashes freshen the breath and clean some debris, but have not proven to be effective antiseptics and are considered nontherapeutic by the ADA (105). An important consideration with the use of mouthwashes is the potential for these agents to disguise and delay treatment of pathologic conditions such as ANUG, purulent oral infections, periodontitis, and respiratory infections (105). The ADA Council on Dental Therapeutics suggests that "if marked breath odor persists after proper toothbrushing, the cause should be investigated" and not masked with mouthwash (105).

Cosmetic mouthwashes can be classified by appearance, alcohol content, and active ingredients. In general, mouthwashes are medicinal or alcoholic, minty (green) or spicy (red); they contain various miscellaneous ingredients. Aromatic oils include thymol, eucalyptol, menthol, and methyl salicylate. These oils are antibacterial and have some local anesthetic activity. Benzoic acid is an antimicrobial agent, and cetylpyridinium chloride is a cationic surfactant capable of bactericidal activity although it does not penetrate plaque well. Domiphen bromide is a bactericidal agent similar to cetylpyridinium. Glycerin is a topical protectant that tastes sweet and is soothing to oral mucosa. Zinc chloride/citrate is an astringent that neutralizes odoriferous sulfur compounds produced in the oral cavity. Phenol is a local anesthetic, antiseptic, and bactericidal agent that penetrates plaque better than either cetylpyridinium or domiphen. The most popular cosmetic mouthwashes are phenolic (medicinal) and minty. Alcohol contributes significantly to the flavor (105). The higher the alcohol content, the higher the "bite" or impact in the mouth. This can contribute to a feeling of greater refreshment (105).

Antiplaque Mouthrinses In the past 5 years, there has been a proliferation of nonprescription antiplaque mouthrinses. Many manufacturers have made antiplaque claims, but, to be accepted by the ADA, data submitted must conform to the aforementioned guidelines. To date, only Listerine has received ADA acceptance as a nonprescription antiplaque/antigingivitis mouthwash (106). Three clinical studies of 6 months or more were submitted to the Council on Dental Therapeutics to demonstrate effectiveness. Final reduction in plaque indices ranged from 14 to 34%, and final reductions in gingival indices ranged from 22 to 34% (106). In all trials, patients rinsed with 20 ml twice daily in addition to their normal oral hygiene regimen. Two independent, 6-month microbiological studies submitted to the council demonstrated no deleterious effects on oral flora. In addition, long-term studies established soft tissue safety and lack of mutagenicity. The active ingredients in Listerine are the aromatic oils and benzoic acid, both of which are antibacterial. Listerine contains 29% alcohol, but in all clinical trials, a hydroalcoholic control was the basis for comparison of effect. Although alcohol exerts a drying effect on oral mucosa, daily alcoholic mouthwash use is not associated with an increased incidence of oral or pharyngeal cancer (107).

Sanguinaria extract in combination with zinc chloride is marketed as Viadent antiplaque rinse. Although effective against plaque-forming bacteria in vitro, results using the rinse alone or in conjunction with Viadent dentifrice have been mixed. Results have ranged from no significant effect with the rinse alone (108, 109) to 50–60% reductions in plaque/gingivitis scores with combined twice daily use of Viadent rinse and dentifrice (110). The sanguinaria dentifrice used alone has not proven to be effective (111). A recent trial using twice daily brushing and rinsing with Viadent produced "20% or greater" reductions in plaque and gingivitis scores over a 28-week period (112).

A definitive assessment of sanguinaria's antiplaque efficacy is not possible based on published data. Other mouthwashes containing cetylpyridinium chloride and domiphen bromide have made antiplaque claims in the past, but these claims have not been substantiated by long-term clinical trials (113).

An entirely new prebrushing plaque-removal rinse called Plax was marketed with claims of removing 300% more plaque than brushing alone. The active antiplaque ingredient in Plax is sodium benzoate. This efficacy claim was based on one short-term clinical trial involving 12 subjects (114). Methods did not approximate normal oral hygiene procedures in this small study. Upon further investigation, use of Plax yielded results comparative to placebo (115–118).

Anticalculus mouthrinses containing the same active ingredients as anticalculus dentifrices are now available. Generally, calculus scores are reduced 15–42% with twice daily rinsing in addition to normal oral hygiene (119, 120).

Fluoridated Mouthwashes Four ADA-accepted nonprescription fluoride rinse products are available: Act, Fluorigard, Ghostbusters Anticavity Dental Rinse, and Kolynos. These mouthwashes are therapeutic in that their common ingredient, 0.05% NaF, is a consistently effective anticaries agent.

Studies in which subjects used 0.05% NaF rinse once daily have demonstrated a significant reduction in caries incidence (16–49%), especially when used by children living in an area with a nonfluoridated water supply (121–123). Likewise, a daily 0.1% stannous fluoride aqueous rinse significantly decreases caries incidence in school children living in a community with a fluoridated water supply (124). A significant problem with fluoride rinsing is that children 3–5 years of age swallow significant amounts of rinse each time they swish (125). A usual dose of 0.05% rinse contains 2 mg fluoride ion and could cause mild fluorosis in a fluoridated area. Therefore, the general recommendation is that children under 6 years of age should not use fluoride rinses. Patient instructions for nonprescription fluoride rinses should read as follows: Swish vigorously around and between teeth for one minute, then spit out. DO NOT SWALLOW. Use once daily (or twice daily for Listermint with fluoride) after cleaning teeth. Do not eat or rinse the mouth for 30 minutes afterward.

Miscellaneous Mouthwashes Dentists may suggest that their patients use oxygenating mouthwashes or drops as an adjunctive treatment of specific conditions or as a postoperative aid to cleaning and relief of dis-

comfort. Oral wound cleansing products have been used in cleansing minor wounds or in relieving minor gum inflammation resulting from minor dental procedures, dentures, orthodontic appliances, accidental injury, or other irritations of the mouth or gums (126). Hydrogen peroxide and carbamide peroxide release molecular oxygen immediately upon contact with tissue enzymes but tissue and bacterial exposure to the oxygen is very brief (127). The mechanical action of the liberated oxygen is useful in loosening particulate matter and cleaning debris from wounds. The efficacy of oxygenating products in killing anaerobic bacteria in the treatment of infections and periodontitis has not been established (127). After a thorough review process, the Food and Drug Administration (FDA) has determined that no ingredient has been found to be generally recognized as safe and effective for use as an over-the-counter (OTC) oral wound healing agent (128). This ruling pertains to allantoin, carbamide peroxide in glycerin, water-soluble chlorophyllins, and hydrogen peroxide in aqueous solution.

Recently, some dentists have undertaken home bleaching of vital teeth using topical 10% carbamide peroxide (Gly-Oxide, Proxigel). Under the supervision of the dentist, patients are instructed to expose extrinsically stained teeth to the peroxide gel by wearing custom-made mouthguards coated with a thin gel film. Anecdotal reports of successful tooth bleaching are now emerging. However, because of safety and efficacy concerns, patients should be strongly discouraged if they attempt this procedure without a dentist's direct supervision.

Prolonged rinsing with oxygenating products could lead to soft tissue irritation, decalcified tooth surfaces, and the development of black hairy tongue (127). An alternative to commercial products is warm salt water which some advocate for its cleansing and soothing properties (129). One teaspoon of salt dissolved in a 6–8 ounce glass of warm water can be used safely as an oral rinse.

Denture Products

Denture Cleansers

Dentures accumulate plaque, stain, and calculus by a process very similar to that which occurs with natural teeth (130). Denture patients are often most concerned that plaque may cause oral malodor and staining. However, a great deal of evidence implicates denture plaque as a major cause of mucosal disease (131, 132). Conditions such as denture stomatitis, inflammatory papillary hyperplasia, and chronic candidiasis can be caused by ill-fitting dentures, trauma, and the lack of denture cleanliness. Therefore, dentures should be thoroughly cleansed once daily to remove unsightly stains, potentially harmful plaque, and debris.

Denture cleansers are either chemical or abrasive in their cleaning action. The three types of chemical cleansers are alkaline peroxides, alkaline hypochlorites, and dilute acids. The abrasive cleaners are available as pastes, gels, or powders.

Alkaline peroxide cleaners are the most commonly used chemical denture cleansers. These powders or tablets become alkaline solutions of hydrogen peroxide when dissolved. The ingredients are alkaline detergents and perborates, the latter of which causes oxygen release for a mechanical cleaning effect. These products are most effective on new plaque and stains when soaked for 4–8 hours. The alkaline peroxides have few serious disadvantages and do not damage the surface of acrylic resins. However, they can bleach acrylic resin with regular use (133).

Alkaline hypochlorites (bleach) remove stains, dissolve mucin, and are both bactericidal and fungicidal. Hypochlorite acts directly on the organic matrix of plaque to dissolve its structure but cannot dissolve calculus (133). The most serious disadvantage of hypochlorite is that it corrodes metal denture components such as chromium-cobalt and gold-plated nickel pins. However, the addition of anticorrosive phosphate compounds has greatly reduced this effect (130). Hypochlorite solutions also bleach acrylic resin (133).

Dilute acids, often 3–5% hydrochloric acid, work by dissolving the inorganic (calcium) phosphate and are effective against calculus and stain on dentures (133). They corrode metal components and are harmful to fabrics, eyes, and skin if spilled during handling (133).

Although many studies have been done on denture cleaning products, only a few comparative trials have been published. One study compared Denalan, Mersene, Kleenite, Efferdent, and Polident in terms of plaque and stain removal after one 10-minute soak (134). Kleenite and Mersene removed 57% of staining and were significantly more effective than Denalan (36%), Polident (34%), or Efferdent (26%). Mersene removed 42% of accumulated plaque and was significantly more effective than Kleenite (19%), Efferdent (11%), Denalan (7%), or Polident (6%). Another study compared Mersene, Polident, Efferdent, and a homemade alkaline hypochlorite combination of 4 ml Clorox and 2 tsp Calgon in 100 ml of tap water in terms of plaque removal after a 15-minute soak (135). Mersene and the homemade hypochlorite were significantly more effective than Polident and Efferdent (90% vs. 35%). The greater effectiveness of Mersene and Clorox/Calgon may be related to a higher pH when compared to that of Polident and Efferdent. Mersene is no longer available commercially. The relative ineffec-

tiveness of all products tested during a short soaking time is often contrary to advertising claims. Plaque removal is increased by brushing the dentures after they soak in cleansers; these instructions are included on some products (133).

The ADA CDMIE has accepted the following denture cleansers as safe and effective: Complete, Dentu-Creme, Dentu-Gel, Efferdent and Efferdent paste, Polident powder and tablets, and Smoker's Polident.

In general, good daily plaque removal can be accomplished with thorough use of a denture brush and low abrasion paste. However, geriatric or handicapped patients may prefer an alkaline peroxide soak solution for daily, overnight cleaning. The hypochlorite bleaches should be used no more than once weekly because of their acrylic resin bleaching. Dilute acids are not suitable for routine patient use because of the care with which they must be handled (133). All denture products should be rinsed off the denture completely before insertion. Contact with oral or other mucous membranes results in tissue irritation or, more seriously, in severe chemical burns from the alkaline or acid products (133). All denture cleansers should be kept out of reach of children because accidental ingestion may cause severe oropharyngeal burns (136, 137). Patients should not soak or clean dentures in hot water or hot soaking solutions because distortion or warping may occur. Stains that are resistant to proper denture brushing and soaking in available solutions should be evaluated by a dentist (133).

Denture Adherents

Denture adhesives may be the most overused dental products purchased by patients. Chronic bone resorption of the mandibular and maxillary ridges that support a denture is a consequence of even the best-fitting denture. Periodic dental examinations are necessary to evaluate bone resorption and ensure proper denture fit. Although denture adhesives may increase denture retention in some persons, the need for adhesives increases as the quality of the denture adaptation to underlying soft tissues deteriorates (138, 139). Furthermore, pathologic changes in soft tissue under the denture, such as ulcers and fibrous lesions, and accelerated bone resorption have been reported with the inappropriate use of denture adhesives and ill-fitting dentures (138, 139). These materials can provide a medium for bacterial and fungal growth, resulting in dangerous infection and inflammation of soft tissues (140). Excessive application of adherents could also cause denture repositioning with resultant malocclusion (138, 139). Patients who believe that daily use of denture adherents is necessary to attain denture security and comfort should be referred to their dentist for reevaluation.

Denture adherents are usually composed of the following: materials that swell, gel, and become viscous, such as karaya, pectin, or methylcellulose; materials that are antibacterial, such as methyl salicylate, sodium borate, or hexachlorophene; and materials that serve as preservatives, fillers, or wetting or flavoring agents, such as propylparaben, magnesium oxide, sodium lauryl sulphate, and petroleum derivatives. Adherent powders have either a vegetable gum base or are composed of synthetic polymers such as long-chain ethylene oxide. Adherent pastes usually contain karaya gum, petroleum jelly, colorings, and flavorings.

The ADA Council on Dental Materials and Devices has accepted some denture adhesive products with the understanding that the labeling indicate that they are to be used only temporarily or upon the recommendation of a dentist. All accepted denture adhesives contain the following warning label:

> [Product name] is acceptable as a temporary measure to provide increased retention of dentures. However, an ill-fitting denture may impair your health—consult your dentist for periodic examination.

The ADA CDMIE has accepted the following denture adherents as safe and effective: Co-Re-Ga, Effergrip, Firmadent, Perma-Grip, Rigident Powder, Rigident Cream, Super Wernet's Powder, Wernet's Adhesive Cream, and Wernet's Powder with Neoseal.

Denture Reliners and Cushions Extended use of reliners or cushions for dentures results in harm to the patient and damage to the denture. Denture reliners and cushions have been associated with bone resorption, tumors, traumatic ulcers, and gingival inflammation of the denture-bearing tissues (141, 142). In addition, these products change the positioning of the denture, which can result in denture distortion, malocclusion, temporomandibular joint problems, decreased mastication function, and altered aesthetics (143). Some dentists requested that the sale of these products be halted (141, 144). The ADA does not accept any of these products and discourages their use. The FDA Bureau of Medical Devices requires the following warning label on these products.

> **WARNING** For temporary use only. Long-term use of this product may lead to faster bone loss, continuing irritation, sores, and tumors. For use only until a dentist can be seen.

In general, any patients who are considering purchasing a denture reliner or cushion because of actual or perceived denture problems should see their dentist as soon as possible.

Denture Repair Kits Broken dentures, like natural dentition, can be evaluated and repaired only by a dentist. Initial fitting and periodic refitting of dentures requires extensive dental knowledge and skill. A cracked, broken, or distorted denture is, for all practical purposes, impossible for a patient to repair properly at home (145). Denture repair kits usually contain methacrylate or other types of glue or acrylic materials. The ADA, as in the case of reliners and cushions, strongly discourages the use of denture repair kits (146). The FDA requires the following label on these products:

> **WARNING** For emergency repairs only. Long-term use of home-repaired dentures may cause faster bone loss, continuing irritation, sores, and tumors. This kit is for emergency use only. See your dentist without delay.

The pharmacist should strongly discourage the use of denture repair kits.

Products for Cold Sores and Canker Sores

Many nonprescription products are available for treatment of cold sores and canker sores. Some of these products provide symptomatic relief, some are irrational and may involve more risk than benefit, and none has been shown conclusively to decrease the recurrence rate of lesions or to be curative. Many products are intended for extraoral use only and are not for intraoral use.

Canker Sore Treatment

The main goals in treating canker sores are to control discomfort and to promote healing, so that the patient can eat, drink, and perform routine home oral care. Topical oral protectants such as Orabase, denture adhesives, or benzoin tincture can be effective in covering lesions and affording symptomatic relief (36, 147). These products can be applied as needed. Both Orabase and benzoin tincture are accepted by the ADA as topical protectants.

Topical application of local anesthetic pastes or gels also affords temporary pain relief. Benzocaine and butacaine are the most common local anesthetics in nonprescription products. Benzocaine is a known sensitizer (allergen) and should not be used by patients with a history of problems with other benzocaine-containing products (82, 148). The FDA has accepted topical local anesthetic products containing benzocaine 5–20%, benzyl alcohol 0.05–0.1%, dyclonine 0.05–0.1%, hexylresorcinol 0.05%–0.1%, menthol 0.04–2%, phenol 0.5–1.5%, phenolate sodium 0.5–1.5% phenol, and salicyl alcohol 1–6% as safe and effective (149). Sustained use of products containing substantial amounts of menthol, phenol, camphor, and eugenol as anesthetic, counterirritant, or antiseptic treatments for canker sores should be discouraged. These agents may cause tissue irritation and damage or systemic toxicity, especially if overused (149). None of these products has been accepted as safe and effective by the ADA for treating canker sores. The value of nascent oxygen-releasing compounds (carbamide peroxide, hydrogen peroxide, and perborates) as effective antiseptics and cleansers of aphthous lesions (small ulcers) has not been established (128), and tissue irritation and black hairy tongue have been reported (127). Oral aspirin or acetaminophen as systemic analgesics afford additional relief of discomfort. Aspirin should not be retained in the mouth before swallowing or placed in the area of the oral lesions because of the high risk of severe chemical burns with necrosis (150). (See *Plate 2–8.*)

Cold Sore Treatment

The primary goal in treating cold sores, as with canker sores, is to control discomfort and promote healing of these self-limiting lesions. The cold sore should be kept moist to prevent drying and fissuring. Cracking of the lesions may render them more susceptible to secondary bacterial infection, may delay healing, and usually increases discomfort. Therefore, products that are highly astringent are best avoided. Bland emollient creams, petrolatum, or protectants such as Orabase can aid in moistening and protecting cold sores (36). If there is evidence of secondary infection of a cold sore, topical application of bacitracin and/or neomycin ointments is recommended along with systemic antibiotics when indicated. Allergic reactions to topical neomycin have been reported. Topical local anesthetics in nondrying bases aid in decreasing pain (36). Oral aspirin or acetaminophen also is effective in controlling discomfort. Patients who associate occurrence of cold sores with sun exposure may benefit from the application of a sunscreen containing 5% para-aminobenzoic acid or various other ultraviolet ray blockers in the form of a lipstick. (See Chapter 34, *Sunscreen and Suntan Products.*)

Numerous other products have been proposed in the treatment of cold sores. Evidence demonstrating efficacy, however, is lacking. Preparations containing *Lactobacillus acidophilus* have not shown any conclusive efficacy in the treatment of cold sores or any other oral lesions (36). Nonoxynol 9, a surfactant–spermicidal agent available in nonprescription contraceptive products, has shown "uniformly enthusiastic" results in one clinical trial (151). However, no well-controlled studies have been conducted to demonstrate its efficacy. The essential amino acid L-lysine in oral daily doses from 300 to 1,200 mg has been touted as "accelerating recovery" and "suppressing recurrence" of cold sores (152). However, subsequent work has produced conflicting results regarding L-lysine's effect on duration, severity, or recurrence rate of cold sores (153–155). An FDA OTC advisory panel has listed L-lysine, *Lactobacillus acidophilus*, and *L. bulgaricus* as safe but not yet proven effective for treatment of herpes simplex labialis (36). Topical application of caustic or escharotic agents such as phenol or silver nitrate are considered contraindicated by the ADA (36). Topical counterirritants, such as camphor, are of unproven efficacy and are not accepted by the ADA. Topical application of 0.5% hydrocortisone creams or ointments or other corticosteroids are contraindicated according to the ADA (156). Although some investigators consider topical steroids of benefit for herpes infections, most now consider them unsafe and contraindicated, because of the possibility of spreading lesions (36, 41).

Products for Toothache

Nonprescription medications for toothache commonly contain eugenol or benzocaine. Eugenol and clove oil are accepted by the ADA for professional use by the dentist. However, these agents are not accepted as safe and effective nonprescription drugs for toothache. They are generally ineffective in the hands of the patient for toothache and can cause soft tissue damage. Benzocaine also is not accepted by the ADA as a safe and effective self-treatment for toothache. Toothache is usually an indication of pathology involving tooth substance, dental pulp, or the supporting periodontium. Even if aspirin or acetaminophen is effective in relieving toothache, the patient should seek professional dental help as soon as possible.

Products for Teething

Teething is the eruption of the deciduous teeth through the gingival tissues. Usually this process is uneventful. However, when teething causes sleep disturbances or irritability, symptomatic treatment should be considered. Topical local anesthetics, such as benzocaine and frozen teething rings, may provide symptomatic relief, although the efficacy of these products is unproven. The ADA has not accepted any product for teething. When teething is accompanied by fever or malaise, a dentist or physician should be contacted to rule out an infectious process.

PATIENT CONSULTATION

After assessing a patient's oral complaint or problem, the pharmacist can advise the patient on the appropriate treatment with a nonprescription product or refer the patient to a dentist. The pharmacist should be able to inform a patient when an oral complaint is usually self-limiting and not severe, or when a problem is likely to be progressive and have serious consequences. An unconcerned patient asking advice about nonprescription medications to treat an oral abscess with accompanying fever, malaise, swelling, lymphadenopathy, and purulent exudate should be immediately referred to a dentist. On the other hand, a concerned patient seeking advice about nonprescription products for a small recurrent cold sore can be reassured that it is usually a self-limiting problem that will resolve with proper self-treatment.

The pharmacist may be the first, last, or only health care professional to advise a patient. The patient must know which nonprescription medications not to use and why, despite the advertising claims. Examples include advising against a "whitening" toothpaste to clean a denture because of excess abrasiveness and advising against applying camphor or phenolic compounds to canker sores because of possible irritation, tissue damage, or systemic toxicity. When counseling a patient on rational self-medication, the pharmacist should do more than just recommend a product. The patient should be informed about how to use the product properly, how long to use the product, what to expect from the product, cautions with the use of the product, and what to do if the product is ineffective. For example, when recommending a sodium fluoride mouthrinse, the patient should know that the fluoride rinse should be used after cleaning the teeth and should be expectorated; that nothing should be taken by mouth for 30 minutes after use; that the mouthrinse can benefit the patient for as long as the patient has natural dentition; that the fluoride is preventive in action and will not cure already carious teeth; and that the product should be kept out of the reach of children because of possible ethanol or fluoride toxicity (157).

Patient counseling about a nonprescription medication should include more than merely explaining if a product is preventive, curative, or palliative in its action. The patient should realize that nonprescription drugs should improve the condition being treated. If the drug results in no change, worsens the condition, or causes another problem, the product should be discontinued and professional help sought. For instance, a properly used benzocaine product applied to canker sores should afford a reasonable amount of symptomatic relief. However, if the canker sores get progressively more inflamed and painful after application of the product, the patient should be informed to stop using the product because of possible benzocaine allergy. Even nonprescription dental products rarely associated with adverse effects should not escape evaluation by the pharmacist when assessing a problem and counseling the patient. Dentifrices, one of the most widely used nonprescription drug products, have been reported to cause desquamation, irritation, and allergic reactions (82). Patients experiencing one of these infrequent effects secondary to a dentifrice should be advised to discontinue use of commercial dentifrices, substitute baking soda or salt water, and see their dentist.

SUMMARY

Because dental disease is the most frequently encountered health care problem in the United States, and because pharmacists see more people with dental problems than dentists do, today's pharmacist needs a sound knowledge of dental products and dental therapeutics. The pharmacist–dentist team can improve oral health. With useful references such as the *Journal of the American Dental Association* and the special annual July dental issue of *Pharmacy Times*, awareness of ongoing FDA and ADA evaluation of dental products, and open lines of communication with dental practitioners, pharmacists can better serve their role as dental health consultants and members of the dental health care team.

REFERENCES

1 "Nutritional Disorders of Children: Prevention, Screening, and Follow-up," U.S. Dept. of Health, Education, and Welfare, DHEW Publication #HSA 76-5612, 1976, p. 82.

2 The Prevalence of Dental Caries in United States Children, The National Dental Caries Prevalence Survey, U.S. Dept. of Health and Human Services, NIH Publication No. 82–2245, Bethesda, Md., December, 1981.

3 D. W. Banting et al., *J. Dent. Res.*, *64*, 1141 (1985).

4 C. W. Douglass et al., *J. Am. Dent. Assoc.*, *107*, 403 (1983).

5 R. G. Rozier et al., *J. Pub. Health Dent.*, *41*, 14 (1981).

6 D. M. Makuc, Institute of Statistics Mimeo Series, no. 1265. Dept. of Biostatistics, University of North Carolina at Chapel Hill, 1980.

7 J. D. Beck et al., *Comm. Dent. Oral Epidemiol.*, *12*, 17 (1984).

8 Council on Dental Health and Health Planning, American Dental Association, *J. Am. Dent. Assoc.*, *105*, 75 (1982).

9 *Drug Store News*, *10 (14)*, Ad Insert (1988).

10 A. A. Dugoni, *Pharm. Times*, *55*, 45 (1989).

11 American Dental Association/American Pharmaceutical Association Liaison Committee, "The Dentist and the Pharmacist," American Dental Association, Chicago, Ill., 1983, p. 1.

12 M. Pader, "Oral Hygiene Products and Practice," 1st ed., Marcel Dekker, New York, N.Y., 1988, p. 101.

13 E. Newbrun, *Science*, *217*, 418 (1987).

14 M. Pader, "Oral Hygiene Products and Practice," 1st ed., Marcel Dekker, New York, N.Y., 1988, pp. 226–228.

15 A. I. Jacknowitz, *U.S. Pharmacist*, *13*, 29–31 (1988).

16 A. Bar, *World Rev. Nutr. Diet.*, *55*, 1–27 (1988).

17 R. G. Campbell and D. D. Zinner, *J. Nutr.*, *100*, 11 (1970).

18 M. Pader, "Oral Hygiene Products and Practice," 1st ed., Marcel Dekker, New York, N.Y., 1988, pp. 45–59.

19 S. M. Adair, "Pediatric Dentistry," 1st ed., W. B. Saunders, Philadelphia, Pa., 1988, p. 20.

20 F. A. Carranza, Jr., "Glickman's Clinical Periodontology," 7th ed., W. B. Saunders, Philadelphia, Pa., 1990, pp. 202–209.

21 A. Hugosen, *J. Periodontal Res.*, Supplement 5, 1 (1970).

22 D. W. Cohen et al., *J. Periodontol.*, *42*, 653 (1971).

23 A. H. Mohamed, Ph.D. Thesis, University of Illinois, Chicago, Ill., 1971.

24 J. Silness and H. Loe, *Acta Odontologica Scand.*, *24*, 747 (1966).

25 "International Conference on Research in the Biology of Periodontal Disease," College of Dentistry, University of Illinois, 1977, p. 227.

26 "International Conference on Research in the Biology of Periodontal Disease," College of Dentistry, University of Illinois, 1977, pp. 247–249, 402.

27 F. A. Carranza, Jr., "Glickman's Clinical Peridontology," 7th ed., W. B. Saunders, Philadelphia, Pa., 1990, pp. 149–159.

28 W. J. Loesche et al., *J. Periodontol.*, *53*, 223–230 (1982).

29 R. J. Genco et al., "Contemporary Periodontics," 1st ed., C. V. Mosby, St. Louis, Mo., 1990, 63–81.

30 R. J. Genco et al., "Contemporary Periodontics," 1st ed., C. V. Mosby, St. Louis, Mo., 1990, pp. 348–359.

31 "Canker Sores and Other Oral Ulcerations," PHS No. 1329, U.S. Government Printing Office, Washington, D.C., 1965, pp. 1–14.

32 E. A. Graykowski et al., *J. Am. Dent. Assoc.*, *69*, 118 (1964).

33 M. F. Barile et al., in "Microbial Protoplasts, Spheroplasts, and L-Forms," L. B. Guze, Ed., Williams and Wilkins, Baltimore, Md., 1967, pp. 444–456.

34 R. N. Shore and W. B. Shelby, *Arch. Dermatol.*, *109*, 400 (1974).

35 T. C. Francis, *Oral Surg.*, *30*, 476 (1970).

36 T. A. Gossel, *U.S. Pharmacist*, *13*, 62–69 (1988).

37 R. S. Rogers III et al., *Arch. Dermatol.*, *109*, 361 (1974).

38 A. E. Dolby, *Immunology*, *17*, 709 (1969).

39 R. A. Lindemann et al., *Oral Surg.*, *60*, 281 (1985).

40 N. K. Wood and P. W. Goaz, "Differential Diagnosis of Oral Lesions," 2nd ed., C. V. Mosby, St. Louis, Mo., 1980, pp. 101–104.

41 E. B. Smith, *J. Am. Med. Assoc.*, *235*, 1731 (1976).

42 R. S. Griffith et al, *Dermatologica*, *156*, 257 (1978).

43 D. W. Kannangara et al., *Oral. Surg.*, *50*, 103–109 (1980).

44 C. B. Sabiston, Jr., and W. A. Gold, *Oral Surg.*, *38*, 187 (1974).

45 C. B. Sabiston, Jr., et al., *Oral Surg.*, *41*, 430 (1976).

46 J. J. Crawford, "Guide to Antibiotic Use in Dental Practice," 1st ed., Quintessence Publishing, Chicago, Ill., 1984, 33–37.

47 T. B. Aufdemonte and M. A. McPherson, *Oral Surg.*, *46*, 776 (1978).

48 T. M. Arendorf and D. M. Walker, *Arch. Oral Biol.*, *25*, 1 (1980).

49 S. Dreizen, *Am. J. Med.*, 28033 (Oct. 30, 1984).

50 R. P. Masella et al., *J. Prosthet. Dent.*, *33*, 250 (1975).

51 L. P. Samaranayake and T. W. MacFarlane, *Arch. Oral Biol.*, *25*, 603 (1980).

52 L. P. Samaranayake et al., *Arch. Oral Biol.*, *25*, 611 (1980).

53 T. W. MacFarlane et al., *Br. Dent. J.*, *144*, 199 (1978).

54 D. P. Lu, *Oral Surg*, *54*, 521–526 (1982).

55 A. Mashberg and A. M. Samit, *Cancer*, *38*, 67 (1989).

56 G. N. Connolly et al., *N. Engl. J. Med.*, *314*, 1020 (1986).

57 J. C. Feldman et al., *Prev. Med.*, *4*, 444 (1975).

58 W. H. Binnie et al., *J. Oral Pathol.*, *12*, 11 (1983).

59 R. C. Wunderlich et al., *J. Am. Dent. Assoc.*, *110*, 929 (1985).

60 W. B. Gillette and R. L. VanHouse, *J. Am. Dent. Assoc.*, *101*, 476 (1980).

61 F. A. Carranza, Jr., "Glickman's Clinical Periodontology," 7th ed., W. B. Saunders, Philadelphia, Pa., 1990, p. 706.

62 B. F. Hawkins et al., *Quintessence Int.*, *17*, 361–365 (1986).

63 J. G. Kreifeldt et al., *J. Dent. Res.*, *59*, 2047 (1980).

64 J. Bratel et al., *Clin. Prev. Dent.*, *10*, 23–26 (1988).

65 C. C. Schifter et al., *Clin. Prev. Dent.*, *5*, 15–19 (1983).

66 F. A. Carranza, Jr., "Glickman's Clinical Periodontology," 7th ed., W. B. Saunders, Philadelphia, Pa., 1990, p. 687.

67 L. Galvind and E. Zeuner, *J. Clin. Periodontol.*, *13*, 135 (1986).

68 L. J. Mueller et al., *Dent. Hygiene*, *13*, 546–550 (1987).

69 E. VanDerLinden et al., Vol. 67, Abstract 2289, 66th Annual Session, International Association for Dental Research, Montreal, PQ, Canada, March 1988.

70 R. L. Boyd et al., Vol. 67, Abstract 2292, 66th Annual Session, International Association for Dental Research, Montreal, PQ, Canada, March 1988.

71 E. J. Coontz, *Comp. Cont. Educ. Dent.*, Supplement 6, 117–122 (1988).

72 "Accepted Dental Therapeutics," 40th ed., American Dental Association, Chicago, Ill., 1984, p. 337.

73 International Conference on Research in the Biology of Periodontal Disease, College of Dentistry, University of Illinois, 1977, pp. 325–326, 371.

74 G. Greenstein, *J. Periodontol.*, *58*, 827–836 (1987).

75 D. M. Lamberts et al., *J. Periodontol.*, *53*, 393 (1982).

76 H. C. Hill et al., *J. Periodontol.*, *44*, 411 (1973).

77 D. A. Perry and G. Pattison, *Dent. Hygiene*, *11*, 16–19 (1986).

78 S. M. Mauriello, *Clin. Prev. Dent.*, *9*, 18–22 (1987).

79 M. Pader, "Oral Hygiene Products and Practice," 1st ed., Marcel Dekker, New York, N.Y., 1988, pp. 426–430.

80 M. Pader, "Oral Hygiene Products and Practice," 1st ed., Marcel Dekker, New York, N.Y., 1988, pp. 430–439.

81 *Consumer Reports*, *51*, 144–149 (1986).

82 W. C. Rubright et al., *J. Am. Dent. Assoc.*, *97*, 215 (1978).

83 M. Pader, "Oral Hygiene Products and Practice," 1st ed., Marcel Dekker, New York, N.Y., 1988, pp. 439–453.

84 *Federal Register*, *45*, 20670 (1980).

85 "Accepted Dental Therapeutics," 40th ed., American Dental Association, Chicago, Ill., 1984, pp. 409–411.

86 W. A. Zacherl, *J. Dent. Res.*, *60*, 577 (1981).

87 B. B. Beiswanger et al., *J. Dent. Res.*, *60*, 577 (1981).

88 Council on Dental Therapeutics, *J. Am. Dent. Assoc.*, *117*, 785 (1988).

89 L. W. Ripa, *J. Am. Dent. Assoc.*, *118*, 85–91 (1989).

90 M. E. Jensen and F. J. Kohout, *J. Am. Dent. Assoc.*, *117*, 829–832 (1988).

91 "Nutritional Disorders of Children: Prevention, Screening, and Follow-up," U.S. Dept. of Health, Education, and Welfare, DHEW Publication #HSA 76-5612, 1976, p. 87.

92 W. W. Briner and M. D. Francis, *Arch. Oral Biol.*, 7, 541 (1962).

93 W. J. Loesche et al., *Caries Res.*, 7, 283 (1973).

94 Council on Dental Therapeutics, *J. Am. Dent. Assoc.*, *112*, 529–532 (1986).

95 B. E. Kohut et al., *Clin. Prev. Dent.*, *11*, 13–15 (1989).

96 M. Kazmierczak et al., Vol. 67, Abstract 1068, 66th Annual Session, International Association for Dental Research, Montreal, PQ, Canada (1988).

97 P. J. White and R. X. Fallen, *Caries Res.*, *21*, 40–46 (1987).

98 C. J. Kleber et al., *J. Am. Dent. Assoc.*, *103*, 723 (1981).

99 T. A. Gossel, *U. S. Pharmacist*, Jan., 29 (1975).

100 W. J. Tarbet et al., *J. Am. Dent. Assoc.*, *105*, 227 (1982).

101 S. H. Y. Wei, "Pediatric Dentistry," 1st ed., Lea and Febiger, Philadelphia, Pa., 1988, p. 31.

102 P. C. Fox et al., *J. Am. Dent. Assoc.*, *110*, 519 (1985).

103 G. Rolla et al., *Scand. J. Dent. Res.*, *89*, 247 (1981).

104 *Federal Register*, *45*, 20671 (1980).

105 M. Pader, "Oral Hygiene Products and Practice," 1st ed., Marcel Dekker, New York, N.Y., 1988, pp. 489–504.

106 Council on Dental Therapeutics, *J. Am. Dent. Assoc.*, *117*, 515–517 (1988).

107 A. Marshberg et al., *J. Am. Dent. Assoc.*, *110*, 731 (1985).

108 K. B. W. Gross et al., *Dent. Hygiene*, *11*, 62–66 (1987).

109 J. Afseth and G. Rolla, *Caries Res.*, *21*, 285–288 (1987).

110 R. A. Miller et al., *J. Clin. Ortho.*, *22*, 304–307 (1988).

111 S. M. Mauriell and J. D. Bader, *J. Periodontol.*, *59*, 238–243 (1987).

112 D. S. Harper et al., Vol. 68, Abstract 1616, American Association for Dental Research, San Francisco, Calif., 1989.

113 T. A. Gossel, *U.S. Pharmacist*, *13*, 46–51 (1988).

114 R. C. Emling and S. L. Yankell, *Comp. Cont. Educ. Dent.*, *6*, 636–645 (1985).

115 E. Grossman, *Clin. Prev. Dent.*, *10*, 3–6 (1988).

116 B. B. Beiswanger et al., Vol. 68, Abstract 1472, American Association for Dental Research, San Francisco, Calif., 1989.

117 M. Kazmierczak et al., Vol. 68, Abstract 1474, American Association for Dental Research, San Francisco, Calif., 1989.

118 N. Sharma, Vol. 68, Abstract 1473, American Association for Dental Research, San Francisco, Calif., 1989.

119 K. N. Rostogi et al., Vol. 68, Abstract 1468, American Association for Dental Research, San Francisco, Calif., 1989.

120 P. Soparkar et al., Vol. 68, Abstract 832, 67th Annual Session, International Association for Dental Research, Dublin, Ireland, 1989.

121 A. J. Rugg–Gunn et al., *Br. Dent. J.*, *135*, 353 (1974).

122 P. Torell and Y. Ericsson, *Acta Odontolog. Scand.*, *23*, 287 (1965).

123 W. S. Driscoll et al., *J. Am. Dent. Assoc.*, *105*, 1010 (1982).

124 "Accepted Dental Therapeutics" 40th ed., American Dental Association, Chicago, Ill., 1984, pp. 407–408.

125 W. H. Wei and M. J. Kanellis, *J. Am. Dent. Assoc.*, *106*, 626 (1983).

126 *Federal Register*, *48*, 33991 (1983).

127 "Accepted Dental Therapeutics," 40th ed., American Dental Association, Chicago, Ill., 1984, pp. 321–322.

128 *Federal Register*, *51*, 26113 (1986).

129 *Federal Register*, *48*, 33985 (1983).

130 T. A. Gossel, *U.S. Pharmacist*, *13*, 56–62, 76 (1988).

131 J. Theilade, *Comm. Dent. and Oral Epidemiol.*, *3*, 115 (1975).

132 E. Budtz-Jorgensen and U. Bertram, *Acta Odontol. Scand.*, *28*, 71 (1970).

133 Council on Dental Materials, Instruments, and Equipment., *J. Am. Dent. Assoc.*, *106*, 77 (1983).

134 R. H. Augsburger and J. M. Elahi, *J. Pros. Dent.*, *47*, 356 (1982).

135 M. Ghalichebaf et al., *J. Pros. Dent.*, *48*, 515 (1982).

136 A. L. Abramson, *Ann. Otol. Rhinol. Laryngol.*, *14*, 102 (1975).

137 A. L. Abramson, *Arch. Otolaryngol.*, *104*, 514 (1978).

138 I. K. Adisman, *J. Pros. Dent.*, *62*, 711–715 (1989).

139 T. A. Gossel, *U.S. Pharmacist*, *12*, 42–51 (1987).

140 G. D. Stafford, *Dent. Practitioner.*, *21*, 17 (1970).

141 J. B. Woelfel and R. L. Curry, *J. Am. Dent. Assoc.*, *71*, 603 (1965).

142 C. R. Means, *J. Prosthet. Dent.*, *14*, 1086 (1964).

143 J. B. Woelfel and J. A. Kreider, *J. Prosthet. Dent.*, *20*, 319 (1968).

144 B. W. Thurgood and L. F. DeCounter, *J. Prosthet. Dent.*, *36*, 17 (1976).

145 A. Samant and W. R. Cinotti, *Clin. Prev. Dent.*, *9*, 14–17 (1987).

146 American Dental Association/American Pharmaceutical Association Liaison Committee, "The Dentist and the Pharmacist," American Dental Association, Chicago, Ill., 1983, p. 8.

147 "Accepted Dental Therapeutics," 40th ed., American Dental Association, Chicago, Ill., 1984, p. 79.

148 "Accepted Dental Therapeutics," 40th ed., American Dental Association, Chicago, Ill., 1984, p. 159.

149 *Federal Register*, *47*, 22809 (1982).

150 Z. Kawashima et al., *J. Am. Dent. Assoc.*, *91*, 130 (1975).

151 H. J. Donsky, *N. Engl. J. Med.*, *300*, 371 (1979).

152 R. S. Griffith et al., *Dermatologica*, *156*, 257 (1978).

153 N. Milman et al., *Acta Dermatovener. [Stockh.]*, *60*, 85 (1978).

154 J. J. DiGiovanna and H. Blank., *Arch. Dermatol.*, *120*, 48 (1984).

155 D. J. Thein and W. C. Hurt., *Oral Surg.*, *58*, 659 (1984).

156 "Accepted Dental Therapeutics." 39th ed., American Dental Association, Chicago, Ill., 1982, p. 40.

157 E. R. Weller-Fahy et al., *Pediatrics*, *66*, 302 (1980).

TOOTHPASTE PRODUCT TABLE

Product (Manufacturer)	Abrasive Ingredient	Relative Abrasivity[a]	Therapeutic Ingredient	Foaming Agent	Other Ingredients
Aim[b] (Lever Bros.)	hydrated silica		sodium monofluorophosphate	sodium lauryl sulfate	alcohol, sorbitol, PEG-32, sodium saccharin, sodium benzoate, cellulose gum, flavor
Aqua-Fresh[b] (SmithKline Beecham)	hydrated silica calcium carbonate calcium glycerophosphate		sodium monofluorophosphate	sodium lauryl sulfate	PEG-8, sorbitol, cellulose gum, sodium benzoate, titanium dioxide, sodium silicate, calcium, carrageenan, flavor
Aqua-Fresh Tartar Control[b] (SmithKline Beecham)	hydrated silica		sodium fluoride, 0.221%	sodium lauryl sulfate	tetrapotassium pyrophosphate, tetrasodium pyrophosphate, sorbitol, glycerin, PEG-8, flavor, xanthan gum, sodium saccharin, sodium benzoate, FD&C red #30, FD&C blue #1, FD&C yellow #10
Chloresium (Rystan)	calcium carbonate dicalcium phosphate		chlorophyllin	sodium lauryl sulfoacetate	glycerin, sorbitol, carrageenan, mineral oil, methylparaben, flavor
Close-Up (Chesebrough Ponds)	hydrated silica		sodium monofluorophosphate	sodium lauryl sulfate	sorbitol, polyols, glycerin, alcohol, sodium saccharin, cellulose gum, sodium benzoate, flavor
Colgate[b] (Colgate-Palmolive)	dicalcium phosphate dihydrate		sodium monofluorophosphate, 0.76%	sodium lauryl sulfate	glycerin, cellulose gum, sodium benzoate, tetrasodium pyrophosphate, sodium saccharin, flavor
Colgate Tartar Control[b] (Colgate-Palmolive)	hydrated silica		sodium fluoride	sodium lauryl sulfate	sorbitol, glycerin, tetrapotassium pyrophosphate, PEG-12, tetrasodium pyrophosphate, cellulose gum, flavor, PVM/MA copolymer, titanium dioxide, sodium saccharin
Crest[b] (Procter & Gamble)	hydrated silica		sodium fluoride	sodium lauryl sulfate	sorbitol, trisodium phosphate, sodium phosphate, titanium dioxide, xanthan gum, carbomer-956, flavor, sodium saccharin
Crest Tartar Control[b] (Procter & Gamble)	hydrated silica		sodium fluoride, 0.243%	sodium lauryl sulfate	glycerin, tetrapotassium pyrophosphate, tetrasodium pyrophosphate, disodium pyrophosphate, sorbitol, PEG-6, flavor, xanthan gum, sodium saccharin, carbomer-956, titanium dioxide, FD&C blue #1
Denquel (Procter & Gamble)	calcium carbonate silica magnesium aluminum silicate		potassium nitrate	sodium lauryl sulfate	glycerin, sorbitol, cellulose gum, sodium saccharin, flavor
Dentagard[b] (Colgate-Palmolive)	hydrated silica		sodium monofluorophosphate, 0.76%	sodium lauryl sulfate	sorbitol, glycerin, PEG-12, flavor, sodium benzoate, titanium dioxide, cellulose gum, sodium saccharin, FD&C red #40

TOOTHPASTE PRODUCT TABLE, continued

Product (Manufacturer)	Abrasive Ingredient	Relative Abrasivity[a]	Therapeutic Ingredient	Foaming Agent	Other Ingredients
Extar (Extar)	magnesium oxide calcium carbonate sodium polymetaphosphate silica gel			sodium lauryl sulfate	tragacanth, sodium saccharin, spralene mint, mint oil, flavor, menthol
Extar Dentifrice Powder (Extar)	sodium polymetaphosphate sodium phosphate				sequestrene, sodium saccharin
Gleem (Procter & Gamble)	calcium pyrophosphate		sodium fluoride, 0.22%	blend of anionic surfactants	glycerin, sorbitol, cellulose gum, flavor
Kolynos (Whitehall)	dicalcium phosphate			sodium lauryl sulfate	
Listerine (Warner-Lambert)	dicalcium phosphate				
Macleans Fluoride Toothpaste[h] (SmithKline Beecham)	calcium carbonate, 38% magnesium aluminum silicate		sodium monofluorophosphate, 0.76%	sodium lauryl sulfate, 1.15%	glycerin, 26%; cellulose gum; flavor; sodium saccharin; sodium silicate; sodium benzoate
Pearl Drops Stainfighting Toothpolish (Carter)	dicalcium phosphate dihydrate dicalcium phosphate			sodium lauryl sulfate	sorbitol, glycerin, cellulose gum, flavor, sodium saccharin, methylparaben
Pearl Drops Stainfighting Toothpolish Gel with Fluoride - Tartar Control (Carter)	hydrated silica		sodium fluoride	sodium lauryl sulfate	sorbitol, tetrapotassium pyrophosphate, tetrasodium pyrophosphate, PEG-12, flavor, cellulose gum, sodium saccharin, FD&C blue #1, FD&C yellow #10
Pearl Drops Stainfighting Toothpolish with Fluoride - Tartar Control (Carter)	hydrated silica		sodium fluoride	sodium lauryl sulfate	sorbitol, glycerin, tetrapotassium pyrophosphate, tetrasodium pyrophosphate, PEG-12, flavor, titanium dioxide, cellulose gum, sodium saccharin
Pearl Drops Toothpolish Gel with Fluoride (Carter)	hydrated silica		sodium monofluorophosphate	sodium lauryl sulfate	sorbitol, glycerin, PEG-12, flavor, cellulose gum, trisodium phosphate, sodium phosphate, sodium saccharin, FD&C blue #1
Pearl Drops Toothpolish with Fluoride (Carter)	aluminum hydroxide hydrated silica		sodium monofluorophosphate	sodium lauryl sulfate	glycerin, PEG-12, flavor, titanium dioxide, cellulose gum, trisodium phosphate, sodium phosphate, sodium saccharin
Pepsodent (Lever Bros.)	hydrated alumina dicalcium phosphate dihydrate hydrated silica			sodium lauryl sulfate	sorbitol, PEG-32, cellulose gum, flavor, sodium saccharin, sodium benzoate
Pepsodent Ammoniated Tooth Powder (Lever Bros.)	hydrated alumina hydrated silica			sodium lauryl sulfate	urea, sodium chloride, PEG-32, carrageenan, sodium saccharin, flavor
Pepsodent Tooth Powder (Lever Bros.)	hydrated alumina hydrated silica			sodium lauryl sulfate	PEG-32, carrageenan, sodium saccharin, flavor

TOOTHPASTE PRODUCT TABLE, continued

Product (Manufacturer)	Abrasive Ingredient	Relative Abrasivity[a]	Therapeutic Ingredient	Foaming Agent	Other Ingredients
Promise[b] (Block)	dicalcium phosphate dicalcium phosphate dihydrate silica	1½	potassium nitrate, 5%	sodium lauryl sulfate	glycerin, sorbitol, hydroxy-ethylcellulose, flavor, sodium saccharin, parabens, FD&C yellow #10, FD&C blue #1
Protect[c] (John O. Butler)		1	dibasic sodium citrate, 2% (in a pleuronic gel)		
Pycopay Tooth Powder (Block)	sodium bicarbonate calcium carbonate magnesium carbonate tricalcium phosphate				flavor sodium chloride
Revelation Tooth Powder (Alvin Last)	calcium carbonate			soap	menthol, wintergreen oil
Sensodyne[b] (Block)	diatomaceous earth silica		strontium chloride hexahydrate	sodium methyl cocoyltaurate	glycerin, sorbitol, hydroxy-ethylcellulose, flavor, guar gum, titanium dioxide, PEG-40 stearate, sodium saccharin, parabens
Sensodyne Mint (Block)	dicalcium phosphate dihydrate dicalcium phosphate silica		potassium nitrate, 5%	sodium lauryl sulfate	glycerin, sorbitol, hydroxy-ethylcellulose, flavor, sodium saccharin, parabens, FD&C yellow #10, FD&C blue #1
Thermodent (Mentholatum)	diatomaceous earth silica		strontium chloride hexahydrate	sodium methyl cocoyltaurate	sorbitol, glycerin, titanium dioxide, hydroxyethylcellulose, flavor, preservative
Topol Smoker's Toothpolish (Jeffrey Martin)	dicalcium phosphate magnesium aluminum silicate			sodium lauryl sulfate	sorbitol, propylene glycol, sodium saccharin, parabens, cellulose gum, flavor
Topol Smoker's Toothpolish with Fluoride (Jeffrey Martin)	insoluble sodium metaphosphate dicalcium phosphate magnesium aluminum silicate silica		sodium fluoride	sodium lauryl sulfate	sorbitol, glycerin, sodium carrageenan, flavor, cellulose gum, sodium saccharin, parabens, titanium dioxide
Ultra Brite (Colgate-Palmolive)	hydrated silica alumina		sodium monofluorophosphate, 0.76%	sodium lauryl sulfate	glycerin, cellulose gum, sodium benzoate, titanium dioxide, sodium saccharin, flavor
Viadent Fluoride (Vipont)	hydrated silica		sodium monofluorophosphate	sodium lauryl sulfate	sanguinaria extract, sorbitol, titanium dioxide, carboxymethylcellulose, flavor, sodium saccharin, citric acid, zinc chloride
Viadent Original (Vipont)	dicalcium phosphate			sodium lauryl sulfate	sanguinaria extract, glycerin, sorbitol, titanium dioxide, zinc chloride, carrageenan, flavor, sodium saccharin, citric acid

[a] *Consumer Reports, 140,* March (1984).
[b] Indicates ADA "Seal of Approval" and acceptance by the Council on Dental Therapeutics.
[c] Indicates provisional ADA approval.

ARTIFICIAL SALIVA PRODUCT TABLE

Product (Manufacturer)	Form Supplied	Ingredients
Moi-Stir (Kingswood Lab)	pump spray bottle	solution: dibasic sodium phosphate; magnesium, calcium, sodium and potassium chlorides; sorbitol; sodium carboxymethylcellulose; parabens; mint flavor
Moi-Stir Swabsticks (Kingswood Lab)	sticks	solution: dibasic sodium phosphate; magnesium, calcium, sodium and potassium chlorides; sorbitol; sodium carboxymethylcellulose; parabens
Moi-Stir 10 (Kingswood Lab)	pump spray	solution: sodium carboxymethylcellulose, potassium chloride, dibasic sodium phosphate, parabens
Orex (Young Dental)	plastic squeeze bottle	solution: monobasic and dibasic potassium phosphates; magnesium, potassium, calcium and sodium chlorides; sodium fluoride; sorbitol solution; sodium carboxymethylcellulose; methylparaben
Saliv-Aid (Copley)	liquid	NS[a]
Saliva Substitute (Roxane)	squirt bottle	solution: sorbitol, sodium carboxymethylcellulose, methylparaben
Salivart (Westport Pharmaceuticals)	aerosol can (nitrogen propellant)	solution: sodium carboxymethylcellulose; sorbitol; sodium, potassium, calcium and magnesium chlorides; dibasic potassium phosphate; nitrogen (as propellant)
Xero-Lube (Scherer)	pump spray or squeeze bottle	solution: monobasic and dibasic potassium phosphates; magnesium, potassium, calcium and sodium chlorides; sodium fluoride; sorbitol solution; sodium carboxymethylcellulose; methylparaben

[a] Ingredients not specified.

MOUTHWASH PRODUCT TABLE

Product (Manufacturer)	Antiseptic	Anesthetic	Astringent	Other Ingredients
Act[a] (Johnson & Johnson)	alcohol, 7% (cinnamon flavor) 8% (mint flavor)			sodium fluoride, 0.05% tartrazine (mint flavor) flavor
Alkaline Aromatic Tablets (Vale)				sodium chloride, 5 gr sodium bicarbonate, 5 gr sodium borate, 5 gr sodium benzoate, 7/24 gr sodium salicylate, 7/24 gr
Amosan (Oral-B)	sodium peroxyborate			saccharin flavor
Cepacol (Lakeside)	alcohol, 14% cetylpyridinium chloride, 1:2000			phosphate buffers aromatics
Chloraseptic Mouthwash/Gargle[b] **and Throat Spray**[b] (Richardson-Vicks)	phenol, 1.4%			saccharin menthol and cherry flavor
Fluorigard Anti-Cavity Fluoride Rinse[a] (Colgate-Palmolive)				sodium fluoride, 0.05%
Gly-Oxide (Marion)	carbamide peroxide, 10%			citric acid flavor glycerin propylene glycol sodium stannate
Green Mint Mouthwash (Block)	alcohol			chlorophyll sorbitol surfactant flavor
Isodettes Sore Throat Spray Cherry & Menthol (Goody's)	phenol sodium phenolate			flavor propylene glycol sodium hydroxide FD&C red #40 D&C yellow #10 (menthol) FD&C blue #1 (cherry)
Lavoris (DEP)	alcohol		zinc chloride	glycerin polysorbate 80 citric acid flavor poloxamer 407 clove oil
Larylgan[b] (Whitehall)	ethyl alcohol			antipyrine, 0.3% pyrilamine maleate, 0.05% sodium caprylate, 0.5% saccharin menthol gentian violet methyl salicylate benzyl alcohol glycerin castor oil parabens other aromatics

MOUTHWASH PRODUCT TABLE, continued

Product (Manufacturer)	Antiseptic	Anesthetic	Astringent	Other Ingredients
Listerine (Warner-Lambert)	alcohol, 26.9%			menthol methyl salicylate eucalyptol thymol
Listermint (Warner-Lambert)	alcohol, 12.8%		zinc chloride	glycerin poloxamer 407 saccharin sodium sodium citrate citric acid flavor sodium lauryl sulfate
Listermint with Fluoride (Warner-Lambert)	alcohol, 6.65%		zinc chloride	sodium fluoride, 0.02% glycerin poloxamer 407 sodium lauryl sulfate sodium citrate flavor sodium saccharin citric acid D&C yellow #10 FD&C green #3
Mouthwash and Gargle (McKesson)	cetylpyridinium chloride alcohol, 14%			saccharin D&C green #5
Odara (Lorvic)	phenol, 2% alcohol, 48%		zinc chloride	glycerin potassium iodide methyl salicylate eucalyptus oil myrrh tincture
Ora Fresh (Cinnamon)[b,c] (A.V.P.)			zinc chloride	sodium benzoate methylparaben propylene glycol saccharin flavor
Ora Fresh (Peppermint)[b,c] (A.V.P.)	phenol sodium phenate			propylene glycol glycerin flavor saccharin
Orasept Throat Spray (Pharmakon)	ethanol, 53.83% methylbenzethonium chloride, 1.04%	benzocaine, 1%		glycerin sorbitol solution, 70% peppermint oil menthol calcium saccharin D&C green #5
Perimed (Olin)	hydrogen peroxide, 1.5% povidone-iodine, 5%			saccharin
Peroxyl Mouthrinse (Colgate-Hoyt)	hydrogen peroxide, 1.5% alcohol, 6%			mint flavor
Scope (Procter & Gamble)	cetylpyridinium chloride, 0.45% domiphen bromide, 0.005% alcohol, 18.5%			tartrazine wintergreen flavor saccharin
Sore Throat Relief Formula (DeWitt)	phenol, sodium phenolate (total phenol 1.4%)			menthol

MOUTHWASH PRODUCT TABLE, continued

Product (Manufacturer)	Antiseptic	Anesthetic	Astringent	Other Ingredients
S.T. 37 (SmithKline Beecham)	hexylresorcinol, 0.1%			glycerin
Sucrets Maximum Strength Mouthwash/Gargle[b] and Throat Spray[b] (SmithKline Beecham)	alcohol, 10%	dyclonine hydrochloride, 0.1%		sorbitol mint flavor
Viadent (Vipont)	alcohol		zinc chloride, 0.2%	sanguinaria extract glycerin polysorbate 80 flavor sodium saccharin poloxamer 407 citric acid

[a] Indicates ADA "Seal of Approval" and acceptance by the Council on Dental Therapeutics.
[b] Sugar free.
[c] Alcohol free.

DENTURE CLEANSER PRODUCT TABLE

Product (Manufacturer)	Ingredients
Complete (Vicks)	calcium carbonate, sodium lauryl sulfate, silica, magnesium aluminum silicate
Denalan (Whitehall)	sodium percarbonate, 30%; sodium tripolyphosphate; sodium sulfate; sodium lauryl sulfate; flavor
Denclenz Liquid Denture Cleaner (Sandoz)	hydrochloric acid and detergents in a brush/bottle applicator
Dentu-Creme Denture Toothpaste (Block)	dicalcium phosphate dihydrate, propylene glycol, calcium carbonate, silica, sodium lauryl sulfate, glycerin, hydroxyethylcellulose, flavor, magnesium aluminum silicate, sodium saccharin, parabens
Divi-Dent Denture Cleanser (Block)	sorbitol, triethanolamine lauryl sulfate, silica, trisodium EDTA
Efferdent Tablets (Warner-Lambert)	potassium monopersulfate, sodium borate perhydrate, sodium carbonate, sodium lauryl sulfoacetate, sodium bicarbonate, citric acid, magnesium stearate, flavor
Effervescent Denture Tablets (Rexall)	sodium bicarbonate, citric acid, sodium perborate, sodium acid pyrophosphate, sodium benzoate, trisodium phosphate, sodium lauryl sulfate, poloxamer 188, sorbitol, silica, peppermint oil, povidone
Extar Denture Cleanser (Extar)	sodium polymetaphosphate, sodium saccharin, parabens, peppermint, sodium phosphate, sequestrene, lactose
K.I.K. (K.I.K. Co)	sodium perborate, 25%; trisodium phosphate, 75%
Kleenite (Vicks)	sodium chloride, trisodium phosphate, sodium perborate, sodium dichloroisocyanurate, sodium lauryl sulfate, disodium EDTA
Mersene Denture Cleaner (Colgate-Palmolive)	troclosene potassium, sodium perborate, trisodium phosphate
Polident Denture Cleanser Powder (Block)	sodium perborate monohydrate, potassium monopersulfate, sodium carbonate, sodium acid pyrophosphate, surfactant, sodium bicarbonate, fragrance
Polident Tablets (Block)	potassium monopersulfate, sodium perborate monohydrate, sodium carbonate, surfactant, chelating agents, proteolytic enzyme, sodium bicarbonate, citric acid, fragrance
Smokers' Polident Denture Cleanser Tablets (Block)	sodium carbonate, potassium monopersulfate, citric acid, sodium bicarbonate, sodium perborate monohydrate, surfactant, chelating agent, proteolytic enzyme, fragrance

DENTURE ADHESIVE PRODUCT TABLE

Product (Manufacturer)	Ingredients
Brace (SmithKline Beecham)	cellulose gum, 25%; methyl vinyl ether-maleic anhydride and/or acid copolymer, 15%; povidone, 10%; petrolatum, 34.9%; mineral oil, 14.9%; flavor, 0.2%
Confident (Block)	carboxymethylcellulose gum, 32%; ethylene oxide polymer, 13%; petrolatum, 42%; liquid petrolatum, 12%; propylparaben, 0.05%
Corega Powder (Block)	karaya gum, 94.6%; water-soluble ethylene oxide polymer, 5%; flavor, 0.4%
Dentrol Liquid Denture Adhesive (Block)	carboxymethylcellulose sodium, ethylene oxide polymer, mineral oil, polyethylene, flavor, propylparaben
Effergrip Denture Adhesive Cream (Warner-Lambert)	carboxymethylcellulose sodium, 39%; cationic polyacrylamide polymer, 10%
Fasteeth (Vicks)	karaya gum, calcium sodium poly(vinyl methyl-ether maleate), carboxymethylcellulose sodium, sodium borate
Fasteeth Extra Hold (Vicks)	calcium sodium poly(vinyl methyl-ether maleate), carboxymethylcellulose sodium
Firmdent (Moyco)	karaya gum, sodium borate, peppermint flavor
Fixodent (Vicks)	calcium sodium poly(vinyl methyl-ether maleate), petrolatum base, carboxymethylcellulose sodium
Orafix (SmithKline Beecham)	karaya gum, 51%; petrolatum, 30%; mineral oil, 13%; peppermint oil, 0.08%
Orafix Medicated (SmithKline Beecham)	benzocaine, 2%; allantoin, 0.2%; karaya gum, 51%; petrolatum, 28%; mineral oil, 13%; peppermint oil, 0.08%
Orafix Special (SmithKline Beecham)	cellulose gum, 25%; methyl vinyl ether-maleic anhydride and/or acid copolymer, 15%; povidone, 10%; petrolatum, 34.9%; mineral oil, 14.9%; flavor, 0.2%
Orahesive Powder (Colgate-Hoyt)	gelatin, 33.3%; pectin, 33.3%; carboxymethylcellulose sodium, 33.3%
Permagrip Denture Adhesive Cream and Powder (Lactona)	carboxymethylcellulose sodium, cationic polyacrylamide
Polident Dentu-Grip (Block)	carboxymethylcellulose gum, 49%; ethylene oxide polymer, 21%; flavor, 0.4%
Poli-Grip (Block)	karaya gum, 51%; petrolatum, 36.7%; liquid petrolatum, 9.4%; magnesium oxide, 2.7%; propylparaben; flavor
Sea-Bond (Combe)	ethylene oxide polymer, sodium alginate
Staze (Commerce)	karaya gum, 46.23%; petrolatum, 48.4%
Super Poli-Grip (Block)	carboxymethylcellulose sodium, ethylene oxide polymer, petrolatum, mineral oil, flavor, propylparaben
Super Poli-Grip Powder (Block)	calcium sodium methyl vinyl ether-maleic anhydride copolymer, carboxymethylcellulose sodium, flavor
Wernet's Cream (Block)	carboxymethylcellulose gum, 32%; petrolatum, 42%; mineral oil, 12%; ethylene oxide polymer, 13%; propylparaben, 0.05%; flavor, 0.5%
Wernet's Powder (Block)	karaya gum, 94.6%; water-soluble ethylene oxide polymer, 5%; flavor, 0.4%

TOOTHACHE/COLD SORE/CANKER SORE PRODUCT TABLE

Product (Manufacturer)	Anesthetic	Other Ingredients
Amosan (Oral-B)		sodium peroxyborate monohydrate; sodium bitartrate; saccharin; peppermint, menthol and vanilla flavors
Anbesol Gel (Whitehall)	benzocaine, 6.3%	phenol, 0.5%; alcohol, 70%; viscous water-soluble base
Anbesol Liquid (Whitehall)	benzocaine, 6.3%	phenol, 0.5%; povidone-iodine (0.04% available iodine); alcohol, 70%
Anbesol, Maximum Strength Gel and Liquid (Whitehall)	benzocaine, 20%	alcohol, 60%
Babee Teething Lotion[a] (Pfeiffer)	benzocaine, 2.5%	cetalkonium chloride, 0.02%; alcohol, 20%; hamamelis water; propylene glycol; sodium benzoate; urea; menthol; camphor
Baby Anbesol Gel (Whitehall)	benzocaine, 7.5%	viscous water-soluble base without alcohol
Baby Orajel (Commerce)	benzocaine, 7.5%	FD&C red #40, flavor, glycerin, polyethylene glycols, sodium saccharin, sorbic acid, sorbitol
Baby Orajel Nighttime Formula (Commerce)	benzocaine, 10%	FD&C red #40, flavor, glycerin, polyethylene glycols, sodium saccharin, sorbic acid, sorbitol
Benzodent (Vicks)	benzocaine, 20% eugenol, 0.4%	hydroxyquinoline sulfate, 0.1%; denture adhesive-like base
Betadine Mouthwash/Gargle (Purdue Frederick)		povidone-iodine, 0.5%; alcohol, 8.8%
Blistex Lip Ointment (Blistex)		camphor, 0.5%; phenol, 0.5%; allantoin, 1%
Butyn Dental Ointment (Abbott)	butacaine, 4% eugenol	benzyl alcohol, ≈ 1%; lanolin; petrolatum; white wax; natural flavor
Campho-Phenique Gel and Liquid (Winthrop)	phenol, 4.7%	camphor, 10.8%
Cankaid (Becton Dickinson)		carbamide peroxide, 10%; anhydrous glycerol
Cold Sore Lotion (Pfeiffer)		gum benzoin, 7%; alcohol, 85%
Dalidyne (Dalin)	benzocaine	methylbenzethonium chloride; tannic acid; camphor; chlorothymol; menthol; benzyl alcohol; alcohol, 61%; aromatic base
Dent's Dental Poultice (C.S. Dent)	benzocaine, 16.6%	oleoresin capsicum, 0.25%; oxyquinoline, 1.82%; thymol, 0.91%; glycerin mineral oil; polyoxyethylene sorbitan monoleate
Dent's 3 in 1 Toothache Relief (C.S. Dent)	eugenol (drops, gum) benzocaine (gel, gum)	alcohol, 60% (drops); chlorobutanol anhydrous, 0.09% (drops)
Dent's Toothache Drops (C.S. Dent)	eugenol	alcohol, 60%; chlorobutanol, 0.09%; propylene glycol
Dent's Toothache Gum (C.S. Dent)	benzocaine eugenol	petrolatum; cotton and wax base
Double-Action Kit (C.S. Dent)	eugenol, 7.5%	denatured alcohol, 60%; chlorobutanol, 0.09%; with acetaminophen tablets, 325 mg
Dr. Hands Teething Gel and Lotion (Roberts)		tincture of pellitory; hamamelis water; alcohol, 10%; clove oil; menthol
Foille Plus Spray (Blistex)	benzocaine, 5%	chloroxylenol, 0.6%

TOOTHACHE/COLD SORE/CANKER SORE PRODUCT TABLE, continued

Product (Manufacturer)	Anesthetic	Other Ingredients
Herpecin-L (Campbell)		pyridoxine hydrochloride, allantoin, padimate 0, titanium dioxide
HVS 1 + 2 (Chemi-Tech)		benzalkonium chloride
Jiffy (Block)	benzocaine eugenol	alcohol, 56.5%
Jiffy Toothache Drops (Block)	benzocaine, 5% eugenol, 9%	menthol, 2%; SD alcohol 38-B, 76%
Kank-A Liquid Professional Strength (Blistex)	benzocaine, 20%	cetyl pyridinium chloride, 0.5%; ethylcellulose film formers
Lip Medex (Blistex)		camphor, 1%; phenol, 0.5%
Lotion-Jel (C.S. Dent)	benzocaine	
Numzident Gel (Goody's)	benzocaine, 10%	flavor; glycerin; PEG-8; PEG-75; sodium saccharin
Numzit Cold Sore Lotion (Goody's)	benzocaine, 6.3% phenol, 0.5%	menthol; clove oil; povidone-iodine; alcohol, 70%
Numzit Gel (Goody's)	benzocaine, 7.5%	PEG-8; PEG-75; sodium saccharin; clove oil; peppermint oil
Numzit Lotion (Goody's)	alcohol, 12% benzocaine, 0.2%	sodium alginate; sodium saccharin; glycerin; methylparaben; FD&C blue #1; FD&C red #40; alcohol, 12%
Orabase-B with Benzocaine (Colgate-Hoyt)	benzocaine, 20%	pectin; gelatin; carboxymethylcellulose sodium; polyethylene; mineral oil
Orabase-O (Colgate-Hoyt)	benzocaine, 20%	polyethylene; mineral oil
Orabase Plain (Colgate-Hoyt)		pectin; gelatin; carboxymethylcellulose sodium; polyethylene; mineral oil
Orajel[a] (Commerce)	benzocaine, 10%	saccharin
Orajel CSM (Commerce)	benzocaine, 10%	tannic acid, 6%; benzalkonium chloride, 0.125%
Orajel-D[a] (Commerce)	benzocaine, 10% eugenol	saccharin
Orajel Maximum Strength (Commerce)	benzocaine, 20%	clove oil; flavor; polyethylene glycols; sodium saccharin; sorbic acid
Orajel Mouth-Aid[a] (Commerce)	benzocaine, 20%	benzalkonium chloride, 0.12%; zinc chloride, 0.1%; allantoin; flavor; polyethylene glycols; propyl gallate; propylene glycol; sodium saccharin; sorbic acid; trisodium EDTA
Orasept Liquid (Pharmakon)	benzocaine, 1.53%	tannic acid, 12.16%; methylbenzethonium chloride, 1.53%; denatured ethyl alcohol 38B, 53.31%; camphor; menthol; benzyl alcohol; spearmint oil; oil of cassia
Peroxyl (Colgate-Hoyt)		hydrogen peroxide, 1.5%; mint flavor
Peroxyl Mouthrinse (Colgate-Hoyt)		hydrogen peroxide, 1.5%; alcohol, 6%; mint flavor
Pfeiffer's Cold Sore (Pfeiffer)		gum benzoin, 7%; camphor; menthol; thymol; eucalyptol; alcohol, 85%

TOOTHACHE/COLD SORE/CANKER SORE PRODUCT TABLE, continued

Product (Manufacturer)	Anesthetic	Other Ingredients
Poloris Dental Poultice (Block)	benzocaine, 7.5 mg/ poultice	capsicum
Proxigel (Reed & Carnrick)		carbamate peroxide, 11%; water-free gel base
Red Cross Toothache Medication (Mentholatum)	eugenol, 85%	sesame oil
Rid-A-Pain Dental Drops[a] (Pfeiffer)	benzocaine, 2.5%	cetalkonium chloride, 0.02%; alcohol, 20%
Rid-A-Pain Gel[a] (Pfeiffer)	benzocaine, 10%	alcohol, 7.5%
Stopzit (Goody's)	denatonium benzoate monohydrate, 0.3%	isopropyl alcohol, butyl acetate, ethylcellulose, SD alcohol
Tanac[a] (Commerce)		benzalkonium chloride, 0.4%; tannic acid, 2.858%
Tanac Liquid[a] (Commerce)	benzocaine, 10%	tannic acid, 6%; benzalkonium chloride, 0.125%; saccharin
Tanac Roll-On[a] (Commerce)	benzocaine, 5%	tannic acid, 6%; benzalkonium chloride, 0.125%; saccharin
Tanac Stick[a] (Commerce)	benzocaine, 7.5%	tannic acid, 6%; benzalkonium chloride, 0.125%; allantoin, 0.2%; octyl dimethyl PABA, 0.75%; saccharin

[a]Sugar free.

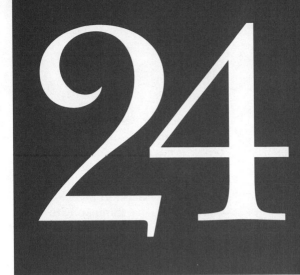

Michael L. Kleinberg
and Melba C. Connors

OSTOMY CARE PRODUCTS

*Q*uestions to ask in patient/consumer counseling

What type of ostomy do you have? Where is it located?

How long have you had the ostomy?

Do you irrigate and/or use a pouch?

What type of appliance are you using?

What is the stoma size?

Do you have problems with the skin surrounding the stoma?

Have you noticed any change in the contents of your fecal discharge or urinary output?

Are you experiencing any problems related to your ostomy such as diarrhea or gas?

Are you having any problems with odor or gas control?

Are you taking any prescription or nonprescription medications?

An ostomy is the surgical formation of an opening, or outlet, through the abdominal wall for the purpose of eliminating waste. It is usually made by passing the colon, small intestine, or ureters through the abdominal wall. The opening of the ostomy is called the stoma. (The anatomy of the lower digestive tract is shown in Figure 1.) Major functions of the digestive system include digestion and absorption of food stuffs and absorption of water. Digestion begins in the mouth and continues in the stomach and small intestine; water absorption takes place in the large intestine. (See Chapter 11, *Antacid Products*, and Chapter 13, *Antidiarrheal and Other Gastrointestinal Products*.)

An understanding of the digestive process is important because ostomy surgery interrupts this process. The particular problems associated with each type of ostomy are directly related to the phase of digestion that is interrupted.

Ostomy surgery necessitates the use of an appliance designed to collect the waste material normally eliminated through the bowel or bladder. Approximately 90,000 ostomies are created annually in the United States, and more than 1 million patients have established stomas (1).

The idea of cutting into the abdominal cavity and creating an artificial opening is not new. This type of surgery was first suggested in 1710 by a French physician, Alexis Littre (2). Since that time, the technique of ostomy surgery has been refined greatly. The surgical creation of a stoma is only the first step in the rehabilitation of an ostomate (a person with an ostomy). Complete recovery depends on how well ostomy patients understand and adjust to their changed medical and physical circumstances.

Because each ostomy patient is different, one patient may benefit from one type of appliance, while another may develop problems with it. The ostomy patient should be familiar with applying and fitting an appliance that affords maximum benefit.

Pharmacists who are involved in ostomy care must be familiar with the various types of ostomies and with the use and maintenance of the appliances for each type of surgery. They should also be prepared to provide patients with information on problems related to ostomy care such as skin care, diet, fluid intake, and drug therapy.

Pharmacy involvement in ostomy care is important. The American Pharmaceutical Association identifies ostomy care as a clinical role for the pharmacist in direct patient care. The American Society of Hospital Pharmacists specifies experience in ostomy care in the accreditation standards for residency training. Procurement and distribution of ostomy supplies and patient counseling are necessary services that can be provided by the pharmacist.

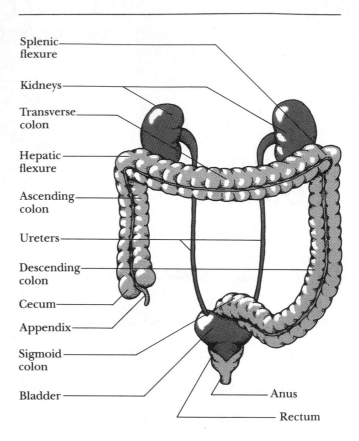

FIGURE 1   Anatomy of the lower digestive and urinary tracts.

TYPES OF OSTOMIES

Several types of ostomies are performed regularly. They include ileostomy, in which the entire colon and possibly part of the ileum are removed; colostomy (ascending, transverse, descending, and sigmoid), in which the colon is partially removed; and urostomy or urinary diversion, in which the bladder may be removed. A discussion of each type follows. Special problems affecting patients often depend on the location of the ostomy. Skin irritation and electrolyte and fluid imbalance cause more problems in ostomates with a fluid or semisoft stoma discharge. This is a factor for ileostomates, for ascending and transverse colostomates, and for those with a urinary diversion. Urostomates and ileostomates may also experience an increased incidence in kidney and gallbladder stone formation. Constipation may be a problem in patients with descending and sigmoid colostomies.

Ileostomy

An ileostomy is a surgically created opening between the ileum and abdominal wall. Reasons to have

ileostomy surgery include ulcerative colitis, Crohn's disease, trauma, familial polyposis, or necrotizing enterocolitis. The two most common disorders requiring ileostomy surgery, ulcerative colitis and Crohn's disease, are inflammatory conditions affecting the intestines. Ulcerative colitis affects the large intestine and rectum. Its clinical course is often prolonged, with the patient experiencing remissions and exacerbations. Crohn's disease may involve any part of the gastrointestinal (GI) tract. As the disease progresses, the bowel wall thickens, causing the lumen to narrow. Obstruction may result, requiring surgery. Patients with these diseases may develop debilitating extraintestinal manifestations. In an acute episode, toxic megacolon and perforation are possible. These conditions require surgery. The entire colon is surgically removed, and the ileum is brought to the surface of the abdomen (Figure 2A).

It should be mentioned that a total proctocolectomy, which results in an ileostomy, is considered a cure for the ulcerative colitis patient. Because of the possibility of recurrence, coupled with the total loss of large bowel function, the same surgical procedure is less often used in Crohn's disease.

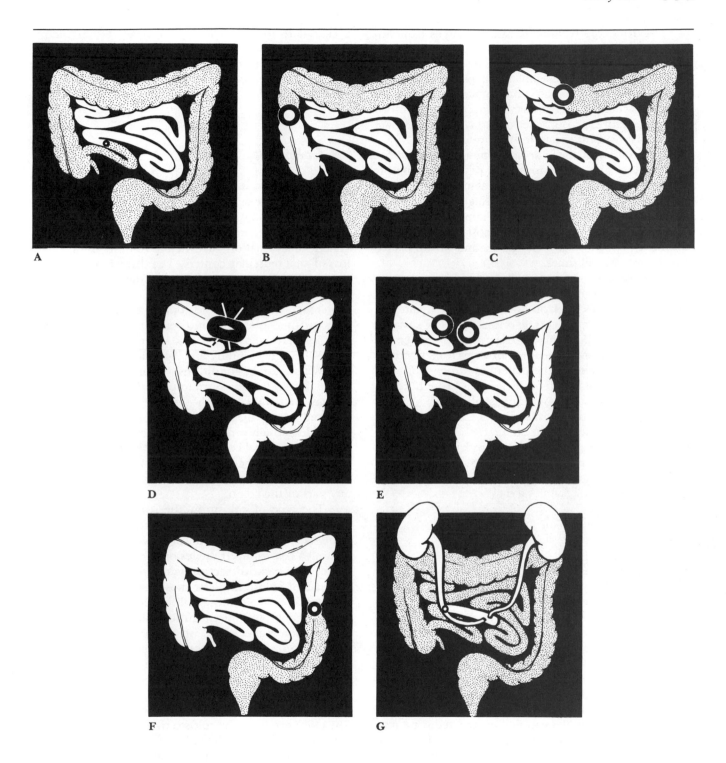

FIGURE 2A-G   Types of ostomies. A, Ileostomy. B, Ascending colon. C, Transverse colostomy. D, Loop ostomy. E, Double-barrel colostomy. F, Descending or sigmoid colostomy. G, Ileal conduit. Adapted from the "Hollister Ostomy Reference Chart," © Copyright 1978, 1979, 1980, Hollister, Incorporated (all rights reserved) and from J. R. Wuest, *J. Am. Pharm. Assoc., NS15*, 626 (1975).

The discharge from an ileostomy ranges from liquid to semisoft because it contains fluid that normally would be absorbed from the large bowel. For this reason, it is especially important for ileostomates to pay close attention to adequate fluid intake. When the colon is removed, the body loses the capacity to reabsorb water. Therefore, ileostomates must maintain adequate fluid intake to compensate for this water loss.

Excoriation of the skin is a common problem for ileostomates. The continuous flow of liquid, semisoft discharge contains active pancreatic enzymes that irritate and digest unprotected skin. Diligent hygiene and special protective measures can help prevent these problems. Patients with standard ileostomies are never continent. The flow is continuous, and an appliance must be worn at all times.

Researchers are continually working on ways to render the ileostomate continent. One procedure, developed by Dr. Nils Kock of Sweden, may be an alternative for those who meet certain criteria (3). The surgeon creates a pouch internally, made from 35–50 cm of ileum. An intussusception of the bowel is used to create a "nipple" that renders the patient continent for stool and flatus. The distal limb of the ileum is brought to the abdomen. A flush stoma is made just above the hairline. The pouch is emptied by inserting a catheter through the nipple into the pouch. At first, the pouch holds approximately 75 ml. It stretches with use so that 6 months postoperatively it can hold 600–800 ml without discomfort or danger. At this time, the pouch needs to be drained only 3 or 4 times a day.

Restorative Proctocolectomy

A newer operation now available involves sparing the rectum of those with ulcerative colitis or familial polyposis. The mucosa is stripped from the rectum, rendering it free of disease. An internal pouch is created from the small bowel, but without a nipple valve. The distal end of the ileum is then pulled through the rectum and is attached. Thus the sphincter is preserved and no ostomy is necessary. Because of the different ways the internal pouch can be constructed, one may hear this operation described as an "S" or "J" pouch. The recipients of this procedure have more frequent bowel movements and may experience some perianal skin irritation.

Because the diseases and conditions requiring ileostomy surgery are found primarily in persons 15–25 years of age, the advantages of these operations are obvious. For those in the prime of their athletic, social, and sexual life, the absence of an external pouch allows a speedy adjustment and rehabilitation. Not everyone is a candidate for this surgery, however. Other factors taken into consideration are the patient's age (between 15 and 50 is believed to be ideal), intelligence, absence of Crohn's disease, motivation, other handicaps, and general health.

Colostomy

A colostomy is the creation of an artificial opening using part of the large intestine or colon. Major indications for performing a colostomy include obstruction of the colon or rectum, cancer of the colon or rectum, genetic malformation, diverticular disease, trauma, and loss of anal muscular control. The three types of colostomies (Figure 3) are named for the portion of the bowel that is brought to the outside of the body to form the stoma: ascending colostomies; transverse colostomies (further subdivided into temporary loop ostomies, double-barrel colostomies, and permanent stoma colostomies); and descending and sigmoid colostomies.

When certain conditions are present in the lower bowel, it may be necessary to perform a temporary colostomy so that the lower bowel can heal. Healing of the diseased bowel may take several weeks, months, or years. Eventually, the colon and rectum are reconnected, and bowel continuity is restored. A permanent colostomy is formed when the rectum is removed. A colostomy, permanent or temporary, may be made in any part of the colon.

The type of colostomy the surgeon will perform depends on the condition being treated. If the disease entity is cancer, the section of bowel may be resected without a colostomy. If the lesion is in the lower rectum, however, the entire rectum is removed, resulting in a permanent colostomy. The most common disease that may result in a colostomy is diverticulitis. It presents as small "balloon-like" areas in the lining of the large intestine. Sometimes these areas become irritated and rupture, resulting in peritonitis, which usually requires emergency surgery. To protect the perforated section and/or the suture line when this area is surgically removed, a temporary colostomy may be performed. This can be made at any point in the bowel above the lesion. The more proximal the colostomy, the more watery and frequent the output will be. When the disease process is resolved and/or the suture line healed, a comparatively minor operation is performed to restore the continuity of the large intestine.

Ascending Colostomy

The ascending colostomy retains the ascending colon but removes or bypasses the rest of the large bowel. This ostomy appears on the right side of the abdomen

(Figure 2B). Its discharge is semiliquid because the fluid has not been reabsorbed. The patient must wear an appliance continuously.

Transverse Colostomy

In a transverse colostomy, an opening is usually created on the right side of the transverse colon (Figure 2C) in one of two ways. One method entails lifting a loop of the transverse colon through the abdominal incision. A rod or bridge then is placed under the loop to give additional support (Figure 2D) and removed after a few days. Another method is to divide the bowel completely and have two openings (double-barrel colostomy) (Figure 2E). In this case, the proximal stoma discharges fecal material, and the distal stoma secretes small amounts of mucus. Although the remaining colon increases its hydrating function with time, the discharge generally stays semisoft. Generally, irrigation does not

produce control in those with transverse colostomies; therefore, an appliance is worn continuously.

Descending and Sigmoid Colostomies

Descending and sigmoid ostomies are on the left side of the abdomen (Figure 2F). They can be made as double-barrel or single-barrel openings. Because the fecal discharge is firm and often can be regulated by irrigation, an appliance may not be needed. However, many patients prefer appliances to irrigation. Several factors that should be considered in connection with the decision to irrigate include (4):

- The capability of the patient to manage the irrigation procedure;

- The prognosis of the patient;

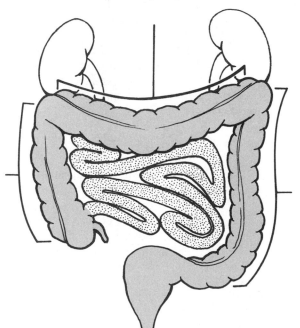

Transverse colon

Colostomy type/duration
usually loop, or double-barrel
and temporary (4-6 weeks)

Stool
soft, unformed; active digestive
enzymes may be present

Ascending colon

Colostomy type/duration
usually loop and temporary
(4-8 weeks)

Stool
liquid to soft; unformed with
active digestive enzymes
present

**Descending or
sigmoid colon**

Colostomy type/duration
usually end matured and
permanent

Stool
formed; usually no digestive
enzymes present

FIGURE 3 Colostomy care based on location and permanence. Copyright© 1977, American Journal of Nursing Company. Adapted with permission from *Am. J. Nurs., 77 (3)*, 443 (1977).

- The presence of either stomal stenosis or peristomal hernia;
- The presence of radiation enteritis.

Urinary Diversions

Urinary diversions are performed as a result of bladder loss or dysfunction usually caused by cancer, neurogenic bladder, or genetic malformation. An ileal or colon conduit is created by implanting the ureters into an isolated loop of bowel, the distal end of which is brought to the surface of the abdomen (Figure 2G). An appliance is worn continuously. Another procedure, a ureterostomy, detaches the ureters from the bladder and brings them to the outside of the abdominal wall. This procedure is performed less frequently because the ureters tend to stenose (narrow) unless they have been dilated permanently by previous disease.

Continent Urostomy

Dr. Kock has now developed an operation to render urinary diversion patients continent. It is very much like the continent ileostomy previously described, except that ureters are inserted into the proximal limb of the ileum leading into the isolated internal ileal pouch and an additional nipple valve is created at the proximal opening of the pouch. This keeps the urine from refluxing back up to the kidneys, thus lessening infection. Other continent urinary operations, such as the "Indiana pouch," are being devised, but they are all similar in that they are drained by a catheter.

APPLIANCES AND ACCESSORIES

The appliance is an extremely important aspect of the ostomate's well-being. The ostomate has lost a normal functioning body process; the appliance takes over that lost function and seemingly becomes a part of the body. The type of appliance depends on the type of surgery performed. Patients with regulated colostomies (who irrigate routinely with no output from the stoma between irrigations) may wear closed-end appliances or a gauze square. Those with unregulated colostomies and ileostomies usually wear open-end appliances to

allow frequent emptying. The ideal appliance should be leak-proof, comfortable, easily manipulated, odor-proof, inconspicuous, inexpensive, and safe (5). Unfortunately, no one appliance meets all these criteria. Major manufacturers of ostomy products and accessories are listed in the appendix to this chapter.

Appliances

In the past, most ostomy appliances were reusable. The advantages of reusable appliances are their durability, availability in many complexities, and relatively low cost. Their disadvantages are that they require cleaning before each use and that they are heavy, tend to retain odor, and often require a separate skin barrier. Reusable appliances may still be the best choice for some patients because of the many modalities available for treatment.

Most ostomates are now fitted with disposable appliances. Most of these appliances incorporate a skin barrier in each flange, eliminating the need for a separate skin barrier. The disposable equipment is available in one- and two-piece systems. The two-piece system allows the patient to center the flange easily and to change the pouch, if desired, without removing the flange from the skin. The one-piece system is very flat, eliminating a ring that might be noticeable through clothes. The one-piece is also easy to apply because it does not require the dexterity needed for the two-piece system. Some manufacturers offer different depths of convexity, which make the two-piece system available to more people. Reusable and disposable appliances are available in both transparent and opaque styles.

Belts

Special belts attached to various appliances give additional support. Belts are made for specific appliances and generally are not interchangeable. Not all ostomates need to wear belts. Indications for use are a deeply convex faceplate, poor wearing time, activity (especially in children), heavy perspiration, and personal preference. Belts may cause ulcers if worn too tight. To be effective, the belt must be kept even with the belt hooks. If the belt slips up around the waist, it may cause poor adherence and possibly a cut of the stoma.

Skin Barriers

Skin barriers are intended to protect the skin immediately adjacent to the stoma and provide a barrier between the skin and the stoma discharge. They also correct imperfections in the skin surface allowing the appliance to fit securely. Except in patients with urinary diversions, a skin barrier should always be used with the appliance. Skin barriers (e.g., Stomahesive wafers, HolliHesive wafers, and Colly-Seals), powders, and pastes are available for special skin problems. The powder is used on weeping skin. The paste (which is not a glue but has a paste consistency) is used to seal around the stoma and to fill in creases in the skin. These products produce a flat surface for application of other skin barriers.

Skin Protective Dressings

A waterproof dressing can be applied to the skin in a thin film, which might be described as a chemical bandage. After application, the product leaves a thin protective layer on the skin that aids in the removal of adhesive tape and absorbs the stress normally applied to the top layers of the skin when the ostomy appliance is removed. Although these dressings promote skin protection, they do not replace skin barriers such as Stomahesive. When the skin is reddened but unbroken, these preparations briefly protect the skin from the contact agent causing the redness. They also can help to waterproof tape around a draining wound. These dressings come in varying forms: gel, bottle (with brush), spray can, roll-on, and wipe-on packets.

Transparent, semipermeable dressings come in many different sizes, from one used for intravenous sites to a complete body wrap. These dressings are transparent, sterile materials that are sticky on one side, which can be used as a dressing, as a second skin to which appliances are affixed, or as a prophylactic for preventing skin irritation. They take some dexterity to apply, however, and two persons may be needed to apply larger pieces. Op Site, Tegaderm, and Bioclusive are examples of these dressings.

Special Skin Care

Several companies manufacture products especially for the incontinent patient or others at high risk of excoriation. The products include a gentle liquid cleaner that renders output odorless, a cream that can be rubbed into the skin and to which the appliance will adhere, and an ointment that is not water soluble and gives high-grade protection to vulnerable areas where pouching is not appropriate.

Tape

Hypoallergenic tape supports appliances. A strip may be applied across the top, bottom, and sides of the faceplate, with half on the faceplate and half on the skin.

Irrigating Sets

A patient having a colostomy distal to the splenic flexure, who gives no history of an irritable bowel, who is not a child, who does not have a disabling handicap, and who wants to maintain control without a pouch, is a candidate for irrigation. To be safe and effective, a colostomy irrigation set, rather than a standard enema set, should be used. This set consists of a reservoir for the irrigating fluid, a tube, graduated clamp, soft catheter, and a dam (or cone) (Figure 4). Perforation of the bowel is a serious complication of irrigation, but it has almost been eliminated by use of a cone, which is inserted ½ to 1 inch into the colostomy. For those who are not able to

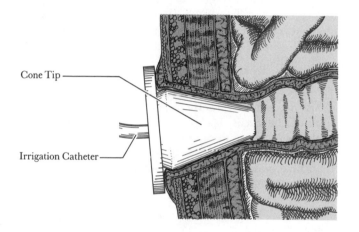

Cone Tip

Irrigation Catheter

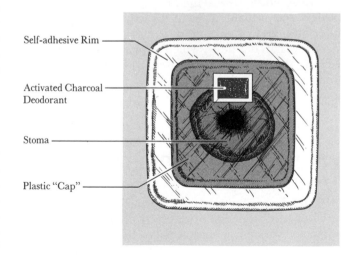

Self-adhesive Rim

Activated Charcoal Deodorant

Stoma

Plastic "Cap"

FIGURE 4 Colostomy irrigation set. A cone-tipped irrigator is preferred to a plain catheter to avoid possibility of false passage and bowel perforation. Copyright © 1978 CIBA-GEIGY Corporation. Adapted with permission from *Clinical Symposia*, illustrated by John A. Craig, M.D. All rights reserved.

use a cone, the catheter should not be inserted more than 2 inches past the dam. Although introducing water into the bowel stimulates peristalsis, control (meaning at least 24 hours without any output) is rarely achieved unless the colostomate instills and holds in a prescribed amount of water. Therefore, the dam, takes the place of the absent sphincter, allowing the patient to hold in the water.

The irrigating set also includes a sleeve that attaches to a faceplate that is held onto the patient by a belt. The distal end of the sleeve is inserted into the toilet. In this way, the returns go into the commode without any waste material to clean up after this procedure. Frequency of irrigation depends somewhat on the colostomate's normal bowel habits. After control, patients may wear a piece of gauze over their stoma or wear a security pouch. The irrigation is not necessary for health. It is merely one method of management.

Deodorizers

Odor control is either local or systemic. Some agents are placed directly in the appliance to mask the odor of the fecal discharge. Liquid concentrates are available as companion products of most ostomy devices; they can be placed directly into the pouch to neutralize odor. Specially formulated bathroom sprays are also available. Ostomates sometimes place aspirin tablets in the pouch for odor control, but this practice should be discouraged because aspirin may irritate the stoma.

In addition to local methods of odor control, other devices are available that fit directly on the pouch to filter and control gas and odors. One commercial device is a charcoal filter, which is placed on the pouch. Newer pouches are formulated with an odor-barrier film.

FITTING AND APPLICATION

Measuring the stoma to determine the proper fit of an appliance is an important part of ostomy care. An appliance with an opening smaller than the stoma may cause abrasion of the stoma and poor wearing time. An appliance with an opening larger than necessary, even with a snug-fitting skin barrier, may allow skin excoriation and hyperplasia formation. Considerations in fitting the appliance include body contour, stoma location, skin creases and scars, and the type of ostomy. The lack of uniformity in types of ostomies and ostomy equipment makes it difficult to give standard instructions for application. Some procedures for applying

different types of appliances and their accessories (Figure 5) are discussed in greater detail in readily available patient-oriented pamphlets (6, 7). An enterostomal therapy (ET) nurse is an excellent resource to aid in the custom fitting of these appliances.

POTENTIAL COMPLICATIONS

Ostomates may experience both psychologic and physical complications. The pharmacist should be prepared to handle these complications or refer the patient to an ET nurse. Preoperatively, a thorough explanation of the type of surgery to be performed, what to expect during the postsurgical recovery period, and the appliances and supplies the patient will use often alleviates the patient's anxiety.

Psychologic Complications

Following ostomy surgery, depending on prior mental status and self-confidence, the patient may be psychologically depressed. There also may be the fear of not being able to engage in former work, participate in sports, perform sexually, or have children. The pharmacist should reassure the patient that the ability to carry out these activities or functions generally remains unchanged. However, the pharmacist should be aware that most males having a radical resection of the rectum or bladder are rendered organically impotent. Penile implants could enable a male to regain part or all of this function. If this is the patient's concern, a referral to his surgeon would be appropriate.

The United Ostomy Association, formed in 1962, is comprised of various ostomy organizations in the United States whose main purpose is to help ostomy patients by giving moral support and supplying information. The United Ostomy Association (36 Executive Park, #120, Irvine, CA 92714, 714-660-8624) sponsors national, regional, and local meetings and publishes a quarterly journal and other literature.

Enterostomal therapy is a comparatively new nursing specialty. Registered nurses with postgraduate education from an accredited school for enterostomal therapy may specialize in ostomy care. A representative listing of ET nurses may be obtained from the Executive Secretary, International Association of Enterostomal Therapy, 2081 Business Center Drive, #290, Irvine, CA 92715, 714-476-0268.

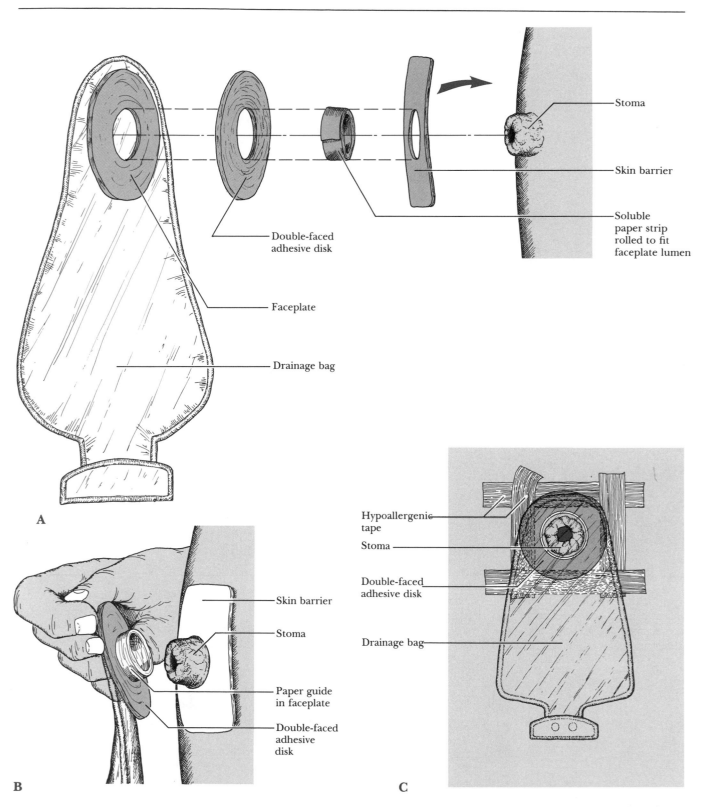

Stoma

Skin barrier

Soluble
paper strip
rolled to fit
faceplate lumen

Double-faced
adhesive disk

Faceplate

Drainage bag

A

Skin barrier

Stoma

Paper guide
in faceplate

Double-faced
adhesive
disk

B

Hypoallergenic
tape

Stoma

Double-faced
adhesive disk

Drainage bag

C

FIGURE 5A-C   Components of an ileostomy appliance. A, Drainable bag and skin barrier. B, After skin barrier is affixed to skin, the appliance is placed, using paper strip guide to align faceplate lumen over stoma. C, Hypoallergenic tape placed around faceplate in "picture frame" fashion.

Physical Complications

Physical complications of ostomies include stenosis of the stoma, fistula formation, prolapse, retraction, and skin irritation. A continuing series of articles concerning physical problems, their assessment, and care have been published in the medical literature (8).

Stenosis

Stenosis, or narrowing of the stoma, is caused by the formation of scar tissue. Excessive scar tissue usually is caused by improper surgical construction, postoperative ischemia, active disease, or alkaline stomatitis or dermatitis. Although dilation of the stoma often is advocated to prevent or palliate this problem, the only cure is revision of the stoma.

Fistula

The formation of an opening, or fistulous tract, from inside the body to the skin most often is a manifestation of inflammatory bowel disease. Other causes of this complication are cancer, abscess formation, foreign body retention, radiation, tuberculosis, and trauma. Treatment includes hyperalimentation and/or surgery.

Prolapse

Prolapse, the abnormal extension of the bowel beyond the abdominal wall, frequently results when the opening in the abdominal wall is too large. The danger of prolapse is the resultant decrease in blood supply to the bowel outside the abdominal cavity. Treatment is surgical correction.

Retraction

Retraction is the recession of the stoma to a subnormal length caused by several factors, including active Crohn's disease. It also may lead to damage of the skin surface. Treatment is surgical correction.

Skin Irritation

Skin irritation can occur from a number of causes, most commonly excoriation from the output, sensitivity to a product, monilial infection, epithelial hyperplasia, alkaline dermatitis, infection, and Crohn's disease.

Output Excoriation   Excoriation, an abrasion of the epidermis by digestive enzymes from output, occurs when an improper pouch is worn, the lumen in the faceplate is too big, or the pouch has leaked without prompt replacement. This allows fecal or urinary output to come in contact with the skin. Fecal output may contain active pancreatic enzymes (especially in the case of an ileostomy) that digest the skin protein. The alkaline nature of the fecal output also is irritating to unprotected skin. Alkaline urine is similarly irritating and causes excoriation. These two conditions are treated differently. After diagnosis and treatment, a skin barrier and pouch may be applied. The pouch should be changed as infrequently as possible to lessen irritation, and treatment should be continued until the skin is clear.

Sensitivity   Preoperative patch testing of patients with a history of allergy, adhesive tape reaction, eczema, psoriasis, and/or those with very fair skin can help prevent skin irritation caused by sensitivity to a product. Patch testing can easily be done by the physician or ET nurse and checked by the patient at home.

Monilial Infection   Yeast manifestation may be a problem in patients wearing appliances continuously. A dark, warm, and moist environment provides an area for growth of species of *Candida*. The primary symptom is itching. If the condition is diagnosed early, an application of nystatin powder is useful. If the infection is allowed to continue unchecked, skin will become denuded, the faceplate will not stick, and additional skin irritation will result from the output. This preparation should be used every other day and for 1 week after skin has become clear.

In treating monoilial infections, it is also important to ascertain whether the ostomate is taking antibiotics. Any antibiotic, but especially a broad-spectrum agent, changes the flora of the skin, and the entrenched monilia become difficult to eradicate. Treatment for ostomy patients taking antibiotics should be given as outlined but continued for 1 month after the yeast is gone.

Hyperplasia   Hyperplasia, the overgrowth of hyperplastic skin, occurs when the faceplate opening is too large. In the early stages, there is no pain, but later the affected skin cells multiply and cause agonizing pain. The condition resembles a mucosal malignancy. To treat the condition, a Colly-Seel is placed over this skin, fitting closely around the stoma. A convex faceplate that fits just $1/16$ inch larger than the stoma is applied, and a snug belt is added. A mild case of hyperplasia generally resolves in 1 week. Severe cases, although treated the same, may take from 1 month to 6 weeks to heal. Other treatment methods are cauterization and surgical removal.

Alkaline Dermatitis   Many patients with urinary diversions have problems with alkaline urine. Although normal urine is not particularly irritating on intact skin, urine that is alkaline may have gross effects on the stoma and skin. It is a major cause of frank blood in the pouch because it renders the stoma extremely friable.

The treatment is to acidify the urine. This can be done by avoiding alkaline ash foods, especially citrus fruits and juices which, although originally acidic, are excreted in alkaline form. Ascorbic acid or cranberry juice acidifies the urine.

The stoma and skin may be soaked with a 50% solution of white vinegar and water. The saturated cloth is renewed with new solution as often as necessary. This treatment must be repeated every 4 hours while the patient is awake. The appliance then can be applied. If the manifestation is mild, this procedure should be conducted once every other day until the skin is clear. Most of the new urinary appliances have an antireflux feature, which keeps the urine from resting on the stoma or exposed skin.

Infection   Ostomates are not affected more often with infection on the peristomal skin, or anywhere else, than nonostomates. A possible exception to this is those with Crohn's disease. However, an infection occurring under the faceplate can be a problem. If the skin is indurated, swollen, and red, it may need incision and draining. At that time, a culture is taken and sent to the lab for culture and sensitivity testing. The appropriate antibiotic then can be prescribed topically and/or systemically. It may be a challenge to devise a way that contains the discharge, yet leaves the affected area accessible for treatment.

Excessive Sweating   Sweating under the faceplate can decrease wearing time and cause monilial infection. Cement and a belt may be necessary to hold the appliance in place. Discomfort from perspiration underneath the collection pouch can be alleviated by purchasing or making a cover or bib to keep the pouch material from touching the skin.

DIET

Diet does not play an important role in management of the ostomy patient. Most patients can eat a liberal diet, including the foods eaten before surgery, if the foods are chewed well. However, it is wise to remain on a diet low in fiber for the first 6 weeks after surgery to allow the intestine to heal and swelling to resolve. After that time, a regular diet can be resumed. Urostomates may want to avoid asparagus or other foods that cause odor. Irrigating colostomates should avoid anything that causes them to have loose stools. (This varies with each individual.) Patients with

ileostomies are more prone to obstruction from high roughage foods eaten in large quantities or exclusive of other food. Certain foods should be chewed well and eaten in small amounts and with other food; these foods include popcorn, nuts, corn on the cob, mushrooms, bran products, citrus fruits, coconut, Chinese vegetables, raw celery, and raw carrots.

Because they have no control over gas passage, fecal ostomates may prefer to cut down on gas-forming foods such as beans, vegetables of the cabbage family, onions, beer, and carbonated drinks.

Odor-producing foods such as cheese, eggs, fish, beans, onions, vegetables of the cabbage family, some vitamins or medications, or asparagus may be avoided.

Patients with a urinary ostomy, ileostomy, or ascending colostomy must include an adequate amount of fluid in their diets to prevent the precipitation of crystals or kidney stones in the urine. Absence of the large bowel may not allow normal absorption of water needed to maintain urinary volume.

USE OF DRUGS

Because part or all of the colon is removed and intestinal transit time may be altered, the ostomate may have difficulty in taking prescription or nonprescription medication (Table 1).

Coated or sustained-release preparations may pass through the intestinal tract without being absorbed, and the patient may receive a subtherapeutic dose. The ostomate should look for any undissolved drug particles in the pouch. Liquid preparations or preparations crushed or chewed before swallowing are best. Patients should be cautioned about drugs that will discolor the urine or feces because ostomates may be more conscious of these discharges.

The ostomate also must be careful in taking antibiotics, diuretics, and laxatives. Antibiotics may alter the normal flora of the intestinal tract, causing diarrhea or fungal infection of the skin surrounding the stoma. If diarrhea occurs, fluid and electrolyte intake should be increased. Antidiarrheal and antimotility drugs may affect ileal excreta (9). The physician may prescribe nystatin powder to treat fungal overgrowth.

Sulfa drugs should be used with caution. Crystallization in the kidney may occur more often in patients having difficulty with fluid balance. To minimize this problem, fluid intake should be increased, and the urine should not be acidified. In ileostomy patients, whose fluid and electrolyte balance is more difficult to maintain, diuretics should be given with care because

TABLE 1 Drug effects on the ostomate

	Colostomate	Ileostomate	Urostomate
DOSAGE FORMS			
Chewable tablets	1	1	1
Enteric-coated tablets	1	3	1
Sustained-release medication	1	3	1
Liquid medication	1	1	1
Gelatin capsules	1	1	1
COMPOUNDS			
Alcohol	1	1	1
Antibiotics (poorly absorbed)	1	2, 3	1, 2
Antidiarrheal agents	1, 2	1	1
Calcium-containing antacids	2	2	2
Corticosteroids	1	2	1
Diuretics	1	2	2
Magnesium-containing antacids	2	2	1
Opiates	1, 2	1	1
Salicylates	1	1	1
Salt substitutes	1	2	1
Stool softeners	1	2	1
Sulfa drugs	1	1	2
Vitamins	1	2	1

1, Probably no adverse effects; 2, may cause an increase in adverse effects, patient should be monitored; 3, may be ineffective, patient should be monitored.

TABLE 2 Drugs that may discolor feces

Drug (brand name)	Effect	Drug (brand name)	Effect
Aluminum antacids	Whitish color or speckling	Phenazopyridine (Pyridium)	Orange red
Antibiotics (oral)	Greenish gray	Phenolphthalein	Red
Anticoagulants (excess)	Pink to red to black (bleeding)	Phenylbutazone (Butazolidin)	Pink to red to black (bleeding)
Bismuth Salts	Black	Pyrvinium	Red
Charcoal	Black	Pamoate (Povan)	
Ferrous salts	Black	Salicylates	Pink to red to black (bleeding)
Heparin	Pink to red to black (bleeding)	Senna (and other anthraquinone derivatives)	Yellow-green to brown
Indomethacin (Indocin)	Green		
Oxyphenbutazone (Tandearil)	Pink to red to black (bleeding)		

Reprinted from S. Strauss, "Your Prescription and You—A Pharmacy Handbook for Consumers," 3rd ed., Medical Business Services, Ambler, Pa., 1978.

additional loss of fluid may cause dehydration and electrolyte imbalance (10). The ileostomate should be monitored for signs of hyponatremia if salt substitutes are prescribed.

Laxatives may be used in colostomy patients, but only under close supervision. Ostomates tend to become obstructed, and the laxative's particular action may cause perforation. If the colostomate is constipated, a stool softener may be recommended. Antacids may also cause problems and should be taken with caution. Calcium-containing products may cause calcium stones in the urostomate; magnesium products may cause diarrhea in the ileostomate; and aluminum products may cause constipation in the colostomate. To alleviate any anxiety, the patient should be counseled on drugs that may discolor the feces (Table 2).

SUMMARY

With proper instructions and equipment, ostomates can lead normal, healthy lives. Pharmacists can help by giving patients the necessary information concerning treatment, ostomy supply services, and appropriate referrals to an ET nurse.

REFERENCES

1 J. R. Benfield et al., *Arch. Surg.*, *107*, 62 (1973).

2 C. D. Cromar, *Dis. Colon Rectum*, *7*, 256 (1968).

3 Z. Cohen and R. Stone, *Ostomy Manag.*, *2*, 4 (1980).

4 R. Watt, *Am. J. Nurs.*, *77*, 442 (1977).

5 M. Sparberg, "Ileostomy Care," Charles C. Thomas, Springfield, Ill., 1971, p. 18.

6 L. Gross, "Ileostomy: A Guide," United Ostomy Association, Inc., Los Angeles, Calif., 1974, p. 28.

7 N. N. Gill et al., "Instructions for the Care of the Ileostomy Stoma," Cleveland Clinic Foundation, Cleveland, Ohio, p. 3.

8 C. Travers, *J. Enterost. Ther.*, *7*, 8 (1980).

9 P. Kramer, *Dig. Dis.*, *22*, 327 (1977).

10 N. D. Gallagher et al., *Gut*, *3*, 219 (1962).

APPENDIX: MAJOR MANUFACTURERS OF OSTOMY PRODUCTS AND ACCESSORIES

Atlantic Surgical Company, Inc.
1834 Landsdowne Avenue
Merrick, Long Island, NY 11566
516-868-4545
Full line of appliances and auxiliary products.

Bard International Division
730 Central Avenue
Murray Hill, NJ 07974
201-277-8000
Full line of appliances and auxiliary products.

Blanchard Ostomy Products
2216 Chevy Oaks Circle
Glendale, CA 91206
213-242-6789
Reversible appliances and karaya wafers.

Convatec
(A Squibb Company)
CN5254
Princeton, NJ 08543-5254
201-359-9200
Appliances and supplies.

Coloplast, Inc.
5610 West Sligh Avenue
Suite 100
Tampa, FL 33634
813-886-5634
800-237-4555
Full line of supplies and auxiliary products.

Cymed, Inc.
3447 Investment Boulevard
Suite #2
Hayward, CA 94545
415-782-7550
Appliances and supplies.

Foxy Enterprises
Plaza 16-E Lancaster Avenue
Ardmore, PA 19003
215-642-6207
Custom-made pouch covers.

Hy Tape Surgical Products Corporation
772 McLean Avenue
Yonkers, NY 10704
914-237-1234
Type L closed-end pouches, tape.

Hollister, Inc.
2000 Hollister Drive
P.O. Box 250
Libertyville, IL 60048
312-642-2001
Pouches and auxiliary products.

Johnson & Johnson Company
501 George Street
New Brunswick, NJ 08903
201-524-0400
Paper tape; transparent, semipermeable dressing.

Marlen Manufacturing and Development Co.
5150 Richmond Road
Bedford, OH 44146
216-292-7060
Full line of appliances and auxiliary products.

Mason Laboratories
119 Horsham Road
Horsham, PA 19044
215-675-6044
Colly-Seel and Colly-Seel appliances.

3M Medical Products Division
3M Center 225-52-01
St. Paul, MN 55144-1000
612-733-1100
Micropore paper tape;
transparent, semipermeable dressing.

Nu-Hope Labs, Inc.
P.O. Box 39348
Los Angeles, CA 90039
213-666-5249
Appliances and supplies.

Palex Medical, Inc.
8807 Northwest 23rd Street
Miami, FL 33172
305-592-1830
800-446-6786
One-piece appliances and skin barriers.

The Perma-Type Company, Inc.
P.O. Box 175
Farmington, CT 06032
203-677-7388
Appliances and supplies.

Perry Products
3803 East Lake Street
Minneapolis, MN 55406
612-722-4783
Nonadhesive appliances.

Robinson Surgical Appliance Company
21 East Main Street
Auburn, WA 98002
206-TE3-3161
Appliances.

H. W. Rutzen and Son
345 West Irving Park Road
Chicago, IL 60618
Appliances.

Torbot Company
1185 Jefferson Boulevard
Warwick, RI 02886
401-739-2241
Appliances and auxiliary supplies.

Smith & Nephew United, Inc.
11775 Starkey Road
Largo, FL 34643
813-392-1261
Auxiliary products.

VPI
P.O. Box 266
Spencer, IN 47460
800-843-4851
One-piece nonadhesive nondisposable
appliances.

OSTOMY PRODUCT TABLE

Product (Manufacturer)	Ingredients
Adhesive Disk Products	
A-D's (Gricks)	NS[a]
HoliHesive Skin Barrier (Hollister)	gelatin, pectin, carboxymethylcellulose sodium, polyisobutylene
HoliSeal Skin Barrier (Hollister)	gelatin, pectin, polyisobutylene
Lan-Tex (Atlantic)	hydrophilic polymer combined with synthetic rubber polymer
Pre-Cut Adhesive Supports (Smith & Nephew United)	rubber-based adhesive
Seal-Tite (Smith & Nephew United)	rubber-based adhesive
Universal Adhesive Gaskets (Smith & Nephew United)	rubber-based adhesive
Cement Products	
Adhesive Formula (Atlantic)	natural rubber, zinc oxide, hexane
Mastisol (Ferndale)	gum mastic
Medical Adhesive (Hollister)	silicone base adhesive, hydrocarbon propellant
Nu-Hope Adhesive (Nu-Hope)	natural rubber, hexane
Skin-Bond (Smith & Nephew United)	natural rubber, hexane
Skin-Bond (nonflammable) (Smith & Nephew United)	natural rubber, 1,1,1-trichloroethane
Skin-Hesive (Smith & Nephew United)	natural rubber, petroleum solvent
Solvent Products	
Atlantic Adhesive Remover (Atlantic)	naptha petroleum
Cleansing Solvent (Nu-Hope)	mineral spirits
Detachol (Ferndale)	paraffin hydrocarbons
Medical Adhesive Remover (Hollister)	chloro-fluoro solvent, hydrocarbon propellant
Uni-Solve (Smith & Nephew United)	naptha, 1,1,1-trichloroethane
Uni-Solve (nonflammable) (Smith & Nephew United)	1,1,1-trichloroethane
Universal Remover (Hollister)	organic solvents, silicone oil, ethyl alcohol

[a] Ingredients not specified.

OSTOMY PRODUCT TABLE, continued

Product (Manufacturer)	Ingredients
Deodorizer Products	
APPLIANCE	
Banish II (Smith & Nephew United)	zinc ricinoleate
Deo-Pel (Gricks)	NS[a]
Odo-Way (Smith & Nephew United)	chlorine-producing tablets
Oxychinol (Ferndale)	potassium oxyquinoline sulfate
QAD Tablets (Atlantic)	quaternary ammonium compound
Super Banish (Smith & Nephew United)	silver nitrate, ethylene thiourea
Uri-Kleen (Smith & Nephew United)	phosphoric acid
INTERNAL	
Charcocaps (Requa)	activated charcoal, 260 mg
Derifil (Rystan)	chlorophyll, 100 mg
Skin Protective Products	
Carbo Zinc (Nu-Hope)	karaya gum powder
Formula A Stretchable Karaya Washers and Sheets (Smith & Nephew United)	karaya gum powder, propylene glycol
Karaya Gum (Various manufacturers)	karaya gum powder
Karaya Powder (Smith & Nephew United)	karaya gum powder
Karaya Seal Ring (Hollister)	karaya gum
Moisture Barrier Skin Ointment (Hollister)	petrolatum, propylparaben, BHA, vitamins A,D,E
Nu-Cream (Nu-Hope)	vitamins A,B,D,E, dl-panthenol, allantoin
Nu-Gard (Nu-Hope)	isopropyl alcohol, butyl ester of PVM/MA copolymer, dimethyl phthalate
Premium Paste (Hollister)	film former, gelatin, pectin
Premium Skin Barrier (Hollister)	gelatin, pectin, carboxymethylcellulose sodium, polyisobutylene
Pro Cute (Ferndale)	stearic acid, cetyl alcohol, forlan-LM, ceraphyl 230, glycerin, triethanolamine, deltyl prime, P.V.P., sorbic acid, cetrimide, silicone, perfume, menthol
Relia-Seal (Davol)	NS[a]

[a] Ingredients not specified.

OSTOMY PRODUCT TABLE, continued

Product (Manufacturer)	Ingredients
Skin Conditioning Creme (Hollister)	aloe juice, isopropyl palmitate, isopropyl myristate, isopropyl stearate, vitamins A,D,E
Skin Gel (Hollister)	glycerin, allantoin, isopropyl alcohol, film formers, plasticizers
Skin-Prep (Smith & Nephew United)	poly MVE/MA *n*-butyl monoester
Stomahesive (Squibb)	NS[a]
Tincture of Benzoin (Various manufacturers)	tincture of benzoin
Uni-Care (Smith & Nephew United)	allantoin, dimethicone, isopropyl palmitate, aloe vera gel
Uni-Derm (Smith & Nephew United)	anhydrous lanolin, petrolatum, isopropyl palmitate
Uni-Salve (Smith & Nephew United)	petrolatum, casein

[a] Ingredients not specified.

Roberta S. Carrier

25

CONTRACEPTIVE METHODS AND PRODUCTS

*Q*uestions to ask in patient/consumer counseling

What type of contraceptive method are you now using?

What contraceptive products have you used before?

What did you like or dislike about your current or previous contraceptive methods?

What does your partner like or dislike about your current contraceptive method?

Are you in a stable relationship now?

Have you discussed contraception and sexual health matters with your physician or another health care provider?

Do you belong to a religious faith that has specific guidelines concerning family planning?

Do you have children?

Do you know the risks of being infected with acquired immune deficiency syndrome (AIDS) or other sexually transmitted diseases (STDs)?

How do you protect yourself from STDs, including AIDS?

Throughout history, people have sought to control their fertility in order to prevent or choose the number and timing of pregnancies. As knowledge of reproductive physiology has increased, a wider variety of safe and reliable methods of contraception has been developed.

The earliest recorded methods of contraception include vaginal pessaries made of crocodile dung, used in ancient Egypt; coitus interruptus, mentioned in the Book of Genesis in the Bible; and a cervical cap made from a lemon half, said to have been used by Casanova (1).

According to the 1987 Ortho Birth Control Study of U.S. women 18–44 years of age who were at risk of an unintended pregnancy, 93% used some method of contraception. Sterilization of either the woman or the man continued to be the most used method, accounting for 36% of those surveyed. The next most prevalent method was the birth control pill used by 32% of the women. Four percent of the women used the diaphragm; 3% relied on the intrauterine device (IUD). IUD use declined considerably from the 1982 figure of 7%, probably because of the decreased availability of these devices. The remaining population at risk (approximately 25%) used nonprescription methods or did not use any contraception (2).

Today, in the United States and worldwide, reliance on nonprescription methods of contraception is widespread. Because of their accessibility, nonprescription products are important methods of contraception for persons who do not have access to or who do not want to use family planning clinics or other organized health care systems.

Even if a prescription contraceptive is chosen as the primary method, low-cost and low-risk nonprescription methods and products may be appropriate at different times throughout a person's reproductive life. Some people use nonprescription methods as their primary means of contraception because of their inability to use or their preference not to use a prescription method of contraception.

Consistent and proper use of a contraceptive, whether prescription or nonprescription, will significantly reduce the incidence of unwanted pregnancies. However, as a recent survey of women undergoing counseling for unplanned pregnancies found, nonuse or improper use of contraceptives was responsible for 74% of unwanted pregnancies (3). It has been estimated that in the United States 51% of pregnancies were unplanned (4); it becomes very clear that much more attention must be paid to family planning and contraceptive counseling services.

Of particular concern is the high risk of pregnancy in the adolescent population. The 1982 National Survey of Family Growth found that 18% of 15-year-old women and 66% of 19-year-old women had experienced sexual intercourse. The high teenage pregnancy rate in the United States (one in ten 15–19 year olds), compared with other developed countries, may have much to do with the fact that the average teen has unprotected intercourse for an average of 1 year before seeking contraceptive advice. Only one in three sexually active teenagers consistently uses contraception. Often contraceptive use doesn't occur until after a young woman becomes pregnant. Efforts to disseminate accurate information on biological reproduction and access to contraceptive products are vital to addressing this serious problem.

CHOICE OF CONTRACEPTIVES

There is no perfect method of birth control. Throughout a woman's life, her contraceptive choice may change along with her reproductive priorities. Before selecting a method, every couple should carefully consider several important factors, including safety, effectiveness, and acceptability.

The method's safety factors include the risk of side effects and the amount of protection against infectious diseases, including human immunodeficiency virus (HIV), the virus implicated in causing AIDS. Another safety consideration is the potential for method-associated effects on future fertility.

The effectiveness of a contraceptive method is reported in two ways (Table 1): the lowest expected accidental pregnancy rate in the first year of use (method-related failure rate), and the typical accidental

pregnancy rate (use-failure rate). The lowest expected rate is very difficult to measure; it indicates the theoretical effectiveness given accurate and consistent use of the method every time intercourse occurs. The more realistic typical, or use-failure, rate includes those pregnancies that may have occurred because of inconsistent or improper use of the method. The effectiveness of a method increases with the age of the population using the method (because of decreased fertility); effectiveness also increases with the length of time the method is used. In addition, couples who use contraception to prevent pregnancy have fewer failures than those who use contraceptives to space the births of their children.

The percentage of people who continue using a given method after 1 year indicates the method's acceptability (Table 1). Important factors in determining a method's acceptability include religious beliefs, future reproductive plans, complexity, degree of interruption of spontaneity, "messiness," partner supportiveness, and cost.

Pharmacists should be aware of the safety, effectiveness, and acceptability of the different methods to help their clients make informed decisions.

Natural Family Planning

Natural family planning methods, also called periodic abstinence or fertility awareness methods, use various techniques to determine a woman's fertility cycles. These techniques are also helpful to the couple wanting to know the optimal time for conception. Natural family planning is widely used around the world and is the only method of contraception approved by the Roman Catholic Church.

Natural family planning is divided into four methods: calendar, basal body temperature (BBT), cervical mucus, and symptothermal. Each method requires the woman to keep detailed records of her menstrual cycles and other symptoms associated with monthly changes in hormone levels. (See Chapter 7, *Menstrual Products*.) Data acquired, such as BBT or the character and quantity of cervical mucus (Figure 1), are recorded on detailed monthly charts. After several months of charting, a woman is usually able to predict her most fertile time; the couple can then choose to abstain from sexual intercourse if they want to avoid pregnancy (5).

Calendar Method

The calendar method, also known as the rhythm method, is based on records of monthly menstrual cycle lengths. Estimated ovulation days, considered to be 14 + 2 days before the onset of menstruation, are used to

TABLE 1 Failure rates during the first year of use of a method and first-year continuation rates in the United States

Method (1)	% of women experiencing an accidental pregnancy in the first year of use			% of women continuing use at one year[d]	
	Lowest expected[a] (2)	Typical[b] (3)	Lowest reported[c] (4)	Exc. preg. (5)	Inc. preg. (6)
CHANCE	89	89			
SPERMICIDES[e]	3	21	0	55	43
PERIODIC ABSTINENCE		20		84	67
Ovulation	8		8[h]		
Symptothermal	6		11[h]		
Calendar	10		14[h]		
Postovulation	2		2[h]		
WITHDRAWAL	4	18	7[h]		
CAP[f]	5	18	8	77	63
SPONGE	5 nullips	18 nullips	14 nullips	73	60
	>8 parous	>28 parous	28 parous	73	<53
DIAPHRAGM[f]	3	18	2	69	57
CONDOM[g]	2	12	4[h]	73	64
IUD		6		74	70
Medicated	1		0.5		
Nonmedicated	2		3		
PILL		3		75	73
Combined	0.1		0		
Progestogen only	0.5		1		
INJECTABLE PROGESTOGEN				70	70
DMPA	0.3	0.3	0		
NET	0.4	0.4	0		
IMPLANTS				90	90
Capsules	0.04	0.04	0		
Rods	0.03	0.03	0		
FEMALE STERILIZATION	0.2	0.4	0		
MALE STERILIZATION	0.1	0.15	0		

[a] Among couples who initiate use of a method (not necessarily for the first time) and who use it perfectly (both consistently and correctly), the authors' best guess of the percentage expected to experience an accidental pregnancy during the first year if they do not stop use for any other reason.

[b] Among *typical* couples who initiate use of a method (not necessarily for the first time), the percentage who experience an accidental pregnancy during the first year if they do not stop use for any other reason.

[c] In the literature on contraceptive failure, the *lowest reported* percentage who experienced an accidental pregnancy during the first year following initiation of use (not necessarily for the first time) if they did not stop use for any other reason. However, see Note h.

[d] Among couples attempting to avoid pregnancy, the percentage who continue to use a method, under the alternative assumptions that no one becomes pregnant (col. 5) and that the proportion becoming pregnant is given by col. 2 (col. 6).

[e] Foams, creams, jellies, and vaginal suppositories.

[f] With spermicidal cream or jelly.

[g] Without spermicides.

[h] Too low, because rate is based on more than 1 year of exposure.

R. A. Hatcher et al., "Contraceptive Technology 1988–1989," 14th ed., Irvington Publishers, New York, N.Y., 1988, p. 151.

determine the woman's fertile period. The fertile period is calculated according to estimates of the viable life of ova and sperm (6). The fertilizable life of the ovum is estimated to be from 6 to 24 hours following ovulation, as measured by peaks in estrogen and luteinizing hormone (LH). Sperm viability is considered to be 72 hours at most. A woman with records of her last 12 months of cycles can determine her fertile period by subtracting 18 days from the shortest cycle to determine the first fertile day, and subtracting 11 days from the longest cycle to determine the last fertile day. For example, if a woman's shortest cycle in the last year was 25 days, and her longest cycle was 30 days, her fertile period would be from day 7 to day 19 of her cycle (Table 2).

The calendar method is considered the least effective of natural family planning methods, primarily because of the normal variations in the length of a woman's menstrual cycle. This method should be used in conjunction with other natural family planning methods; it is no longer recommended that it be used alone by natural family planners. The calendar method is still widely practiced; however, the results are many unintended pregnancies (5, 6).

Basal Body Temperature Method

In the BBT method, the woman measures her body temperature every day before arising and charts this temperature. The time of ovulation may be predicted from a study of these temperature charts. The BBT usually drops 12–24 hours before ovulation and then shows a sharp rise of about 0.3° C (0.4–0.8° F) above the lowest point or nadir over a 24–48-hour period (5–7). This sharp rise, called the thermal shift, is caused by high progesterone levels. The "safe" (infertile) period is considered to start after 3 days of postnadir temperature elevation and last until the start of the next cycle (menstruation). Because of the method's inaccuracy in predicting when ovulation occurs, the postmenstrual or preovulatory safe period is difficult to determine, and those who engage in intercourse during this period have a higher pregnancy rate.

A mercury or electric thermometer calibrated in 0.1° increments enables the detection of small changes in body temperature. Electronic digital thermometers are more accurate than mercury thermometers and have a shorter recording time (45–90 sec). Mercury thermometers must be shaken down each night because shaking the thermometer in the morning may cause the woman's body temperature to change. The temperature must be taken before any activity and at a standard time every day. Oral, rectal, or vaginal temperature may be used, but an individual should use one method (site) consistently.

Poor correlation of the thermal shift with ovulation reduces the accuracy of the BBT method. Furthermore, some women have monophasic cycles and don't have a definite temperature dip or rise. Temperature changes are difficult to interpret during the postpartum period and just before and during menopause. Stress, fever, lactation, and use of an electric blanket may also affect temperature changes (7). At these times, it is best for a couple to use an alternate method.

Cervical Mucus Method

The cervical mucus method, also called the Billings method, is based on the rather consistent changes in cervical mucus that take place during a normal menstrual cycle. Every day the woman observes mucus at the vulva (vaginal orifice) and charts the character and amount produced (Figure 1). On days after menstruation, most women notice a sensation of dryness at the vaginal orifice. As estrogen levels rise, the cervical mucus increases in quantity and elasticity (stretchability) and becomes clear, resembling raw egg white (5–7). The "peak" symptom, considered to be the last day of the clear, stretchy, estrogenic mucus, has been shown to be within a day of ovulation for most women. With the postovulatory rise in progesterone, the mucus becomes thick and sticky or is absent. The woman is considered fertile from the first day of detectable mucus after menstruation until 72 hours after the peak symptom. With experience, a woman learns to differentiate other vaginal secretions, such as an infectious discharge or seminal fluid, from normal mucus. Most women become adept in the use of this method after three cycles. When using this method of contraception, the couple must abstain from sexual intercourse for an average of 17 days each month (5). This method has the distinct ad-

TABLE 2	How to calculate the interval of fertility		
If the shortest cycle has been (no. of days)	The first fertile (unsafe) day is	If the longest cycle has been (no. of days)	The last fertile (unsafe) day is
21*	3rd day	21	10th day
22	4th	22	11th
23	5th	23	12th
24	6th	24	13th
25	7th	25	14th
26	8th	26	15th
27	9th	27	16th
28	10th	28	17th
29	11th	29	18th
30	12th	30	19th
31	13th	31	20th
32	14th	32	21st
33	15th	33	22nd
34	16th	34	23rd
35	17th	35	24th

* Day 1, first day of menstrual bleeding.

Reprinted with permission from R. A. Hatcher et al., "Contraceptive Technology 1980–1981," 10th ed., Irvington Publishers, New York, N.Y., 1980, pp. 100–115.

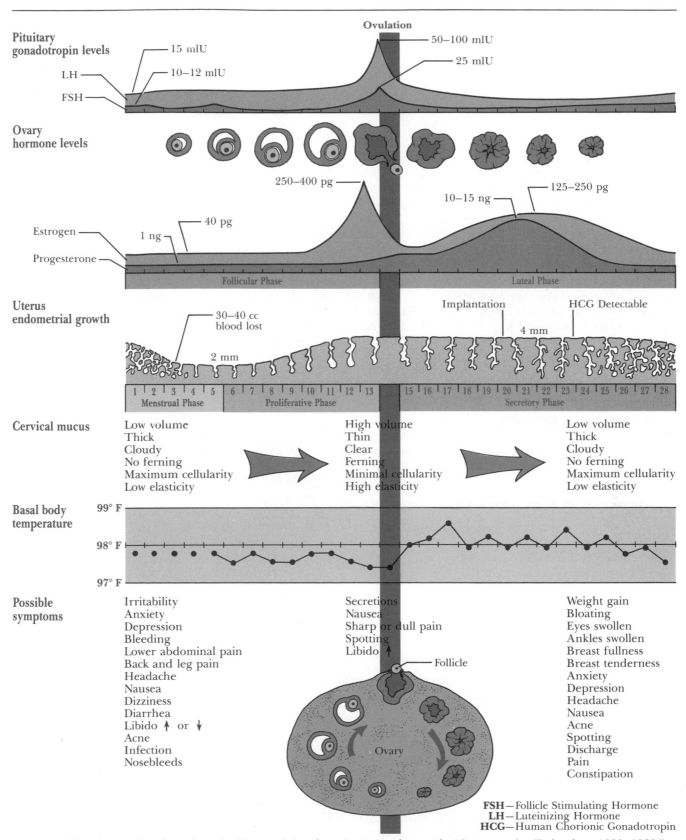

Pituitary gonadotropin levels

Ovulation

15 mlU
50–100 mlU
25 mlU

LH
10–12 mlU
FSH

Ovary hormone levels

250–400 pg
10–15 ng
125–250 pg

Estrogen
40 pg
1 ng
Progesterone

Follicular Phase
Luteal Phase

Uterus endometrial growth

Implantation
HCG Detectable

30–40 cc blood lost
4 mm
2 mm

| 1 | 2 | 3 | 4 | 5 | 6 | 7 | 8 | 9 | 10 | 11 | 12 | 13 | 15 | 16 | 17 | 18 | 19 | 20 | 21 | 22 | 23 | 24 | 25 | 26 | 27 | 28 |

Menstrual Phase | Proliferative Phase | Secretory Phase

Cervical mucus

Low volume
Thick
Cloudy
No ferning
Maximum cellularity
Low elasticity

High volume
Thin
Clear
Ferning
Minimal cellularity
High elasticity

Low volume
Thick
Cloudy
No ferning
Maximum cellularity
Low elasticity

Basal body temperature

99° F

98° F

97° F

Possible symptoms

Irritability
Anxiety
Depression
Bleeding
Lower abdominal pain
Back and leg pain
Headache
Nausea
Dizziness
Diarrhea
Libido ↑ or ↓
Acne
Infection
Nosebleeds

Secretions
Nausea
Sharp or dull pain
Spotting
Libido ↑

Follicle

Ovary

Weight gain
Bloating
Eyes swollen
Ankles swollen
Breast fullness
Breast tenderness
Anxiety
Depression
Headache
Nausea
Acne
Spotting
Discharge
Pain
Constipation

FSH—Follicle Stimulating Hormone
LH—Luteinizing Hormone
HCG—Human Chorionic Gonadotropin

FIGURE 1 The menstrual cycle. Adapted with permission from R. A. Hatcher et al., "Contraceptive Technology 1988–1989," 14th ed., Irvington Publishers, New York, N.Y., 1989, p. 4.

vantage of being useful for postpartum lactating women and those nearing menopause. Another advantage is that women who use this method are likely to detect any abnormalities in their normal mucus patterns caused by infections, and can seek early treatment.

Symptothermal Method

The symptothermal method combines BBT charting with notation of other cyclical signs of ovulation (Figure 1). These signs include breast tenderness, intermenstrual pain (mittelschmerz), labial edema, cervical mucus peak symptoms, and changes in the character and position of the cervix. Most studies of the effectiveness of this method use the thermal shift of the BBT method to determine the postovulatory safe period and the cervical mucus or calendar calculation to determine the end of the preovulatory or postmenstrual infertile period (7). Combinations of these methods have good predicted effectiveness; the lowest reported failure rate is 11% (Table 1).

Hormone Assays for In-Home Use

Investigators in Australia have been working on home urine assays for estrogen and pregnanediol as measures of the beginning and the end of the fertile phase (5). These urine assays may become available as a nonprescription method for use in family planning.

Advantages of Natural Family Planning

Natural family planning methods have a positive effect by encouraging communication within a relationship and may be the only truly "shared" contraceptive method. The cost of monitoring symptoms is minimal. Because no chemicals are used in preventing conception, there are no risks to the fertility or health of the couple, nor to the fetus should pregnancy occur.

Disadvantages of Natural Family Planning

A couple must also consider the disadvantages of natural family planning. First, these techniques have higher pregnancy rates than other methods of contraception. Second, these techniques provide no protection against STDs. Because of the discipline that these techniques require, however, couples who practice them tend to be in stable, long-term, monogamous relationships and, therefore, are at low risk for STDs. The third and most controversial risk is that of increased abnormal pregnancy outcomes, such as birth defects or fetal wastage, in the event of unintentional pregnancy. This risk may be related to conception with aged gametes (either sperm or ovum). Comparative studies

have found a relative risk of 1.0:5.2 for birth defects or spontaneous abortion among those practicing natural family planning at the time of conception. Although the present evidence for an increased risk of abnormal pregnancy outcomes is not conclusive, additional information on this controversial issue should become available as surveillance continues (8).

The Pharmacist's Role

Natural family planning methods, especially the BBT and cervical mucus methods, require extensive training and support. The pharmacist may supply BBT thermometers and monitoring charts. The pharmacist should be supportive and be able to answer questions or refer the couple to certified trainers in natural family planning. The couple should be advised that some medications may interfere with physical signs and symptoms that are to be observed and charted. For example, phenothiazines or aspirin may alter body temperature, and vaginal creams or douches will interfere with cervical mucus determinations. A pharmacist with the proper training and environment should consider counseling in natural family planning as a unique practice possibility.

Vaginal Contraceptives

Vaginal contraceptives (spermicides) use surface active agents to immobilize (kill) sperm. The spermicides approved as Class I agents by the Food and Drug Administration (FDA) include nonoxynol 9, octoxynol 9, and menfegol (Table 3). Most currently available products use nonoxynol 9 (see product tables).

Spermicides come in a variety of forms: foam, cream, jelly, suppository, and film. Spermicides, when used alone, appear to have the highest contraceptive failure rate among typical first-year users (Table 1) (9). Use-effectiveness greatly improves if spermicides are used in conjunction with other barrier methods such as diaphragms, cervical caps, or condoms. Of these products, foam appears to be most effective if used consistently. If the woman desires to douche, she should wait 8 hours after intercourse.

Advantages

Spermicides are easy to use and readily available without prescription; most forms are inexpensive. Unit-dose containers of foam or suppositories can be discretely carried in a purse. Spermicides are useful as a backup to other contraceptive products, such as condoms, or may be used if a birth control pill has been missed. Spermicidal creams or jellies are a good choice if lubrication is desired. There is also a growing body of literature suggesting that spermicides are effective in vitro for inhibiting growth of HIV and many other STD-causing organisms, and that they are possibly protective in vivo for many STDs, including chlamydiosis and gonorrhea (10–12).

Disadvantages

As previously mentioned, the low use-effectiveness rate of spermicides is their major disadvantage. Each product has very specific directions for use, both in terms of quantity, and most importantly, timing with respect to coital activity. Users must be reminded to follow the directions for each product. Some people are sensitive (allergic) to the components, and others find spermicides messy. There has been concern about a possible association between spermicide use and birth defects or miscarriage; however, after reviewing two large population studies (13, 14), the FDA has concluded that no increased risk of birth defects can be attributed to spermicides (15).

Spermicides Designed for Use with Diaphragms or Cervical Caps

Vaginal jellies and creams designed for use with diaphragms and cervical caps have lower concentrations of spermicide. Because of the lower concentration of spermicide, these products should not be used alone. Products designed for use alone, which contain a higher concentration of spermicide, may also be used with a diaphragm. The woman should fill the diaphragm or cervical cap one-third full with spermicide and position

| TABLE 3 | FDA categorization of active ingredients of vaginal contraceptives | |

Ingredient	Category
Dodecaethyleneglycol monolaurate	III
Laureth IOS	III
Menfegol	I
Methoxypolyoxyethyleneglycol laurate-550 and nonoxynol 9	III
Nonoxynol 9	I
Octoxynol 9	I
Phenylmercuric acetate and phenylmercuric nitrate	II

Federal Register, 45, 82017 (1980)

it over the cervix, carefully checking its placement, as previously instructed by her health care provider. The diaphragm or cervical cap with the spermicide may be inserted up to an hour before intercourse. The diaphragm is to be left in place at least 6 hours after intercourse; if coitus is repeated within 6 hours, additional cream or jelly should be inserted without removing the diaphragm. If 6 hours have elapsed, the diaphragm should be removed, washed, and filled with new spermicide (16). A recent study found that contraceptive jelly retained spermicidal activity for up to 12 hours; the cream was effective for up to 24 hours after application (17). If this finding is confirmed, the recommended times for insertion before intercourse and reapplication of spermicide for repeated intercourse may be liberalized.

The cervical cap need not be removed if intercourse is repeated and may be left in place for up to 48 hours. In the event of repeated intercourse, it is advisable to reapply spermicide vaginally in order to ensure full protection (18).

Vaginal Cream and Jelly Spermicides

When vaginal creams or jellies are used without a diaphragm or cervical cap, care should be taken to choose a product with a higher concentration of spermicide than in those designed for use with barriers. Creams have better lubricating and spreading qualities, and gels may be less messy. A full applicator of cream or jelly should be deposited high in the vagina, near the cervix. These products are immediately effective and may be inserted up to 30–60 minutes in advance of intercourse. Applications should be repeated if intercourse is repeated. Douching should be delayed for 8 hours after the last act of intercourse. Although rare, allergic reactions may be experienced by either partner. Couples having oral–genital sex may find the taste of some of these products unpleasant (9).

Vaginal Suppositories

Vaginal suppositories are solid or semisolid dosage forms that dissolve when activated by the moisture in the woman's vaginal tract. They must be inserted high up in the vagina at least 10–15 minutes before intercourse. Occasionally the suppository will not completely dissolve, resulting in an unpleasant, gritty sensation during intercourse. Although most medicated suppositories require refrigeration, vaginal suppositories can be stored at room temperature. As with other medicated suppositories, there is a risk that the user may forget to unwrap the product or choose the wrong orifice for insertion; therefore, the pharmacist should make certain the couple understands the directions.

Contraceptive Foams

When used alone, contraceptive foams appear to have better efficacy rates than do other vaginal contraceptives, possibly because of better adherence to the cervical area and vaginal walls. The availability and ease of use also make foam an excellent product to use in combination with condoms, as a backup method for women who use oral contraceptives, and by those with newly inserted IUDs. Attention must be paid to the directions for use for each product because some products require two applicatorsful while others require only one for an effective dose. For convenience, applicators may be filled up to 7 days before use. Prefilled applicators are also commercially available. Foam is immediately effective upon insertion and, as with the other vaginal preparations, should be placed as close to the cervix as possible. If desired, contraceptive foam, like creams and jellies, may be inserted up to an hour before coitus. Douching should be delayed for 8 hours after intercourse to allow adequate time for the spermicide to act.

Contraceptive Film

Vaginal contraceptive film has been approved by the FDA for nonprescription marketing in the United States. It is made in England and has been used in Europe for about 10 years. The active ingredient is nonoxynol 9, and the film is available in packets of 3, 6, or 12 paper-thin 2 x 2 in. sheets. The film, which is activated by vaginal secretions, is inserted on the tip of a finger and placed at the cervix, where it should be allowed to dissolve for at least 5 minutes before intercourse. It is effective for 2 hours. The film has an advantage of being portable and discreet (9). It is unknown how widely marketed or used this product is, or how effective the film is in relation to other products.

Contraceptive Sponge

The contraceptive sponge, approved by the FDA in 1983, is a small, circular (2.5 cm thick, 5.5 cm in diameter), disposable polyurethane sponge that is permeated with 1 g of nonoxynol 9. The sponge is moistened with about 2 tbsp of water to activate the spermicide and is inserted into the vagina so that the concave side covers the cervix. The sponge is believed to prevent conception in three ways: as a mechanical barrier, by the direct action of the spermicide, and by absorbing the semen. The sponge is considered effective for 24 hours, regardless of the number of times intercourse is repeated. As with the diaphragm, it should be kept in place for 6 hours after coitus. A woven polyester loop is attached to the convex side to facilitate removal of the sponge.

Typical failure rates for the contraceptive sponge range from 13.4 to 28.3 pregnancies per 100 women in the first year of use (19, 20). When data from the U.S. multicenter study were analyzed according to different patient characteristics, it was found that whether the women had previously given birth was a major factor in predicting effectiveness. Women who had not given birth (nulliparous) had an accidental pregnancy rate of 13.9%, not statistically different from the diaphragm users studied; women who had given birth (parous) had 28.3% risk of accidental pregnancy (20). Proposed theories for this discrepancy include a poor fit in women who have delivered vaginally, or the possibility that the parous women had different contraceptive objectives—that is, they were spacing their pregnancies rather than preventing conception. At this time, it may be prudent to recommend the sponge only to women who have not yet had children.

Advantages

The contraceptive sponge is safe, portable, and widely available without prescription. As with other products containing nonoxynol 9, in vitro research has found that the sponge elute inactivates high titers of HIV at concentrations that should be much lower than those expected to be attained in vaginal fluid (21). Several studies in populations at risk for STDs found that use of the contraceptive sponge decreased the risk of gonorrhea and chlamydiosis (22, 23).

Disadvantages

The contraceptive sponge has several disadvantages. The sponge may be dislodged during intercourse. A woman must be able to locate her cervix and be comfortabe with inserting the sponge. Some women have difficulty removing the sponge, and this product has been known to fragment on removal. Contraindications to use include spermicide sensitivity, anatomic abnormalities of the vagina, and a history of toxic shock syndrome (TSS). Although the toxin-producing bacteria responsible for TSS are apparently inhibited in vitro by contraceptive sponges (24), the Centers for Disease Control have identified an increased risk of about the same magnitude as that for tampon users (25). The relative risk of TSS for tampon users has been estimated at 8–30 times baseline; for the sponge, the TSS risk is estimated to be 7.8–40 times baseline. For this reason, the woman should take special care to wash her hands before inserting the sponge, and she should not use the sponge during menstruation or post partum; women should be advised not to exceed the 24-hour recommended retention time. (See Chapter 7, *Menstrual Products*.) The user should also be advised to make sure that the whole sponge is removed because fragments left in the vagina may serve as a focus for infection. A small increase in the incidence of yeast infection has also been reported among sponge users (23).

Condoms

The condom, also known as a rubber, sheath, prophylactic, safe, skin, or French letter, is the most important contraceptive device in this era of deadly sexually transmitted infectious diseases. Originally described in the 16th century by Fallopius as a means of protecting the wearer from syphilis (1), the condom is still the most important means, besides sexual abstinence, of protection against STDs.

The sheath described by Fallopius was made of linen, but modern materials are much more comfortable for the users and their partners. Latex condoms come in a variety of colors and styles, ranging in thickness from 0.02 mm to approximately 0.1 mm. Other variations include reservoir tips and ribbed, studded, lubricated, and spermicidally lubricated styles (26). Condoms made from lamb cecum (skins) are more expensive and provide less protection from infectious diseases than latex condoms. Skin condoms should be recommended only for those who are allergic to rubber (27) or who are not at risk for STDs, such as those in a long-term, mutually monogamous relationship.

Since 1976, condom quality has been under the scrutiny of the FDA. The Center for Devices and Radiological Health is responsible for monitoring the quality of condoms produced in and imported into the United States (28, 29). In 1987, the testing program was expanded because of concerns about protection from the AIDS virus. The United States uses a water-leak test as the standard. The failure rate per batch is not to exceed 4 condoms per 1,000. Of batches that met the quality guidelines, the average failure rate was 2.3 per 1,000 tested (29).

The typical use-failure rate for condoms is 10–13 pregnancies per 100 women during the first year of use (9, 26). The most common cause of use-failure with condoms (as with all other contraceptive methods) is the lack of consistent, proper use. An important part of being able to effectively use a product entails understanding the directions for use. A recent review of the printed instructions included in condom packaging found that condom instructions are written at a high-school reading level and above (30); however, many Americans do not have high-school reading skills.

The pharmacist should stress to the condom user the importance of using only lubricants that do not harm the integrity of the condom. Condom users should avoid any oil-based lubricants, including Vase-line, Vaseline Intensive Care lotion, baby oil, or corn oil (31, 32). These products cause rapid deterioration in the latex and may lead to breaks in the condom. If lubrication is desired, the appropriate water-based products include K-Y jelly, Ortho Personal Lubricant, or any of the spermicidal creams or jellies.

Excessive heat or exposure to ozone at levels found in metropolitan areas will significantly decrease the integrity of the latex within 6 hours; therefore, proper storage of condoms is important. Pharmacists should emphasize that condoms should be protected from light and excessive heat (33). The shelf life of condoms under optimal conditions as packaged by the manufacturers is 3–5 years; the user should always check for discoloration, brittleness, or stickiness; if found, the condom should be discarded (29).

Proper Use

Condoms should be placed on the erect penis before any genital contact because precoital urethral secretions may contain sperm and semen. Rather than interrupting foreplay, many couples find it pleasurable to incorporate condom use into foreplay by having the partner put it on (26). If the condom doesn't have a reservoir tip, a half-inch space should be left at the tip. Air should be squeezed from this reservoir as the condom is unrolled its full length. To minimize tears, care should be taken with rings and fingernails, and adequate lubrication should be ensured before vaginal or anal entry. If the condom breaks, it must be replaced immediately. If ejaculation has occurred, a spermicidal product may be inserted, although the protective value of this procedure is uncertain. Once ejaculation has occurred, the user should withdraw the penis while still erect, holding on to the base of the condom to prevent it from slipping off and spilling semen. Spermicidal condoms or the use of vaginal spermicides may minimize the risk should leakage occur.

The incidence of condom breakage is unknown. Various reports have included a rate of 1 break per 164 acts of intercourse in a general population of health care workers (26); 0.5% breakage rate for anal intercourse and 0.8% breakage rate for vaginal intercourse in a study conducted in brothels in Australia (34); 5% breakage rate in a Danish study of both female prostitutes and hospital personnel (35); and an 8% incidence of tearing or slippage during anal intercourse among Dutch homosexuals (36).

Disadvantages

For the vast majority of people, condoms are an effective, acceptable, inexpensive, safe, and nontoxic method of birth control. The most frequent complaint is decreased sensitivity of the glans penis, resulting in decreased sexual pleasure. Strategies for countering this complaint might include the use of lambskin condoms, very thin condoms, or ridged condoms.

Condom dermatitis, which may occur in either partner, is very rare. The sensitizers are usually antioxidants or accelerators used in processing the rubber (27). Because different manufacturers use different processes, changing brands may alleviate the problem; lamb cecum condoms may also be used.

Withdrawal

Coitus interruptus (withdrawal), although used by only a small percentage of couples in the United States, is commonly practiced in some European countries (37) and other parts of the world. The practice entails coital activity until ejaculation is imminent, then withdrawal of the penis and ejaculation away from the vagina or vulva. The accidental pregnancy rate is about 18% in the first year of use (37). Method failures (pregnancy even when the method is used correctly and consistently) may occur because preejaculation fluid may contain millions of sperm. Disadvantages of this method include a higher pregnancy rate, a lack of protection against STDs, the requirement of considerable self-control by the man, and the potential for diminished pleasure for the couple because of interrupted intercourse. Although this method should not be recommended, it is certainly better than no method.

Douching

Vaginal douches should *not* in any way be considered a method of contraception. Under favorable conditions in the female reproductive tract, active sperm have been found in the cervical crypts and oviducts within 5 minutes of ejaculation (6). Postcoital douching has no effect in removing sperm from the upper reproductive tract and might, in fact, force sperm higher in the reproductive tract. Because consistent users of douches have a higher incidence of pelvic infections and ectopic pregnancies (38), it is questionable whether this practice even for personal hygiene is beneficial to health. (See Chapter 27, *Personal Care Products*.)

AIDS AND SEXUALLY TRANSMITTED DISEASES

As health care practitioners in a position to offer much-needed health information, pharmacists must keep current in their knowledge of all aspects of prevention and treatment of STDs, especially with respect to AIDS infections.

AIDS and HIV Infections

In the United States and worldwide, more than 80% of HIV infections are transmitted through sexual intercourse (39). The known routes of transmission include blood and blood products, via transfusions, sharing contaminated needles, or accidental sticks from contaminated needles; mucous-membrane exposures, through saliva, seminal fluid, and vaginal fluids including menstrual blood; and perinatal and peripartum transmission to infants. Table 4 outlines guidelines for "safer sex" activities. Sexual abstinence or a mutually monogamous relationship with an uninfected individual are the only sure ways to prevent infection with the AIDS virus through sexual contact. If neither of these options is feasible, a latex (not natural membrane) condom should be used for any oral, anal, or vaginal intercourse (Table 2) (40). In populations at risk, individuals who have consistently used condoms have a rate of seroconversion (an indication of infection with the AIDS virus) significantly lower than those who do not use condoms (41, 42). It is very important, however, to emphasize that condom use cannot guarantee safe sex, because of the possibility of condom breakage (35, 36). Accumulating laboratory data suggest that the spermicide, nonoxynol 9, is effective in killing the HIV virus and might offer additional protection when used with condoms (29, 42, 43). It is possible, although not yet proven, that spermicides alone or as a component of the contraceptive sponge may also offer some protection from HIV infections.

Because compliance with safe sex practices, especially with regard to condom use, is poor even among those at risk, other behavioral factors aimed at lowering risk should be stressed (44). These changes include changes in lifestyle and sexual practices.

Other Sexually Transmitted Diseases

There are more than 20 STDs, both bacterial and viral, that may have severe long-term consequences on the health and reproductive capabilities of those infected. Chlamydiosis is now the most common STD in the United States, causing pelvic inflammatory disease, cervicitis, and infertility in women; urethritis and epididymitis in men; and conjunctivitis and pneumonia in

TABLE 4	"Safer sex" practices suggested for reducing the risk of acquiring HIV infection

Safe activities
Massage
Hugging
Body rubbing
Friendly kissing (dry)
Masturbation
Hand-to-genital touching (hand job) or mutual masturbation

Possibly safe activities
Kissing (wet)
Vaginal or anal intercourse using latex condom (use with spermicide even safer)
Oral sex on a man using a latex condom
Oral sex on a woman who does not have her period or a vaginal infection with discharge

Unsafe Activities
Any intercourse without a latex condom
Oral sex on a man without a latex condom
Oral sex on a woman during her period or a vaginal infection with discharge
Semen in the mouth
Oral–anal contact
Sharing sex toys or douching equipment
Blood contact of ANY kind, including menstrual blood and sharing needles

Reprinted from R. A. Hatcher et al., "Contraceptive Technology 1988–1989," 14th ed., Irvington Publishers, New York, N.Y., 1988, p. 4.

neonates (45). Gonorrhea, herpes simplex virus, genital warts, and syphilis are still major problems (39, 46). Tactics to prevent transmission by using latex condoms and spermicides, along with changes in sexual practices as described for AIDS, are recommended and can have a major effect on the prevalence of these STDs (10).

As previously mentioned, spermicidal contraceptive sponges appear to be protective against chlamydiosis and gonorrhea (12, 23, 46) and may add to the protective effects of condom use. Because some of these diseases (e.g., syphilis, herpes) may be spread through skin lesions, condoms and spermicides may not be effective in preventing these types of infection (39).

CONTRACEPTIVE COUNSELING

Not many decisions in life are more personal or more important than the choice of a contraceptive. Optimally, the decision should be made by the couple, not just one partner. Because no single method is likely to be suitable through one's entire reproductive life, all of the options should be presented in a clear and nonjudgmental manner. All people not in a mutually monogamous relationship should be aware of how they will protect themselves and their partners from AIDS and other STDs, and choose their contraceptive method accordingly.

The pharmacist can promote opportunities for consultation by removing barriers that may prevent discussion. The pharmacist should stock contraceptive products and information in an area where the consumer can browse and the pharmacist can easily interact with the customer—such as next to or directly in front of the prescription counter. A private area for consultation is a high priority if adequate discussion is to take place.

The pharmacist should make special efforts to offer contraceptive information and services to adolescents. This population group is especially likely to be noninformed or misinformed about reproductive matters. Pharmacists who are uncomfortable with discussing reproductive health with young people should refer adolescents to a clinic that specializes in such services. Adolescents, especially, need clear and accurate information on all aspects of reproductive health. Because written instructions often are written above the reading level of most students, verbal instructions are very important. Nonprescription methods particularly useful for the impulsive adolescent might include condoms, contraceptive foam in prefilled applicators, or the contraceptive sponge.

Condom use should be stressed as a method of disease prevention for all, including individuals who use prescription methods of contraception. Reservoir-tip and spermicidally lubricated condoms add additional protection against STDs and rupture.

Condoms and spermicides offer excellent backup protection in combination with other methods, including oral contraceptives and periodic abstinence.

Diaphragms, cervical caps, or natural family planning methods may be most appropriate for couples in stable relationships because these methods require special fitting or training. In addition to stocking spermicidal products and BBT thermometers, pharmacists may serve as referral centers for couples wanting to use these methods of family planning.

Further information on reproductive health and AIDS information may be found by contacting the organizations listed in Appendixes 1 and 2.

Pharmacists can be invaluable in contributing to the reproductive health and knowledge in their communities. Reproductive health and contraceptive information may be one of the most challenging areas of a pharmacist's practice; this information may also have the most profound impact on the well-being of clients.

REFERENCES

1 B. C. Eichhorst, *Primary Care, 15 (3),* 437 (1988).

2 J. Darroch Forrest and R. R. Fordyce, *Fam. Plan. Perspect., 20 (3),* 112 (1988).

3 A. M. Sophocles, Jr., and E. M. Brozovich, *J. Fam. Pract., 22 (1),* 45 (1986).

4 J. G. Dryfoos, *Fam. Plan. Perspec., 14,* 81 (1982).

5 J. B. Brown et al., *Obstet. Gynecol., 157,* 1082.

6 H. Klaus, *Obstet. Gynecol. Survey, 37,* 128 (1982).

7 B. A. Gross, *Clin. Reprod. Fertil., 5,* 91 (1987).

8 R. H. Gray and R. T. Kambic, *Human Reprod., 3,* 693 (1988).

9 R. A. Hatcher et al., "Contraceptive Technology 1988–1989," 14th ed., Irvington Publishers, New York, N.Y., 1988, pp. 323–330.

10 K. M. Stone et al., *Am. J. Obstet. Gynecol., 155,* 180 (1986).

11 B. Voeller, *Lancet, 1 (8490),* 1153 (1986).

12 W. C. Louv et al., *J. Infect. Dis., 158,* 518 (1988).

13 J. L. Mills et al., *Fertil. Steril., 43,* 442 (1985).

14 S. Harlap et al., *Teratology, 31,* 381 (1985).

15 *FDA Drug Bull., 16,* 21 (1986).

16 R. A. Hatcher et al., "Contraceptive Technology 1988–1989," 14th ed., Irvington Publishers, New York, N.Y., 1988, pp. 308–310.

17 W. S. Leitch, *Contraception, 34,* 381 (1986).

18 R. A. Hatcher et al., "Contraceptive Technology 1988–1989," 14th ed., Irvington Publishers, New York, N.Y., 1988, pp. 314–320.

19 D. A. Edelman and B. B. North, *Am. J. Obstet. Gynecol., 157,* 1164 (1987).

20 S. L. McIntyre and J. E. Higgins, *Am. J. Obstet. Gynecol., 155,* 796 (1986).

21 B. Polsky et al., *Lancet, 1 (8600),* 1456 (1988).

22 M. J. Rosenberg et al., *Sex. Transm. Dis., 14,* 147 (1987).

23 M. J. Rosenberg et al., *J. Am. Med. Assoc., 257,* 2308 (1987).

24 K. M. Remington et al., *Obstet. Gynecol., 69,* 563 (1987).

25 G. Faich et al., *J. Am. Med. Assoc., 255,* 216 (1986).

26 R. A. Hatcher et al., "Contraceptive Technology 1988–1989," 14th ed., Irvington Publishers, New York, N.Y., 1988, pp. 332–353.

27 A. A. Fisher, *Cutis, 39,* 281 (1987).

28 G. C. Provencher and P. J. Miller, *Am. J. Nurs., 88,* 640 (1988).

29 *Morbid. Mortal. Weekly Rep., 37,* 133 (1988).

30 G. A. Richwald et al., *Public Health Rep., 103,* 355 (1988).

31 B. Voeller et al., *Contraception, 39,* 95 (1989).

32 N. White et al., *Nature, 335,* 19 (1988).

33 L. J. Clark et al., *Contraception, 39,* 245 (1989).

34 J. Richters et al., *Lancet, 2,* 1487 (1988).

35 P. C. Gotzsche and M. Hording, *Scand. J. Infect. Dis., 20,* 233 (1988).

36 G. J. P. Van Griensven et al., *Genitourin. Med., 64,* 344 (1988).

37 R. A. Hatcher et al., "Contraceptive Technology 1988–1989," 14th ed., Irvington Publishers, New York, N.Y., 1988, pp. 368–370.

38 R. A. Hatcher et al., "Contraceptive Technology 1988–1989," 14th ed., Irvington Publishers, New York, N.Y., 1988, pp. 186–187, 326.

39 R. A. Hatcher et al., "Contraceptive Technology 1988–1989," 14th ed., Irvington Publishers, New York, N.Y., 1988, pp. 3–5, 15.

40 *N.Y. State J. Med., 88,* 264 (1988).

41 E. N. Ngugi et al., *Lancet, 2,* 887 (1988).

42 P. J. Feldblum and J. A. Fortney, *Am. J. Public Health, 78,* 52 (1988).

43 C. A. M. Rietmeijer et al., *J. Am. Med. Assoc., 259,* 1851 (1988).

44 K. Henry and M. T. Osterholm, *Am. J. Public Health, 78,* 1244 (1988).

45 L. L. Sanders et al., *J. Am. Med. Assoc., 255,* 1750 (1986).

46 B. B. North, *J. Reprod. Med., 33,* 307 (1988).

APPENDIX 1: FAMILY PLANNING INFORMATION

■ Planned Parenthood Federation of America, Inc.
810 Seventh Avenue
New York, NY 10019

Offers family planning services, infertility therapy, pregnancy counseling, abortion and sterilization services or referral for such services, education for marriage and sex education, prenatal care, and a variety of special programs. Patient-level pamphlets cover all methods or individual ones (some in Spanish). Teaching aids, posters, and subscription periodicals are offered.

■ The Population Council
Office of Communications
1 Dag Hammarskjold Plaza
New York, NY 10017

Publishes the bimonthly *Studies in Family Planning* and quarterly *Population and Development Review,* as well as books and monographs. The Council endeavors to advance knowledge in the broad field of population by fostering research, training, and technical consultation and assistance in the social and biomedical sciences. Works to develop and improve contraceptive methods, as well as analyze the causes of population change, their societal implications, and appropriate policy responses.

■ Zero Population Growth, Inc.
1346 Connecticut Avenue, N.W.
Washington, DC 20036

Works to mobilize broad public support for population stabilization in the United States and worldwide through public policy advocacy and population education. Actively supports access by all people to safe, legal contraception methods and family-planning services. Publishes *ZPG Reporter* (bimonthly), *ZPG Activist, Media Targets, Teachers PET Term Paper,* action alerts, factsheets, and brochures.

■ The Alan Guttmacher Institute
111 Fifth Avenue
New York, NY 10003

Publishes *Family Planning Perspectives* (bimonthly), *International Family Planning Perspectives* (quarterly), and *Planned Parenthood Washington Memo.* The Institute has several publications to assist administrators and program officials in developing a statewide approach to family planning programs that will meet federal and state requirements.

■ Population Information Program
The Johns Hopkins University
624 North Broadway
Baltimore, MD 21205

Publishes *Population Reports,* an excellent series that provides an accurate and authoritative overview of important developments in the population and family planning field.

■ Population Information Program
The Rockefeller Foundation
1133 Avenue of the Americas
New York, NY 10036

Strives towards the goal of improved population policies through support of research and training programs in biomedicine and demography.

■ Special Programme of Research, Development and Research Training in Human Reproduction
World Health Organization
Avenue Appia
1211 Geneva 27, Switzerland

The objectives are geared to meet the expressed needs of member states for improved methods for family planning, study of their safety and efficacy, and the diagnosis, prevention, and treatment of infertility. The Programme also supports the strengthening of research capabilities in these areas of research in developing countries.

APPENDIX 2: AIDS INFORMATION

■ AIDS Action Council
729 Eighth Street, S.E.
Suite 200
Washington, DC 20003
Phone: 202-547-3101

■ American Association of Physicians for Human Rights
P.O. Box 14366
San Francisco, CA 94114
Phone: 415-558-9535

■ Centers for Disease Control
Public Inquiries Office
1600 Clifton Road, N.E.
Building 1, Room B63
Atlanta, GA 30333
Phone: 404-639-3534

■ Gay Men's Health Crisis
P.O. Box 274
132 West 24th Street
New York, NY 10011
Phone: 212-807-6655

■ Hispanic AIDS Forum
c/o APRED
853 Broadway, Suite 2007
New York, NY 10003
Phone: 212-870-1902

- Literature Search Program
  Reference Section
  National Library of Medicine
  8600 Rockville Pike
  Bethesda, MD 20894

- Local Red Cross or
    American Red Cross
  AIDS Education Office
  1730 D Street, N.W.
  Washington, DC 20006
  Phone: 202-373-8300

- Los Angeles AIDS Project
  1362 Santa Monica Boulevard
  Los Angeles, CA 90046
  Phone: 213-871-AIDS

- Minority Task Force on AIDS
  c/o New York City Council of Churches
  475 Riverside Drive, Room 456
  New York, NY 10115
  Phone: 212-749-1214

- Mothers of AIDS Patients
  c/o Barbara Peabody
  3403 E Street
  San Diego, CA 92102
  Phone: 619-234-3432

- National AIDS Network
  729 Eighth Street S.E., Suite 300
  Washington, DC 20003
  Phone: 202-546-2424

- National Association of
    People with AIDS
  P.O. Box 65472
  Washington, DC 20035
  Phone: 202-483-7979

- National Coalition of Gay Sexually
    Transmitted Disease Services
  c/o Mark Behar
  P.O. Box 239
  Milwaukee, WI 53201
  Phone: 414-277-7671

- National Council of Churches
    AIDS Task Force
  475 Riverside Drive, Room 572
  New York, NY 10115
  Phone: 212-870-2421

- National Gay Task Force
  AIDS Information Hotline
  Phone: 800-221-7044
         212-807-6016 (NY state)

- National Sexually Transmitted
    Diseases Hotline
  American Social Health Association
  Phone: 800-227-8922

- Public Health Service AIDS Hotline
  Phone: 800-342-AIDS
         800-342-2437

Reprinted from R.A. Hatcher et al., "Contraceptive Technology 1988–1989," 14th ed., Irvington Publishers, New York, N.Y., 1988.

SPERMICIDE PRODUCT TABLE

Product (Manufacturer)	Dosage Form	Spermicide	Other Ingredients
Anvita (A. O. Schmidt)	suppositories	phenylmercuric borate, 1:2,000	boric acid aluminum potassium sulfate thymol chlorothymol aromatics cocoa butter
Because (Schering)	foam	nonoxynol 9, 8%	benzethonium chloride, 0.2%
Conceptrol (Ortho)	gel	nonoxynol 9, 5.56%	
Conceptrol Disposable (Ortho)	gel	nonoxynol 9, 4%	
Delfen (Ortho)	foam	nonoxynol 9, 12.5%	
Emko (Schering)	foam	nonoxynol 9, 8%	benzethonium chloride, 0.2% stearic acid triethanolamine glyceryl monostearate poloxamer 188 polyethylene glycol 600 substituted adamantane dichlorodifluoromethane dichlorotetrafluoroethane
Emko Pre-Fil (Schering)	foam	nonoxynol 9, 8%	
Encare (Thompson Medical)	suppositories	nonoxynol 9, 2.27%	
Intercept (Ortho)	suppositories	nonoxynol 9, 100 mg	
Koromex (Schmid)	foam	nonoxynol 9, 12.5%	acetic acid propylene glycol isopropyl alcohol laureth-4 cetyl alcohol polyethylene glycol stearate fragrance sodium acetate propellant 12
Koromex (Schmid)	jelly	nonoxynol 9, 3%	propylene glycol cellulose gum boric acid sorbitol starch simethicone fragrance
Ramses (Schmid)	jelly	nonoxynol 9, 5%	
Semicid (Whitehall)	suppositories	nonoxynol 9, 100 mg	polyethylene glycol base
Shur-Seal Gel (Milex)	jelly	nonoxynol 9, 2%	
Today Sponge (Whitehall)	sponge	nonoxynol 9, 1,000 mg	

SPERMICIDE PRODUCT TABLE, continued

VAGINAL SPERMICIDES USED WITH A DIAPHRAGM

Product (Manufacturer)	Dosage Form	Spermicide	Other Ingredients
Gynol II (Ortho)	jelly	nonoxynol 9, 2%	
Koromex (Schmid)	cream	octoxynol, 3%	boric acid polysorbate 60 propylene glycol sorbitan stearate stearic acid fragrance
Koromex Crystal Clear (Schmid)	gel	nonoxynol 9, 2%	boric acid cellulose gum propylene glycol simethicone sorbitol
Ortho-Creme (Ortho)	cream	nonoxynol 9, 2%	
Ortho-Gynol (Ortho)	jelly	octoxynol 9, 1%	

CONDOM PRODUCT TABLE

Brand Name (Supplier)	Type
Conture (Ansell)	rubber-shaped, packaged with lubricant
Excita Extra (Schmid)	rubber-ribbed, packaged with spermicidal lubricant
Excita Fiesta (Schmid)	rubber-ribbed, packaged with lubricant in assorted colors
Fourex (Schmid)	lamb cecum, packaged pre-moistened
Guardian (Youngs)	rubber-reservoir end, packaged with lubricant
Hugger (Ansell)	rubber-reservoir end, packaged with lubricant
Koromex (Schmid)	rubber-reservoir end, packaged with spermicidal lubricant
Magnum (Carter)	rubber-reservoir end, textured interior surface, tapered shape, packaged with lubricant
Mentor (Carter)	rubber-reservoir end, adhesive seal, packaged with lubricant and removable protective sleeve
Mentor Plus (Carter)	rubber-reservoir end, adhesive seal, packaged with spermicidal lubricant
Naturalamb (Youngs)	lamb cecum-regular end, packaged with lubricant
Nuda (Ansell)	rubber-shaped/thin, packaged with lubricant
Prime (Ansell)	rubber-reservoir end, packaged with lubricant
Prime, Non-lubricated (Ansell)	rubber reservoir end, packaged dry
Ramses Extra (Schmid)	rubber-reservoir end, packaged with spermicidal lubricant
Ramses Extra For Her (Schmid)	rubber-reservoir end, packaged with spermicidal lubricant
Ramses Extra Ribbed (Schmid)	rubber-ribbed, packaged with spermicidal lubricant
Ramses Extra Strength (Schmid)	rubber-reservoir end, packaged with spermicidal lubricant
Ramses Nuform (Shaped) (Schmid)	rubber-reservoir end, packaged with lubricant
Ramses Regular (Schmid)	rubber-reservoir end, packaged dry
Ramses Sensitol (Schmid)	rubber-reservoir end, packaged with lubricant
Rough Rider (Ansell)	rubber-studded, packaged with lubricant
Sheik Elite (Schmid)	rubber-reservoir end, packaged with spermicidal lubricant
Sheik Regular (Schmid)	rubber-plain end, packaged dry rubber-reservoir end, packaged dry
Sheik Ribbed (Schmid)	rubber-reservoir end, packaged with lubricant

CONDOM PRODUCT TABLE, continued

Brand Name (Supplier)	Type
Sheik Sensi-Creme (Schmid)	rubber-reservoir end, packaged with lubricant
She's Sheik (Schmid)	rubber-reservoir end, packaged with spermicidal lubricant
Stimula (Ansell)	rubber-ribbed, packaged with lubricant
Sultan (Ansell)	rubber-ribbed, packaged with lubricant
Tahiti (Ansell)	rubber-colored, packaged with lubricant
Today (Whitehall)	rubber-reservoir end, contoured shape, packaged with or without spermicidal lubricant
Trojan (Carter)	rubber-plain end, packaged dry
Trojan-Enz, Lubricated (Carter)	rubber-reservoir end, packaged with lubricant
Trojan-Enz, Non-lubricated (Carter)	rubber-reservoir end, packaged dry
Trojan-Enz with Spermicidal Lubricant (Carter)	rubber-reservoir end, packaged with spermicidal lubricant
Trojan Extra Strength (Carter)	rubber-reservoir end, colored, packaged with lubricant
Trojan For Women (Carter)	rubber-reservoir end, packaged with lubricant
Trojan For Women with Spermicidal Lubricant (Carter)	rubber-reservoir end, packaged with spermicidal lubricant
Trojan Naturalube (Carter)	rubber-reservoir end, contoured shape, ribbed/textured, packaged with lubricant
Trojan Plus (Carter)	rubber-reservoir end, contoured shape, colored, packaged with lubricant
Trojan Plus 2 (Carter)	rubber-reservoir end, contoured shape, packaged with spermicidal lubricant
Trojan Ribbed (Carter)	rubber-reservoir end, ribbed/textured, colored, packaged with lubricant
Trojan Ribbed with Spermicidal Lubricant (Carter)	rubber-reservoir end, ribbed/textured, packaged with spermicidal lubricant

Benjamin Hodes

26

HEMORRHOIDAL PRODUCTS

*Q*uestions *to ask in patient/consumer counseling*

What is the nature of the symptoms? What improves or worsens the symptoms?

How long have the symptoms been present? Do they recur? Are they associated with straining at a bowel movement?

Have you noticed any bleeding? Describe the bleeding.

Have you treated the symptoms without the use of medication?

Have you previously used any nonprescription or prescription drugs for these symptoms?

Have you recently changed your diet or amount of fluid intake?

Do you take laxatives regularly? If so, which ones and how frequently?

What other medications do you take?

Are you pregnant or have you recently been pregnant?

Do you frequently experience constipation or diarrhea?

Do you have any other medical conditions such as heart failure, liver disease, inflammatory disease of the intestine, or varicose veins?

Anorectal disease, including hemorrhoids, is an annoying and uncomfortable disorder. Several diseases affecting the anorectal area are not amenable to self-treatment; however, many symptoms of anorectal disease may be self-treated. Numerous nonprescription products are available for relief of the burning, pain, itching, inflammation, irritation, swelling, and general discomfort of hemorrhoids.

CLINICAL CONSIDERATIONS

In addition to hemorrhoids, anorectal disease encompasses other disorders, some of which may be serious. The pharmacist should carefully evaluate symptoms reported by the patient before recommending a product for self-medication. Some anorectal disorders require immediate medical attention.

Anatomy and Physiology

With respect to anorectal diseases, three parts of the body are of concern: the perianal area, the anal canal, and the lower portion of the rectum (Figure 1).

Perianal Area

The perianal area (about 7 cm in diameter) is the portion of the skin and buttocks immediately surrounding the anus. The presence of sensory nerve endings makes the perianal area very sensitive to pain.

Anal Canal

The anal canal (about 4 cm long) is the channel connecting the end of the gastrointestinal (GI) tract (rectum) with the outside of the body. The lower two-thirds of the canal is covered by modified anal skin, which is structurally similar to the skin covering other parts of the body. The canal contains sensory nerve endings as well as pressure receptors that allow the perception of distention pain.

The point in the mid-upper canal at which the skin lining changes to mucous membrane is the dentate or pectinate line.

Two sphincters encircling the anal canal control passage of fecal material. The external (anal) sphincter, located at the bottom of the anal canal, is a voluntary muscle. The internal sphincter, which allows passage into the anal canal, is an involuntary muscle. Both sphincters lie under the tissues of the anal canal and extend downward. Under normal conditions the external sphincter is closed and prevents the involuntary passage of feces and/or discharges.

In healthy individuals, the skin covering the anal canal serves as a barrier against absorption of substances into the body. Therefore, treatment applied to this area of the anal canal can be expected to manifest only local effects. If disease is present, the loss of protective oils or breaks in the surface may alter the character of the skin covering the canal; consequently, the ability of the skin to serve as a protective barrier is diminished.

Anal crypts are normal pocket-like formations located at the internal side of the dentate line. They face upward and, because of their position, sometimes retain small amounts of fecal material that may cause irritation. This irritation may lead to infections and stimulate the development of anorectal disease. Investigators commonly distinguish between rectal mucosa and anal mucosa and consider the anorectal ring to be the end of the anal canal (1). For the purposes of this discussion, the appearance of the mucosal region will mark the beginning of the rectal area.

Rectum

The rectum (about 12–15 cm long) is the lower end of the GI tract that extends from the dentate line up to the sigmoid colon. It is lined with semipermeable mucous membranes, is highly vascularized, and contains no sensory pain fibers. Like the anal canal, it contains pressure receptors. The skin of the anal canal and the mucous membrane in the rectum of individuals without anorectal disease protect the body from invasion by the bacteria present in the feces.

Substances absorbed through the mucous membrane may exert systemic effects because of the plexus of hemorrhoidal vessels beneath the mucosa and the paths followed by the blood returning to the heart through the hemorrhoidal veins. This process may allow some substances to enter the systemic circulation without passing through the liver. This effect is important in evaluating the potential systemic toxicity of locally applied drugs. The rectal pH, ranging from neutral to basic, is important in determining the extent to which substances in the rectum are absorbed.

The most prominent parts of the vasculature in the region above and below the pectinate line are the three hemorrhoidal arteries and the accompanying veins. Veins and arteries above the pectinate line are referred to as internal and those below as external.

Description

Hemorrhoids (also known as "piles") are abnormally large or symptomatic conglomerates of vessels, supporting tissues, and overlying mucous membrane or skin of the anorectal area. They may be classified according to either their degree of severity or their location (2) (Figure 1).

External Hemorrhoids

The two types of external hemorrhoids, thrombosed and cutaneous, occur below the dentate line.

Thrombosed   A thrombosed hemorrhoid is a hemorrhoidal vessel either in the anal canal or adjacent to the anus that contains a blood clot or thrombus. The clot may vary in size from that of a pea to a walnut.

Cutaneous (Skin Tags)   Cutaneous hemorrhoids consist of fibrous connective tissue covered by anal skin and are located outside the anal sphincter at any point on the circumference of the anus. They may result from a previously thrombosed external hemorrhoid in which the clot has become organized and been replaced by connective tissue (3) or from uneven skin healing after hemorrhoidectomy.

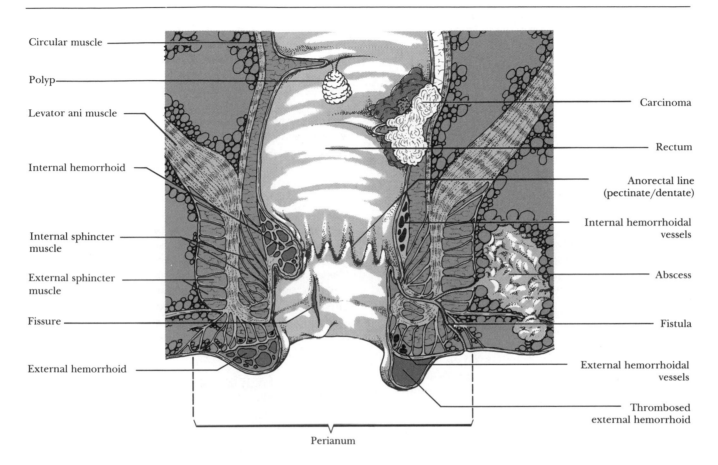

Circular muscle

Polyp

Levator ani muscle

Internal hemorrhoid

Internal sphincter muscle

External sphincter muscle

Fissure

External hemorrhoid

Carcinoma

Rectum

Anorectal line (pectinate/dentate)

Internal hemorrhoidal vessels

Abscess

Fistula

External hemorrhoidal vessels

Thrombosed external hemorrhoid

Perianum

FIGURE 1   Selected disease states in anorectal region.

Internal Hemorrhoids

Internal hemorrhoids occur above the dentate line. Occasionally, because of its size and distention, an internal hemorrhoid descends below the dentate line and outside the anal sphincter. It is then referred to as a prolapsed hemorrhoid.

Internal–External Hemorrhoids

Internal and external hemorrhoids sometimes occur together. Also known as mixed hemorrhoids, they appear as baggy swellings. The following types occur:

- Prolapsed—in rare cases, a hemorrhoid that is characterized by pain until the prolapse is reduced; blood, which is bright red, may or may not be present;

- Without prolapse—a hemorrhoid that may be characterized by bleeding, but not pain;

- Strangulated—a hemorrhoid that has prolapsed to such a degree and for so long that its blood supply is occluded by the anal sphincter's constricting action; very painful and usually becomes thrombosed.

Other Anorectal Disorders

Some potentially serious disorders, including fissures, fistulas, inflammatory bowel diseases, and tumors, may also present hemorrhoidal symptoms and should not be self-medicated. Patients should be referred to a physician if any of the following conditions are suspected:

- Abscess—a painful swelling in the perianal or anal canal area caused by bacterial infection and resulting in the formation of a localized area of pus; usually, *Staphylococcus* is the primary organism involved;

- Anal fistula—a channel-like lesion near the anus with swelling, pain, and pruritus; anorectal abscess usually results in an anal fistula;

- Anal fissure—a slitlike ulcer in the anal canal lining; this common condition, which may be painful, may exist alone or in conjunction with hemorrhoids;

- Condyloma latumi—one of the secondary lesions of syphilis; its symptoms are similar to those of an external hemorrhoid;

- Condyloma acuminata—venereal warts that appear as multiple, polymorphic lesions in the genital or perianal region; they are usually sexually transmitted;

- Cryptitis—inflammation and hypertrophy of the anal crypts; the main symptom is pain aggravated by defecation; the condition probably originates in an anal gland;

- Malignant neoplasm—a serious disease often characterized by constipation; bleeding and pain may be associated with malignant anal tumors (the most common of which is squamous cell carcinoma), which are usually unnoticeable and located in the rectum;

- Polyps—benign or malignant tumors of the rectum that are characterized by bleeding and, rarely, by protrusion of a mass through the anus or a feeling of fullness or pressure in the rectum.

Etiology

Hemorrhoidal disease appears with the greatest frequency in persons 20–50 years of age (2). It has been estimated that, in the United States, 58% of people over 40 years of age have hemorrhoids to some extent (4). Many factors have been implicated in the etiology of hemorrhoidal disease (5), including erect posture, diet, constipation, sneezing, portal hypertension, and anal infection (6). Symptomatic hemorrhoids develop only in susceptible individuals; socioeconomic and cultural factors and pregnancy are precipitating causes (7).

Internal Hemorrhoids

Internal hemorrhoids are classified according to location: left lateral, right posterior, and right anterior. These hemorrhoids occur when the three "cushions" that are considered normal anatomic structures (8) become engorged and protrude into the anal canal. Aging and other factors cause deterioration of connective tissue; therefore, these cushions become loosened from their submucosal anchoring and gradually become

elongated and descend toward the anus (9). Because of this weakening, the veins also become distended. As the loose anal lining descends, the hemorrhoids and weakened cushions become increasingly exposed and susceptible to increased pressure from straining or trauma resulting from constipated stools. Eventually, engorgement of the blood vessels may result in clot formation, swelling, and the erosion of the lining and vessel wall with bleeding (9). In support of this etiology, microscopic analysis of hemorrhoidectomy specimens revealed fragmented supportive connective tissue (10). After repeated episodes of straining with a relaxed sphincter, the hemorrhoids dilate and ultimately prolapse out of the anus. Eventually this will lead to hemorrhoids that are permanently prolapsed and enlarged.

Heredity also is considered a factor in hemorrhoidal formation, although this is controversial (11). Dietary and cultural patterns may also predispose persons to hemorrhoids (12). Low-fiber diets and inadequate fluid intake contribute to hard stools and constipation. Constipation leads to straining at defecation, which in turn leads to increased pressure within the hemorrhoidal vessels, thereby precipitating formation of hemorrhoids.

Hemorrhoids may also be precipitated by chronic diarrhea, cardiac failure, obesity, coughing, sneezing, vomiting, pregnancy, pelvic tumors, physical exertion, and anal infection. There is some question about whether portal hypertension is a precipitating cause of hemorrhoids (13).

Pregnancy is by far the most common cause of hemorrhoids in young women. The gravid uterus causes increased pressure in the middle and interior hemorrhoidal vessels. Labor may also intensify the hemorrhoidal condition and produce intense symptoms after delivery. Pelvic tumors may give rise to hemorrhoids by a similar process. Another possible cause of anorectal disorders is an infection initially occurring in the anal crypts and spreading to the tissue nearby, causing inflammation that may result in a fistula or abscess.

External Hemorrhoids

External hemorrhoids are recognized as a swelling of the skin and associated blood vessels around the rim of the anus (14). External hemorrhoids are covered by highly innervated skin, and when this skin is stretched by a thrombosis, sudden and severe pain can result.

Symptoms

Itching, burning, pain, inflammation, irritation, swelling, and discomfort are symptoms of anorectal disease. These symptoms may be relieved by self-medication if they are not manifestations of more serious anorectal disease. Bleeding, seepage, protrusion, prolapse, and thrombosis should not be self-medicated because a more serious disorder may be masked, and because no appropriate nonprescription therapy is available.

Itching

Itching, or pruritus, occurs as a manifestation of mild inflammation associated with many anorectal disorders. Pruritus ani refers to persistent itching in the anal and perianal area that occurs even in people with good hygiene.

Itching is one of the most common symptoms of anorectal disease and may be secondary to swelling, irritation caused by dietary factors, or moisture in the anal area.

Itching is rarely symptomatic of hemorrhoidal disease, except where there is mucous discharge from prolapsing internal hemorrhoids. Sensitivity to fabrics, dyes and perfumes in toilet tissue, detergents, local treatment, and fecal contents are common causes of itching. Fungal infections, parasites, allergies, and associated anorectal pathologic lesions may also cause itching. Broad-spectrum antibiotic therapy may trigger itching as a result of infection secondary to overgrowth of yeast organisms. Chronic use of mineral oil can lead to pruritus ani. Sometimes itching may be attributed to a psychologic cause.

Burning

Burning, a common symptom of anorectal disease, represents a somewhat greater degree of irritation of the anorectal sensory nerves than itching. The burning sensation may range from a feeling of warmth to a feeling of intense heat and may be constant or associated with defecation.

Pain

Acute inflammation of the anal tissue can cause pain. Hemorrhoidal pain is steady and aching, and is usually worsened by standing or defecation. Pain is experienced with acute external hemorrhoids. Chronic external hemorrhoids often exhibit no pain. Because of the absence of sensory nerve endings above the dentate line, uncomplicated internal hemorrhoids rarely cause pain. However, when strangulation, thrombosis, or ulceration occurs, pain may be severe (3). Patients with severe persistent pain should be referred to a physician.

Inflammation

Inflammation is a tissue reaction distinguished by heat, redness, pain, and swelling. Inflammation often is caused by trauma, allergy, or infection. The inflammation itself, but not the underlying cause, may be relieved by self-medication.

Irritation, Swelling, and Discomfort

Irritation is a response to stimulation of the nerve ending and is characterized by burning, itching, pain, or swelling. Swelling is caused by an accumulation of excess fluid associated with engorged hemorrhoids or hemorrhoidal tissue. Discomfort, a vague and generalized uneasiness, may result from any or all of these symptoms.

Bleeding

Bleeding is almost always associated with internal hemorrhoids and may occur before, during, or after defecation. The amount of bleeding experienced is often variable and is not related to the amount of hemorrhoidal tissue present. When bleeding occurs from an external hemorrhoid, it is due to an acute thrombosis accompanied by rupture. Pain often accompanies the bleeding in this case, although a patient may experience some relief of the pain with the onset of the bleeding. Blood from hemorrhoids is usually bright red and covers the fecal matter. Bleeding is stimulated by defecation but may occur as an "oozing," soiling underclothes.

The chronic blood loss associated with bleeding hemorrhoids infrequently produces severe anemias. Bleeding may indicate the presence of serious anorectal disease and should not be self-medicated.

Seepage

Seepage, the involuntary passing of fecal material or mucus, is caused by an anal sphincter that does not close completely. This symptom cannot be self-medicated, and the patient should be referred to a physician.

Protrusion

Protrusion is a frequent sign or symptom of uncomplicated internal and external hemorrhoids and is defined as the projection of hemorrhoidal or rectal tissue outside the anal canal. The rectal protrusion may vary in size and usually appears after defecation, prolonged standing, or unusual physical exertion. It is painless except when thrombosis, infection, or ulceration is present. Strangulation of a protruding hemorrhoid by the sphincter may lead to thrombosis. Self-treatment is not appropriate.

A prolapsed hemorrhoid is an internal hemorrhoid that, because of distention, is located below the dentate line and outside the anal sphincter.

A painful lump may develop when the anal sphincter contraction interferes with blood flow from a prolapsed internal or mixed hemorrhoid, resulting in thrombosis. If this prolapsed hemorrhoid returns to above the anal sphincter before thrombosis occurs, the pain and lump usually disappear. However, when defecation occurs later, both lump and pain are likely to recur. Permanently prolapsing internal hemorrhoids cause a mucoid discharge, which in turn may lead to perianal irritation.

Thrombosis

Thrombosis, or blood clotting, within a hemorrhoid is a common complication. Abrupt onset of severe, constant pain in the anal area, accompanied by a grape-sized lump, is a sign that thrombosis of a mixed or external hemorrhoid may have occurred. If untreated, the burning pain persists about 5–7 days, diminishing in intensity after the first day. A hard, tender lump at the site of the pain also appears; after the second day this lump slowly dissipates and eventually leaves a skin tag.

If the thrombosed hemorrhoid resides entirely above the dentate line (pure internal hemorrhoid), there may be minimal pain because of the lack of sensory nerve supply. Patients are likely to be unaware of the presence of this type of hemorrhoid unless there are sudden changes in bowel habits.

If thrombosed hemorrhoids persist, gangrene and ulcers may develop on the hemorrhoid surface. This condition may lead to an oozing of blood as well as hemorrhaging, particularly when the patient is defecating or standing. If the clot remains exposed, infection may occur, and an abscess or fistula may result.

ASSESSMENT

By questioning the patient, the pharmacist should be able to determine whether self-medication is desirable and, if so, which nonprescription drug product is suitable.

The pharmacist should recommend an appropriate nonprescription product for treatment of minor anorectal symptoms (itching, burning, pain, swelling, or discomfort). The patient should be referred to a physician if a lump, bleeding, seepage, prolapse, or severe and persistent pain is present, or if symptoms worsen or do not improve after 7 days of self-treatment.

TREATMENT

Nonprescription products for symptomatic treatment of anorectal disease are available in many dosage forms, as discussed later in this chapter.

Pharmacologic Agents

The pharmacologic agents used for relief of anorectal disease symptoms include local anesthetics, vasoconstrictors, protectants, counterirritants, astringents, wound-healing agents, antiseptics, analgesics, anesthetics, antipruritics, keratolytics, and anticholinergics. Products containing an excessive number of agents may not be optimally effective because of potential interaction among ingredients.

Local Anesthetics

Topical anesthetics temporarily relieve pain, burning, itching, discomfort, and irritation by preventing the transmission of nerve impulses. They should be used in the perianal region or the lower anal canal; symptoms within the rectum generally are not relieved by topical anesthetics because there are no rectal sensory nerve fibers (15, 16).

Because local anesthetics may be rapidly absorbed through the rectal mucosa and cause potentially toxic systemic effects, their application should be limited to the area below the rectum (17, 18). Absorption through the perianal skin, even if abraded, would not be particularly rapid.

Local anesthetics may produce allergic reactions, both locally and systemically (19, 20). Such reactions may cause burning and itching that are indistinguishable from symptoms of the anorectal disease being treated. If symptoms return after cessation of therapy, a physician should be contacted.

Recommended Anesthetics   Of the local anesthetics used in hemorrhoidal preparations, only benzocaine and pramoxine hydrochloride are currently recommended for use in the perianal or lower anal canal regions.

- Benzocaine—Benzocaine, when used externally in the base form, is effective in concentrations of 5–20% applied up to 6 times a day. The dosage should not exceed 2.4 g in 24 hours (21–23). Because absorption through the skin is poor, the possible systemic effects are minimized. The most common adverse reaction to topical benzocaine is sensitization (24, 25). Polyethylene glycol ointment is the recommended vehicle; other vehicles may not release benzocaine as well (26).

- Pramoxine hydrochloride—Pramoxine hydrochloride, when used externally, is considered effective in a cream or jelly water-miscible base at a 1% concentration applied up to 5 times a day not to exceed 100 mg in 24 hours (27). Adverse effects are rare, and pramoxine hydrochloride exhibits less cross-sensitivity than other local anesthetics because of its distinct chemical structure (28).

Proposed Anesthetics   A recent decision by the Food and Drug Administration (FDA) not to require final formulation testing of anorectal drug products (29) has enabled local anesthetics previously classified as Category III (available data are insufficient to classify as safe and effective) to be tentatively proposed as Category I (safe and effective). The local anesthetics tentatively being reclassified as Category I for external use are benzyl alcohol, dibucaine, dibucaine hydrochloride, dyclonine hydrochloride, lidocaine, tetracaine, and tetracaine hydrochloride (30).

The recommended concentrations are benzyl alcohol, 1–4%; dyclonine hydrochloride, 0.5–1%; lidocaine, 2–5%; tetracaine and tetracaine hydrochloride, 0.5–1% (31).

Dibucaine and dibucaine hydrochloride are considered pharmacologically equivalent (32) and are proposed as being safe and effective for external use in concentrations of 0.25–1% up to 3 or 4 times a day (33).

Anesthetics Not Recommended   Other local anesthetics used in hemorrhoidal preparations are not recommended because they are not generally recognized as safe and effective. Additional evidence is required to demonstrate the effectiveness of diperodon used externally or intrarectally. Phenacaine hydrochloride is considered unsafe because of the possibility of adsorption leading to systemic toxicity (34). Additional evidence is required to show that the following anesthetics are effective intrarectally: benzocaine, benzyl alcohol, dibucaine, dibucaine hydrochloride, dyclonine hydrochloride, lidocaine, pramoxine hydrochloride, tetracaine, and tetracaine hydrochloride (34).

Vasoconstrictors

Vasoconstrictors are chemical agents structurally related to the naturally occurring catecholamines, epinephrine and norepinephrine, that function as transmitters of messages from nerves to receptors. Applied locally in the anorectal area, they stimulate the alpha-adrenergic receptors in the vascular beds, causing constriction of the arterioles. Although it has been demon-

strated that there is a prompt altering of the blood supply to the mucosa when vasoconstrictors are applied locally, the FDA advisory review panel does not recognize or approve the use of vasoconstrictors for the control of minor bleeding (35, 36). In view of the fact that rectal bleeding may be a sign of more serious disease, a physician should be consulted.

Vasoconstrictors relieve itching because they also produce a slight anesthetic effect by an unknown mechanism (37). Conclusive evidence that vasoconstrictors reduce swollen hemorrhoids is lacking, even though they constrict arterioles in skin and mucous membranes in other parts of the body and may prevent fluid accumulation and swelling.

Adverse Effects   The FDA advisory review panel concluded that potentially serious side effects, including elevation of blood pressure, cardiac arrhythmia, nervousness, tremor, sleeplessness, and aggravation of symptoms of hyperthyroidism, are less likely to occur when vasoconstrictors are used locally in recommended safe dosages (36). Because of the possibility of systemic adverse reactions, vasoconstrictors should not be used in patients who have diabetes, hyperthyroidism, hypertension, difficulty in urination due to prostate enlargement, and cardiovascular disease, and in those who are taking monoamine oxidase inhibitors. Some users of vasoconstrictors may experience nervousness, tremor, sleeplessness, nausea, and loss of appetite.

Recommended Vasoconstrictors   Three vasoconstrictors are recommended for external use: aqueous solutions of ephedrine sulfate, epinephrine hydrochloride, and phenylephrine hydrochloride. Ephedrine sulfate and phenylephrine hydrochloride solutions are also recommended for internal use (intrarectal) (38). Epinephrine base has recently been tentatively placed in Category I for external use (39) in doses of 0.005–0.01%. These agents are not commercially available for anorectal use in a solution dosage form. Epinephrine undecylenate and epinephrine hydrochloride have been classified as ineffective for intrarectal use. Additional data are needed to establish the safety and effectiveness of epinephrine base for external and intrarectal use and epinephrine undecylenate for external use.

- Ephedrine sulfate—Ephedrine sulfate (aqueous solution), which is readily absorbed through mucous membranes in the rectum, has a more prolonged effect than epinephrine and acts on both alpha- and beta-adrenergic receptors. Because ephedrine antagonizes the effects of phenothiazines, it is contraindicated in patients receiving such therapy (40). The hypertensive effects of ephedrine are potentiated by monoamine oxidase inhibitors, as well as tricyclic antidepressants. Combined use through the oral route can lead to serious, even lethal, effects (41). Its onset of action ranges from a few seconds to 1 minute, its duration of action is 2–3 hours, and it is effective in the relief of itching and swelling. The recommended dosage is 0.1–1.25% applied up to 4 times a day and not to exceed 100 mg in 24 hours (42).

- Epinephrine hydrochloride—Epinephrine hydrochloride (aqueous solution) is effective in the relief of itching and swelling only when used externally because epinephrine is inactivated at the pH of the rectum (43). Epinephrine is absorbed from the mucous membrane and acts on both alpha- and beta-adrenergic receptors. In a solution dosage form, epinephrine hydrochloride applied externally is effective for the temporary relief of itching and swelling (42). The recommended dosage is 0.005–0.01% applied up to 4 times a day and not to exceed 0.8 mg in 24 hours.

- Phenylephrine hydrochloride—Phenylephrine hydrochloride (aqueous solution) is believed to relieve itching caused by histamine release and reduces congestion in the anorectal area (42, 44). It acts primarily on the alpha-adrenergic receptors and produces vasoconstriction by a direct effect on receptors rather than by norepinephrine displacement. The recommended dosage is 0.25% applied up to 4 times a day and not to exceed 2 mg in 24 hours (42).

Protectants

Protectants prevent irritation of the anorectal area and water loss from the stratum corneum skin layer by forming a physical barrier on the skin. Little or no absorption is expected from protectants. Protection of the perianal area from irritants such as fecal matter and air leads to a reduction in irritation and concomitant itching.

Absorbents, adsorbents, demulcents, and emollients are included in the protectant classification. Many substances classified as protectants also are used as vehicles, bases, and carriers of pharmacologically active substances.

Adverse reactions to protectants as a class are minimal. Wool alcohols do cause allergies and are probably responsible for most cases of lanolin allergy (45).

Recommended Protectants   The protectants recommended for use are aluminum hydroxide gel (in moist conditions only), calamine, cocoa butter, cod liver oil, glycerin in aqueous solution, kaolin, lanolin, mineral oil, shark liver oil, starch, white petrolatum, petrolatum, and zinc oxide. All of these protectants are rec-

ommended for external and internal (intrarectal) use, with the exception of glycerin, which is recommended for external use only. Of the recommended protectants, petrolatum is probably the most effective (46).

If a protectant is used in a nonprescription preparation, it should comprise at least 50% of the dosage unit; if two to four protectants are used, their total concentration should be at least 50%. These dosages were arrived at by determining the amount of protectant required to provide adequate thickness to prevent water loss from the epidermis (47). Any protectant ingredient, except cod liver oil and shark liver oil, used in combination should contribute at least 12.5% by weight. Cod liver oil and shark liver oil should be of sufficient amount to provide 10,000 USP units of vitamin A and 400 USP units of cholecalciferol in a 24-hour period. Calamine should not exceed 25% by weight per dosage unit.

Protectants Not Recommended   The bismuth salts found in some hemorrhoidal products are not recommended as protectants. Bismuth subnitrate is not considered safe because it may be absorbed, producing toxic symptoms from the bismuth ion as well as the nitrate ion (48). The effectiveness of bismuth oxide, bismuth subcarbonate, wool alcohols (lanolin), and bismuth subgallate as protectants in the anorectal area has not been established.

Counterirritants

Counterirritants distract from the perception of pain and itching by stimulating cutaneous receptors to evoke a feeling of comfort, warmth, cooling, or tingling. Because the rectal mucosa contains no sensory nerve endings, counterirritants exert no effect in this area and are recommended for external use only and not for intrarectal use. (See Chapter 32, *External Analgesic Products.*)

There are no currently recommended counterirritants. Menthol, camphor, and juniper tar have been reclassified as analgesics, anesthetics, and antipruritics, and will be discussed under that section. Neither hydrastis nor oil of turpentine is considered safe; both lack demonstrated effectiveness (49, 50).

Astringents

Applied to the skin or mucous membranes for a local and limited effect, astringents coagulate the protein in the skin cells, thereby protecting the underlying tissue and decreasing the cell volume. When appropriately used, astringents lessen mucus and other secretions and help relieve local anorectal irritation and inflammation (51).

Calamine and zinc oxide in concentrations of 5–25% are recommended as astringents for both external and internal use. The heavy metal zinc in these compounds acts as a protein precipitant and provides an astringent effect. Witch hazel (hamamelis water) in a concentration of 10–50% is recommended as an astringent for external use in anorectal disorders; its effectiveness is due primarily to its alcohol content. The FDA advisory review panel concluded that hamamelis water provides temporary relief of itching and burning and is safe and effective for external use (52). Witch hazel is incorporated in commercially available pads or wipes that are advertised as being useful for hemorrhoids. Recommended products are limited to those containing the appropriate quantity of astringent.

Tannic acid is not safe for anorectal use because it is well absorbed and may cause liver damage (53).

Wound-Healing Agents

Several ingredients in nonprescription hemorrhoidal products are claimed to be effective in promoting wound healing or tissue repair in anorectal disease. In particular, the substance skin respiratory factor (SRF), a water-soluble extract of brewer's yeast also referred to as live yeast cell derivative, is the subject of considerable controversy. Although some tests have supported manufacturer claims, there currently is insufficient evidence that products containing SRF promote the healing of diseased anorectal tissue (54). However, the FDA is evaluating new data concerning the effectiveness of SRF (54). The FDA advisory review panel on over-the-counter (OTC) hemorrhoidal drug products studied data on cod liver oil, peruvian balsam, shark liver oil, vitamin A, and vitamin D and found them lacking in demonstrated effectiveness as wound healers (55).

Antiseptics

Antiseptics generally inhibit the growth of microorganisms. Some nonprescription anorectal products contain compounds intended for use as antiseptics. However, because of the large numbers of microorganisms in feces, it is unlikely that the use of antiseptics in the anorectal area will provide a degree of antisepsis greater than that achieved by washing with soap and water. There is no convincing evidence that using antiseptics prevents infection in the anorectal area.

Compounds claimed to have antiseptic properties are boric acid, boric acid glycerite, hydrastis, phenol, resorcinol, and sodium salicylic acid phenolate. Boric acid and boric acid glycerite are not considered safe because of boric acid toxicity (56). Hydrastis, phenol, resorcinol (used intrarectally), and sodium salicylic acid phenolate (56) are not considered safe for use in the anorectal area (49, 50, 57). Evidence is lacking to clearly demonstrate the effectiveness of resorcinol as an external antiseptic, although it is considered safe at concentrations of 0.5–2.5% per dosage unit (58). Benzethonium, 8-quinolinol benzoate, secondary amyl tricresols, 8-hydroxyquinoline sulfate, cetylpyridinium, and chlorothymol have been used as antiseptics in products intended for use in the anorectal area. The safety and efficacy of these compounds in treating the symptoms of anorectal disease remain to be evaluated.

Keratolytics

Keratolytics cause desquamation and debridement or sloughing of the epidermal surface cells. By loosening surface cells, keratolytics may help to expose underlying skin tissue to therapeutic agents. Used externally, they are useful in reducing itching, although their mechanism of action is unknown. Because mucous membranes contain no keratin layer, the intrarectal use of keratolytics is not justified and may cause harm.

The two keratolytics recommended for external use only are aluminum chlorhydroxy allantoinate (alcloxa) and resorcinol. The dosage ranges established by the FDA advisory review panel are up to six 2-g applications per day of a 0.2–2.0% ointment for alcloxa and of a 1.0–3.0% ointment for resorcinol (59). Precipitated and sublimed sulfur are not effective for intrarectal use as keratolytics.

Resorcinol is not safe when used intrarectally as a keratolytic. Additional evidence is required to determine whether precipitated and sublimed sulfur are effective as keratolytics when used externally. Although evidence exists that allantoin is effective as a keratolytic and protectant, the safety and effectiveness of allantoin in treating the symptoms of anorectal disease remain to be evaluated (60).

Anticholinergics

Anticholinergics inhibit or prevent the action of acetylcholine, the transmitter of cholinergic nerve impulses. Because anticholinergics act systemically, they are not effective in ameliorating the local symptoms of anorectal disease.

Atropine, which is included in some products designed for anorectal use, is not safe because systemic toxicity may result from the absorption of the alkaloid through diseased skin and through the rectal mucosa if the product is applied intrarectally (60).

Analgesics, Anesthetics, and Antipruritics

To promote consistency in the rulemaking process, the FDA has redesignated as "analgesic, anesthetic, and antipruritic" several ingredients that were formerly classified as "counterirritants" (61). This nomenclature was adopted to conform with the FDA pharmacologic designations of the active ingredients despite the inherent redundancy of the terms "anesthetic" and "antipruritic" as defined in this section.

In the anorectal area, a topically applied drug that relieves pain by depressing cutaneous sensory receptors is defined as an analgesic, anesthetic drug. Similarly, a topically applied drug that relieves itching by depressing cutaneous sensory receptors is defined as an antipruritic drug (62).

Menthol (0.1–1%), juniper tar (1–5%), and camphor (0.1–3%) have been proposed as safe and effective for external use in the anorectal area (61). (See Chapter 32, *External Analgesic Products*.)

Hydrocortisone

Topically applied hydrocortisone-containing products have the potential to reduce itching, inflammation, and discomfort by vasoconstriction, lysosomal membrane stabilization, and antimitotic activity (63). The FDA has proposed the nonprescription use of hydrocortisone and hydrocortisone acetate in concentrations of 0.25–0.5% for anal itching (64).

Hydrocortisone and hydrocortisone acetate, 0.5%, for topical application are available on a nonprescription basis and are indicated for temporary relief of itching genital and anal areas.

Bulk-Forming Laxatives

Because constipation is a precipitating factor in hemorrhoidal disease, patients may be advised to consider the use of bulk-forming laxatives. (See Chapter 15, *Laxative Products*.) Ingredients commonly found in these products include barley malt extract, methylcellulose, and psyllium hydrocolloid. Patients must follow directions with each product for proper fluid intake to prevent impaction and to increase efficacy. Adequate fluid intake in general should also be encouraged.

Miscellaneous

Collinsonia (stoneroot), *Escherichia coli* vaccines, lappa (burdock), leptandra (culver's root), and mullein are ingredients in nonprescription products that do not fall within the previously discussed pharmacologic classifications. With the exception of *E. coli* vaccines, these compounds are remnants of herbal medicine. There is no evidence that they are effective in treating symptoms of anorectal disease. The safety and effectiveness of *E. coli* vaccines also are unproven (65).

Dosage Forms

Drugs for treatment of anorectal disease symptoms are available in many dosage forms. For intrarectal use, suppositories, creams, ointments, gels, and foams are available. Applicators, fingers, and pile pipes are used to facilitate their application. Creams, ointments, gels, pastes, wipes, pads, liquids, and foam are used externally.

Ointments and Suppositories

Although there are considerable pharmaceutical differences among ointments, creams, pastes, and gels, the therapeutic differences are not significant. (See Chapter 28, *Topical Anti-infective Products*.) "Ointment" will be used to refer to all semisolid preparations designed for external or intrarectal use in the anorectal area. A suppository is defined as a solid dosage form and differs very little from semisolids in its vehicle formulation.

Ointments are vehicles for drugs used in treating anorectal disease symptoms and also possess inherent protectant and emollient properties. The primary function of an ointment base is the efficient delivery of the active ingredients. Applying an ointment may have a beneficial psychologic effect on patients with anorectal disorders (66). When used externally, ointments should be applied as a thin covering to the perianal area and the anal canal.

For intrarectal use, pile pipes and fingers can be used to apply ointments. Pile pipes have the advantage over fingers in that the drug product may be introduced into the rectal mucosa where a finger cannot reach. For most efficient use, the pile pipe should have lateral openings, as well as a hole in the end, to allow the drug product to cover the greatest area of rectal mucosa. The pile pipe should be lubricated before insertion by spreading the ointment around the pipe tip. The potential for systemic absorption is greatest from the rectal mucosa.

The lubricating effect of a suppository may ease straining at the stool. The insertion of a suppository may also provide a beneficial psychologic effect. However, because of their many disadvantages, suppositories are not recommended as a dosage form in treating anorectal disease symptoms. In prone patients, suppositories may leave the affected region and ascend into the rectum and lower colon (67). If the patient remains prone after inserting a suppository or an ointment, the active ingredients may not be evenly distributed over the rectal mucosa. Suppositories and ointments are relatively slow acting because they must melt to release the active ingredient.

Foams

Foam products present no proven advantage over ointments; however, theoretically, they provide more rapid release of active ingredients. Their disadvantages include the difficulty in establishing that the foam remains in the affected area and the fact that the size of the foam bubbles determines the concentration of active ingredient available (68).

Anal Hygiene

Cleansing the anorectal area with mild and unscented soap and water on a regular basis and after each bowel movement is helpful in relieving hemorrhoidal symptoms and may prevent recurrence of perianal itching. Practical means of cleansing after a bowel movement include the use of commercially available hygienic wipes or pads. Patients should be advised to blot or pat rather than rub the irritated perianal area with these wipes. This advice also applies to the use of toilet tissue, which should be unscented and uncolored.

Sitz baths are useful in relieving hemorrhoidal symptoms and in promoting good hygiene. Patients should sit in warm water (110°–115°F) 2–3 times a day for 15 minutes (69). Plastic sitz baths, which fit over the toilet rim for convenient patient use, are easily cleaned and available at pharmacies.

Surgical Treatment

Modern surgical treatments for hemorrhoids include injection of sclerosing agents, rubber band ligation, dilatation of anal canal and lower rectum, cryosurgery, hemorrhoidectomy, and laser coagulation (2).

PRODUCT SELECTION GUIDELINES

Patient Considerations

Knowledge of a patient's present condition, medical history, and medication profile is necessary to deter-
mine how an individual may respond to self-medication. First, the pharmacist must determine whether the patient has symptoms amenable to self-medication.

Conditions such as diarrhea and constipation will complicate, if not render impossible, the self-treatment of anorectal disease symptoms. If a patient is confined to bed, a suppository dosage form is probably not appropriate. Patients with cardiovascular disease, diabetes, hypertension, and hyperthyroidism should not use a product containing a vasoconstrictor. Patients experiencing difficulty in urination and/or taking monoamine oxidase inhibitors should not use an anorectal product containing a vasoconstrictor. Patients taking phenothiazines should avoid anorectal products containing ephedrine. Individuals with a tendency toward skin allergies should avoid lanolin and benzocaine in anorectal products.

Pregnant and nursing women should use only products recommended for external use; only the recommended protectants should be used internally or intrarectally. Children with hemorrhoids or other anorectal disease should be referred to a physician (70).

Product Considerations

Nonprescription anorectal preparations are intended to provide symptomatic relief for the burning, itching, pain, swelling, irritation, and discomfort of anorectal disorders. However, a wider range of more powerful steroidal products is available by prescription for use in treating anorectal disease.

In recommending an appropriate nonprescription product, the pharmacist should consider the type and amount of ingredients and the dosage form. A product containing recommended ingredients in appropriate combination at effective dosage levels should be offered. For intrarectal use the only approved ingredients are protectants and astringents. Currently, no commercially available products containing vasoconstrictors are recommended. A pile pipe of appropriate length (2 inches), with a well-lubricated and flexible tip, and with holes on the sides, may be used to apply an ointment-type product. Suppositories are not recommended for use as a dosage form for the self-treatment of anorectal conditions.

As a general rule, products containing the least number of recommended ingredients should be suggested. These products are most likely to minimize undesirable interactions and maximize effectiveness. In general, scented and tinted products should also be avoided.

Biopharmaceutical Considerations

The bioavailability of drugs from anorectal dosage forms is a result of complex interplay among physicochemical, physiologic, manufacturing, dosage form, dosage, and application variables. The precise relationship between theoretical bioavailability considerations and therapeutic effectiveness of anorectal dosage forms remains to be established. Absorption from anorectal dosage forms involves release from the vehicle, dissolution into surrounding medium, diffusion to a membrane, and penetration of the membranes. For oleaginous bases, diffusion from the base is the rate-limiting step in the release of a drug from its vehicle (71). Most drugs used in hemorrhoidal products are basic amines (local anesthetics and vasoconstrictors). The un-ionized base is soluble in lipid ointment bases; the salt form is not soluble in lipid ointment bases. The un-ionized form penetrates the lipid tissue barriers such as nerve membranes. Salt forms from weak bases are converted to the un-ionized base at tissue pH.

The solubility of the drug and its partitioning in a vehicle determine to a large extent its release rate from that vehicle.

If a drug has a greater affinity for the vehicle than the surrounding medium, a relatively slow release rate is expected. Conversely, if a drug has a greater affinity for the surrounding medium than the vehicle, a relatively rapid release rate occurs. Ephedrine sulfate dissolved in an oleaginous base such as cocoa butter is released relatively rapidly into a surrounding aqueous medium.

In the case of oleaginous bases, the rate-limiting step in absorption seems to be the rate at which the drug leaves the vehicle and dissolves in the surrounding fluid (72). The rate at which a drug diffuses from its base depends on a number of factors, including the vehicle pH, the drug concentration, the dissociation constant of the drug, the presence of surfactants, and the drug's particle size (73, 74).

For a water-soluble or water-miscible base (polyethylene glycol), a water-soluble drug form is preferred to facilitate absorption because the absorption rate appears to be controlled by the transfer of the drug through the mucosa.

In ointments, creams, and suppositories, additives such as viscosity-increasing agents and/or surfactants are often required to achieve a high-quality product. Surfactants may increase or decrease drug absorption (75).

The absorption rate of an anorectal product may be affected by the manufacturing process. For example, the release rates associated with cocoa butter may vary according to the temperature at which the cocoa butter was melted. This effect may be explained by the polymorphic nature of cocoa butter.

PATIENT CONSULTATION

The pharmacist should emphasize the importance of good anal hygiene in helping to prevent and alleviate symptoms. Specific advice should include the following:

- For maximum effect, nonprescription anorectal products should be used after, rather than before, bowel movements.

- If seepage, bleeding, or protrusion occurs, a physician should be contacted as soon as possible.

- Products designed for external use only should not be inserted into the rectum.

- If insertion of a product in the rectum causes pain, use of the product should be discontinued and a physician consulted.

- Products to be used externally should be applied sparingly.

- If possible, before any nonprescription anorectal product is applied, the anorectal area should be washed with soap and warm water, rinsed thoroughly, and gently dried by patting or blotting with toilet tissues or soft cloth.

- If symptoms worsen or do not improve after 7 days, a physician should be consulted.

Cleansing the anorectal area with a moistened unscented and uncolored toilet tissue or cotton ball after defecation is recommended. Sitz baths are an alternative nondrug therapy for symptoms of uncomplicated anorectal disease. Moreover, the importance of maintaining normal bowel function by eating properly, drinking adequate amounts of fluid, and avoiding excessive laxative use should be emphasized as a means of preventing anorectal disease. A diet high in fiber and fluid will promote the formation of large, easily passed stools, thereby preventing constipation and accompanying straining. A well-controlled study in patients with symptomatic hemorrhoids demonstrated a significant reduction in bleeding and pain within 6 weeks among patients receiving psyllium (76). Stool softeners may also be useful to prevent straining that may lead to hemorrhoids. (See Chapter 13, *Antidiarrheal Products*, and Chapter 15, *Laxative Products*.)

SUMMARY

For external use, an ideal formulation would contain, in addition to one to four protectants totaling at least 50% of the formulation composition, three recommended ingredients, each from a separate pharmacologic category chosen from the following: local anesthetics, analgesics, anesthetics, antipruritics, astringents, vasoconstrictors, and keratolytics. A combination containing a suitable local anesthetic, protectant, and astringent should be effective in relieving the itching, irritation, burning, discomfort, and pain associated with anorectal disease.

For internal/intrarectal use a model product would contain from one to four protectants totaling at least 50% of the dose and an appropriate astringent and/or vasoconstrictor. An ointment-type dosage form applied with the suitable pile pipe is recommended. This product should relieve the itching, swelling, discomfort, irritation, and pain of anorectal disease.

Products containing benzocaine (20%) in a polyethylene glycol base would be expected, when used externally, to be effective in relieving itching, burning, and pain. For intrarectal use, a product consisting of 100% petrolatum is appropriate to recommend and is safe for use by pregnant women.

The pharmacist should make clear to the patient that if symptoms worsen or do not improve after 7 days or if bleeding, protrusion, and/or seepage occurs, a physician should be consulted as soon as possible.

REFERENCES

1   R. L. Holt, "A Cure and Preventative: Hemorrhoids," California Health, Laguna Beach, Calif., 1977, p. 22.

2   M. P. Bubrick and R. B. Benjamin, *Post Grad. Med., 77,* 165 (1985).

3   R. T. Shackelford, in "Diseases of the Colon and Anorectum," R. Turrell, Ed., W. B. Saunders, Philadelphia, Pa., 1969, p. 896.

4   Z. Cohen, *Can. J. Surgery, 28,* 230–231 (1985).

5   L. E. Smith, *Gastroenter. Clin. of N. Am., 16,* 81 (1987).

6   D. Driscoll et al., *U.S. Pharmacist, 5,* (50) 43–44 (1981).

7   L. Hyams and J. Philpot, *Am. J. Proctol., 21,* 177 (1970).

8   W. H. F. Thompson, *Br. J. Surgery, 62,* 542–552 (1975).

9   A. R. Dennison et al., *Surg. Clin. N. Am., 68* (6), 1403 (1988).

10   L. E. Smith, *Gastroenter. Clin., of N. Am., 16,* 83 (1987).

11   E. Granet, "Manual of Proctology," Yearbook, Chicago, Ill., 1954, p. 115.

12   R. L. Holt, "A Cure and Preventative: Hemorrhoids," California Health, Laguna Beach, Calif., 1977, pp. 50–69.

13   D. M. Jacobs et al., *Dis. Colon Rectum, 23,* 567–569 (1980).

14   A. R. Dennison et al., *Surg. Clin. N. Am., 68* (6), 1402 (1988).

15   L. Van Dam, Statement to FDA Advisory Review Panel on OTC Hemorrhoidal Drug Products, May 1, 1976.

16   J. C. White, Statement to FDA Advisory Review Panel on OTC Hemorrhoidal Drug Products, May 1, 1976.

17   "The Pharmacological Basis of Therapeutics," 6th ed., A. G. Gilman et al., Eds., Macmillan, New York, N.Y., 1980, p. 311.

18   J. Adriani and D. Campbell, *J. Am. Med. Assoc., 162,* 1527 (1956).

19   E. Epstein, *J. Am. Med. Assoc., 198,* 517 (1966).

20   C. G. Lange and R. Luifart, *J. Am. Med. Assoc., 146,* 717 (1951).

21   H. Dalili and J. Adriani, *Clin. Pharmacol. Ther., 12,* 913 (1971).

22   J. Adriani and P. Zipernich, *J. Am. Med. Assoc., 188,* 711 (1964).

23   J. Adriani and H. Dalili, *Curr. Res. Anesth. Analg., 50,* 834 (1971).

24   H. Wilson, *Practitioner, 197,* 673 (1966).

25   *Med. Lett. Drugs Ther., 11,* 70 (1969).

26   *Federal Register, 45,* 35609–10 (1980).

27   *Med. Lett. Drugs Ther., 23,* 100 (1981).

28   "The Pharmacological Basis of Therapeutics," 6th ed., A. G. Gilman et al., Eds., Macmillan, New York, N.Y., 1980, p. 310.

29   *Federal Register, 53,* 30776 (1988).

30   *Federal Register, 53,* 30777 (1988).

31   *Federal Register, 53,* 30778 (1988).

32   *Federal Register, 53,* 30759 (1988).

33   *Federal Register, 53,* 30761 (1988).

34   *Federal Register, 45,* 35613 (1980).

35   O. Thulesius and J. E. Gjores, *Acta Chir. Scand., 139,* 476 (1973).

36   *Federal Register, 45,* 35621 (1980).

37   F. M. Melton and W. B. Shelly, *J. Invest. Dermatol., 15,* 325 (1950).

38   *Federal Register, 45,* 35622 (1980).

39   *Federal Register, 53,* 30778 (1988).

40   "The Pharmacological Basis of Therapeutics," 6th ed., A. G. Gilman et al., Eds., Macmillan, New York, N.Y., 1980, pp. 414

41   "The Pharmacological Basis of Therapeutics," 6th ed., A. G. Gilman, L. S. Goodman, and A. Gilman, Eds., Macmillan, New York, N.Y., 1980, pp. 427, 430.

42   *Federal Register, 45,* 35623–25 (1980).

43   E. Granet, "Manual of Proctology," Yearbook, Chicago, Ill., 1954, p. 59.

44   F. M. Melton and W. B. Shelley, *J. Invest. Dermatol., 15,* 325 (1950).

45   *Federal Register, 45,* 35635 (1980).

46   G. K. Steigleder and W. P. Raab, *J. Invest. Dermatol., 38,* 129 (1962).

47   *Federal Register, 45,* 356 (1980).

48   J. M. Arena, "Poisoning," Charles C. Thomas, Springfield, Ill., 1979, p. 391.

49   K. Genest and D. W. Hughes, *Can. J. Pharm. Sci., 4,* 4145 (1969).

50   W. B. Deichman and H. W. Gerarde, "Toxicology of Drugs and Chemicals," Academic, New York, N.Y., 1969, p. 448.

51 E. M. Boyd, in "Pharmacology in Medicine," 4th ed., V. A. Drill, Ed., McGraw-Hill, New York, N.Y., 1971, p. 1034.

52 *Federal Register, 45,* 35646 (1980).

53 B. Korpassy and K. Kovacs, *Br. J. Exp. Pathol., 30,* 266 (1949).

54 *Federal Register, 53,* 30765 (1988).

55 *Federal Register, 45,* 35650 (1980).

56 M. A. Valdes-Dapena and J. B. Arey, *J. Pediatr., 61,* 531 (1962).

57 "AMA Drug Evaluations—1973," 2nd ed., American Medical Association, Chicago, Ill., 1973, p. 893.

58 *Federal Register, 45,* 35663 (1980).

59 *Federal Register, 45,* 35665 (1980).

60 D. W. Melxell and S. B. Mecca, *J. Am. Pod. Assoc., 56,* 357 (1966).

61 *Federal Register, 53,* 30779 (1988).

62 *Federal Register, 53,* 30781 (1988).

63 "AMA Drug Evaluations—1980," 4th ed., John Wiley and Sons, New York, N.Y., 1980, pp. 1009–1052.

64 *Federal Register, 53,* 30766 (1988).

65 "The Pharmacological Basis of Therapeutics," 6th ed., A. G. Gilman et al., Eds., Macmillan, New York, N.Y., 1980, p. 126.

66 *Federal Register, 45,* 35669 (1980).

67 *Federal Register, 45,* 35589 (1980).

68 L. Augsberger and R. T. Shangraw, *J. Pharm. Sci., 57,* 624 (1968).

69 E. W. Martin, "Techniques of Medication," J. B. Lippincott, Philadelphia, Pa., 1969, p. 181.

70 *Federal Register, 45,* 35599 (1980).

71 "Evaluations of Drug Interactions," 2nd ed., American Pharmaceutical Association, Washington, D.C., 1976.

72 W. A. Ritschel, "Biopharmaceutical Development and Evaluation of Rectal Dosage Forms, Applied Biopharmaceutics II," University of Cincinnati, College of Pharmacy, Cincinnati, Ohio, 1973, p. 1160.

73 N. A. Allawalla and S. Riegelman, *J. Am. Pharm. Assoc. Sci. Ed., 42,* 267 (1953).

74 J. Anschel and H. A. Lieberman, in "The Theory and Practice of Industrial Pharmacy," 2nd ed., L. Lachman et al., Eds., Lea and Febiger, Philadelphia, Pa., 1976, pp. 245–269.

75 S. Riegelman and W. J. Crowell, *J. Am. Pharm. Assoc. Sci. Ed., 47,* 115 (1958).

76 F. Moesgaard et al., *Diseases of Colon and Rectum, 25,* 454 (1982).

HEMORRHOIDAL PRODUCT TABLE

Product (Manufacturer)	Application Form	Anesthetic	Antiseptic	Astringent	Protectant	Other Ingredients
A-Caine Rectal (A.V.P.)	ointment	diperodon hydrochloride, 0.25%		zinc oxide, 5% bismuth subcarbonate, 0.2%	cod liver oil and petrolatum base	phenylephrine hydrochloride, 0.25% pyrilamine maleate, 0.1%
Americaine (DuPont Critical Care)	ointment	benzocaine, 20%	benzethonium chloride, 0.1%			
Anocaine Hemorrhoidal (Hauck)	suppository	benzocaine		zinc oxide bismuth subgallate balsam Peru	vegetable oil	
Anumed (Major)	suppository			bismuth subgallate, 2.25% bismuth resorcin compound, 1.75% benzyl benzoate, 1.2% zinc oxide, 11% balsam Peru, 1.8%	hydrogenated vegetable oil	
Anusol (Parke-Davis)	ointment	pramoxine hydrochloride, 1%		zinc oxide, 11% balsam Peru, 1.8%		benzyl benzoate, 1.2% polyethylene wax mineral oil
Anusol (Parke-Davis)	suppository			zinc oxide, 11% balsam Peru, 1.8% bismuth subgallate, 2.25% bismuth-resorcin compound, 1.75%	vegetable oil base	benzyl benzoate, 1.2%
Balneol (Reid-Rowell)	cleansing lotion					mineral oil; propylene glycol; glyceryl stearate/PEG-100 stearate; laureth-4, PEG-4 dilaurate; lanolin oil; sodium acetate; carbomer 934; triethanolamine; methylparaben; docusate sodium; fragrance; acetic acid
BiCozene (Sandoz)	cream	benzocaine, 6%			cream base	resorcinol, 1.67%

HEMORRHOIDAL PRODUCT TABLE, continued

Product (Manufacturer)	Application Form	Anesthetic	Antiseptic	Astringent	Protectant	Other Ingredients
Calmol 4 (Mentholatum)	cream suppository			zinc oxide, 5% (cream), 10% (suppository) bismuth subgallate (suppository)	cocoa butter, 80% (suppository)	
CPI (Century)	suppository			bismuth subgallate, 2.25% bismuth resorcin compound, 1.75% benzyl benzoate, 1.2% zinc oxide, 11% balsam Peru, 1.8%	hydrogenated vegetable oil	
Fleet Relief Anesthetic Hemorrhoidal (Fleet)	ointment	pramoxine hydrochloride, 1%				
Formulation R (G & W)	ointment				shark liver oil, 3%	live yeast cell derivative phenylmercuric nitrate, 1:10,000
Gentz Wipes (Roxane)	pads	pramoxine hydrochloride, 1%	cetylpyridinium chloride, 0.05%	hamamelis water, 50% aluminum chlorhydroxy allantoinate, 0.2%	propylene glycol, 10%	fragrance
Hemet Hemorrhoidal (Halsey)	suppository	benzocaine		zinc oxide bismuth subgallate balsam Peru	vegetable oil base	
Hemet Rectal (Halsey)	ointment	diperodon hydrochloride, 0.25%		bismuth subcarbonate, 0.2% zinc oxide, 5%	cod liver oil petrolatum	pyrilamine maleate, 0.1% phenylephrine hydrochloride, 0.25%
Hemocaine (Hauck)	ointment	diperodon hydrochloride, 0.25%		bismuth subcarbonate, 0.2% zinc oxide, 5%	cod liver oil petrolatum	pyrilamine maleate, 0.1% phenylephrine hydrochloride, 0.25%
Hemorrin (Jeffrey Martin)	ointment suppository			bismuth subgallate, 2.25% bismuth resorcin compound, 1.75% balsam Peru, 1.8% zinc oxide, 11%		
Hem-Prep (G & W)	suppository	benzocaine		bismuth subgallate zinc oxide	shark liver oil	phenylmercuric nitrate 1:10,000
Lanacane (Combe)	cream	benzocaine, 6%	benzethonium chloride, 0.1%		water-washable base	

HEMORRHOIDAL PRODUCT TABLE, continued

Product (Manufacturer)	Application Form	Anesthetic	Antiseptic	Astringent	Protectant	Other Ingredients
Medicone Rectal (Medicone)	ointment	benzocaine, 2%	menthol, 0.4%	zinc oxide, 10% balsam Peru, 1.26%	castor oil, 1.26% petrolatum-lanolin, 83.6%	hydroxyquino-line sulfate, 0.5%
Medicone Rectal (Medicone)	suppository	benzocaine, 130 mg	hydroxyquin-oline sulfate, 16 mg menthol, 9 mg	zinc oxide, 195 mg balsam Peru, 65 mg	vegetable and petroleum oil base	
Mediconet (Medicone)	pads		benzalkonium chloride, 0.02%	hamamelis water, 50%	ethoxylated lanolin, 0.5% glycerin, 10%	alkylaryl polyether methylparaben, 0.15% perfume
Non-Steroid proctoFoam (Reed & Carnrick)	foam	pramoxine hydrochloride, 1%			mineral oil	
Nupercainal (Ciba)	ointment	dibucaine, 1%			lanolin, white petrolatum, light mineral oil	acetone sodium bisulfite
Nupercainal Suppositories (Ciba)	suppository			zinc oxide	cocoa butter	acetone sodium bisulfite bismuth subgallate
Pazo (Bristol-Myers Products)	ointment suppository	benzocaine, 0.8% (ointment) 15.44 mg (suppository)	camphor, 2.18% (ointment) 42.07 mg (suppository)	zinc oxide, 4% (ointment) 77.2 mg (suppository)		ephedrine sul-fate, 0.2% (ointment) 3.86 mg (suppository)
Peterson's (Peterson's Health & Beauty Inc.)	ointment	camphor, 4.86% phenol, 3.16%		tannic acid, 2.16% zinc oxide, 6.5%	petrolatum beeswax	
Pontocaine (Winthrop)	cream ointment	tetracaine hydrochloride (equivalent to 1% base) (cream) tetracaine base, 5% (ointment)	menthol, 0.5% (ointment)		white petrola-tum (ointment) white wax (ointment)	methylparaben (cream) sodium bisulfite (cream)
Preparation H (Whitehall)	cream ointment suppository		phenylmercuric nitrate, 0.01%		shark liver oil, 3%	live yeast cell derivative (supplying 2000 units of skin respira-tory factor)/oz
Preparation H Cleansing, Regular & Medicated (Whitehall)	pads			hamamelis water, 30% (regular) 50% (medicated)	glycerin	alcohol, 7.4% methylparaben octoxynol-9 (medicated)

HEMORRHOIDAL PRODUCT TABLE, continued

Product (Manufacturer)	Application Form	Anesthetic	Antiseptic	Astringent	Protectant	Other Ingredients
Primaderm-B (Arrow Medical)	ointment	benzocaine		zinc oxide	cod liver oil petrolatum-lanolin base	
Rectagene Medicated (Pfeiffer)	ointment	benzocaine, 3%		bismuth subgallate, 1% zinc oxide, 1.5%	polyethylene glycol base	phenylephrine hydrochloride, 0.2% pyrilamine maleate cetalkonium chloride
Tronolane (Ross)	cream suppository	pramoxine hydrochloride, 1%			water-miscible base (cream) vegetable oil triglyceride (suppository)	
Tucks (Parke-Davis)	cream ointment pads			hamamelis water, 50%	glycerin, 10% (pads)	alcohol, 7% (cream & ointment)
Vaseline Pure Petroleum Jelly (Chesebrough Ponds)	ointment				white petrolatum, 100%	
Wyanoid Relief Factor (Wyeth)	suppository		boric acid	zinc oxide bismuth subcarbonate bismuth oxyiodide balsam Peru	cocoa butter beeswax	belladonna extract, 15 mg ephedrine sulfate, 3 mg

Donald R. Miller and Mary Kuzel

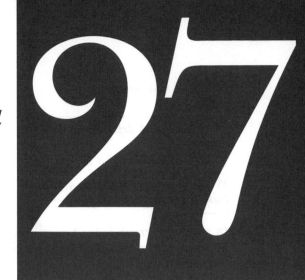

PERSONAL CARE PRODUCTS

*Q*uestions to ask in patient/consumer counseling

Feminine Cleansing Products

Have you noticed any difference in your vaginal discharge? Are you having pain or itching?

Are there any sores in the vaginal area?

Have you had this condition before?

How long has the condition been present?

Have you ever seen a physician for this condition or treated it yourself?

Do you douche? If so, how frequently?

Are you taking any prescription drugs? Are you using any nonprescription feminine cleansing or deodorant products?

Do you currently use an IUD? Have you ever used one?

Are you pregnant?

Do you have any medical problems such as diabetes?

Antiperspirant and Deodorant Products

Do you want to purchase an antiperspirant, a deodorant, or a combination of both types?

Do you perspire heavily even in cool temperatures? Do you perspire heavily when you are nervous and excited?

Do you feel that you need an extra-strength product? Why?

Do the palms of your hands and the soles of your feet perspire heavily?

Has the amount of perspiration changed recently?

Have you ever had an allergic reaction to any antiperspirant or deodorant product?

Skin-Bleaching Agents

Have you been using a skin-bleaching product? If so, for how long?

For what type of freckle or "skin spot" do you use it?

How long has it been present?

Has it changed color or increased in size?

Do you have any medical problems?

Is there any possibility that you are pregnant?

Are you taking any medications, including birth control pills?

Depilatories

Why do you want to use a depilatory?

Are you currently taking any medications?

Is your skin very sensitive?

TABLE 1	Classification of vaginitis	
Type	**Organism**	**Age group affected**
INFECTIOUS		
Atrophic (senile)	Coliforms *Staphylococcus* *Streptococcus*	Postmenopausal Prepubertal, rarely
Bacterial	*Gardnerella vaginale** Coliforms *Staphylococcus* *Streptococcus*	All
Gonorrhea	*Neisseria gonorrhoeae*	Adult
Herpes II	Herpes II	All
Monilial	*Candida albicans*	Adult (especially if pregnant or diabetic)
Mycoplasma	*Mycoplasma*	All
Preadolescent (childhood vulvovaginitis)	Helminths Coliforms *Staphylococcus* *Streptococcus*	Prepubertal
Trichomonal	*Trichomonas vaginalis*	Adult Prepubertal, rarely
Tuberculous	*Mycobacterium tuberculosis*	All
NONINFECTIOUS		
Allergic and chemical		All (when foreign chemicals are instilled vaginally)
Postirradiation		All (when irradiation is used for treatment of cervical carcinoma)
Traumatic		All

*Gardnerella vaginale (formerly *Hemophilus vaginalis* and *Corynebacterium vaginale*) is frequently considered by itself because it is the most frequent pathogen in nonspecific bacterial vaginitis.

these organisms (9). Although childhood vulvovaginitis is relatively uncommon, it usually has the same cause and manifestations as atrophic vaginitis. Vaginal discharge in prepubertal girls or presence of a foreign object in the vagina should arouse suspicion of sexual abuse (10). Candidal and trichomonal infections may occur simultaneously, and both organisms may be present in the normal, healthy vagina (11, 12). Trichomonal vaginitis is transmitted primarily through sexual contact.

Symptoms

The symptoms of vaginitis, leukorrhea, and pruritus may cause a woman to seek medical attention or to self-medicate. Offensive odor may be caused by discharge associated with trichomonal or gardnerella organisms. The description of a purulent vaginal discharge should alert the pharmacist to the possibility of vaginitis and the need for a specific diagnosis and prescribed therapy. In postmenopausal women, a thin watery discharge accompanied by pruritus indicates possible atrophic vaginitis or malignancy. The pharmacist should determine whether vaginitis symptoms are present, how long they have persisted, and whether predisposing factors exist. The patient also should be asked whether any previous attempts at self-treatment have been made, because symptoms may be caused by an adverse reaction to a nonprescription product.

Pruritus with or without a malodorous discharge may occur in conditions other than vaginitis, such as cystitis, urethritis, chemical irritation, sexually transmitted disease, and carcinoma of the cervix, endometrium, or vagina. Regardless of the cause, these symptoms are an indication for diagnostic evaluation by a physician, especially if they are persistent, severe, or recurrent. Patients should be told not to bathe or douche immediately before visiting a physician for an examination for vaginitis (13).

Depending on the specific diagnosis of vaginitis, the physician may prescribe antitrichomonal, antimonilial (antifungal), or antibacterial therapy. Metronidazole, 500 mg taken orally for 7 days, remains the treatment of choice for bacterial vaginosis and is also highly effective against trichomonal organisms (7). In atrophic vaginitis, however, systemic or local estrogenic hormone therapy may be prescribed because estrogen stimulates vaginal epithelium, increasing its thickness and resistance to infection. In cases of vaginitis, nonprescription feminine cleansing and deodorant products should be used only on a pharmacist's or physician's advice.

Vaginal Douches

Douches may exert cleansing effects by lowering surface tension and promoting mucolytic and proteolytic action; however, standards for evaluating these effects have not been established (12). Douche products are available as liquids, liquid concentrates to be diluted in water, powders to be dissolved in water, and powders (insufflations) to be instilled as powders. (The term "douche" is not limited to a stream of water.) Within

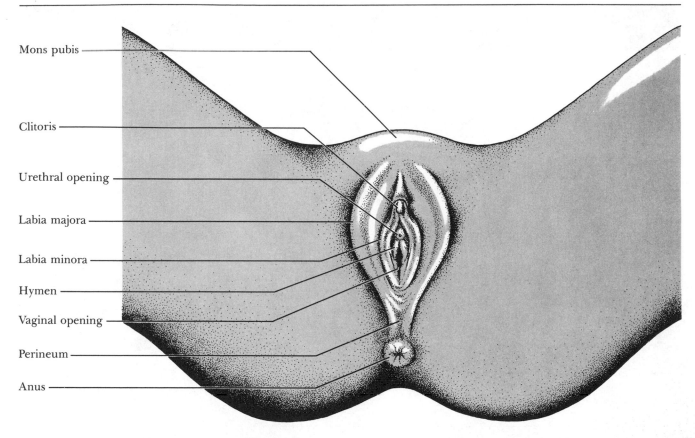

FIGURE 2   External genitalia of the adult female.

the past few years, premixed douche liquids in disposable applicators have become available and are widely advertised. Disposable applicators are convenient to use and eliminate the care and cleansing procedures that nondisposable douche equipment requires.

Ingredients

Recommended concentrations for many ingredients in feminine cleansing and deodorant products are listed in Table 2; however, many manufacturers do not list concentrations.

Antimicrobial Agents   Most antimicrobial agents in douche products are present in concentrations that provide preservative properties but no therapeutic activity. They include benzethonium and benzalkonium chlorides, chlorothymol, hexachlorophene, and parabens. Other compounds such as boric acid, cetylpyridinium chloride, eucalyptol, menthol, oxyquinoline, phenol, sodium perborate, and thymol may be included for purported antiseptic or germicidal activity. However, the value of these ingredients as antimicrobials is questionable, depending in some cases on the

concentration used. Because many manufacturers do not list concentrations of ingredients when the products are considered cosmetics, it is impossible to assess their efficacy. The possibility of local irritation or sensitization exists with many antimicrobial agents found in douches; if these effects are encountered, the patient should be instructed to discontinue use of the product and to consult a physician.

Counterirritants   Counterirritant compounds such as eucalyptol, menthol, phenol, methyl salicylate, and thymol are included in douche products for their anesthetic or antipruritic effects; however, the efficacy of these agents has not been substantiated. Eucalyptol and methyl salicylate may mask odors by their fragrances. Aromatic agents (chlorothymol, eucalyptol, menthol, thymol, or methyl salicylate) may be added for the general effect of producing a soothing and refreshing feeling. (See Chapter 32, *External Analgesic Products*.)

Astringents   Astringent substances such as ammonium and potassium alums and zinc sulfate are included in some douches to reduce local edema, inflammation, and exudation. Micronized aluminum powder also has

TABLE 2 Categories of active ingredients in feminine cleansing and deodorant products

Ingredient	Recommended concentration[a]	Indication			
		Relief of minor irritation	Alters pH	Astringent	Lowers surface tension and mucolytic
Acetic acid	0.375%		III(E)		III(E)
Alkyl aryl sulfonate	0.1%				III(E)
Allantoin	0.33%	III(E)			
Aloe vera, stabilized	90%	III(E)			
Alum	0.037–0.06%			III(E)	
Benzalkonium chloride	0.1%	III(S,E)			
Benzethonium chloride	0.2–0.5%	III(S,E)			
Benzocaine	0.2–0.65%	III(E)			
Boric acid	1%	III(S,E)	III(S,E)	III(S,E)	III(S,E)
Boroglycerin		III(S,E)	III(S,E)	III(S,E)	III(S,E)
Calcium and sodium propionate[b]	up to 20%				
Citric acid	0.1–0.5%		III(E)		
Docusate	0.002%				I
Edetate disodium	0.01–0.33%	III(S,E)			
Edetate sodium	4.4%	III(S,E)			
Hexachlorophene		II			
Lactic acid	0.4–1.3%		III(E)		
Nonoxynol 9	0.0176–0.2%	III(E)			I
Octoxynol 9	0.088%	III(E)			I
Oxyquinoline citrate	2%	III(S,E)			
Oxyquinoline sulfate	2%	III(S,E)			
Papain	0.005%				III(E)
Phenol	0.31–1.5%	II			
Phenolate		II			
Potassium sorbate[b]	1–3%	I			
Povidone–iodine	0.15–0.3%	I			
Sodium bicarbonate			III(E)		
Sodium borate		III(S,E)	III(S,E)	III(S,E)	III(S,E)
Sodium carbonate	1 tsp/l		III(S,E)		
Sodium lactate			III(E)		
Sodium lauryl sulfate	0.01–0.02%				I
Sodium perborate		III(S,E)	III(S,E)	III(S,E)	III(S,E)
Sodium salicylate		II			
Sodium salicylic acid phenolate		II			
Tartaric acid	0.047%		III(E)		
Zinc sulfate	0.02%			III(E)	

[a] Recommended concentrations for Category I and III ingredients.
Concentration not specified for some ingredients.
[b] FDA will not allow marketing in OTC products at this time.
Category I = safe (S) and effective (E) for OTC use;
Category II = neither safe nor effective for OTC use;
Category III = safety and/or effectiveness not yet established.
Reprinted with permission from T. A. Gossel, *U.S. Pharmacist, 11* *(5)*, 24 (1986).

been used as an astringent douche (3). The astringent concentration is important because many astringents are irritants in moderate or high concentrations (14).

Proteolytics At least one proteolytic agent, papain, is used in a douche product to remove excess vaginal discharge. Papain may elicit allergic reactions.

Surfactants Docusate sodium, nonoxynol 4, and sodium lauryl sulfate are used to facilitate the douche's spread over vaginal mucosa and penetration of mucosal folds (rugae) (2). Cetylpyridinium chloride, benzalkonium chloride, and benzethonium chloride also have surface-active properties.

Substances Affecting pH Many vaginal douche products are buffered or contain substances that purposely render them either acidic or alkaline. For example, sodium perborate and sodium bicarbonate provide alkalinity, and lactic acid and citric acid provide acidity. The significance of pH and buffering is discussed in the section on advisability of douching.

Miscellaneous Ingredients Other ingredients occasionally found in douches are emollients, emulsifiers, keratolytics, and substances intended to raise the preparations' osmolarity. Liquid vehicles are alcohol, propylene glycol, water, or combinations of these substances. Talc is used as a vehicle for douche powders intended to be instilled as powders (insufflations). Lactose may be added as a bacterial nutrient. Many gynecologists believe that a simple douche consisting of small amounts of white vinegar and tap water (2 tablespoons of vinegar per quart of water) is as good as commercially available products. Premixed vinegar douches are commercially available.

Types of Syringes

Several types of syringes are used for douching. The water bottle–syringe combination (fountain syringe) and the folding feminine syringe are held above hip level while the douche liquid is instilled into the vagina by gravity. These syringes are supplied with the necessary tubing and tips for use with douches or with enemas. Patients should be advised of the difference between douche and enema tips and that they are not interchangeable. Interchanging douche and enema tips may lead to infection. The main advantage to the combination (fountain) and folding feminine syringes is that fluids are instilled with gentle gravity force only, thereby minimizing the chance of excessive fluid force.

Bulb-type feminine syringes also may be used with douche liquids. The main advantage of bulb-type feminine syringes is ease of handling because it is not necessary to use tubing or to hold the syringe at an elevated level. Care must be exercised, however, to avoid excessive squeezing and excessive fluid force on instillation of the douche. Excessive force may introduce fluid into the cervix, which may cause an inflammatory response depending on the degree of uterine involvement.

Douching Techniques

To avoid the possible dangers of improper douching, several investigators recommend procedures to ensure safe instillation (9, 15–17):

- Douches should never be instilled with excessive pressure. The force of gravity is sufficient if a bag, tube, and nozzle are used. The douche bag should not be more than 60 cm (about 24 inches) above the hips. If a syringe is used, minimum pressure should be applied.

- Most douches should be instilled while the patient is lying down with the knees drawn up and the hips raised. For convenience, a bathtub is the preferred location; a toilet may also be used.

- Water used to dilute powder or douche solutions should be lukewarm, not hot.

- Douching equipment should be cleansed thoroughly before and after use. Sterilization by boiling is recommended. (The use of disposable douche products eliminates this inconvenience.)

- Douches should not be used during pregnancy.

- Douches should not be used when using the cervical mucus method of contraception, so that test results are not altered. (See Chapter 25, *Contraceptive Methods and Products*.)

Recommendations concerning the frequency of douching vary widely. One study found that 175 women douching daily had higher vaginal epithelial glycogen concentrations than 199 women douching less often, implying that more frequent douching produced a beneficial effect. Water and a medicinal powder douche were used, but the ingredients and nature of the medicinal powder were not stated (18).

Some studies indicate that routine douching should be avoided entirely (16, 19, 20). A common recommendation, however, is that women who prefer routine douching should not do so more than twice a week unless otherwise advised by the physician or pharmacist. The potential for harm from frequent douching depends in part on the formulation and the technique of instillation, both of which may be incorrect. Properly prepared and properly instilled, a douche used twice a week should cause no harm, but it has not been proven that twice-weekly or even less frequent douching is necessary at all.

An alternative self-bathing method for vaginal and perineal areas has been studied for benefits and possible adverse effects in more than 500 women, including 180 with symptoms or diagnosis of vaginitis. The technique involves gentle washing, with the fingers, of the vulvar, perineal, and anal regions and the vagina, using only lukewarm water and a mild soap. The technique was effective as a cleansing practice and was 94% effective in clearing the symptoms of vaginitis, which had a recurrence rate of slightly more than 5% (21).

Patient Consultation

Evaluating whether a woman should use a douche for routine vaginal cleansing is difficult; both sides of the conflict are well represented in the literature. The position of the Food and Drug Administration (FDA) regarding safety and efficacy of vaginal douching is that there are no standards for evaluating or substantiating claims (22). Further, patients with repeated bouts of incapacitating vaginitis are frequently susceptible to suggestions for untested and ineffective treatments, such as bizarre diets or yogurt douches (23). Evaluating a patient's degree of frustration should be part of the overall assessment.

Adverse effects of douches on vaginal pH, flora, and cytology have been cited as potential hazards of routine douching. However, the effects of acidic, alkaline, and vinegar douches on vaginal pH and vaginal mucosal cytology are not significant (4, 24). An alkaline douche is considered to be more effective than an acidic douche for removing vaginal discharge and relieving pruritus, and it is effective as adjunctive therapy in vaginitis (24–26).

Other reports also support douching as a safe, effective cleansing mechanism that does not alter vaginal pH significantly if the douche preparation is unbuffered (2, 3, 27); acidic rather than alkaline douches are advised, however, because shifts toward alkalinity may inhibit normal flora and promote pathogen growth (2, 3). Of course, care should be taken that the douche is not excessively acidic, causing irritation or injury.

In one study, douching caused no significant alterations in normal vaginal flora. Moreover, significant increases in vaginal epithelial glycogen content were observed in women who douched. It was concluded that douching was not only harmless but even beneficial to vaginal and cervical epithelium (18). Other studies have also attested to the safety of routine douching carried out according to physician instructions (28, 29). No evidence was found that douche ingredients may be absorbed systemically in significant quantities. Boric acid and phenylmercuric acetate may be absorbed. Use of boric acid should be discouraged because the FDA advisory panel on over-the-counter (OTC) vaginal drug products has placed it in Category III. Numerous reports of toxicity and poisoning from boric acid have been reported (30).

On the other hand, available evidence shows that povidone–iodine is absorbed from the vagina in significant amounts (31). This poses a particular hazard to pregnant women, in whom amniotic fluid may contain total iodine levels 10–150 times the control values (32). It seems unlikely that a single application of povidone–iodine during pregnancy would affect the fetus; however, repeated application may result in iodine-induced goiter and hypothyroidism in the fetus, with sequelae such as airway obstruction, mental and physical retardation, and neurologic disturbances (31). The vagina is a highly absorptive organ, and during pregnancy it becomes hyperemic, having the potential for exaggerated absorption of toxic substances. Therefore it seems wise to avoid douching with anything that contains potentially toxic chemicals during pregnancy. Pregnant women may also be at risk for fetal complications or other hazards of douching.

A significant number of case reports described adverse effects, suggesting that douching may be unwise without specific indication. Five cases were studied in which salpingitis, endometritis, or pelvic inflammatory disease was associated with douching. Instillation pressure of the douche fluid was implicated in each case (17). Douching may increase the incidence of ectopic pregnancy. A recent study reported that women who douched at least weekly had twice the risk of tubal ectopic pregnancy than women who never douched (33).

Ninety percent of 101 patients with pelvic inflammatory disease were reported as being "vigorous" douchers (34). Other conditions linked to douching are infection, hemorrhage, trauma, embolism, and chemical peritonitis (15, 16, 21, 35).

Perhaps the most frequent adverse effects of douches are direct, primary mucosal/dermal irritation or allergic contact sensitivity from specific ingredients. No well-controlled clinical studies of these effects on vaginal mucosa after douching could be found, but many ingredients of douche preparations have been implicated in these dermal effects. Dermal irritants or sensitizers may affect the vaginal epithelium similarly. Compounds incorporated into douche products that cause direct chemical effects, especially allergic contact sensitivity, include benzalkonium and benzethonium chlorides, benzocaine, chlorhexidine hydrochloride, chloroxylenol, parabens, phenol, propylene glycol monostearate, and triethanolamine (36–41).

Potential hazards must be weighed against the questionable value of routine douching in the absence of symptoms. According to one investigator, despite reported adverse effects, "a douche properly prepared and administered is harmless" (17). The key words in this statement are "properly prepared and administered." This is where the pharmacist can help by proper counseling.

Douche products should not be considered contraceptive agents. Douches of normal volume, properly instilled, are ineffective in removing seminal fluid for contraceptive purposes (20). Precoital douches also are ineffective as contraceptives (17). Postcoital douching is preferred by some women, but the benefits are probably psychologic or placebo because the superiority of douching over cleansing with soap and water has not been conclusively demonstrated. Douching should be delayed for 6–8 hours after the use of a vaginal spermicide because spermicidal agents may be removed in the douching process. (See Chapter 25, *Contraceptive Methods and Products*.)

Feminine Deodorant Sprays

Feminine deodorant sprays are aerosol products in mist or powder form intended for use on the external genital area to reduce or mask objectionable odor. A typical formula includes an antimicrobial agent, an emollient carrier, a perfume, and a propellant. Talc is added to spray powders. The FDA considers these products cosmetic and prohibits references to "hygiene" by manufacturers (42). The sprays do not possess therapeutic or medicinal properties. They may have only a placebo effect.

Ingredients

Some concentrations of feminine deodorant spray ingredients may be safe for external skin but not necessarily for vaginal mucosa.

Perfumes Fragrances or perfumes, the main ingredients of feminine deodorant sprays, are responsible for deodorant activity. Fragrances are characterized as mild or strong, short- or long-lasting, sweet, medicinal, and floral, among other categories (43). Some products contain encapsulated perfumes that are released slowly on contact with moisture. They should be selected with care because some may be irritating to perineal and vaginal mucosa (44).

Antimicrobials Antimicrobial compounds in sprays include benzalkonium and benzethonium chlorides, chloroxylenol, and hexachlorophene. These and similar compounds are preservatives rather than therapeutic agents. Although a deodorant action may be achieved by inhibiting or eradicating vulvoperineal bacteria, the sprays do not deodorize by this mechanism. Properly used, they do not alter normal vulvovaginal flora (45). Holding the spray too close to the body may result in an excessively high surface concentration of the antimicrobial agent or may cause the agent to enter into the vagina, where the concentration also may be excessive.

Emollients A number of emollient substances are included in these formulations as vehicles and for their soothing effect on the skin. The most commonly used are fatty alcohols, esters such as isopropyl myristate, and polyoxyethylene derivatives of fatty esters. Unfortunately, some of these substances also may be sensitizers (37, 39, 43).

Propellants If the spray is held too close to the body and the propellant reaches the skin, the chilling effects or even tissue freezing when the spray evaporates may cause irritation and edema (43, 46, 47). With proper application, propellants are not likely to be irritants. The fluorinated hydrocarbon propellants previously used have been largely replaced by aliphatic hydrocarbons such as propane and isobutane. These have low toxicity potential and a vapor pressure similar to fluorocarbons (48). Furthermore, they appear to be less hazardous to the environment.

Proper Application of Sprays

Most manufacturers recommend that sprays be held at least 20 cm (about 8 inches) from the body during application. By following this direction, premarketing evaluations of sprays consistently demonstrate safety. The most frequent adverse effect resulting from applying a spray held too closely is irritation as a result of evaporation and "chilling" from propellants inappropriately reaching the skin, excessive concentrations of ingredients on cutaneous surfaces, or accidental penetration of ingredients into the vagina from the force of the spray (ingredients are intended only for external use).

The relationship between frequency of use and the incidence of adverse effects has not been described well in the literature. It is reasonable to assume, however, that frequent application, perhaps several times a day, may elicit more frequent local reactions than less frequent use. If women are fully informed of the possibility and nature of side effects, they can, with the help of the pharmacist, determine a desirable frequency of application for themselves.

Patient Consultation

As with douche products, the advisability and benefits of using feminine deodorant sprays are controversial. Their efficacy even as deodorants has been questioned, and adverse effects have been reported (49). When the sprays are used as directed, however, manufacturers report that extensive testing fails to demonstrate adverse effects.

A feminine deodorant spray was evaluated in 1,400 women after more than 200,000 test applications by direct application and patch testing (50). The study findings supported the position that sprays were non-irritating and nonsensitizing. However, the results of the study are difficult to evaluate because many details were not provided. It was also reported that in one group of 300 women, 8% of the control group experienced erythema from soap and water, but only 3% of those using sprays experienced this effect. The study results provided no other explanations for consumer complaints of vulvar irritation after the use of these sprays. It was suggested that close-fitting and/or non-absorbent undergarments cause vulvar irritation even if no spray is applied; that the symptoms might appear if sprays are used immediately after intercourse; or that the sprays are held too close to the body when applied.

Despite reports that these aerosol products are not hazardous when evaluated in controlled studies and when properly used, there is evidence that hazards do exist. Physicians in private practice reported vulvar irritation in some of their female patients, and feminine deodorant sprays were strongly suspected as being the cause (51, 52). The FDA receives many reports of adverse local reactions, all locally severe and all attributed to the use of these products (53). In most of these cases, systemic steroid treatment was required even when the sprays were discontinued. The specific ingredients responsible for adverse effects, however, were not identified. Four positive patch-test reactions to specific ingredients were reported after 30 women and 2 men were tested with the individual ingredients in 12 different sprays (43). The ingredients eliciting positive responses were benzethonium chloride, chlorhexidine, isopropyl myristate, and perfume. Ingredients in douches that cause either direct primary irritation or allergic contact sensitization also are found frequently in feminine deodorant sprays. Women who use sprays immediately before sexual intercourse also may exhibit local reactions (42).

Most evidence criticizing feminine deodorant spray use is from case reports or complaints received by manufacturers, physicians, and the FDA; most evidence in defense of these products is cited by the authors as the findings of controlled studies. However, in controlled studies, subjects are given instructions on proper application. The use of sprays throughout the population is uncontrolled, and it is especially difficult to assess the incidence of improper application. It seems that feminine deodorant sprays are harmless to most users, but reports of adverse effects are too frequent to be ignored, and the significant potential hazards must be considered. Furthermore, the superiority of these sprays over soap and water has been questioned (54, 55). In the absence of conclusive demonstrations of prominent adverse effects, feminine deodorant sprays continue to be marketed.

Miscellaneous Products

Although their uses and ingredients are similar to the douche or spray formulations, some nonprescription vaginal products are available as suppositories, powders, premoistened towelettes, and local anesthetic creams.

Premoistened towelettes are used for their deodorant, cleansing, or cosmetic properties. Except for the propellants in sprays, ingredients of these towelettes are similar to those of aerosols. Women who are sensitive to aerosol propellants might be informed of the towelette formulations. Direct irritation or sensitization from other towelette ingredients may occur.

One vaginal product contains benzocaine as the local anesthetic and resorcinol for antimicrobial effects. Concentrations of benzocaine and resorcinol in this cream are not provided, so efficacy cannot be readily determined. Either ingredient may cause local irritation or sensitization (14, 36, 37). The intended purpose and use of this product present another significant hazard: the masking of vaginitis symptoms. In the presence of symptoms possibly indicating vaginitis, the pharmacist should not recommend a vaginal cream or similar local anesthetic vaginal product without concurrent recommendation by the woman's physician.

Nonprescription hydrocortisone products are now available. A possibility of increased mucosal absorption of the hydrocortisone exists. Patients should be instructed to use hydrocortisone products with caution because they could mask vaginitis symptoms. These products should not be used intravaginally.

Product Selection Guidelines

The pharmacist should determine persistence, recurrence, and severity of any symptom or ascertain signs of infection or disease before attempting to recommend a product. Patient history or medication profiles may reveal predisposing factors to vaginitis such as pregnancy, diabetes, and chronic use of steroids (including oral contraceptives) or antibiotics (especially tetracyclines). If local infection or systemic diseases are suspected, medical diagnosis and treatment are always indicated.

When satisfied that a nonprescription product may be used safely, the pharmacist should make the following recommendations:

■ Douches used routinely in the absence of symptoms should be acidic or as nearly physiologic as possible.

■ If a douche is used to remove excessive discharge, an alkaline douche may be more effective.

- Use of douches and sprays should be avoided before coitus.

- Douches are not contraceptive and should be used after coitus only for cleansing. If spermicidal agents are used, douching should be delayed at least 6–8 hours following intercourse.

- Proper application techniques should be followed.

- If irritation occurs, the product should be discontinued.

- Regardless of the reasons for seeking a vaginal product, thorough cleansing with soap and water may be equally or more effective.

ANTIPERSPIRANTS AND UNDERARM DEODORANTS

Commercial products to alleviate body odor have been sold since the late 1800s. Today, Americans spend more than three-quarters of a billion dollars annually on products to decrease or prevent underarm odor and wetness (56). Nearly every adult in North America uses one of the many antiperspirants, deodorants, or deodorant soaps available. However, many consumers are unaware of the difference between antiperspirants and deodorants, and they may buy one product expecting the other's effect. Therefore, pharmacist input into the selection of a product is desirable.

Anatomy and Physiology of Sweat Glands

Commercial products may be aimed at affecting the products of two types of sweat glands—eccrine and apocrine. Eccrine, or true sweat glands, are simple coiled tubular glands lying deep in the dermis, unrelated to hair follicles. They are distributed over most of the skin surface, but particularly on the palms, soles, face, and axillae. Eccrine glands consist of a secretory coil in the lower dermis and subcutaneous tissue and a duct that travels in a helical manner to the skin surface (Figure 3). The duct contains an intraepidermal unit that modifies composition of the sweat. Constituents of eccrine secretion are water, sodium, potassium, chloride, urea, lactate, and very small amounts of glucose. The secretion is hypotonic and has a pH of 4–6.8.

Adequate eccrine gland function is vital to maintenance of normal body temperature. Heat can be dispelled by evaporation of moisture on the skin surface. However, the cooling function of sweat is provided by glands all over the body and therefore inhibition of sweating in just one area, such as the axillae, is not harmful (57). Although perspiration contains "waste products" such as urea and lactate, perspiring is not important in purification of the blood. People who live in cool environments do not suffer from lack of perspiration (57).

The eccrine glands are unusual because they are cholinergic in function but supplied with sympathetic nerves. Intact innervation is necessary for function. Activity of the glands' nervous stimulation is controlled by three stimuli: Thermal stimulation produces sweating mainly on the face and upper trunk; emotional stimulation causes perspiration mainly on the palms, soles, and axillae; and sensory stimulation can produce local perspiration (hot, spicy food causes sweating around the

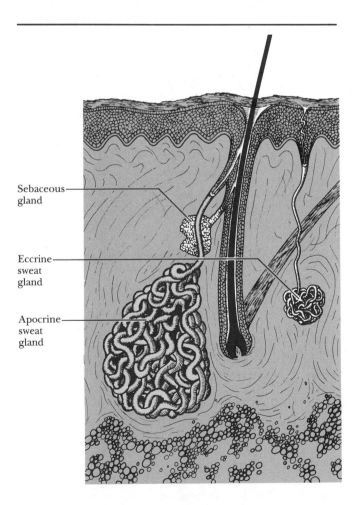

FIGURE 3 Glandular appendages of the epidermis.

face). Eccrine glands in the axillae are unique in being responsive to both thermal and emotional stimulation. Thermal stimulation has a latent period before sweating starts, but emotional and sensory stimulation cause an immediate response. In the normal adult, the quantity of eccrine perspiration varies from negligible under basal conditions to 12 l in 24 hours at maximal stimulation (57). The average production is about a liter a day, but this varies with race, age, sex, conditioning, and acclimatization to heat. Eccrine sweat is normally odorless, although food and drug substances may be excreted with it.

Apocrine glands produce a scanty, milky substance that is odorless upon secretion but becomes odoriferous upon bacterial decomposition. Apocrine glands are confined mainly to the axilla, the areola, groin, and perineum. They are poorly developed in children and begin to enlarge at puberty. Each consists of a coiled secretory tubule and a duct that normally opens into the neck of the hair follicle above the sebaceous gland (Figure 1). The secretion serves no known useful purpose but it may have evolved as a mechanism for sexual attraction (57). Apocrine secretion is intermittent and produced at a very slow rate. There are differences in apocrine activity among races. Secretion rate is indifferent to thermal stimulation but responds to emotional stress and mechanical stimulation. Again, apocrine secretion in the axillae may be unique in its responsiveness to heat or the combination of heat and emotional stimulation (58).

Disorders of Sweat Glands

Some underarm moisture (hidrosis) or odor (bromhidrosis) is normal but is ingrained into our culture as being offensive. Excess wetness may be embarrassing as well as damaging to clothes. Odor and wetness are related but distinct problems. Wetness is caused by eccrine glands, while odor is primarily caused by bacterial decomposition of apocrine secretion. It is hard to determine which causes more concern because most people consider the problems to be inseparable (56).

Wetness is caused by water being secreted faster than it evaporates. The axillae normally retain moisture because evaporation is retarded there. Transient hyperhidrosis is a physiologic response to heat or emotion. Pathologic hyperhidrosis may be caused by certain medical disorders such as thyrotoxicosis, anxiety, fever, abnormalities in the autonomic system, or disorders of the sweat glands themselves (59). Hyperhidrosis caused by disorders of the sweat glands usually presents as a sym-

metrical problem involving the axillae, soles, or palms (causing moist handshakes). Hyperhidrosis more often affects young women (60).

In contrast to hyperhidrosis, anhidrosis may be caused by hypothermia, local lesions in the autonomic nervous system, or malfunction of the sweat gland itself. Compensatory hyperhidrosis occurs in the remaining normal sweat glands when those elsewhere are not functioning (61).

Prickly heat (miliaria rubra) involves closure of the pores of the eccrine sweat glands and blockage of sweat delivery. Closure of the pores causes sweat to enter the surrounding epidermis with consequent irritation. (See Chapter 31, *Diaper Rash and Prickly Heat Products.*)

The immediate cause of body odor is the growth of bacteria in the secretion of apocrine sweat glands. The odor of freshly collected perspiration may be mild but not generally objectionable. The odor varies with the individual, activity, emotional state, and diet (62). Both eccrine and apocrine secretions are sterile and initially odorless. When left to stand, perspiration undergoes considerable change, mainly because of bacterial degradation of apocrine secretions (63). It is not clear which component actually causes the odor, but degradation of apocrine secretions produces short-chain fatty acids such as isovaleric acid (which cause a typical acidic "sweaty" odor) (64), mercaptans, indoles, ammonia, amines, and hydrogen sulfide. The presence of hair increases axillary odor because it acts as a collecting site for secretions, debris, and bacteria. Wetness from eccrine secretion promotes bacterial growth and dispersion of apocrine secretion. Oddly enough, however, excessive watery eccrine sweat may wash away apocrine sweat so that no odor is present (65). Conversely, patients with axillary odor may have no problem with wetness (65).

Because bacterial decomposition of apocrine secretion is required for odor, differences in flora between subjects have been examined. Data suggest that subjects with pungent body odor are relatively few in number and that they have a much higher number of lipophilic diphtheroids in their microflora than subjects without strong body odor (64). In most cases the body odor is not caused by biologic dysfunction but is simply a matter of personal hygiene. Presence of sebum, perspiration, and debris greatly increase axillary odor. Regular removal of debris by bathing will reduce odor, but washing alone does not remove all products of degraded perspiration and cannot remove many of the resident bacteria on the skin. Therefore some individuals must use additional measures.

In assessing the appropriate method of dealing with perspiration problems, the pharmacist must first determine whether the person is more concerned about wetness or odor. Second, the pharmacist should determine if the problem is psychologic or pathologic. In pathologic hyperhidrosis, patients will complain of constant heavy perspiration inappropriate to the climate and situation and will complain of palmar or plantar sweating more frequently than axillary (59). Nonprescription antiperspirants are not adequate to relieve pathologic hyperhidrosis. Patients with such a problem should be referred to a physician for diagnosis and treatment.

Wetness problems that do not respond to nonprescription products may be treated in several ways. Stronger concentrations of aluminum chloride in absolute ethanol (Drysol and Xerac-AC) are available by prescription. These preparations are applied to the hyperhidrotic areas at bedtime; the area may be covered with a plastic wrap, then the residue is washed off in the morning (66). Systemic anticholinergics may be prescribed to reduce perspiration flow. Rarely, in refractory cases of hyperhidrosis, radiotherapy or various operative procedures, including sympathectomy, liposuction, excision, or curettage of eccrine glands, and cryotherapy, may be attempted (59, 67).

More recently, the technique of iontophoresis (passing an electrical current through the area of the sweat glands) has been used (67–69). This technique may work by producing keratotic plugs within sweat glands that temporarily block flow (70). A battery-run device called the Drionic is available for home use. However, some authorities believe the Drionic is no more effective than topical antiperspirants (69,70).

Treatment of Perspiration Problems

Disorders of perspiration can be approached in multiple ways. A substance can be applied to reduce the amount of eccrine perspiration secreted (no product can effectively reduce apocrine secretion). Such substances are labeled antiperspirants, and are classified as drugs by the FDA because they are intended to influence a physiologic body process. In addition, a substance may prevent, mask, or change perspiration odor without attempting to block its flow. These preparations are termed deodorants and are regarded as cosmetics. Deodorants may contain perfumes to mask odor, germicides to inhibit bacterial growth, or powders to absorb moisture. Many commercial products are combinations of antiperspirants and deodorants. However, any product labeled as a "deodorant" cannot make any antiperspirant claims.

The fact that numerous products are marketed for these purposes speaks for their popularity. Plain antiperspirants tend to be the least acceptable because their action is relatively hard to notice, while the failure of a deodorant product to do its job is much more obvious.

Another approach to preventing odor is good hygiene. Shaving the affected area may be helpful by removing hair that serves to retain moisture, which acts as a substrate for bacteria.

Pharmacologic Agents

The FDA advisory review panel on OTC antiperspirant drug products issued a tentative monograph in October 1978 (57). The FDA then issued a tentative final monograph in August 1982 (71). The FDA decided that aluminum chlorohydrates, aluminum chloride, buffered aluminum sulfate, and aluminum zirconium chlorohydrates were safe and effective as topical antiperspirants in the appropriate concentration. However, only aluminum chlorohydrates had sufficient safety data to permit their use in aerosolized dosage form (71).

Currently used ingredients have evolved from the empirical use of astringent metal salts, many of which were tried and discarded because of undesirable properties such as staining or irritation. Although their action in reducing flow of eccrine perspiration can be measured objectively, their mechanism of action has been a subject of intense debate that is still unresolved. The oldest theory attributes their action to simple astringency, causing shrinkage of the pore. It was speculated that antiperspirants acted on sweat glands to produce inflammation and swelling around the duct, thereby contracting its orifice. However, a number of chemicals that are strong astringents have minimal antiperspirant activity. Another theory was that antiperspirants increased the permeability of the sweat duct, causing reabsorption of sweat (the "leaky hose" theory) (72).

Studies have indicated that a physically demonstrable obstruction of the duct accounts for anhidrosis (73, 74). After stripping the stratum corneum from the skin, antiperspirant activity still remains; thus, obstruction is more than superficial. A plug may be caused by keratin precipitated by the antiperspirant. However, the keratin plug is probably a late, nonspecific reaction to injury, while the initial plug is caused by an amorphous, aluminum-containing cast that extends down the length of the duct. There is no inflammation (73). The individual sweat duct remains physically occluded until it is replaced by normal cell renewal in 2–3 weeks. Thus, antiperspirants have a prolonged action (57). The degree to which antiperspirants decrease wetness is relatively feeble and could not be enough to cause an appreciable decrease in odor (57). Antiperspirants are also strong antibacterials and, therefore, may be effective deodorants (66, 75).

For maximum decrease in wetness, prescription products must be used. Ideally, the product should be applied at night when sweat glands are inactive, and after application, the affected area should be occluded for 2–8 hours. A high degree of acidity may be desirable to help deposit the aluminum salts deep in the epidermis. Dry skin also enhances penetration (59, 76).

Because acidity is irritating to the skin and damaging to clothing, nonprescription antiperspirant formulations may be buffered by the addition of urea or glycine in 5–10% concentrations. Buffers do not appreciably increase the pH of a preparation or act as alkalis to precipitate aluminum hydroxide, which would reduce antiperspirant activity. However, at ironing temperatures, urea decomposes to ammonia and neutralizes acidity to protect clothing (62).

The most common adverse effect of nonprescription antiperspirants is skin irritation (tingling, stinging, or burning), which is caused by a chemical reaction between antiperspirants and the skin; sensitization is very rare (57). Normally irritation can be reduced by decreasing the frequency or amount used. Antiperspirants should not be applied to freshly shaved skin. If erythema or papules develop, discontinuation of the product should be advised for a few days. During this period, a deodorant can be applied instead. The patient can usually return to the same antiperspirant later, using it in lesser amounts. The contents of all products are fully labeled so that a user who is sensitive to a specific ingredient can choose a different formulation.

There is no evidence that antiperspirants cause permanent harm to sweat glands. Normal sweating resumes a week after discontinuing use. There also is no evidence of systemic toxicity caused by topical application of antiperspirants. However, antiperspirants should not be applied to broken or irritated skin, because axillary granulomas have been reported (77).

Aluminum Chloride

Aluminum chloride, $AlCl_3$, hydrolyzes in water to aluminum hydroxide and hydrochloric acid, forming strongly acidic solutions. This high acidity tends to damage fabrics in contact with treated skin and is very irritating to the skin at higher concentrations. Therefore the FDA advisory review panel on OTC antiperspirant drug products has recommended that only concentrations of 15% or less (in aqueous solution) should be considered both effective and safe. Although alcoholic solutions of aluminum chloride are available by prescription, there are no data on the safety of this formulation for unsupervised use. Solutions of aluminum chloride show significantly greater efficacy compared to less irritating antiperspirant compounds (57).

Aluminum Chlorohydrates

Aluminum chlorohydrates are available commercially in several different forms that differ in the ratio of aluminum to chlorine. The empirical formulas of the most widely used ingredients are $Al_2(OH)_4Cl_2$ and $Al_2(OH)_5Cl$, which are known as ⅔ basic and ⅚ basic aluminum chloride, respectively. Aluminum chlorohydrates are also available as polyethylene glycol or propylene glycol complexes. These complexes are formulated to provide greater alcohol solubility and do not affect the safety or efficacy of the salts from which they are prepared (57). The advantage of chlorohydrate salts over aluminum chloride is their lower acidity. The greater the aluminum-to-chloride ratio in the salt, the less acidic is the solution.

The panel found that aluminum chlorohydrates are safe and effective when applied topically to the underarms in concentrations of 25% (anhydrous) or less. These concentrations have produced very little skin irritation, in patch testing or in market experience.

Aluminum Zirconium Chlorohydrates

Salts of zirconium enjoyed a brief period of popularity until they were discovered to cause skin and lung granulomas. However, they apparently are safer when combined with aluminum salts. Aerosol products containing zirconium have been banned (78). Skin changes have been found in rabbits injected with zirconium aluminum glycine complex, but the panel did not consider this serious enough to disallow nonprescription use in nonaerosol form (57).

Aluminum zirconium salts vary in their ratio of aluminum to zirconium to chlorine. These complexes are also acidic, with solutions having a pH of about 4. They are recommended for nonprescription use in concentrations of not more than 20% anhydrous weight, applied topically to the axillae.

Buffered Aluminum Sulfate

Aluminum sulfate itself produces a high degree of irritation. However, it is available as an 8% solution buffered with 8% sodium aluminum lactate. This preparation is effective and virtually nonirritating (57).

Glutaraldehyde

Glutaraldehyde 2% in buffered solution is available without prescription. It is used to treat hyperhidrosis of the palms and soles, but not the axillae (79). A drawback is that brown staining of the skin occurs (69). It is thought to act by occluding the sweat ducts.

Antibacterials

Deodorants may contain perfumes and colognes to mask body odor, or they may prevent it by inhibiting bacterial action.

The antibiotic neomycin has excellent broad-spectrum topical activity. However, it may sensitize the skin to further applications. Boric acid has also been used, but it can be absorbed through the skin and cause toxicity. Quaternary ammonium compounds such as benzalkonium chloride have a broad spectrum of activity. However, they are swiftly inactivated by the skin and are incompatible with soaps or anionic surfactants.

The phenolic compounds are longer lasting and compatible with soaps. Hexachlorophene was the most widely used before it was banned from nonprescription use. Triclosan and trichlorocarbanilide are frequently found in deodorants and deodorant soaps such as Dial and Coast. The astringent aluminum salts also have antiseptic properties. Compounds of metals other than aluminum are used as deodorants. Zinc phenolsulfonate is useful in liquid products; zinc oxide, peroxide, or stearate is used in powders (62).

Sodium bicarbonate is a time-honored deodorant; besides absorbing moisture, its alkalinity may be inhibitory to bacteria.

Others

Chlorophyll is another product that has been reported anecdotally to have deodorant properties. However, there is no evidence that chlorophyll, either applied topically or taken systemically, is effective as a deodorant (80).

Dosage Forms

The ideal antiperspirant or deodorant should apply conveniently, dry quickly, not stain clothing, be nonirritating, and last all day after a single application. The variety of products available indicates that they are far from ideal.

Creams were the first available form of antiperspirant but were largely abandoned for more convenient forms. Aerosols became immensely popular in the 1960s, capturing up to 85% of the market. However, their use plummeted after publicity about adverse effects on the lungs and on the environment. Furthermore, their effectiveness is low.

All dosage forms are not equally effective. Table 3 gives the range of perspiration reduction in laboratory hot rooms based on data submitted to the FDA. Several points are illustrated by these data:

- No nonprescription product inhibits wetness completely in the axillae; during normal use only 20–40% reduction can be expected (56).

- Minor variations in formulation may have a critical effect on a product's activity (81); thus, two similar products may be quite different in effectiveness.

- There is extreme individual variability in response to antiperspirants; some subjects actually perspire more after some applications (78).

The FDA advisory review panel believed that a 20% reduction in wetness was the minimum required to be noticeable by the user. Therefore, the FDA has suggested but not required that an average reduction of 20% be ensured for each final formulation (71).

Powders are not listed in Table 3 because these are generally deodorants that absorb moisture. To be active, antiperspirant ingredients must be in solution or aerosol (62).

Labeling Claims

The panel believed there were insufficient data on nonprescription antiperspirants for certain label claims to be allowed. Unless appropriate data are submitted for each product, the FDA would prohibit claims of "long-lasting" or "all day" effectiveness, and claims of being effective for "emotional" or "troublesome" perspiration. Claims about "extra strength" would be disallowed entirely because concentration does not necessarily correlate with effectiveness. The only claim allowed will be a statement to the effect that the product reduces underarm wetness (71).

TABLE 3 Efficacy of antiperspirant application forms

Application form	Average sweat reduction
Aerosols	20–33%
Creams	35–47%
Liquids	15–54%
Lotions	38–62%
Roll-ons	14–70%
Sticks	35–40%

Reprinted from the *Federal Register, 43,* 46694 (1978).

Patient Consultation

The pharmacist should be sure that the consumer understands the difference between deodorants and antiperspirants. Deodorants are not a substitute for cleanliness; their use should follow bathing. Antiperspirants reduce but do not stop wetness, especially during thermal or emotional stress. Antiperspirants are not effective immediately after application. Repeated applications over time are needed to achieve the maximal effect (57).

Before applying antiperspirants, the user should let the underarm dry. This reduces discomfort from moisture-induced hydrolysis of aluminum salts to hydrochloric acid by moisture. In addition, the antiperspirant effect is completely abolished if the subject is perspiring during application (72). Antiperspirants should not be applied to open, broken, abraded, or freshly shaved skin.

Finally, the patient should be advised of the marked variation in response to antiperspirants from person to person and product to product. If one product does not perform satisfactorily, it is quite reasonable to try others.

SKIN-BLEACHING PRODUCTS

Hyperpigmentation of the skin may result from a variety of causes. It is usually asymptomatic and of no medical consequence, although it occasionally may signify systemic illness. Hyperpigmentation, particularly on the face, however, can be a source of cosmetic disability and mental distress. Thus, agents that can bleach away excess pigment when applied topically have a large market among all racial and ethnic groups around the world. Most of the skin-bleaching products are available without a prescription. Although they serve a cosmetic function, it is important to emphasize that these products are drugs and have potential toxicity.

Physiology of Skin Pigmentation

Normal skin color is contributed by melanocytes in the basal layer of the epidermis, which produce pigment granules called melanosomes (Figure 4). These pigment granules contain a complex protein called melanin, a brown-black pigment. Melanocytes can be viewed as

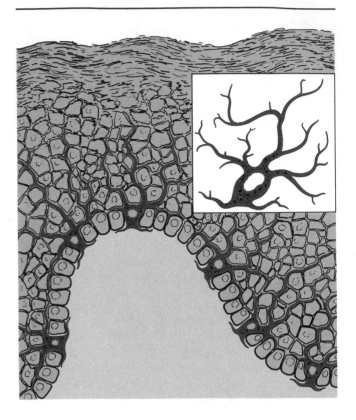

FIGURE 4 Melanocytes in the epidermis. The melanin-forming cells are situated among the basal cells. They have long branching cell processes of tubes through which the pigment granules are carried to be injected into the remaining nonmelanin-forming cells of the epidermis. The inset shows a single melanocyte with its elaborate branches.

Adapted with permission from D. M. Pillsbury, "A Manual for Dermatology," W. B. Saunders. Philadelphia, Pa., 1971, pp. 22, 30.

tiny one-celled glands with long projections to pass pigment particles into the keratinocytes, which synthesize skin keratin. As keratinocytes migrate upward, they carry the pigment with them and deposit it on the surface of the skin as they die. (See Chapter 28, *Topical Anti-infective Products.*) Melanocytes are also present in the hair bulb cells and pass pigment granules on to the hair (82).

Melanin is the most efficient sunscreen known. It prevents damaging ultraviolet (UV) rays from the sun from entering deeper parts of the skin. When UV radiation strikes the skin, not all of it is absorbed. Some reaches the deeper layers and may cause sunburn. Solar radiation also stimulates melanocytes to provide more melanin. This results in gradual skin darkening or a "tan." The various human races have roughly the same number of melanocytes, but dark-skinned peoples have more active cells.

Hyperpigmentation Syndromes

Certain systemic diseases and skin diseases cause pigment cells to become overactive, resulting in darkening of the skin, or to become underactive with resultant lightening of the skin.

Endocrine imbalances, caused by Addison's disease, Cushing's disease, hyperthyroidism, pregnancy, or estrogen therapy (including oral contraceptives), and skin cancer (melanoma) will affect skin pigmentation. Metabolic alterations affecting the liver and certain nutritional deficiencies can be associated with diffuse melanosis (83). Physical trauma or inflammatory dermatoses may cause a postinflammatory pigmentation. Also, certain drugs such as chlorpromazine and hydroxychloroquine have an affinity for melanin and may cause hyperpigmentation. Thus, the pharmacist must inquire about concurrent drug therapy and systemic illnesses before recommending a nonprescription product. Diffuse pigmentation disorders and those caused by systemic factors should never be self-medicated without prior evaluation by a physician. Similarly, lesions that are changing in size, shape, or color may be cancerous and should never be self-treated.

Several causes of hyperpigmentation are amenable to self-medication (82–85). These include freckles, melasma, and lentigines. Freckles are simply spots of uneven pigmentation that are exacerbated by the sun. Melasma (also called chloasma) is a condition in which blotchy patches occur on the face, usually because of a hormonal imbalance; it is often caused by pregnancy ("the mask of pregnancy") or oral contraceptives, and sun exposure is necessary for its development. Lentigines are hyperpigmented spots that may appear at any age anywhere on the skin or mucous membranes and are caused by an increased deposition of melanin and an increased number of melanocytes. They are darker than freckles and not induced by UV radiation. Solar or "senile" lentigines, commonly but incorrectly known as "liver spots," appear on the exposed surfaces of fair-skinned people and are induced by UV radiation.

Treatment

The intensity of localized hyperpigmentation in producing freckles, melasma, lentigines, or postinflam-matory pigmentation may be decreased by topical non-prescription skin-bleaching agents. Specific systemic therapy is required for diffuse systemic pigmentation disorders.

Nonprescription products are directed at suppression of melanin formation within the skin. The importance of avoiding excessive exposure to sunlight and of using sunscreen agents or protective clothing must be emphasized to patients.

Physician-directed management of hyperpigmentation may include more effective prescription agents such as ointments formulated with 0.1% tretinoin (retinoic acid), 5% hydroquinone, and 0.1% dexamethasone (86). Monobenzone should not be used because it produces irreversible depigmentation of normal as well as darkened skin. Light cryosurgical freezing with liquid nitrogen may also be used.

Pharmacologic Agents

Historically, a number of topical agents have been used in skin-bleaching preparations. These have included hydroquinone, the monobenzyl and monomethyl ethers of hydroquinone, ammoniated mercury, ascorbic acid, and peroxides (87). Only preparations containing hydroquinone were submitted to the FDA advisory review panel on skin-bleaching agents (83).

Hydroquinone

The FDA in a tentative final monograph has recommended that only hydroquinone (*p*-dihydroxybenzene) in concentrations of 1.5–2.0% be available for OTC use (84). Hydroquinone and its derivatives are extensively used by industry as antioxidants.

Hydroquinone produces reversible depigmentation of the skin and hair of mice, guinea pigs, and humans by a complex mechanism of action. Hydroquinone and its derivatives are oxidized by tyrosinase to form highly toxic, free radicals that cause selective damage to the lipoprotein membranes of the melanocyte, thereby reducing conversion of tyrosine to dopa and subsequently to melanin (88). However, experiments on guinea pigs also indicate that it has toxic effects at the subcellular level in both follicular and nonfollicular melanocytes. It disrupts membranous cytoplasmic organelles, affecting formation, melanization, and degradation of melanosomes.

Several studies demonstrate that topical preparations of 2–5% hydroquinone are effective in producing cutaneous depigmentation (83). The 2% concentration is safer and has produced results equal to higher concentrations (86).

The effectiveness of hydroquinone varies among patients. The results are best on lighter skin and on lighter lesions. In blacks the response to hydroquinone depends on the amount of pigment present (89). The earlier it is used to treat minor skin blemishes, the more likely results will be satisfactory. When depigmentation does occur, melanin production is reduced by about one-half (83). Hyperpigmented areas fade more rapidly and completely than surrounding normal skin (85). Treatment may not lead to complete disappearance of hypermelanosis, but results are often satisfactory enough to reduce self-consciousness about hyperpigmentation.

When beginning treatment, melanin excretion may transiently increase. A decrease in skin color usually becomes noticeable in about 4 weeks; however, the time of onset varies from 3 weeks to 3 months. Eighty percent of patients with melasma improve within 8 weeks (85). Depigmentation lasts for 2–6 months but is reversible. Darker lesions repigment faster than lighter lesions. Because the ability of the sun to darken lesions is much greater than that of hydroquinone to lighten them, strict avoidance of sunlight is imperative. Although sunscreens may help, even visible light may cause some darkening and sun protection should preferably be opaque (86). Some hydroquinone products are available in an opaque base (Eldopaque) or together wth a sunscreen (Ambi). (See Chapter 34, *Sunscreen and Suntan Products.*)

Side effects of topical hydroquinone are mild when used in low concentrations. Tingling or burning on application and subsequent erythema and inflammation were observed in 8% of patients using a 2% concentration and 32% of patients using a 5% concentration of hydroquinone (86). Higher concentrations frequently irritate the skin and if used for prolonged periods cause disfiguring effects including epidermal thickening, pitch-black pigmentation, and colloid milium (yellowish papules associated with colloid degeneration) (83, 90).

In some cases lesions become slightly darker before fading. A transient inflammatory reaction may develop after the first few weeks of treatment. Occurrence of inflammation makes subsequent lightening more likely, although inflammation can occur without the development of depigmentation. Appearance of mild inflammation need not be considered an indication to stop therapy except in the patient whose reaction increases in intensity (sensitization should be considered). Topical hydrocortisone may be used temporarily to alleviate the reaction. Contact with the eyes should be avoided. A patch test can be done to test for allergy to hydroquinone; however, the majority of reactions are irritant and not allergic in nature.

Reversible brown discoloration of nails has been reported occasionally following application of 2% hydroquinone to the back of the hand (91). The discoloration is probably caused by formation of oxidation products of hydroquinone.

If hydroquinone is accidentally ingested, it seldom produces serious systemic toxicity (83). However, oral ingestion of 5–15 g doses has produced tremor, convulsions, and hemolytic anemia (92).

Hydroquinone is easily oxidized in the presence of light and air. Any discoloration or darkening of the cream is an indication of deterioration in the strength of available hydroquinone (83). Thus, the preferable method of packaging it is in small squeeze tubes.

The dosage of hydroquinone is a thin application of 1.5–2% concentration rubbed into affected areas twice daily. Because of lack of safety data, it is not recommended for children under 12, except with the supervision of a physician. If no improvement is seen within 3 months, the use of hydroquinone should be discontinued and the advice of a physician sought (84). Once the desired benefit is achieved, hydroquinone can be applied as often as needed to maintain depigmentation of the skin.

Ammoniated Mercury

Ammoniated mercury, also known as ammoniated mercuric chloride, was in common use as a skin-bleaching agent before monobenzone became available. No products with this ingredient were submitted for review by the panel, probably because of recognized concern for its safety. Chronic application can cause systemic mercury intoxication, and sensitization is common. There also is a lack of efficacy data. Therefore, the panel on skin-bleaching products has recommended that ammoniated mercury not be made available on a nonprescription basis.

Monobenzone

The monobenzyl ether of hydroquinone is restricted to prescription-only use. Its actions and onset time are similar to hydroquinone except that depigmentation may be permanent. Monobenzone should never be used to treat hyperpigmentation because it permanently depigments both the hyperpigmented and the normal skin (85). Its use is restricted to depigmenting residual areas of normal skin in patients with extensive vitiligo (condition resulting in patches of depigmentation, possibly with hyperpigmented borders).

Secondary Ingredients

Because hydroquinone is oxidized by contact with air, additional antioxidants such as sodium bisulfite may be added to the formulation. Hydroquinone is incompatible with alkali or ferric salts because of the ease of oxidation (92). Iodochlorhydroxyquin or oxyquinolone sulfate may be added as antimicrobial preservatives (83).

The inclusion of a sunscreen agent, such as an aminobenzoic acid ester, is rational and appropriate, provided that combination products are advertised as skin-bleaching agents with added sunscreen and not primarily as sunscreens.

Patient Consultation

Before selecting a nonprescription product, the pharmacist should be sure that a physician has confirmed the need for using it. These products should be used only in areas of brownish color. Reddish or bluish areas, such as diffuse port wine stains, are not amenable to treatment. These products should not be used on areas that are changing in size, shape, or color. Skin-bleaching products are intended to lighten only limited areas of hyperpigmented skin. If the product is effective, the results should be noticeable within 2 to 3 months. It will not permanently injure the skin. Hydroquinone may be applied to a small area of unbroken skin and assessed for 24 hours to observe for irritation or allergic reactions. It should never be applied near the eyes or to cut, abraded, or sunburned skin.

DEPILATORIES

Although the biologic significance of hair is minute, its cosmetic importance is considerable. Any discrepancy between cosmetic standards and normal biologic range may be embarrassing. Excessive growth of facial or body hair has been a common complaint among women for centuries (93). Some remedies used in the past for hair removal include arsenic trisulfide ointment, hot leeches, ants' eggs, and the blood of yellow frogs (93, 94).

Physiology of Normal and Abnormal Hair Growth

Racial and cultural factors affect both the type of normal hair growth and people's attitude about it. In American culture any hair except on the scalp is consid-

ered a masculine trait. However, the growth of upper lip and preauricular hair soon after puberty is a normal racial characteristic among females of some ethnic groups. It is attributed to sensitivity of the skin to androgens (94). Excessive hair growth of essentially normal distribution is termed hypertrichosis; a change in hair growth distribution inconsistent with sex and racial background is called hirsutism (94). Either condition may be caused by a change in one of two distinct features of hair growth: cycle or pattern.

The hair growth cycle comprises successive stages of growth (anogen) and rest (telogen). During the rest period, the fully developed hair is retained in the follicle for a while and then shed. If the rest phase is long and hair is shed well before the next growth phase for that follicle, the skin appears relatively hairless. If the rest phase is short, the succeeding hair appears in the follicle shortly after or even before the earlier hair is gone, and the skin appears hairy. Androgens influence the growth cycle by increasing the length of the growth phase, which decreases the length of the rest phase.

The hair growth pattern refers to the type of hair made by the follicle, either "vellus" or "terminal." Follicles over most of the body produce only fine, fuzz-like vellus hair; however, follicles can be transformed to produce longer, coarser, pigmented terminal hair. In both sexes, androgens cause terminal hair to replace vellus in the pubic area and axillae. Additional androgen stimulation causes transformation of follicles on the face, chest, and abdomen.

Hirsutism can usually be traced to an endocrine origin (94). It may be caused by the virilizing effects of excessive androgen or progestin production or by excessive adrenal corticosteroids. Hypertrichosis may be caused by drugs such as acetazolamide, chlorpromazine, diazoxide, cyclosporine, minoxidil, penicillamine, or phenytoin (95, 96). The central issue in determining whether self-medication is advisable is separating the infrequent instances of endocrine or drug-induced disease from the vast majority of cases in which excess hair is purely a cosmetic problem. Whenever the signs of virilization are present, or the pattern of hair growth has changed markedly, the patient should be referred to a physician for assessment. The menstrual history can be valuable. If menstruation is completely normal, the patient is unlikely to have serious endocrinopathy.

Methods of Hair Removal

Medical demands for hair removal are rare. Occasionally ingrown beard hairs need to be removed and surgeons still remove hair from operative sites (97). Pseudofolliculitis barbae is a frequent condition in blacks in whom the sharp tips of shaven beard hairs curve in an 180° arc toward the epidermis and penetrate the skin, causing papules and pustules. Chemical depilatories can be useful in this condition because hair is cleanly removed at the skin surface to produce a blunt tip, which is less likely to penetrate skin than a shaved hair (98).

There is no way to increase or decrease the number of hair follicles in the skin; these are fixed at birth. However, hair can be removed either at the surface (depilation) or at the roots (epilation). Because epilation removes the hair at a deeper point it has to be repeated less often. All practical methods except electrolysis are temporary (Table 4).

Women often shave hair from their legs and trunk, but find shaving the face repugnant. There is no evidence that shaving makes hair grow faster or coarser (93, 94). Local epilation by plucking is usually not harmful and probably the best method of removing a few strong hairs. If removal of the hair is complete and includes the hair bulb, hair is not noticeable again for 3–6 weeks. However, damage to the follicles may sometimes cause infection.

Wax epilation is essentially a form of mass plucking. A wax of low melting point (or adhesive semisolid applied on a backing material) rapidly solidifies and enmeshes hair. It is then pulled quickly off the skin, against the direction of hair growth, along with embedded hairs. If not done skillfully this technique can be painful, and allergic reactions to the adhesives can occur. The patient should be cautioned to make sure that the wax is not too hot prior to use. Moreover, hair must be at least 1 mm long in order to be grasped by the wax.

Permanent removal of hair by electrolysis (galvanic or short-wave diathermy) can be very tedious and expensive, even on facial hair, because only a few nonadjacent hairs should be done at one time. It is useful for women with a few coarse hairs. Galvanic electrolysis is less traumatic but slower than wax epilation (97). Even with good technique, the 15–25% of hairs in telogen phase regrow and the operation has to be done again. Although somewhat painful (the needle must be inserted into the bulb of the hair shaft), some dermatology experts feel that competent operators can produce excellent results (99). However, self-operated electrolysis is not advisable because significant scarring occurs if the follicle is not destroyed correctly.

Depilatory creams and lotions are thus a logical and convenient alternative for hair removal. Most chemical depilatories are based on substituted mercaptans used in the presence of alkaline-reacting materials (calcium thioglycolate with calcium hydroxide). This combination has generally supplemented the sulfides of barium, strontium, and calcium, which are faster acting but are poisonous and have strong odors.

TABLE 4 Methods of hair removal

Method	Implement or process
DEPILATION (action on the hair shaft)	
Shaving	Razor or electric shaver
Abrasion	Pumice or fiber
Dissolving	Chemicals, enzymes
Bleaching	Peroxides, organic acids
EPILATION (action on the hair root)	
Extraction	Tweezers, wax, adhesives, powered devices for home use (e.g., Epilady)
Toxins	Metabolic—endocrine or nutritional disorders
	Disease—infection, immune deficiency
	Poison—metals, drugs
Destruction	Electrolysis—galvanic
	Cautery—short-wave
	Chemical—phenol, acid
	Ionization—X-rays or gamma rays

Adapted with permission from H. B. Spoor, *Cutis*, *21*, 283 (1978).

Chemical depilatories act by reducing disulfide bonds between cystine molecules in hair keratin. Increasing osmotic pressure within the hair fiber results in swelling and deterioration to a soft plastic mass which is easily wiped off the skin in 5–15 minutes. To some extent, skin is subject to the same degradation as hair because cystine makes up 15% of keratin in hair and 2% in skin (100). Although thioglycolate is a known contact allergen (100), its preparations seldom cause skin reactions; when reactions do occur, they are usually irritant reactions rather than allergic. Hair that regrows is less bristly than after shaving, so there is less itching during regrowth. Coarse, highly pigmented hair is harder to remove than vellus hair. Chemical depilatories also have bactericidal properties (101).

Pharmacologic Agents

Thioglycolates

Thioglycolates make up the large majority of commercial preparations and are available as pastes, lotions, or creams. A 2–4% concentration is sufficient; higher concentrations do not work appreciably faster

(102). Increasing the concentration of alkali increases the depilation rate but also increases skin irritation. Thioglycolates are safe topically and have little systemic toxicity if absorbed (102); they have only a mild odor. These preparations are oxidized by air and therefore should not be kept too long, and they should be kept in a tightly covered container.

Alkaline Sulfides

Barium, calcium, or strontium sulfides act two to three times faster than thioglycolate (102) but are more irritating. They have a strong odor caused by hydrolysis of hydrogen sulfide and are poisonous if ingested. Sulfides are indicated for men with thick beard hair because thioglycolates act too slowly in such cases (100).

Application

The depilatory may be tested by applying to a small patch of normal skin for 15 minutes and then washing off. If no reaction occurs within 24 hours, a thick layer of depilatory is applied with the enclosed plastic glove or applicator against the direction of hair growth. The depilatory is left on for 5–15 minutes (the length of application varies with the formulation; package directions should be followed carefully). The depilatory is removed with a spatula or tissue (avoiding contact with water to minimize odor). The skin is washed with soap and water. Some manufacturers provide an emollient lotion to soothe the skin and prevent dryness. If necessary, 1% hydrocortisone cream can be applied to counteract irritation. The treatment is repeated as needed, normally every 2–4 weeks.

NONMEDICATED SHAMPOOS

In contrast to body hair, scalp hair has long been a source of beauty and social distinction. Interestingly, it has only been in this century that much attention has been paid to cleansing it (103).

Originally, shampoos were made of soaps; today synthetic detergents are used almost exclusively in commercial products. The success of modern shampoos is based not only on their cleansing properties, but also on the cosmetics that impart luster, beauty, and manageability to hair. A good shampoo makes hair feel clean, provides it with a gloss or sheen, and does not leave it "frizzy" or unmanageable (does not adversely affect its physical properties). Shampoos are often formulated to emphasize special properties, such as minimizing eye sting, conditioning, adding body, or having an appealing fragrance.

Hair

Hair has three layers: the medulla, which receives nourishment from the root; the cortex, which contains pigment, and the cuticle, which is a thin translucent layer that lets color shine through to the outside. Normal hair varies in thickness (texture) from coarse to fine.

Hair soil includes natural skin secretions, skin debris, dirt from the environment, and residue of hair-grooming products. The scalp normally secretes enough oil to keep the hair glossy and the scalp comfortable. However, a build-up of oil between shampoos makes the hair limp and stringy. On the other hand, too little oil makes hair dull, lifeless, "flyaway," and easily breakable.

Specialty Shampoos

Today's shampoos may stress any number of special components or properties. However, their main benefit is still cleansing. Manufacturers must be careful about therapeutic claims because such products would be considered drugs by the FDA.

A conditioner is a product applied to hair to restore oils, sheen, elasticity, and manageability. It is useful on dry, damaged, or over-processed hair. Many shampoos include conditioners in the formulation, but conditioners are best applied after the shampoo.

A cream rinse is a product used after a shampoo to smooth the cuticle, eliminate tangles, and make hair manageable.

Protein shampoos are excellent for fine, limp, or damaged hair. Hair strands can be increased in bulk with a protein shampoo, by conditioning, or by coloring. Protein shampoos are not necessary for normal hair; they do not help dry hair and can make oily hair limp sooner after shampooing. The protein does not become a permanent part of the hair; it is only absorbed temporarily and washed off again at the next shampoo.

Because hair is dead tissue, no product can "feed" hair to make it healthier.

Herbal shampoos contain saponins from natural products, such as quillaja bark or soaproot, that foam well and have good cleansing properties.

Baby shampoos contain nonirritating detergents, and few, if any, additives such as perfumes that could irritate eyes.

Ingredients

Soaps are sodium or potassium salts of fatty acids. Unfortunately, during washing they tend to form insoluble mineral salts, which leave a dulling scum on hair especially in areas with hard water. Sequestering agents can be added to bind calcium and magnesium ions or soaps and detergents. However, there are no longer any major soap-based shampoos on the market (104).

In synthetic detergents, the carboxyl group of the fatty acid is replaced with another hydrophilic group, thus avoiding their negative properties. Detergents tend to be classified by their hydrophilic groups (anionic, cationic, amphoteric, or nonionic). Adult shampoos are usually anionic, while those for children are more likely to be amphoteric or nonionic in composition. Cationic materials are more likely to be found in hair rinses and conditioners. By far the most widely used detergent in shampoos is the anionic agent, sodium lauryl sulfate (a sulfated derivative of lauryl alcohol). It and other alkyl sulfates are completely effective in hard water, provide excellent foam, and leave hair feeling smooth and soft. They also are easily perfumed, easily rinsed out, and do not become rancid (103). Sodium salts were used originally, but now ammonium or tri- and diethanolamine salts are often used because they are less drying to hair.

Nonionic and amphoteric detergents also are popular. They have low foaming properties but are especially mild to the eyes. Many shampoos contain a combination of soaps and detergents to balance their desirable characteristics. Most complaints about shampoos are about skin or eye irritation, but occasionally users may have an allergic skin reaction to a specific ingredient or additive (105).

Additives

As perusal of any label will verify, many secondary ingredients are routinely added to shampoos.

Conditioning agents are added to coat hair with a very small amount of lubricating material because most surfactants cleanse hair so well that it becomes unmanageable. These are emollients such as lanolin and its derivatives, glycerol, propylene glycol, and lauryl or octyl sarcosines. Cationic materials are added to reduce the electrostatic charge on hair (but are irritating to the

eyes). They are adsorbed onto hair and retained after rinsing.

Foam builders and stabilizers (fatty acid amides) make the product more pleasing to use although lots of foam is not a prerequisite to good cleansing. Thickeners, which may be simple salts (sodium chloride) or methylcellulose derivatives, also make the product more aesthetically acceptable. Sequestering agents prevent formation of calcium, magnesium, and iron soaps. These include ethylenediaminetetraacetic acid (EDTA), citric acid, and pyrophosphates. Short-chain alcohols act as clarifying agents and increase rinsability. In creams and lotions, stearate and palmitate salts are added as opacifying agents. Finally, the formulation may include preservatives, antioxidants, buffering agents, perfumes, and dyes.

Formulations

Shampoos are available in clear liquids, lotions, pastes, and gels, allowing for great latitude in physical and performance capabilities. Dry shampoos are valuable to ill or incapacitated persons who cannot wet their hair. Dry shampoos are mixtures of absorbent powders and mild alkalis that pick up soil from hair and scalp. After leaving them in hair for a period, they are brushed or combed out.

Product Selection Guidelines

Most modern shampoos work very well, with little to distinguish among them in consumer acceptability (106). The more effective a shampoo is in cleansing, the harsher it will be on hair. Those who shampoo more regularly should choose a gentle shampoo. Teenagers tend to have oily hair and should avoid conditioning shampoos, although a cream rinse will aid in combing and provide manageability. Shampoos for dry or oily hair vary in the amount of detergent and conditioners in the formulation.

One sudsing and rinse is enough for frequent shampooing. Hair should be rinsed very well to remove all traces of shampoo. For best results, hair should be gently dried with a towel or blow dryer set at low temperatures.

SUMMARY

The psychologic benefits of using personal care products are unquestionable. However, such products may be misused in terms of selection, frequency of use, or technique of application. Many products can cause direct contact irritation or allergic sensitivity, but perhaps the greatest hazards are with the user and inadequate counseling, rather than with the product. The incidence of adverse effects is small, but, in almost all cases, the benefits are only cosmetic.

The available literature is not convincing that vaginal cleansing and deodorant products are advisable for routine use. Antiperspirants and underarm deodorants, skin-bleaching agents, depilatories, and non-medicated shampoos are appropriate for routine use if the user understands what can be reasonably expected from the product. The pharmacist's advice in product selection and education can be of great value.

REFERENCES

1 J. D. McCue, *Arch. Intern. Med.*, *149*, 565 (1989).

2 K. J. Karnaky, *Am. J. Surg.*, *101*, 456 (1961).

3 K. J. Karnaky, *Am. J. Obstet. Gynecol.*, *115*, 283 (1973).

4 R. Glynn, *Obstet. Gynecol.*, *20*, 369 (1962).

5 H. J. Palacios, *Ann. Allergy*, *37*, 110 (1976).

6 *Drug Ther. Bull.*, *18(14)*, 55 (1980).

7 C. H. Weaver and M. B. Mengel, *J. Fam Pract.*, *27*, 207 (1988).

8 M. G. Gravett et al., *J. Am. Med. Assoc.*, *256*, 1899 (1986).

9 F. Sadik, *J. Am. Pharm. Assoc.*, *NS12*, 565 (1975).

10 T. Novothy, *Postgrad. Med.*, *73*, 303 (1983).

11 T. D. De and N. V. Tu, *Am. J. Obstet. Gynecol.*, *87*, 92 (1965).

12 L. A. Gray and M. L. Barnes, *Am. J. Obstet. Gynecol.*, *92*, 125 (1963).

13 R. Landesman, *Drug Ther.*, *9(1)*, 185–186 (1979).

14 "Remington's Pharmaceutical Sciences," 16th ed., A. Osol, Ed., Mack, Easton, Pa., 1980, p. 720.

15 J. Barnes, *Practitioner*, *184*, 668 (1960).

16 J. F. Byers, *Am. Fam. Physician*, *10*, 135 (1974).

17 D. V. Hirst, *Am. J. Obstet. Gynecol.*, *64*, 179 (1952).

18 J. H. Long et al., *West. J. Surg. Obstet. Gynecol.*, *71*, 122, (1963).

19 "Summary Minutes of the FDA OTC Panel on Contraceptives and Other Vaginal Drug Products," Rockville, Md., Feb. 7–8, 1975.

20 H. A. Kaminetzky, *J. Am. Med. Assoc.*, *191*, 154 (1965).

21 L. McGowan, *Am. J. Obstet. Gynecol.*, *93*, 506 (1965).

22 "Summary Minutes of the FDA OTC Panel on Contraceptives and Other Vaginal Drug Products," Rockville, Md., Sept. 20–21, 1974.

23 J. D. Solbel, *Ann. Int. Med.*, *101*, 90 (1984).

24 R. Glynn, *Obstet. Gynecol.*, *22*, 640 (1963).

25 M. H. Gotlib and D. N. Adler, *Med. Times*, *96*, 902 (1968).

26 R. S. Cohen et al., *Curr. Ther. Res.*, *15*, 839 (1973).

27 W. A. Abruzzi, *J. Am. Med. Women's Assoc.*, *21*, 406 (1966).

28 R. J. Stock et al., *Obstet. Gynecol.*, *42*, 141 (1973).

29 C. A. D. Ringrose, *N. Engl. J. Med.*, *295*, 1319 (1976).

30 T. A. Gossel, *U.S. Pharmacist*, *11(5)*, 20 (May 1986).

31 H. Vorherr et al., *J. Am. Med. Assoc.*, *244*, 2628 (1980).

32 N. Etling et al., *Obstet. Gynecol.*, *53*, 376 (1979).

33 W.-H. Chow et al., *Am. J. Obstet. Gynecol.*, *153*, 727–729 (1985).

34 H. H. Neumann and A. De Cherney, *N. Engl. J. Med.*, *295*, 789 (1976).

35 G. F. Egenolf and R. McNaughton, *Obstet. Gynecol.*, *7*, 23 (1956).

36 F. H. Downer and C. J. Stevenson, *Adverse Drug React. Bull.*, *42*, 136 (1973).

37 C. D. Calnan, *Proc. Roy. Soc. Med.*, *55*, 39 (1962).

38 *Med. Lett. Drugs Ther.*, *10*, 27 (1968).

39 A. A. Fisher et al., *Arch. Dermatol.*, *104*, 286 (1971).

40 A. A. Fisher and M. A. Stillmann, *Arch. Dermatol.*, *106*, 169 (1972).

41 E. Schmunes and E. J. Levy, *Arch. Dermatol.*, *106*, *169* (1972).

42 *Federal Register*, *40*, 8926 (1975).

43 G. Carsch, *Soap Chem. Spec.*, *47*, 38 (1971).

44 A. A. Fisher, *Arch. Dermatol.*, *108*, 801 (1973).

45 J. Meyer-Robin and V. Kassebart, *Kosmetologie*, *4*, 159 (1971).

46 F. Sadik, *Pharmindex*, *22*, 11 (1980).

47 J. A. Cella, *Am. Cosmet. Perfum.*, *86(10)*, 84 (1971).

48 P. A. Sanders, in "Modern Pharmaceutics," G. S. Banker and C. T. Rhodes, Eds., Marcel Dekker, New York, N.Y., 1979, pp. 591–647.

49 G. McBride, *J. Am. Med. Assoc.*, *219*, 449 (1972).

50 G. S. Kass et al., "Feminine Hygiene Deodorant Sprays," Paper presented at XIV International Congress of Dermatology, Venice, Italy, May 22, 1972.

51 A. Kantner, *Am. Cosmet. Perfum.*, *87*, 31 (1972).

52 B. A. Davis, *Obstet. Gynecol.*, *36*, 812 (1970).

53 J. M. Gowdy, *N. Eng. J. Med.*, *287*, 203 (1972).

54 *Med. Lett. Drugs Ther.*, *12*, 88 (1970).

55 M. Morrison, *FDA Consumer*, *7*, 16 (1973).

56 I. L. Chavkin, *Cutis*, *23*, 24 (1979).

57 *Federal Register*, *43*, 46694 (1978).

58 H. J. Hurley, in "Dermatology in General Medicine," T. B. Fitzpatrick et al., Eds., McGraw-Hill, New York, N.Y., 1987, p. 697.

59 W. J. Cunliffe and S. G. Tan, *Practitioner*, *216*, 149 (1976).

60 A. E. Elkhouly and R. T. Yousef, *J. Pharm. Sci.*, *63*, 681 (1974)

61   W. B. Shelley and R. Florence, *N. Engl. J. Med.*, *263*, 1056 (1960).

62   S. Plechner, in "Cosmetics: Science and Technology," 2nd ed., Vol. 2, M. S. Balsam and E. Sagarian, Eds., Wiley-Interscience, New York, N.Y., 1972, pp. 373–416.

63   W. B. Shelley et al., *Arch. Dermatol. Syphilol.*, *68*, 430 (1953).

64   J. N. Lubows et al., in "Principles of Cosmetics for the Dermatologist," P. Frost and S. N. Horwitz, Eds., C. V. Mosby, St. Louis, Mo., 1982, pp. 89–97.

65   H. J. Hurley, *J. Am. Med. Assoc.*, *250*, 419 (1983).

66   *Med. Lett. Drugs Ther.*, *19*, 20 (1977).

67   W. P. Coleman, *J. Dermatol. Surg. Oncol.*, *14*, 1085 (1988).

68   R. L. Dobson, *Arch. Dermatol. 123*, 883 (1987).

69   J. W. White, *Mayo Clin. Proc.*, *61*, 951 (1986).

70   *Med. Lett. Drugs Ther.*, *28*, 109 (1986).

71   *Federal Register*, *47*, 36492 (1982).

72   C. M. Papa and A. M. Kligman, *J. Invest. Dermatol.*, *49*, 139 (1967).

73   E. Holzle and A. M. Kligman, *J. Soc. Cosmet. Chem.*, *30*, 279 (1979).

74   S. A. McWilliams et al., *Br. J. Dermatol.*, *117*, 617 (1987).

75   W. B. Shelley and H. J. Hurley, *J. Am. Med. Assoc.*, *244*, 1956 (1980).

76   E. Holzle and A. M. Kligman, *J. Soc. Cosmet. Chem.*, *30*, 357 (1979).

77   S. Williams and A. J. Freemont, *Br. Med. J.*, *288*, 1651 (1984).

78   *Federal Register*, *42*, 41374 (1977).

79   "AMA Drug Evaluations," 6th ed., American Medical Association, Chicago, Ill., 1986, p. 1524.

80   R. Blake, *J. Am. Podiatry Assoc.*, *58*, 109 (1968).

81   P. A. Majors and J. E. Wild, *J. Soc. Cosmet. Chem.*, *25*, 139 (1974).

82   J. A. Parrish, "Dermatology and Skin Care," McGraw-Hill, New York, N.Y., 1975, pp. 29–31.

83   *Federal Register*, *43*, 51546 (1978).

84   *Federal Register*, *47*, 39108 (1982).

85   K. A. Arndt, "Manual of Dermatologic Therapeutics," 2nd ed., Little, Brown, Boston, Mass., 1978, pp. 118–126.

86   K. A. Arndt and T. B. Fitzpatrick, *J. Am. Med. Assoc.*, *194*, 965 (1965).

87   S. S. Bleehan, *J. Soc. Cosmet. Chem.*, *28*, 407 (1977).

88   K. Jimbow et al., *J. Invest. Dermatol.*, *62*, 436 (1974).

89   M. C. Spencer, *J. Am. Med. Assoc.*, *194*, 962 (1965).

90   R. A. Hoshow et al., *Arch. Dermatol.*, *121*, 105 (1985).

91   R. J. Mann and R. M. Harman, *Br. J. Dermatol. 108*, 363 (1983).

92   "AHFS Drug Information 89," American Society of Hospital Pharmacists, Bethesda, Md., 1989, p. 2011.

93   *Lancet*, *1*, 488 (1967).

94   J. H. Casey, *Aust. N.Z. J. Med.*, *10*, 240 (1980).

95   R. N. Earheart et al., *South. Med. J.*, *70*, 442 (1977).

96   A. McQueen, in "Iatrogenic Diseases," 2nd ed., P. F. D'Arhy and J. P. Griffin, Eds., Oxford University Press, New York, N.Y., 1979, pp. 77–91.

97   H. B. Spoor, *Cutis*, *21*, 283 (1978).

98   J. F. Dunn, *Am. Fam. Physician*, *38 (3)*, 169 (1988).

99   *Med. Lett. Drugs Ther.*, *23*, 44 (1981).

100   A. J. Natow, *Cutis*, *38 (2)*, 91 (1986).

101   S. J. Powis et al., *Br. Med. J.*, *2*, 1166 (1976).

102   R. H. Barry, in "Cosmetics: Science and Technology," 2nd ed., Vol. 2, M. S. Balsam and E. Sagarian, Eds., Wiley-Interscience, New York, N.Y., 1972, pp. 39–72.

103   D. H. Powers, in "Cosmetics: Science and Technology," 2nd ed., Vol. 2, M. S. Balsam and E. Sagarian, Eds., Wiley-Interscience, New York, N.Y., 1972, pp. 73–116.

104   R. L. Goldenberg, in "Principles of Cosmetics for the Dermatologist," P. Frost and S. N. Horwitz, Eds., C. V. Mosby, St. Louis, Mo., 1982, pp. 13–15.

105   N. Van Haute and A. Dooms-Goossens, *Contact Dermatitis*, *9*, 169 (1983).

106   *Consumer Reports*, *33*, 529 (1968).

PERSONAL CARE PRODUCT TABLE

Product (Manufacturer)	Antimicrobial	Local Anesthetic/ Antipruritic/Counterirritant	Other Ingredients
Acu-dyne Douche (Acme United)	povidone-iodine		
Betadine Antiseptic Gel (Purdue Frederick)	povidone-iodine, 10%		
Betadine Douche (Purdue Frederick)	povidone-iodine		
Betadine Vaginal Suppositories (Purdue Frederick)	povidone-iodine, 10%		
CondomMate Inserts (Upsher-Smith)			polyethylene glycol blend surfactant glyceride
Cortef Feminine Itch Cream (Upjohn)		hydrocortisone, 0.5%	aloe vera cetyl palmitate glyceryl monostearate polyethylene glycol stearamidoethyl diethylamine parabens
Crème de la Femme (Especially)			mineral oil white petrolatum
Femidine Douche (A.V.P.)	povidone-iodine		
Feminique Disposable Douche (Schmid)			sodium benzoate sorbic acid lactic acid octoxynol-9
Feminique Vinegar & Water Disposable Douche (Schmid)			vinegar
Gynecort Creme (Combe)		hydrocortisone, 0.5%	
K-Y Jelly (Johnson & Johnson)	chlorhexidine gluconate		glucono delta lactate sodium hydroxide glycerin hydroxyethylcellulose
Lubrin Inserts (Upsher-Smith)			caprylic/capric triglyceride glycerin laureth-23
Massengill Baking Soda Disposable Douche (SmithKline Beecham)			sodium bicarbonate
Massengill Disposable Douche: Scented and Unscented (SmithKline Beecham)	cetylpyridinium chloride diazolidinyl urea		EDTA SD alcohol 40 lactic acid octoxynol-9 fragrance colors
Massengill Douche Powder: Floral and Unscented (SmithKline Beecham)		methyl salicylate phenol thymol menthol eucalyptus oil	ammonium alum sodium chloride PEG-8

PERSONAL CARE PRODUCT TABLE, continued

Product (Manufacturer)	Antimicrobial	Local Anesthetic/ Antipruritic/Counterirritant	Other Ingredients
Massengill Liquid (SmithKline Beecham)		methyl salicylate eucalyptol menthol thymol	SD alcohol 40 lactic acid sodium lactate octoxynol-9 aromatics
Massengill Medicated Disposable Douche (SmithKline Beecham)	povidone-iodine, 0.3%		
Massengill Medicated Liquid (SmithKline Beecham)	povidone-iodine, 0.3%		
Massengill Medicated Towelette (SmithKline Beecham)	diazolidinyl urea	hydrocortisone, 0.5%	DMDM hydantoin isopropyl myristate parabens polysorbate 60 propylene glycol sorbitan stearate steareth-2
Massengill Towelette Baby Powder and Unscented (SmithKline Beecham)	cetylpyridinium chloride		lactic acid sodium lactate potassium sorbate octoxynol-9 EDTA
Massengill Vinegar & Water Disposable Douche (SmithKline Beecham)	cetylpyridinium chloride diazolidinyl urea		EDTA vinegar
Massengill Vinegar & Water Disposable Douche Extra Mild (SmithKline Beecham)			vinegar
Maxilube Jelly (Mission)			silicone oil glycerin carbomer 934 triethanolamine sodium lauryl sulfate parabens
New Freshness Disposable Douche (Fleet)			vinegar octoxynol-9 sorbic acid
Norforms (Personal Labs)	methylbenzethonium chloride		PEG-20 PEG-6 PEG-20 palmitate methylparaben lactic acid
Norforms Herbal (Personal Labs)	methylbenzethonium chloride		PEG-2 PEG-6 PEG-20 palmitate methylparaben lactic acid
Operand Douche (Redi)	povidone-iodine (1% iodine)		

PERSONAL CARE PRODUCT TABLE, continued

Product (Manufacturer)	Antimicrobial	Local Anesthetic/ Antipruritic/Counterirritant	Other Ingredients
Personal Lubricant Gel (Ortho)			glycerin propylene glycol sodium carboxy-methylcellulose sodium alginate sorbic acid methylparaben
PMC Douche Powder and Disposable Douche (Thomas & Thompson)	boric acid, 82%	thymol, 0.3% phenol, 0.2% menthol	ammonium aluminum sulfate, 16% eucalyptus oil peppermint oil
Replens (Columbia)			glycerin mineral oil polycarbophil carbomer 934P hydrogenated palm oil glyceride methylparaben sorbic acid
Summer's Eve Herbal and White Flowers Scent (Fleet)			octoxynol-9 citric acid sodium benzoate sodium citrate fragrance
Summer's Eve Hint of Musk (Fleet)	diazolidinyl urea		citric acid octoxynol-9 sodium benzoate fragrance sodium citrate
Summer's Eve Medicated Disposable Douche (Fleet)	povidone-iodine, 0.3% (when mixed)		
Summer's Eve Post-Menstrual Disposable Douche (Fleet)			sodium lauryl sulfate monosodium & disodium phosphates sodium chloride EDTA
Summer's Eve Regular Disposable Douche (Fleet)			citric acid sodium benzoate sodium citrate
Summer's Eve Vinegar & Water Disposable Douche (Fleet)			vinegar water
Trichotine Liquid and Powder (Reed & Carnrick)			sodium perborate (powder) sodium borate (liquid) aromatics sodium lauryl sulfate alcohol, 8% (liquid) sodium chloride (powder)
Trimo-San Jelly (Milex)	oxyquinoline sulfate, 0.025%		boric acid, 1% sodium borate, 0.7% sodium lauryl sulfate glycerin

PERSONAL CARE PRODUCT TABLE, continued

Product (Manufacturer)	Antimicrobial	Local Anesthetic/ Antipruritic/Counterirritant	Other Ingredients
Triva Douche Powder (Boyle)	oxyquinoline sulfate, 2%		EDTA, 0.33% alkyl aryl sulfonate, 35% sodium sulfate, 53% lactose, 9.67%
Vaginex Cream (Schmid)		tripelennamine hydrochloride	
Zonite (SmithKline Beecham)	benzalkonium chloride, 0.2%	menthol, 0.08% thymol, 0.08%	propylene glycol, 5% buffer

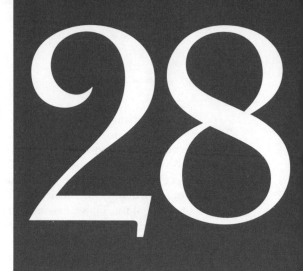

Michael R. Jacobs and Paul Zanowiak

TOPICAL
ANTI-INFECTIVE
PRODUCTS

Questions to ask in patient/consumer counseling

What area of the skin is affected? How extensive is the area involved?

Is the skin broken? Is there pus? Is it painful?

How long have you had this condition? Have you ever had it before? Are any other members of your family also affected?

Has the condition developed as the result of a previous rash or skin problem?

Has the condition worsened?

Do you have a fever or any flulike symptoms?

Do you have diabetes? Do you have any other medical conditions?

Do you have any allergies to topical medications?

What treatments have you tried for this condition? Were they effective?

What oral or topical medications are you presently using? Have they been effective?

Topical anti-infectives are used to counteract local infection of tissue (mucous membranes and the skin). The active ingredients of these products are antimicrobials; most are antibacterial or antifungal. Because this product classification is so broad, discussion is limited to antimicrobial products for use in prevention and self-treatment of skin infections.

SKIN ANATOMY
AND PHYSIOLOGY

The skin is the body's largest organ and is involved in numerous physical and biochemical processes (1). Normal skin thickness is 3–5 mm; the thickest skin is on the palms and soles, and the thinnest skin is on the eyelids and parts of the genitals. The skin is divided into three main layers (Figure 1). The outermost layer (epidermis), which is compact and nonvascular, consists of stratified squamous epithelial cells. The next layer (the dermis or corium) is formed of vascular and connective tissue. These two layers are not similar in composition but adhere firmly to each other. The hypodermis, or subcutaneous layer, is the innermost layer.

The epidermis is composed of several distinct sublayers. The innermost, in close association with the dermis, is the stratum germinativum, which consists of columnar/cuboidal epithelial cells. Above this is the prickle cell unit (stratum spinosum), composed of polygonal epithelial cells, which is thicker in the palms than in hairy skin. These two epidermal sublayers are involved in mitotic processes of epidermal regeneration and repair. The prickle cells are produced by cellular division and contain keratinocytes, the pigment-forming melanocytes that contain melanin precursors and melanin granules. As the keratinocytes migrate to the skin surface, they change from living cells to dead, thick-walled, flat, nonnucleated cells containing keratin, a fibrous protein.

Above the prickle cells is the granular sublayer (stratum granulosum), which is actually several thicknesses of flattened polygonal cells. These cells contain granules of keratohyaline, which are changed to keratin in the outermost portion (stratum corneum, or horny outer layer of the epidermis). The clear area (stratum lucidum), present only in thick skin, is between the granular unit and the stratum corneum. It is a narrow band of flattened, closely packed cells believed to contain eleidin, a possible derivative of keratohyaline. The stratum corneum is composed of flat, scaly dead (keratinized) tissue. Its outermost cells are flat (squamous) plates that are constantly shed (desquamated).

The dead cells lost from the outer surface of the epidermis are replaced by new cells generated by the mitotic processes of the stratum spinosum and stratum germinativum. The newer cells push older ones closer to the surface. In the process they become flattened, lose their water content, fill with keratin, and gradually die, taking their place on the skin surface.

The dermis, which supports the epidermis and separates it from the lower fatty layer, consists mainly of collagen and elastin embedded in a mucopolysaccharide substance. Fibroblasts and mast cells are found throughout. The dermis also contains a network of nerves and capillaries that comprise the neurovascular supply to the dermal appendages (hair follicles, sebaceous glands, and sweat glands). The main sublayers of the dermis are the papillary and reticular units. The papillary sublayer, adjacent to the epidermis, is very rich in blood vessels, and the papillae probably act as conduits to bring blood nutrients near the avascular epidermis. The reticular sublayer, below the papillae, contains coarser tissue that connects the dermis with the hypodermis.

The hypodermis, composed of relatively loose connective tissue of varying thickness, provides necessary pliability for the skin. In most areas, this layer also includes a fatty unit (panniculus adiposus), which facilitates thermal control, food reserve, and cushioning or padding.

Skin Appendages

Hair Follicle

A hair shaft is generated by a hair germ at the base of a follicle. The follicle is basically an inward tubular folding of the epidermis into the dermis. The hair within the follicle is a fiber of keratinized epithelial cells that increase as a result of multiplication of cells in the hair germ.

Sebaceous Glands

Most sebaceous or sebum-producing glands are located in the same area as the hair because they are usually appendages of the follicles. Sebaceous glands not associated with hair follicles may be found in the genital areas, around the nipples of the breast, and on the edge of the lips. The ducts of the glands are lined with epithelial cells that are continuous with the basal layers of the epidermis. The sebaceous glands are holocrine, because the gland cells from which the sebum is derived are destroyed in its production. Sebum covers the hair and skin surface and is a mixture of free fatty acids (mainly palmitic and oleic), triglycerides, waxes, cholesterol, squalene, other hydrocarbons, and traces of fat-soluble vitamins. With sweat it forms an emulsion that includes surface waste products of cutaneous cells.

Sweat Glands

Two types of sweat glands are identified in association with dermal anatomy: the eccrine and apocrine glands. Both are considered exocrine because their secretions (sweat) reach the skin surface through distinct ducts. They are not holocrine, and differ anatomically in their distribution over body surface and in the character of their secretions.

Eccrine Glands Eccrine glands are independent of hair follicles and develop from the epithelium of the skin surface, extending in a coil to the dermis. The secretory epithelium is located in the hypodermis, and the ducts ascend through the epidermis as wavy or curved channels. They are present over most of the body surface, except for the genital areas and legs, and are especially numerous on the palms and soles.

Eccrine glands are cholinergically innervated, although the nerve fibers are sympathetic. Eccrine sweat production is controlled by the heat regulatory centers of the hypothalamus. Emotional stress and cholinergic drugs also can trigger eccrine sweating. Eccrine sweat is basically an electrolyte solution with pH of approximately 5. It is devoid of fats, carbohydrates, and proteins. The volume produced (several liters per day) is much greater than that of apocrine sweat.

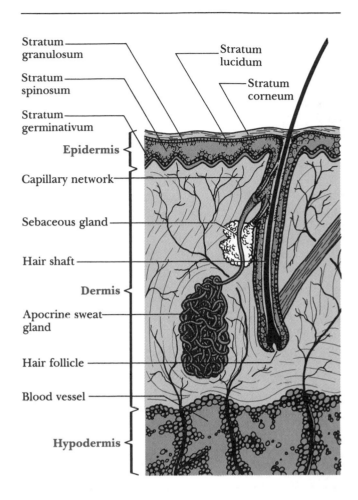

Stratum granulosum

Stratum spinosum

Stratum germinativum

Epidermis

Capillary network

Sebaceous gland

Hair shaft

Dermis

Apocrine sweat gland

Hair follicle

Blood vessel

Hypodermis

Stratum lucidum

Stratum corneum

FIGURE 1   Cross section of human skin.

Apocrine Glands   An apocrine sweat gland generally is attached to a hair follicle by a duct, leading down into a coiled, secretory glandular tubule. These tubules are covered with myoepithelium, allowing contraction to adrenergic stimulation. Such stimulation, as in stress, releases a milky secretion that contains proteins, sugars, and lipids. This secretion is odorless until skin bacteria act upon its contents, producing the characteristic pungent odor of apocrine sweat. (See Chapter 27, *Personal Care Products*.)

Apocrine glands are present around the nipples, in the axillae, and in the anogenital region. They are much larger than eccrine glands but produce much less volume of sweat. They do not function in body temperature regulation but are responsive to hormone secretion. Consequently, the onset of action of these glands is associated with puberty.

Nails

The nails are modifications of the keratinized layer of the epidermis. The nail bed on which the nail plate lies derives from the basal epidermal layers. The body of the plate, at its periphery, is surrounded by the nail root. The root is derived from the nail groove, which is a process of the basal epidermal unit. The white area at the base is called the lunula, and the part of the nail groove that enfolds the plate at its margin is the eponychium. The hyponychium is a thick layer of stratum corneum immediately beneath the plate of the nail's distal tip.

Skin Surface

The secretions that accumulate at the skin surface are weakly acidic with a pH of 4.5–5.5 (the acid mantle) (1). The pH varies slightly from individual to individual and among different areas of the body; it is somewhat higher in areas where perspiration evaporates slowly (2). It differs in the sexes.

Various microorganisms live on the surface of intact skin. The individual species that make up the flora exist in a normal ecologic balance. The flora of the various skin areas is diverse, including aerobic and anaerobic species of *Staphylococcus, Corynebacterium,* and *Sarcina* and occasional Gram-negative rods. The number of organisms on various areas of the skin differs. Changes in the kind and number of organisms occur during different periods of life and during different seasons. Flora population varies among individuals, some having a constantly high microbial population.

NORMAL SKIN FUNCTION

The skin acts as a barrier between the environment and the body, protecting the body from harmful external agents, such as pathogenic organisms and chemicals (3). Its ability to carry out this function depends on a variety of factors including the age of the individual, underlying disease states, use of certain oral or topical medications, and preservation of an intact stratum corneum (4). The skin also contributes to sensory experiences and is involved in temperature control, development of pigment, and synthesis of some vitamins. It is important in hydroregulation because it controls moisture loss from the body and moisture penetration into the body.

Except for the stratum corneum, the cells of all layers use nutrients and oxygen and excrete water and carbon dioxide. Most oxygen is supplied from the blood, although a small amount is supplied from the external environment. Similarly, carbon dioxide is removed from the tissues mainly by the blood, but small amounts are discharged directly to the atmosphere.

Dermal hydration is important to the health and normal function of the skin. If the corneal layer becomes dehydrated, it loses elasticity and permeation characteristics become altered. Returning water to the skin is the only means by which dryness can be reversed. The stratum corneum can be hydrated by water transfer from the lower layers and by water accumulation (perspiration) induced by occlusive coverings, such as tight, impervious bandages (plastic wrap) or oleaginous pharmaceutical vehicles (petrolatum). Generally, such moisture accumulation seems to "open" the compactness of the stratum corneum for renewed suppleness and more effective penetration by drug molecules. (See Chapter 30, *Dermatitis, Dry Skin, Dandruff, Seborrhea, and Psoriasis Products*.)

The acid mantle has been postulated to be a protective mechanism because microbes tend to grow better at pH 6–7.5. Infected areas have higher pH values than those of normal skin. Several fatty acids found in sweat and sebum (propionic, caproic, and caprylic) inhibit microbial and fungal growths. Therefore, the importance of the acid mantle concept is not solely in the inherent pH, but more likely in the specific compounds responsible for the acidity.

The buffer capacity of skin surface secretions is another protective mechanism. When the pH is raised or lowered, the skin readjusts to a normal pH. Moreover, the normal skin flora acts as a defense mechanism by controlling the growth of potential pathogenic organisms and their possible invasion of the skin and body.

Percutaneous Absorption Factors

A drug must be released from its base if it is to exert an effect at the desired site of activity (either the skin surface, the epidermis, or the dermis). The release of a topical drug from its base occurs at the interface between the skin surface and the applied layer of product. The physical–chemical relationship between the drug and the base determines the rate and amount of drug released. Considerations such as the solubility of the drug in the base, its diffusion coefficient in the base, and its partition coefficient into sebum and the stratum corneum are significant to its efficacy (5). A drug with a strong affinity for the base is released less readily than one whose solubility in the base is lower. Likewise, a drug with a proper balance of polar and hydrocarbon moieties (a partition coefficient approaching 1) penetrates the stratum corneum more readily than drugs that are either highly polar or highly lipoidal, because

that portion of the skin possesses both hydrated proteins and lipids. Other factors influencing drug release include the degree of hydration of the stratum corneum, the pKa of the drug, the pH of the base and of the skin surface, the drug concentration, the thickness of the applied layer, and the temperature. In the latter case, the blood flow is altered dramatically according to the temperature of the zone of application. As the temperature increases, blood flow in the area increases as well as the rate of percutaneous absorption. These factors are applicable to drug release from all topical dosage forms: medicated powders, ointments, pastes, emulsified cream or lotion bases, gels, suspensions, and solutions.

Greasy, hydrocarbon bases such as petrolatum are occlusive, promote hydration, and generally increase molecular transport. Hydrous emulsion bases are less occlusive; water-soluble bases (polyethylene glycols) are nonocclusive. The latter, in fact, may attract water from the stratum corneum, thereby decreasing drug transport. Powders with hydrophilic ingredients also decrease hydration because they promote evaporation from the skin by absorbing available water and increasing its surface area.

Substances are transported from the skin surface to the general circulation through percutaneous absorption. Minor routes of such transport involve passage between the keratinized units of the stratum corneum and through the skin's appendages (hair follicles, sweat glands, and sebaceous glands). The major route is by passive diffusion through the stratum corneum, followed successively by transfer through the deeper epidermal layers and the papillary dermis.

After application of a topical drug product, transport of the drug cannot begin until the surface of the stratum corneum is "charged" with the drug. A delay period occurs while a drug is transferring from its vehicle (base) into and through the sebum, and then into the stratum corneum.

Depending on the physical–chemical properties of a drug and those of sebum and the various skin layers, the drug movement into and through the skin meets with varying degrees of resistance. The sebum, when present, can be a minor barrier to drug transfer, depending on the partition coefficient of the drug. The stratum corneum provides the greatest resistance and therefore is a rate-limiting barrier to percutaneous absorption. Because it is nonliving tissue, the stratum corneum may be viewed as having the general characteristics of an artificial and semipermeable membrane, and molecular passage through it is completely passive (bulk diffusion). Once a molecule has crossed the stratum corneum, there is much less resistance to its transfer across the rest of the epidermis into the dermis.

When the corneum is hydrated extensively, drug diffusion in general is accelerated. Because occlusion (with a plastic covering) increases the hydration of the stratum corneum from within the skin, it fosters the transfer of all drugs. This occurs because the hydration swells the stratum corneum, loosening its normally tight, densely packed arrangement, thereby making such diffusion easier. Likewise, the increased amount of water present under such conditions probably further enhances the transfer of polar molecules.

Wounds, burns, chafed areas, and extensive lesions of various dermatoses alter the integrity of stratum corneum and result in artificial shunts of the percutaneous absorption process. Scarring and inflammation also can alter the process. Drug absorption in such instances essentially is uncontrolled and could lead to potentially dangerous systemic concentrations. Extreme care must be used in applying topical medication to damaged skin, especially when large areas are involved. (See Chapter 33, *Burn and Sunburn Products*.)

CUTANEOUS INFECTIONS

Cutaneous infections may be caused by bacteria, fungi, viruses, or parasites. (See Chapter 23, *Oral Health Products*, Chapter 36, *Insect Sting and Bite Products*, and Chapter 29, *Acne Products*.) Many bacterial and fungal infections are amenable to topical therapy. Careful assessment of the condition must be made before appropriate treatment can be recommended.

Bacterial Infections

Some bacterial skin infections are classified as pyodermas because pus is usually present. They are caused principally by species of beta-hemolytic *Streptococcus* and hemolytic *Staphylococcus* (4). The lesions result from external infection or reinfection and may be superficial or involve deeper dermal tissue. These pyodermic infections may be either primary (in which no previous dermatoses exist) or secondary (in which a predisposing dermal problem preceded the infection). Other organisms may be present in secondary pyodermas, including Gram-negative bacteria (*Pseudomonas aeruginosa*), which are especially prevalent on warm moist skin such as axillae, ear canals, and interdigital spaces.

Infections by pathogenic organisms are related to the breakdown of the skin's "disinfecting" protective mechanisms or to the development of an abundance of colonies of pathogenic organisms (4). A breakdown of the normal ecological balance may be enhanced by alterations in the skin's other defense mechanisms.

Normally, the stratum corneum has only about 10% water content, which ensures elasticity but is generally below that needed to support luxuriant microbial growth (4). An increase in moisture content may allow microbial growth, leading to infection.

A break in the intact surface has a deleterious effect on the skin's defensive properties, allowing large numbers of pathogenic organisms to be introduced into the inner layers.

In addition, infection may be predisposed by excessive scrubbing of the skin (especially with strong detergents), excessive exposure to water, occlusion, increasing the skin temperature, excessive sweating or bathing, and injury (4, 6–8). Therefore, the presence and severity of microbial skin infection generally are dependent on the condition of the skin's defense mechanisms, the number of pathogenic organisms present, and the supportive nutrient environment for those organisms.

The main pyodermic infections are impetigo, folliculitis, furuncles (boils), carbuncles, erysipelas, ecthyma, and pyonychia.

Impetigo

Impetigo, caused by species of *Streptococcus* and/or *Staphylococcus*, probably is the most superficial of the pyodermas, mainly involving the surface areas. Direct contact with the lesions or infected exudate generally is required for its transmission. The lesions initially are small red spots that rapidly evolve into characteristic vesicles (tiny sacs or blisters) filled with amber fluid (9). Exudate collects and forms yellow or brown crusts on the skin's surface, which are surrounded by a zone of erythema. The eruptions may be circular with clear central areas and may occur in groups. The exposed parts of the body are most easily affected, but no area of the skin is immune if autogenous reinfection is not controlled. (See *Plate 4–16*.) Impetigo is most common in children and is contagious.

Generally, in primary impetigo (impetigo vulgaris) the responsible bacteria cause the infection directly. Some forms, however, occur secondarily to the presence of other infections, injury, or the general breakdown of skin defenses. Bockhart's impetigo usually occurs in association with other conditions (furuncles, discharging ears, or wounds). Lesions are characteristically tiny follicular pustules around hair shafts and may be encircled by narrow red rings (areolae).

Ecthyma

Ecthyma is similar to impetigo in that the same organisms are involved, but the lesion is much deeper.

In contrast to facial impetigo, the legs most commonly are affected, and the lesions occur singularly and tend to be localized. The lesion begins as an erythematous pustule that rapidly erodes and become crusted. This condition often occurs as a secondary infection to mild trauma or injury to the skin. In humid tropical environments, the lesions may become quite destructive.

Erysipelas

Erysipelas, caused by species of beta-hemolytic *Streptococcus*, is characterized by a rapidly spreading, red, and edematous plaque. This superficial infection has sharply established borders and a glistening surface (9). It occurs most often on the scalp and face, and the organisms enter through a break in the skin. (See *Plate 4–17.*) It is usually accompanied by fever, chills, and malaise.

Folliculitis

Follicular pustules may be superficial or deep, depending on the pathogen or the site involved. They involve only the hair shafts; surrounding tissue is not affected. Usually the superficial forms are very similar to Bockhart's impetigo and may be secondary infections. Skin areas regularly exposed to water, grease, oils, tars, and other contaminants seem most susceptible to folliculitis.

Furuncles and Carbuncles

Furuncles and carbuncles are generally staphylococcal infections located in or around hair follicles. In these pyodermas, the lesion may start as a superficial folliculitis but develops into a deep nodule. (See *Plate 4–18.*) The fully established furuncle has elevated swelling, is erythematous, and is very painful. Furuncles are most common in males. Hairy areas and areas subject to maceration and friction (collar, waist, buttocks, and thighs) seem most vulnerable. The initial erythema and swelling stage is followed by thinning of the skin around the primary follicle, centralized pustulation, destruction of the pilosebaceous structure, discharge of the core (plug), and central ulceration. Scarring often occurs. Furunculosis is common, with new lesions appearing intermittently for months or years.

Furuncles may be secondary infections to other dermatoses or diseases. Diabetes mellitus or agammaglobulinemia may predispose an individual to furuncles or carbuncles. Chronic cases of these pyodermas should be referred to a physician for evaluation of a possible underlying disease.

Carbuncles begin in a manner similar to furuncles and may have similar etiologies. Carbuncles involve clusters of follicles with deeper and broader penetra-

tion over a larger area than furuncles. Furuncles may develop into carbuncles by infiltration or infection of adjacent follicles.

Paronychia

Paronychia is a pyogenic infection of the nails, accompanied by swelling and tenderness of the surrounding tissue. Paronychia is caused primarily by beta-hemolytic species of *Streptococcus* and *Staphylococcus*. Moderate pressure may force a pus exudate, and the nail may develop with irregularities. (See *Plate 4–19.*) It is important that this condition be differentiated from candidal or other fungal infections.

Otitis Externa

Otitis externa, an inflammation of the external ear, may be a secondary infection and may be associated with seborrheic scaling of the scalp. Increase in the moisture content of the external ear over long periods gradually leads to changes in the types of organisms present. External heat, humidity, or swimming may play a role in the development of this condition. The most common initial complaint is itching. With increasing severity, however, edema, crusting, and oozing may occur. (See Chapter 22, *Otic Products.*)

Fungal Infections

Fungal infections, often called dermatomycoses, are among the most common cutaneous disorders (10, 11). Characteristically, they exhibit single or multiple lesions that may have mild scaling or deep granulomas (inflamed nodules). Superficial infections affect the hair, nails, and skin and are generally caused by three genera of fungi: *Trichophyton, Miscrosporum,* and *Epidermophyton*. Species of *Candida* may also be involved (12). Fungal infections of hairless skin are generally superficial, and the organisms are found in or on the uppermost skin layers. In fungal infections of areas covered with heavy hair, the infections are much deeper because of hair follicle penetration.

Tinea Pedis

Tinea pedis, also known as athlete's foot or ringworm of the feet, is caused by several species of fungi. (See Chapter 37, *Foot Care Products.*)

Tinea Capitis

Transmitted by direct contact with infected persons or animals, tinea capitis is caused by species of

Microsporum and *Trichophyton*. Most cases of this infection occur in children. Depending on the causative organism, the clinical presentation varies from noninflamed areas of hair loss to deep, crusted lesions, which may lead to scarring and permanent hair loss. (See *Plate 4-20.*) These large lesions, similar to carbuncles in appearance, are called kerions.

Tinea Cruris

Tinea cruris (also called jock itch) is caused by *Epidermophyton floccosum, Trichophyton rubrum,* and *Trichophyton mentagrophytes*. It occurs on the medial and upper parts of the thighs and the pubic area, and is more common in males. The lesions have specific margins that are elevated slightly and are more inflamed than the central parts; small vesicles are found at the margins. Acute lesions are bright red and turn brown in chronic cases; they may scale. This condition is generally bilateral with severe pruritus.

Tinea Corporis

Species of *Trichophyton* and *Microsporum* are the causative organisms of tinea corporis. There is a higher incidence of tinea corporis among persons living in humid climates. The lesions involve glabrous (smooth and bare) skin and begin as small, circular, erythematous scaly areas. They spread peripherally and the borders may contain vesicles or pustules. Tinea corporis should be differentiated from noninfectious dermatitis because the lesions may be similar in appearance.

Other Fungal Infections

Moniliasis or candidiasis, caused mainly by *Candida albicans,* usually occurs in intertriginous areas such as the groin, axillae and interdigital spaces, under breasts, and at the corners of the mouth. Involvement of the mucous membranes is known as thrush, vaginal candidiasis, or pruritus ani, depending on the area affected. Candidal paronychia is most common in people whose activities involve routine immersion of the hands in water. Systemic diseases such as diabetes, infection, and malignancy may lower general resistance and allow candidal infections to flourish. Certain drugs, including oral antibiotics and steroids, may also contribute to candidal infection. Pregnancy is often a predisposing cause of vaginal candidiasis because of changes in vaginal pH and flora.

Other fungal skin infections include tinea barbae (barber's itch or ringworm of the beard); tinea manuum (hands); tinea versicolor, in which the lesions are brown; tinea circinata, generally ringed, red lesions that can agglomerate into polycyclic configurations; and tinea unguium (onychomycosis), in which the nail may become hypertrophic, discolored, and scaly (12). (See *Plate 5-21A* and *B.*)

Viral Infections

Viral infections may occur directly in or on the skin and present as warts, molluscum contagiosum, or herpes simplex (13). (See Chapter 23, *Oral Health Products,* and Chapter 37, *Foot Care Products.*) Herpes zoster infections also present with cutaneous manifestations and affect a nerve or group of nerves of the same area.

Chickenpox and measles are systemic viral diseases that also present with important diagnostic dermatologic manifestations.

Herpes Simplex

Herpes simplex is a viral infection of the skin and mucous membranes. The causative agent is a fairly large virus, *Herpesvirus hominis* (HVH). (See *Plate 5-22.*) There are two strains: herpesvirus type 1 (herpes labialis or cold sores), which is commonly found on the lips, and herpesvirus type 2, which generally occurs as genital lesions and is sexually transmitted.

Herpes Zoster

Herpes zoster, neurotropic in humans, is caused by the zoster-varicella virus, which is the same virus that causes chickenpox. The highly contagious, generalized, and usually benign chickenpox will develop in the nonimmune host, while the localized and painful zoster (shingles) will develop in the partially immune host. Children with leukemia or on long-term therapy with corticosteroids and patients who are immunosuppressed because of disease or medications are extremely vulnerable to the zoster virus. The different clinical manifestations of these two diseases reflect the interaction between this virus and the host immune mechanisms.

Zoster probably results from reactivation of a latent virus, which resides in the dorsal root or cranial nerve ganglion cells. It is mainly a disease of adults who have usually had chickenpox. Lesions appear suddenly and acutely along the course of a nerve or group of nerves on one side of the body as reddened, swollen, round plaques ranging in size from about 5 mm to areas larger than a hand; the spinal ganglia seem to be the primary site. The plaques may be painful after lesions form, and it is possible for them to appear as successive "showers" or crops over several days. The lesions develop into fairly large blisters that become crusty in 1–2 weeks. (See *Plate 5-23A* and *B.*) The regional lymph nodes are generally tender.

Molluscum Contagiosum

Molluscum contagiosum is a viral tumor caused by a poxvirus containing deoxyribonucleic acid (DNA). The disease is contracted by direct contact with an infected person, fomites, or autoinoculation.

The virus is manifested by small (3–5 mm), pink, slightly raised lesions usually found on the abdomen, inner thigh, or perianal areas. The mature lesion has a slight depression on the top and has a soft core that can be easily expressed. They may occur in groups or as a single lesion. Erythema does not usually accompany the lesion unless there is a secondary bacterial infection.

EVALUATION

Before recommending a topical product for self-medication of various cutaneous infections, the pharmacist should ascertain what type of infection exists. The pharmacist should also be aware of noninfectious processes such as contact dermatitis, psoriasis, or drug-induced eruptions (14). Antimicrobial agents generally should be considered only in the case of an infectious etiology.

The pharmacist can play an important role by preventing erroneous self-medication and by recommending medical attention if the condition calls for it. Incorrect self-medication may cause a delay in healing, possible progression of the disease, toxicity, obvious discomfort, and unnecessary cost. Immediate medical attention should be sought if the following circumstances exist:

- There is doubt as to the causative factor or organism (organic or some other process; bacteria or fungi).

- Appropriate treatment has not been successful and the condition is getting worse.

- Applications of drug products have been used for several days over large areas, especially on denuded skin (potential for systemic toxicity).

- Drainage is excessive and has occurred for several days.

- Improper cleaning of infectious exudate has led to widespread infection.

- There is predisposing illness, such as diabetes or systemic infection, or symptoms of such illness.

- Fever and/or malaise occurs.

- A primary dermatitis (allergic dermatitis, psoriasis, or seborrhea) exists and has developed a secondary infection that is difficult to treat with nonprescription products.

- Lesions are deep and extensive.

- Lancing is needed to aid drainage.

The use of nonprescription topical antimicrobial products should be limited to superficial conditions that involve minimal areas, when no predisposing illnesses exist. Self-administered topical products should be viewed as extensions of supportive treatment (proper cleaning, proper hygiene, and clean bandaging), and not as "miracle" treatments. Medical attention should be sought in all but the most superficial, uncomplicated skin infections, especially if it appears that systemic medication is needed. Deep-seated and complicated secondary infections require medical attention. Improper lancing as self-treatment may cause scarring and spreading of the infected exudate.

As noted, only the most superficial, minor cutaneous infections are amenable to topical anti-infective therapy. In more severe cases of bacterial infection, widespread fungal infection, or infections of the nails, systemic therapy is required. Medical treatment will be directed by the patient's clinical presentation and, when necessary, cultures of the lesion to determine the infecting organism. Minor surgical procedures such as debridement, curettage, and liquid nitrogen are indicated in the treatment of some dermatoses. Such procedures must be performed by a dermatologist.

DRUG AND PRODUCT CATEGORIES

The various antimicrobial nonprescription drugs used to prevent skin infection include antibiotics, antifungals, and antiseptics. Individual antimicrobial agents for such uses are discussed within these categories in the following section. Two Food and Drug Administration (FDA) advisory review panels on over-the-counter (OTC) antimicrobial drugs (antimicrobial I and II) have evaluated these drugs for safety and therapeutic efficacy. A detailed review of the FDA and advisory review panel activities was presented in the eighth edition of this text. A final ruling has been made for first-aid antibiotic drug products (15), but not for antiseptic or antifungal drug products. Antibiotics are discussed in the following section on pharmacologic agents.

PHARMACOLOGIC AGENTS

Various topical antibiotics, antifungal agents, and antiseptics have been used in nonprescription products for dermal conditions.

Antibiotics

The topical nonprescription antibiotics included in the FDA's first-aid antibiotic monograph are bacitracin zinc ointment, chlortetracycline hydrochloride ointment, neomycin sulfate ointment, and polymyxin sulfate in combination with neomycin and/or bacitracin (15). Oxytetracycline, in combination with polymyxin, is also included. Polymyxin, neomycin, and bacitracin may also be used in combination with local anesthetic active ingredients. The rationale for their use in combination is to help prevent infection and to temporarily relieve the discomfort of minor cuts, burns, and abrasions.

Bacitracin

Bacitracin, including its zinc salt, is a polypeptide antibiotic that is generally bactericidal. Specifically, bacitracin acts to inhibit cell-wall synthesis. Topically, the drug is not absorbed to any significant extent, whether applied to wounds, mucous membranes, or denuded or intact skin; systemic toxicity is rare. However, hypersensitivity reactions, ranging from localized itching and swelling to anaphylactic reactions, may occur. The drug is active against Gram-positive organisms. The development of resistance in previously sensitive organisms is rare. Topical nonprescription preparations usually contain 400–500 units per gram of ointment and are applied 1–3 times a day. Bacitracin may be used topically in both infants and children (15).

Neomycin

Neomycin, an aminoglycoside antibiotic, is effective against many Gram-negative organisms and some staphylococci. Resistant organisms may develop. The mechanism of action appears to be that of inhibiting protein synthesis by irreversibly binding to the 30S ribosomal subunit. It is considered to be bactericidal. Neomycin has the highest rate of development of hypersensitivity, with reactions occurring in 5–8% of patients (16). Although not absorbed when applied to intact skin, application to large areas of denuded skin has been known to cause systemic toxicity (ototoxicity and nephrotoxicity) (16).

For topical use, neomycin is available in cream and ointment forms, alone or in combinations. The con-

centration commonly used in nonprescription products is 3.5 mg/g (equivalent to 5 mg/g of neomycin sulfate). Applications are made 1–3 times a day. Neomycin is most frequently used in combination with polymyxin and bacitracin to prevent the development of neomycin-resistant organisms.

Polymyxin B Sulfate

Polymyxin B sulfate is effective against Gram-negative bacteria but not against Gram-positive bacteria or fungi. Fewer resistant organisms develop than with neomycin. It is presumed to produce its antibacterial property by altering the permeability of the bacterial membrane. Toxicity rarely occurs with topical therapy. Concentrations of 5,000 units per gram and 10,000 units per gram are available in nonprescription combination preparations. Applications are usually made 1 or 2 times a day.

Tetracyclines

Tetracycline, chlortetracycline, and oxytetracycline are broad-spectrum antibiotics. They are presumed to exert their bacteriostatic effect by binding to the 30S ribosomal subunit and thus inhibit protein synthesis. Three-percent ointments of tetracycline and chlortetracycline are available; toxicity is rare when applied topically. Long-term use may lead to overgrowth of nonsusceptible bacteria or fungi. Oxytetracycline is included in the FDA's proposed monograph for use only in combination with polymyxin B sulfate. These products are applied 1–3 times a day.

Antifungal Agents

Agents used for cutaneous skin infections are found in ointments, creams, powders, and aerosols. However, not all of these agents have been recommended as safe and effective by the FDA advisory review panel on OTC antifungal drug products (17).

Chloroxylenol

In 0.5–3.75% concentrations, chloroxylenol (parachlorometaxylenol) was classified as safe for use for up to 13 weeks for the treatment of athlete's foot, jock itch, or ringworm. However, additional safety data (for long-term uses) and clinical effectiveness data are needed before the FDA can place it in the monograph (17).

Undecylenic Acid

Undecylenic acid has the greatest antifungal activity of the fatty acids. It may cause irritation and sensitization and should be discontinued if these side effects occur. It is basically a fungistatic agent, requiring long exposure at high concentrations to be effective. It is used with its zinc, calcium, or copper salts in ointment, cream, powder, and aerosol forms (2–5% acid, 20% salt) for an additive antifungal effect.

Haloprogin

Haloprogin offers another effective alternative for the treatment of athlete's foot, jock itch, and ringworm. The compound has significant antibacterial activity against several species of *Trichophyton* as well as *Streptococcus*, *Staphylococcus*, and *Candida* (18).

Haloprogin has been shown to be superior to placebo (19) and equally effective with tolnaftate (19, 20). One investigator has shown higher cure rates and fewer relapses with haloprogin compared to tolnaftate based on laboratory criteria (KOH slide preparations and cultures), although clinical cure rates were equal (21). Side effects of the drug applied topically are relatively rare and minor. They include burning, itching, and scaling of the skin. Should these side effects occur, the preparation should be discontinued.

Prescription products include haloprogin 1% cream and solution. Although recommended for nonprescription use by the FDA advisory review panel, no nonprescription products have yet been marketed.

Miconazole

Miconazole nitrate is another topical antifungal recommended for nonprescription use. This agent was originally approved for use by prescription but has been reclassified as nonprescription. It, too, is included in the proposed monograph. Miconazole demonstrates activity against both fungi and Gram-positive bacteria, but has no activity against Gram-negative bacteria (22).

Miconazole does demonstrate a low rate of recurrent infections when therapy is continued for at least 2 weeks (23, 24). However, the onset of recurrence simply may be delayed. There is little information on the comparative efficacy of miconazole, tolnaftate, and haloprogin. Side effects occur rarely and are usually self-limiting with discontinuation of the preparation.

Miconazole is available as a 2% cream, powder, and spray.

Selenium Sulfide

Selenium sulfide is effective in the treatment of tinea versicolor and seborrheic dermatitis of the scalp. It is used in nonprescription topical products to control dandruff, usually as a detergent suspension. Contact with the eyes and sensitive skin areas should be avoided because it is a potential irritant. Although not absorbed significantly when applied to the skin, it is hazardous if swallowed, producing central nervous system effects and respiratory and vasomotor depression. In the treatment of tinea versicolor, the agent should be applied to the affected areas, allowed to stand overnight, and washed off in the morning. This is repeated once weekly for 4 weeks. Alternatively, applications may be made nightly for 15–20 minutes, for several weeks.

Tolnaftate

Tolnaftate is a topical nonprescription antifungal agent effective against most species of fungi (except *C. albicans*) that cause cutaneous infections. Complete clearing of cutaneous lesions may take more than a month of therapy. The mechanism of action appears to be through inhibition of squalene epoxidation (25). Tolnaftate is used in the treatment of all forms of tinea; however, tinea unguium responds poorly to therapy unless the infection is very superficial. Topically, tolnaftate has a low incidence of toxicity. However, if local irritation occurs, treatment should be discontinued. Tolnaftate is available as a 1% cream, powder, solution, gel, and spray. (See Chapter 37, *Foot Care Products*.) It usually is not effective alone in disease states involving areas with hair follicles (e.g., scalp, beard) or nails.

Iodochlorhydroxyquin

Iodochlorhydroxyquin has both antifungal and antibacterial properties. Its antibacterial properties have been used to treat dermal infectious conditions such as pyoderma, folliculitis, and impetigo; its antifungal properties have been used to treat mucocutaneous mycotic conditions such as athlete's foot, jock itch, ringworm (tinea), and moniliasis (26). It is mildly irritant and may cause initial stinging or itching. If these effects persist, discontinuation of the product is recommended. Several dosage forms (lotion, cream, ointment) contain both this drug and hydrocortisone. These are prescription-only products; however, they have been used at times for noninfectious dermal conditions such as contact dermatitis and atopic dermatitis (27). Therapeutic success derived in such cases may be due only to the hydrocortisone.

In October 1989, the FDA approved the marketing of clotrimazole as a nonprescription antifungal agent. This drug previously had been available only by prescription. It is now available as both a prescription (Lotrimin) and nonprescription (Lotrimin AF) drug. Note should be taken of this event, for it constitutes the presence on the market of a drug product, in the same strength and dosage form, that is both a prescription and nonprescription drug (28).

Antiseptics

Antiseptics inhibit growth and development of microorganisms, but may not eradicate the organism. Many nonprescription drug products contain antiseptics. However, not all of these have been classified as safe and effective by FDA's OTC review panel (29).

Ethanol

Ethanol has good bactericidal activity in a 20–70% concentration and acts relatively quickly but has little residual effect. In concentrations above 80%, however, its bactericidal effect is low. It rapidly denatures cellular protein of microorganisms, lowers the surface tension of bacteria to help in their removal, and has a solvent effect on sebum. It is not an effective antiviral agent, nor does it kill spores. It is not a desirable wound antiseptic because it irritates already damaged tissue. The coagulum formed may, in fact, protect the bacteria.

Ethanol usually contains denaturants. Although not recognized as a skin sensitizer, excessive exposure in high concentrations can dehydrate the corneum. Systemic ingestion produces usual alcoholic intoxication and severe gastrointestinal (GI) distress. The GI symptoms will be exacerbated if denatured alcohol is ingested.

Isopropyl Alcohol

Isopropyl alcohol has somewhat stronger bactericidal activity and lower surface tension than ethanol. In general, it is used like ethanol solutions for its cleansing and antiseptic effects on the skin. It can be used undiluted or as a 70% aqueous solution. Denaturants are not added because isopropyl alcohol itself is not potable. Isopropyl alcohol has a greater potential for drying the skin because its lipid solvent effects are stronger than those of ethanol.

Iodine

Solutions of elemental iodine or those that release iodine from chemical complexes are used as presurgical skin antiseptics and as wound antiseptics. Their antimicrobial effect is attributed to their ability to oxidize microbial protoplasm. Caution must be taken that strong iodine solution (Lugol's) not be used as an antiseptic. Iodine solution USP (2% iodine, 2.5% sodium iodide) is used as an antiseptic for superficial wounds. Iodine tincture USP (2% iodine, 2.5% sodium iodide, and about 50% alcohol) is less preferable than the aqueous solution because it is irritating to the tissue.

In general, bandaging should be discouraged after iodine applications to avoid tissue irritation. Iodine solutions stain skin, may be irritating to tissue, and may cause sensitization in some people.

Iodophors

Iodophors are organic complexes of iodine. Two of these complexes are povidone–iodine and poloxamer iodine. Free iodine is released slowly from these preparations and is probably responsible for the antiseptic effects of these agents. The percentage of active ingredient varies according to the product type from 0.5 to 1% in ointments to 0.75% in shampoos and skin antiseptics. Iodophors are less irritating, nonstaining, and less sensitizing than iodine solutions.

Chlorhexidine Gluconate

Chlorhexidine gluconate did not fall within the purview of the FDA's advisory review antimicrobial I and II panels. Recognized as an effective antimicrobial agent, chlorhexidine has been used in Europe and Canada. FDA approval for topical antiseptic use in the United States was granted in 1976 through the new drug application procedure (30). Chlorhexidine gluconate is structurally a biguanide and resembles quaternary ammonium salts (30). It is effective against both Gram-positive and Gram-negative bacteria and some fungi. It exhibits residual adherence to skin surfaces.

Some surfactants and serum protein can reduce the antiseptic potential of chlorhexidine gluconate; it exhibits low potential for sensitization and irritation (30). A prominent warning against use in the ear appears on the labeling of nonprescription products containing this compound.

Mercurial Compounds

Several mercurial compounds have antiseptic properties. In general, however, they are considered poor antiseptics for wounded skin because serum and tissue proteins reduce their antimicrobial potency. If these compounds are used extensively or on large areas of abraded skin, mercury may be absorbed and may become a systemic poison. Their use should be discouraged in such conditions.

Inorganic salts of mercury are tissue irritants. Such toxic properties are reduced when the mercury is incorporated into an organic compound. Some investigators believe that the alcoholic component of mercurial tinctures has greater antimicrobial effect than the mercurial component (31).

Merbromin Merbromin is less effective as a skin antiseptic than the other organic mercurials. However, it is used in some cases as a preoperative germicide (2%, aqueous). Serous fluids reduce its antimicrobial potency.

Nitromersol Nitromersol is more effective as an antiseptic than soluble inorganic compounds of mercury but is less effective than ethanol. It is not a serious tissue irritant and is available as a tincture in a dilution of 1:200.

Thimerosal Thimerosal has antibacterial and antifungal properties, but it is less effective than ethanol. It is found in several types of topical products, including aqueous solutions, tinctures, ointments, creams, and aerosols. Systemic toxicity occurs less frequently with thimerosal than with other mercurials because the mercury in thimerosal is tightly bound to the organic configuration. The usual concentration is 0.1%.

Hydrogen Peroxide

Hydrogen peroxide (3% solution), also not reviewed or classified by the antimicrobial I and II panels, is the most widely used antimicrobial oxidizing agent; sodium and zinc peroxides also are used. Enzymatic release of oxygen from hydrogen peroxide occurs when it comes into contact with blood and tissue fluids. The mechanical release (fizzing) of the oxygen has a cleansing effect on a wound, but organic matter reduces its effectiveness. The duration of action is only as long as the period of active oxygen release. Using peroxide on the intact skin is of doubtful value, because release of the nascent oxygen is too slow.

This compound must be used only where the released gas can escape; therefore, it should never be used in abscesses, nor should bandages be applied too soon after its use.

Phenolic Compounds

Phenol In very dilute solutions, phenol is an antiseptic and disinfectant. It has local anesthetic activity and is claimed to be an antipruritic in concentrations of 1:100 to 1:200, as in phenolated calamine lotion. In aqueous solutions of more than 1%, it is a tissue irritant and should not be used on skin, except as a keratolytic or peeling agent.

Oleaginous Phenolic Solutions Oily solutions of phenol and camphor are often used as nonprescription antiseptics in the treatment of minor cuts, insect bites, athlete's foot, fever blisters, and cold sores. Such products contain relatively high concentrations of phenol (4%) and must be used with caution. If applied to moist areas, partitioning of the phenol out of the oleaginous vehicle into the water present results in caustic concentrations of phenol on the skin. To avoid such damaging effects, these products should be applied only to dry skin.

Substituted Phenols Substituted phenols include the halogenated phenols (hexachlorophene) and the al-kyl-substituted phenols (cresols and resorcinol). Halogenation of a phenolic compound increases antiseptic properties. Dihalogenated and trihalogenated forms have greater potency but are less water soluble than monohalogenated phenols.

Triclosan Triclosan is used in soap bars at concentrations up to 0.5% (31), although the usual maximum concentration is 0.3% (32). It has been placed by the FDA advisory review panel on OTC antimicrobial I drug products in Category III for such use, as well as for use as a skin antiseptic and skin-wound protectant. Subsequent to the panel's recommendations, the FDA proposed that it may be effective and placed it in Category III for use as a health care personnel handwash, patient handwash, patient preoperative skin preparation, and surgical hand scrub.

Cresols Cresols are alkyl derivatives of phenol. Three isomers (ortho, meta, and para) have disinfectant properties. Because cresol irritates the skin, use is limited to disinfection of inanimate objects and surfaces. The isomers are more potent bactericides than phenol but are at least as toxic.

Resorcinol Resorcinol is much less potent than phenol as an antimicrobial agent, but its systemic effects are similar. As an extemporaneously prepared ointment (2% or more), it is used in antifungal therapy (e.g., ringworm). However, other topical agents, such as tolnaftate, are more effective for such use.

Resorcinol monoacetate Resorcinol monoacetate exerts an even milder antibacterial effect than resorcinol, but has a longer duration of action because it releases resorcinol slowly. Both resorcinol and the monacetate are used in acne preparations for their keratolytic effect and mild antibacterial effect. (See Chapter 29, *Acne Products.*)

Hexylresorcinol Hexylresorcinol is more effective than phenol as an antibacterial agent and is less toxic. It has been used in mouthwashes. The FDA advisory review panel on OTC antimicrobial I drug products has judged it safe and effective (Category I) as a skin-wound cleanser (29). It is used in low concentrations (0.1%) and may be irritating.

Thymol and Chlorothymol Thymol and chlorothymol are also alkyl derivatives of phenol with minor antimicrobial and antifungal properties.

Parachlorometaxylenol Parachlorometaxylenol in 2% concentration is more effective than phenol. It is an ingredient in nonprescription products used for seborrhea and acne. However, more information relative to its percutaneous absorption is needed before it can be assigned Category I status (29, 31).

Quaternary Ammonium Compounds Quaternary ammonium compounds are cationic surfactants that have antimicrobial activity on Gram-positive and Gram-negative bacteria but not on spores. Gram-negative bacteria are more resistant than Gram-positive ones; thus, they need a longer period of exposure. Quaternary ammonium compounds are sometimes included in topical anti-infective products. In addition to their antiseptic properties, these agents are used for their cleansing properties. Quaternary ammonium compounds emulsify sebum and have a detergent effect to remove dirt, bacteria, and desquamated epithelial cells. Their antimicrobial activity is caused by disrupting the membranes and denaturing lipoproteins of microbes. The "quats" can be inactivated by various anionic adjuvant ingredients (e.g., soaps, viscosity building agents).

The FDA proposed monograph includes benzalkonium chloride, benzethonium chloride, and methylbenzethonium chloride (29). These compounds are formulated as creams, dusting powders, and aqueous or alcoholic solutions. Concentrates are available for dilution to proper concentration for topical use.

If used undiluted, these concentrates may cause serious irritation. Quaternary compounds are irritating to the eyes, so caution must be used when applying them to skin near the eyes. For use on broken or diseased skin, concentrations of 1:5,000 to 1:20,000 may be used. For use on intact skin and minor abrasions, a concentration of 1:750 is recommended.

Methylbenzethonium chloride is effective against microorganisms that split urea to form ammonia. It is used as a diaper rinse and for applications to areas subject to irritation from ammonia formation (groin, thighs, and buttocks). (See Chapter 31, *Diaper Rash and Prickly Heat Products*.)

PRODUCT SELECTION GUIDELINES

Once the pharmacist has evaluated the patient's condition, medical referral or appropriate self-medication should be recommended. Topical self-medication with anti-infective products must be reserved for superficial, uncomplicated infections. More serious infections should be referred to a physician for systemic therapy. Additionally, although many anti-infective nonprescription products are available, few have been studied under controlled conditions. Studies comparing agents within a class are also limited in number. It is difficult, therefore, to recommend one product over another in the treatment of superficial infections.

For the treatment of impetigo, the compounds most studied are neomycin, bacitracin, and polymyxin, either alone or in combination. Although the topical nonprescription preparations are effective, they lead to

delayed clearing of lesions compared with systemic antibiotics. Topical agents seem to be most effective when the lesions are not extensive (33). Cleaning the area with soap and water and gently removing loose crusts should improve response to topical therapy. Systemic streptococcal infections can occur in the presence of impetigo. Some physicians, therefore, treat all impetigo infections systemically, as well as topically.

Although less objective information is available for other bacterial skin infections (erysipelas, ecthyma, and folliculitis), treatment with the medications listed above may be effective as long as the infection is not extensive. Furuncles and carbuncles may require lancing, which should be done only under the direction of a physician. Bacterial infections of the nails are rare and may require drainage and treatment with systemic antibiotics; therefore, these infections should also be treated by a physician.

Some superficial fungal infections, such as tinea corporis or tinea cruris, respond well to topical antifungal agents. However, success of therapy increases when the lesions are small. If the lesions are extensive or involve beard, scalp, or nails, topical therapy is generally ineffective; systemic therapy should be considered upon referral to a physician. In the case of tinea pedis, product selection may be guided by patient preference and cost to the patient. Patients with fungal dermal infections should be advised to use the product for at least 2–4 weeks, even if symptoms and lesions disappear. Patients who seek aid from recurrent infections should be questioned about the duration of prior treatment and advised accordingly.

The use of first-aid antibiotics helps prevent infection in minor cuts, burns, and abrasions. Although the use of topical antimicrobials seems desirable in theory, there is little evidence to support their routine use in such cases. Cleaning the wound with soap and water or with hydrogen peroxide, followed by an appropriate dressing may be the only "treatment" necessary. Should the area become inflamed or painful, or should pus develop, a physician should be consulted.

CONSULTATION

The pharmacist should explain the proper use of the suggested product. For infections, intermittent applications are considered poor therapy; regular applications are preferable. If increased irritation occurs, the patient should be instructed to contact a physician. The appropriate "thickness" of applications should be suggested to avoid overmedication or undermedication. The pharmacist must make sure that the patient understands that none of these topical anti-infectives are to be used internally.

In addition to the information about nonprescription drug usage, the pharmacist may also provide information that will help eradicate the infection and possibly prevent future infections. This information would include proper cleaning of the infected area, avoiding the use of tight fitting or "occlusive" clothing, and avoiding situations that could lead to recurring infections.

Moreover, the patient should be informed of the expected duration of therapy and those conditions that, if they occur, would result in the need for physician-directed care (e.g., the development of a secondary bacterial infection). In general, the patient should see substantial improvement in 1 week; if this does not occur, the patient should be referred to a physician. Recurring skin infections may be a sign of undiagnosed diabetes or other organic problem(s). A pharmacist who is aware of recurring infections should refer the patient to a physician.

SUMMARY

Topical antimicrobials are used to treat and prevent cutaneous infections caused by bacteria, fungi, and viruses. Knowledge of design and formulation aspects of topical antimicrobial products is important in selecting appropriate therapeutic agents and products. A patient interview is essential to determine whether self-medication or medical attention is indicated. If self-medication is appropriate, the pharmacist should instruct the patient in the use of nonprescription drugs and other supportive procedures. The outcomes and recommendations of the FDA's OTC advisory review panel should be followed to ascertain the status of the various topical antimicrobial ingredients as to safety and therapeutic efficacy, as well as for all other nonprescription ingredients and products.

REFERENCES

1   G. F. Odlan, "Structure of the Skin in Biochemistry and Physiology of the Skin," L. A. Goldsmith, Ed., Oxford University Press, Oxford, Eng., 1983, pp. 3–63.
2   J. S. Jellinek, "Formulation and Function of Cosmetics," 2nd ed., Wiley, New York, N.Y., 1970, pp. 4–14.
3   W. D. Stewart et al., "Dermatology: Diagnosis and Treatment of Cutaneous Disorders," 4th ed., C. V. Mosby, St. Louis, Mo., 1978, p. 3.
4   R. R. Roth and W. D. James, J. Am. Acad. Dermatol., 20, 367–390 (1989).
5   P. J. Cascella and J. E. Powers, U.S. Pharmacist, 13 (12), 26 (1988)
6   M. T. Hojyo-Tomoka et al., Arch. Dermatol., 107, 723 (1973).
7   L. F. Montes and W. H. Wilborn, Br. J. Dermatol., 81, 23 (1969).
8   R. R. Marples, "Skin Bacteria and Their Role in Infection," H. I. Maibach and G. Hildrick-Smith, Eds., McGraw-Hill, New York, N.Y., 1965, pp. 33–42.
9   B. M. Barker and F. Prescott, "Antimicrobial Agents in Medicine," Blackwell Scientific Publications, London, Eng., 1973, pp. 18–149.
10   E. L. Laden, "Modern Dermatologic Therapy," T. H. Sternberg and V. D. Newcomer, Eds., McGraw-Hill, New York, N.Y., 1959, pp. 374–377, 386–403.
11   M. B. Sulzberger and J. Wolfe, "Dermatology: Diagnosis and Treatment," 2nd ed., Yearbook Medical, Chicago, Ill., 1961, pp. 277–356.
12   J. T. Scrafani, U.S. Pharmacist, 26 (1978).
13   W. D. Stewart et al., "Dermatology: Diagnosis and Treatment of Cutaneous Disorders," 4th ed., C. V. Mosby, St. Louis, Mo., 1978, p. 293.
14   W. Bruinsma, "A Guide to Drug Eruptions," Excerpta Medica, Amsterdam, The Netherlands, 1973, pp. 45–48, 87–103.
15   Federal Register, 52, 47312–24 (1987).
16   M. A. Sande and G. L. Mandell, "The Pharmacological Basis of Therapeutics," 6th ed., A. G. Gilman et al., Eds., Macmillan, New York, N.Y., 1980, p. 1177.
17   Federal Register, 47, 12480 (1982).
18   S. Seki, et al., "Antimicrobial Agents Chemotherapy," 1963, p. 569.
19   H. W. Hermann, Arch. Dermatol., 106, 839 (1972).
20   R. Katz and B. Cahn, Arch. Dermatol., 106, 837 (1972).
21   V. H. Carter, Curr. Ther. Res., 14, 307 (1972).
22   G. Hildick-Smith, Adv. Biol. Skin, 12, 303 (1972).
23   S. J. Mandy and T. C. Garrott, J. Am. Med. Assoc., 230, 72 (1974).
24   J. E. Fulton, Jr., Arch. Dermatol., 111, 596 (1975).
25   K. J. Barrett-Bee et al., J. Med. Vet. Mycol., 24, 155–160 (1986).
26   S. C. Harvey, "Remington's Pharmaceutical Sciences," 17th ed., A. R. Gennaro, Ed., Mack Publishing, Easton, Pa., 1985, p. 1227.
27   "Physician's Desk Reference," 39th ed., B. B. Huff, Ed., Medical Economics, Oradell, N.J., 1985, p. 876.
28   The Green Sheet, 38 (A50), 3 (1989).
29   Federal Register, 43, 1210–49 (1978).
30   D. R. Ward, Stuart Pharmaceuticals, Wilmington, Del.; FDA's Summary for Basis of Approval, NDA 17–768 (Hibiclens), and laboratory data developed as part of NDA requirements, personal communication.
31   "AMA Drug Evaluations," 4th ed., Wiley, New York, N.Y., 1980, p. 1017–1026.
32   S. Spainhour, CIBA-Geigy Corporation, Greensboro, N.C., personal communication, 1989.
33   H. C. Dillon, Int. J. Dermatol, 19, 443 (1980).

TOPICAL ANTI-INFECTIVE PRODUCT TABLE

Product (Manufacturer)	Antiseptic	Antifungal Agent	Antibiotic	Other Ingredients
Achromycin Ointment (Lederle)			tetracycline hydro-chloride, 3%	
ACU-dyne (Acme United)	available iodine, 1%			
Aftate Gel, Powder and Spray Powder for Jock Itch (Schering-Plough)		tolnaftate, 1%		alcohol, 14% (spray powder) talc (powder)
Antifungal (Major)		tolnaftate, 1%		
Argyrol S.S. (Iolab)	mild silver protein, 10%			
Aureomycin Ointment (Lederle)			chlortetracycline, 3%	
Baciguent Ointment (Upjohn)			bacitracin, 500 units/g	
Bacitracin (Various manufacturers)			bacitracin, 500 units/g	
Bactal Soap (Whittaker General)	triclosan, 0.5%			anhydrous soap, 10%
Bactine (Miles)	benzalkonium chloride, 0.13%			lidocaine hydrochloride, 2.5%
Bactine First Aid Antibiotic (Miles)			polymyxin B sulfate, 5000 units/g bacitracin, 500 units/g neomycin sulfate, 5 mg/g	mineral oil white petrolatum
Benza (Century)	benzalkonium chloride, 1:750			
Benzalkonium Chloride (Various manufacturers)	benzalkonium chloride, 17% or 17.5%			
Betadine Solution, Microbicidal Applicator, Swab Aid, Swab Sticks, Gauze Pads and Whirlpool Concentrate (Purdue Frederick)	povidone-iodine, 10%			
B.F.I. Powder (SmithKline Beecham)	bismuth formic iodide boric acid			zinc phenolsulfonate bismuth subgallate potassium alum eucalyptol menthol thymol amol
Biodine Topical 1% (Major)	iodine, 1%			

TOPICAL ANTI-INFECTIVE PRODUCT TABLE, continued

Product (Manufacturer)	Antiseptic	Antifungal Agent	Antibiotic	Other Ingredients
Blis-To-Sol Liquid (Chattem)		undecylenic acid salicylic acid		
Blis-To-Sol Powder (Chattem)		salicylic acid benzoic acid		
Beezee Mist Aerosol (Pedinol)	aluminum chlorhydrate	undecylenic acid		menthol
Caldesene (Pharmacraft)		calcium undecylenate, 10%		
Campho-Phenique (Winthrop)	phenol, 4.7%			camphor, 10.8%
Castaderm (Lannett)	resorcin boric acid acetone phenol			basic fuchsin alcohol, 9%
Castel Minus (Syosset)	resorcinol, 10% acetone			basic fuchsin hydroxyethylcellulose alcohol, 10%
Castel Plus (Syosset)	resorcinol, 10% acetone			basic fuchsin hydroxyethylcellulose alcohol, 10%
Clorpactin WCS-90 Powder (Guardian)	available chlorine, 3-4%			
Clorpactin XCB (Guardian)	available chlorine, 4-4.9%			
Cruex Medicated Cream (Fisons)		undecylenic acid, 3% zinc undecylenate, 20%		
Cruex Powder (Fisons)		calcium undecylenate, 10%		
Cruex Spray Powder (Fisons)		undecylenic acid, 2% zinc undecylenate, 20%		
Dakin's Solution (Century)	sodium hypochlorite, 0.5%			
Dakin's Solution ½ Strength (Century)	sodium hypochlorite, 0.25%			
Decylenes (Rugby)		undecylenic acid zinc undecylenate		
Desenex Antifungal Foam (Fisons)		undecylenic acid, 10%		alcohol, 29%
Desenex Cream (Fisons)		zinc undecylenate, 20% undecylenic acid, 3%		
Desenex Liquid (Fisons)		undecylenic acid, 10%		alcohol, 40%

TOPICAL ANTI-INFECTIVE PRODUCT TABLE, continued

Product (Manufacturer)	Antiseptic	Antifungal Agent	Antibiotic	Other Ingredients
Desenex Ointment and Powder (Fisons)		zinc undecylenate, 20% undecylenic acid, 5% (ointment) 2% (powder)		
Efodine (Fougera)	available iodine, 1%			
Enzactin (Whitehall)		triacetin, 250 mg/g		
Fungacetin (Blair)		triacetin, 25%		
Fungi-Nail (Kramer)	resorcinol, 1% parachlorometaxylenol, 2% acetic acid, 2.5%	salicylic acid, 2%		benzocaine, 0.5% propylene glycol hydroxypropyl methylcellulose alcohol, 0.5%
Genaspor (Goldline)		tolnaftate, 1%		
Gentian Violet (Various manufacturers)		gentian violet, 1% or 2%		
Germicin (CMC)	benzalkonium chloride, 50%			
Iodex-P (Medtech)	povidone-iodine, 10%			
Iodex Regular (Medtech)	iodine, 4.7%			oleic acid
Iodochlorhydroxy-quin Cream and Ointment (Various manufacturers)		iodochlorhydroxy-quin, 3%		
Iodine, Strong Solution (Lugol's Solution) (Various manufacturers)	iodine, 2% potassium iodide, 10%			
Iodine Swabs (Various manufacturers)	iodine, 2%			alcohol, 47%
Iodine Topical Solution (Various manufacturers)	iodine, 2% sodium iodide, 2.4%			
Iodine Tincture (Various manufacturers)	iodine, 2% sodium iodide, 2.4%			alcohol, 47%
Iodine Tincture, Strong (Various manufacturers)	iodine, 7% potassium iodide, 5%			alcohol, 83%
Isodine Antiseptic Solution (Blair)	povidone-iodine, 10%			

TOPICAL ANTI-INFECTIVE PRODUCT TABLE, continued

Product (Manufacturer)	Antiseptic	Antifungal Agent	Antibiotic	Other Ingredients
Lagol Oil (Alvin Last)	8-hydroxyquinoline			mineral oil cottonseed oil
Lanabiotic Ointment (Combe)			polymyxin B sulfate, 10,000 units/g bacitracin, 500 units/g neomycin sulfate, 5 mg/g	
Lotrimin AF Cream and Solution (Schering-Plough)		clotrimazole, 1%		
Lubraseptic Jelly (Guardian)	o-phenylphenol, 0.1% p-tert-pentylphenol, 0.02% phenylmercuric nitrate, 0.007%			
Mallisol (Hauck)	povidone-iodine, 10%			
Medi-Quik (Mentholatum)			bacitracin, 500 units/g neomycin, 3.5 units/g polymyxin B sulfate, 5000 units/g	mineral oil petrolatum
Mercurochrome (Various manufacturers)	merbromin, 2%			
Mercurochrome II (Becton Dickinson)	benzalkonium chloride isopropyl alcohol, 5%			lidocaine hydrochloride menthol
Merlenate Ointment (Vortech)		zinc undecylenate, 20% caprylic acid, 5% sodium propionate, 2%		
Mersol (Century)	thimerosal, 1:1000			alcohol, 52.5%
Merthiolate Solution and Tincture (Lilly)	thimerosal, 1:1000			alcohol, 50% (tincture)
Micatin Cream, Powder and Spray (Ortho)		miconazole nitrate, 2%		
Myciguent Cream and Ointment (Upjohn)			neomycin sulfate, 5 mg/g	
Mycitracin (Upjohn)			polymyxin B sulfate, 5000 units/g bacitracin, 500 units/g neomycin sulfate, 5 mg/g	
N.B.P. (Forest)			polymyxin B sulfate, 5000 units/g bacitracin, 400 units/g neomycin base, 3.5 mg/g	
Neo-Castaderm (Lannett)	boric acid resorcin acetone phenol			alcohol, 9%

TOPICAL ANTI-INFECTIVE PRODUCT TABLE, continued

Product (Manufacturer)	Antiseptic	Antifungal Agent	Antibiotic	Other Ingredients
Neomixin (Hauck)			polymyxin B sulfate, 5000 units/g zinc bacitracin, 400 units/g neomycin base, 3.5 mg/g	
Neomycin (Various manufacturers)			neomycin sulfate, 0.5%	
Neosporin Cream (Burroughs Wellcome)			polymyxin B sulfate, 10,000 units/g neomycin, 3.5 mg/g	
Neosporin Ointment (Burroughs Wellcome)			polymyxin B sulfate, 5000 units/g bacitracin zinc, 400 units/g neomycin 3.5 mg/g	white petrolatum
Neosporin Ointment, Maximum Strength (Burroughs Wellcome)			polymyxin B sulfate, 10,000 units/g bacitracin zinc, 500 units/g neomycin, 3.5 mg/g	
Neo-Thrycex (Commerce)			polymyxin B sulfate, 5000 units/g bacitracin, 400 units/g neomycin base, 3.5 mg/g	
New Skin (Medtech)	8-hydroxyquinoline, 1%			clove oil, 1% pyroxylin (collodion), 98%
NP-27 Aerosol Powder, Cream and Solution (Thompson Medical)		tolnaftate, 1%		alcohol, 14.9% (aerosol powder)
Obtundia (Otis Clapp)	cresol-camphor complex			
Obtundia First Aid Spray (Otis Clapp)	cresol-camphor complex			
Oil-O-Sol (Health Care Industries)	hexylresorcinol, 0.1%			corn oil, 52% castor oil, 40.8% camphor oil, 6.8%
Osti-Derm (Pedinol)	phenol	zinc oxide		magnesium carbonate aluminum acetate solution camphor glycerin
Oxyzal Wet Dressing (Gordon)	benzalkonium chloride, 1:2000 oxyquinoline sulfate			
Paladine Solution (Hauck)	povidone-iodine, 10%			
Polydine (Century)	povidone-iodine			

TOPICAL ANTI-INFECTIVE PRODUCT TABLE, continued

Product (Manufacturer)	Antiseptic	Antifungal Agent	Antibiotic	Other Ingredients
Polysporin Aerosol (Burroughs Wellcome)			polymyxin B sulfate, 200,000 units/90 g zinc bacitracin, 10,000 units/90 g	
Polysporin Ointment & Powder (Burroughs Wellcome)			polymyxin B sulfate, 10,000 units/g bacitracin zinc, 500 units/g	white petrolatum
Povadyne (Acme/Chaston)	povidone-iodine			
Poviderm Ointment & Solution (Vortech)	povidone-iodine, 10% (ointment) 7.5% (solution)			
Povidone-Iodine (Various manufacturers)	povidone-iodine, 10%			
Prophyllin (Rystan)		sodium propionate, 1% (solution) 5% (ointment)		chlorophyll, 0.0025% (solution) 0.0125% (ointment)
Quinsana Plus (Mennen)		undecylenic acid, 2% zinc undecylenate, 20%		
Sal-Dex (Scrip)	isopropyl alcohol, 40%	undecylenic acid, 10% salicylic acid, 15%		propylene glycol
Salicylic Acid Soap (Stiefel)		salicylic acid, 3.5%		
Salicylic Acid and Sulfur Soap (Stiefel)		salicylic acid, 3% sulfur, 10%		
Sea Breeze (Clairol)				alcohol, 48% peppermint oil clove oil eucalyptus oil eugenol camphor
Sea Breeze Extra Strength (Clairol)				alcohol, 60% peppermint oil clove oil eucalyptus oil eugenol camphor
Septa (Circle)			polymyxin B sulfate, 5000 units/g bacitracin, 400 units/g neomycin base, 3.5 mg/g	
S.T. 37 (SmithKline Beecham)	hexylresorcinol, 0.1%			glycerin
Terramycin Ointment with Polymyxin B Sulfate (Leeming)			oxytetracycline hydrochloride, 33.4 mg/g polymyxin B sulfate, 10,000 units/g	

TOPICAL ANTI-INFECTIVE PRODUCT TABLE, continued

Product (Manufacturer)	Antiseptic	Antifungal Agent	Antibiotic	Other Ingredients
Thimerosal (Various manufacturers)	thimerosal, 1:1000			alcohol, 50%
Tinactin (Schering)		tolnaftate, 1%		
Ting Cream (Fisons)		tolnaftate, 1%		
Ting Powder (Fisons)		tolnaftate, 1%		cornstarch talc
Ting Spray Liquid (Fisons)		tolnaftate, 1%		alcohol, 41%
Ting Spray Powder (Fisons)		tolnaftate, 1%		alcohol, 14% talc
Torofor (Torch)		iodochlorhydroxy- quin, 3%		
Trimycin (Halsey)			polymyxin B sulfate, 5000 units/g bacitracin, 400 units/g neomycin base, 3.5 mg/g	diperodon hydro- chloride, 10 mg/g
Triple Antibiotic (Various manufacturers)			polymyxin B sulfate, 5000 units/g bacitracin, 400 units/g neomycin base, 3.5 mg/g	
Triple Antibiotic DP (Rugby)			polymyxin B sulfate, 5000 units/g bacitracin, 400 units/g neomycin base, 3.5 mg/g	diperodon hydro- chloride, 10 mg/g
Triple Antibiotic Ointment (Vortech)			polymyxin B sulfate, 5000 units/g bacitracin, 400 units/g neomycin sulfate, 5 mg/g	
Undecylenic Acid Compound (Various manufacturers)		undecylenic acid, 5% zinc undecylenate, 20%		
Undoguent (Torch)		undecylenic acid, 5% zinc undecylenate, 20%		
Vaseline First Aid Carbolated Petro- latum Jelly (Chesebrough Ponds)	chloroxylenol, 0.5%			petroleum
Vioform Cream and Ointment (Ciba)		iodochlorhydroxy- quin, 3%		
Whitfield's (Various manufacturers)		benzoic acid, 6% salicylic acid, 3%		
Whitsphill (Full Strength) (Torch)		benzoic acid, 12% salicylic acid, 6%		

TOPICAL ANTI-INFECTIVE PRODUCT TABLE, continued

Product (Manufacturer)	Antiseptic	Antifungal Agent	Antibiotic	Other Ingredients
Zeasorb-AF Powder (Stiefel)		tolnaftate, 1%		talc
Zephiran Chloride Solution and Spray (Winthrop)	benzalkonium chloride, 0.13%			
Zephiran Towelettes (Winthrop)	benzalkonium chloride chlorothymol			alcohol, 20% perfume

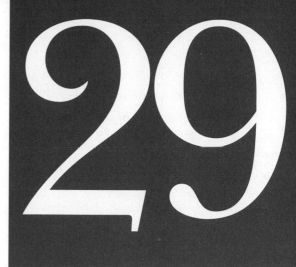

ACNE PRODUCTS

Joye Ann Billow

Questions to ask in patient/consumer counseling

How long have you had acne?

Are the blemishes whiteheads and blackheads? Are there also swollen lumps under the skin? Are the blemishes painful?

Does the problem seem to be only in areas where your clothes rub (e.g., hats, headgear, shoulder pads, etc.)?

Have you recently been in a hot and humid environment?

Does the sunlight in summer help to clear the acne?

What type of cosmetics, including aftershave lotions, do you use?

Are you exposed to oils in the atmosphere (e.g., cooking oils)?

Do you use any hair oils or creams? How often do you shampoo your hair?

Are you currently using any prescription or nonprescription medications? If so, what are they?

Have you already tried any medications, scrubs, diets, or other treatments? How effective were they?

Have you been to a physician for treatment of this condition? How long ago? What treatment did the physician suggest? How long did you follow the treatment?

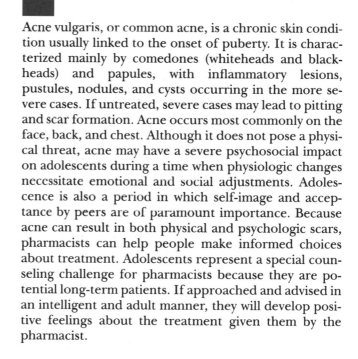

Acne vulgaris, or common acne, is a chronic skin condition usually linked to the onset of puberty. It is characterized mainly by comedones (whiteheads and blackheads) and papules, with inflammatory lesions, pustules, nodules, and cysts occurring in the more severe cases. If untreated, severe cases may lead to pitting and scar formation. Acne occurs most commonly on the face, back, and chest. Although it does not pose a physical threat, acne may have a severe psychosocial impact on adolescents during a time when physiologic changes necessitate emotional and social adjustments. Adolescence is also a period in which self-image and acceptance by peers are of paramount importance. Because acne can result in both physical and psychologic scars, pharmacists can help people make informed choices about treatment. Adolescents represent a special counseling challenge for pharmacists because they are potential long-term patients. If approached and advised in an intelligent and adult manner, they will develop positive feelings about the treatment given them by the pharmacist.

INCIDENCE

The incidence of acne in adolescents is nearly universal. In one study of 1,555 young people 8–18 years of age, all had recognizable acne at the ages of maximal incidence—14 years for females and 16 years for males (1). Moreover, 50% of the girls and 78% of the boys had acne severe enough to be termed clinical.

Acne may also occur in prepubertal children and in older persons. Subclinical lesions were noted in about one-third of the 8- and 9-year-olds. In females acne may not occur until the 20s or 30s, may be milder than that of males, and may be exacerbated by cosmetics (acne cosmetica).

ETIOLOGY

Acne vulgaris has its origin in the pilosebaceous units in the dermis (Figure 1). These units, consisting of a hair follicle and the associated sebaceous glands, are connected to the skin surface by a duct (the infundibulum) through which the hair shaft passes. The sebaceous glands produce sebum, a mixture of fats and waxes. The sebum passes to the skin surface through the infundibulum and then spreads over the skin to retard water loss and maintain hydration of skin and hair. Because the sebaceous glands are most common on the face, back, and chest, acne tends to occur most often in these areas. (See Chapter 28, *Topical Anti-infective Products*.)

At puberty, the production of androgenic hormones increases in both sexes. The increasing influx of circulatory testosterone is taken up by the sebaceous gland and converted by the enzyme 5-alpha-reductase to dihydrotestosterone, which is considered to be the tissue androgen responsible for acne. The sebaceous glands, under the influence of increased androgen levels, increase in size and activity, producing larger amounts of sebum. At the same time, keratinization of the follicular walls increases and causes mechanical blockage of the sebum flow, resulting in dilation of the follicle and entrapment of sebum and cellular debris. This lesion is a microcomedo, the initial pathologic lesion (Figure 2).

Although androgens are the major stimulus to sebaceous gland development and sebum secretion, patients with acne do not necessarily have abnormal androgen levels. It is theorized that acne-prone patients have increased end-organ sensitivity to normal levels of androgens, facilitating the hypertrophic changes (2, 3).

The epithelial tissue, an extension of the surface epidermis, forms the lining of the infundibulum and becomes thinner as it extends into the deeper portions of the duct. Normally, the epithelial tissue continually sheds cells that are carried to the skin surface by the flow of sebum. However, in acne, the shed epithelial cells are more distinct and durable, and they stick together to form a coherent horny layer that blocks the follicular channel (4). This impaction plugs and distends the follicle to form a microcomedo (Figure 2).

As more cells and sebum are added, the microcomedo enlarges and becomes visible (white-

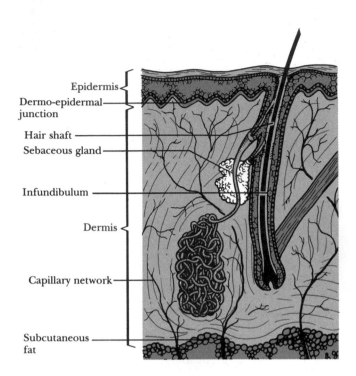

FIGURE 1   Normal pilosebaceous unit.

head); it is called a closed comedo (its contents do not reach the surface of the skin) (Figure 2). Two processes may follow, one leading to noninflammatory acne and the other to inflammatory acne. Most patients have a combination of noninflammatory and inflammatory acne.

If the plug enlarges and protrudes from the orifice of the follicular canal, it is called an open comedo (its contents open to the surface) (Figure 2). Acne characterized by the presence of closed and open comedones is called noninflammatory acne. (See *Plate 6–24*.) The tip of the plug may darken (blackhead) because of melanin produced by the epithelial cells lining the infundibulum (not dirt or oxidized fat) (5). Open comedones may be carefully expressed with a cleaned comedo extractor. Care should be taken to avoid dirty fingers or dirty extractors, both possible sources of infection.

Inflammatory acne is characterized by inflammation around the comedo, which can rupture to form a papule (Figure 2). Papules are inflammatory lesions appearing as raised, reddened areas on the skin. These lesions may enlarge to form pustules, which are inflammatory lesions also appearing as raised, reddened areas but filled with pus. The pustules may rupture

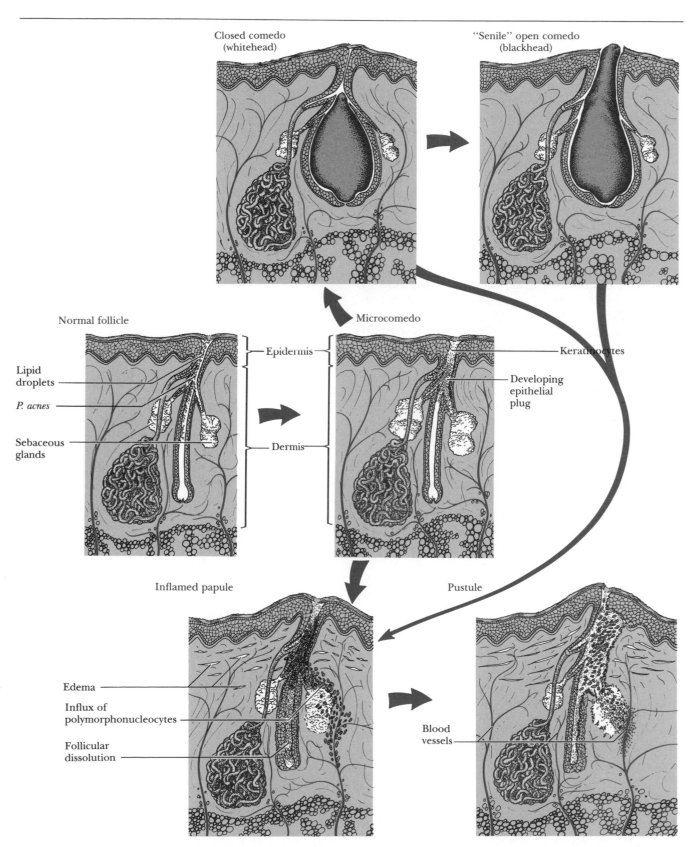

Closed comedo
(whitehead)

"Senile" open comedo
(blackhead)

Normal follicle

Microcomedo

Epidermis

Keratinocytes

Lipid
droplets

P. acnes

Sebaceous
glands

Dermis

Developing
epithelial
plug

Inflamed papule

Pustule

Edema

Influx of
polymorphonucleocytes

Follicular
dissolution

Blood
vessels

FIGURE 2   Pathogenesis of acne. Adapted with permission from J. E. Fulton and S. Bradley, *Cutis, 17,* 560 (1976).

spontaneously. More extensive penetration into surrounding tissue produces nodulocystic lesions.

Inflammatory acne typically begins with closed comedones. As the microcomedo develops, it distends the follicle so that the cellular lining of the walls is spread and thinned. At this stage, primary inflammation of the follicle wall may develop, with disruption of the epithelial lining and lymphocyte infiltration into and around the follicular wall (6).

However, if the follicle wall ruptures or is ruptured by picking or squeezing, and the contents are discharged into the surrounding tissue, a more severe inflammatory reaction results. The epithelial cells, the sebum, and any microorganisms present represent foreign substances capable of eliciting an inflammatory reaction. The results may be abscesses, which, in the process of healing, may cause scars or pits.

Current theories explaining the development of inflammatory acne suggest that the initial inflammation of the follicle wall results from the presence of free fatty acids derived from the sebum (6). In the presence of bacterial lipolytic enzymes, triglycerides in the sebum are split, releasing the fatty acids. The normal bacterial flora in the sebaceous duct produce the enzymes responsible for splitting the triglycerides.

The main microorganisms found in the sebaceous duct are an anaerobic rod, *Propionibacterium acnes* (*Corynebacterium acnes*), and one or two species of *Staphylococcus*. These organisms are the predominant flora that normally inhabit the skin. They are not considered to be pathogens and die rapidly if the follicle wall is ruptured and they are released into the surrounding tissues. *P. acnes* generally is regarded as the source of the lipolytic enzymes responsible for free fatty acid formation in the sebum. The effectiveness of oral tetracycline and topical antibiotics in treating inflammatory acne is due to their ability to suppress the normal bacterial population of the sebaceous duct, thus reducing free fatty acid concentrations (7).

The hair in the follicle may play an important role in comedo development. If the hair shaft is thin and small, it may not be able to maintain an open channel and then becomes entrapped in the plug. The heavier hair of the scalp and beard typically pushes the developing plug to the surface, thus preventing comedo formation. In adult life, acne may disappear spontaneously. This may be because the cells lining the follicles become less susceptible to comedogenic materials (5).

The presence of pustules or cysts indicates inflammatory acne, which is more likely to cause permanent scarring than noninflammatory acne. (See *Plate 6–25*.) Picking or squeezing inflamed follicles or attempting to express closed comedones may produce inflammatory lesions by rupturing the follicle walls. Inflammatory acne should be treated by a physician. Treatment requires prescribed medication, such as tretinoin and isotretinoin, and possibly excision and drainage of inflammatory lesions.

CLASSIFICATION

Although a number of studies considered by the Food and Drug Administration (FDA) advisory review panel classify improvement in terms of total lesions, a more convenient grading scale for comedonal and papulopustular acne is based on the number of lesions on one side of the face (Table 1). The scale ranges from least severe (Grade I) to most severe (Grade IV).

PREDISPOSING FACTORS

Many women with acne experience a premenstrual flare-up of symptoms. (See Chapter 7, *Menstrual Products*.) The flare-up cannot be explained on the basis of hormone levels alone, although the change in the progesterone level has been implicated. Changes in sebaceous activity have been claimed to be responsible. It also has been suggested that the premenstrual flare-up, seen in 60–70% of women with acne, is caused by a reduction in the size of the orifice of the pilosebaceous duct, resulting in obstruction (8). A corollary to these findings is that oral contraceptives with high androgenic activity also have been implicated in the production of acne.

Hydration also decreases the size of the pilosebaceous duct orifice, a change that is reversible (9). This reduction explains the exacerbation of acne in conditions of high humidity or in situations where frequent and prolonged sweating occurs.

Local irritation or friction may increase the incidence of acne symptoms. Rough or occlusive clothing, headgear straps, and pieces of equipment used in athletics often aggravate acne. Resting the chin or cheek on the hand frequently or for long periods creates localized conditions conducive to lesion formation in acne-prone individuals.

Acne cosmetica is a low-grade form of acne on the face, cheek, and chin. The lesions of acne cosmetica typically are closed, noninflammatory comedones and cannot be distinguished from similar lesions of acne vulgaris. In some instances, an inflammatory lesion is seen. This form of acne was found in about one-third of adult women who were examined, but not in adult men (10). Furthermore, half of the cosmetic cream bases

TABLE 1	Grading scale for comedonal and papulopustular acne based on number of lesions on one side of the face	
Grade	Comedonal lesions	Papulopustular lesions
I	10	10
II	10–25	10–20
III	25–50	20–30
IV	>50	>30

Adapted from G. Plewig and A. M. Kligman, "Acne: Morphogenesis and Treatment," Springer-Verlag, New York, N.Y., 1975.

GOALS OF TREATMENT

Acne is rarely cured, but it can be controlled. In most cases, available therapeutic regimens and patient compliance will reduce symptoms and minimize permanent scarring. Because acne persists for long periods, frequently from adolescence to the early 20s or beyond, treatment must be long-term and consistent. Remission or reduction in severity of lesions may occur, but treatment should be resumed when necessary.

Acne treatment includes the following objectives:

- Relieving discomfort;

- Removing excess sebum from the skin with proper cleansing;

- Preventing closure of the pilosebaceous orifice;

- Using irritants to unblock ducts;

- Minimizing conditions conducive to acne, such as the presence of physical irritants and the use of oil-based cleansers and cosmetics;

- Educating the individual in the proper use of and patience with the treatment regimen.

used by these women were comedogenic in rabbit ear tests and on the skin of human volunteers. However, the condition responded readily to topical treatment with tretinoin.

Pomade acne, commonly seen in blacks and manifested by comedones along the hairline on the forehead and temples, was reported to be caused directly by the long-term use of hair dressings that contain petrolatum or liquid petrolatum (11).

Exogenous sources of corticosteroids, both systemic and topical (prescription and nonprescription), may also induce hypertrophic changes by sensitizing the follicle and producing "steroid acne." These lesions are characterized by uniform red papules succeeded by closed comedones and, finally, open comedones (2).

Other drugs known to precipitate acne eruptions include androgens, bromides, ethionamide, haloperidol, halothane, iodides, isoniazid, lithium, phenytoin, and trimethadione. Cobalt irradiation and hyperalimentation therapy also have been implicated (2, 12).

Little is known to support a direct relationship between diet and acne (13). Although several studies demonstrated that chocolate does not affect acne (14), some clinicians remain unconvinced and suggest that it be removed from the diet. Other clinicians feel that dietary restrictions for individuals with acne are unwarranted because no convincing evidence has been presented to implicate nuts, fats, colas, or carbohydrates. However, an indirect relationship between acne and a diet high in fat and refined carbohydrates and low in fiber has been proposed, suggesting that dietary habits may be a risk factor in acne as well as more serious illnesses (15).

Controlling or decreasing the levels of *P. acnes*, suppressing or altering hormonal activity, correcting disfiguring effects, and using the newer approaches for treating acne must be directed by a physician (16). However, pharmacists play a very effective role in all aspects of acne treatment.

The starting point in the treatment of acne is the practice of proper skin hygiene to remove excess sebum. The preferred method of removing excess sebum from the skin is a conscientious program of daily washing. The affected areas should be thoroughly washed at least twice daily with warm water, soap, and a soft washcloth and then patted dry. More frequent washing is appropriate if the skin is oily. Scrubbing should not be vigorous because it may worsen acne and cause "acne mechanica." The purpose of washing is to produce a mild drying of the skin and, perhaps, mild erythema (17). Washing should cause barely visible peeling that can loosen comedones. If washing produces a feeling of tautness in the skin, the intensity and frequency of washings should be reduced. Switching to a less drying soap should also be considered.

Ordinary facial soaps that do not contain moisturizing oils are usually satisfactory. Soaps containing antibacterial agents have been suggested for controlling acne, but no conclusive evidence has been presented to indicate their value. Although sulfur, salicylic acid, and sulfur–resorcinol combinations have been accorded status as Category I agents by the review panel, their benefit as ingredients in soaps is questionable because little, if any, residue is left on the skin after thorough washing (18).

Soap substitutes containing surfactants (ionic or nonionic) have been suggested for acne because they are less drying to the skin. However, because a mild degree of drying is desirable, an ordinary facial soap should be tried first. Some cleansing preparations contain pumice, polyethylene, or aluminum oxide particles to add abrasive action to the cleansing effect. Buf-Puf is a polyester cleansing sponge that assists in the removal of the outer layer of dead skin cells by gentle abrasion. Used gently, these agents may be helpful in noninflammatory acne. Abrasives should be avoided in inflammatory acne because of increased irritation. If it is inconvenient to wash during the day, a cleansing pad that contains alcohol, acetone, and a surfactant may be used.

Because acne treatment begins with removing excess sebum from the skin, topically applied products such as cosmetics and hair dressings should be water based, rather than oil based. Frequent hair shampooing should be encouraged because acne usually is accompanied by an oily scalp.

TOPICAL NONPRESCRIPTION PRODUCTS

Benzoyl Peroxide

Benzoyl peroxide is one of the most effective topical nonprescription medications available for acne (19). Benzoyl peroxide possibly acts in several ways. It causes irritation and desquamation, which prevents closure of the pilosebaceous orifice. The irritant effect causes an increased turnover rate of the epithelial cells lining the follicular duct, which increases sloughing (17). This increase results in a looser structure of the follicular plug and promotes resolution of the comedones (20). The oxidizing potential of benzoyl peroxide may contribute to bacteriostatic and bacteriocidal activity, suppressing the local population of *P. acnes* and reducing free fatty

acids. Benzoyl peroxide also exhibits irritant, drying, peeling, and comedolytic effects.

Benzoyl peroxide is available in concentrations of 2.5%, 5%, and 10% and is formulated as a lotion, gel, or cream. It is also available in 5% and 10% concentrations as liquid and bar cleansers and is found in many combination products. The irritant properties of the various concentrations and formulations are not equivalent. For example, the drying effect of the alcohol gel base can enhance its effectiveness; therefore, it is superior to a lotion of the same concentration. Some products, mainly the gels, are available by prescription only, which ensures physician supervision.

Patient instructions for use of topical nonprescription benzoyl peroxide suggest that the affected area be gently cleansed with a nonmedicated soap and then dried before the product is applied. A small quantity of the preparation should be smoothed over affected areas once or twice daily. Because some individuals are sensitive to benzoyl peroxide, the initial applications may be limited to one or two small areas to determine whether discomfort or reaction will occur. Fair-skinned individuals should initiate therapy with the 5% strength and apply it only once daily during the first few weeks of therapy. Pharmacists should warn patients that benzoyl peroxide:

- Should not be used around the eyes, mouth, lips, and inside of nose;

- Should not be used concurrently with other topical products;

- Is for external use only;

- May cause stinging and burning;

- May bleach clothing.

If excessive stinging and burning occur after application, the preparation should be removed with soap and water and not reapplied until the next day. Other sources of irritation, such as sunlamps and excessive exposure to the sun, should be avoided. Most people tolerate benzoyl peroxide lotions, but about 1–3% are hypersensitive to the ingredient.

Sulfur

Sulfur generally is used in the precipitated or colloidal form at 2–10% concentrations. The higher concentrations produce a more intense effect. Other forms of sulfur such as zinc sulfide and sodium thiosulfate are milder. Although sulfur helps resolve comedones, evidence suggests that it may also promote the development of new ones (21). Sulfur (but not thiosulfate or sulfide) was found to be comedogenic in rabbit ear tests and, on long exposure, on the backs of human subjects (21), although other evidence refutes this observation (22). Sulfur has met the criteria of the FDA review panel for topical over-the-counter (OTC) antibacterial acne products. It is generally accepted as being an effective agent for promoting the resolution of acne lesions. Sulfur lotions are applied in a thin film to the affected area once or twice daily. However, they have a noticeable color and odor, characteristics the pharmacist must consider when recommending their selection and use.

Salicylic Acid

Salicylic acid is available in nonprescription acne products in concentrations of 0.5–2%. Its pharmacologic action is dependent on the concentration: deep keratolytic (sloughing) action at concentrations greater than 5%, a surface keratolytic action at 1–4%, and an acidifying effect at 0.1% and greater. The keratolytic effect and possible enhanced absorption of other agents provide the rationale for the topical use of salicylic acid (18); however, its safety is questionable when it is used over large areas for prolonged periods of time.

Resorcinol

Although resorcinol is not regarded as efficacious in the treatment of acne, it is still offered for that purpose in concentrations of 1–2%. Resorcinol may produce a dark brown scale on some darker skinned individuals, who should be forewarned (22). The reaction is reversible when the medication is discontinued. There is some question as to whether resorcinol absorption may precipitate systemic toxicity. It is advisable to caution patients to apply resorcinol-containing products only to affected areas and not over extensive areas of the body.

Combination Products

Assorted nonprescription combinations of benzoyl peroxide, sulfur, salicylic acid, and resorcinol are available to treat acne. The efficacy of these combinations over the single ingredient products has not been clearly demonstrated; concomitant use of multiple irritants is generally not recommended.

TOPICAL PRESCRIPTION PRODUCTS

Tretinoin

Tretinoin (vitamin A acid or retinoic acid) is a topical medication proven effective in treating acne. It is available as a cream and a liquid in a concentration of 0.05%. A lower concentration gel (0.025%) is also available and may reduce the irritation associated with tretinoin use. Tretinoin, which acts as an irritant to increase epithelial cell proliferation and ultimately reduce comedo formation, apparently is more irritating than benzoyl peroxide, particularly in the early stages of treatment (23). Tretinoin not only changes follicular keratinization but also decreases the number of normal cell layers of the stratum corneum from 14 to 5. This decreased depth of the barrier layer may allow other topical agents to penetrate the skin more readily. Tretinoin should be reserved for use in moderate to severe acne after treatment with milder agents such as benzoyl peroxide has proven unsuccessful. It may be used alone for comedonal acne; as an adjunct for inflammatory papulopustular acne; or as an adjunct for acne secondary to steroids, ionizing radiation, tars, and chlorinated hydrocarbons.

Individuals using tretinoin for the first time should be cautioned that the skin will become red and peel, usually within a week of initiating therapy. This condition will last approximately 3 or 4 weeks. An exacerbation of the acne can be expected to occur during the initial 4–6 weeks. Severe irritation may require alternate day therapy. Patients should be reassured that this exacerbation is temporary and that 3 months of therapy may be required for clearing of comedones. Inflammatory lesions generally improve more rapidly. Eight to 12 weeks are required before the effectiveness of therapy can be assessed. Also, because the drug can increase susceptibility to sunburn, prolonged or excessive exposure to the sun should be avoided. An effective sunscreen should be used if exposure cannot be avoided. (See Chapter 34, *Sunscreen and Suntan Products*.)

Antibiotics

Acne is not an infection. The inflammation found in some cases is the result of a foreign body reaction to follicular contents. The microorganisms involved are the nonpathogenic normal flora found deep within the follicles and out of the reach of the usual antibacterial agents applied to the skin surface. Therefore, most topically applied antibacterial agents have not been of value in treating acne.

An exception is the use of fat-soluble derivatives of erythromycin, tetracycline, meclocycline, and clindamycin (24, 25). These derivatives are applied either as dilute solutions in organic solvents or as creams. Their effectiveness is due to their ability to diffuse through the fatty contents of the sebaceous follicle to reach the *P. acnes* in the lower segments of the follicle. They suppress the activity of these organisms, which reduces the production of comedogenic free fatty acids from the sebum.

Metronidazole

Metronidazole in a 0.75% gel formulation is approved for the treatment of adult acne (acne rosacea). The mechanism of action is unknown but may be due to antibacterial or anti-inflammatory action (26).

SYSTEMIC TREATMENT

Antibiotics

Oral tetracycline, erythromycin, minocycline, and clindamycin are effective in treating inflammatory acne. These drugs suppress the growth of normal cutaneous flora (*P. acnes*), which decreases formation of free fatty acids and consequently decreases inflammation.

Oral antibiotic therapy may produce some adverse effects; however, these are usually minor. Gastrointestinal upset is the most common problem. Candidiasis may occur in young females. Less common is the occurrence of a Gram-negative folliculitis caused by species of *Klebsiella* or *Proteus*.

An ad hoc study committee of the American Academy of Dermatology recognized oral tetracycline as a rational, effective, and relatively safe drug for use with inflammatory acne (27). Tetracycline is the drug of choice because it is the least costly and exhibits the fewest side effects. It is effective in low doses because high concentrations are achieved in the sebaceous follicle. However, tetracycline is not effective for the resolution of noninflammatory comedones.

Pseudomembranous colitis, secondary to treatment with clindamycin, has been reported; however, the connection has not been confirmed in more recent studies (28).

It is recommended that once clearing is achieved with oral antibiotic therapy, maintenance therapy with topical agents may be sufficient.

Isotretinoin

Isotretinoin (13-*cis*-retinoic acid) is an oral medication that effectively treats severe nodulocystic acne that is resistant to other forms of therapy. The precise mechanism of action has not been elucidated; however, effects observed include inhibition of sebum production and follicular keratinization with a consequent reduction in the concentration of *P. acnes* on the skin surface. A temporary exacerbation of the condition may be noted when therapy is initiated, but resolution occurs with continued therapy. Prolonged remission may persist following the course of therapy.

Adverse reactions include mucocutaneous effects that are frequently experienced during therapy, for example, cheilitis (inflammation of the lips). These effects occur in over 90% of the patients treated with this drug. Affected persons may obtain relief with the use of lip balms.

Because isotretinoin appears to share many of the toxicities observed with other retinoids, the patient treated with isotretinoin should be advised not to use vitamin A or other retinoids concurrently (29).

A significant portion of the patient population likely to use isotretinoin for acne treatment consists of females of reproductive age. Retrospective studies clearly indicate a link between use of isotretinoin early in pregnancy and a high risk of either spontaneous abortion or congenital malformations (30). Recognizing the hazards associated with isotretinoin, the manufacturer has developed an extensive program to prevent the use of the drug during pregnancy. Materials provided include patient brochures and a consent form for use by the prescribing physician. When dispensing isotretinoin, the pharmacist should make a special effort to ensure that female patients understand the dangers of becoming pregnant while taking the drug.

Zinc Sulfate

The treatment of acne with oral zinc sulfate has been suggested by work reported in Sweden (31). Other studies, however, have not noted any significant differences between patients given zinc or placebo (32, 33).

Estrogen Therapy

Very severe or otherwise unresponsive cases of acne in young women may be treated by estrogen therapy. The effectiveness of estrogen in this case is due to its inhibition of androgens at the adrenal gland. Oral contraceptives with high estrogenic and low androgenic activities are the most common sources of estrogens for this purpose.

Therapies under Investigation

The combination of oral ibuprofen, a nonsteroidal anti-inflammatory agent, and tetracycline for the treatment of acne vulgaris is under investigation (34). Ketaconazole, an antifungal agent that inhibits testosterone synthesis, is being investigated as a treatment for acne in women (35).

OTHER TREATMENTS

Ultraviolet Radiation

Exposure to sunlight often is beneficial in acne; consequently, improvement is often noted during the summer. The improvement is believed to result from the irritant properties of the ultraviolet wavelengths of sunlight (UV-B, 290–320 nm), which stimulate increased proliferation of the epithelium. (See Chapter 33, *Burn and Sunburn Products*, and Chapter 34, *Sunscreen and Suntan Products*.) Ultraviolet lamps produce the same effect, but they generally are not recommended because of the difficulty in determining and regulating the amount of limited exposure necessary to produce the required mild erythema. If a sunlamp is used, care must be taken to protect the eyes from the light's damaging effect. It also may be wise to time the exposure to avoid the danger of falling asleep under the lamp. In general, the use of artificial ultraviolet radiation should be avoided, especially in persons being treated with tetracyclines or retinoid derivatives.

Cosmetic Repair

Some patients who have severe scarring and pitting as the result of acne may seek cosmetic repair. The initial approach was dermabrasion. Intralesional injection of corticosteroids or bovine collagen has been used (36). Silicone implants are being investigated (37). None of these processes seem to be entirely satisfactory, and they can be costly.

FORMULATION CONSIDERATIONS

The formulation carrying topical acne medication to the skin can influence the drug's effectiveness. Therefore, the pharmacist should pay particular attention to this aspect of product selection when advising a patient.

Suspensions, lotions, creams, and gels are the vehicles generally used for antiacne preparations. Lotions and creams should have a low fat content so that they do not counteract drying and peeling. Nonfatty gels dry slowly if formulated in a completely aqueous base. Ethyl or isopropyl alcohol added to liquid preparations and gels hastens their drying to a film. Use of the volatile solvents may enhance the effectiveness of the preparation because of the drying effect, but that effect may be cosmetically unacceptable to the patient. (See Chapter 28, *Topical Anti-infective Products*.)

Thickening agents in preparations should not dry to a sticky film. The solids in most preparations leave a film that is not noticeably visible and does not need coloring to blend with the skin. However, some products are intended to hide blemishes by depositing an opaque film of insoluble masking agents such as zinc oxide on the skin. These products are tinted to improve their cosmetic effect.

A general guideline might be to recommend cream formulations for patients with fair complexions and gels for those with dark complexions.

COUNSELING GUIDELINES

A variety of therapeutic approaches may be used to treat acne. Familiarity with these approaches will help the pharmacist in advising individuals whether to self-medicate or consult a physician. One study found that only 10 to 11% of the subject group of high school students sought medical help for acne, but about 60% were self-medicating (38). The size of the self-medicating group emphasizes the opportunity for pharmacist counseling.

Before offering advice, the pharmacist should examine the patient's medication history, including previous measures taken to control the acne; which medications were used, when, and for how long; and the degree of success and personal acceptance of the preparations tried. Subjective data on a patient's attitude toward treatment and willingness to actively participate in a skin care program involving a continued daily regimen of washing affected areas and applying medication should be determined.

The pharmacist should clearly explain the basis for the recommendation given the patient: Comedonal and mild papular acne can usually be successfully self-medicated, whereas moderately severe papular acne and pustular and cystic acne require the attention of a physician.

Once the decision to self-medicate or consult a physician has been made, the pharmacist should clearly explain the treatment program and acne process and correct any misconceptions. The pharmacist should advise the patient about scalp and hair care, the use of cosmetics, and, above all, the need for long-term, conscientious care. Positive moral support often is necessary to reduce patient concern.

Acne patients should be aware of the following:

- Picking at or squeezing comedones increases the likelihood of infection, inflammation, and scarring.

- The skin should be kept clean, but scrubbing may exacerbate the condition.

- Only water-based makeup and cosmetics should be used.

- Moisturizers should be noncomedogenic.

- Diet plays an important role in maintaining health; however, some of the old "folklore" dietary restrictions are not necessary.

- Stressful situations may play a role in acute flare-ups of acne, but do not cause acne.

- Sexual activity plays no role in the occurrence or worsening of acne.

- Treatment only controls acne; it does not cure it and must continue even after acute flare-ups have cleared.

SUMMARY

Acne vulgaris occurs almost universally in young adults from their early teens to middle 20s and occasionally appears in prepubertal and older people. Generally, acne cannot be cured, but it may be controlled to improve appearance and to prevent the development of severe acne with its resultant scarring. With empathy and reassurance, acne patients may understand that the condition is not irreparable and that care must be given to the affected areas for a long time for improvement to occur.

REFERENCES

1 J. L. Burton et al., *Br. J. Dermatol.*, *85*, 119 (1971).

2 "Manual of Dermatologic Therapeutics with Essentials of Diagnosis," 2nd ed., K. A. Arndt, Ed., Little, Brown and Co., Boston, Mass., 1978, pp. 3–15.

3 M. A. Quan et al., *J. Fam. Pract.*, *11*, 1041 (1980).

4 A. M. Kligman, *J. Invest. Dermatol.*, *62*, 268 (1974).

5 D. Blair and C. A. Lewis, *Br. J. Dermatol.*, *82*, 572 (1970).

6 R. K. Frienkel, *N. Engl. J. Med.*, *280*, 1161 (1969).

7 R. K. Frienkel et al., *N. Engl. J. Med.*, *273*, 850 (1965).

8 W. J. Cunliffe and M. Williams, *Lancet*, *2*, 1055 (1973).

9 M. Williams et al., *Br. J. Dermatol.*, *90*, 631 (1974).

10 A. M. Kligman and O. H. Mills, *Arch. Dermatol.*, *106*, 843 (1972).

11 G. Plewig et al., *Arch. Dermatol.*, *101*, 580 (1970).

12 L. E. Cluff et al., "Clinical Problems with Drugs," Vol. 86, W. B. Saunders, Philadelphia, Pa., 1975.

13 J. E. Rasmussen, *Int. J. Dermatol.*, *16*, 488 (1977).

14 J. E. Fulton et al., *J. Am. Med. Assoc.*, *210*, 2071 (1969).

15 E. W. Rosenberg and B. S. Kirk, *Arch. Dermatol.*, *117*, 193 (1981).

16 S. B. Frank, "Acne Vulgaris," Charles C. Thomas, Springfield, Ill., 1971, p. 175.

17 R. M. Reisner, *Pediatr. Clin. N. Am.*, *20*, 851 (1973).

18 *Federal Register*, *50 (10)*, 2172–82 (1985).

19 J. Fulton et al., *J. Cutan. Pathol.*, *1*, 191 (1974).

20 P. Vasarenish, *Arch. Dermatol.*, *98*, 183 (1968).

21 O. H. Mills and A. M. Kligman, *Br. J. Dermatol.*, *86*, 620 (1972).

22 J. S. Strauss et al., *Arch. Dermatol.*, *114*, 1340 (1978).

23 B. S. Belnap, *Cutis*, *23*, 856 (1979).

24 J. E. Fulton, *Arch. Dermatol.*, *110*, 83 (1974).

25 S. B. Frank, *Postgrad. Med.*, *61*, 92 (1977).

26 *Am. Pharm.*, *NS29*, 425 (1989).

27 Ad Hoc Committee on the Use of Antibiotics in Dermatology, *Arch. Dermatol.*, *111*, 1630 (1975).

28 P. Dantzig, *Arch. Dermatol.*, *112*, 53 (1976).

29 "American Hospital Formulary Service—Drug Information 85," G. K. McEvoy, Ed., published by authority of the Board of Directors of the American Society of Hospital Pharmacists, Bethesda, Md., 1985, pp. 1648–1652.

30 P. M. Fernhoff and E. J. Lammer, *J. Pediatr.*, *105*, 595 (1984).

31 G. Michaelsson et al., *Arch. Dermatol.*, *113*, 31 (1977).

32 I. Orris et al., *Arch. Dermatol.*, *114*, 1018 (1978).

33 V. M. Weimar et al., *Arch. Dermatol.*, *114*, 1776 (1978).

34 R. C. Wong et al., *J. Am. Acad. Dermatol.*, *11*, 1076 (1984).

35 P. Ghetti et al., *Arch. Dermatol.*, *122*, 629 (1986).

36 R. L. Cahn, *Postgrad. Med.*, *67*, 129 (1980).

37 N. G. Popovich, *Pharm. Internat.*, *7*, 71 (1986).

38 R. J. Schachter et al., *N.Y. State J. Med.*, *71*, 2886 (1971).

ACNE PRODUCT TABLE

Product (Manufacturer)	Application Form	Benzoyl Peroxide	Sulfur	Resorcinol/ Salicylic Acid	Other Ingredients
Acne-Aid (Stiefel)	cream	10%			
Acne-Aid Cleansing Bar (Stiefel)	bar				surfactant blend, 6.3%
Acnederm (Lannett)	lotion		5%		zinc sulfate, 1% zinc oxide, 10% isopropyl alcohol, 21%
Acno Cleanser (Baker/Cummins)	liquid				isopropyl alcohol, 60% laureth-23 tetrasodium EDTA
Acno Lotion (Baker/Cummins)	lotion		3%		salicylic acid, 2%
Acnomel (SmithKline Beecham)	cream		8%	resorcinol, 2%	alcohol, 11% bentonite titanium dioxide
Acnophill (Torch)	ointment		5%		zinc oxide, 10% potassium, 5% zinc sulfides-polysulfides
Acnotex (C & M Pharm.)	lotion		8%	salicylic acid, 2.25%	methylbenzethonium chloride isopropyl alcohol, 22% acetone
Aveeno Cleansing Bar For Acne (Rydelle Labs)	bar			salicylic acid, 2%	colloidal oatmeal, 51% sodium cocoyl isethionate purified water glycerin lactic acid sodium lactate potassium sorbate magnesium aluminum silicate titanium dioxide PEG-14M
Ben-Aqua 5 (Syosset)	lotion	5%			
Ben-Aqua 10 (Syosset)	lotion	10%			
Benoxyl 5 (Stiefel)	lotion	5%			
Benoxyl 10 (Stiefel)	lotion	10%			
Bensulfoid (Poythress)	cream		8% (colloidal)	resorcinol, 2%	alcohol, 10% zinc oxide, 6% thymol, 0.5%
Betadine Skin Cleanser (Purdue Frederick)	cleanser				povidone-iodine, 7.5%
Brasivol (Stiefel)	abrasive cleanser (fine, medium and rough)				aluminum oxide particles in a surfactant cleansing base sodium lauryl sulfate
Brasivol Base (Stiefel)	liquid				surfactant base with neutral soaps and polyoxyethylene lauryl ether

ACNE PRODUCT TABLE, continued

Product (Manufacturer)	Application Form	Benzoyl Peroxide	Sulfur	Resorcinol/ Salicylic Acid	Other Ingredients
Buf-Bar (3M Personal Care)	bar		3%		titanium dioxide
Clear By Design (SmithKline Beecham)	gel	2.5%			carbomer 940 dioctyl sodium sulfosuccinate sodium hydroxide EDTA
	pads			salicylic acid, 1%	citric acid cocamphodiacetate dimethicone copolyol disodium laureth- sulfosuccinate fragrance SD alcohol 40B, 16% sodium carbonate
Clearasil Adult Care (Vicks)	cream stick		3% 8%	resorcinol, 2% resorcinol, NS[a]	alcohol, 10%
Clearasil Antibac- terial Bar (Vicks)	soap				triclosan, 0.75%
Clearasil Benzoyl Peroxide (Vicks)	tinted & vanishing creams lotion	10% 10%			
Clearasil Double Clear Pads (Vicks)	medicated pads			salicylic acid, 1.25% (regular strength) 2% (maximum strength)	alcohol, 40%
Clearasil Medi- cated Astringent (Vicks)	liquid			salicylic acid, 0.5%	alcohol, 43%
Cuticura (DEP Corp.)	ointment		0.5% (precipitated)		phenol, 0.1% oxyquinoline, 0.05% petrolatum mineral oil mineral wax isopropyl palmitate synthetic beeswax pine oil rose geranium oil
Cuticura Acne Cream (DEP Corp.)	cream	5%			
Del Aqua-5 (Del-Ray)	gel	5%			polyoxyethylene lauryl ether
Del Aqua-10 (Del-Ray)	gel	10%			polyoxyethylene lauryl ether
Dry and Clear (Whitehall)	cream lotion	10% 5%			
Drytex Lotion (C & M Pharm)	liquid			salicylic acid, NS[a]	acetone, 10% isopropyl alcohol, 40% polysorbate 20 methylbenzethonium chloride

ACNE PRODUCT TABLE, continued

Product (Manufacturer)	Application Form	Benzoyl Peroxide	Sulfur	Resorcinol/ Salicylic Acid	Other Ingredients
Finac Lotion (C & M Pharm)	lotion		2%		methylbenzethonium chloride isopropyl alcohol, 8%
Fostex 5% BPO (Westwood)	gel	5%			
Fostex 10% BPO (Westwood)	bar cream gel tinted cream wash	10%			
Fostex Medicated Cleansing Bar (Westwood)	bar		2%	salicylic acid, 2%	boric acid docusate sodium urea
Fostex Medicated Cover-up (Westwood)	cream		2%		
Fostril (Westwood)	lotion	2%			laureth-4 zinc oxide talc
Ionax Astringent Skin Cleanser (Owen)	liquid			salicylic acid, NS[a]	allantoin acetone polyoxyethylene ethers isopropyl alcohol, 48%
Ionax Foam (Owen)	aerosol foam				benzalkonium chloride, 0.2% polyoxyethylene ethers soapless surfactant
Ionax Scrub (Owen)	paste				benzalkonium chloride, 0.2% granular polyethylene polyoxyethylene ethers alcohol, 10%
Komed (Barnes-Hind)	lotion			salicylic acid, 2%	isopropyl alcohol, 22% sodium thiosulfate, 8% menthol camphor colloidal alumina
Komex (Barnes-Hind)	cleanser				sodium borate tetrahydrate decahydrate granules
Liquimat (Owen)	lotion		5%		alcohol, 22% tinted bases
Listerex Golden Lotion (Warner-Lambert)	cleanser			salicylic acid, 2%	polyethylene granules surface-active cleansers
Listerex Herbal Lotion (Warner-Lambert)	cleanser			salicylic acid, 2%	polyethylene granules surface-active cleansers
Loroxide (Dermik)	lotion	5.5%			tinted base
Lotio Alsulfa (Doak)	lotion		colloidal sulfur, 5%		colloidal clays, 95%
Medicated Face Conditioner (MFC) (Mennen)	liquid			salicylic acid, 1%	alcohol, 55%

ACNE PRODUCT TABLE, continued

Product (Manufacturer)	Application Form	Benzoyl Peroxide	Sulfur	Resorcinol/ Salicylic Acid	Other Ingredients
Neutrogena Acne Mask (Neutrogena Dermatologics)	oil-absorbing clay mask	5%			
Noxzema Antiseptic Skin Cleanser - Regular Strength (Noxell)	cleanser				alcohol, 63%
Noxzema Antiseptic Skin Cleanser - Extra Strength (Noxell)	cleanser				ethyl alcohol, 36% isopropyl alcohol, 34%
Noxzema Antiseptic Skin Cleanser - Sensitive Skin (Noxell)	cleanser				benzalkonium chloride, 0.13%
Noxzema Clear-Ups Acne Medicated Anti-Acne Gel (Noxell)	gel			salicylic acid, 0.5%	
Noxzema Clear-Ups Acne Medicated Maximum Strength (Noxell)	lotion	10%			
Noxzema Clear-Ups Medicated Skin Cleansing Pads - Maximum & Regular Strength (Noxell)	medicated pads			salicylic acid, 0.5% (regular) 2% (maximum)	alcohol, 63% (regular) 64% (maximum)
Noxzema On-the-Spot Treatment-Tinted & Vanishing (Noxell)	lotion	10%			
Oxy-5 (SmithKline Beecham)	lotion	5%			
Oxy-10 (SmithKline Beecham)	lotion	10%			
Oxy Clean Maximum Strength Medicated Cleanser & Pads (SmithKlineBeecham)	cleanser pads			salicylic acid, 2%	alcohol, 50% citric acid menthol sodium lauryl sulfate
Oxy Clean Medicated Cleanser & Pads (SmithKlineBeecham)	cleanser pads			salicylic acid, 0.5%	alcohol, 40% citric acid menthol sodium lauryl sulfate
Oxy Clean Medicated Soap (SmithKlineBeecham)	soap			salicylic acid, 3.5%	sodium borate
Oxy Wash (SmithKline					

ACNE PRODUCT TABLE, continued

Product (Manufacturer)	Application Form	Benzoyl Peroxide	Sulfur	Resorcinol/ Salicylic Acid	Other Ingredients
PanOxyl Bar 5 (Stiefel)	cleanser	5%			mild surfactant base
PanOxyl Bar 10 (Stiefel)	cleanser	10%			mild surfactant base
Pernox Lotion (Westwood)	lotion		2%	salicylic acid, 1.5%	surfactants polyethylene granules
Pernox Regular and Lemon (Westwood)	cleanser		2%	salicylic acid, 1.5%	surfactants polyethylene granules
pHisoAc (Winthrop)	cream		6% (colloidal)	resorcinol, 1.5%	alcohol, 10%
pHisoAc BP (Winthrop)	cream	10%			bronopol calcium sulfate dimethicone docusate sodium solution glyceryl stearate and PEG-100 stearate hydroxyethylcellulose laureth-4 light mineral oil stearamide MEA-stearate white petrolatum
Propa P.H. Liquid Acne Soap (Commerce)	liquid	10%			
Propa P.H. Medicated w/Aloe (Commerce)	cleansing pads cream stick			salicylic acid, 0.5% (pads) 2% (cream and stick)	aloe (pads and stick) bentonite (stick) alcohol, 25% (pads)
RA Lotion (Medco Labs)	lotion			resorcinol, 3%	calamine starch alcohol, 43% sodium borate bentonite
Rezamid (Dermik)	lotion		5%	resorcinol, 2%	tinted base alcohol, 28.5% chloroxylenol, 0.5%
SalAc Cleanser (GenDerm)	liquid			salicylic acid, 2%	
Salicylic Acid Soap (Stiefel)	bar			salicylic acid, 3.5%	
Salicylic Acid and Sulfur Soap (Stiefel)	bar		10% (precipitated)	salicylic acid, 3%	
Saligel Acne Gel (Stiefel)	gel			salicylic acid, 5%	hydroalcoholic gel (alcohol, 14%)
Sastid AL (Stiefel)	cleanser		1.6%	salicylic acid, 1.6%	aluminum oxide, 20% surfactants
Sastid Plain Therapeutic Shampoo and Wash (Stiefel)	cleanser		1.6%	salicylic acid, 1.6%	surfactant base
Sastid Soap (Stiefel)	cleanser		10%	salicylic acid, 3%	

ACNE PRODUCT TABLE, continued

Product (Manufacturer)	Application Form	Benzoyl Peroxide	Sulfur	Resorcinol/ Salicylic Acid	Other Ingredients
Seale's Lotion Modified (C & M Pharm)	lotion		6.4%		zinc oxide bentonite sodium borate acetone
Seba-Nil (Owen)	solution				alcohol, 49.7% polysorbate 80
Seba-Nil Cleansing Mask (Owen)	cleanser				polyethylene granules
Sebasorb (Summers)	liquid		2%	salicylic acid, 2%	attapulgite, 10% polysorbate 80
Stri-Dex Lotion (Glenbrook)	lotion			salicylic acid, 0.5%	simethicone emulsion sodium carbonate sodium dodecylbenzene sulfonate sodium xylenesulfonate fragrance citric acid alcohol, 28%
Stri-Dex Maximum Strength Medicated (Glenbrook)	medicated pads			salicylic acid, 2%	ammonium xylenesulfonate sodium dodecylbenzene sulfonate fragrance simethicone emulsion sodium carbonate citric acid alcohol, 44%
Stri-Dex Maximum Strength Treatment (Glenbrook)	cream	10%			bronopol calcium sulfate dimethicone docusate sodium solution glyceryl stearate and PEG-100 stearate hydroxyethylcellulose laureth-4 light mineral oil stearamide MEA-stearate white petrolatum
Stri-Dex Medicated (Glenbrook)	medicated pads			salicylic acid, 0.5%	dodecylbenzene sulfonate sodium xylene sulfonate fragrance citric acid alcohol, 28%
Sulforcin (Owen)	lotion		5%	resorcinol, 2%	alcohol, 11.65%
Sulfur Soap (Stiefel)	cleanser		10% (precipitated)		
Sulpho-Lac (Bradley)	soap		5%		

ACNE PRODUCT TABLE, continued

Product (Manufacturer)	Application Form	Benzoyl Peroxide	Sulfur	Resorcinol/ Salicylic Acid	Other Ingredients
Sulray (Alvin Last)	bar cream		5% 3%		sulfurated lime solution zinc sulfate glyceryl stearate laureth-23 PEG-8 stearate glycerin silica parabens
Therac (C & M Pharm)	lotion		4%	salicylic acid, 2.35%	
Tyrosum Packets (Summers)	cleanser				alcohol, 50% acetone, 10% polysorbate 80, 2%
Vanoxide (Dermik)	lotion	5%			
Xerac Alcohol Gel (Person & Covey)	gel		4%		alcohol, 44%
Xerac BP 5 (Person & Covey)	gel	5%			laureth-4
Xerac BP 10 (Person & Covey)	gel	10%			laureth-4
Zinc Sulfide Compound Lotion, Improved (Paddock)	lotion		sulfur, 48 mg/ml (as sulfide, polysulfides, and thiosulfate)		zinc, 27 mg sodium borate boric acid aluminum hydroxide

a Quantity not specified.

Joseph R. Robinson

30

DERMATITIS, DRY SKIN, DANDRUFF, SEBORRHEIC DERMATITIS, AND PSORIASIS PRODUCTS

*Q*uestions to ask in patient/consumer counseling

How long have you had this condition? Is the condition itchy or painful?

Which area of the skin is affected? Is the condition patchy or uniformly distributed?

Do you have the condition all the time or does it come and go?

Are you taking any medications? Are you taking any new medication or have you changed the dosage on any drug you are taking?

What seems to make the condition worse?

Is your skin exposed to detergents or chemicals at home or at work? What types of cosmetics do you use? Does the environment in which you live or work usually have low or high relative humidity?

Have you recently made any changes in products for personal use (soap, deodorant, or shampoo)?

Do you have a family history of skin disease, asthma, or hay fever?

Have you consulted a dermatologist? What was recommended?

What treatments have you used? How effective were they?

Considering the skin's exposure to a wide variety of chemicals and environmental insults, it demonstrates remarkable resiliency and recuperative ability. (See Chapter 28, *Topical Anti-infective Products*.) However, under certain conditions the skin's defenses break down, and drug therapy may be beneficial. Conditions such as dermatitis, dry skin, dandruff, seborrheic dermatitis (seborrhea), and psoriasis must be considered from both the cosmetic and pathologic points of view so that the pharmacist can advise patients on the appropriate use of nonprescription products.

DERMATITIS

Dermatitis is a noninfectious, inflammatory dermatosis in which the affected skin is erythematous. It is a pattern of skin manifestations rather than a specific disease and can be either acute or chronic.

The term "eczema" was used formerly for a large group of inflammatory skin disorders of unknown etiology, many of which are now called by more specific names, such as seborrhea and psoriasis. When the cause of a particular skin condition was elucidated, the disease was given a different name, and the eczema nomenclature was dropped or modified. Today most dermatologists use the more current term "dermatitis" and define it as "skin inflammation from whatever cause."

Dermatitis may be precipitated by external (exogenous) or internal (endogenous) sources.

The main symptoms of dermatitis are pruritus (itching) and weeping of the skin. The itching may convert to pain over time, and the weeping may diminish, giving way to a dry, scaly condition; at no time does the epidermal tissue appear normal. Symptoms may include redness, papules, vesicles, and edema. (See Table 1 for a definition of selected dermatologic terms.) The lesions may be patchy in distribution. In the acute stages, there is a uniform pattern of papular vesicles on an erythematous base.

In the chronic form of the condition, weeping may be absent, but epidermal thickening and scaling are present. Excoriations, crusting, and secondary infections may occur as sequelae to the pruritus (1).

Exogenously Induced Dermatitis

The conditions of exogenously induced dermatitis are grouped under the general heading of contact dermatitis (Table 2). They include irritant dermatitis, caused by primary or secondary irritants, and allergic dermatitis. Skin diseases are the most common of all reported occupational diseases; the majority of these cases are caused by contact dermatitis. Agricultural and manufacturing workers face the greatest risk (2). The offending substance irritates the skin on first or multiple exposure or may generate an allergic response. In either case, the result is skin inflammation.

Irritant Dermatitis

A primary irritant, such as a strong acid, generally elicits a response on first exposure; secondary irritants such as soaps, cosmetics, topical medications, and detergents cause an inflammatory response only if the agent is repeatedly applied or if certain ancillary circumstances are met.

The symptoms of irritant dermatitis range from mild erythema accompanied by pruritus to actual necrosis and skin ulceration. Primary irritants cause pruritic erythema or perhaps ulceration; secondary irritants, which often generate low-grade inflammation for a long period, tend to produce symptoms more closely related to chronic dermatitis (Table 2).

Generally, the factors influencing skin irritation are the chemical itself, the climate, and biologic variation in the host. The degree of skin irritation from an applied substance is a function of the intrinsic irritation potential of the test material, its concentration, its ability to remain bound to the skin, and the texture of the exposed skin.

TABLE 1 Definition of selected dermatologic terms

Term	Definition
Crust (scab)	Dried remains of exudate from erosive or ulcerated skin lesions
Erythema	A reddening of the skin caused by congestion of the dermal vasculature
Ulceration	An erosion of the epidermis extending into the dermis
Macule	A small, discolored patch or spot on the skin
Necrosis	Death of a cell or group of cells that form part of the living body
Papule	A solid, circumscribed elevation of the skin, varying roughly from 1 mm to 1 cm in size
Pustule (superficial abscess)	A circumscribed collection of free pus in the skin
Scale	Accumulation of loose, horny fragments of stratum corneum
Vesicle (blister)	A sharply circumscribed collection of free fluid in the skin
Plaque	A papular lesion greater than 1 cm in size

Adapted from S. L. Moschella et al., "Dermatology," W. B. Saunders, Philadelphia, Pa., 1975.

Applying a strong acid or base to the cutaneous skin surface causes irritation and a subsequent inflammatory reaction. Similarly, the irritant properties of topical drugs such as camphor, coal tar, menthol, and resorcinol are well known, but classification of these agents as primary or secondary irritants is a function of their concentration. Very high camphor concentrations are needed to produce the same degree of irritation as that achieved with relatively low coal tar levels. Agents such as bithionol and hexachlorophene, which are bound to the epidermal layer, cause irritation with repeated application. Some substances used to treat certain skin conditions, such as psoriasis, may be irritating to the affected skin.

Environmental conditions play a role in skin texture and its resistance to irritant substances. High humidity allows greater skin hydration and thus faster penetration. Occlusion also keeps the skin hydrated.

Factors such as age and skin color also are influential in irritant dermatitis. Aged skin is less prone to irritation than youthful skin, presumably because penetration is more difficult. Darker skinned races seem to be less susceptible than lighter skinned individuals, although the evidence to prove this observation is scant.

Concomitant administration of more than one substance may induce skin irritation. A secondary irritant that is not irritating to the skin when applied alone may cause irritation in combination with an agent that promotes absorption, such as a surfactant or keratolytic. Damaged skin also encourages skin irritation.

One of the most common forms of irritant dermatitis that the pharmacist will confront is hand dermatitis or "dishpan hands." This condition often is caused by repeated exposure to mild primary irritants such as soap and water. It is marked by erythema, dryness, chapping, and pruritus of the dorsa of the hands.

Allergic Dermatitis

Allergic reactions are classified as immediate (anaphylactic), intermediate (Arthus), cytotoxic, and delayed (tuberculin) (Table 3). Most cases of allergic contact dermatitis fall into the category of delayed hypersensitivity reactions. Common contact allergens include nickel, chromate, the catechols of poison ivy and poison oak, synthetic chemicals, and topical drugs such as antibiotics, antihistamines, and "caine" types of local anesthetics (3). (See Chapter 35, *Poison Ivy and Poison Oak Products*, and Chapter 28, *Topical Anti-infective Products*.) Components of cosmetics may also serve as contact allergens; the most common offenders include lanolin, parabens, perfumes, and dyes.

True allergic reactions cannot occur on first exposure to an allergen. Some individuals react abnormally, with appropriate skin manifestations, to common substances such as mushrooms, strawberries, or shellfish, but the changes do not appear to be mediated by antibodies or delayed sensitivity mechanisms, and they usually occur on first exposure. Thus they are not allergies but rather idiosyncrasies caused by an intrinsic factor or defect in the tissues. (See *Plate 6–26*.)

Immediate (Anaphylactic) Reaction In an immediate allergic reaction, the antibody sensitizes tissue cells passively. Subsequent administration of exogenous antigen reaches the sensitized cells, causing cell injury and release of endogenous agents such as histamine, kinins, and prostaglandins. These agents cause further local changes, which usually include contraction of smooth muscle, increased vascular permeability, and edema. The cell injury from this type of reaction is transient, and most of the cells recover. However, cell death may occur. Antihistamines suppress or modify the tissue changes in species of animals in which hista-

---

TABLE 2 Exogenously induced dermatitis

Characteristic	Weak or secondary irritant dermatitis[a]	Irritant dermatitis[b]	Allergic dermatitis[c]
Mechanism	Abrasion, desiccation, trauma, dryness, soreness, and fissures precede eruption	Direct insult to tissue, no preceding dryness or fissuring	Immunologic; initial contact sensitizes; subsequent contact elicits a response; no preceding eruption
Onset	Slow; over days, months, or years	Sudden; response in 30 minutes to several days after exposure	Sudden; response in 24–28 hours after exposure
Symptoms	Hyperkeratosis, erythema, vesicles, and fissuring	Erythema, vesicles, exudation, and sometimes necrosis	Erythema, vesicles, edema, and necrosis
Usual location	Hands	Hands	Hands and face
Patch test	Negative	Positive	Positive

[a] Cumulative insults are required.
[b] Single exposure to an offending agent is sufficient.
[c] Multiple exposures are usually required.

TABLE 3   Types of allergic reactions in the skin

	Anaphylaxis	Arthus reaction	Cytotoxic reaction	Delayed reaction
Response mediator	Sensitizing antibody	Precipitating antibody	Antibody or cell	Cell
Skin test	Immediate wheal or flare	Arthus reaction with polymorph infiltration, appearing in 2–4 hours but may progress to necrosis for hours or days	Immediate wheal and flare, granulomatous lesions with or without polymorphs, first appearing in 2–6 hours	Delayed, tuberculin response
Clinical manifestation	Erythema	Serum sickness	Eczema	Eczema
Skin or vascular changes	Urticaria; angioneurotic edema	Allergic vasculitis; nodular vasculitis	Purpura; homograft rejection	Contact dermatitis; homograft rejection

Adapted from W. E. Parrish, "An Introduction to the Biology of the Skin," Blackwell Scientific, Oxford, Eng., 1970.

mine is the most active agent. They do not prevent the antigen–antibody reaction but rather occupy the histamine receptor sites on the effector cells.

Intermediate (Arthus) Reaction   In an intermediate allergic reaction, the antigen combines with the antibody in tissue spaces or in the circulation to produce a type of complex, which causes secondary changes to the tissue, depending on concentration and composition. The primary change is massive infiltration of the extravascular tissue; this usually occurs 2–4 hours after exposure to the antigen. Corticosteroid administration suppresses full development of the Arthus reaction.

Cytotoxic Reaction   A cytotoxic reaction is an allergic reaction in which cells are damaged. In the allergic classification, it is restricted to cell damage caused by delayed sensitivity specific for the antigen in the susceptible target cell. The lysis of red blood cells by antibodies specific for the red cells is an example of the reaction of an antibody with an antigen acquired by the cell. The cell that has adsorbed the antigen usually is damaged.

Delayed (Tuberculin) Reaction   A delayed allergic reaction may take 24–48 hours to reach a maximum response and occurs in the absence of demonstrable globulin antibody. The lesion produced is a diffuse reaction characterized by erythema and accumulation of fluid (edema). The allergic response may be inhibited by corticosteroids but is not altered by antihistamines. The essential features of the delayed sensitivity reaction are its mediation by cells only and its passive transfer to normal subjects by cells only.

Delayed hypersensitivity is the major mechanism involved in allergic contact dermatitis. Contact sensitization may occur 7–10 days after the first contact with a potent allergen, or it may develop after several years of repeated exposure to weaker allergens. Once the reaction is initiated, it builds in severity for 4–7 days; healing may occur in several weeks to a month. Susceptibility to allergic contact dermatitis may last a lifetime, although in certain cases hypersensitivity is lost.

Infective Dermatitis

Infective dermatitis is a skin condition caused by the presence of microorganism toxins, not by the organism's specific pathogenic activity. The mechanism of action for this type of dermatitis has not been established, but it is known that inoculating the skin of susceptible individuals with a bacterial culture or filtrate causes the condition. It is presumed that bacterial toxins or antigens elicit the unfavorable response. The condition responds favorably to systemic antibiotics. Topically applied agents such as neomycin also may be used. Many of these drugs, however, have considerable sensitizing potential, particularly when they are used chronically. Caution must therefore be exercised in their use.

Endogenously Induced Dermatitis

Atopic dermatitis and neurodermatitis are conditions with unknown internal causes. Symptoms generally last longer (years) than those of exogenously induced dermatitis.

Atopic Dermatitis

Atopic dermatitis occurs primarily during childhood and early adulthood, usually in the folds of the arms or knees, and is one of the most common dermatologic problems seen in children. It may begin shortly after birth and last many years, or it may disappear after 1 or 2 years. The symptoms are erythema, scaling, and weeping, accompanied by severe pruritus. Patients are often intolerant to sudden changes and extremes of temperature and humidity. Unfortunately, secondary or associated infections are common, making diagnosis and treatment difficult. The etiology of the condition is unknown, but patients often have associated asthma or hay fever. Because skin sensitivity to a wide range of agents is common, skin tests are not reliable diagnostic aids.

Atopic dermatitis sometimes is associated incorrectly with anaphylactic allergy. In both cases affected individuals show positive skin tests and develop allergic signs after exposure. However, normal treatment for allergy, such as avoiding contact with allergens and administration of antihistamines, seldom brings relief to the patient with atopic dermatitis.

Neurodermatitis

Neurodermatitis, a chronic form of eczema, is found more often in women and is generally localized in the nape of the neck, legs, genitoanal region, and forearms (4). The areas of involvement are highly lichenified (the skin thickens and hardens, and normal markings are exaggerated) and become worse when continually rubbed or scratched. Because lichenified skin is more itchy than normal skin, a vicious cycle develops. Emotional stress plays a role in this disorder (5). Scratching actually becomes a conditioned response, leading to the development of a scratch–lichenification cycle. Minor tranquilizers, sedatives, and especially counseling are useful in treating this disorder.

Assessment of Dermatitis

Because treatment of dermatitis is often different from that of other cutaneous disorders, assessment of the condition is important before initiating therapy. By noting the location and distribution of the lesions and taking a careful history of the patient's occupational and leisure activities, the pharmacist may be able to diagnose contact dermatitis. Atopic dermatitis should be considered in light of the patient's age, family history of atopy, and duration of the eruption.

Contact Dermatitis

In most cases of contact dermatitis, an accurate assessment is readily made on the basis of the eczematous character, configuration, and location of the rash and itching. Lesions are often asymmetric in distribution, reflecting where contact with the offending substance occurred. A rash on the backs and sides of the fingers and hands, eyelids, groin, wrists, and feet often suggests contact dermatitis. Seborrhea, however, also must be considered in cases of genitoanal or eyelid involvement. Tinea cruris (jock itch) and tinea pedis (athlete's foot) are other possibilities. (See Chapter 28, *Topical Anti-infective Products*, and Chapter 37, *Foot Care Products*.)

By asking questions about the patient's environment (home, work, medications, and clothes), the pharmacist may be able to identify a possible irritant or allergen. Patch testing by a physician also is useful in diagnosis of allergic reactions. It is important to identify the offending substance because its removal will result in improvement of the condition (6–8).

In some cases of dermatitis (especially eruptions of the hands), there is a mixture of infectious eczematoid, atopic, and contact dermatitis. With contact dermatitis, once the skin reacts to one substance, it may be more vulnerable to other substances, making diagnosis and treatment more complicated. Allergic or primary irritant dermatitis may be a secondary eruption caused by an agent used in therapy, complicating one of the other forms of dermatitis. Common offenders include benzocaine, neomycin, and ethylenediamine.

Atopic Dermatitis

Because atopic dermatitis is primarily a disease of the young, the age of the patient is important in diagnosis. By taking a medical history, the pharmacist may determine if the patient has a history of atopic disorders. The possibility of contact dermatitis must also be explored. Inquiries should be made regarding the onset and duration of the eruption. Atopic dermatitis is marked by remissions and exacerbations and, unlike contact dermatitis, single eruptions may last for months or years. Finally, the location and distribution of the lesions should be taken into account. The classic case of childhood atopic dermatitis involves the cheeks and extensor surfaces of the forearms and legs. (See *Plate 6-27A, B*, and *C*.) Unlike seborrhea and psoriasis, the disease generally does not involve the groin, and scalp involvement is limited to infants (9). Lesions are typically symmetric in distribution. If atopic dermatitis is suspected, a physician should be consulted.

Treatment of Dermatitis

Dermatitis therapy must be approached cautiously to prevent deterioration of the condition. In some forms of dermatitis, the patient is sensitive to a wide variety of agents, and therapeutic entities may aggravate inflamed skin. In atopic dermatitis, therapy is needed for long periods. In contact dermatitis, however, the duration of therapy is much shorter, because withdrawal of the allergen or irritant improves the condition. Before recommending any product for the treatment of contact dermatitis, the pharmacist should help the patient identify the offending substance(s). Prevention of further exposure is the key to effective therapy.

In general, nonprescription products used to treat dermatitis should not be used on children under 2 years of age, except under the advice and supervision of a physician. The Food and Drug Administration (FDA) advisory review panel on over-the-counter (OTC) miscellaneous drug products has made this recommendation because very young children have a higher body surface area to weight ratio than older individuals and therefore are at increased risk for systemic toxicity from topically applied drugs. This is accentuated by the fact that infants under 6 months of age have underdeveloped hepatic enzyme systems for metabolizing absorbed drugs (10). (See Minichapter B, *Nonprescription Drug Use in Children*.)

General Measures

For most forms of dermatitis, it is worthwhile to protect the lesions from clothing and fingernails, especially in small children. Clothing worn next to the skin should be absorbent, light, and nonirritating (such as cotton), laundered with bland soaps and double rinsed (11). Wool, silk, and any rough clothing should be avoided. It may be necessary to loosely bandage the area and cut the patient's fingernails to prevent scratching. Oral antihistamines may be beneficial in alleviating itching.

The patient should be instructed to avoid known or suspected irritants and allergens, particularly in acute dermatitis. If repeated exposure to the substance occurs, the area should be immediately and thoroughly irrigated with water. The use of soaps containing fragrances and dyes also should be discouraged (12, 13). Cetaphil lotion, Lowila, or Neutrogena soap are suitable alternatives. Occlusive agents or covers should not be applied when weeping is present; rather, during the acute weeping stage, saline, tap water, or Burow's solution compresses may be applied.

As an alternative to applying compresses, the patient may bathe 2 or 3 times a day using saline or tap water. Exposure should be limited to 30 minutes. Oatmeal-based products may be added to the bath for cleansing. Oatmeal contains 50% starch (a demulcent) with about 25% protein and 9% oil (14). It is claimed to be soothing and antipruritic, but controlled studies are lacking. If the use of compresses or bathing does not improve the weeping in 1–3 days, a physician should be consulted.

Once vesiculation subsides, topical hydrocortisone (0.5%) may be useful to decrease inflammation. The pharmacist may instruct the patient to apply a thin film of the preparation every 4 hours. If improvement is not seen in several days, a physician should be consulted.

The eczematous lesion may progress to a dry, scaly stage. To moisturize the skin and alleviate attendant pruritus, the patient should be instructed to apply an emollient such as petrolatum 3 or more times a day. Presoaking the affected area in warm water for 5–10 minutes may enhance this effect by moisturizing the skin and alleviating attendant pruritus. Topical hydrocortisone ointment may be useful for acute flare-ups during this stage.

The pharmacist often will be confronted with cases of "dishpan hands." To aid the patient with mild hand dermatitis, the following instructions may be given (15):

- Wear vinyl gloves when doing dishes and handling fresh fruits. (Rubber gloves may be sensitizing.) Remember that wearing a glove with a hole in it will trap irritants next to the skin and is worse than wearing no gloves at all. Thin white cotton liners worn under the vinyl gloves may prevent irritation from the vinyl and absorb perspiration.

- When washing the hands, use lukewarm water and a minimal amount of soap.

- Apply a bland moisturizer such as white petrolatum or Eucerin after each handwashing and at numerous other times during the day. Many nonprescription hand creams and lotions contain perfumes and parabens. These products should be avoided because the allergenic components may irritate the skin or cause sensitivity reactions.

- Use a topical hydrocortisone ointment if the condition does not respond to moisturizers, barring the presence of an infection. (An ointment should be selected because of its emollient effect.) Apply the medication after each handwashing and frequently throughout the day. It should be applied thinly and massaged in thoroughly. If the skin is very dry, a thin layer of white petrolatum may be applied *after* rubbing in the hydrocortisone ointment, or cosmetic gloves may be worn.

- After the condition subsides, continue to apply a bland moisturizer or hydrocortisone ointment at least 4 times a day until the skin condition has healed completely.

Pharmacologic Agents

Ingredients in nonprescription products for dermatitis include astringents, antipruritics, protectants, and hydrocortisone. Keratolytics usually are avoided in dermatitis unless extensive lichenification has occurred. These agents and those that reduce the mitotic activity of the epidermis, such as tars and anthralin, should be used cautiously because of their irritant properties.

Astringents Mild astringents are sometimes needed to reduce the weeping that may occur in dermatitis. These agents are defined as substances that check oozing, discharge, or bleeding when applied to the skin or mucous membranes and work by coagulating protein (16). They generally have a low cell penetrability, which results in their activity being limited to the cell surface and interstitial spaces. The permeability of the cell membrane and capillary endothelium is reduced, resulting in a drying of the affected area (17). The protein precipitate that forms may serve as a protective coat, allowing new tissues to grow underneath (16). The tissue often appears wrinkled and blanched as a result of astringent activity.

The FDA advisory review panel on OTC miscellaneous external drug products has identified two astringent solutions as being safe and effective: aluminum acetate (Burow's solution) and witch hazel (Hamamelis water). Numerous other ingredients, including alum and zinc oxide, have been promoted as astringents. However, data demonstrating their safety and effectiveness as astringents are lacking, resulting in a Category II rating by the advisory review panel (16).

Aluminum acetate solution USP (4.8–5.8%) may be used as a soak or local compress to help dry weeping areas. The solution first must be diluted with 10–40 parts of water. Patients may soak the affected area in the solution 2–4 times daily for 15–30 minutes or loosely apply a compress of washcloths or small towels soaked in the astringent solution. Such dressings should be rewetted with solution, as often as every 15–30 minutes throughout the period of application. Isotonic saline solution, tap water, or diluted white vinegar (¼ cup per pint of water) may also be used in this fashion (18).

Witch hazel is no longer listed in the official compendia, but has been used for centuries as an astringent solution. It is a natural product prepared from the twigs of *Hamamelis virginiana* and contains tannins, trace amounts of volatile oils (which give it a characteristically pleasant odor), and 14–15% alcohol, all of which may contribute to its astringent activity. The product may be applied as often as necessary in the treatment of minor skin irritations (16).

Calamine lotion, aluminum hydroxide gel (0.15–5%), kaolin (4–20%), and other powder-based aqueous products that dry weeping through water adsorption or astringency should be used with caution.

These agents have a tendency to crust, and removing the crusts may cause bleeding and potential infections.

Antipruritics The itching associated with dermatitis may be mediated through several different mechanisms, which may explain the usefulness of three major classes of pharmacologic agents as antipruritics: local anesthetics, antihistamines, and steroids. Cooling the area through application of a soothing, bland lotion may also reduce the extent of pruritus, but is only transitory in its effect.

The itching sensation is mediated by the same nerve fibers that carry pain impulses. Local anesthetics block conduction along axonal membranes, thereby relieving itching, as well as pain. Agents such as benzocaine (5–20%) may be applied to the affected area 3 or 4 times daily. Certain local anesthetics such as dibucaine, lidocaine, and tetracine can cause serious systemic side effects such as convulsions and myocardial depression. For this reason they should not be used in large quantities, particularly if the skin is raw or blistered. Two of the safest topical anesthetics appear to be dyclonine and benzocaine. (See Chapters 36, *Insect Sting and Bite Products*, and 33, *Burn and Sunburn Products*.)

Itching may be mediated by a variety of endogenous substances, including histamine. On this basis, topical antihistamines such as diphenhydramine hydrochloride (1–2%) and tripelennamine hydrochloride (0.5–2%) have been used as antipruritic agents. Their activity stems from an ability to compete with histamine at H_1 receptor sites and to exert a topical anesthetic effect. Local anesthesia may be the more important mechanism of action because the cause of itching in many conditions such as atopic dermatitis has not been established and may not be related to histamine at all (19).

Diphenhydramine and tripelennamine both are considered safe and effective for use as nonprescription external analgesics. These agents may, however, act as haptenes and produce sensitization reactions after prolonged use. The FDA advisory review panel on OTC external analgesic drug products does not recommend topical use of these agents for more than 7 days except under the advice and supervision of a physician (20).

Protectants A skin protectant is defined as a substance that protects injured or exposed skin or mucous membrane surfaces from harmful or annoying stimuli (21). Zinc oxide (1–25%) is one of the most widely used and clinically accepted skin protectants. It may be applied as a paste (Lassar's), ointment, or lotion (calamine) and is claimed to be mildly astringent and antiseptic as well as protective in its activity.

If the affected area is weeping, astringents and adsorbents such as calamine and aluminum hydroxide gel may be used as skin protectants, as discussed above.

If the affected area is dry, bland moisturizing agents such as petrolatum and cocoa butter may be applied, as is presented in detail under the discussion of dry skin. Patients should be cautioned, however, that covering the lesions or applying a product with an occlusive barrier may increase the degree of tissue maceration and prevent heat loss, resulting in discomfort. In general, if the condition worsens or does not improve within 7 days, a physician should be consulted.

Bismuth subnitrate, boric acid, tannic acid, and sulfur have been used as skin protectants, but data supporting their efficacy are lacking. Indeed, sulfur may further irritate the affected area by virtue of its keratolytic properties. Bismuth subnitrate and boric acid have been linked with fatalities in infants. Tannic acid may cause hepatotoxity. For these reasons, these agents have been placed in Category II by the FDA advisory review panel on OTC skin-protectant drug products. (See Table 4 for a list of the other tentative recommendations of the advisory review panel.)

Topical Hydrocortisone Hydrocortisone (0.25–0.5%) is one agent available for nonprescription treatment of dermatitis. Its principal use is to relieve itching. This activity stems from a generalized anti-inflammatory effect. The official indications for its use include temporary relief of itching associated with minor skin irritations, inflammation, and rashes caused by dermatitis, insect bites, poison ivy, poison oak, poison sumac, soaps, detergents, cosmetics, and jewelry. It is also indicated for external genital, feminine, and anal itching. (See Chapters 36, *Insect Sting and Bite Products*; 35, *Poison Ivy and Poison Oak Products*; 26, *Hemorrhoidal Products*; and 27, *Personal Care Products*.) Hydrocortisone acts prophylactically to prevent further inflammation. It does not reverse existing inflammation.

Various studies provide strong documentation for the efficacy of hydrocortisone as an antipruritic and anti-inflammatory agent in the 0.5–5% dosage range. Several studies using a 0.25% concentration have also shown favorable results (22). Hydrocortisone generally should be applied 3 or 4 times a day. If the emollient effect of the steroid vehicle is desired, or if the agent is likely to be washed off, such as in hand dermatitis, more frequent applications may be necessary. Application to the scalp may be made once a day because the drug usually is not rubbed off (22).

Many patients do not use topical steroid preparations properly; some tend to apply far too much per application and others may apply the product too infrequently. Therefore, the pharmacist should instruct the patient to apply only a thin film and to massage it into the skin thoroughly. Proper frequency of application should be stressed. The pharmacist may also suggest washing or soaking the area just before application to help promote drug absorption.

Compound	Category
Allantoin	I
Aluminum hydroxide gel	I
Bismuth subnitrate	II
Boric acid	II
Calamine	I
Cocoa butter	I
Dimethicone	I
Glycerin	I
Kaolin	I
Petrolatum	I
Shark liver oil	I
Sulfur	II
Tannic acid	II
White petrolatum	I
Zinc acetate	I
Zinc carbonate	I
Zinc oxide	I

TABLE 4 Tentative FDA classifications of nonprescription ingredients used as skin protectants

Excerpted from *Federal Register, 48,* 6381 (1983).

Before recommending a hydrocortisone product, the pharmacist must be certain that the area of application is not infected. Signs of bacterial infection include redness, heat, pus, and crusting. Fungal infections may be marked by erythema and scaling; vaginal infections may be accompanied by a discharge. Topical hydrocortisone may mask the symptoms of these dermatologic infections while the infection progresses in severity.

Use of systemic steroids has been associated with many adverse effects. Topical hydrocortisone, however, generally will not produce systemic complications, because absorption is minimal. Approximately 1% of a hydrocortisone solution applied to normal skin on the forearm is absorbed systemically (23). Absorption increases in the presence of skin inflammation or with the use of occlusive agents. Certain adverse local effects such as skin atrophy may arise with prolonged use because of the antimitotic/antisynthetic effect of hydrocortisone on cells. In practice, however, clinically detectable atrophy rarely occurs with hydrocortisone in the concentrations available without a prescription. This problem may occur with the newer, fluorinated products. In general, continued and frequent use of topical hydrocortisone products should be discouraged. If the patient's condition worsens, or if symptoms persist for more than 7 days or clear up and occur again within a few days, a physician should be consulted. The FDA advisory review panel on OTC external analgesic drug products has placed hydrocortisone in Category I as an antipruritic agent.

Dimers of Linoleic Acid Dimers of linoleic acid are being investigated as prophylactic agents to reduce irritation from various detergents and allergens such as poison ivy (24). Encouraging results have been obtained after topical application of these agents, but they are not available for use in the United States.

Product Selection Guidelines for Dermatitis

When deciding on which product to recommend for the control of dermatitis, the pharmacist must evaluate not only the various active ingredients found in nonprescription products, but also the vehicle itself. The type of vehicle (ointment, cream, lotion, gel, solution, or aerosol) has a significant effect on dermatitis. The following simple guidelines may be used to choose an appropriate vehicle (25):

- If a drying effect is desired, solutions and gels should be recommended. It must be noted, however, that components of these systems may quickly diffuse into the underlying tissue and possibly cause irritation.

- If slight lubrication is needed, creams and lotions are adequate.

- If the lesion is very dry and fissured, ointments are the vehicle of choice. However, they should be avoided in intertriginous areas because of their maceration potential.

- In an acute process, ointments may cause further irritation because of their occlusive effect.

- Aerosols, gels, or lotions may be recommended when the dermatitis affects a hair-covered area of the body.

Topical nonprescription products come in various package sizes. The pharmacist must be able to recommend an appropriate amount of drug to treat a given condition. Table 5 lists the amount of drug needed to cover a given area of the body. By being aware of details such as this, the pharmacist can serve the patient economically as well as therapeutically.

DRY SKIN

Almost everyone has had dry or chapped skin. In some people it is a seasonal occurrence; in others the condition is chronic. Although dry skin is not life threatening, it is annoying and uncomfortable because of the attendant pruritus and, in some cases, pain and inflammation. In addition, dry skin is more prone to bacterial invasion than normal skin.

Symptoms

Dry skin is characterized by one or more of the following symptoms:

- Roughness and flaking;
- Loss of flexibility;
- Fissures;
- Hyperkeratosis;
- Inflammation;
- Pruritus.

The condition tends to appear on the lower legs, the back of the hands, and the forearms. Dry skin is especially prevalent during the winter months. It is known to be secondary to other disease states, prolonged detergent use, malnutrition, and physical damage to the stratum corneum.

TABLE 5 Grams of cream or ointment required for four sparing applications in 1 day

Part of the body	Grams
Face and ears	5
Neck	5
Upper extremity	10
Lower extremity	20
Anterior trunk	15
Posterior trunk	15

Excerpted from E. Epstein, "Common Skin Disorders—A Manual for Physicians and Patients," Medical Economics Company, Oradell, N.J., 07649, 1979, p. 5.

Factors in Skin Hydration

The cardinal characteristic of a dry skin condition is inadequate moisture content in the stratum corneum. It is a common misconception that dry skin is caused by a lack of natural skin oils; on the contrary, dry skin is caused by a lack of water. The pathophysiology of dry skin therefore can be described by examining the factors involved in skin hydration.

Age

Dry skin occurs commonly in elderly individuals. As skin ages, the entire epidermal layer thins and the skin's hygroscopic substances decrease in quantity, decreasing its ability to retain moisture. Hormonal changes that accompany aging result in lowered sebum output and therefore lowered skin lubrication (26). In addition, keratin cross-linking induced by long-term exposure to ultraviolet (UV) radiation causes skin to harden. This cross-linking also is associated with increased surface dryness and general pruritus.

Other Disease States

A number of systemic and dermatologic disorders may lead to a dry skin condition. Examples of such systemic disorders include hypothyroidism and dehydration.

Dermatologic conditions marked by scaling and dryness include contact dermatitis, atopic dermatitis, and psoriasis. In psoriatic lesions, transepidermal water loss may be as high as 0.48 mg/cm²/hr as compared with 0.18 mg/cm²/hr in control subjects (27). Neighboring skin, however, is not affected (28). These dermatologic disorders may be differentiated from a simple dry skin condition on the basis of other attendant symptoms.

Two dermatologic conditions difficult to differentiate from simple dry skin are asteatotic eczema and dominant ichthyosis vulgaris. Asteatotic eczema is characterized by dry and fissured skin, inflammation, and pruritus. Sebaceous secretions are scanty or absent. It is more common during dry winter weather and in elderly individuals; it apparently is an extension of the dry skin condition.

Dominant ichthyosis vulgaris affects 0.3–1.0% of the population. It is a genetic disorder that should be suspected when a patient complains of a familial tendency to excessive dryness and chapping. Patients also may have an associated history of atopic disease. Symptoms include dryness and roughness of the skin, accompanied by small, fine, white scales. The condition tends to appear on the extensor aspects of the arms and legs. Dryness of the cheeks, heels, and palms also may be noted. In severe forms of the disease, a classic fish scale-like appearance of the stratum corneum arises (27, 29).

Weather Conditions

Relative humidity is important in maintaining normal skin hydration. Keratin (the horny skin layer) softens when the stratum corneum's moisture content is about 10%. This level occurs at 60% relative humidity. In a normal indoor climate, moisture content is 10–15%; at 95% relative humidity, the stratum corneum's moisture content increases to 65%. With low temperature and relative humidity, however, the outer skin layer dries out (30, 31), becomes less flexible, and may crack when flexed, increasing the rate of moisture loss. High wind velocity also causes this condition.

Integrity of Stratum Corneum Cell Membranes

One theory states that water retention in the stratum corneum depends on the presence of hygroscopic substances within the corneum cells (32). These substances are contained by cell membranes permeable to water but not to electrolytes. Physical disruption, extraction of lipids with solvents, or prolonged detergent use may damage cell membranes, allowing the hygroscopic substances to be lost and reducing the ability of the stratum corneum to retain water (33–36).

Natural Moisturizing Factor

Moisture is diffused rapidly to the keratin layer from lower skin layers, about 50–100 times faster than it is lost from the epidermal surface to the environment. However, water movement through the keratin itself is relatively slow. A hydrophilic substance called natural moisturizing factor may influence keratin moisture retention (37). Several components of this substance, including lactate, polypeptides, hexosamines, pentoses, urea, pyrrolidine, carboxylic acids, and inorganic ions, have been isolated and identified (38–40). However, when they are applied to the skin surface, only temporary hydration results. It is thought that natural moisturizing factor, because of its natural hygroscopicity, increases the amount of water the stratum corneum absorbs at any given relative humidity but that it does not interact significantly with the protein itself in the horny layer (41).

Many of the components of natural moisturizing factor are water soluble and easily removed from the skin. Perhaps this is why excessive bathing may lead to a dry skin condition; hygroscopic substances may be leached from the skin, especially if soaps are present to disrupt stratum corneum cell membranes.

Integrity of the Stratum Corneum

To maintain normal skin hydration, the water content of the stratum corneum must remain at approximately 10%. Water is lost from the skin through perspiration (as much as 2 l per hour under extreme thermal stress) and transepidermal diffusion, a relatively constant process. Because human skin is such an effective barrier, only about 120 ml of water per day is lost from the average adult skin surface (2 m²) through transepidermal diffusion (42). Removal of the stratum corneum barrier increases the water loss rate about 50 times (43, 44).

Physical damage to the stratum corneum dramatically increases the transepidermal water loss, but within 1 or 2 days a temporary parakeratotic barrier (a barrier consisting of incompletely keratinized, nucleated cells) provides 50% of the normal function, and total function is restored in 2 or 3 weeks.

Assessment of Dry Skin

When assessing a dry skin condition, the pharmacist should consider several factors before suggesting a therapeutic program that will eliminate or counteract any causative factors. A useful series of such measures has been outlined in the *Manual of Dermatologic Therapeutics* (45). The temperature and relative humidity of the home and work environment should be considered; keeping room temperatures low and using humidifiers may be beneficial. A history of the work environment also is useful to determine whether the problem may be caused by repeated exposure to detergents; dishpan hands may be relieved by the use of vinyl gloves. Frequency of bathing also should be considered. Excessive bathing (more than once every 1 or 2 days) may have a drying effect on the skin.

Dry skin may be the manifestation of another disease state. By obtaining a medical history, the pharmacist may be able to uncover a primary disorder triggering the dry skin condition such as hypothyroidism or atopic disease. Psoriasis and contact dermatitis are other possibilities. A drug history should be taken to investigate the possibility of a drug eruption or dehydration secondary to diuretic use. If any of these primary events is suspected or if signs of an infection are present (redness, heat, and pus), a physician should be consulted.

Asteatotic eczema and dominant ichthyosis vulgaris are difficult to differentiate from a simple dry skin condition. If the condition is severe enough to be associated with inflammation and pruritus, asteatotic eczema may be the correct diagnosis. If the pharmacist elicits a positive history of atopic disease or a familial tendency toward dry skin, or if the normal markings in the patient's palms and soles are clearly accentuated, dominant ichthyosis vulgaris is a possibility. Fortunately, misdiagnosis is not of great consequence, because simple dry skin, asteatotic eczema, and dominant ichthyosis vulgaris are treated similarly.

Treatment of Dry Skin

The main objectives in treating dry skin are to raise the stratum corneum's moisture level and to reestablish its integrity. Water is the only true plasticizer for human stratum corneum, but simply adding water to the skin is not a useful approach unless the stratum corneum can retain it (37). If hydrated skin is not covered immediately with an occlusive substance (e.g., petrolatum) or with a plastic covering, it dehydrates quickly. There are several methods of treating dry skin (46):

- Lubricating the skin;

- Moisturizing (hydrating and thickening) the skin;

- Chemically softening the keratinous epidermal layer;

- Using topical hydrocortisone if inflammation is present.

Lubricating the Skin

A lubricant is any substance that lessens friction. It does not necessarily raise the stratum corneum moisture level. Rather, the use of a lubricant is more psychologic—the skin feels smooth. Various nonprescription cosmetic products in an assortment of vehicles serve as lubricants. Those most heavily promoted in advertisements include bath oils and products containing natural vegetable and animal oils.

Bath Oils Bath oils generally consist of a mineral or vegetable oil plus a surfactant. Mineral oil products are adsorbed better than vegetable oil products (47). Adsorption onto and absorption into the skin increase as temperature and oil concentration increase. Bath oils, which are applied at a high temperature but unfortunately at a low oil concentration, are moderately effective in improving a dry skin condition. Part of their effect is caused by the slip or lubricity they impart to the skin, which may be more important to the patient than are the occlusive properties. When applied as wet compresses, however, bath oils are effective in treating dry skin (48). Patients may also be instructed to mix 1 tsp of bath oil per ¼ cup warm water and use this as a rubdown. In this way, excessive bathing may be avoided.

Patients using bath oils should be cautioned that these products may make the tub slippery, creating a safety hazard, especially for the elderly. Moreover, they make cleansing of the skin with soaps more difficult.

Natural Products Attempts have been made to formulate products that duplicate the normal oil mantle of the skin as a means of treating dry skin. Because sebum and skin surface lipids contain a relatively high concentration of fatty acid glycerides, vegetable and animal oils such as avocado, cucumber, mink, peanut, safflower, sesame, turtle, and shark liver have been used. These oils are included in dry skin products presumably because of their unsaturated fatty acid content. However, sebum is not an effective barrier against moisture loss from the skin. Although the use of these oils contributes to skin flexibility and lubricity, their occlusive effect is less than that of petrolatum. There is a great psychologic appeal to products containing these oils. However, their actual value in treating a dry skin condition is not documented. Squalene, another ingredient that has been used, is a normal component of skin lipids and serves as a reasonably effective barrier against moisture loss.

Moisturizing Agents

An ideal moisturizer should fulfill certain conditions (40). It should regulate and maintain the stratum corneum water level above the critical level (10%) but not to such a degree as to induce superhydration or maceration. Superhydration of the stratum corneum reduces its barrier efficiency, making it more susceptible to invasion by microorganisms, irritants, and allergens. In addition to this most important characteristic, the effectiveness of a moisturizing agent should be independent of environmental changes, and continued application should not cause damage to the stratum corneum by the removal of or interference with its natural moisturizers. The product should be nonirritating, nonsensitizing, and stable in cosmetic formulations. The agents used most commonly as nonprescription moisturizers are humectants and occlusives.

Humectants Humectants are defined as substances that promote retention of water because of their hygroscopicity. The most commonly used humectants in dermatology include glycerin and propylene glycol. Theoretically, the humectant acts by being absorbed into the skin to help replace any missing hygroscopic substances, or if absorption does not occur, the humectant on the skin surface attracts water from the atmosphere and serves as a reservoir for the stratum corneum. In the case of glycerin, however, these theoretical mechanisms of action do not apply.

Products containing 50% glycerin (glycerin and rose water) often are used to treat a dry skin condition. Glycerin does not penetrate into the skin, and high humidity is needed for it to attract water from the environment. (The incidence of dry skin is lowest when relative humidity is high.) Glycerin also increases the transepidermal moisture loss rate, an effect opposite to what is usually desirable. Despite these limitations, glycerin is effective in treating dry skin.

A partial explanation for glycerin's mechanism of action is that it accelerates moisture diffusion from the dermal tissue to the surface and holds water in intimate contact with the skin. Through this mechanism it brings moisture from the dermal region to the parched stratum corneum. In addition, glycerin provides lubrication to the skin surface. The FDA advisory review panel on OTC skin-protectant drug products tentatively has recommended that diluted glycerin (20–45%) be given Category I status as a skin protectant (Table 4). Undiluted glycerin, however, may have a dehydrating effect on the skin and is not considered by the panel to be an effective skin protectant.

Occlusive Agents Occlusives are substances that promote retention of water because of their hydrophobicity; moisture in the skin cannot pass through the occlusive barrier. These agents, also known as emollients, often are used in combination with a humectant in dry skin formulations. The most commonly used occlusives include petrolatum, lanolin, cocoa butter, mineral oil, and silicones such as dimethicone.

Occlusives have several mechanisms of action in correcting a dry skin condition. First, they prevent moisture evaporation from the skin surface. Some researchers believe that the prevention of normal transepidermal water loss is not sufficient to maintain normal hydration (40). Therefore, the pharmacist should instruct the patient to soak the affected area in water for 5–10 minutes and then immediately apply the occlusive agent (49). In this way, more moisture will be trapped in the skin.

Occlusives also may act by reestablishing the integrity of the stratum corneum. It is believed that prolonged occlusion (a plastic film used 6–14 nights) enhances the metabolic rate in the epidermis, thereby increasing production of protein and low molecular weight, water-soluble materials that become part of the stratum corneum (50). Substances that restore damaged keratin quickly are preferable to occlusives with long-term action.

Frequency of application depends on the severity of the dry skin condition as well as the hydration efficiency of the occlusive agent. In the case of dry hands, the patient may need to apply the occlusive agent after each hand-washing and at numerous other times during the day. Care must be exercised to avoid excessive hydration or maceration. In addition, although most commercial formulations generally are bland, contact with the eye or with broken or abraded skin should be avoided because irritation from formulation ingredients is possible in these cases. This is especially true with emulsion systems because the surfactants in these systems may denature protein. Moreover, recent studies imply that so-called "inert" vehicles may have an effect on wound healing, either accelerating or retarding it, depending on the vehicle used (51, 52).

Petrolatum seems to be the most effective occlusive agent and tentatively has been given Category I status as a skin protectant. Unfortunately, it is not well accepted by the consumer because of its greasiness and staining properties. Mineral oil is not as effective a barrier as petrolatum, and silicones are even less effective than mineral oil (53, 54). Because of its high occlusive ability, petrolatum should not be applied over puncture wounds, infections, or lacerations because maceration and further inflammation may occur under the seal. The same precaution should be taken with dimethicone.

Lanolin is found in many nonprescription moisturizing products. It is a natural product, derived from sheep wool. Some patients develop an allergic reaction to this substance, presumably because of its wool wax fraction. For this reason, lanolin has been omitted from many ointment preparations. Patients with a previous history of allergic reactions to topical medications apparently have a greater risk of developing an allergic reaction to lanolin. Through examining the patient's medication history, the pharmacist may identify such patients and advise accordingly.

There is a general lack of consumer appeal for oleaginous products because of the greasy texture and difficulty of spreading. In most cases, the less effective but more esthetic oil-in-water emulsions are preferred. These agents help alleviate the pruritus associated with dry skin by virtue of their cooling effect as the water evaporates from the skin surface. Moreover, there is sufficient oil in most oil-in-water emulsions to form a continuous occlusive film on the skin surface with the aid of waxes, gums, and other formulating agents (55). This film forms after the water has evaporated.

The second type of emulsion system is the water-in-oil emulsion. These products feel greasier than oil-in-water emulsions. Whether one emulsion form is safer and more effective than the other has not been determined. The thickness of the oil film on the skin from an oil-in-water emulsion is less than that from a water-in-oil emulsion because the former product contains less oil. However, other ingredients in the product may contribute to correcting the dry skin condition (33, 56).

Keratin-Softening Agents

Chemically altering the keratin layer softens the skin and cosmetically improves its appearance. This treatment approach does not need substantial addition of water, but all of the attendant dry skin symptoms may not be alleviated unless water is added to the keratin layer. Agents used as softeners in nonprescription dry skin products are urea, lactic acid, and allantoin (46).

Urea (Carbamide) Urea (10–30%) is mildly keratolytic and increases water uptake in the corneum, giving it a high water-binding capacity (57, 58). Moreover, this small molecule apparently has a direct effect on stratum corneum elasticity because of its ability to bind to skin protein (59). Urea accelerates fibrin digestion at about 15% concentration and is proteolytic at 40%. It is considered safe and has been recommended for use on crusted necrotic tissue. Concentrations of 10% have been used on simple dry skin; 20–30% systems have been used for treating difficult dry skin conditions, such as those seen in podiatric practice. Urea-containing creams are claimed to produce good hydration and help remove scales and crusts (49). They also have the advantage of being less greasy than some occlusive preparations. In some instances, urea preparations cause stinging and burning and may be irritating to sensitive patients. Animal or human urine has been used for centuries in treating dry skin, presumably because of the urea content.

Lactic Acid Lactic acid (2–5%) is an alpha-hydroxy acid that has been useful in the treatment of dry skin conditions. Lactic acid apparently increases the hydration of human skin and may act as a modulator of epidermal keratinization rather than as a keratolytic agent (60). The carboxyl group of the molecule seems to be indispensible for keratinization control, and structure–activity relationships for various alpha-hydroxy acids have been established (61). It is thought that alpha-hydroxy acids may serve as natural regulators of epithelial function and therefore have the potential of being ideal pharmacologic agents (24).

Allantoin Allantoin (0.5–2.0%) and allantoin complexes are claimed to soften keratin by disrupting its structure. Allantoin is a product of purine metabolism and is considered a relatively safe compound but apparently is less effective than urea. It may be useful for individuals sensitive to various topical preparations because it is purported to form complexes with a variety of sensitizing agents, rendering them nonsensitizing (62). The advisory review panel has tentatively recommended that allantoin be considered safe and effective as a skin protectant for adults, children, and infants when applied in concentrations of 0.5–2.0%.

Topical Hydrocortisone

Topical hydrocortisone (0.5%) may be used in the treatment of dry skin if inflammation and its attendant pruritus are present. An ointment should be selected because of its emollient effect. However, the inflammation and pruritus associated with dry skin are best treated by alleviating their cause (restoring normal skin hydration). Therefore, a more direct approach to the problem is to use moisturizers and keratin-softening ingredients.

Secondary Formulation Ingredients

The main active ingredients contained in nonprescription dry skin products are simply water and oil. However, an overwhelming number of secondary ingredients are added to enhance product elegance and stability:

- **Emulsifiers**
  Cholesterol
  Magnesium aluminum silicate
  Polyoxyethylene lauryl ether (Brij)
  Polyoxyethylene monostearate (Myrj)
  Polyoxyethylene sorbitan monolaurate (Tween)
  Propylene glycol monostearate
  Sodium borate plus fatty acid
  Sodium lauryl sulfate
  Sorbitan monopalmitate (Span)
  Triethanolamine plus fatty acid

- **Emulsion stabilizers (thickening agents)**
  Carbomer
  Cetyl alcohol
  Glyceryl monostearate
  Methylcellulose
  Spermaceti
  Stearyl alcohol

- **Preservatives**
  Cresol
  Parabens

Many secondary formulation ingredients have the potential for producing contact dermatitis, either through an irritant or sensitizing effect. For example, sodium lauryl sulfate, polysorbates, and sorbitan esters may serve as dermal irritants; ethylenediamine, parabens, or naturally occurring fatty substances may generate allergic reactions. From a toxicity standpoint, these ingredients cannot be assumed inert.

Product Selection Guidelines for Dry Skin

When deciding on which product to recommend for a dry skin condition, the pharmacist should consider three factors: the efficacy of individual products, the area to which the agent will be applied, and patient acceptance. One of the most efficacious products for dry skin care is petrolatum. Moreover, many elderly patients seem to tolerate it better than some of the more elegant preparations (49). Other effective alternatives include Eucerin, Nivea Cream, Purpose Dry Skin Cream, and urea-containing products such as Aquacare/HP. Urea products not only are effective, but have the advantage of being less greasy than many of the occlusive agents.

A large number of cosmetic dry skin formulations are available on the market. These may contain natural oils, vitamins, or a variety of fragrances that have a psychologic appeal. However, the fragrances and dyes found in many of these formulations may be irritating to sensitive dry skin.

Efficacy may need to be sacrificed to achieve patient acceptance of a product. Greasy products may be unacceptable if they are applied to the face, hands, feet, or intertriginous (skin fold) areas. In such cases, gels or oil-in-water emulsions may be useful. Gels and lotions also may be used if the area of application is quite hairy. The pharmacist should recommend the most efficacious product that the patient will accept.

DANDRUFF

Dandruff is a chronic, noninflammatory scalp condition characterized by excessive scaling of scalp tissue (63). Subjective estimates of its incidence range widely (2.5–70% of the population) (64, 65). However, on the basis of visual observation and objective corneocyte count, about 18% of the population has moderately severe dandruff or worse, and another 18% has mild dandruff (66, 67).

Dandruff is not a disease; rather, it is a normal physiologic event much like growth of hair and nails, except that the end product is visible on the scalp and has substantial cosmetic and social impact. It appears at puberty, when many skin activities are altered, reaches a peak in early adulthood, levels off in middle age, and declines in advancing years. The process correlates with the proliferative activity of the epidermis.

Symptoms

Dandruff is characterized by accelerated epidermal cell turnover (epidermopoiesis), an irregular keratin breakup pattern, and the shedding of cells in large flakes. Pruritus may also occur. It is normal for epidermal cells on the scalp to continually slough off just as on other parts of the body. However, the epidermal cell turnover rate in normal individuals is greater on the scalp than on other parts of the body and involves the infundibulum of the hair follicle (68, 69). In dandruff patients, the epidermal cell turnover rate is about twice that in individuals without dandruff.

Flaking seems to be the only visible manifestation of dandruff. This is a result of an increased rate of horny substance production on the scalp and the sloughing of large scales (squamae). Dandruff flakes often appear around a hair shaft because of the epithelial growth at the base of the hair, which restricts elimination of sloughed keratin. The flakes appear white because of air in the clefts between the cellular fragments. This phenomenon does not occur in the normal condition because the horny substance breaks up in a much more uniform fashion (63). The scalp horny layer in normal individuals consists of 25–35 fully keratinized, closely coherent cells per square millimeter arranged in an orderly fashion. However, in dandruff, the intact horny layer has fewer than 10 normal cells per square millimeter and nonkeratinized cells are common. With dandruff, crevices occur deep in the stratum corneum, resulting in cracking, which generates large flakes. If the large clumps or flakes can be broken down to smaller units, the visibility of dandruff decreases.

As the rate of keratin cell turnover increases, the number of incompletely keratinized cells (parakeratotic cells) increases. Parakeratosis is characterized by retention of nuclei in keratin layer cells. The number of these cells helps distinguish dandruff from psoriasis or seborrhea; there are more cells in psoriasis and seborrhea than in the dandruff condition. Parakeratotic cells in dandruff appear in clusters, possibly as a result of tiny inflammation foci that are incited when capillaries squirt a load of inflammatory cells into the epidermis, causing accelerated epidermal growth in a small area (70). These microfoci are found in all scalps but are increased proportionately in dandruff.

The specific cause of the accelerated cell growth seen in dandruff is unknown. It is not due, as had been earlier theorized, to microorganisms. For many years it was assumed that dandruff was a result of elevated microorganism levels, particularly of the yeast, *Pityrosporom ovale*, on the scalp (65, 71). However, the presence of these organisms does not lead to dandruff, nor does their elimination influence the condition (72). Their accelerated growth occurs as a result of the dandruff condition, which provides a favorable growth medium. Despite the absence of a causative link between microorganisms and dandruff, certain antidandruff products contain antimicrobial ingredients such as benzalkonium chloride, povidone–iodine, and diiodo-

hydroxyquin. The questionable statement, "to prevent secondary infections," is not altogether acceptable as a rationale for inclusion of these agents.

Assessment of Dandruff

Dandruff is a trivial medical problem, and treatment is fairly straightforward. Some characteristic features may help the pharmacist in distinguishing dandruff from other, more serious skin conditions such as seborrhea and psoriasis (66):

- Dandruff is seasonal; it is mild in the summer months and most severe from October through December.

- Unlike seborrhea and psoriasis, dandruff is considered noninflammatory and is limited to the scalp.

- Dandruff is uniform and diffuse in its distribution. Patchiness occurs only as a result of brushing the hair, which dislodges adherent flakes.

- Dandruff is a very stable process and is not subject to sudden shifts in severity from week to week. It is less subject to outside stress than psoriasis and seborrhea.

- Although poor hygiene does not cause dandruff in a nondandruff patient, it can exacerbate existing symptoms.

Table 6 lists distinguishing features of dandruff, seborrhea, and psoriasis. In addition to these rather general differences, there are more elaborate cytologic differences (73). For the pharmacist without access to extensive laboratory diagnostic aids, the site of the condition, the influence of external factors, and the overall severity of the condition are often useful in distinguishing the conditions.

Treatment of Dandruff

There is no cure for dandruff, only control of the condition. Total removal of hair eliminates the dandruff condition, but this approach is obviously rather drastic and generally unacceptable. Washing the hair and scalp frequently, perhaps daily, often is sufficient to control dandruff. Nonprescription dandruff products contain specific agents to reduce epidermal turnover rate, lyse keratin aggregates, disperse scales into smaller subunits, relieve itching, and serve as antimicrobials.

To control a dandruff condition, patients may change from one antidandruff product to another. This is rational as long as the patient changes to a product with a different mechanism of action.

Cytostatic Agents

Using cytostatic agents is the most direct approach to controlling dandruff. By increasing the time necessary for epidermal turnover, it is possible to bring about a dramatic decline in visible scurf. Selenium sulfide and zinc pyrithione at concentrations of 1 to 2% reduce cell turnover rate significantly. This cytostatic activity is not restricted to conditions where the rate of epidermal turnover is great, but also is observed in normal skin, where application of these compounds proportionately lengthens turnover time. Each product has its own mechanism of action for accomplishing this. Selenium sulfide is thought to have a direct antimitotic effect on epidermal cells, whereas zinc pyrithione's action is more likely due to a nonspecific toxicity for epidermal cells. The pyrithione moiety is apparently the active part of the molecule (74). Zinc pyrithione is considered by some to be slower acting than selenium sulfide, but this suggestion has not been proven (66, 69). At nonprescription concentrations, both products are safe and effective in controlling dandruff, and have been placed into Category I by the FDA advisory review panel on OTC miscellaneous external drug products. (See Table 7 for a list of the other tentative recommendations of the panel.)

The product's effectiveness is influenced by several factors. Zinc pyrithione is strongly bound to both hair and the external skin layers, and the extent of binding correlates with clinical performance (75). The drug does not penetrate into the dermal region. Its absorption increases with contact time, temperature, concentration, and frequency of application. Before using one of these products, the patient may be advised to shampoo with a cleansing agent to remove dirt and scale. This may be followed by a zinc pyrithione shampoo, worked into the scalp vigorously for 5–10 minutes, and repeated 2 or 3 times weekly.

Long-term use of 1 to 2% zinc pyrithione shampoos has not been associated with toxicity. This may be related to the fact that zinc pyrithione is relatively insoluble in water and is not easily absorbed through the skin or mucous membranes. Nevertheless, pharmacists should caution against using this agent on broken or abraded skin. Rare cases of contact dermatitis have been reported.

Selenium sulfide, like zinc pyrithione, is more effective with longer contact time and should be applied in a similar manner. This product must be rinsed from

---

TABLE 6 Distinguishing features of dandruff, seborrhea, and psoriasis

Characteristic	Dandruff	Seborrhea	Psoriasis
Location	Scalp	Scalp and other areas of the body, for example, axilla	Scalp and other areas of the body, particularly those prone to stress (elbows, knees, scalp, and face)
Influence of external factors	Generally a stable condition, does not fluctuate from week to week	Influenced by many external factors, notably stress	Influenced by irritation and other external stress
Inflammation	Absent	Present	Present
Epidermal hyperplasia	Absent	Present	Present
Epidermal kinetics	Turnover rate is two times faster than normal[a]	Turnover rate is about five to six times faster than normal[a]	Turnover rate is about five to six times faster than normal[a]
Percentage of parakeratotic cells	Rarely exceeds 5% of total corneocyte count[b]	Commonly makes up 15–25% of corneocyte count[b]	Commonly makes up 40–60% of corneocyte count[a]

[a]Adapted from K. J. McGinley et al., *J. Invest. Dermatol.*, *53*, 107 (1969).
[b]Adapted from A. M. Kligman et al., *J. Soc. Cosmet. Chem.*, *25*, 73 (1974).

TABLE 7 Tentative FDA classifications of OTC ingredients used for the treatment of dandruff, seborrheic dermatitis, cradle cap, and psoriasis[a]

Compound	Category	Uses[b]
Alkyl isoquinolinium bromide	III	D
Allantoin	III	D,S,P
Benzalkonium chloride	III	D
Benzethonium chloride	III	D,C
Benzocaine	II	P
Borate preparations	II	D,S
Captan	III	D
Chloroxylenol	III	D,S
Coal tar preparations	I, III[c]	D,S,P
Colloidal oatmeal	II	D
Cresol	II	P
Ethohexadiol	III	D
Eucalyptol	III	D
Hydrocortisone preparations	III	D,S,P
Juniper tar	III	D,S,P
Lauryl isoquinolinium bromide	III	D
Menthol	III	D,S,P
Mercury oleate	II	P
Methylbenzethonium chloride	III	C
Methyl salicylate	III	D
Phenol and phenolate sodium	III	S,P
Pine tar preparations	III	D,S,P
Povidone–iodine	III	D,S
Resorcinol	II	S,P
Salicylic acid	I	D,S,P
Selenium sulfide	I	D
Sodium salicylate	III	D,S
Sulfur	I	D
Thymol	III	D
Undecylenate preparations	III	D,S,P
Zinc pyrithione	I	D,S

[a] Excerpted from *Federal Register, 47,* 54655-6 (1982).

[b] C = Cradle cap, D = Dandruff, S = Seborrheic dermatitis, P = Psoriasis

[c] Category I for use in shampoos only. Category III for other uses.

the hair thoroughly or discoloration may result. Frequent use of selenium sulfide tends to leave a residual odor and make the scalp oily. The pharmacist may advise the patient to follow the selenium sulfide shampoo with a cream rinse or conditioner to help counteract any undesirable effects. This, however, may reduce the efficacy of the therapeutic shampoo (76, 77).

In general, cytostatic toxicity is minimal. Selenium sulfide, however, has been associated with several adverse effects; skin burns, particularly under the fingernails, and some cases of conjunctivitis have been reported. Pharmacists should caution the patient to avoid

contact with the eyes and broken skin. Selenium sulfide is highly toxic if ingested orally.

Keratolytic Agents

Keratolytic agents are used in dandruff products to loosen and lyse keratin aggregates, which facilitates their removal from the scalp in smaller particles. They presumably act by dissolving the cement that holds epidermal cells together. There are many types of keratolytics, with distinctly different modes of action. Resorcinol is presumed to act as a keratolytic by its irritant effect, which causes vesicle formation in the stratum corneum. Sulfur is believed to function by an inflammatory process, causing increased sloughing of cells. Salicylic acid lowers skin pH, causing increased hydration of keratin and thus facilitating its loosening and removal. Allantoin also is claimed to have chemical debriding properties.

Vehicle composition, contact time, and concentration are important considerations to the success of a keratolytic. Salicylic acid functions best as a keratolytic when used in an oil-in-water emulsion base (78–81), whereas sulfur shows its best activity in a nonemulsion base. Contact time is minimal in a shampoo. Therefore, significant absorption/adsorption of the agent by the skin cannot occur. Ointments applied a few times per day and left on are naturally much more effective. However, because ointments and pastes are difficult to use on the hairy scalp, aqueous and alcoholic preparations are preferred.

The keratolytic concentrations in nonprescription scalp products are not sufficient to impair the normal skin barrier but do affect the abnormal parakeratotic stratum corneum (82). Salicylic acid at a concentration of 10–15% shows a keratolytic effect in 2 or 3 days; 3–5% concentrations take 7 days; and 1% concentrations (the usual concentration in nonprescription shampoos is 1 to 2%) take 10 days. Sulfur acts similarly. A 10–20% concentration is keratolytic after 1 or 2 days, 5% in 7 days, 3% in 8 or 9 days, and 1% in 14 days. The *Medical Letter* has classified antidandruff keratolytic products as being moderately effective in controlling dandruff (77).

Keratolytic agents are associated with several adverse side effects, and the pharmacist should counsel the patient accordingly. These agents have a primary irritant effect, particularly on mucous membranes and the conjunctiva of the eye. Toxic manifestations after application of resorcinol to broken or abraded skin have been reported (83, 84). These agents also have the potential of acting on hair keratin as well as skin keratin, and hair appearance may suffer as a result.

The advisory review panel has recommended that salicylic acid (2–3%) and sulfur (2–5%) be placed in Category I for dandruff treatment. This rating also applies to products containing both ingredients. Resorcinol, allantoin, and sodium salicylate all are considered to be safe, but efficacy data are lacking.

Detergents

Detergents normally are not considered to be active ingredients in nonprescription dandruff products. However, for mild forms of dandruff, vigorous washing with a nonmedicated shampoo at frequent intervals (every 1–3 days) may help control excess scaling. Massaging the scalp produces an immediate dispersion of scales into smaller, less visible subunits. Detergents may contribute to this effect by virtue of their surfactant activity. The detergent residue left on the scalp after shampooing is thought to interrupt the lipid-horny cell layer structure at the keratin layer surface, causing subsequent sloughing of keratin in smaller subunits. Detergents found in shampoos include sodium lauryl sulfate, polyoxyethylene ethers, triethanolamine, and quaternary ammonium compounds such as benzalkonium chloride, benzethonium chloride, and isoquinolinium bromides.

Patients should be instructed to massage the scalp vigorously during shampooing and to allow the shampoo to remain on the scalp for several minutes. This is followed by a thorough rinse because, although a detergent residue is beneficial to a point, soaps and other components of shampoos may act as a "glue," joining together small flakes to make larger, more visible ones.

Tar Products

Coal tars may have been used since ancient times for their antidandruff properties. Their activity seems to be dependent on dispersion of scales (66) and an ability to reduce the number and size of epidermal cells produced. Various mechanisms of action for these therapeutic effects have been proposed and reported (10). The advisory review panel has concluded that coal tar shampoos are both safe and effective in controlling dandruff.

Although traditional dermatologic agents, coal tars have undesirable side effects such as photosensitization and staining of the skin and hair, especially in patients with blonde, bleached, or gray hair. For further information regarding side effects of coal tar, please see the corresponding section under the discussion of psoriasis. In general, the color, odor, and staining properties of these products tend to make them cosmetically unacceptable.

Antipruritics

Many aromatic substances have been included in nonprescription dandruff products for their alleged antipruritic activity. It is thought that they act as counterirritants or by substituting a cool sensation for that of itching. Menthol (0.04–1.5%), eucalyptol (0.09%), juniper tar (up to 5%), resorcinol (2%), phenol (up to 1.2%), methylsalicylate (0.06%), and pine tar (0.3–8%) fall into this category. All are considered to be safe when applied to the scalp in the specified concentrations. However, they may cause local irritation, and patients should be instructed to avoid contact with the eyes and rinse their eyes immediately should this occur. They also may be dangerously toxic if ingested orally.

The advisory review panel believes that the temporary relief of itching does not amount to effective control of dandruff (10). Because efficacy data are lacking, each of these substances has been placed into either Category II or III.

Topical hydrocortisone (0.25–1%) has been promoted for the temporary relief of itching. Numerous controlled and uncontrolled studies provide strong evidence for its efficacy as an antipruritic agent when used in concentrations of 1% or more. However, data are lacking to demonstrate effectiveness in treating dandruff at the lower concentrations used in nonprescription products. For this reason, the advisory review panel has recommended that topical hydrocortisone be placed in Category III. Because dandruff is a noninflammatory condition, the use of topical hydrocortisone should be discouraged.

Antimicrobials

Despite the absence of a causative link between microorganisms and dandruff, certain antidandruff products contain antimicrobial ingredients such as quaternary ammonium compounds, povidone–iodine, diiodohydroxyquin, boric acid, captan, and aromatic compounds including chloroxylenol, cresol, and thymol among others. The value of some of these agents may be due more to dispersion of flakes than to other activity. Because a definitive relationship between microbial reduction and controlling dandruff has not been established, each of these substances has been placed into Category II or III by the advisory review panel. Boric acid has the additional problem of being unsafe because of potential significant absorption through damaged skin. The questionable statement, "to prevent secondary infection," is not altogether acceptable as a rationale for inclusion of any of these agents.

Product Selection Guidelines for Dandruff

When deciding on which product to recommend for dandruff, the pharmacist may follow these simple guidelines:

- The patient first should increase the frequency of shampooing to once every 1–3 days, using the usual product. The hair should be rinsed thoroughly after shampooing.

- If increased frequency of shampooing does not control the condition, a zinc pyrithione-containing product may be used 2 or 3 times per week. Selenium sulfide is a suitable alternative. Improvement may be noted within several weeks. Because their activity increases with longer contact time, medicated shampoos should be left on the scalp for 5–10 minutes before rinsing.

- Keratolytic agents and other medicated shampoos may be used, but do not appear to have any advantage over the more effective cytostatic agents.

Dandruff is a normal physiologic event, and total control using therapeutic agents may not be possible. The patient must be reassured that the condition eventually runs its course and will decline in severity.

SEBORRHEIC DERMATITIS

Seborrheic dermatitis (seborrhea) is a general term for a group of eruptions that occur predominantly in the areas of greatest sebaceous gland activity (the scalp, face, and trunk). Nonprescription therapy is effective in many cases. Through an understanding of the symptoms of seborrhea and the appropriate therapy, the pharmacist may play a key role in its management.

Symptoms

Seborrhea is marked by accelerated epidermal proliferation and sebaceous gland activity. The distinctive characteristics of the disorder are its common occurrence in hairy areas (especially the scalp), the appearance of well-demarcated, dull yellowish-red lesions, and the associated presence of greasy or dry scales (85). Pruritus is not uncommon. Seborrhea may occur in children, but it is more common in middle-aged groups and the elderly, particularly males. The most common form is seborrhea capitis, which is characterized by greasy scales on the scalp, frequently extending to the middle one-third of the face with subsequent eye involvement. (See *Plate 7–28*.) Lesions also may appear in the external auditory canal and around the ear. When seborrhea capitis occurs in newborns and infants dur-

ing the first 12 weeks of life, it is referred to as "cradle cap." Pruritus generally does not accompany cradle cap, and the condition often clears spontaneously by 8–12 months of age. (86).

Etiology

The cause of seborrhea is unknown. A constitutional predisposition seems to exist, and emotional or physical stress may serve as aggravating factors (87). Proposed etiologic factors have included vitamin B deficiency, food allergies, autoimmunity, and climate changes (88). The characteristic accelerated cell turnover and enhanced sebaceous gland activity give rise to the prominent scale displayed in the condition, although there is no quantitative relationship between the degree of sebaceous gland activity and susceptibility to seborrhea. Hence, predisposing factors are complex.

It is almost universally accepted that seborrhea is merely an extension of dandruff. Some researchers, however, dissent from this view, offering evidence that seborrhea is a separate condition from simple dandruff (66). Nucleocytes (parakeratotic cells) commonly make up 15–25% of the corneocyte count in seborrheic dermatitis but rarely exceed 5% in dandruff. This evidence and other distinguishing features of the two conditions are shown in Table 6.

Assessment of Seborrhea

The differential diagnosis of seborrheic dermatitis is not always simple. Other disorders that need to be considered include dandruff, psoriasis, atopic dermatitis, and fungal infections. Fortunately, misdiagnosis of the seborrheic condition as dandruff is not of great consequence because both involve accelerated epidermal turnover with scaling as the principal manifestation. Therefore, treatment is generally the same in both cases. However, some unique aspects of seborrheic capitis are worth noting. Dandruff is considered a relatively stable condition, whereas seborrhea fluctuates in severity, often as a result of stress. Involvement of eyebrows and eyelashes with associated eyelid problems, such as blepharitis, is common in seborrhea but not in dandruff. Another distinguishing feature is the fact that dandruff is a noninflammatory condition, whereas seborrhea is accompanied by erythema and sometimes by crusting (89).

The best distinguishing characteristic to differentiate seborrhea from psoriasis is the location of the lesions. Seborrhea commonly involves the face and generally is not found on the extremities, whereas psoriasis is rarely found on the face and has a tendency to appear on the elbows and knees. The scalp generally is involved in both conditions, and if this is the only site of involvement, differential diagnosis is difficult. The term "seborrhiasis" has been coined to describe this condition. The appearance of the scales may help to distinguish the two disorders; seborrhea usually is marked by greasy, thick yellow scales, and psoriatic scales are generally dry and silvery in appearance.

Atopic dermatitis, like psoriasis, may be distinguished from seborrhea on the basis of scale appearance and location of the lesions; atopic dermatitis commonly occurs in the folds of the arms or knees and itching is generally more intense than in seborrhea. Moreover, patients presenting with atopic dermatitis often have a history of atopic disease, such as asthma or hayfever. Thus, by taking a medical history, the pharmacist may help determine the probable etiology of the condition.

Fungal infections constitute a fourth condition that may be mistaken for seborrhea. Proper diagnosis is important, for seborrheic therapy using hydrocortisone may worsen fungal infections. If the lesion is located in the groin, tinea cruris (jock itch) must be considered, especially during warm weather. Scalp lesions must be evaluated for the possibility of tinea capitis (ringworm of the scalp). Tinea capitis spreads peripherally and leads to partial alopecia.

Treatment of Seborrhea

The treatment of seborrhea capitis is generally the same as the treatment of dandruff. Both conditions respond to keratolytic preparations, tars, selenium sulfide (1–2%), and zinc pyrithione (1–2%). After an initial cleansing shampoo to remove scales, one of these agents may be applied to the scalp vigorously for 5–10 minutes. This may be repeated 2 or 3 times a week for best results.

Frequent use of selenium sulfide tends to make the scalp oily and may actually aggravate the seborrheic condition. If the patient has a very oily scalp, a more drying shampoo such as Sebulex (2% salicylic acid and 2% sulfur) may be beneficial (88).

If the seborrhea spreads to the ear canal or the eyelids, a physician should be consulted for appropriate therapy. Control of the scalp condition as well as the use of specific otic and ophthalmic agents is warranted.

The main difference between the treatment of dandruff and seborrhea is the use of topical steroids in the latter. Hydrocortisone lotions for scalp dermatitis are now available without a prescription. These products are not indicated for the dandruff condition, but they

may play a useful role in seborrhea management.

The use of topical hydrocortisone in seborrhea capitis should be reserved for those cases that have not responded to therapy with shampoos. The patient may be instructed to apply the hydrocortisone product once a day at the onset of therapy and then intermittently to control acute exacerbations of the disease.

The pharmacist should instruct the patient in the proper technique of applying the hydrocortisone lotion to the scalp. The hair should be parted and the product applied directly to the scalp and massaged in thoroughly. This process is repeated until desired coverage is achieved. The absorption of medication into the scalp will be enhanced if the lotion is applied after shampooing, for skin hydration will promote drug absorption.

Frequent and continued use of hydrocortisone in the treatment of seborrhea capitis is to be discouraged, for topical steroids are capable of producing a rebound dermatitis when therapy is discontinued. If the condition worsens or if symptoms persist for more than 7 days, a physician should be consulted. The patient should be instructed to rely primarily on shampooing to control the disease, and to use hydrocortisone only when necessary (88).

The treatment of cradle cap should be under a physician's direction because of the young age of the patients involved. Frequent shampooing and scrubbing with products that contain sulfur and salicylic acid generally is satisfactory. Removal of thick, adherent scales may be facilitated by applying slightly warmed mineral oil (86).

Benzethonium chloride (0.065–0.2%) and methylbenzethonium chloride (0.07%) are quaternary ammonium compounds contained in several nonprescription products used in treating cradle cap. Although both are considered to be safe when used in the specified concentrations, the statement "to prevent infection of cradle cap lesions by susceptible microorganisms" is not altogether acceptable as a rationale for inclusion. Efficacy data for the use of these two antiseptics in treating cradle cap is insufficient, hence a Category III rating.

In general, nonprescription products used to treat seborrhea, with the exception of those proven safe in treating cradle cap, should not be used on children under 2 years of age, except under the advice and supervision of a physician. The advisory review panel has made this recommendation because of toxicity concerns, as discussed earlier (10).

Product Selection Guidelines for Seborrhea

Seborrhea capitis often can be controlled with nonprescription products. When deciding on which product to recommend to the patient, the pharmacist may follow these simple guidelines:

- To initiate therapy, a zinc pyrithione-containing product may be used 2 or 3 times a week. Selenium sulfide and keratolytic preparations are suitable alternatives. Improvement should be seen within 2 weeks.

- If the condition fails to respond to these agents, a tar-containing shampoo may be used. Alternatively, a coal tar gel or a tar oil bath additive may be applied sparingly to the lesions 3–8 hours before shampooing (89).

- If the condition still is refractory, a hydrocortisone lotion, or gel may be applied sparingly once a day and worked into the scalp thoroughly. Improvement should be seen within 7 days.

- Recalcitrant cases and cases involving large areas of the body or children under 2 years of age should be referred to a physician for evaluation.

PSORIASIS

Psoriasis accounts for approximately 5% of all visits to dermatologists in the United States (85). Its annual cost to Americans is estimated at $248 million (90). Of particular interest to pharmacists is the fact that nonprescription drug products represent $100 million of this total figure. A thorough understanding of the symptoms of psoriasis as well as its pathophysiology, assessment, and treatment is therefore warranted.

Symptoms

Psoriasis is a papulosquamous skin disease marked by the presence of small elevations of the skin as well as scaling. Lesions are flat-topped, pink or dull red in color, and covered with silvery scales. The edge of the lesion is sharply delineated, and individual diameters may vary from a few mm to 20 cm or more (91). When psoriatic scales are removed mechanically, small bleeding points appear (Auspitz sign). Psoriatic skin is more permeable to many substances than normal skin. For example, it may lose water 8–10 times faster than normal skin. In fact, when large areas of the body surface

are involved, whole body skin water loss may be as much as 2 to 3 liters per day, in addition to normal perspiration loss. Evaporation of this volume of water requires over 1,000 calories. For this reason, psoriatic patients may show increased metabolic rates at the expense of tissue catabolism and muscle wasting (92).

Psoriatic lesions have a tendency to appear on the scalp, elbows, knees, fingernails, and the genitoanal region. Lesions frequently develop in sites of vaccination or skin tests, scratch marks, or surgical incisions, and have been reported to be produced by shock and noise. In fact, the response to skin trauma is so predictable (Koebner's phenomenon) that it can be used in diagnosis. For example, when scaling is not evident, diagnosis is difficult. However, scales may be induced by light scratching. It has been shown that both the epidermis and dermis must be damaged before the reaction occurs, and the response generally occurs in 6–18 days following the injury (93, 94).

Psoriasis assumes several different pathologic forms. Acute guttate psoriasis accounts for about 17% of psoriatic cases. It is characterized by many small lesions distributed more or less evenly over the body. These lesions may later coalesce to form large characteristic plaques. (See *Plate 7–29A, B, and C.*) Psoriasis in children is usually of the guttate variety and may be precipitated by various systemic diseases such as streptococcal tonsillitis. Acute attacks of guttate psoriasis also have been noted to occur at puberty and following childbirth. When the psoriatic condition is initiated by a guttate attack, the disease carries a better prognosis than that of a slower and more diffuse onset.

A second type of psoriasis is known as "pustular psoriasis." This type may or may not be a true form of psoriasis. It is marked by localized pustules on the palms and soles.

Psoriasis is basically a disease of the skin. The only tissues besides skin known to be clinically involved are the synovium and nails. In many patients with coexisting joint disease and psoriasis, the arthritic component is not easily distinguishable from rheumatoid arthritis. Certain psoriatic patients, however, have a unique form of arthritis, which has been dubbed psoriatic arthritis. Psoriatic arthritis is distinguished from rheumatoid arthritis in several respects. First, its onset is often in the distal rather than the proximal joints of the fingers or toes, and this involvement is almost always associated with psoriasis of the nails. Second, psoriatic arthritis is often asymmetric in its joint involvement and generally affects a fewer number of joints (95).

The duration of psoriasis is variable. A lesion may last a lifetime, or it may disappear quickly. When lesions disappear, they may leave the skin either hypopigmented or hyperpigmented. The disease course is marked by spontaneous exacerbations and remissions and tends to be chronic and relapsing.

Pathophysiology

When one examines the natural history of psoriasis in patients, several points of interest emerge. For example, there seems to be an inherited predisposition to psoriasis, because about 40% of psoriatic patients show an associated family history (96). Evidence supports an autosomal dominant mode of inheritance, and genetic markers as determined by the major histocompatibility locus antigen (HLA) system have been identified (97). In the case of psoriasis, HLA-B17 has been associated with the disease (98). Environmental factors, however, are not to be downplayed. Hot weather and sunlight have been noted to improve the condition; cold weather worsens it. Many investigators agree that emotional stress also affects psoriasis adversely (99). Another factor involved in the pathogenesis of psoriasis is endocrine function. For example, psoriasis has been noted to improve or clear during pregnancy and reappear after parturition. The bulk of information supports a multifactorial inheritance of psoriasis because both genetic and environmental components play a role in the disease.

A natural history of psoriasis goes on to reveal that no age is exempt from the condition; most cases develop in individuals 10–50 years of age. Psoriasis is approximately three times more prevalent in white people than it is in nonwhites; it is rarely found in Afro-Americans, Japanese, and American Indians. It is distributed almost equally between men and women.

The pathophysiology of the psoriatic lesion is very complex, involving not only the epidermis, but also the dermis and the body's immune system. The major pathophysiologic events involved in the disease process are accelerated epidermal proliferation and metabolic activity, proliferation of capillaries in the dermal region, and invasion of the dermis and epidermis by inflammatory cells. An understanding of these three basic processes is fundamental to an appreciation of psoriasis therapy.

Accelerated epidermal proliferation is one hallmark of psoriasis, leading to excessive scaling of the skin. Normal epidermal turnover is 25–30 days; in psoriatic plaque skin it is ≤3–4 days (100). There are two schools of thought on this phenomenon; both deal with cell cycle kinetics. The first theory is that the accelerated epidermal proliferation is due to a shortening of cell division cycle time. Data have been collected showing that the germinative cell cycle of the psoriatic cell is 12 times faster than normal (37.5 versus 457 hours) (101). These data, however, have been disputed (102). The second theory is that the germinative layer in human epidermis is composed of three distinct populations of epidermal cells. In normal skin, only one of these populations is actively cycling, but in psoriasis all three populations are recruited into active proliferation (103).

Accelerated epidermal proliferation is aided by the fact that the psoriatic lesion demonstrates extensive infolding of the dermal-epidermal junction. The greatly expanded surface area that results and the presence of 2 or 3 basal cell layers lead to a greatly exaggerated mitotic growth and epidermal thickness. The keratin produced has many parakeratotic cells, and the granular layer is absent in severe cases.

When one considers the extent of epidermal proliferation present in psoriasis, it logically follows that an expanded vascular system is needed to satisfy increasing metabolic requirements. In psoriasis, proliferation of capillaries in the dermal region occurs. The resultant capillary loops are arranged vertically at the center of the plaque and are responsible for the bleeding (Auspitz sign). It has been postulated that the psoriatic plaque may generate an angiotactic substance responsible for this capillary proliferation, enabling the lesion to expand (104, 105).

The third major pathophysiologic event in psoriasis is invasion of the dermis and epidermis by inflammatory cells. Mononuclear cells and polymorphonuclear (PMN) leukocytes can be found in the dermis; PMN leukocytes also tend to infiltrate the epidermis (106). Extracts of psoriatic scale have been shown to contain factors that can induce directed migration (chemotaxis) of these inflammatory cells (106). Moreover, mononuclear cells and PMN leukocytes from psoriatic patients have been shown to exhibit enhanced responsiveness to chemoattractants (107, 108). Lithium carbonate increases the total mass of circulating PMN leukocytes in patients and also has been associated with an induction or exacerbation of psoriatic symptoms (109, 110). The presence of inflammatory cells in psoriatic skin may induce epidermal proliferation and has led to many postulations about the possible role of the immune system in the pathogenesis of psoriasis.

The mononuclear infiltrate found in psoriatic dermal tissue is largely composed of T-lymphocytes and macrophages (111). The T-lymphocytes are thought to be responsible for cell-mediated immunity and also can suppress or assist the stimulation of antibody production. It has been postulated that there is a T-cell defect in psoriasis. More specifically, there may be a lack of suppression of the humoral immune system, leading to autoantibody production against skin antigens (112). Various data have been collected in support of an autoimmune theory of psoriasis (113).

Although much research has been done recently on the causes of psoriasis (113–118), the specific biochemical event triggering psoriatic skin formation remains unknown. Prostaglandins and polyamines as well as cyclic nucleotides are being investigated as having a possible role. It is possible that cyclic adenosine 3′:5′-monophosphate (AMP) mediates the regulation of epidermal proliferation and that there is a defect in the adenylcyclase–cyclic AMP system in psoriatic skin (119–124). It originally was thought that cyclic AMP levels were lowered in the psoriatic lesion and that this contributed to enhanced epidermal proliferation. Conflicting data, however, have been obtained, and the precise role of cyclic AMP in the pathogenesis of psoriasis has yet to be clarified (123).

Assessment of Psoriasis

Diagnosis usually is straightforward for simple psoriasis. Sites of involvement, the dry silvery appearance of the scale, and a small area of bleeding (Auspitz sign) after scale removal are characteristic. Pruritus and joint involvement also may be present. Precipitating factors such as a recent vaccination, disease, pregnancy, or trauma are useful evidence in a preliminary diagnosis.

It is important not to confuse psoriasis with other disease that may have similar symptoms but call for different treatment. When the scalp or the flexural and intertriginous areas are involved, psoriasis must not be mistaken for moniliasis or seborrhea. Identifying the fungal organism from lesion scrapings proves the presence or absence of moniliasis. Seborrhea and psoriasis sometimes are distinguished by their scale appearance and color. Psoriasis of the scalp generally produces silvery, dry, patchy, adherent scales; seborrhea usually is manifested as a yellowish, oily scale (seborrhea oleosa) and tends to be more diffuse. Moreover, in psoriasis the plaque has a full, rich, red color with a particular depth of hue and opacity not normally seen in seborrhea or dermatitis. In dark-skinned races this quality is lost. If lesions are present in the groin, axilla, and inframammary region, diagnosis based on visual inspection may be difficult. More elaborate histologic and pathologic diagnosis may be done by a physician (125–127).

Other skin diseases whose symptoms resemble those of psoriasis are localized neurodermatitis, particularly in the genitoanal region, and fungal conditions with circular or annular lesions. When psoriasis alternates with or is complicated by other diseases, such as seborrhea, diagnosis is much more difficult.

Treatment of Psoriasis

There is no cure for psoriasis, only a reduction in severity. Different stages of the disease are treated by different methods. Acute psoriatic onset characterized by severely erythematous lesions calls for soothing local therapy such as a bland, nonmedicated cream. Tars, salicylic acid, and aggressive UV radiation therapy must be avoided at this stage, because of their potential irritant effect. As the acute process subsides and the usual thick-scaled plaques appear, more potent therapy with agents such as keratolytics may be used. Many patients respond well to simple measures, but others are refractory to the most formidable treatment.

There is consensus that "guerilla tactics are better than a frontal assault," with the more powerful agents held in reserve (84). In eruptive or unstable forms of the disease, even mild sunlight may provoke a Koebner-type exacerbation. The advisory review panel recommends that only mild cases of psoriasis be self-treated. Individuals with severe cases involving large areas of the body should be under a physician's care (10). Nonprescription drugs may be an efficacious part of the physician's armamentarium, and the pharmacist must be a knowledgeable consultant. Nonprescription therapy may take the following approach:

- Discussion with the patient as to the nature of the condition (acceptance of the disease may reduce stress or emotional instability);

- Simple local measures such as bland emollients or creams and mild keratolytic products;

- Sunlight (UV radiation in suberythemal doses) and tar products;

- Topical hydrocortisone.

In addition to nonprescription products, several prescription-only medications are available. The use of these medications sometimes necessitates day care or hospitalization of the patient.

Topical Agents

Drug penetration of diseased skin is facilitated if a portion of the psoriatic plaque is removed before therapy; the area is first soaked in water, or an occlusive bandage is used after the drug is applied. Occlusion with a plastic film also alters the skin cell metabolic rate and allows reformation of the granular layer in the psoriatic plaque. Daily baths containing oil emulsions and use of bland emollients are helpful in removing scales (128). Psoriatic skin is more permeable to many substances than normal skin, resulting in rapid drug entrance. Thus, in the early stage, the disorder responds rapidly to local treatment, and then the improvement rate slows as the skin barrier approaches normalcy.

The nonprescription agents most commonly found in topical products for treatment of psoriasis are coal tar, keratolytics, and bland emollients either individually or in combination. In general, combination therapy consists of applying coal tar at night and using a keratolytic during the day. An addition to the nonprescription armamentarium is topical hydrocortisone. The advisory review panel's standard of effectiveness for these medications is their ability to permeate the skin barrier and control excessive shedding and flaking (10). As with other dermatoses, these agents are not to be used in children under 2 years of age except as directed by a physician.

Tar Products Tar products have been a very popular treatment for psoriasis over the years, and many nonprescription products are available. Crude coal tar consists of a heterogeneous mixture of many different compounds. Its mechanism of action is not known, but coal tar has been attributed with being antiseptic, antipruritic, keratoplastic (capable of building up horny substance), and photosensitizing (129).

Crude coal tar (1–5%) and UV radiation therapy have been used in the treatment of psoriasis since 1925 in a method known as the Goeckerman regimen (130). A therapeutic benefit of both the tar alone and the irradiation alone has been demonstrated, but the combination is more effective than either agent by itself, and remissions lasting up to 12 months have been reported after 2–4 weeks of therapy (131, 132). The coal tar is removed from the skin before irradiation takes place. Otherwise, the UV radiation will not reach the skin. For many years, the therapeutic response with this form of therapy was believed to be caused by phototoxicity, but this theory has been challenged (133–136). Now it is thought that the mechanism of coal tar may lie in its ability to cross-link with deoxyribonucleic acid (DNA) (90). Coal tar in combination with UV radiation also may increase prostaglandin synthesis in the skin, which may be related to its beneficial effect (90). Combinations of 1% crude coal tar with long-wavelength UV radiation and of 6% crude coal tar with UV radiation have been shown to be equally effective (137). Hence, only modest levels of coal tar are needed. Moreover, crude coal tar from high- and low-temperature sources seems equally effective (138).

Coal tar is available in many different kinds of pharmaceutical vehicles. Creams, ointments, pastes, lotions, bath oils, shampoos, soaps, and gels are available. This wide variety of products has in part resulted from an attempt to develop a cosmetically acceptable product, one that masks the unpleasant odor, color, and staining properties of crude coal tar. *Liquor carbonis detergens* (LCD) is a 20% tincture of coal tar that has been useful in the development of cosmetically acceptable tar products. It is used in concentrations of 3–15%.

Tar gels represent a unique dosage form that appears to deliver the beneficial elements of crude coal tar in a form both convenient to apply and cosmetically acceptable (90). These gels are nongreasy and nonstaining because they do not rub off on clothing. They also have the advantage of being nearly colorless. The pharmacist should caution the patient, however, that these gels may have a drying effect on the skin, necessitating use of an emollient (129).

Certain side effects are associated with the use of coal tar. These include folliculitis, staining of the skin and hair, photosensitization, and dermatitis due to irritation (139). Certain patients may even show a worsening of the condition when exposed to coal tar products.

The active photosensitizers of coal tar include acridine, anthracene, and pyridine. If the patient is currently using other photosensitizing drugs such as tetracyclines, phenothiazines, or sulfonamides, the pharmacist should give appropriate warnings. Moreover, the patient should not use extensive exposure to sunlight or sunlamps to simulate the Goeckerman regimen. This procedure requires careful monitoring of UV radiation exposure by a physician. Indeed, patients should be cautioned that the use of coal tar may increase their tendency to sunburn for up to 24 hours after application (10).

Crude coal tar and UV radiation both are thought to have carcinogenic potential particularly in the anogenital area. However, there have been no reports of an increased frequency of skin cancer in psoriatic patients treated for many years with coal tar and UV radiation (128). Nevertheless, the advisory review panel has recommended that topical coal tar products be placed in Category III for safety considerations. In the event that these agents are reclassified in Category I, the panel recommends the following label warning: "Do not use this product in or around the rectum or in the genital area or groin except on the advice of a physician" (10).

An exception for categorization was made for coal tar shampoos. Because contact time with the skin is minimal, coal tar shampoos were deemed safe enough to be placed in Category I.

Anthralin (Dithranol) Anthralin is an effective topical agent that may cause a more rapid resolution of psoriatic plaques than crude coal tar. Remissions may last for weeks to as long as 2 years. Anthralin is structurally related to acridine and is thought to act by reducing deoxyribonucleic acid (DNA) synthesis due to its intercalation between DNA base pairs (128).

Anthralin (0.2–0.8%) is used in combination with a daily coal tar bath and UV radiation exposure in a procedure known as the Ingram technique (139). Anthralin is most effective when incorporated into a stiff paste allowing prolonged adherence to the skin. These pastes, however, can be difficult to apply and have the disadvantage of not being water soluble, thereby making removal from the skin difficult (128).

Anthralin is irritating to the skin and should not be applied to normal skin, the face, genitalia, or areas of acute eruption. It also has a propensity to stain clothing and skin a purple-brown color (139). A derivative of anthralin, triacetoxyanthracene, lacks the burning and staining effects of anthralin but is less effective.

Keratolytics Keratolytics, by definition, are chemical substances that loosen keratin, thereby facilitating desquamation. They are useful in psoriasis when very thick scales are present. One of the most commonly used nonprescription keratolytics is salicylic acid (2–10%). It has been suggested that salicylic acid acts by decreasing corneocyte to corneocyte cohesion in the abnormal horny layer found in psoriatic lesions (140). Salicylic acid also has been classified as being antiseptic, photoprotective, astringent, antipruritic, anti-inflammatory, and antiepidermoplastic (141, 142). Other nonprescription keratolytics include sulfur, allantoin, and resorcinol. Salicylic acid has emerged as the most effective and least toxic of the keratolytics (139). Many patients respond to salicylic acid in cream or ointment form, applied several times per day. The advisory review panel has recommended that salicylic acid (1.8–3%) be placed in Category I for treatment of psoriasis.

Proper therapy with salicylic acid calls for consultation with the pharmacist. The patient should be told that salicylic acid is more effective if the psoriatic area is first soaked in warm water for 10–20 minutes (128). An occlusive dressing may be used. Extensive body application of concentrated salicylic acid preparations (>5%) must be avoided, or systemic toxicity may occur (90). The patient should be warned that the initial signs of systemic toxicity include nausea, vomiting, hearing changes, or mental confusion (139). Because salicylic acid is an irritant, there is concern about worsening of the psoriatic condition. Keratolytics therefore should be applied at a low concentration initially, and the dose should be increased as patient tolerance develops.

Salicylic acid is useful in the treatment of psoriasis when combined with other agents. Because it has a keratin-softening effect, it may aid the penetration of these agents into the skin (141). It has been suggested that the efficacy of salicylic acid could be improved if it were available in a slow-release vehicle or one maintaining close proximity of the compound to the skin (24).

Antipruritics Pruritus associated with psoriasis may be related to the dry skin condition that accompanies the disease. Bland emollients such as petrolatum and Aquaphor are effective hydrating agents. Moreover, the use of white petrolatum may inhibit the development of Koebner's phenomenon (94). Because many occlusives are greasy, patients may prefer the less effective, more esthetic oil-in-water emulsion creams or lotions such as Nivea, Albolene, and Lubriderm (27).

It has been suggested that the attendant pruritus of psoriasis may be alleviated with systemically administered antihistamines. However, it has yet to be established whether the itching of psoriasis is histamine mediated. Perhaps antihistamines are serving as no more than sedatives in these patients. Although sedation may be beneficial, a more direct therapy for pruritus should be sought.

Antihistamines also have been used topically to alleviate pruritus. This type of therapy should be discouraged, because of its questionable efficacy and the possibility of producing an allergic contact dermatitis.

Benzocaine has been included in several psoriasis products, presumably because of its anesthetic/antipruritic activity. However, such activity does not control the psoriatic condition, and the advisory review panel consequently has placed benzocaine into Category II. For further information regarding antipruritic agents, please see the corresponding section under the discussion of dandruff.

Topical Corticosteroids Topical corticosteroids play an important role in the management of psoriasis. These agents have several effects on cellular activity, including anti-inflammatory, antimitotic/antisynthetic, antipruritic, vasoconstrictor, and immunosuppressive effects (143). Efficacy may be enhanced by use of fluorinated compounds or an occlusive dressing. Continued use of topical steroids beyond 2 or 3 weeks may render the drug less effective in psoriasis (tachyphylaxis may occur) (139).

Certain adverse effects are associated with the use of topical steroids. These include local atrophy of the skin after prolonged use and the aggravation of certain cutaneous infections. The possibility of systemic sequelae exists and is enhanced by the use of fluorinated compounds, occlusive dressings, or application to large areas of the body (139). Because children have a greater surface area to body mass ratio, they are at greater risk of developing systemic complications. In general, however, the concentrations of hydrocortisone available in nonprescription preparations are unlikely to cause systemic sequelae.

Another problem with hydrocortisone is that there is usually a prompt rebound of psoriasis when topical steroid therapy is discontinued. The psoriasis may reappear as the more severe pustular form (128). Relapse occurs more quickly after topical corticosteroids than after tar or anthralin therapy.

Pharmacists may play a vital role in patient care by prudently advising patients about the use of nonprescription topical hydrocortisone preparations products. The patient may be instructed to apply the hydrocortisone as a thin film 2–4 times a day at the onset of therapy, and intermittently thereafter to control exacerbations. The medication should be massaged into the skin thoroughly. Continued and frequent use of hydrocortisone is to be discouraged because topical steroids may become less effective with prolonged use, promote local rebound, have potentially adverse local effects, and, most importantly, do not induce remissions of psoriasis (128). The patient should be instructed to rely primarily on other treatments, such as tars and keratolytics, for psoriasis and to use topical hydrocortisone only when necessary.

The FDA advisory review panel on OTC miscellaneous external drug products has recommended that hydrocortisone (0.25–1%) be placed in Category III for treatment of psoriasis and seborrheic dermatitis. This rating is due to a lack of efficacy data for hydrocortisone concentrations of less than 1%, and a lack of safety data for using 1% products on a nonprescription basis.

Mercurials Mercurial ingredients are included in nonprescription drug products as topical antimicrobials. Ammoniated mercury (5–10%), with or without keratolytic, and mercury oleate both have been used in the treatment of psoriasis. Their beneficial effect is doubtful, and a propensity toward causing allergic contact dermatitis and potential nephrotoxicity should restrict their use. The advisory review panel has consequently placed these agents into Category II (10, 144).

Colchicine Application of colchicine (1%) in hydrophilic ointment for several weeks has been tried. This approach is still experimental, and the possibility of toxic side effects such as tissue necrosis may limit its usefulness (145, 146).

Systemic Agents

PUVA Therapy An increasingly important mode of therapy is the use of systemic or topical psoralens in combination with UV radiation (147–153). This photochemotherapeutic process has the acronym, PUVA, which stands for psoralen (P) and long-wave UV radiation (UV-A) (320–340 nm). The most common psoralen employed in this process is 8-methoxypsoralen (8-MOP, methoxsalen), which is used in oral doses of 0.65 mg/kg, followed 2 hours later by carefully monitored exposure to long-wave UV radiation (128). This timing corresponds with the attainment of peak serum levels of the psoralen (139). Treatments are repeated 2 or 3 times weekly until clearing of the lesion occurs (an average of 20 treatments). Patients then receive weekly or biweekly maintenance therapy. Remissions averaging 22 weeks, however, have been reported even without the use of maintenance therapy (154).

Instead of oral administration, methoxsalen may be used as a 0.15–1% topical suspension applied to lesions 1 or 2 hours before UV exposure (139). Topical application, however, enhances the risk of blistering, and patients must be cautioned to avoid any sun exposure after application of the product. The topical preparation has the advantage of being clean, nonstaining, and odorless.

The mechanism of action of PUVA therapy remains elusive. It has been suggested that, under the influence of long-wave UV radiation, psoralens bind to thymidine in DNA and form interstrand cross-links, thereby inhibiting DNA replication and cell multiplication (139, 155). Another theory is that PUVA inhibits the chemotactic activity of psoriatic scale, suppressing the migration of PMN leukocytes into the lesion (156).

PUVA therapy has demonstrated its efficacy in the treatment of psoriasis. However, the safety of the procedure must also be considered. Immediate side effects that may occur include nausea, pruritus, erythema, and occasional blistering. Concomitant use of other dermal irritants may aggravate dermal toxicity, and special cautions have been called for in the treatment of patients who are using other photoactive drugs such as sulfonamide-based diuretics. A prospective study of patients receiving PUVA therapy failed to demonstrate a significantly increased rate of severe, acute toxicity in patients concomitantly using other photoactive drugs (157). However, this study was not tightly controlled, and the photoactive drugs being used by many of the patients were diuretics. Controlled studies using a balanced cross-sampling of photoactive drugs are needed to draw a general conclusion about the safety of using such drugs during PUVA therapy. Until that time, it is prudent for the pharmacist to give appropriate warnings to these patients.

Long-range side effects that may occur include the development of cataracts or cutaneous carcinoma. One study demonstrated that PUVA-treated patients had an observed incidence of cutaneous carcinoma 2.6 times that expected for an age, sex, and geographically matched population (158). This increased incidence, however, may be due to other carcinogens to which this population had been exposed, and the relative importance of PUVA for the development of these tumors is difficult to assess. Nevertheless, PUVA therapy has a potential for serious long-range side effects and should be restricted to patients with severe, recalcitrant, disabling psoriasis that is not adequately responsive to other forms of therapy.

Retinoids Retinoids consist of a group of compounds including vitamin A and its analogs. Vitamin A is believed to be involved in epidermal activity, particularly the physiologic control of keratinization. Consensus, however, is that it is ineffective in treating psoriasis. Preliminary results on topically applied tretinoin (vitamin A acid) are encouraging, but additional work is needed. Tretinoin has the disadvantage of producing considerable irritation when applied topically.

Vitamin A analogs represent a new frontier in the management of psoriasis (159–162). These agents may act by helping to normalize cell differentiation in the psoriatic lesion. An investigational oral retinoid, etretinate has been shown to be a potent antipsoriatic agent and has been used in combination with PUVA therapy (159). The combination therapy of etretinate and PUVA decreases the total energy of UV radiation required for PUVA alone, accelerates the response of psoriasis to PUVA, and is effective in certain patients who have been considered PUVA failures (161).

Side effects associated with the use of etretinate include alopecia, elevated serum transaminase levels, and dryness of the lips, mouth, and nose (160). Combination therapy employing lower doses of etretinate may decrease the incidence of such side effects.

Methotrexate   Accelerated epidermal proliferation has been cited as one pathophysiologic event of psoriasis. Methotrexate has been employed in the therapy of psoriasis because it serves as an antimitotic agent. Specifically, it is thought to inhibit DNA synthesis by blocking dihydrofolate reductase. The serious potential side effects and toxicity of systemic methotrexate are well known. Strict supervision of patients receiving methotrexate, including frequent blood analysis and regular liver biopsy, is essential (163). Results of a survey of dermatologists showed that methotrexate, hydroxyurea, and azaribine were used in chemotherapy for psoriasis by 50%, 10%, and 2% of the dermatologists polled (164). Despite this relatively high usage of methotrexate, only a small percentage of the patients were given liver biopsy and creatinine tests.

It has been postulated that topical administration of methotrexate could perhaps minimize the undesirable side effects associated with systemic therapy. Topical therapy, however, has proven ineffective. One study suggests that methotrexate acts directly on psoriatic plaque rather than systemically at some distant site (165). Therefore topical therapy is potentially efficacious. Therapeutic failures up to this point may be related to slow partitioning of the active form of the drug from experimental vehicle formulations.

Systemic Corticosteroids   The systemic use of corticosteroids is contraindicated in all but the most severe forms of psoriasis. This restricted use is due to the undesirable side effects accompanying systemic use of steroids as well as the fact that after therapy is stopped, the disease is almost certain to be worse than it was initially (166).

Product Selection Considerations for Psoriasis

When deciding on which product to recommend for a psoriatic condition, the pharmacist must consider the area to which the agent is going to be applied. The response to topical medications shows striking regional variation. The following guidelines may be used by the pharmacist to choose an appropriate product (167):

Scalp Psoriasis

Elaborate psoriasis shampoos are not necessary to control psoriasis of the scalp. Frequency of shampooing rather than the product itself is the key to effective therapy. The patient may be instructed to shampoo using any type of product. The resultant removal of scales is the goal of therapy. Tar oil bath additives or coal tar solutions may be painted sparingly to the lesions 3–12 hours before each shampoo. Tar gels also may be useful in this approach. Hydrocortisone has been claimed to have little impact on psoriasis of the scalp.

Psoriasis of the Body, Arms, and Legs

Coal tar products may be applied to the body, arms, and legs at bedtime. Because coal tar often stains clothing, the pharmacist should advise the patient to use old sheets and bed clothing. This therapy may be followed by a bath in the morning to help remove the coal tar as well as psoriatic scale.

Topical hydrocortisone may be applied to the lesions 2 or 3 times during the day. The medication should be applied sparingly and massaged into the skin thoroughly. Continued and frequent use of hydrocortisone should be discouraged.

A product containing salicylic acid may be useful if thick scales are present. It may be applied several times during the day. The pharmacist may instruct the patient to soak the area of application in warm water for 10–20 minutes before application of the medication.

Intertriginous Psoriasis

Intertriginous areas such as the armpits and genitoanal region are sensitive to irritants such as coal tar and salicylic acid. Therefore, these agents should not be used to treat psoriasis in these areas. Rather, hydrocortisone cream may be applied sparingly 2 or 3 times a day and used less frequently as improvement occurs.

Psoriasis is not a trivial medical problem, and psoriatic patients should be under a physician's care. The pharmacist's role in the management of psoriasis is that of a knowledgeable consultant.

SUMMARY

Many patients are afflicted with dermatitis, dry skin, dandruff, seborrhea, and psoriasis. It is important that patients suffering from these dermatologic problems be assessed properly before self-medication is recommended. Therapy effective in one disorder may exacerbate another. The pharmacist can perform a valuable service by helping patients determine the nature of their problem and the most effective therapy to alleviate it.

REFERENCES

1 "Textbook of Dermatology," 3rd ed., Vol. 1, A. Rook et al., Eds., Blackwell Scientific Publications, London, Eng., 1979, pp. 299–349.

2 C. L. Wang, *Lab. Rev.*, Feb., 1979, p. 17.

3 *J. Invest. Dermatol.*, *73*, 414 (1979).

4 "Textbook of Dermatology," 2nd ed., Vol. 2, A. Rook et al., Eds., Blackwell Scientific Publications, Oxford, Eng., 1975, pp. 289–290.

5 H. Baker, *Br. Med. J.*, *4*, 544 (1973).

6 D. Munro-Ashman, *Br. J. Clin. Pract.*, *17*, 537 (1963).

7 L. Fry, *Update Int.*, *1*, 113 (1974).

8 D. G. C. Presbury, *Update Int.*, *1*, 334 (1974).

9 A. M. Margileth, *Ped. Ann.*, *8*, 495 (1979).

10 *Federal Register*, *47*, 54646–84 (1982).

11 K. A. Arndt, "Manual of Dermatologic Therapeutics with Essentials of Diagnosis," Little, Brown and Co., Boston, Mass., 1978, p. 53.

12 R. B. Stoughton, *Arch. Dermatol.*, *92*, 281 (1965).

13 I. Sarkany, *Nurs. Times*, *1211*, 1212 (1971).

14 K. A. Arndt, "Manual of Dermatologic Therapeutics with Essentials of Diagnosis," Little, Brown and Co., Boston, Mass., 1978, p. 333.

15 E. Epstein, *Med. Times*, *108*, 36 (1980).

16 *Federal Register*, *47*, 39444–8 (1982).

17 S. C. Harvey, in "Remington's Pharmaceutical Sciences," 15th ed., Mack Publishing, Easton, Pa., 1975, p. 716.

18 S. A. Davis, *Med. Times*, *108*, 54 (1980).

19 *Br. J. Dermatol.*, *102*, 113 (1980).

20 *Federal Register*, *44*, 69768–866 (1979).

21 *Federal Register*, *48*, 6820–33 (1983).

22 E. Epstein, "Common Skin Disorders—A Manual for Physicians and Patients," Medical Economics, Oradell, N.J., 1979, p. 5.

23 K. A. Arndt, "Manual of Dermatologic Therapeutics with Essentials of Diagnosis," Little, Brown and Co., Boston, Mass., 1978, p. 293.

24 *J. Invest. Dermatol.*, *73*, 473 (1979).

25 E. Epstein, "Common Skin Disorders—A Manual for Physicians and Patients," Medical Economics, Oradell, N.J., 1979, pp. 3–4.

26 R. M. Handjani-Vila et al., *Cosmet. Perfum.*, *90*, 39 (1975).

27 "Dermatology," Vol. 2, S. L. Moschella et al., W. B. Saunders, Philadelphia, Pa., 1975, pp. 1062–1064.

28 G. Rajka and P. Thune, *Br. J. Dermatol*, *94*, 253 (1976).

29 "Textbook of Dermatology," 3rd ed., Vol. 2, A. Rook et al., Eds., Blackwell Scientific Publications, London, Engl., 1979, pp. 1273–1275.

30 R. H. Wildnaur et al., *J. Invest. Dermatol.*, *56*, 72 (1971).

31 J. D. Middleton and B. M. Allen, *J. Soc. Cosmet. Chem.*, *24*, 239 (1973).

32 J. D. Middleton, *Br. J. Dermatol.*, *80*, 437 (1968).

33 M. Mezei et al., *J. Pharm. Sci.*, *55*, 584 (1966).

34 H. Baker, *J. Invest. Dermatol.*, *50*, 283 (1968).

35 J. D. Middleton, *J. Soc. Cosmet. Chem.*, *20*, 399 (1969).

36 I. H. Blank and E. B. Shapiro, *J. Invest. Dermatol.*, *25*, 391 (1975).

37 I. H. Blank, *J. Invest. Dermatol.*, *18*, 433 (1952).

38 O. K. Jacobi, *Proc. Sci. Sect. Toilet Goods Assoc.*, *31*, 22 (1959).

39 K. Laden, *Am. Perfum. Cosmet.*, *82*, 77 (1967).

40 S. J. Stianse, *Cosmet. Perfum.*, *89*, 57 (1974).

41 B. F. VanDuzee, *J. Invest. Dermatol.*, *71*, 140 (1978).

42 A. M. Kligman, in "The Epidermis," W. Montagna and W. C. Lobitz, Jr., Eds., Academic, New York, N.Y., 1964.

43 D. Spruit and K. W. Malton, *J. Invest. Dermatol.*, *45*, 6 (1952).

44 D. Monash and I. H. Blank, *Arch. Dermatol.*, *78*, 710 (1958).

45 K. A. Arndt, "Manual of Dermatologic Therapeutics with Essentials of Diagnosis," Little, Brown and Co., Boston, Mass., 1978, p. 76.

46 R. L. Goldenberg, *Skin Allerg. News*, *5*, 20 (1974).

47 E. A. Taylor, *J. Invest. Dermatol.*, *37*, 69 (1961).

48 I. I. Lubowe, *West. J. Med.*, *1*, 45 (1960).

49 K. A. Arndt, "Manual of Dermatologic Therapeutics with Essentials of Diagnosis," Little, Brown and Co., Boston, Mass., 1978, p. 77.

50 R. L. Anderson et al., *J. Invest. Dermatol.*, *61*, 375 (1974).

51 W. H. Eaglstein and P. M. Mertz, *J. Invest. Dermatol.*, *74*, 90 (1980).

52 N. S. Penneys et al., *Br. J. Dermatol.*, *103*, 257 (1980).

53 G. Barnett, in "Cosmetics: Science and Technology," 2nd ed., M. S. Balsam and E. Sagarin, Eds., Wiley, New York, N.Y., 1972.

54 G. K. Steigleder and W. P. Raab, *J. Invest. Dermatol.*, *38*, 129 (1962).

55 E. M. Seiner et al., *J. Am. Podiatr. Assoc.*, *63*, 571 (1973).

56 S. Rothman, "Physiology and Biochemistry of the Skin," University of Chicago Press, Chicago, Ill., 1954, p. 26.

57 H. Ashton et al., *Br. J. Dermatol.*, *84*, 194 (1971).

58 D. P. Nash, *J. Am. Podiatr. Assoc.*, *61*, 382 (1971).

59 B. F. VanDuzee, *J. Invest. Dermatol.*, *71*, 140 (1978).

60 E. J. Van Scott and R. J. Yu, *Arch. Dermatol.*, *110*, 586 (1974).

61 E. J. Van Scott and R. J. Yu, in "The Ichthyoses," R. Marks and P. J. Dykes, Eds., Spectrum Publications, New York, N.Y., 1978, p. 3.

62 *Federal Register, 43,* 34634 (1978).

63 A. B. Ackerman and A. M. Kligman, *J. Soc. Cosmet. Chem., 20,* 81 (1969).

64 S. Bourne and A. Jacobs, *Br. Med. J., 1,* 1268 (1956).

65 F. C. Roia and R. W. Vanderwyk, *J. Soc. Cosmet. Chem., 20,* 113 (1969).

66 A. M. Kligman et al., *J. Soc. Cosmet. Chem., 25,* 73 (1974).

67 K. J. McGinley et al., *J. Invest. Dermatol., 53,* 107 (1969).

68 H. Goldschmidt and A. M. Kligman, *Arch. Dermatol., 88,* 709 (1963).

69 G. Plewig and A. M. Kligman, *J. Soc. Cosmet. Chem., 20,* 767 (1969).

70 A. M. Kligman, *Cosmet. Perfum., 90,* 16 (1975).

71 F. C. Roia and R. W. Vanderwyk, *J. Soc. Cosmet. Chem., 15,* 761 (1964).

72 J. J. Leyden et al., *Arch. Dermatol., 112,* 333 (1976).

73 H. Goldschmidt and M. A. Thew, *Arch. Dermatol., 106,* 476 (1972).

74 G. C. Priestly and J. C. Brown, *Acta Dermatovener.* (Stockh.), *60,* 145 (1980).

75 T. Okumura et al., *Cosmet. Perfum., 90,* 101 (1975).

76 C. A. Bond, in "Applied Therapeutics for Clinical Pharmacists," 2nd ed., M. A. Koda-Kimble et al., Eds., Applied Therapeutics, San Francisco, Calif., 1978, p. 857.

77 *Med. Lett. Drugs Ther., 19,* 63 (1977).

78 E. Strokosch, *Arch. Dermatol. Syphilol., 47,* 16 (1943).

79 E. Strokosch, *Arch. Dermatol. Syphilol., 47,* 216 (1943).

80 E. Strokosch, *Arch. Dermatol. Syphilol., 48,* 384 (1943).

81 E. Strokosch, *Arch. Dermatol. Syphilol., 48,* 393 (1943).

82 "Textbook of Dermatology," 3rd ed., Vol. 2, A. Rook et al., Eds., Blackwell Scientific Publications, London, Eng., 1979, p. 2310.

83 "The United States Dispensatory," 27th ed., Lippincott, Philadelphia, Pa., 1973, p. 1018.

84 K. W. Chesterman, *J. Am. Pharm. Assoc., NS12,* 576 (1972).

85 "Textbook of Dermatology," 3rd. ed., Vol. 1, A. Rook et al., Eds., Blackwell Scientific Publications, London, Eng., 1979, pp. 308–312.

86 S. Hurwitz, *Clin. Pediatr. Dermatol.,* W. B. Saunders Company, Philadelphia, Pa., 1981, p. 13.

87 K. A. Arndt, "Manual of Dermatologic Therapeutics with Essentials of Diagnosis," Little, Brown and Co., Boston, Mass., 1978, p. 173.

88 D. L. Cram, *Med. Times, 108,* 74 (1980).

89 E. Epstein, "Common Skin Disorders—A Manual for Physicians and Patients," Medical Economics, Oradell, N.J., 1979, p. 86.

90 *J. Invest. Dermatol., 73,* 402 (1979).

91 J. W. Burnett and H. M. Robinson, Jr., "Clinical Dermatology for Students and Practitioners," Yorke Medical, New York, N.Y., 1978, p. 178.

92 "Textbook of Dermatology," 3rd ed., Vol. 2, A. Rook et al., Eds., Blackwell Scientific Publications, London, Eng., 1979, p. 1333.

93 L. Stankler, *Br. J. Dermatol., 81,* 534 (1969).

94 J. S. Comaish and J. S. Greener, *Br. J. Dermatol., 94,* 195 (1976).

95 M. A. Krupp and M. J. Chatton, "Current Medical Diagnosis and Treatment," Lange Medical, Los Altos, Calif., 1981, p. 499.

96 E. M. Farber and M. L. Nall, *Dermatologica, 148,* 7 (1974).

97 L. E. Cutler et al., *Arch. Dermatol., 116,* 718 (1980).

98 R. C. Williams et al., *Br. J. Dermatol., 95,* 163 (1976).

99 R. H. Seville, *Br. J. Dermatol., 97,* 301 (1977).

100 G. Weinstein, *Br. J. Dermatol., 92,* 229 (1975).

101 G. Weinstein and P. Frost, *J. Invest. Dermatol., 50,* 254 (1968).

102 M. Duffill et al., *Br. J. Dermatol., 94,* 355 (1976).

103 S. Gelfant, *Br. J. Dermatol., 95,* 577 (1976).

104 F. S. Glickman and Y. Rapp, *Arch. Dermatol., 112,* 1789 (1976).

105 J. E. Wolf, Jr., and W. R. Hubler, Jr., *Arch. Dermatol., 113,* 1458 (1977).

106 M. V. Dahl et al., *J. Invest. Dermatol., 71,* 402 (1978).

107 G. G. Krueger et al., *J. Invest. Dermatol., 71,* 195 (1978).

108 A. Wahba et al., *Acta Dermatovener.* (Stockh.), *59,* 441 (1979).

109 I. Skoven and J. Thormann, *Arch. Dermatol., 115,* 1185 (1979).

110 G. Lazarus and R. Gilgor, *Arch. Dermatol., 115,* 1183 (1979).

111 J. R. Bjerke et al., *J. Invest. Dermatol., 71,* 340 (1978).

112 D. N. Sauder et al., *Arch. Dermatol., 116,* 51 (1980).

113 J. J. Guilhou et al., *Br. J. Dermatol., 95,* 295 (1976).

114 K. Aso et al., *J. Invest. Dermatol., 63,* 375 (1975).

115 G. Mahrle and C. E. Orfanos, *Br. J. Dermatol, 93,* 495 (1975).

116 P. D. Mier and J. Van Den Hurk, *Br. J. Dermatol., 94,* 219 (1976).

117 J. J. Guilhou et al., *Br. J. Dermatol., 94,* 501 (1976).

118 G. Mahrle and C. E. Orfanos, *Br. J. Dermatol., 95,* 591 (1976).

119 J. J. Voorhees and E. A. Duell, *Arch. Dermatol., 104,* 352 (1971).

120 R. K. Wright et al., *Arch. Dermatol., 107,* 47 (1973).

121 M. M. Mui et al., *Br. J. Dermatol., 92,* 255 (1975).

122 S. Wadskov et al., *Acta Dermatovener.* (Stockh.), *59,* 525 (1979).

123 K. Adachi et al., *J. Invest. Dermatol., 74,* 74 (1980).

124 C. L. Marcelo et al., *J. Invest. Dermatol., 72,* 20 (1979).

125 "Dermal Pathology," J. H. Graham et al., Eds., Harper and Row, New York, N.Y., 1972, pp. 325–332.

126 M. Gordon et al., *Arch. Dermatol., 95,* 402 (1967).

127 E. J. Van Scott and T. M. Ekel, *Arch. Dermatol., 88,* 373 (1963).

128 W. Watson, *Rat. Drug. Ther., 13,* 4 (1979).

129 C. Grupper, in "Psoriasis—Proceedings of the International Symposium at Stanford University," 1971, E. M. Farber and A. J. Cox, Eds., Stanford University Press, Stanford, Calif., 1971, p. 354.

130 W. H. Goeckerman, *Northwest Med., 24,* 299 (1925).

131 P. Frost et al., *Arch. Dermatol., 115,* 840 (1979).

132 D. L. Cram, *Hosp. Form., 11,* 596 (1976).

133 L. Tanenbaum et al., *Arch. Dermatol., 111,* 467 (1975).

134 L. Tanenbaum et al., *Arch. Dermatol., 111,* 395 (1975).

135 J. A. Parrish et al., *J. Invest. Dermatol., 70,* 111 (1978).

136 P. Frost et al., *Arch. Dermatol., 115,* 840 (1979).

137 A. R. Marisco et al., *Arch. Dermatol., 112,* 1249 (1976).

138 R. S. Chapman and O. A. Finn, *Br. J. Dermatol., 94,* 71 (1976).

139 B. G. Bryant, *Am. J. Hosp. Pharm., 37,* 814 (1980).

140 D. L. Roberts et al., *Br. J. Dermatol., 103,* 191 (1980).

141 E. G. Weirich, *Dermatologica, 151,* 268 (1975).

142 E. G. Weirich et al., *Dermatologica, 151,* 321 (1975).

143 *Br. J. Dermatol., 101,* 599 (1979).

144 *Federal Register, 47,* 436–42 (1982).

145 K. H. Kaidbey et al., *Arch. Dermatol., 111,* 33 (1975).

146 P. M. Gaylarde and I. Sarkany, *Arch. Dermatol., 112* (1976).

147 H. Schaefer et al., *Br. Jr. Dermatol., 94,* 363 (1976).

148 J. W. Petrozzi et al., *Arch. Dermatol., 113,* 292 (1977).

149 *Arch. Dermatol., 112,* 35 (1976).

150 T. Lakshmipathi et al., *Br. J. Dermatol., 96,* 587 (1977).

151 K. W. Wolff et al., *Arch. Dermatol., 112,* 943 (1976).

152 J. W. Melski et al., *J. Invest. Dermatol., 68,* 328 (1977).

153 J. W. Petrozzi and J. O. Barton, *Arch. Dermatol., 115,* 1061 (1979).

154 A. H. Siddiqui and R. H. Cormane, *Br. J. Dermatol., 100,* 247 (1979).

155 R. S. Cole, *Biochem. Biophys. Acta, 217,* 30 (1970).

156 N. Mizuno et al., *J. Invest. Dermatol, 72,* 64 (1979).

157 R. S. Stern et al., *Arch. Dermatol., 116,* 1269 (1980).

158 R. S. Stern et al., *N. Engl. J. Med., 300,* 809 (1979).

159 A. Lassus, *Br. J. Dermatol., 102,* 195 (1980).

160 H. J. Van Der Rhee et al., *Br. J. Dermatol., 102,* 203 (1980).

161 P. O. Fritsch et al., *J. Invest. Dermatol., 70,* 178 (1978).

162 G. Heidbreder and E. Christophers, *Arch. Dermatol. Res., 264,* 331 (1979).

163 L. E. King, Jr., *Arch. Dermatol., 111,* 131 (1975).

164 R. G. Bergstresser et al., *Arch. Dermatol., 112,* 977 (1976).

165 A. E. Newburger et al., *J. Invest. Dermatol., 70,* 183 (1978).

166 G. M. Lewis and C. E. Wheeler, "Practical Dermatology," 3rd ed., W. B. Saunders, Philadelphia, Pa., 1967, pp. 207–218.

167 E. Epstein, "Common Skin Disorders—A Manual for Physicians and Patients," Medical Economics, Oradell, N.J., 1979, p. 133.

DERMATITIS AND PSORIASIS PRODUCT TABLE

Product (Manufacturer)	Application Form	Keratolytic/ Keratin Softener	Tar Product	Other Ingredients
Alphosyl (Reed & Carnrick)	cream lotion	allantoin, 1.7%	crude coal tar extract, 5%	
Ammoniated Mercury (Various manufacturers)	ointment			ammoniated mercury, 5%
Aquatar (Herbert)	gel		coal tar extract, 2.5%	
Bactine (Miles)	cream			hydrocortisone, 0.5%
Balnetar (Westwood)	bath oil		coal tar, 5% (equivalent)	mineral oil; lanolin oil; PEG-4-dilaurate
CaldeCORT (Fisons)	cream light cream spray			hydrocortisone acetate (equivalent to hydrocortisone, 0.5%)
Cetaphil (Owen)	cleanser			cetyl and stearyl alcohol; propylene glycol; sodium lauryl sulfate; parabens
Coal Tar (Various manufacturers)	solution		coal tar, 20%	
Cortaid (Upjohn)	cream lotion ointment spray			hydrocortisone, 0.5%; aloe (cream, ointment)
Cortizone-5 (Thompson Medical)	cream ointment			hydrocortisone, 0.5%
Delacort (Mericon)	lotion			hydrocortisone, 0.5%
Denorex (Whitehall)	shampoo		coal tar solution, 9%	menthol, 1.5%; alcohol, 7.5%
Dermacort (Reid-Rowell)	lotion			hydrocortisone, 0.5%
Denorex Extra Strength (Whitehall)	shampoo		coal tar solution, 12.5%	menthol, 1.5%
DermiCort (Republic)	cream			hydrocortisone, 0.5%
Dermolate (Schering)	cream			hydrocortisone, 0.5%
Dermtex HC (Pfeiffer)	cream			hydrocortisone, 0.5%
DHS Tar (Person & Covey)	shampoo		coal tar, 0.5%	cleansing agents
DHS Tar Gel (Person & Covey)	shampoo		coal tar, 0.5%	
DHS Zinc (Person & Covey)	shampoo			zinc pyrithione, 2%

DERMATITIS AND PSORIASIS PRODUCT TABLE, continued

Product (Manufacturer)	Application Form	Keratolytic/ Keratin Softener	Tar Product	Other Ingredients
Dr. Gordshell's Salve (Thomas & Thompson)	ointment		rosin	lard; tallow; beeswax; elder flowers; bayberry; sassafras oil; benzoic acid
Duplex T (C & M)	shampoo		coal tar solution, 10%	sodium lauryl sulfate, 15%
Estar (Westwood)	gel		coal tar, 5%	alcohol, 13.8%
FoilleCort (Blistex)	cream			hydrocortisone acetate, 0.5%
H₂ Cort (Vangard)	cream			hydrocortisone, 0.5%
Hydrocortisone (Various manufacturers)	cream lotion			hydrocortisone, 0.5%
Hydro-Tex (Syosset)	cream			hydrocortisone, 0.5%
Hytone (Dermik)	cream			hydrocortisone, 0.5%
Iocon (Owen)	shampoo		coal tar solution	alcohol, 2.1%
Ionil T (Owen)	shampoo	salicylic acid, 2%	coal tar solution, 4.25%	polyoxyethylene ethers; benzalkonium chloride; alcohol; isopropyl alcohol; EDTA
Ionil T Plus (Owen)	shampoo		tar distillate, 2%	sodium laureth sulfate; lauramide DEA; quaternium-22; laureth-23; talloweth-60 myristyl glycol; TEA lauryl sulfate; glycol distearate; laureth-4; TEA-abietoyl hydrolyzed collagen; DMDM hydantoin; EDTA; fragrance; FD & C blue #1; Ext D & C yellow #7
Kay-San (Commerce)	cream	allantoin, 0.5% resorcinol, 0.4%	coal tar, 0.5%	sodium salicylate, 0.6%; parachlorometaxylenol, 0.25%
Lanacort (Combe)	cream			hydrocortisone acetate, 0.5%
Lavatar (Doak)	bath oil		tar distillate, 25%	
L.C.D. (Schieffelin)	cream		coal tar solution, 5.8%	
Lipoderm (Spirt)	capsule			pancreas, 500 mg; pyridoxine hydrochloride, 3 mg
Medotar (Medco)	ointment		coal tar, 1%	polysorbate 80, 0.5%; octoxynol-5; zinc oxide; starch; white petrolatum

DERMATITIS AND PSORIASIS PRODUCT TABLE, continued

Product (Manufacturer)	Application Form	Keratolytic/ Keratin Softener	Tar Product	Other Ingredients
Neutrogena T/ Derm (Neutrogena Dermatologics)	body oil		coal tar, 5% (equivalent)	emollient oil base
Neutrogena T/Gel (Neutrogena Dermatologics)	shampoo		coal tar, 2% (equivalent)	shampoo base
Neutrogena T/Gel (Neutrogena Dermatologics)	conditioner		coal tar, 1.5% (equivalent)	conditioner base
Neutrogena T/Gel Scalp Solution (Neutrogena Dermatologics)	emollient	salicylic acid, 2%	coal tar, 2% (equivalent)	water-washable emollient base
Neutrogena T/Sal (Neutrogena Dermatologics)	shampoo	salicylic acid, 2%	coal tar, 2% (equivalent)	shampoo base
Oxipor VHC (Whitehall)	lotion	salicylic acid, 1%	coal tar solution, 48.5%	benzocaine, 2%; alcohol, 81%
Packer's Pine Tar (Rydelle)	shampoo soap		pine tar, 0.82% (shampoo) 5.87% (soap)	
Pentrax (GenDerm)	shampoo		coal tar, 8.75%	highly concentrated detergents
Pharma-Cort (Purepac)	cream			hydrocortisone acetate, 0.5%
Polytar (Stiefel)	shampoo soap		polytar, 1%	conditioners (shampoo)
Pragmatar (SmithKline)	cream	salicylic acid, 3% precipitated sulfur, 3%	cetyl alcohol-coal tar, 4%	emulsion base
P&S Plus (Baker Cummins)	gel	salicylic acid, 2%	coal tar solution, 8%	
Psorex (DEP)	shampoo		coal tar, 1%	
Psorigel (Owen)	gel			alcohol; laureth-4; fragrance; propylene glycol; hydroxyethylcellulose
Racet SE (Lemmon)	cream			hydrocortisone, 0.5%
Rhulicort (Rydelle)	cream lotion			hydrocortisone, 0.5% (equivalent)
Sulfur-8 (Schering-Plough)	ointment	sulfur, 2%		menthol, 1%; triclosan, 0.1%; mineral oil
Tar-Doak (Doak)	lotion		tar distillate, 5%	doak oil, 10%
Tarpaste (Doak)	paste		tar distillate, 5%	zinc oxide
Tarsum Shampoo/ Gel (Summers)	shampoo	salicylic acid, 5%	coal tar solution, 10%	

DERMATITIS AND PSORIASIS PRODUCT TABLE, continued

Product (Manufacturer)	Application Form	Keratolytic/ Keratin Softener	Tar Product	Other Ingredients
Tegrin (Block)	cream lotion shampoo	allantoin, 1.7% (cream and lotion)	coal tar solution, 5%	emollient base (cream and lotion); surfactant (shampoo)
Tegrin (Block)	soap		coal tar solution, 5%	soap base
Tersa-Tar (Doak)	shampoo		tar distillate, 3%	
Vanseb-T Cream Tar Dandruff Shampoo (Herbert)	shampoo	sulfur, 2% salicylic acid, 1%	coal tar, 5%	sodium lauryl sulfate; sodium stearate; fatty alkylolamide condensate; hydrolyzed animal protein; hydrochloric acid; PEG-75 lanolin; dimethicone copolyol; imidazolidinyl urea; fragrance
Vanseb-T Lotion Tar Dandruff Shampoo (Herbert)	shampoo	sulfur, 2% salicylic acid, 1%	coal tar, 5%	sodium dodecylbenzenesulfonate; sodium C14-16 olefin sulfonate; titanium dioxide; bentonite; hydrolyzed animal protein; quaternium-33; ethyl hexanediol; imidazolidinyl urea; perfume; dimethicone copolyol
Vaseline Pure Petroleum Jelly (Chesebrough Ponds)	gel			white petrolatum, 100%
Zetar (Dermik)	shampoo		whole colloidal coal tar, 1%	chloroxylenol, 0.5%

DRY SKIN PRODUCT TABLE

Product (Manufacturer)	Application Form	Keratin Softener	Humectant	Other Ingredients
Acid Mantle (Dorsey)	cream lotion		glycerin	aluminum acetate; cetyl-stearyl alcohol; sodium lauryl sulfate; petrolatum (cream); synthetic beeswax (cream); mineral oil (cream); methylparaben
Allercreme Skin (Owen)	lotion		glycerin	mineral oil; petrolatum; lanolin; lanolin oil; lanolin alcohols; triethanolamine; cetyl alcohol; stearic acid; parabens
Allercreme Ultra Emollient (Owen)	cream		glycerin	mineral oil; petrolatum; lanolin; lanolin alcohol; lanolin oil; glyceryl stearate; PEG-100 stearate; squalane; cetyl alcohol; sorbitan laurate; quaternium-15; parabens
Alpha Keri (Westwood)	bath oil body oil			mineral oil; lanolin oil; PEG-4-dilaurate; benzophenone-3; fragrance
Alpha Keri Soap (Westwood)	soap		glycerin	sodium tallowate; sodium cocoate; mineral oil; PEG-75; titanium dioxide; lanolin oil; sodium chloride; BHT; EDTA
Alpha Keri Spary (Westwood)	spray			mineral oil; lanolin oil; alcohol, 28%; PPG-15 stearyl ether; C12-15 alcohols benzoate; PEG-4-dilaurate; polysorbate 85
Aveeno (Rydelle)	lotion		glycerin	colloidal oatmeal, 1%; allantoin, 0.5%; distearyldimonium chloride; petrolatum; isopropyl palmitate; cetyl alcohol; dimethicone; sodium chloride; benzyl alcohol
Aveeno Bath Treatment Regular (Rydelle)	powder			colloidal oatmeal, 100%
Aveeno Bath Treatment Oilated for Dry Skin (Rydelle)	powder			colloidal oatmeal, 43%; mineral oil; calcium silicate; laureth-4; lanolin alcohol
Aveeno Cleansing Bar Dry Skin (Rydelle)	bar		glycerin	colloidal oatmeal, 51%; sodium cocoyl isethionate; vegetable oil (hydrogenated); vegetable shortening; PEG-75; lauramide DEA; lactic acid; sodium lactate; sorbic acid; titanium dioxide
Aveeno Cleansing Bar Normal to Oily Skin (Rydelle)	bar		glycerin	colloidal oatmeal, 51%; sodium cocoyl isethionate; lactic acid; sodium lactate; petrolatum; magnesium aluminum silicate; potassium sorbate; titanium dioxide; PEG-14M
Aveeno Colloidal Oatmeal (Rydelle)	treatment			natural colloidal oatmeal
Aveeno Shower & Bath (Rydelle)	oil			colloidal oatmeal, 5%; mineral oil; glyceryl stearate; PEG-100 stearate; laureth-4; preservative; anti-caking agent; benzaldehyde
Balmex Emollient (Macsil)	lotion			lanolin oil, silicone, balsam Peru
Candermyl (Owen)			glycerin	oleic/palmitoleic triglycerides; polyaminoacid; sodium lactate methylsilanol; propylene glycol; polyglyceryl-3 hexadecylether; cholesterol; dicetyl phosphate; triethanolamine; carbomer 940; imidazolidinyl urea; hydrolyzed mucopolysaccharides; honey; hexylene glycol; phenoxyethanol; usnic acid; 18-beta-glycyrretinic acid; citric acid, methylchloroisothiazolinone; methylisothiazolinone; propyl gallate; parabens; fragrance

DRY SKIN PRODUCT TABLE, continued

Product (Manufacturer)	Application Form	Keratin Softener	Humectant	Other Ingredients
Carmol 10 (Syntex)	lotion	urea, 10%		nonlipid base
Carmol 20 (Syntex)	cream	urea, 20%		nonlipid base
Cetaphil (Owen)	cleanser			cetyl and stearyl alcohol; propylene glycol; sodium lauryl sulfate
Clocream (Upjohn)	cream			vitamins A and D, vanishing cream base
Complex 15 (Baker/Cummins)	cream lotion		glycerin	mineral oil; glyceryl stearate; lecithin; cetyl acetate; dimethicone; stearic acid; glycol stearate; lanolin alcohol acetate; triethanolamine; cetyl alcohol; magnesium aluminum silicate; imidazolidinyl urea; parabens; carbomer 934; EDTA
Corn Huskers (Warner-Lambert)	lotion		glycerin, 6.7%	SD alcohol 40; algin; TEA-oleoyl sarcosinate; methylparaben; guar gum; calcium sulfate; calcium chloride; TEA-fumarate; TEA-borate
Curel Moisturizing (Rydelle)	cream lotion		glycerin	quaternium-5; petrolatum; isopropyl palmitate; 1-hexadecanol; dimethicone; parabens
Cutemol (Summers)	cream			liquid petrolatum; acetylated lanolin; lanolin alcohols extract; isopropyl myristate wax; allantoin, 0.2%; sorbitan sesquioleate
Dermassage (Kendall)	lotion	urea		mineral oil; lanolin; menthol, 0.11%; TEA-stearate; propylene glycol; stearic acid; diammonium phosphate; triclosan; parabens
DOB (Person & Covey)	bath oil			mineral oil; acetylated lanolin; acetylated lanolin alcohol; isopropyl myristate; laureth-4; sorbitan sesquioleate
Domol (Miles)	bath oil			di-isopropyl sebacate; isopropyl myristate; mineral oil
Eclipse After Sun (Dorsey)	lotion		glycerin	petrolatum; oleth-3 phosphate; carbomer 934; imidazolindinyl urea; benzyl alcohol; cetyl esters wax
Emollia (Gordon)	lotion			mineral oil; cetyl alcohol; propylene glycol; white wax; sodium lauryl sulfate; oleic acid; parabens
Esoterica (SmithKline Beecham)	lotion			propylene glycol dicaprylate/dicaprate; propylene glycol; TEA-stearate; mineral oil; isocetyl stearate; glyceryl stearate; cetyl esters wax; hydrolyzed animal protein; dimethicone; TEA carbomer 941; fragrance; parabens; quaternium-15
Eucerin (Beiersdorf)	lotion			mineral oil; lanolin acid glycerin ester; lanolin alcohol; isopropyl myristate; PEG-40 sorbitan peroleate; sorbitol; propylene glycol; beeswax; magnesium sulfate; aluminum stearate
E-Vital (Pasadena)	cream			vitamins E & D; 5670 IU/60 g each; vitamin A, 14,175 IU/60 g, panthenol, 2%; allantoin, 0.2%
E-Vitamin (Forest)	ointment			vitamin E, 30 mg/g
Gordo-Vite E (Gordon)	cream			vitamin E, 50 mg/g
Gormel (Gordon)	cream	urea, 20%		
Hydrisinol (Pedinol)	cream lotion			sulfonated hydrogenated castor oil, hydrogenated vegetable oil

DRY SKIN PRODUCT TABLE, continued

Product (Manufacturer)	Application Form	Keratin Softener	Humectant	Other Ingredients
Jeri-Bath (Dermik)	bath oil			dewaxed oil-soluble fraction of lanolin; mineral oil; nonionic emulsifier
Keri Creme (Westwood)	cream			mineral oil; talc; sorbitol; ceresin; lanolin alcohol/mineral oil; magnesium stearate; glyceryl oleate/propylene glycol; isopropyl myristate; parabens; fragrance; quaternium-15
Keri Facial Cleanser (Westwood)	lotion		glycerin	squalane; propylene glycol; glyceryl stearate/PEG-100 stearate; stearic acid; steareth-20; lanolin alcohol; magnesium aluminum silicate; cetyl alcohol; beeswax; PEG-20-sorbitan beeswax; parabens; quaternium-15; fragrance
Keri Facial Soap (Westwood)	soap		glycerin	sodium tallowate; sodium cocoate; mineral oil; octyl hydroxystearate; fragrance; titanium dioxide; PEG-75; lanolin oil; dioctyl sodium sulfosuccinate; PEG-4 dilaurate; propylparaben; PEG-40 stearate; glyceryl monostearate; PEG-100 stearate; sodium chloride; BHT; EDTA
Keri Light Lotion (Westwood)	lotion		glycerin	stearyl alcohol/ceteareth-20; cetaryl octanoate; stearyl heptanoate; stearyl alcohol; squalane; carbomer 934; fragrance; sodium hydroxide; parabens; quaternium-15
Keri Lotion (Westwood)	lotion (scented and unscented)			mineral oil; propylene glycol; glyceryl stearate; PEG-40 stearate; PEG-100 stearate; PEG-4-dilaurate; laureth-4; lanolin oil; parabens; carbomer 934; triethanolamine; dioctyl sodium sulfosuccinate; quaternium-15
Keri Silky Smooth (Westwood)	lotion		glycerin	petrolatum; dimethicone; steareth-2; cetyl alcohol; benzyl alcohol; laureth-23; carbomer 934; magnesium aluminum silicate; fragrance; quaternium 15; sodium hydroxide
Lacti-Care (Stiefel)	lotion	lactic acid sodium PCA		mineral oil; isopropyl palmitate; stearyl alcohol ceteareth-20; sodium hydroxide; glyceryl stearate; PEG-100 stearate; myristyl lactate; cetyl alcohol; carbomer 940; imidazolidinyl urea; dehydroacetic acid
Lanoline (Burroughs Wellcome)	cream			lanolin w/solid and liquid petrolatum
Lanolor (Squibb)	cream			lanolin oil; glyceryl stearates; propylene glycol; isopropyl palmitate; cetyl alcohol; sodium lauryl sulfate; simethicone; PEG monostearate; cetyl esters wax; sorbic acid; methylparaben
Lobana (Ulmer)	lotion			mineral oil; triethanolamine stearate; stearic acid; lanolin; cetyl alcohol; potassium stearate; propylene glycol, parabens, fragrance
Lobana Derm-Ade (Ulmer)	cream			vitamins A, D, E in cream base with moisturizers; emollients; silicone
Lowila Cake (Westwood)	cleanser bar	urea	lactic acid	dextrin; sodium lauryl sulfoacetate; boric acid; sorbitol; mineral oil; PEG-14M; dioctyl sodium sulfosuccinate; cellullose gum; fragrance
LubraSol (Pharmaceutical Specialties)	bath oil			mineral oil; lanolin oil; PEG-200 dilaurate; oxybenzone

DRY SKIN PRODUCT TABLE, continued

Product (Manufacturer)	Application Form	Keratin Softener	Humectant	Other Ingredients
Lubriderm (Warner-Lambert)	cream lotion		glycerin (cream)	cream: mineral oil; petrolatum; glyceryl stearate; PEG-100 stearate; hydrogenated polyisobutene; lanolin; lanolin alcohol; lanolin oil; cetyl alcohol; sorbitan laurate; fragrance; parabens; quaternium-15 lotion: mineral oil; petrolatum; sorbitol; lanolin; lanolin alcohol; stearic acid; triethanolamine; cetyl alcohol; fragrance; parabens; sodium chloride
Lubriderm Lubath (Warner-Lambert)	bath oil			mineral oil, PPG-15 stearyl ether, oleth-2, nonoxynol-5
Mammol (Abbott)	ointment			bismuth subnitrate, 40%; castor oil, 30%; anhydrous lanolin, 22%; ceresin wax, 7%; peruvian balsam, 1%
Moisturel Cream (Westwood)	cream lotion		glycerin	cream: petrolatum, PG dioctanoate; cetyl alcohol; steareth-2; dimethicone; PVP/hexadecene copolymer; laureth-23; magnesium aluminum silicate; diazolidinyl urea; carbomer 934; sodium hydroxide; kathon CG lotion: petrolatum; dimethicone; steareth-2; cetyl alcohol; benzyl alcohol; laureth-23; carbomer 934; magnesium aluminum silicate; quaternium-15; sodium hydroxide
Moisturel Sensitive Skin (Westwood)	cleanser			sodium laureth sulfate and laureth 6 carboxylic acid and disodium laureth sulfosuccinate; methyl gluceth 20; cocamidopropyl betaine; diazolidinyl urea; kathon CG
Neutrogena Body (Neutrogena)	lotion oil			lotion: glyceryl stearate; isopropyl myristate; PEG-100 stearate; butylene glycol; imidazolidinyl urea; carbomer 934; parabens; sodium lauryl sulfate; triethanolamine; cetyl alcohol oil: isopropyl myristate; sesame oil; PEG-40 sorbitan peroleate; parabens
Nivea Moisturizing (Beiersdorf)	cream lotion		glycerin (cream)	cream: mineral oil; petrolatum; lanolin alcohol; microcrystalline wax; paraffin; magnesium sulfate; decyl oleate; octyl dodecanol; aluminum stearate; citric acid; magnesium stearate lotion: mineral oil; lanolin; isopropyl myristate; cetearyl alcohol; glyceryl stearate; acrylamide/sodium acrylate copolymer simethicone; methylchloroisothiazolinone; methylisothiazolinone
Nivea Skin (Beiersdorf)	oil			mineral oil; petrolatum; lanolin; lanolin acid; glycerin ester; lanolin alcohol; sodium borate; methylchloroisothiazolinone; methylisothiazolinone
Nutraderm (Owen)	bath oil cream lotion			bath oil: mineral oil; lanolin oil; PEG-4 dilaurate; benzophenone-3; butylparaben cream and lotion: mineral oil; sorbitan stearate; stearyl alcohol; sodium lauryl sulfate; cetyl alcohol; carbomer 940; parabens; triethanolamine; fragrance
Nutraderm 30 (Owen)	lotion		lactic acid malic acid sodium PCA glycerin	petrolatum; cetearyl alcohol; ceteareth-20; dimethicone; C10-30 cholesterol/lanosterol esters; cyclomethicone; cetyl alcohol; sodium lactate; cetyl lactate; C12-C15 alcohols lactate; xanthan gum; sodium hydroxide; parabens; diazolidinyl urea; fragrance
Nutraplus (Owen)	cream lotion	urea, 10%		glyceryl stearate; acetylated lanolin alcohol; isopropyl palmitate; stearic acid; cetearath-5; petrolatum; parabens; carbomer 940
NutraSpa (Owen)	liquid			mineral oil; PEG-4-dilaurate; lanolin oil; butylparaben; benzophenone-3; fragrance

DRY SKIN PRODUCT TABLE, continued

Product (Manufacturer)	Application Form	Keratin Softener	Humectant	Other Ingredients
Oilatum Soap (Stiefel)	soap			polyunsaturated vegetable oil, 7.5%
Panscol (Baker Cummins)	lotion ointment			salicylic acid, 3%; phenol, 0.5%
Pedi-Bath (Pedinol)	bath salts			colloidal sulfur; sodium bicarbonate; pine needle oil
Pedi-Vit-A (Pedinol)	cream			vitamin A, 100,000 IU/30 mg
Pen•Kera (Ascher)		urea	glycerin	octyl palmitate; mineral oil; lanolin alcohol; polysorbate 60; sorbitan stearate; carbomer 940; triethanolamine; wheat germ glycerides; diazolidinyl urea; polyamino sugar condensate; dehydroacetic acid
Plexolan (Alvin Last)	ointment			petrolatum; lanolin, 15.5%; mineral oil; ozokerite; PEG-400-distearate; fragrance; zinc oxide; methylparaben
Polysorb Hydrate (Fougera)	cream			sorbitan sesquioleate; wax & petrolatum base
Pretty Feet & Hands (SmithKline Beecham)	lotion			paraffin; TEA-palmitate; TEA-stearate; magnesium aluminum silicate; fragrance; palmitic acid; stearic acid; methylparaben; propylparaben
Pro-Cute (Ferndale)	lotion		glycerin	cetyl alcohol; stearic acid; forlan-LM; deltyl prime; ceraphyl 230; silicone; triethanolamine; povidone; sorbic acid; dowicil 200; menthol
Purpose Dry Skin (Ortho Derm)	cream		lactic acid	mineral oil; petrolatum; almond oil; propylene glycol; glyceryl stearate; sodium lactate; steareth-20; cetyl alcohol; cetyl esters wax; steareth-2; xanthan gum; sorbic acid
Rea-Lo (Whorton)	cream lotion	urea, 30% (cream) 15% (lotion)		oil base (lotion)
RoBathol (Pharmaceutical Specialties)	bath oil			cottonseed oil; alkyl aryl polyether alcohol
Saratoga (Blair)	ointment			zinc oxide, 14%; boric acid, 1.75%; eucalyptol, 1.1%; white beeswax; white petrolatum
Sardo (Schering-Plough)	bath oil			mineral oil; isopropyl palmitate
Sardoettes (Schering-Plough)	towelettes			mineral oil; isopropyl palmitate
Sarna (Stiefel)	lotion			0.5% each of camphor, menthol and phenol in an emollient base
Shepard's (Dermik)	cream lotion		glycerin	sesame oil; SD alcohol 40-B; stearic acid; propylene glycol; ethoxydiglycol; triethanolamine; glyceryl stearate; cetyl alcohol; simethicone; parabens; vegetable oil; monoglyceride citrate; BHT; citric acid
Shepard's Skin (Dermik)	cream ·	urea	glycerin	glyceryl stearate; ethoxydiglycol; propylene glycol; stearic acid; isopropyl myristate; cetyl alcohol; lecithin; parabens
Sofenol 5 (C & M)	lotion		glycerin	mineral oil; petrolatum; allantoin; dimethicone; soluble collagen; cetyl-stearyl alcohol; PEG-40-stearate; sodium borate; kaolin; steareth-20 methacrylate; sorbic acid

DRY SKIN PRODUCT TABLE, continued

Product (Manufacturer)	Application Form	Keratin Softener	Humectant	Other Ingredients
Soft 'N Soothe (B.F. Ascher)	cream			benzocaine; menthol; natural oat protein; lanolin oil; mineral oil; lanolin alcohol
Surfol Post-Immersion (Stiefel)	bath oil			mineral oil; isopropyl myristate; isostearic acid; PEG-40; sorbitan peroleate
Ultra Derm (Baker Cummins)	bath oil lotion		glycerin (lotion)	bath oil: mineral oil; lanolin oil; octoxynol-3 lotion: mineral oil; petrolatum; lanolin oil; glyceryl stearate; propylene glycol; PEG-50-stearate; propylene glycol stearate SE; cetyl alcohol; sorbitan laurate; potassium sorbate; phosphoric acid; tetrasodium EDTA.
Ultra Mide Moisturizer (Baker Cummins)	lotion	urea, 25%		
Ureacin-10 (Pedinol)	lotion	urea, 10%		vegetable oil base
Ureacin-20 (Pedinol)	cream	urea, 20%		vegetable oil base
Vaseline Dermatology Formula (Chesebrough Ponds)	cream lotion			white petrolatum; mineral oil; dimethicone
Vaseline Intensive Care, Extra Strength (Chesebrough Ponds)	lotion		glycerin	white petrolatum; zinc oxide
Vaseline Pure Petroleum Jelly (Chesebrough Ponds)	gel			white petrolatum
Vitamin E (Various Manufacturers)	cream liquid oil			vitamin E
Vitec (Pharmaceutical Specialties)	cream			vitamin E
Wibi (Owen)	lotion		glycerin	SD alcohol 40; PEG-4; PEG-6-32; stearate; glycol stearate; carbomer 940; PEG-75; methylparaben; triethanolamine; menthol; fragrance
Wondra (Procter & Gamble)	lotion		glycerin	petrolatum; lanolin acid; stearyl alcohol; cyclomethicone; EDTA; hydrogenated vegetable glycerides phosphate; cetyl alcohol; isopropyl palmitate; stearic acid; PEG-100-stearate; carbomer 934; dimethicone; titanium dioxide; imidazolidinyl urea; parabens

DANDRUFF AND SEBORRHEA PRODUCT TABLE

Product (Manufacturer)	Application Form	Keratolytic	Cytostatic Agent	Other Ingredients
Anti-Dandruff Brylcreem (SmithKline Beecham)	shampoo		pyrithione zinc, 1%	mineral oil, propylene glycol, paraffin wax, excipients
Betadine (Purdue Frederick)	shampoo			povidone-iodine, 7.5%
Breck One (Breck)	cream lotion shampoo		pyrithione zinc, 1%	anionic surfactants, 15.6%
Danex (Herbert)	shampoo		pyrithione zinc, 1%	sodium methyl cocoyl taurate, hydrolyzed animal protein, lauramide DEA, sodium cocoyl isethionate, magnesium aluminum silicate, sodium phosphate, citric acid, quaternium-15, fragrance, mixed tocopherols
Denorex, Regular (Whitehall)	shampoo			coal tar solution, 9% menthol, 1.5% alcohol, 7.5%
DHS Tar (Person & Covey)	shampoo			coal tar, 0.5%
DHS Zinc (Person & Covey)	shampoo		pyrithione zinc, 2%	
Diaparene Cradol (Glenbrook)	liquid			methylbenzethonium chloride, 1:1500 petrolatum
Diasporal (Doak)	cream	colloidal sulfur, 3% salicylic acid, 2%		isopropyl alcohol, 95%
Duplex T (C & M)	shampoo			coal tar solution, 10% sodium lauryl sulfate, 15%
Fostex Medicated Cleansing (Westwood)	shampoo	sulfur, 2% salicylic acid, 2%		
Glover's Medicated Ointment (Glover)	ointment	salicylic acid, 3% sulfur, 5%		petrolatum, mineral oil, glyceryl tribehenate, archidyl propionate, fragrance, polysorbate-20, propylparaben, iron oxides, talc
Head & Shoulders (Procter & Gamble)	shampoo		pyrithione zinc, 1%	
Iocon (Owen)	shampoo			coal tar solution alcohol, 2.1%
Ionil (Owen)	shampoo	salicylic acid, 2%		polyoxyethylene ethers, benzalkonium chloride, alcohol, tetrasodium edetate

DANDRUFF AND SEBORRHEA PRODUCT TABLE, continued

Product (Manufacturer)	Application Form	Keratolytic	Cytostatic Agent	Other Ingredients
Ionil Plus (Owen)	shampoo	salicylic acid, 2%		sodium laureth sulfate, lauramide DEA, quaternium-22, talloweth-60, myristyl glycol, laureth-23, TEA lauryl sulfate, glycol distearate, laureth-4, TEA-abietoyl hydrolyzed collagen, DMDM hydantoin, tetrasodium EDTA, sodium hydroxide, fragrance, FD&C blue #1
Ionil T (Owen)	shampoo	salicylic acid, 2%		coal tar solution, 5% benzalkonium chloride, 0.2% polyoxyethylene ethers isopropyl alcohol, 4% alcohol, 12%
Ionil T Plus (Owen)	shampoo			crude coal tar, 2%
Metasep (MiLance)	shampoo			parachlorometaxylenol, 2% isopropyl alcohol, 9%
Meted (GenDerm)	shampoo	sulfur, 3% salicylic acid, 2%		highly concentrated detergents
Meted 2 (GenDerm)	shampoo	colloidal sulfur, 2.3% salicylic acid, 1%		
Neutrogena T/Gel (Neutrogena)	shampoo			coal tar extract, 2%
Ogilvie (Ogilvie)	shampoo			monoundecylenamido MEA-sulfosuccinate disodium
Packer's Pine Tar (Rydelle)	shampoo			pine tar, 0.82%
Pentrax (GenDerm)	shampoo			crude coal tar, 4.3% conditioning agent
Pernox (Westwood)	shampoo			sodium laureth sulfate, lauramide DEA, quaternium-22, PEG-75 lanolin/hydrolyzed animal protein, sodium chloride, lactic acid
pHisoDan (Winthrop)	shampoo	precipitated sulfur, 5% sodium salicylate, 0.5%		entsufon sodium, lanolin, cholesterols, white petrolatum, diethanol lauramide, disodium EDTA, fragrance, polyoxyethylene (2), sodium chloride
Polytar (Stiefel)	shampoo			polytar, 1% conditioners
P&S (Baker Cummins)	liquid			phenol mineral oil glycerin
	shampoo	salicylic acid, 2%		

DANDRUFF AND SEBORRHEA PRODUCT TABLE, continued

Product (Manufacturer)	Application Form	Keratolytic	Cytostatic Agent	Other Ingredients
Psorex (DEP)	shampoo			coal tar, 1%
Rezamid Tinted (Dermik)	lotion	sulfur, 5% resorcinol, 2%		chloroxylenol, 0.5%; alcohol, 28.5%
Scadan (Miles)	lotion			cetrimonium bromide, 1% stearyl dimethyl benzyl ammonium chloride, 0.1%
Sebaquin (Summers)	shampoo			iodoquinol, 3%
Sebex (Rugby)	shampoo		pyrithione zinc, 2%	
Sebex-T (Rugby)	shampoo	colloidal sulfur, 2% salicylic acid, 2%		coal tar solution, 5%
Sebucare (Westwood)	lotion	salicylic acid, 1.8%		laureth-4, 4.5%; alcohol, 61%; butyl ether; dihydroabietyl alcohol
Sebulex Conditioning Shampoo with Protein (Westwood)	shampoo	salicylic acid, 2% sulfur, 2%		sodium octoxynol-3 sulfonate, sodium lauryl sulfate, lauramide DEA, acetamide MEA, amphoteric-2, hydrolyzed animal protein, magnesium aluminum silicate, propylene glycol, methylcellulose, PEG-14M, fragrance, disodium EDTA, dioctyl sodium sulfosuccinate, FD & C Blue #1, D & C Yellow #10
Sebulex Medicated Shampoo (Westwood)	shampoo	sulfur, 2% salicylic acid, 2%		surfactants
Sebulon (Westwood)	shampoo		pyrithione zinc, 2%	acetamide MEA, benzyl alcohol, cocamide DEA, D & C Green #5, disodium oleamido PEG-2 sulfosuccinate, FD & C Green #3, fragrance, guar gum, magnesium aluminum silicate, quaternium-15 TEA lauryl sulfate
Sebutone (Westwood)	shampoo	sulfur, 2% salicylic acid, 2%		tar, 0.5%; surfactants, cleansers, wetting agents
Selenium Sulfide (Various manufacturers)	lotion-shampoo		selenium sulfide, 1%	
Selsun Blue (Ross)	shampoo		selenium sulfide, 1%	surfactants
SLT Lotion (C & M)	lotion	salicylic acid, 3%		coal tar solution, 2% lactic acid, 5% isopropyl alcohol, 65% benzalkonium chloride

DANDRUFF AND SEBORRHEA PRODUCT TABLE, continued

Product (Manufacturer)	Application Form	Keratolytic	Cytostatic Agent	Other Ingredients
Sulfur-8 Light Hair and Scalp Conditioner (Schering-Plough)	ointment	sulfur, 2%		menthol, triclosan
Sulfur-8 Shampoo (Schering-Plough)	shampoo			triclosan
Sulray (Alvin Last)	cream soap	sulfur, 3% (cream) 5% (soap)		cream: sulfurated lime solution, zinc sulfate, water, glyceryl stearate, laureth-23, PEG-8 stearate, glycerin, silica, parabens
Sulray (Alvin Last)	shampoo	sulfur, 2%		sodium lauryl sulfate, lauramide DEA, glycol stearate, DMDM hydantoin, methylparaben, propylparaben, citric acid
Tarlene (Medco Labs)	lotion	salicylic acid, 2.5%		refined coal tar, 2% propylene glycol oleth-3 oleth-20
Tarsum (Summers)	shampoo	salicylic acid, 5%		coal tar solution, 10%
Tegrin Medicated (Block)	shampoo			coal tar extract, 5%
Vanseb (Herbert)	cream lotion shampoo	sulfur, 2% salicylic acid, 1%		proteins, surfactants
Vanseb-T (Herbert)	shampoo	sulfur, 2% salicylic acid, 1%		coal tar solution, 5%
X-seb (Baker Cummins)	shampoo	salicylic acid, 4%		
X-seb T (Baker Cummins)	shampoo	salicylic acid, 4%		coal tar solution, 10%
Zetar (Dermik)	shampoo			whole colloidal coal tar, 1%; chloroxylenol, 0.5%
Zincon (Lederle)	shampoo		pyrithione zinc, 1%	surfactants
ZNP Bar (Stiefel)	bar		pyrithione zinc, 2%	

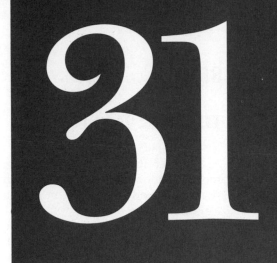

Gary H. Smith

DIAPER RASH AND PRICKLY HEAT PRODUCTS

*Q*uestions to ask in parent/consumer counseling

Diaper Rash

Do you use disposable diapers or a diaper service?

Do you use cloth diapers? How do you launder them?

Where does the rash occur, and what does it look like?

Do you use double diapers or plastic pants?

How often do you change the baby's diapers?

How do you clean the baby's skin during a diaper change?

What products have you already tried for the rash?

Does the baby have a fever?

Has the baby had diarrhea recently?

Has the baby ever had a yeast infection?

Is there a family history of allergic disorders?

Has any new food recently been added to the baby's diet?

Prickly Heat

Where is the rash located and what does it look like?

How long has the rash been present?

Does the patient sleep in a very warm and humid room?

How much clothing does the patient wear during the day and night?

What products have you already tried for the rash?

Diaper rash and prickly heat (miliaria rubra) are acute, transient, inflammatory skin conditions that occur in many infants and young children. Both conditions cause burning and itching that can result in restlessness, irritability, and sleep interruption. Most cases can be reversed easily by simple home remedies; however, prevention is the best treatment.

The skin of most adults is about 2 mm thick, but infant skin is about 1 mm thick and therefore more delicate. The epidermis (the outermost skin layer) represents about 5% of the total skin thickness; therefore, the external barrier that protects the infant from the environment is very thin (1). (See Chapter 28, *Topical Anti-infective Products*, for a discussion of skin anatomy.) For the skin to function most efficiently, it should remain dry and smooth and maintain a slightly acidic pH.

DIAPER RASH

Diaper rash, or diaper dermatitis, is one of the most common dermatitides in infants. One study reported an incidence of 17% in 1-week-old infants (2). In a recent survey of 1,089 infants 1–20 months of age, the frequency of diaper rash approached 65%, with the majority of cases reported as slight or mild. Only about 5% of the infants had severe dermatitis; the remainder of the cases were classified as moderate. The incidence of the rash peaked between 9 and 12 months of age (3).

The Food and Drug Administration (FDA) advisory review panel on OTC miscellaneous external drug products did not classify any individual ingredients in those drug products intended to treat diaper rash or prickly heat. Therefore, in 1982 FDA announced intent to propose an advance notice of proposed rulemaking and reopened four administrative records (antimicrobial, external analgesic, skin protectant, and antifungal) for drug product ingredients for use in the treatment of diaper rash or prickly heat. The FDA published the panel's statement as follows: "Diaper rash is a common skin problem of infancy, caused by contact with urine and feces, worsened by occlusion with plastic pants, and often secondarily infected with *Candida albicans*. It has an excellent prognosis for permanent cure after an infant is toilet trained. Incontinent adults may get similar irritant contact dermatitis" (4–8).

Etiology

Urine and feces have long been implicated as contributing to the development of diaper rash. Normal newborns begin urinating within 24 hours after birth. Urination occurs up to 20 times a day until 2 months of age and as many as 8 times a day from 2 months to 8 years of age. Defecation also occurs several times a day in infants (9). Breast-fed infants tend to urinate less frequently and have a lower incidence of dermatitis than bottle-fed infants. Furthermore, the urine and feces tend to be less alkaline and therefore less irritating than that of bottle-fed infants (3, 10, 11).

The distribution of diaper rash may be positional. If the baby lies on the stomach, the rash may be ventral; if the baby lies on the back, the rash may be dorsally located. It may spread to the entire diaper area, depending on the promptness of therapy and what causes the rash. The diaper area is vulnerable to inflammation because the skin is warm and moist and is exposed to irritants and bacteria. Ammonia probably plays a role in irritating a previously existent condition, but it is also possible that certain foods in the diet of the baby may be a contributing factor. High-protein foods may make the urine and stools more acidic and produce an "acid scald" (12). Secondary infections caused by various microorganisms and other complications may occur.

The pathologic changes vary with the causative factors and the severity of the dermatitis. Diaper rash may range from mild erythema with or without maceration and chafing, to vesicles, pustules, or bullae. Deeper nodular and infiltrated lesions may develop depending on the primary cause of the dermatitis. Seborrhea, psoriasis, and atopic dermatitis may predispose to irritation and infection.

Ammonia

Until recently, the most widely accepted theory of the etiology of diaper rash was the presence of ammonia and other irritating end products of the enzymatic breakdown of urine. Ammoniacal dermatitis was first described in 1886 (13), and other reports followed in the early 1900s (14, 15). It was later learned that ammonia in the diaper area is produced by urea-splitting bacteria found in the stool (16). The causative organism, *Brevibacterium ammoniagenes*, was isolated from stool samples of 31 children with diaper rash. Other ammonia-liberating organisms include *Micrococcaceae*, the aerobic diphtheroids, lactose-fermenting gram-negative rods, and species of *Proteus* and *Pseudomonas*. These organisms are saprophytic and can ferment urea to produce ammonia as follows:

$$CO(NH_2)_2 + 2H_2O \rightleftharpoons (NH_4)_2CO_3 \rightleftharpoons 2NH_3 + H_2O + CO_2$$

It was theorized that ammonia causes diaper rash by raising the skin pH. Moreover, it may form soap after combining with constituents of natural skin oils.

One study found a close correlation between urine's odor and its ability to produce erythema, regardless of the urinary pH (17). This study showed that malodorous, putrescent materials, in the absence of ammonia and high pH, may cause erythema. These materials also are produced by enzymatic degradation of urine.

More recent studies have not shown this relationship (18). One study failed to demonstrate erythema or other changes in the skin of the buttocks of 10 infants after the application of a 24-hour occlusive dressing containing 1.6% ammonia in urine. This ammonia concentration was five times the mean concentration found in 26 infants with diaper rash. It was further noted that in the 26 infants with diaper dermatitis, 44.4% had organisms capable of liberating ammonia in 4–6 hours; 52.3% of 82 control infants without diaper rash had ammonia-liberating organisms present. *Brevibacterium ammoniagenes* was isolated in a total of 5 of the 26 infants, of which only 3 had diaper rash. This study casts doubt on the importance of this organism and ammonia as a causative factor in diaper dermatitis.

It has been confirmed that infant urine does not cause skin irritation for up to 48 hours, but that skin damage can occur after 10 days of continuous exposure. Although specific irritants have not been identified, the ammonia found in the diaper area now appears to promote irritation by increasing the pH of the area, which in turn increases the activities of fecal proteases and lipases that can damage skin. Feces in the absence of urine or ammonia have been shown to cause skin irritation. Therefore, the presence of feces in the diaper area is more responsible for the promotion of diaper rash than urine, which explains the increased occurrence of diaper rash in infants with diarrhea or frequent stools (3, 19–21). The role of urine in diaper rash may simply be a function of hydration of the skin in the diaper area. One study concluded that wet skin is more permeable to low molecular-weight compounds than dry skin, therefore rendering it more susceptible to irritation (22).

Sweat Retention

If a soiled diaper is not changed promptly, the stratum corneum in the diaper area becomes waterlogged. This saturation causes keratotic plugging of the sweat glands, which results in sweat retention and may cause vesicles (23).

Mechanical and Chemical Irritants

Tightly fitting diapers covered with plastic pants increase the humidity and temperature in the diaper area and prevent air from circulating around the skin, producing an environment conducive to irritation and secondary infection. Irritation results from the diaper's constant rubbing against the skin. Eroded skin is more susceptible to infection. If diapers are changed frequently, irritation may be prevented.

Chemical irritants from various sources may precipitate a rash in the diaper area. Feces remaining in contact with the skin cause irritation, especially if the infant's diet promotes the elimination of irritating substances and unabsorbed foodstuffs, or causes diarrhea. (See *Plate 8-31*.) Preparations commonly applied to the diaper area, such as proprietary antiseptic agents and harsh soaps containing mercury, phenol, tars, salicylic acid, or sulfur, also may cause diaper rash. Diapers rinsed inadequately after washing may retain residues from detergents or bleach that can irritate the diaper area or cause irritant and/or allergic reactions. Precautions should be taken to avoid exposing the sensitive skin of infants and young children to these irritating substances (23, 24).

Complications

Yeast and bacterial infections are the most common complications of diaper rash. These cutaneous infections are often secondary to untreated or improperly treated diaper dermatitis. The moist, warm, alkaline environment created by unchanged diapers is conducive to the development and multiplication of pathogenic bacteria and yeast (18). Most bacteria and yeast do not produce lesions on normal skin. However, if the skin is eroded or macerated or if the normal balance of the skin's bacterial flora is disturbed, these organisms may become pathogenic and cause infection in the diaper area (10).

Yeast infections are caused most commonly by *Candida albicans*, an organism that may be part of the normal colonic flora. Infections caused by *C. albicans* are the most frequent cause of diaper rash complications. The feces are the most common source of this organism (18, 25, 26); a strong correlation exists between the presence of *C. albicans* in the stool and the severity of the diaper dermatitis. Candidal infections of the diaper area have been believed to be a secondary complication of diaper dermatitis, but recent evidence suggests that they may be a primary cause. Therefore, candidal infections should be considered in all cases of severe dermatitis (3, 26). The only precise method of diagnosis is culturing *C. albicans* from scrapings or swabs of the skin lesions; now a potassium hydroxide prep from skin scrapings may be highly suggestive (23, 27). In newborns under 2 weeks of age, candidal diaper dermatitis usually is accompanied by oral thrush. Both conditions probably result from the presence in the mother of a candidal vaginal infection before and during delivery. The lesions are usually erythematous and are surrounded by characteristic satellite pustules. They may become eroded and weeping. A physician should be consulted for appropriate treatment of this condition. The systemic use of some antibiotics, especially amoxicillin, may predispose the infant to diaper candidiasis caused by overgrowth of *C. albicans* in the stool. Infants with severe diaper dermatitis who are concurrently receiving amoxicillin or other broad-spectrum antibiotics should be evaluated for candidiasis by a physician (28). Infectious complications of diaper rash caused by other dermatophytes have also been reported, including *Epidermophyton floccosum* (29–31) and *Trichophyton rubrum* (32).

Bacterial infection of the diaper area is caused most commonly by *Staphylococcus aureus* and is often a form of folliculitis. Classic lesions are follicular micropustules that enlarge with those adjacent to form lakes or pustules. Occasionally, bullous or encrusted impetigo, characterized by large blister-like lesions or honeycomb crusting, respectively, may occur. In some cases, group A *Streptococcus pyogenes* may be the pathogen. An infant with a suspected bacterial infection in the diaper area should be referred to a physician for appropriate diagnosis and therapy (4, 18, 33).

Herpetiform diaper dermatitis has recently been reported and should be considered when a parent of an infant has an active herpes simplex infection (34, 35). Other rare complications include granuloma gluteale infantum (36) and Kawasaki syndrome (37–39). Kawasaki syndrome should be suspected if erythematous, desquamating perineal rash appears in diapered infants or young children who also have symptoms such as fever, lymphadenopathy, or a rash elsewhere, especially on the ears and fingertips.

Ulceration of the penile meatus may be a painful complication of diaper rash in circumcised babies. The pain associated with this condition may lead to reflex inhibition of micturition and secondary distention of the bladder (40, 41).

In the FDA's reopening notices for diaper rash (5–8), the FDA advisory review panel further recommended: The skin under the diaper is macerated by prolonged wetness. Disposable diapers with a plastic backing, or plastic plants used over regular diapers, keep in heat and moisture, causing miliaria (prickly heat) and more maceration than occurs with the use of cloth diapers alone. Bacteria proliferate in this warm, moist environment, thrive on nutrients in feces, and metabolize urine to produce ammonia, an irritant. *C. albicans*, often present in feces, also proliferates to produce a characteristic, bright red, sharply marginated rash with satellite pustules and erosions. Other exacerbating factors are mechanical irritation (chafing), which is caused by rough cloth or tight or stiff plastic, and chemical irritation, which is caused by detergent or bleach in diapers, soap used to cleanse the baby, diarrhea, and heat.

PRICKLY HEAT (MILIARIA)

The lesions associated with this acute dermatitis result from obstruction of the sweat gland pores. Retained sweat causes the dilation and rupture of the epidermal sweat pores, producing swelling and inflammation. (See *Plate 8-32*.) The term "prickly heat" was coined because the lesions usually produce itching and stinging. Prickly heat occurs primarily during hot, humid weather or during a febrile illness with profuse sweating. It also may occur as a result of excessive clothing, polyester clothing, and overcovering, especially at night in warm, humid rooms. Prickly heat may occur during infancy, childhood, or adulthood.

In infants, the lesions most often appear in intertriginous areas and under plastic pants, diapers, and adhesive tape. In children and adults, the dermatitis is seen on areas of skin that have been heavily occluded with clothing. The lesions, which are erythematous papules, may become pustular and are usually localized to the sites of occlusion (13, 42, 43).

PATIENT ASSESSMENT

In general, if the diaper dematitis is confined to the diaper area and does not present symptoms of fungal or bacterial infections, the pharmacist may recommend a nonprescription product. If the infant has had diaper rash for only a few days, self-treatment may be recommended. The pharmacist should determine whether laundry detergents containing irritants are being used. If diaper rash persists 1 week or more after the infant has been treated with protectants and has been changed frequently, or if the rash recurs frequently, the rash may be caused by a problem other than the diaper, and a physician should be consulted. If the infant has had persistent diarrhea, appears irritable, or has a fever, or if the rash is resistant to nonprescription treatment, a physician should be consulted because the problem may be more serious than simple diaper rash.

If the rash is more widespread than the diaper area (groin, intergluteal fold, or lower abdomen), a condition such as atopic dermatitis, psoriasis, seborrheic dermatitis, allergic contact dermatitis, or scabies may be present; these infants should be diagnosed by a physician for appropriate treatment. Candidal and bacterial infections also require a definitive diagnosis by a physician. If the lesions are follicular micropustules or bullous or if they look like impetigo, a bacterial infection may be the cause.

The pharmacist may be able to recognize the cause of many conditions by questioning the parents. In addition to explaining the steps that must be taken to prevent diaper rash and prickly heat, the pharmacist may recommend several products suited to the child's condition. If the pharmacist ascertains that the rash has persisted and appears to be complicated by infection or another process, it should be suggested that the child be taken to a physician.

TREATMENT

The treatments for diaper rash and prickly heat may be considered together, but modifications and additional measures may be required for each condition. The active treatment of diaper rash involves removing the source of irritation, reducing the immediate skin reaction, relieving discomfort, and preventing secondary infection and other complications. The treatment plan should be individualized for both diaper rash and prickly heat. The area should be kept as dry and clean as possible. The diaper should be loose, well ventilated, and changed as quickly as possible after becoming soiled. Plastic pants should be avoided. Products helpful in treatment include skin protectants, antimicrobials (i.e., antiseptics), antifungal agents, and external analgesics. The advisory review panel (5–8) stated that ordinary mild diaper rash, characterized by erythema of the buttocks, perineum, and lower abdomen, responds to very frequent diaper changes, cleansing with water, and removal of plastic occlusion (switching to cloth diapers, often two at the same time). Most treatments, such as talc and zinc oxide ointment and paste, help by protecting the skin, acting as a physical barrier to irritants, and absorbing moisture. The pharmacist should be able to advise parents about which products should be used for a particular kind of dermatitis and the specific care required. As with most forms of therapy, the simplest regimen is the one most likely to be followed consistently. A baby's skin is sensitive, and many babies may be irritated by or allergic to some available products.

In treating mild forms of diaper rash, the best remedy is changing diapers as soon as they are soiled and completely drying the diaper area before a new diaper is used. Plain water should be used to cleanse the diaper area to avoid sensitizing chemicals in soaps and commercial wipes. The parent may be advised to place the infant on an opened diaper during the nap to avoid soiling bed clothes. This practice may prove to be impractical but may work in some cases. A mattress protector may prevent soiling of the bedding or play yard. The condition of infants with ammoniacal dermatitis can improve when they are exposed to air as often as possible. Cornstarch was once thought to serve as a culture medium for microorganisms and to encourage bacterial overgrowth (44). However, cornstarch has recently been shown to be both rational and safe as a dusting powder and does not cause growth of *C. albicans* (45). Use of an incandescent lamp with a 25-watt bulb as a heat source may speed healing (46, 47). This practice, however, may subject the infant to the risk of burning and should not be advised routinely. Careful use of a hair blow-dryer on a low setting is effective in drying the area and safer than a heat lamp. The use of a good protective agent such as zinc oxide paste (Lassar's paste) or white petrolatum provides a barrier to protect the skin from moisture.

In the treatment of prickly heat, the primary goal is to reduce sweating. The clothing should be made of light material and should not cause any rubbing of the skin. Light clothing and covering are recommended to allow air to reach the skin. Air conditioning the environment helps lower humidity and temperature. Maceration and irritants may be reduced by frequent baths or sponge baths at least 2 times a day and the use of a bland talc dusting powder. Oatmeal (1 cup of Aveeno Colloidal Oatmeal in a tub of warm water) and soy protein (1 packet of protein colloidal bath powder in a tub of warm water) may help in treating prickly heat. Frequent diaper changes and the elimination of any excessive soap or chemical irritants help reduce discomfort associated with prickly heat (48).

Treatment of diaper dermatitis with a light application of 0.5–1% topical hydrocortisone after each diaper change for a limited period has been recommended (49, 50). One investigator has recommended application of 2.5% hydrocortisone in highly inflammatory diaper rash. However, it should be noted that corticosteroids may alleviate symptoms of diaper rash but do not eliminate the cause.

Because occlusive dressings facilitate the absorption of topically applied steroids, they should not be used in the diaper area (49). When steroids are applied topically to inflamed or abraded skin, systemic levels may be higher than when they are applied to normal skin because of increased absorption (51). Also, the use of patent fluorinated steroids (e.g., 0.1% triamcinolone cream) can cause thinning of the skin, with resultant striae and easy bruising (5–8).

Recognition of the value of topical hydrocortisone for diaper dermatitis by the medical community does not warrant its use for infants on a nonprescription basis. Because 0.5% hydrocortisone cream is available for nonprescription use, pharmacists should caution parents concerning the use of this product for diaper rash. Hydrocortisone is not recommended for use on children under 2 years of age except under the advice and supervision of a physician. Furthermore, it has been suggested that hydrocortisone should be reserved for cases in which zinc oxide ointment or similar products and standard preventive measures have not been sufficient (52). With this in mind, advice to use hydrocortisone topically for the infant patient without physician intervention does not appear warranted. (See Chapter 35, *Poison Ivy and Poison Oak Products*, for a more complete discussion of hydrocortisone.)

Secondary Complications

Various antiseptic agents have been used to treat staphylococcal- and streptococcal-induced infections. Nonprescription topical antibiotics have an adjunct role at best in the treatment of these bacterial infections. Systemic antibiotics are the treatment of choice for impetigo (53). Quaternary ammonium compounds are included as antibacterial agents in commercial products; however, their effectiveness has been questioned because these cationic surfactants are inactivated by organic matter such as urine and feces. In addition, these compounds may act as irritants in some cases, exacerbating the inflammation, and causing discomfort when applied (54). Antibiotic ointments, especially neomycin, should be used only when clearly indicated because they may cause hypersensitivity reactions (55). Secondary infections that may be caused by bacteria or species of *Candida* should be diagnosed and treated by a physician.

In candidal diaper rash, the use of anticandidal agents may be necessary. Aluminum acetate (Burow's) solution compresses may be used for severe dermatitis. A clean cotton flannel cloth or a facecloth is soaked in warm solution and wrung out for about 1 minute. The cloth is then removed, rinsed, and reapplied 10–12 times. This procedure can be followed by the application of nystatin dusting powder or ointment at a concentration of 100,000 units per gram (27, 56). The use of oral nystatin (100,000 units 4 times daily) along with the topical application of the cream has also been evaluated. The oral administration failed to provide any advantage over the cream alone (57). A 2% amphotericin B ointment also is effective (58). More recently, topical 2% miconazole nitrate cream and 1% haloprogin cream have been shown to be effective in treating candidal diaper rash (59, 60). Hydroxyquinoline can be applied topically for its antibacterial and antifungal activity. A combination of nystatin (100,000 units/g), chlorhexidine (1%), and hydrocortisone (1%) has been favorably evaluated for both fungal and bacterial infections (61). Calcium undecylenate is used for its antifungal activity. Nystatin, amphotericin B, miconazole nitrate, clotrimazole, haloprogin cream, and hydroxyquinoline are prescription-only products; aluminum acetate solution, chlorhexidine, and calcium undecylentate are available without prescriptions.

Avoidance of Dietary Irritants

The theory that various foods and food additives cause a higher incidence of diaper rash has not been substantiated. In a study of 1,184 infants, there was no significant difference in diaper rash between infants fed an iron-fortified formula and those fed formulas without iron (62). If a certain food appears to cause problems, it may be discontinued for a trial period. The nutrients provided by the food, however, should be provided by another food.

Prophylaxis

Good prophylactic practices depend on parental cooperation and responsibility. Common sense is perhaps the best guide for preventive therapy.

A diaper should be changed as soon as it is soiled; leaving a wet diaper on for several hours increases the chances of diaper rash. The apparently unsoiled part of the diaper should never be used to wipe the baby. This spreads microorganisms over the skin that will proliferate when the child next urinates. If frequent changes are impossible, the infant should be kept belly down to reduce the tendency for feces and urine to become compressed under the gluteal area. Diapers should be made of soft material and fastened loosely to prevent rubbing. Plastic pants should be used as seldom as possible because they are occlusive and impede the passage of air through the diaper. The use of plastic pants at night and for extended periods should be discouraged. The only disposable diapers that are occlusive are those with elasticized sides. The elasticized leg diapers should probably be avoided in most cases because they may contribute to prickly heat and diaper rash.

Infants often urinate soon after they are put to bed for the night. Parents can reduce the time a child is exposed to a wet diaper and the amount of urine accumulated at night by changing the diaper within several hours after putting the child to bed.

The diaper area should be cleaned at each diaper change. Mild soap (Oilatum or a commerical baby soap) should be used for cleaning the diaper area and for bathing. It is important that skin folds that entrap perspiration and feces be cleaned thoroughly and rinsed well with clean water. Various diaper wipe products are now available and may be used for cleaning the diaper area. These products may contain antiseptics, soap, and lanolin that may contribute to the rash. Convenience may dictate their use, but caution should be exercised because of the possible presence of irritants. The diaper area should be completely dry before a clean diaper is put on. Exposing the diaper area to warm, dry air for a few minutes between changes helps to keep the skin dry. A bland ointment or dusting powder (such as zinc oxide ointment, cornstarch, or talcum powder) may be recommended after washing.

Several reports have dealt with the use of antibacterial compounds in laundering cloth diapers. If home-laundered diapers are used, they can be soaked in a solution of Borax (½ cup Borax per gallon of water) before washing (47). Another antibacterial compound that can be used to presoak diapers, to reduce odor, and to disinfect diapers is a diluted sodium hypochlorite solution, provided the infant is not sensitive to bleach. Diapers should be washed with mild soap. The use of harsh detergents and water softeners should be avoided. After they are washed, the diapers should be rinsed thoroughly. Air drying diapers in the sun helps kill bacteria. Ironing dry, washed diapers will destroy any surviving bacteria.

The addition of a disinfectant during the washing process is an effective means of reducing bacterial count. A 5.25% sodium hypochlorite bleach (Clorox), properly diluted, reduced the number of organisms from $277/in^2$ to $2/in^2$ (63). The use of clorophene (*o*-benzyl-*p*-chlorophenol) in the first rinse of diapers in a concentration of 1 part clorophene to 2,500 parts water also is effective in treating and preventing ammoniacal diaper dermatitis (64). Acidification of diapers may also be helpful. This effect can be accomplished by a final rinsing of diapers in a solution made by adding 1 cup of vinegar to a half-filled washing machine tub. The diapers are then added and soaked for 30 minutes. This is a more economical alternative (65).

Over the past 10–15 years, there has been a trend away from use of cloth diapers. A recent survey of parents showed that less than 5% used cloth diapers exclusively. The majority (53%) always used disposable, and 42.7% used both (3). Several studies have been conducted to compare the incidence of diaper rash in infants diapered with cloth and the different types of disposable diapers (3, 66–73).

An early study found that diapers cleaned by a diaper service were associated with the lowest incidence of diaper rash (24.4%), disposable diapers showed a similar low incidence (25%), and home-laundered diapers were associated with the greatest incidence (35.6%) (66). The home-laundered diapers were not rinsed with a bacteriostatic agent. These reports show the necessity of using a bacteriostatic agent either in the rinse water or in the diaper pail. Diapers containing fecal material should be rinsed well in the toilet before they are placed in the diaper pail. Commercial diaper services provide essentially sterile diapers.

Another study (67) compared home-laundered diapers with a commercial paper diaper in 146 1-month-old infants. The incidence of severe rash was greater (16.1%) with the commercial disposable diaper than that seen with home-laundered cloth diapers (3.3%). The manufacturer of the disposable diaper has responded with evidence that "types and severity of rash do not differ significantly" between infants diapered in cloth or commercial or disposable diapers (68). A more recent study compared two different brands of disposable diapers with home-laundered cloth diapers; it showed a slightly greater incidence of diaper rash in the cloth diaper group (65).

A survey of 1,089 infants showed a significant inverse correlation between the incidence of diaper rash and the use of disposable diapers. Those infants diapered solely with disposable diapers had a lower level of diaper rash than those diapered with cloth (3).

In 1985, a new disposable diaper (Ultra Pampers)

was introduced that contains absorbent gelling material (AGM) that consists of cross-linked sodium polyacrylate. Diapers containing AGM are designed to absorb moisture and tightly bind it to a gel matrix, to provide a buffering system with its partially neutralized carboxylic acid structure, and to reduce the potential for urine and feces to mix, thereby providing a better pH control. One randomized blinded study compared the AGM disposable, conventional disposable, and home-laundered diapers for skin wetness, skin pH, and diaper dermatitis extent, frequency, and severity. The results showed that infants wearing the AGM diapers were substantially drier and exhibited lower pH values; moreover, their subjective diaper rash grades were lower by a statistically significant reading when compared with infants wearing either conventional disposable or home-laundered diapers.

Home-laundered diapers were the least beneficial in the areas of pH control and wetness. However, there appeared to be no significant difference in the degree of diaper rash between the cloth and conventional disposable diapers (71). Other recent studies comparing AGM diapers with conventional disposable and home-laundered cloth diapers have revealed similar results; infants diapered with AGM diapers consistently have a reduced frequency of and/or less severe diaper dermatitis than infants wearing cloth or conventional disposable diapers. In each case the results were statistically significant, and in no case did the cloth diapers prove to be better than the disposable (70, 73).

In a study in day care centers, 180 children wearing conventional disposable or AGM disposable diapers were evaluated for frequency of diarrhea, antibiotic use, and diaper dermatitis. The children with diarrhea and diapered with AGM diapers had a statistically significantly lower mean grade of diaper rash than infants diapered with conventional diapers. Diaper dermatitis in children taking antibiotics and in children with diarrhea and taking antibiotics was less with the AGM diapers than the conventional diapers, but in neither case was the difference statistically significant (72).

Overall, the recent studies appear to favor AGM diapers but fail to reveal any statistical difference between conventional disposable diapers and home-laundered cloth diapers. No comparison was made in any study with commercial diaper service, nor were mothers of the infants in the cloth diaper groups given any specific washing instructions. The cost benefit of the more expensive AGM diapers must be weighed against the slightly increased benefit in the prevention of diaper dermatitis. In addition, disposable diapers are not biodegradable and may present an ecological hazard. It seems that the prompt changing of diapers when soiled or wet is still the best prevention of diaper rash, irrespective of the type of diaper used.

Prophylaxis with powders and ointments is not

necessary for all babies. Just because an infant wears diapers does not mean that powders and ointments should be applied. If a problem occurs, it should be treated. If it recurs, prophylaxis is warranted. However, most babies who develop diaper rash will respond to treatment and not need prophylaxis. Babies who require continued prophylaxis should have it stopped periodically to determine if it is still necessary (7).

Pharmacologic Agents

As stated above, the FDA advisory review panels did not review or classify any individual ingredients for the treatment of diaper rash or prickly heat. The FDA reopened the administrative records for the four types of products—antimicrobial (5), external analgesic (6), skin protectant (7), and antifungal (8) drug products—to be used in the treatment of diaper rash or prickly heat. In an attempt to make the review as extensive as possible, the FDA compiled a list of ingredients recognized through historical use or use in marketed products as active ingredients for diaper rash or prickly heat. The 50 ingredients are alkyldimethyl benzylammonium chloride, allantoin (5-ureidohydantoin), aluminum acetate, aluminum hydroxide, amylum, balsam peru, benzethonium chloride, benzocaine, bicarbonate of soda, bismuth subnitrate, boric acid, calamine, calcium carbonate, camphor, casein, cod liver oil, cysteine hydrochloride, dibucaine, diperodon hydrochloride, glycerin, hexachlorophene, 8-hydroxyquinoline, iron oxide, lanolin, menthol, methapyrilene, methionine, methylbenzethonium chloride, oil of eucalyptus, oil of lavender, oil of peppermint, oil of white thyme, panthenol, *para*-chloromercuriphenol, petrolatum, phenol, pramoxine hydrochloride, salicylic acid, silicone, sorbitan monostearate, talc, tetracaine, vitamin A, vitamin A palmitate, vitamin D, vitamin D_2, vitamin E, white petrolatum, zinc oxide, and zinc stearate.

Hexachlorophene is included in the list; however, the use of hexachlorophene as a component of nonprescription drug products is restricted to prescription uses by 21 CFR 250.250 (8).

In 1989, the FDA advised a manufacturer of diaper rash preparations about two protocols designed to determine the effectiveness of the preparations in the treatment and prevention of diaper rash (74). The FDA advised that the etiology of diaper rash may not be comparable across an age group of 24 months or younger. In immobile infants, generally under 6 months of age, the rash is almost exclusively caused by the chemical irritation of macerated skin. In the mobile infant, whether crawling or walking, the rash can be caused by the mechanical exacerbation (friction) of the chemical irritation. Therefore, the effectiveness of the various treatments may differ. The FDA further advised that if more than one ingredient is claimed as active, the protocol must be designed to demonstrate the contribution of each ingredient to the effect claimed. In addition, effectiveness ratings of three levels of clinical observations would be sufficient: no rash, mild erythema, and moderate erythema. The FDA pointed out that variables may affect the outcome of the studies; these variables include the type of diaper to be used (disposable or cloth, single or multiple-layered, occluded or plain), frequency of diaper changes, type of cleansing agent to be used, method and frequency of cleansing, and frequency of bowel movements. Some of these variables can be addressed by providing the mother with written instructions on how to treat the infant with the assigned product at each diaper change. Instructions should include the type and amount of cleansing agent, type of treatment applicator, and the amount of product.

Zinc oxide, an excellent protectant found in many products used to treat diaper rash, is a mild astringent with weak antiseptic properties. Many preparations contain various concentrations of zinc oxide and petrolatum. Zinc oxide paste USP, the simplest of these formulations, contains 25% zinc oxide, 25% cornstarch, and 50% white petrolatum. Parents should be informed that this is most easily removed with mineral oil. This combination serves as a highly water-immiscible base. Many preparations contain zinc oxide in a higher concentration than Lassar's paste contains (Desitin contains 40% zinc oxide). Most of the preparations also contain one or more of various other medications such as cod liver oil, vitamins A and D, lanolin, peruvian balsam, and silicone.

In general, these various products are popular and are promoted primarily for the treatment of diaper rash. Only recently have there been controlled studies with these products (75, 76). Reports from Leeming/Pacquin (75) showed Desitin Ointment to be superior to bland soap and unmedicated talcum powder in the treatment of diaper rash. Only two reports have compared one product with the other (76, 77). Lantiseptic Ointment (Corona) [*p*-chloromercuriphenol (1:1,500) in a lanolin and petrolatum base] in a controlled study was shown to be equal or superior to vitamin A and D ointment in the treatment of diaper rash. Although several anecdotal reports indicate that vitamin A and D ointment or cod liver oil-containing ointments may be beneficial in preventing and treating diaper rash (78–81), no evidence exists that indicates any of these products is superior to zinc oxide paste or white petrolatum. One randomized, double-blind study compared two skin care regimens in 114 newborns. One regimen contained vitamin A, Lassar's plain zinc paste, lanolin, and petrolatum. The second regimen contained all the ingredients except vitamin A. Subjects were evaluated during an 11-month period for the incidence of diaper rash. There was no difference between the groups with respect to the frequency or severity of diaper rash, indicating that vitamin A did not prevent diaper rash to any greater degree than the other ingredients (77). Therefore, zinc oxide paste or white petrolatum should be recommended as a protectant and as initial treatment for diaper rash. Use of these products avoids subjecting the infant to compounds, such as peruvian balsam, that may cause skin sensitization.

Powders

The powdered agents used in treating diaper rash and prickly heat are talc, cornstarch, calcium carbonate, kaolin, zinc stearate, microporous cellulose, and magnesium stearate. Talc is a natural hydrous magnesium silicate that allays irritation, prevents chafing, and absorbs sweat. Talc is similar to ointments and creams in that it adheres well to the skin. It is a finely milled powder that will not cake in the folds and cause maceration by friction. Magnesium stearate is included in some dusting powders promoted for infant use because of its ability to adhere to the skin and to serve as a mechanical barrier to irritants. Calcium carbonate, cornstarch, kaolin, zinc stearate, and microporous cellulose are also included in products for their moisture-absorbing properties. When applied after each changing, these products serve primarily to keep the diaper area dry. However, they should be used cautiously because inhalation of the dust by the infant may be harmful and could lead to chemical pneumonia. A recent report substantiates the potential hazards of powders (82). They should be applied with a cotton fluff to spread evenly. Powders should never be applied to an acute oozing dermatitis because they may promote secondary crusting and infection.

Antiseptics

In the past, boric acid has been used extensively for its bacteriostatic and fungistatic activity in diaper dermatitis and prickly heat treatment. It has been incorporated into ointments in concentrations of as much as 3% and into dusting powders. However, there have been reports of toxicity and, in two instances, death associated with boric acid use (83, 84). In one quantitative study of 16 infants, urinary boron levels in infants treated with 3% boric acid/borate ointments were reported to be twice the levels of infants in the control group (85). Concern about boron toxicity has prompted the American Academy of Pediatrics Committee on Drugs to recommend to the FDA that products containing boric acid be reformulated, eliminating

boric acid as an ingredient. The FDA advisory review panel on OTC topical antiseptic drug products concluded that boric acid is not safe for nonprescription use because of the possibility of systemic absorption and toxicity (86).

Other antiseptic compounds are found in diaper rash products. Quaternary ammonium compounds such as benzalkonium chloride, benzethonium chloride, methyl benzethonium chloride, and cetylpyridium chloride are included in several products. These compounds have not been shown to be of any benefit in the treatment of diaper rash. Their inclusion in products is primarily aimed at reducing bacterial flora and preventing infection. However, they are irritating substances and may aggravate or even induce a rash. Because the presence of ammonium-producing bacteria has not been shown to correlate with diaper rash and because the efficacy of the quaternary ammonium compounds is questionable, it is suggested that products containing these substances be avoided (87).

PRODUCT SELECTION GUIDELINES

Pharmacists should advise parents about the correct use of any product they recommend. Some general precautions should be mentioned, such as use of products prior to their expiration dates (when dated) and care in applying topical preparations that might sting or smart already irritated skin. If powders are recommended, parents should be instructed to apply them carefully to prevent the infant from inhaling the powder, which could lead to chemical pneumonia. When soaks and solutions (such as aluminum acetate solution) are used, the unused portion should be discarded after each use; that is, only fresh preparations should be used each time.

Above all, pharmacists should caution parents about the general use of any medication for a baby's skin. The best therapy for diaper dermatitis is to keep the skin clean and dry.

Few infants escape diaper rash. The pharmacist may help by teaching parents the proper procedures for preventing diaper rash and prickly heat. Parents should understand that using medications indiscriminately is not the proper way to treat either condition and is ill advised. Drugs alone cannot stop or prevent diaper rash or prickly heat. Many newborns, infants, and young children may be hypersensitive to various medications, and more harm than good can result from their use.

SUMMARY

Pharmacists should be prepared to offer sound advice on a good prophylactic program and to recommend therapy for uncomplicated, uninfected cases of diaper dermatitis and prickly heat. They also should be prepared to assess the severity of the rash and to be able to recommend appropriate action, either referral to a physician or a treatment plan.

Diaper dermatitis and prickly heat are the two most common afflictions of newborns, infants, and young children, but the incidence and severity may be reduced by following the proper procedures. If the dermatitis does not respond within 1 week to frequent diaper changes, frequent exposure to air, and application of a good protectant, such as zinc oxide paste, a physician should be consulted.

REFERENCES

1 W. L. Weston, "Practical Pediatric Dermatology," Little, Brown, Boston, Mass., 1979, pp. 1–2.

2 G. Weipole, *Klin. Paediatr., 186,* 259 (1974).

3 W. E. Jordan et al., *Pediatr. Dermatol., 3,* 198 (1986).

4 J. J. Leyden and A. M. Kligman, *Arch. Dermatol., 114,* 56 (1978).

5 *Federal Register, 47,* 39407 (1982).

6 *Federal Register, 47,* 39413 (1982).

7 *Federal Register, 47,* 39439 (1982).

8 *Federal Register, 47,* 39465 (1982).

9 K. S. Shepard, "Care of the Well Baby," Lippincott, Philadelphia, Pa., 1968, p. 2310.

10 D. R. Marlow, "Textbook of Pediatric Nursing," W. B. Saunders, Philadelphia, Pa., 1973, pp. 136–137.

11 P. J. Koblenzer, *Clin. Pediatr., 12,* 386 (1973).

12 *Clinical Pediatrics, 3,* 409 (1964).

13 L. Jacquet, *Rev. Mens. Mal. Enf., 4,* 208 (1886).

14 T. S. Southworth, *Arch. Pediatr., 30,* 730 (1913).

15 J. Zahorsky, *Am. J. Dis. Child., 10,* 436 (1915).

16 J. V. Cooke, *Am. J. Dis. Child., 22,* 481 (1921).

17 G. W. Rapp, *Arch. Pediatr., 72,* 113 (1955).

18 J. L. Leyden et al., *Arch. Dermatol., 113,* 1678 (1977).

19 R. Hayakawa and K. Matsunaga, *Pediatrician, 14* (suppl. 1), 18 (1986).

20 R. W. Berg et al., *Pediatr. Dermatol., 3,* 102 (1986).

21 K. W. Buckingham and R. W. Berg, *Pediatr. Dermatol., 3,* 107 (1986).

22 R. E. Zimmerer et al., *Pediatr. Dermatol., 3,* 95 (1986).

23 L. M. Solomon and N. E. Esterly, "Neonatal Dermatology: Major Problems in Clinical Pediatrics," Vol. 9, W. B. Saunders, Philadelphia, Pa., 1973.

24 M. D. Lewis, *Med. J. Aust., 2,* 83 (1976).

25 R. F. Pittillo, *J. Dermatol., 12,* 245 (1973).

26 A. Rebora and J. J. Leyden, *Brit. J. Dermatol., 105,* 551 (1981).

27 P. J. Kozinn, *Antibiot. Annu.,* 910 (1958/1959).

28 P. J. Honig et al., *J. Amer. Acad. Dermatol., 19,* 275 (1988).

29 G. F. Hayden, *Pediatr. Infect. Dis., 4,* 289 (1985).

30 H. Congly, *Can. Med. Assoc. J., 129,* 410 (1983).

31 M. Kahana et al., *Clin. Pediatr., 26,* 149 (1987).

32 R. M. Cavanaugh and J. D. Greeson, *Arch. Dermatol., 118,* 446 (1982).

33 L. F. Montes et al., *Arch. Dermatol., 103,* 400 (1971).

34 R. A. C. Graham-Brown et al., *Br. J. Dermatol., 114,* 746 (1986).

35 H. B. Jenson and E. D. Shapiro, *Pediatr. Infect. Dis. J., 12,* 1136 (1987).

36 S. S. Walsh and W. J. Robson, *Arch. Emerg. Med., 5,* 113 (1988).

37 E. C. Baptist and G. G. Martinez-Torres, *South. Med. J., 81,* 942 (1988).

38 J. P. Farriaux and J. L. Dhondt, *Amer. J. Dis. Child., 142,* 1136 (1988).

39 B. S. Friter and A. W. Lucky, *Arch. Dermatol., 124,* 1805 (1988).

40 S. Swift, *Pediatr. Clin. N. Am., 3,* 759 (1956).

41 J. Brennemann, *Am. J. Dis. Child., 21,* 38 (1921).

42 H. L. Barnett, "Pediatrics," Appleton-Century-Crofts, New York, N.Y., 1968, pp. 1808–1809.

43 E. Holzle and A. M. Kligman, *Br. J. Dermatol., 99,* 117 (1978).

44 K. Arndt, "Manual of Dermatologic Therapeutics," 2nd ed., Little, Brown, Boston, Mass., 1978, p. 68.

45 J. J. Leyden, *Pediatr. Dermatol., 1,* 322 (1984).

46 M. M. Alexander and M. S. Brown, "Pediatric Physical Diagnosis for Nurses," McGraw-Hill, New York, N.Y., 1974, pp. 22–23.

47 D. A. Humphries, Master of Nursing Thesis, University of Washington, Seattle, Wash., 1966.

48 W. E. Nelson, "Textbook of Pediatrics," 2nd ed., W. B. Saunders, Philadelphia, Pa., 1979, p. 1885.

49 R. D. Carr and W. M. Tarnowski, *Acta Derm. Venereol., 48,* 417 (1968).

50 R. B. Scoggins and B. Kliman, *N. Engl. J. Med., 273,* 831 (1965).

51 R. J. Feldman and H. I. Maibach, *Arch. Dermatol., 91,* 661 (1965).

52 A. Kligman and A. Kaidberg, *Cutis, 22,* 232 (1978).

53 T. Mochizuki, *Hosp. Pharm., 12,* 260 (1977).

54 E. Shmunes and E. J. Levy, *Arch. Dermatol., 105,* 91 (1972).

55 J. Patrick et al., *Arch. Dermatol., 102,* 532 (1970).

56 P. J. Kozinn, *J. Pediatr., 59,* 76 (1961).

57 D. Munz, K. R. Powell, and C. H. Pai, *J. Pediatr., 101,* 1022 (1982).

58 P. J. Kozinn, *Antibiot. Annu.,* 128 (1956/1957).

59 R. M. Mackie and E. Scott, *Practitioner, 222,* 124 (1979).

60 L. F. Montes and H. W. Hermann, *Cutis, 21,* 410 (1978).

61 J. J. Grimshaw and R. S. Rivlin, *Br. J. Clin. Pract., 36,* 363 (1982).

62 W. W. Grant, L. Street, and R. G. Fearnow, *J. Pediatr., 81,* 973 (1972).

63 H. S. Whitehouse and N. W. Ryan, *Am. J. Dis. Child., 112,* 225 (1967).

64   W. Friend, *Calif. Med.*, *87*, 56 (1962).

65   A. H. Jacobs, *Pediatr. Clin. N. Am.*, *25*, 209 (1978).

66   W. W. Grant, L. Street, and R. G. Fearnow, *Clin. Pediatr.*, *12*, 714 (1973).

67   F. Weiner, *J. Pediatr.*, *95*, 422 (1979).

68   W. E. Jordan, *J. Pediatr.*, *96*, 957 (1980).

69   H. Stein, *J. Pediatr.*, *101*, 721 (1982).

70   J. L. Seymour et al., *J. Amer. Acad. Dermatol.*, *17*, 988 (1987)

71   R. L. Campbell et al., *J. Amer. Acad. Dermatol.*, *17*, 978 (1987).

72   R. L. Campbell et al., *Pediatr. Dermatol.*, *5*, 83 (1988).

73   A. P. Austin et al., *J. Pediatr. Health Care*, *2*, 295 (1988).

74   Letter from W. E. Gilbertson, Food and Drug Administration, to D. C. Oppenheimer, Pfizer, Inc.; LET092, Docket no. 75N-0183, FDA Dockets Management Branch, Rockville, Md., June 6, 1989.

75   Leeming/Pacquin Pharmaceutical Co., research report, 1974.

76   W. S. James, *J. Med. Assoc. Ga.*, *64*, 133 (1975).

77   J. M. Bosch-Banyeras et al., *Clin. Pediatr.*, *27*, 448 (1988).

78   H. T. Behram et al., *Ind. Med. Surg.*, *18*, 512 (1949).

79   C. B. Heimer et al., *Arch. Pediatr.*, *68*, 382 (1951).

80   P. M. Kruschner et al., *J. Am. Osteopath. Assoc.*, *53*, 215 (1953).

81   H. G. Grayzel et al., *N.Y. State J. Med.*, *53*, 2233 (1953).

82   H. C. Mofenson et al., *Pediatrics*, *68*, 265 (1981).

83   W. T. Maxon, *J. Ky. Med. Assoc.*, *52*, 423 (1954).

84   *Brit. Med. J.*, *2*, 603 (1970).

85   P. Jensen, *Nord. Med.*, *86*, 1425 (1971).

86   *Federal Register*, *45*, 34642 (1978).

87   *Federal Register*, *43*, 1237 (1978).

DIAPER RASH AND PRICKLY HEAT PRODUCT TABLE

Product (Manufacturer)	Application Form	Protectant	Powdered Agent	Antimicrobial	Other Ingredients
A and D Ointment (Schering)	ointment				fish liver oil petrolatum anhydrous lanolin base
Ammens Medicated Powder Regular Fragrance (Bristol-Myers Products)	powder	zinc oxide, 9.1%	talc cornstarch	8-hydroxyquinoline 8-hydroxyquinoline sulfate isostearic acid	PPG methyl glucose ether
Ammens Medicated Powder Shower Fresh Scent (Bristol-Myers Products)	powder	zinc oxide, 9.1%	talc cornstarch	isostearic acid	fragrance PPG-20 methyl glucose ether
Ammorid Dermatologic (Kinney)	ointment	zinc oxide		benzethonium chloride	lanolin
Ammorid Diaper Rinse (Kinney)	powder			methylbenzethonium chloride	edetate disodium
Aveeno Bar (Rydelle)	cleanser			colloidal oatmeal, 50% mild sudsing agent (soap free) lanolin	
Aveeno Colloidal Oatmeal (Rydelle)	powder				oatmeal derivatives
Aveeno (Rydelle)	lotion			colloidal oatmeal, 10% nonionic surfactants emollients	
Aveeno Oilated (Rydelle)	liquid				colloidal oatmeal, 43% lanolin fraction liquid petrolatum
Baby Magic (Mennen)	lotion			benzalkonium chloride, 0.1%	lanolin refined sterols
	oil				mineral oil lanolin
	powder			methylbenzethonium chloride, 0.1%	
Balmex Baby (Macsil)	powder	zinc oxide	talc cornstarch calcium carbonate		peruvian balsam (refined oil)
Balmex Emollient (Macsil)	lotion				peruvian balsam (refined oil) purified silicone lanolin fraction

DIAPER RASH AND PRICKLY HEAT PRODUCT TABLE, continued

Product (Manufacturer)	Application Form	Protectant	Powdered Agent	Antimicrobial	Other Ingredients
Balmex (Macsil)	ointment	zinc oxide bismuth subnitrate			vitamins A and D peruvian balsam (refined oil) benzoic acid beeswax mineral oil silicone synthetic white wax purified water
B-Balm Baby (Vortech)	ointment	zinc oxide, 10% compound benzoin tincture, 0.005 ml/g			phenol, 2.17 mg/g methyl salicylate, 0.67 mg/g
Borofax (Burroughs Wellcome)	ointment			boric acid, 5%	lanolin
Caldesene Medicated (Fisons)	ointment	zinc oxide	talc		cod liver oil lanolin petrolatum
	powder	calcium undecyclenate, 10%	talc		
Comfortine (Dermik)	water-repellent ointment	zinc oxide, 12%			lanolin vitamins A and D
Dalicreme (Dalin)	cream			methylbenzethonium chloride, 0.1%	vitamins A and D diperodon hydro-chloride, 0.25% scented greaseless base
Dalisept (Dalin)	ointment			methylbenzethonium chloride, 0.1% hexachlorophene, 1%	vitamin A, 750 units/g vitamin D, 75 units/g diperodon hydro-chloride, 1% petrolatum-lanolin base
Desitin (Leeming)	ointment	zinc oxide, 40%	talc		cod liver oil petrolatum lanolin
Diaparene Baby (Lehn & Fink)	powder	magnesium carbonate, 3.5%	cornstarch, 96%	methylbenzethonium chloride	fragrance
Diaparene Cushies (Lehn & Fink)	cloth wipe				fragrance SD alcohol 40 surfactant lanolin
Diaparene Medicated (Lehn & Fink)	cream			methylbenzethonium chloride, 1:1,000	petrolatum glycerin
Diaparene Peri-Anal Medicated (Lehn & Fink)	ointment	zinc oxide, 20%		methylbenzethonium chloride, 1:1,000	cod liver oil, 5% water-repellent base

DIAPER RASH AND PRICKLY HEAT PRODUCT TABLE, continued

Product (Manufacturer)	Application Form	Protectant	Powdered Agent	Antimicrobial	Other Ingredients
Dyprotex (Blistex)	ointment on pads	micronized zinc oxide, 40% dimethicone, 2.5%	zinc stearate	propylparaben	petrolatum, 37.6% cod liver oil aloe extract
Flanders Buttocks (Flanders Inc.)	ointment	zinc oxide			boric acid castor oil peruvian balsam
Johnson's Baby Corn Starch (Johnson & Johnson)	powder	cornstarch, 95%			tricalcium phosphate fragrance
Johnson's Baby (Johnson & Johnson)	cream	dimethicone, 2%			water mineral oil paraffin sodium borate lanolin white beeswax ceresin glyceryl stearate propylparaben fragrance
	powder		talc		fragrance
Mediconet (Medicone)	cloth wipe			benzalkonium chloride, 0.02%	hamamelis water, 50% glycerin, 10% ethoxylated lanolin, 0.5% methylparaben, 0.15% perfume
Mexsana Medicated (Schering-Plough)	powder	zinc oxide, 10.8%	cornstarch kaolin	triclosan, 0.1%	camphor euclyptus oil
Oilatum Soap (Stiefel)	cleanser				polyunsaturated vegetable oil, 7.5%
Panthoderm (Jones Medical)	lotion				dexpanthenol, 2% water-miscible base
Plexolan (Alvin Last)	ointment				water petrolatum lanolin, 15.5% mineral oil ozokerite PEG-400 distearate fragrance zinc oxide methylparaben
Spectro-Jel (Recsei)	gel			cetylpyridinium chloride, 0.1%	glycol-polysiloxane, 1% isopropyl alcohol, 15% methylcellulose, 1.5%
Taloin (Adria)	ointment	calamine, 3.6%		methylbenzethonium chloride, 0.13%	eucalyptol, 0.3% silicone base, 1%
Vaseline Pure Petroleum Jelly (Chesebrough-Pond's)	gel				white petrolatum, 100%

DIAPER RASH AND PRICKLY HEAT PRODUCT TABLE, continued

Product (Manufacturer)	Application Form	Protectant	Powdered Agent	Antimicrobial	Other Ingredients
ZBT Baby (Glenwood)	powder		talc magnesium stearate		mineral oil propylene glycol BHT fragrance
Zeasorb (Stiefel)	powder		microporous cellulose carbohydrate acrylic copolymer talc		

Arthur I. Jacknowitz

EXTERNAL ANALGESIC PRODUCTS

32

*Q*uestions to ask in patient/consumer counseling

How long has the pain been present? How did it first appear? How often does it occur?

Can you relate the pain to any specific event, such as an accident, overwork, or a sports-related activity?

Is the pain in a joint or in the muscle?

If the pain is in a joint, is the joint red, swollen, or warm to the touch?

Is the pain worse when you get up in the morning, and does it tend to subside as the day goes on?

Does the pain move to other areas of the body?

Do you have a fever or any "flu" symptoms?

External analgesics are topically applied substances that may have either local analgesic, local anesthetic, local antipruritic, or counterirritant effects. It is important to differentiate these four groups. The topical analgesic, anesthetic, and antipruritic agents depress cutaneous sensory receptors for pain, burning, and itching and act directly on the skin to diminish or obliterate these symptoms caused by burns, cuts, abrasions, insect bites, and other cutaneous lesions. (See Chapters 36, *Insect Sting and Bite Products*, and 33, *Burn and Sunburn Products*.) Topical counterirritants are included among the external analgesics because they are applied to the intact skin for the relief of pain. They differ from the analgesics, anesthetics, and antipruritic agents, however, in that the pain relief they produce results from stimulation of cutaneous receptors to induce sensations such as cold, warmth, and sometimes itching (1). These induced sensations distract from the deep-seated pain in muscles, joints, and tendons, which are distant from the skin surface where the ingredient is applied. In this manner, deep-seated pain is indirectly relieved. Some counterirritant agents actually depress cutaneous receptors in a manner similar to local anesthetics, analgesics, and antipruritics when present in low concentrations. For example, menthol depresses cutaneous receptors in concentrations below 1.0% and stimulates them in concentrations above 1.25%. Percutaneous absorption of active ingredients is not desired with counterirritant external analgesic products and, therefore, they are a distinct class of analgesic products.

Editor's Note: This chapter is based in part upon the chapter by the same title that appeared in the 8th edition but was authored by Nancy E. Lublanezki and Robert W. Cleary.

ETIOLOGY OF MUSCULAR PAIN

Pain is one of the most common ailments for which consumers seek advice and help from health care providers. Although everyone is familiar with the sensation of pain, a definition that is accepted by pain clinicians and researchers was developed only a decade ago. The International Association for the Study of Pain defines pain as an "unpleasant sensory and emotional experience associated with actual or potential tissue damage or described in terms of such damage" (2). It is a multidimensional experience that involves both a discriminative capacity and an interpretation of a stimulus in terms of present and past encounters.

Twenty-five years ago, the gate-control theory of pain integrated physiologic components of pain (3). It postulated that a neural mechanism in the spinal cord acts like a gate that can control the transmission of pain impulses to the brain. According to the gate-control theory, pain signals are carried from specialized pain receptors to the spinal cord via two types of nerve fibers: small nonmyelinated fibers and large myelin-containing nerve cells. The small fibers conduct impulses slowly and are associated with dull, aching, and lingering pain. The large fibers are linked with immediate pain characterized as sharp and precise with a pricking sensation.

Small and large nerve fiber impulses can oppose each other. In fact, mild stimulation of large fibers can attenuate pain felt as a result of activation of the small fibers, a finding that helps to explain the efficacy of topical counterirritants. An example is the effect of applying an external analgesic (stimulating large fibers) to diminish the pain caused by a sports-related knee injury (activation of small fibers).

Pain receptors are present in most areas of the body, including skeletal muscles. Stimuli activating these receptors cause sensory impulses to be transmitted via the nerve fibers to the brain, which may integrate and evaluate the signals as a perception of pain (4).

Skeletal muscle pain is quite common, especially among persons who are not accustomed to strenuous exercise. Motivated by a heightened awareness of the beneficial effects of exercise, more Americans than ever are exercising regularly. With this increased participation, exercise-induced injuries have become more common and are caused by equal and opposite reactions, which result either in macrotrauma or microtrauma (5). Macrotrauma, a sudden catastrophic injury, occurs when an equal and opposite force exceeds the inherent tensile strength of a body structure, such as a bone, ligament, muscle, or tendon, causing the structure to collapse. In contrast, microtrauma is a microscopic,

subclinical injury that results from repeated activity, which, over a period of time, overwhelms the tissue's ability to repair itself. By definition, this pain and dysfunction is described as "overuse syndrome" and is most frequently encountered in the form of tendinitis (6). In addition, bursae, cartilage, bone, and nerves can break down because of repetitive microtrauma from exercise-related activities.

Another overuse injury, described as the new industrial epidemic (7), involves occupational repetition strain injuries. These muscle and tendon injuries of the upper limbs, shoulder girdles, and neck are caused by an overload on particular muscles due to awkward working postures or repeated use; assembly-line workers and typists are likely candidates for this type of strain injury. The overload on these muscles causes pain, fatigue, and a decline in work performance. This condition has become a major cause of disability in industry and has had considerable social and economic consequences (8).

"Sprain," "bruise," and "strain" are terms used to characterize injury to soft tissue. Specifically, a sprain is defined as a partial or complete rupture of a ligament; a bruise, as a rupture of tissue resulting in a hematoma; and a strain, as a partial tear of muscles (9). When these injuries occur, the muscles become sore and painful and movement becomes difficult.

Acute, temporary stiffness and muscle pain can also result from cold, dampness, rapid temperature changes, and air currents. In some cases, visceral stimuli resulting from cardiovascular disease (such as angina pectoris) or gastrointestinal complaints (such as disorders of the gallbladder and esophagus) are felt as referred pain in the skeletal muscles of the shoulder. These episodes tend to be sudden in onset yet self-limiting. Elimination of the cause and/or symptomatic treatment generally provide relief (4).

Because of its pendulous structure, the shoulder area is subject to continuous gravitational pull and, therefore, is subject to more stress and strain than any other articulation of the body. Thus, the prehensile grasp—which raised humans above their ancestors—has resulted in the development of a shoulder girdle that sacrifices stability for mobility and is a major cause of muscular pain (10). Although painful conditions affecting the shoulder are more prevalent in the elderly, they frequently occur in athletes (11) and in certain occupational groups where the arms are used vigorously and repetitively (12).

Tendinitis, resulting from a strain or injury of tendons, is frequently seen at times of maximum physical effort, such as during athletic competition. Three distinct pathologic phases have been described (13). The first phase includes the development of the acute inflammatory response. As inflammation continues and remains untreated, excessive proliferation of connective tissue occurs. Microscopically, the tissue changes in this second phase are characterized by the development of young, vascular elements with fibroblastic growth. In the third phase, persistent and chronic inflammation results in further overgrowth of connective tissue plus tendon degeneration, which may lead to rupture. The pathologic changes occurring in each of the three phases appear to be related primarily to repetitive intrinsic tension overload in the muscle–tendon unit.

Although tendinitis in the shoulder area is a major cause of pain, athletes often suffer injury of tendons in other areas of the body. In fact, it has been said that Achilles tendinitis is the most common injury in sports (6). (See Chapter 37, *Foot Care Products*.) Other examples of this common injury include biceps tendinitis, which occurs in the "throwing athlete," such as a football quarterback or baseball pitcher; patellar tendinitis, which occurs in the volleyball and basketball player; and iliotibial-band tendinitis, which occurs in the runner.

Many factors contribute to the production of an overuse injury such as tendinitis. In industry, these include poorly designed tools, awkward working positions, lack of job variation, inadequate rest breaks, and bonuses for high work rates and overtime (14). In athletics, contributing factors can include the athlete's age, poor technique, exercise of prolonged intensity or duration, improper conditioning, and poorly designed equipment for specific activities (such as poor cushioning of athletic shoes) (5).

Bursae are sacs formed by two layers of synovial tissue that are located at sites of friction between tendon and bone or skin and bone. The bursae enable the motion of the tendons and muscles over bony prominences. With overuse, repetitive trauma from either friction of the overlying tendon or external pressure may cause the bursa to become inflamed with resultant fluid buildup in the bursal wall. This condition, termed "bursitis," is a common cause of localized pain, tenderness, and swelling, which is worsened by any movement of the structure adjacent to the bursa. It may be an acute pain due to either macrotrauma or microtrauma, or it may be chronic pain, in which case an infectious cause should be suspected. Infection or trauma can be documented by appropriate studies of aspirated fluid. Bursitis is a common cause of joint pain and frequently results in limited motion of adjacent joints, especially when the inflamed bursa is superficial and obvious redness and swelling are present. Symptoms of bursitis that mimic arthritic pain can be distinguished by a physical examination. For instance, in contrast to arthritis, direct pressure over the joint capsule of the shoulder does not cause pain in bursitis. (See Chapter 5, *Internal Analgesic Products*.)

Arthritic pain may be caused by rheumatoid arthritis, which may involve almost all peripheral joints, tendons, bursae, and the cervical spine; or by osteoarthritis, which involves degeneration of cartilage with secondary changes in joints. Although both types of rheumatic disorders are chronic systemic diseases, local treatment of painful joints coupled with rest may give temporary symptomatic relief.

Just as the prehensile grasp has imposed a stress upon our shoulder girdles unknown to our ancestors, so has our erect posture predisposed our lower spine to the painful twinge of an aching back. At least 70% of the population will experience lower back pain at some time in their lives. Lower back pain rivals the common cold as the leading cause of absenteeism from industry (15). However, this regional musculoskeletal disorder, unlike the overuse injuries described previously, is due primarily to a sedentary lifestyle (particulary when disrupted by bursts of activity), as well as poor posture, improper shoes, excess body weight, poor mattresses and sleeping posture, and improper technique in lifting heavy objects. Thus, back pain is primarily a disease of living, although most victims recover within a few days to a few weeks with conservative treatment. Low back pain has a significant likelihood of recurrence if the initial episode of low back pain is severe; advancing age also increases the risk of recurrence.

In addition to injuries, the causes of backache include congenital anomalies, osteoarthritis, spinal tuberculosis, and referred pain from diseased kidneys, pancreas, liver, or prostate. Emotional factors including tension, anxiety, repressed anger, and other manifestations of "psychosocial prestress" have been postulated to correlate with the occurrence of low back pain, but a comprehensive review of the literature did not confirm a relationship between low back pain and temperament (16).

MECHANISM OF COUNTERIRRITANT ACTION

Counterirritation, the paradoxical pain-relieving effect achieved by producing less severe pain to counter a more intense one, has been known for centuries. The Greeks, and probably the Egyptians, knew about these effects and referred to them in numerous manuscripts (17). Today, pain sufferers produce bearable pain to counter pain of pathologic origin by biting their lips, clenching their fists, digging their nails into the palms of their hands (18), or using counterirritants.

Counterirritants are medications applied to the skin at pain sites in order to produce a mild local inflammatory reaction. The objective is to provide relief at another site usually adjacent to, or underlying, the skin surface being treated. The intensity of response depends on the irritant employed, its concentration, the solvent in which it is dissolved, and the length of its contact with the skin (18).

Pain is only as intense as it is perceived to be, and the perception of other sensations caused by the counterirritant or its application, such as massage, warmth, or redness, causes the sufferer to disregard the sensation of pain. Several theories have been proposed to explain the action of irritant drugs:

- Stimulation of sensory nerve endings in the skin causes reflexive stimulation of vasomotor fibers to the viscera. These reflexes are mediated through the cerebrospinal axis and dilate the visceral vasculature (19).

- Stimulation of sensory nerve endings in the skin causes axon reflexes, resulting in stimulation of the nerves enervating branches of arterioles to produce vasodilation in the muscles. This action produces an increase in the blood flow to the muscles (20).

- Summation of pain stimuli produces intense stimulation of the areas of pain interpretation of the brain, partly abating visceral pain stimuli. According to this theory, stimuli originating in the viscera or muscles are transmitted over fibers in a common pathway, along with sensations from the skin, and are referred to the same area of the spinal cord as the stimuli from the skin (Figure 1). If the intensity of the stimulation from the skin is increased by a drug's irritant action, the character of the visceral or muscle pain is modified. With intense skin stimulation, the referred pain stimuli may be partly or completely obliterated insofar as the sensorium is concerned. The patient's attention is diverted from the muscular or visceral structure by the application of the counterirritant drug (21).

An additional effect of some products is to produce vasodilatation of cutaneous vasculature. These drugs, known as rubefacients, produce reactive hyperemia; it is hypothesized that this increase in blood pooling and/or flow is accompanied by an increase in localized skin temperature. The increase in localized skin temperature then may act by the counterirritant effect. This positive thermal response for some agents has been documented by thermography (22). The degree of irritation must be controlled, however, as strong irritation may cause erythema and blistering. There is no evidence that the risk of adverse reactions to counterirritants increases when the application site is lightly bandaged. However, there is an increased risk of irritation, redness, or blistering with tight bandaging or occlusive dressing (23).

Undoubtedly, the action of counterirritants in relieving pain has a strong psychologic component; indeed, they may exert a placebo effect through pleasant aromatic odors or from the sensation of warmth or coolness that they produce on the skin.

Some topical analgesics act by overcoming the stimulus that causes the pain. To do this, they must first be percutaneously absorbed. The effects following this absorption are then systemic; the action is the same as that of an internal analgesic. (See Chapter 5, *Internal Analgesic Products.*) Relief of any deep-seated pain is the result of a systemic effect that follows percutaneous absorption if the interstitial fluid drug concentration obtained is sufficiently high (24).

PATIENT ASSESSMENT AND TREATMENT

The pharmacist should appropriately assess the patient's condition before recommending a nonprescription counterirritant preparation. Certain questions should be asked of the patient before deciding whether to recommend a nonprescription product. It is important for the pharmacist to ask the following questions:

- How long has the pain been apparent? What kind of pain is it? Is it debilitating? Conditions amenable to nonprescription treatment are self-limiting (the condition will resolve with or without treatment in a short time). Pain that has been apparent for longer than 7 days may indicate a more serious underlying condition. These patients should be evaluated by a physician. Furthermore, prolonged use can increase the sensitivity to and decrease the effectiveness of external analgesic products (22).

- Is there any apparent cause of the pain? Often muscular or joint pain can be brought on by simple overexertion, such as unaccustomed exercise or other physical activity; such pain is a valid indication for these agents.

- Can the patient locate and describe the pain? If the pain can be specifically located and is of mild intensity, it may be appropriate to recommend a nonprescription product. If, however, the patient has difficulty in locating the origin of the pain, it may be referred pain. For example, pain in the lumbar area may be referred from pelvic viscera and may be an early manifestation of disease in these organs. If the pain is of severe intensity, nonprescription treatment should not be recommended.

- If the pain is in a joint, is the joint red, swollen, and tender to the touch? If so, there may be a fracture or rupture of ligaments or tendons or arthritic involve-

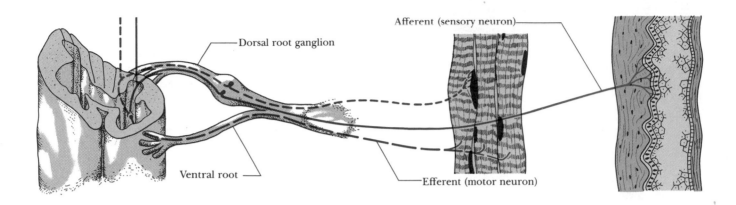

FIGURE 1   Reflex pathways showing the afferent (sensory) fibers, efferent (vasomotor) fibers, and their synapse in the spinal cord. Adapted from F. H. Netter, "The Ciba Collection of Medical Illustrations," Ciba Pharmaceutical Company, New York, N.Y., 1962, p. 65.

ment. Nonprescription products used in this condition would delay an accurate diagnosis.

- Has the patient been diagnosed by a physician as having any type of arthritic condition? If the patient has been diagnosed and is under medical supervision for any type of arthritic condition, it may be appropriate to recommend only a counterirritant preparation as adjunctive treatment. Arthritic conditions should not be self-diagnosed or self-treated. (See Chapter 5, *Internal Analgesic Products*.)

If the pharmacist determines that the condition is minor and that there are no serious underlying conditions, it may be appropriate to recommend a nonprescription preparation. The pharmacist should advise the patient that if the symptoms persist or are not relieved by the preparation within 7 days, or if the symptoms clear up and occur again within a few days (25), the medication should be discontinued and a physician should be consulted.

A follow-up consultation should be arranged by the pharmacist to review the patient's condition. This may prevent prolonged ineffective self-medication that allows a more serious underlying disease to progress.

Pharmacologic Agents

The following ingredients have been recognized as safe and effective counterirritants by the Food and Drug Administration (FDA) advisory review panel on over-the-counter (OTC) topical analgesics. Table 1 classifies these agents by their relative potencies.

Allyl Isothiocyanate

Allyl isothiocyanate, also known as volatile oil of mustard and essence of mustard, is derived from powdered seeds of the black mustard plant and other species of mustard. It can also be prepared synthetically or by distillation after expression of the fixed oil.

In high concentrations, allyl isothiocyanate is absorbed rapidly from intact skin as well as from all mucous membranes. Because penetration into the skin is rapid, ulceration may occur if the agent is not removed soon after application. A poultice, erroneously termed a "mustard plaster," has often been used as a home remedy. It is prepared by mixing equal parts of powdered mustard and flour and moistening with water to form a paste. The paste is then spread on a towel or piece of material and placed on the affected area. The continuous release of allyl isothiocyanate by the presence of water and body heat may cause the inflammatory action to go beyond redness to blistering; therefore, the poultice should not remain on the skin for more than a few minutes. Allyl isothiocyanate is considered to be safe and effective for nonprescription use in concentrations of 0.5–5.0%. It should be applied to the affected areas no more than 3 or 4 times a day.

When preparing a mustard plaster, care should be taken to avoid inhalation of this powerful irritant. This concentration is for adults and children over 2 years of

TABLE 1	Relative potencies of counterirritants	
Group	Characteristics	Ingredients
A	Cause redness, irritation; are relatively more potent than other counterirritants	Allyl isothiocyanate, stronger ammonia water, methyl salicylate, turpentine oil
B	Produce cooling sensation; have organoleptic properties	Menthol, camphor, eucalyptus oil
C	Vasoactive substances, vasodilator	Histamine dihydrochloride, methyl nicotinate
D	Produce irritation without rubefaction, although approximately equal in potency to Group A	Capsaicin, capsicum, capsicum oleoresin

Reprinted from the *Federal Register, 44*, 69784 (1979).

age. There is no recommended dose for children under 2 years of age except under the advice and supervision of a physician (22). In February 1983, the FDA issued a proposed rulemaking on external analgesic products, which indicates that "although it is true that by 6 months of age a child's skin is similar to an adult's with regard to any absorption, there are enough other differences between adults and children under 2 years of age to require different standards of practice in the use of drugs" (22).

Stronger Ammonia Water

Stronger ammonia water is also known as strong ammonia solution. Because it is caustic and the vapors are irritating, it should be handled with care and the vapors should not be inhaled. Inhalation of ammonia vapor causes sneezing and coughing and, in high concentrations, can cause pulmonary edema. Asphyxia has been reported following edema or spasm of the glottis. In addition, ammonia vapor is an eye irritant and can cause weeping, conjunctival swelling, and temporary blindness (26). Stronger ammonia water is an aqueous solution of ammonia containing 27–30% by weight of ammonia (NH_3). It must be diluted before use as a topical agent because of its caustic nature. The concentration considered to be safe and effective for topi-

cal use by adults and children over 2 years of age is a 1.0–2.5% solution of available ammonia. It should be applied to the affected area no more than 3 or 4 times a day (27).

Several liniments containing ammonia can be extemporaneously prepared by adding diluted ammonia water to a combination of oleic acid and sesame oil. The oleic acid reacts with ammonia to form an emulsifying agent for the water and sesame oil. White liniment is such an emulsion. The concentrations of ammonia range from approximately 0.5–2.65%.

Aromatic ammonia spirit ("smelling salts") derived from stronger ammonia water is used for its respiratory stimulant properties. The content of available ammonia is low enough that it may be administered orally in small doses or held near the nostrils for inhalation of volatile vapor.

Eucalyptus Oil

Eucalyptus oil is a naturally occurring volatile oil with a characteristic aromatic, camphoraceous odor. One of the chief constituents of eucalyptus oil is eucalyptol. Both have been categorized as flavors and have mild irritant and rubefacient actions causing a sensation of warmth. Marketing experience of a topical analgesic product containing small amounts of eucalyptus oil produced no evidence of lack of safety. However, a recent case report (28) emphasized the profound central nervous system depression experienced after accidental ingestion. The recommended topical dosage for adults and children over 2 years of age is a 0.5–3.0% concentration applied to the affected area not more than 3 or 4 times a day.

Methyl Salicylate

Methyl salicylate occurs naturally as wintergreen oil or sweet birch oil; gaultheria oil and teaberry oil are other names for the natural compound. Synthetic methyl salicylate is prepared by the esterification of salicylic acid with methyl alcohol. In either form, methyl salicylate is the most widely used counterirritant and has been categorized as safe and effective for use as a nonprescription analgesic when used in the appropriate dosage (29). At very low concentrations, methyl salicylate is used in oral preparations for its pleasant flavor and aroma. Indeed, it has been used as a flavoring agent in candies, cough drops, lozenges, chewing gum, toothpastes, and mouthwashes. Ingestion of more than small amounts of the substance is hazardous because of its high salicylate content. Although the average lethal dose of methyl salicylate is estimated to be 10 ml for children and 30 ml for adults (30), as little as 4 ml has caused death in infants and 5 ml has caused death in children (31).

A survey by the FDA advisory review panel considering methyl salicylate found that oral ingestion of this ingredient from products formulated as ointments caused no deaths and that few cases manifested severe symptoms (32). Nevertheless, regulations require the use of child-resistant containers for liquid preparations containing more than 5% methyl salicylate (33). Even though the agent possesses a high degree of safety for topical use and has had a long marketing history, a recent case report (34) emphasizes the importance of avoiding the use of a heating pad in conjunction with counterirritants containing methyl salicylate. The heating pad produced the elevated temperature, vasodilation, and occlusion necessary to greatly enhance percutaneous absorption of menthol and methyl salicylate, which caused full-thickness skin and muscle necrosis as well as persistent interstitial nephritis.

In addition, a recent study (35) was undertaken to determine the effects of exercise and heat exposure on the percutaneous absorption of methyl salicylate in six healthy volunteers. The results indicated that a three-fold increase in systematic availability of salicylate occurred under heat exposure and exercise as judged by plasma and urine data. The authors cautioned that if individuals were subjected to extreme heat or strenuous physical activity, the resultant increase in absorption of topically applied preparations could lead to adverse systemic reactions.

Therefore, patients should be told not to use heating pads in conjunction with topically applied external analgesics and not to apply these products after strenuous exercise, especially during hot and humid weather.

The rate and extent of percutaneous absorption of various commercially available methyl salicylate preparations were studied after the agents were left in place for 10 hours under occlusive dressing (36). It was found that only about 12–20% of the amount of salicylate applied to the skin is absorbed into the systemic circulation during this period. Furthermore, both the skin permeability coefficient for methyl salicylate and percentage of salicylate absorbed decrease when applied to different areas of the body in this order: abdomen > forearm > instep > heel > plantar. The slower absorption from the foot regions was primarily attributed to fewer hair follicles and a thicker stratum corneum. The authors concluded that topical application of products containing methyl salicylate results in low plasma salicylate concentrations and that the usefulness of these preparations is limited to their local effects.

The recommended topical dosage of methyl salicylate for adults and children over 2 years of age is a 10–60% concentration applied to the affected area no more than 3 or 4 times a day (37). Because of the possibility of percutaneous absorption, this product should be used with caution in individuals who are sensitive to aspirin or who suffer from severe asthma or nasal polyps. In an isolated case report (38), a patient sensitive to aspirin experienced allergic symptoms when exposed to various products containing methyl salicylate, including candy, toothpaste, and liniment. The patient reacted to all products, experiencing throat discomfort and soreness with the oral products and marked swelling and itching with the topical preparation. However, the author concluded that the case was a coincidence rather than the result of cross-reactivity because the patient did not previously report allergic reactions when methyl salicylate and aspirin were used together. Nevertheless, patients who report an allergy to aspirin should be cautioned to avoid products containing methyl salicylate.

Turpentine Oil

Turpentine oil is commonly misnamed "turpentine." Turpentine oil for medicinal use must be of higher quality than commercial turpentine oil. Medicinal turpentine oil, known as spirits of turpentine or rectified turpentine oil, is prepared by steam distillation of turpentine oleoresin collected from various species of pine trees.

Several human fatalities from the ingestion of turpentine oil have been reported. An oral dose of 140 ml in adults (15 ml in children) may be fatal. Turpentine oil is both a primary irritant and a sensitizer. As an irritant, it usually acts by defatting the skin, causing dryness and fissuring. It is often used as a cleanser for removing paints and waxes and can cause hand eczema by irritating sensitive skin.

Turpentine oil has been used as an ingredient in counterirritant preparations with a long history of safety and efficacy. The recommended dosage for adults and children over 2 years of age is a 6–50% concentration applied to the affected area no more than 3 or 4 times a day (39). Application of turpentine liniments to the skin in greater amounts may cause vesicular eruption, urticaria, and vomiting in susceptible individuals (40).

Menthol

Menthol is extracted from peppermint oil or prepared synthetically. The fatal dose of menthol in humans is approximately 2 g/kg (41). It may be used safely in small quantities as a flavoring agent and has found wide acceptance in candy, chewing gum, cigarettes, cough drops, toothpaste, nasal sprays, and liqueurs. Menthol has had extensive use in inhalant preparations for the relief of nasal congestion.

Menthol causes sensitization in certain individuals, although the sensitization index is low (42). Symptoms include urticaria, erythema, and other cutaneous lesions, such as contact dermatitis. A review of reactions to menthol has recently been published (43).

When menthol is used in topical preparations in concentrations of 0.1–1.0%, it depresses sensory cutaneous receptors and acts as an antipruritic. When used in higher concentrations of 1.25–16%, it acts as a counterirritant. When applied to the skin, menthol stimulates the nerves for the perception of cold, while depressing those that perceive pain. Topical application of counterirritant concentrations of menthol initially produces a feeling of coolness that is soon followed by a sensation of warmth. A recent study (44) demonstrated that exposure to 2.0% menthol solution caused the threshold for warmth to rise significantly whereas the threshold for heat pain was unchanged. Although masking of sensations of warmth by menthol-induced sensations of cold may explain the results, a direct effect of the menthol molecule on warmth receptors (i.e., inhibition or desensitization) was considered by the author to be a more likely explanation.

Menthol is usually combined with other ingredients with antipruritic or analgesic properties, such as camphor (45).

The recommended dosage for menthol when used as a counterirritant for adults and children over 2 years of age is 1.26–16% applied to the affected area no more than 3 or 4 times a day (46).

Camphor

Although camphor is naturally occurring and is obtained from the camphor tree, approximately three-fourths of the camphor used is prepared synthetically. The natural product is dextrorotatory; the synthetic product is optically active. In concentrations exceeding 3%, particularly when combined with other counterirritant ingredients, camphor stimulates the nerve endings in the skin and induces relief of pain and discomfort by masking moderate to severe deeper visceral pain with a milder pain arising from the skin at the same level of innervation (47). When applied vigorously, it produces a rubefacient reaction.

The recommended concentration for external use as a counterirritant for adults and children over 2 years of age is 3–11%. Higher concentrations are not more effective as counterirritants and can cause more serious adverse reactions if accidentally ingested (22). In concentrations of 0.1–3.0%, camphor depresses cutaneous receptors and is used as a topical analgesic, anesthetic, and antipruritic. Application should be made no more than 3 or 4 times a day. In children under 2 years of age, there is no recommended dosage except under the advice and supervision of a physician.

Because of its systemic toxicity in high concentrations when taken internally, preparations with camphor concentrations exceeding 11%—such as camphorated oil (camphor liniment), which is a solution of 20% camphor in cottonseed oil—are not considered safe for nonprescription use, and commercial camphor products have been removed from the market (48).

Histamine Dihydrochloride

As a Category I external analgesic agent, histamine dihydrochloride in a 0.025–0.10% concentration is considered to be a safe and effective counterirritant when applied no more than 3 or 4 times a day. Application of products containing histamine dihydrochloride results in vasodilatation and causes percutaneous absorption of histamine from an ointment vehicle containing other medicinal agents. Aqueous vehicles seem to be superior to ointments for percutaneous absorption (49).

Methyl Nicotinate

Methyl nicotinate when used in a 0.25–1.0% concentration is a safe and effective counterirritant when applied no more than 3 or 4 times a day. Although nicotinic acid is inactive topically, this ester possesses a marked power of diffusion and readily penetrates the cutaneous barrier. Vasodilation and elevation of skin temperature result from very low concentrations. It has been shown that indomethacin, ibuprofen, and aspirin significantly depress the skin's vascular response to methyl nicotinate. Because these three drugs suppress prostaglandin biosynthesis, it was concluded that the vasodilator response to methyl nicotinate is mediated at least in part by prostaglandin biosynthesis (50). Susceptible persons who apply methyl nicotinate over large areas may experience a drop in blood pressure and pulse rate and syncope due to generalized vascular dilatation (37). In this regard, a study was undertaken to explore the possibility of age and racial differences in methyl-nicotinate-induced vasodilation of human skin (51). The results indicated an equivalent response among young white and black subjects (26–30 years of age) and elderly white subjects (63–80 years of age) when calculating time-to-peak response, the area under the time–response curve, and the time for the response to decline to 75% of its maximum value. These results were unexpected because differences in percutaneous absorption between black and white human skin have been described in several studies (52).

Capsicum Preparations

Capsicum preparations (capsaicin, capsicum, and capsicum oleoresin) are derived from the fruit of various species of plants of the nightshade family. Capsaicin is the major pungent ingredient of hot pepper. When applied to normal skin, it elicits a transient feeling of warmth. More concentrated solutions produce a sensation of burning pain. However, as a result of tachyphylaxis, this local effect diminishes with repeated applications. Capsicum preparations do not cause blistering or reddening of the skin, even in high concentrations, because of their lack of action upon capillaries or other blood vessels.

To determine the reason for this feeling of warmth, investigators applied a solution of capsaicin to the skin, followed by an intradermal injection of histamine to test for chemical responsiveness (53). Although the capsaicin-treated sites responded with the development of a wheal and itch, the flare response did not occur. This latter response, also known as axon reflex vasodilation, is postulated to be under the control of a neurotransmitter—substance P—which is thought to function in the passage of painful stimuli from the periphery to the spinal cord and higher structures (54). High concentrations of substance P are also present in sensory nerves supplying sites of chronic inflammation (55).

Capsaicin appears to primarily affect substance P by depleting it from sensory neurons that have been implicated in mediating cutaneous pain. Local application of capsaicin to the peripheral axon results in depletion of substance P, both peripherally and centrally—presumably the result of impulse initiation. When substance P is released, the initial burning pain and redness occurs, but this phenomenon abates with repeated applications. The net effect may be analogous to cutting a nerve or ligating it, which also depletes the substance P content of the neuron (56).

Substance P is one of the many neuropeptides that have been isolated from peripheral nerve cells; its depletion by capsaicin has assumed an increasing role in the treatment of certain cutaneous disorders, including postherpetic neuralgia (57, 58), psoriasis (59), postmastectomy pain (60), reflex sympathetic dystrophy, and diabetic neuropathy (54, 61).

Because of capsaicin's use in postherpetic neuralgia, the manufacturer petitioned the FDA in January 1988, to add the following claim to the Category I external analgesic indications for capsaicin: "For symptomatic relief of pain (neuralgia) following episodes of shingles (herpes zoster) after open lesions have healed." However, as reported recently (62), FDA's director of the OTC Drug Evaluation Division responded that "without further information to support such use the claim . . . would be inappropriate for OTC drug labeling because herpes zoster and postherpetic neuralgia are not conditions amenable to self-diagnosis and treatment by a lay person." The director further stated that if the claims were substantiated, "professional labeling could be included in the monograph for this ingredient." Subsequently in early 1990, the use of topical capsaicin as an analgesic, after open zoster lesions have healed, was approved by the FDA.

The recommended dosage for adults and children over 2 years of age is a concentration of capsicum preparation that yields 0.025–0.25% capsaicin, applied to the affected area no more than 3 or 4 times a day (63). It appears that efficacy decreases and local discomfort increases when capsaicin is applied fewer than 3 times daily. Pain relief is usually noted within 14 days after therapy is begun, but occasionally relief will be delayed as much as 4–6 weeks following the start of therapy. It should also be noted that because of variations between lots of capsicum, the concentration range for this drug cannot be expressed as a percentage and must be calculated for each lot.

Trolamine Salicylate

Trolamine salicylate, formerly known as triethanolamine salicylate, although a salicylate salt, is not a counterirritant analgesic. The exact mechanism by which salicylates produce their analgesic effect is not known, but it is generally conceded that they act in part centrally, and in part peripherally as anti-inflammatory agents by inhibition of prostaglandins with subsequent relief of pain. Although data exist to show that trolamine salicylate is absorbed from the skin (64), the FDA concluded after a recent review of submitted documents that the data were still insufficient to support general recognition of effectiveness of trolamine salicylate as an OTC external analgesic (65).

Although the review of data by the FDA in 1983 indicated that trolamine salicylate studies submitted up to that time did not show any significant differences between active drug and placebo, several recent reports suggest that trolamine may be effective in alleviating neuralgia caused by unaccustomed strenuous exercise (66) and muscle soreness induced by a reproducible program of weight training (67). Subsequent studies should help clarify the use of this agent as an external analgesic.

Rationale for Combinations of Ingredients

Two or more safe and effective active ingredients may be combined when each active ingredient contributes to the claimed effect and when the combination does not decrease the safety or effectiveness of any of the individual active ingredients. There are four separate chemical and/or pharmacologic groups of counterirritants that provide four qualitatively different types of irritation. Many preparations marketed use at least two such effects when greater potency is desired. Table 1 lists the individual ingredients and classifies them according to their relative potency. Many products will combine active ingredients from one group of counterirritants with one, two, or three other active ingredients, provided that each active ingredient is from a different group. Menthol (Group B) is often combined with one, two, or three active ingredients from different groups. General guidelines for nonprescription drug combination products state that Category I active ingredients from the same therapeutic category should not ordinarily be combined unless there is some benefit over the single ingredient in terms of enhancing effectiveness, safety, patient acceptance, or quality of formulation (68). In this case, combination products containing only camphor and menthol as the active ingredients have been identified (69).

It is irrational to combine counterirritants with local anesthetics, topical antipruritics, or topical analgesics. These agents depress sensory cutaneous receptors, and their effects would be opposed by the counterirritants, which stimulate cutaneous sensory receptors. It is also irrational to combine counterirritants with skin protectants because the protectants act in opposition to the counterirritants and may nullify their effects (70).

Dosage Forms

The vehicles used to formulate the finished product containing counterirritants are important because percutaneous absorption of counterirritant drugs is generally undesirable. The finished product should consist of ingredients and vehicles that keep skin penetration at or near zero. The FDA urged manufacturers to list all inactive ingredients voluntarily (71), and this listing is now being implemented. The nonprescription counterirritant preparations are usually available as liniments, gels, lotions, and ointments. (See Chapter 28, *Topical Anti-infective Products.*)

Liniments

Solutions or mixtures of various substances in oil, alcoholic solutions of soap, or emulsions are called liniments. They are intended for external application and should be so labeled. They are applied to the affected area with friction and rubbing of the skin, the oil or soap base providing ease of application and massage. Liniments with an alcoholic or hydroalcoholic vehicle are useful in instances where rubefacient or counterirritant action is desired; oleaginous liniments are used primarily when massage is desired. By their nature, oleaginous liniments are less irritating to the skin than alcoholic liniments (72).

Liniments should not be applied to skin that is broken or bruised. The vehicle for a liniment is selected on the basis of the kind of action of the desired components (72).

Gels

Gels used for the delivery of counterirritants are more appropriately classified as jellies because they are generally clear, are composed of water-soluble ingredients, and are of a more uniform, semisolid consistency. A greater sensation of warmth is experienced with a gel than with equal quantities of the same product in a dosage form such as lotion or ointment. Products formulated as gels promote a more rapid and extensive penetration of the medication into the skin and hair follicles. Patients should be advised against using excessive amounts of gels or vigorously rubbing them into the skin because increased penetration may cause an unpleasant burning sensation (72).

Lotions

Lotions, liquid suspensions or dispersions, are applied to the skin, usually without friction, for the protective or therapeutic value of the constituents. Depending on the ingredients, they may be alcoholic or aqueous and are often emulsions. Their fluidity allows rapid and uniform application over a wide surface area and makes them especially suited for application to hairy body areas. Lotions are intended to dry on the skin soon after application, leaving a thin layer of their active ingredients on the skin's surface. Because lotions tend to separate while standing, the label should include the instruction to shake the product before each use.

Ointments

Ointments are semisolid preparations intended for external application to the skin or mucous membranes. Ointments are applied to the skin to elicit one of these general effects: a surface activity, an effect within the stratum corneum, or a more deep-seated activity requiring penetration into the epidermis and dermis. These semisolid dosage forms are particularly desirable for counterirritants because these agents are applied with massage (73).

Clinical Considerations

The dosage forms referred to as "greaseless" are oil-in-water formulations, are therefore "water washable," and are usually preferred for daytime use. In the past, many formulations contained lanolin or anhydrous lanolin as a vehicle. However, because both of these vehicles are obtained from wool fat (to which many people are allergic), these animal waxes are no longer used in contemporary formulations.

The longer any dosage form remains in contact with the skin, the longer the duration of action. There seems to be little agreement on how long the preparations should be left in contact with the skin for optimal results, although a practical guideline is that preparations should be used no more than 3 or 4 times a day. Although it is desirable to protect clothing from stains by covering the application site, the covering should not be tightly applied. Tight bandages increase risks of irritation, redness, and blistering.

Labeling of Counterirritant Preparations

Labeling approved by the FDA advisory review panel on topical analgesics identifies the product as an "external analgesic," "topical analgesic," or "pain relieving" cream, lotion, or ointment and may not necessarily be similar to advertising claims (74). The pharmacist can provide accurate and unbiased information about specific products.

Labeling of preparations must list the active ingredients, including their concentrations, and be identified by their officially recognized "established" names. Recently, manufacturers have voluntarily listed inactive ingredients on the label. The manner of usage and the frequency of applications should also be indicated (74).

The labeling for indications states that these preparations should be used "for the temporary relief of minor aches and pains of muscles and joints." In addition, the labeling recommended by the majority of the panel includes claims for "simple backache, strains, bruises, and sprains" (75). These terms were selected because they would be readily and easily understood by the general population.

It is acceptable to use terms describing certain physical or chemical qualities of the counterirritant preparations, as long as these terms do not imply that any therapeutic effects occur. Terms such as "nongreasy," "soothing," "cooling action," "penetrating relief," "warming relief," and "cool comforting relief" are considered acceptable in labeling.

As with all nonprescription drug products, external analgesics are intended to achieve a beneficial effect within a reasonable period of time. However, claims related to product performance are unacceptable unless they can be substantiated by scientific data. Claims such as "fast," "quick," "prompt," "swift," "immediate," and "remarkable" are misleading and would not signal any property that is important to the safe and effective use of these products (76).

Warnings on counterirritant preparations are as follows:

- For external use only.
- Avoid contact with the eyes.
- If condition worsens, or if symptoms persist for more than 7 days or clear up and occur again within a few days, discontinue use of this product and consult a physician.
- Do not use on children under 2 years of age except under the advice and supervision of a physician.
- Do not apply to wounds or damaged skin.
- Do not bandage tightly.

Safety of Counterirritants

The oral toxicity of the counterirritant preparations is variable; some agents such as capsicum preparations have a low oral toxicity, while other agents such as methyl salicylate and camphor are highly toxic when ingested orally. Although some percutaneous absorption occurs with the topical application of the counterirritants, the amounts absorbed are insignificant when the ingredients do not exceed the maximum recommended effective concentrations and the environmental conditions are normal (i.e., the counterirritant is not applied after strenuous exercise during high outdoor heat).

Self-medication with nonprescription counterirritant preparations may result in harm if directions are not followed exactly. Some individuals overreact to the irritant properties of counterirritants and develop rashes and blisters. In addition to irritation, counterirritants also may produce sensitization, in which case immunologic phenomena are involved. It may be difficult to distinguish between direct topical irritation and topical sensitization. Therefore, the labeling of preparations must indicate prompt discontinuation if excessive skin irritation develops.

Physical Methods of Counterirritation

Although the nonprescription preparations do have their own merit as therapeutic agents, there are simple physical methods of inducing counterirritation. Perhaps the most frequently employed method is heat applied by means of a heat lamp, hot-water bottle, heating pad, or moist steam pack. Heat helps to restore the elastic property of collagen by increasing the viscous flow. Under normal conditions, collagen recoils like a spring once the load is released. After a stretching injury, the collagen tissue does not return to its resting length. Heat also acts selectively on free nerve endings in the tissue and on peripheral nerve fibers to increase the pain threshold. This results in an analgesic effect (77). As recently reported (34), the application of heat should be used with extreme caution if at all in conjunction with a counterirritant preparation. Severe burning or blistering of skin, muscle and skin necrosis, and interstitial nephritis have resulted from the simultaneous use of a counterirritant preparation and heat.

Massaging the painful area is another method of producing counterirritation. The therapeutic benefits of massage have been known for centuries. It is possible that the beneficial effects of some counterirritants used in treating musculoskeletal disorders may be due largely to the rubbing and massage involved in the application of the medication. Massage increases the flow of blood and lymph in the skin and underlying structures.

Studies comparing massage with other modalities are nonexistent because it is difficult to prepare protocols for conducting controlled objective clinical studies on the therapeutic effectiveness of massage techniques. Many clinicians have found that massage is therapeutically beneficial in select situations and use it extensively.

SUMMARY

Counterirritant external analgesic agents provide a method of decreasing the pain and discomfort associated with many minor aches and pains of muscles and joints. However, they must be used correctly to be safe and effective.

Pharmacists can play an important role in patient education by instructing patients on the proper use of these agents. Because external analgesic drug products temporarily relieve only minor pain, patients should understand the degree of relief that can reasonably be expected and the amount of time that it takes for relief to occur. Patients should also be advised when self-medication is not indicated and a physician should be consulted.

REFERENCES

1 *Federal Register, 48,* 5867 (1983).

2 H. Merskey, *Pain, 6,* 249–252 (1979).

3 R. Melzack and P. D. Wall, *Science, 150,* 971–979 (1965).

4 A. G. Lipman, in "Clinical Pharmacy and Therapeutics," 4th ed., E. T. Herfindal et al., Eds., Williams and Wilkins, Baltimore, Md., 1988, pp. 945–949.

5 J. C. Puffer and M. S. Zachazewski, *Am. Fam. Phys., 38,* 225–232 (1988).

6 S. A. Herring and K. C. Nilson, *Clin. Sports Med., 6,* 225–239 (1987).

7 D. Ferguson, *Med. J. Aust., 140,* 318–319 (1984).

8 C. D. Brown et al., *Med. J. Aust., 140,* 329–332 (1984).

9 *Drug Ther. Bull., 14,* 66–67 (1976).

10 R. E. Booth, Jr., and J. P. Marvel, Jr., *Orthop. Clin. North Am., 6,* 353–379 (1975).

11 F. W. Jobe and C. M. Jobe, *Clin. Orthop. Rel. Res., 173,* 117–124 (1983).

12 N. M. Halder, *Arthritis Rheum., 20,* 1019–1025 (1977).

13 R. P. Nirschi, in "Symposium on Upper Extremity Injuries in Athletes," F. A. Petron, Ed., C. V. Mosby, St. Louis, Mo., 1986, pp. 322–336.

14 G. Evans, *Br. Med. J., 294,* 1569–1570 (1987).

15 R. J. Quinet and N. M. Hadler, *Semin. Arth. Rheum., 8,* 261–287 (1979).

16 S. Crown, *Rheumatol. Rehabil., 17,* 114–124 (1978).

17 K. Kane and A. Taub, *Pain, 1,* 125–138 (1975).

18 T. A. Gossel, *U.S. Pharmacist, 12 (8),* 26 (1987).

19 E. A. Swinyard and M. A. Pathak "The Pharmacological Basis of Therapeutics," A. G. Goodman et al., Eds., Macmillan, New York, N.Y., 1980, p. 950.

20 B. S. Post, *Arch. Phys. Med. Rehabil., 42,* 791 (1961).

21 "Krantz and Carr's Pharmacological Principles of Medical Practice," 8th ed., D. M. Aviado, Ed., William and Wilkins, Baltimore, Md., 1972, p. 891.

22 D. W. Lewis and P. J. Verhonick, *Appl. Radiol., 6,* 114 (1977).

23 *Federal Register, 48,* 5864 (1983).

24 *Federal Register, 44,* 69784 (1979).

25 *Federal Register, 48,* 5865 (1983).

26 "Martindale: The Extra Pharmacopoeia," 29th ed., J. E. F. Reynolds, Ed., The Pharmaceutical Press, London, England, 1989, p. 1542.

27 *Federal Register, 44,* 69792–3 (1979).

28 S. Patel and J. Wiggins, *Arch. Dis. Child., 55,* 405–406 (1980).

29 *Federal Register, 44,* 68930 (1979).

30 W. B. Deichman and H. W. Gerarde, "Toxicology of Drugs and Chemicals," Academic Press, New York, N.Y., 1969, p. 662.

31 "Martindale: The Extra Pharmacopoeia," 29th ed., J. E. F. Reynolds, Ed., The Pharmaceutical Press, London, England, 1989, p. 27.

32 *Federal Register, 44,* 68831 (1979).

33 K. Trapnell, *J. Am. Pharm. Assoc., NS16,* 147 (1976).

34 M. C. Y. Heng, *Cutis, 39,* 442–444 (1987).

35 A. Danon et al., *Eur. J. Clin. Pharmacol., 31,* 49–52 (1986).

36 M. S. Roberts et al., *Aust. N.Z. J. Med., 12,* 303–305 (1982).

37 *Federal Register, 44,* 69830–1 (1979).

38 F. Speer, *Ann. Allergy, 43,* 36–37 (1979).

39 *Federal Register, 44,* 69840–1 (1979).

40 "Martindale: The Extra Pharmacopoeia," 29th ed., J. E. F. Reynolds, Ed., The Pharmaceutical Press, London, England, 1989, p. 1067.

41 "Martindale: The Extra Pharmacopoeia," 29th ed., J. E. F. Reynolds, Ed., The Pharmaceutical Press, London, England, 1989, p. 1586.

42 C. Papa and W. Shelley, *J. Am. Med. Assoc., 547,* 189 (1964).

43 A. A. Fisher, *Cutis, 38,* 17–18 (1986).

44 B. G. Green, *Physiol. Behav., 38,* 833–838 (1986).

45 *Federal Register, 48,* 5857 (1983).

46 *Federal Register, 44,* 69828 (1979).

47 W. J. Phelam III, *Pediatrics, 57,* 428–431 (1976).

48 T. A. Gossel, *U.S. Pharmacist, 8 (4),* 12, 14, 16 (1983).

49 *Federal Register, 44,* 69812–3 (1979).

50 J. K. Wilkin et al., *Clin. Pharmacol. Ther., 38,* 273–277 (1985).

51 R. H. Guy et al., *J. Amer. Acad. Dermatol., 12,* 1001–1006 (1985).

52 K. E. Anderson and H. I. Maibach, *J. Amer. Acad. Dermatol., 1,* 276–1282 (1979).

53 J. E. Bernstein et al., *J. Invest. Dermatol., 76,* 394–395 (1981).

54 J. E. Bernstein, *Semin. Dermatol., 7,* 304–309 (1988).

55 F. Lembeck et al., *Neuropeptides, 1,* 175–180 (1981).

56 M. Fitzgerald, *Pain, 15,* 109–130 (1983).

57 J. E. Bernstein et al., *J. Am. Acad. Dermatol., 17,* 93–96 (1987).

58 C. P. N. Watson et al., *Pain, 33,* 333–340 (1988).

59 J. E. Bernstein et al., *J. Am. Acad. Dermatol., 15,* 504–507 (1986).

60 C. P. N. Watson et al., *Pain, 38,* 177–186 (1989).

61 F. T. Todd and R. J. Vavipapa, *N. Engl. J. Med., 321,* 474–475 (1989).

62 *F.D.C. Reports, 51 (9),* T&G 12 (February 27, 1989).

63 *Federal Register, 44,* 69804–5 (1979).

64 J. L. Rabinowitz et al., *J. Clin. Pharmacol., 22,* 42–48 (1982).

65 *Federal Register, 48,* 5855 (1983).

66 V. Politano et al., *Curr. Ther. Res., 38,* 321–327 (1985).

67 D. W. Hill and J. D. Richardson, *J. Orthop. Sports Phys. Train., 11,* 19–23 (1989).

68 *Federal Register, 48,* 5856 (1983).

69 *Federal Register, 48,* 5857 (1983).

70 *Federal Register, 44,* 69786–7 (1979).

71 *Federal Register, 48,* 5859 (1983).

72 J. G. Nairn, in "Remington's Pharmaceutical Sciences," 17th ed., Mack, Easton, Pa., 1985, pp. 1492–1517.

73 E. A. Swinyard and W. Lowenthal, in "Remington's Pharmaceutical Sciences," 17th ed., Mack, Easton, Pa., 1985, pp. 1301–1306.

74 *Federal Register, 44,* 69784 (1979).

75 *Federal Register, 44,* 69841 (1979).

76 *Federal Register, 48,* 5861 (1983).

77 M. Sherman, *J. Am. Pharm. Assoc., NS20,* 46 (1980).

EXTERNAL ANALGESIC PRODUCT TABLE

Product (Manufacturer)	Application Form	Counterirritant	Other Ingredients
Absorbine Arthritic Pain (W.F. Young)	lotion	methyl salicylate, 10%; camphor, 3.25%; menthol, 1.25%; methyl nicotinate, 1%	
Absorbine, Jr. (W.F. Young)	liniment	menthol, 1.27%; chloroxylenol, 0.5%	acetone
Act-On Rub (Keystone)	lotion	methyl salicylate, 10.4%; menthol, 1.5%; camphor, 1.5%; eucalyptus oil, 1.4%; mustard oil, 0.4%	emulsifying wax, isopropyl myristate, glyceryl stearate, lanolin, methyl paraben
Anabalm (Central)	lotion	methyl salicylate, 10%; camphor, 3%; menthol, 1.25%	greaseless nonstaining emulsion base
Analgesic Balm (Various manufacturers)	ointment	methyl salicylate, menthol	
Argesic (Econo Med)	cream	methyl salicylate	triethanolamine, nongreasy vanishing cream base
Aspercreme (Thompson Medical)	lotion cream		triethanolamine salicylate, 10% greaseless base (cream)
Avalgesic (Various manufacturers)	lotion	methyl salicylate, menthol, camphor, methyl nicotinate, capsicum oleoresin	dipropylene glycol salicylate, oil of cassia, ginger oleoresin
Banalg Muscle Pain Reliever (Forest Pharm.)	lotion	menthol, 1%; methyl salicylate, 4.9%; camphor, 2%	greaseless base
Banalg Arthritic Pain Reliever (Forest Pharm.)	lotion	methyl salicylate, 14%; menthol, 3%	greaseless base
Bangesic (Various manufacturers)	liniment	methyl salicylate, camphor, menthol, eucalyptus oil	greaseless base
Baumodyne (Vortech)	gel ointment	gel: menthol, 1.5%; methyl salicylate, 11.35%; eucalyptus oil ointment: methyl salicylate, 15.2%; menthol, 3.12%; eucalyptus oil	methylparaben, propylparaben, greaseless base (gel)
Ben-Gay (Leeming)	lotion	methyl salicylate, 15%; menthol, 7%	emulsion lotion base
Ben-Gay Arthritis Rub, Extra Strength (Leeming)	ointment	methyl salicylate, 30%; menthol, 8%	greaseless nonstaining emulsion base
Ben-Gay Children's Vaporizing Rub (Leeming)	cream	camphor, 5%; menthol, 4%	emulsion ointment base
Ben-Gay Clear (Leeming)	gel	methyl salicylate, 15%; menthol, 7%	hydroalcoholic gel base
Ben-Gay Greaseless/ Stainless (Leeming)	ointment	methyl salicylate, 15%; menthol, 10%	greaseless nonstaining emulsion base
Ben-Gay Original (Leeming)	ointment	methyl salicylate, 18.3%; menthol, 16%	oleaginous base
Ben-Gay Sports (Leeming)	gel	methyl salicylate, 15.0%; menthol, 10.0%	hydroalcoholic gel base
Ben-Gay Sports Balm, Extra Strength (Leeming)	cream	methyl salicylate, 28%; menthol, 10%	greaseless nonstaining emulsion base
Ben-Gay Warming Ice (Leeming)	gel	menthol, 2.5%	hydroalcoholic gel base

EXTERNAL ANALGESIC PRODUCT TABLE, continued

Product (Manufacturer)	Application Form	Counterirritant	Other Ingredients
Betuline (Ferndale)	lotion	methyl salicylate, camphor, menthol	peppermint oil, water soluble base
Counterpain Rub (Squibb)	ointment	methyl salicylate, menthol, eugenol	greaseless base
Deep-Down (SmithKline Beecham)	rub	methyl salicylate, 15%; methyl nicotinate, 0.7%; menthol, 5%; camphor, 0.5%	
Dencorub (Alvin Last)	cream	methyl salicylate, 20%; camphor, 1%; eucalyptus oil, 0.5%; menthol, 0.75%	stearic acid, beeswax, paraffin, petrolatum, glyceryl stearate, mineral oil, triethanolamine, glycerin, lanolin, fragrance, salicylic acid
Dermal-Rub (Hauck)	balm	methyl salicylate, camphor, racemic menthol, cajuput oil	greaseless base
Dermolin (Hauck)	liniment	methyl salicylate, camphor, racemic menthol, mustard oil	isopropyl alcohol, 8%; greaseless base
Doan's Backache (DEP)	spray	methyl salicylate, 15%; menthol, 8.4%; methyl nicotinate, 0.6%	isopropyl alcohol, 12%
Doan's Rub (DEP)	cream	methyl salicylate, 15%; menthol, 10%	
Emul-O-Balm (Fisons)	lotion	menthol, 2.2%; methyl salicylate, 2.2%; camphor, 1.1%	greaseless base
epi-derm (Pedinol)	balm	methyl salicylate, menthol	propylene glycol, isopropyl alcohol
Exocaine Medicated (Commerce)	rub	methyl salicylate, 25%	
Exocaine Odor Free (Commerce)	cream		triethanolamine salicylate, 10% greaseless base
Exocaine Plus (Commerce)	rub	methyl salicylate, 30%	
Flex-all 454 (Chattem)	gel	menthol, methyl salicylate, eucalyptus oil	aloe vera, alcohol, allantoin, boric acid, carbomer 940, diazolidinyl urea, glycerin, iodine, peppermint oil, polysorbate 60, potassium iodide, propylene glycol, parabens, thyme oil, triethanolamine
Foot Medic (Bristol-Myers Products)	gel	menthol	
Ger-O-Foam (Geriatric)	aerosol	methyl salicylate, 30%	benzocaine, 3%; oil emulsion
Gordogesic (Gordon)	cream	methyl salicylate, 10%	propylene glycol, cetyl alcohol, mineral oil, stearic acid, white wax, triethanolamine, sodium lauryl sulfate, methyl paraben, propylparaben
Heet (Whitehall)	lotion spray	lotion: methyl salicylate, 15%; oleoresin capsicum, (as capsaicin, 0.025%); camphor, 3.6% spray: methyl salicylate, 25%; menthol, 3%; camphor, 3%; methyl nicotinate, 1%	lotion: alcohol, 70%; acetone spray: isopropyl alcohol
Icy Hot (Richardson-Vicks)	balm rub	balm : methyl salicylate, 29%; menthol, 7.6% rub: methyl salicylate, 12%; menthol, 9%	

EXTERNAL ANALGESIC PRODUCT TABLE, continued

Product (Manufacturer)	Application Form	Counterirritant	Other Ingredients
Infra-Rub (Whitehall)	cream	methyl salicylate, 35%; menthol, 15%	
Mentholatum (Mentholatum)	ointment	camphor, 9%; menthol, 1.3%	titanium dioxide, fragrance, petrolatum
Mentholatum Deep Heating (Mentholatum)	lotion rub	lotion: methyl salicylate, 20%; menthol, 6% rub: methyl salicylate, 12.7%; menthol, 5.8%	lotion: carbomer 941, lanolin oil, mineral oil, polysorbate 60, sorbitan stearate, trolamine rub: chloroxylenol, fragrance, glyceryl stearate, sodium lauryl sulfate, lanolin
Mentholatum Deep Heating Arthritis Formula (Mentholatum)	cream	methyl salicylate, 30%; menthol, 8%	glyceryl stearate, sodium lauryl sulfate, isoceteth-20, poloxamer 407, quaternium-15, sorbitan stearate
Methagual (Gordon)		methyl salicylate, 8% guaiacol, 2%	petrolatum, white wax, parabens
Minit-Rub (Bristol-Myers Products)	cream	methyl salicylate, 15%; menthol, 3.5%; camphor, 2.3%	anhydrous lanolin, lanoline, calcium benzoate, polysorbate 20, sodium alginate, sorbitol
Mobisyl (B.F. Ascher)	cream		triethanolamine salicylate, 10%
Musterole Deep Strength (Schering-Plough)	ointment	methyl salicylate, 30%; menthol, 3%; methyl nicotinate, 0.5%	
Musterole Regular and Extra Strength (Schering-Plough)	ointment	camphor, menthol	
Myoflex (Rorer)	cream		trolamine salicylate, 10%; greaseless base
Omega Oil (Block)	liniment	methyl salicylate, 17.5%; methyl nicotinate, 0.27%; capsicum oleoresin, 0.24%; histamine dihydrochloride, 0.02%	isopropyl alcohol, 50%
Panalgesic Gold (Poythress)	liniment	methyl salicylate, 55%; camphor, 3%; menthol, 1.25%	emollient oils, 19%; alcohol, 22%
Panalgesic (Poythress)	cream	methyl salicylate, 35%; menthol, 4%	greaseless base
Pronto (Commerce)	gel	methyl salicylate, 15.9%; menthol, 1%; camphor, 1%; methyl nicotinate, 0.25%	isopropanol, 46%
Rid-A-Pain (Pfeiffer)	liniment	methyl nicotinate, 0.5%; methyl salicylate, 10%	washable base
Sloan's (Warner-Lambert)	liniment	turpentine oil, 46.76%; pine oil, 6.74%; camphor oil, 3.35%; methyl salicylate, 2.66%; capsicum oleoresin, 0.62%	
Soltice Quick Rub (Chattem)	cream	menthol, 5%; camphor, 5%	greaseless base
Sportscreme (Thompson)	cream gel		triethanolamine salicylate, 10%; greaseless base
Stimurub (Otis Clapp)	ointment	menthol, methyl salicylate, capsicum oleoresin	

EXTERNAL ANALGESIC PRODUCT TABLE, continued

Product (Manufacturer)	Application Form	Counterirritant	Other Ingredients
Surin (McKesson)	ointment	methyl salicylate, 1.14%; menthol, 0.285%; camphor, 0.475%	methacholine chloride, 0.25%;greaseless base
ThermoRub (Republic)	lotion ointment	lotion: methyl salicylate, camphor, menthol, oleoresin capsicum, eucalyptus oil ointment: methyl nicotinate, 0.5%, histamine dihydrochloride, 0.05%, capsicum oleoresin	ointment: salicylamide, dipropylene, glycol salicylate
Vicks VapoRub (Richardson-Vicks)	rub	camphor, 4.73%, menthol, 2.6%, eucalyptus oil, 1.2%; spirits of turpentine, 4.5%	
Wonder Ice (Pedinol)	gel	menthol	
Yager's Liniment (Yager)	liniment	turpentine oil, camphor	aqua ammonia, 0.5%; ammonium oleate base

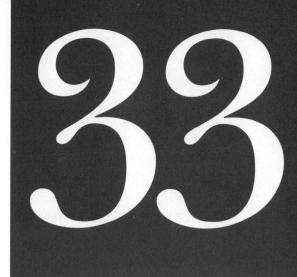

Chester A. (CAB) Bond

BURN AND SUNBURN PRODUCTS

Questions to ask in patient/consumer counseling

What caused the burn—chemicals, sun exposure, or heat?

How severe is the burn? Is the skin broken and/or blistered?

How long ago did the burn occur?

Where is the burn? Does it affect the eyes, genitalia, face, hands, or feet?

Is the burn oozing?

Is the burn painful?

How large is the burned area?

Do you have any other medical problems?

Do you have any other injuries?

What treatments have you used?

Each year in the United States, an estimated 5.6 million fire-related incidents occur (1), resulting in approximately 2 million major burn accidents (2). Because of these accidents, 100,000 persons require hospitalization, spending over 2 million days in hospitals (3). Costs associated with hospitalizations secondary to burns are estimated to exceed $1.5 billion a year. Annually, 12,000 deaths are secondary to burn-related accidents (2). Burn injuries can be broken down by age: under 17 years of age, 33%; between 17 and 44 years, 45%; 45 years and older, 23%. Adjusting the number of burns for the population shows that serious burns are most common in individuals under 17 years of age. Although these figures appear high, the mortality rate has decreased slowly since 1920, with a rapid reduction since 1950 (1, 4). This decrease in mortality emphasizes the effectiveness of fire control measures, flame retardant clothing, and improved safety standards for housing. Additionally, improved systemic and topical therapies, better understanding of the pathophysiology of the burn wound, and the establishment of easily accessible specialized burn centers have reduced morbidity and mortality associated with serious burns.

Confronted with a patient having a small minor burn or sunburn, the pharmacist should render basic first aid, if necessary, and assess whether to recommend physician referral or self-medication for the patient.

ETIOLOGY OF BURNS

Most burns occur in the home; injuries related to heating and cooking account for more than a third of burn injuries (5). In a review of 789 patients admitted to the burn unit of the University Hospital in Uppsala, Sweden, the most common cause of injury was scalding (34%), followed by fire (32%), hot objects (17%), electricity (7%), and chemical agents (4%) (6). In children under 3 years of age, the most common cause of a severe burn is scalding. In children 3–14 years of age, flame burns caused by ignited clothing predominate; in persons 15–60 years of age, industrial accidents account for the largest percent of burns; in those over 60 years of age, accidents associated with momentary blackouts, smoking in bed, or house fires are the most common causes of burns. Alcohol consumption is present in 50% of all burn-related fatalities. Burns are also more common in nonwhites and members of lower socioeconomic groups and in rural areas where space heaters or fireplaces are used for heat. With conventional military warfare, 10–30% of all combat deaths follow thermal injuries (7).

Of the 2 million burn-related accidents occurring annually in the United States, less than 5% are severe enough to require hospitalization. Over 80% of minor burns occur in the home; scalds and contact and fabric burns account for 89% of these household burns (7). Sixty-three percent of household burns are on the hands and arms, and 34% are on the face and legs. Most of these burns do not require medical assistance and may be managed by the patient with appropriate care and nonprescription products. Of the minor burns that occur outside the home, sunburn is the most common. Sunburn has been underrated in most burn surveys because the public often does not consider sunburn in the same context as thermal burns.

SKIN ANATOMY AND PHYSIOLOGY

The skin is the largest organ in the human body and constitutes approximately 17% of the average person's body weight. Figure 1 depicts a cross-section of the normal anatomy of the skin and the depth of burns

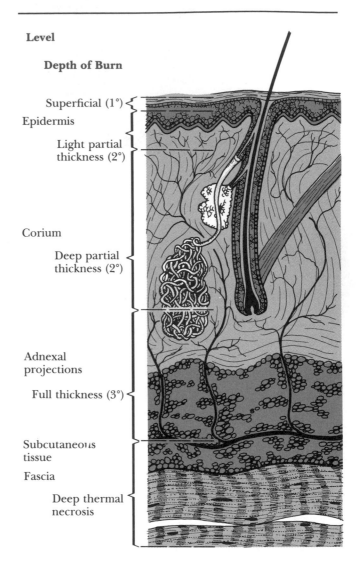

FIGURE 1 Cross-section of skin showing depth of burns.

when thermal damage occurs. The skin's major function is to protect the underlying organ systems from trauma, temperature variations, harmful penetrations, moisture, humidity, radiation, and invasion by microorganisms. In addition, the skin produces secretions from its exocrine glands; is involved in carbohydrate, protein, fat, and vitamin D metabolism; operates its own delayed hypersensitivity reactions; and provides the body with the sense of touch. (See Chapter 28, *Topical Anti-infective Products*.)

PATHOPHYSIOLOGY OF BURNS

Burn damage in the skin causes cellular death, varying degrees of capillary injury, and coagulation of protein. Capillary injury is manifested by increased capillary permeability, resulting in the wet or weepy appearance of second- and third-degree burns. Immediately after a moderate to severe burn, there is cessation of blood flow to the affected area, caused primarily by thrombosis and persisting for 3 to 4 weeks in full-thickness burns. In partial-thickness burns, arterial and venous circulation is restored within 48–72 hours of initial occlusion. Should drying of the wound or infection occur, circulation is not reestablished, and a partial-thickness burn can be converted to a full-thickness burn (8, 9). Therefore, drying of the burn should be prevented. When the blood supply is interrupted, delivery of systemically administered antibiotics to the infection site is prevented and both humoral and cellular defense mechanisms are effectively impeded, thus increasing the risk of infection.

With large deep burns, large amounts of body fluids and electrolytes leave the vascular compartment to extravascular spaces. This fluid redistribution is compounded by the loss of large amounts of body fluids and electrolytes through the burn wound itself. As a result, the cardiac output falls and the patient may go into shock. To prevent this, massive amounts of colloids and intravenous fluids are required during the first 2–4 days of hospitalization. Should the patient experience a respiratory burn from inhaled hot gases, endotracheal intubation and mechanical ventilatory assistance may be required. Complete epithelialization following burns depends on burn depth, the immediate care given to the wound, and whether an infection occurs (10, 11).

Categorization of Burn Injuries

Determining the area and the degree of the burn is not simple even for burn specialists. The American Burn Association has identified three treatment categories for burn patients (11):

- Major Burn Injuries—second-degree burns with a body surface area greater than 25% in adults (20% in children); all third-degree burns with a body surface area of 10% or greater; all burns involving hands, face, eyes, ears, feet, and perineum; all inhalation injuries; electrical burns; complicated burn injuries involving fractures or other major trauma; and burns on all poor-risk patients (elderly patients and those with debilitating diseases);

- Moderate, uncomplicated burn injuries—second-degree burns with a body surface area of 15–25% in adults (10–20% in children); third-degree burns with a body surface area of 2–10%; and burns not involving eyes, ears, face, hands, feet, or perineum;

- Minor burn injuries—second-degree burns with a body surface area of less than 15% in adults (10% in children); third-degree burns with a body surface area of less than 2%; and burns not involving eyes, ears, face, hands, feet, or perineum; excludes electrical injuries, inhalation injuries, and burns on all poor-risk patients.

Determination of Burned Area

The percentage of the body surface that has been burned can be estimated by the "rule of nines" (Figure 2), which divides the body into 11 areas, each representing about 9% of the total. The rule of nines must be adjusted for children under 10 years of age because their bodies have different proportions. Generally, the child's head is 19% of the body surface at birth. Each year the percentage decreases by 1%, which is added in equal amounts to each of the lower limbs.

As a general rule, the area of one side of the hand is 1% of the body surface of an adult. This rule allows quick estimation of the surface area covered by a burn. If the burn is second-degree or greater and covers more than 1% of the body surface, a physician should be consulted.

Determination of Clinical Severity

Determining the severity of the burn is a matter of clinical judgment depending on the burn thickness (Table 1). Burn injury may evolve over the first 24–48 hours, making it somewhat difficult to accurately estimate the severity of serious burns during this time.

First-degree burns These burns affect the epidermis and are characterized by erythema and pain, but no blistering. First-degree burns generally heal within 3 or 4 days with no scarring. First-degree burns are superficial and are considered partial-thickness burns because they affect only the top layer of the skin.

Second-degree burns These burns affect the epidermis and some dermis tissue. They are characterized by erythema, blistering, oozing, and more severe pain. If the second-degree burn is superficial, healing will occur within 3 weeks with no scarring. If the second-degree burn is deep, a firm thick scar with loss of hair, sweat glands, and skin pigmentation will result. Healing

All burns greater than second degree should be evaluated by a physician to prevent infection and other complications. Minor second-degree burns may be treated by the pharmacist, but patients with severe or extensive second-degree burns (> 1% of the body surface) should be sent to a physician for evaluation and treatment. If the degree or severity of the burn is difficult to determine, the patient should be referred to a physician.

Infection

Infection secondary to burns is dangerous and difficult to treat because the burned dead skin provides an ideal growth medium for bacteria, and the avascular burned tissue hinders effective delivery of antimicrobials. The sequence of events leading to clinically significant infections following burn injury has been elucidated. For a very brief period after a severe burn, the wound surface is sterile. Shortly thereafter, colonization occurs by a mixed flora in which Gram-positive organisms predominate (*Staphylococcus* and *Streptococcus*). By the third postburn day, this bacterial population becomes dominated by Gram-negative organisms (*Pseudomonas aeruginosa, Klebsiella, Enterobacter, Proteus*) and the fungi *Candida* (12). By the fifth postburn day, invasion of tissue well beneath the burn surface may occur. These organisms then can proliferate and eventually invade adjacent unburned tissue, causing burn-wound sepsis (13).

To help prevent burn-wound sepsis of severe burns, mafenide, silver nitrate, silver sulfadiazine, and

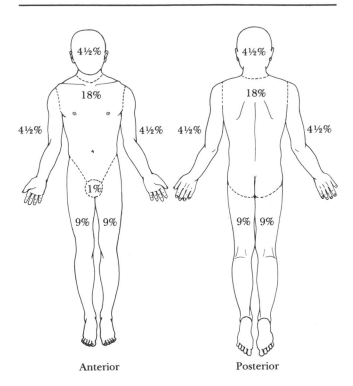

4½%

18%

4½%   4½%   4½%   4½%

1%

9% 9%   9% 9%

Anterior   Posterior

FIGURE 2   Rule of nines, first devised by E. J. Pulaski, M.D., and C. W. Dennison, M.D., is a widely accepted method of quickly estimating the percentage of the body surface burned. For example, an adult with a burn area of one arm (9%), the front of the trunk (18%), and half of one leg (9%) would total a 36% burn. Adapted with permission from "The Guide to Fluid Therapy," Baxter Laboratories, Division of Travenol Laboratories, Inc., Deerfield, Ill., 1969, p. 111.

may take 1 month or more. Second-degree burns are considered partial-thickness burns because they do not affect all layers of the skin. Second-degree burns may become full-thickness burns if they are not adequately cared for.

Third-degree burns These burns affect the full skin thickness, do not blister, have a leathery, white mottled appearance, and are less painful than first- and second-degree burns. Pain often is absent or diminished with third- and fourth-degree burns because of destruction of nervous tissue. Healing occurs very slowly over several months.

Fourth-degree or char burns These burns affect the full-skin thickness and underlying subcutaneous tissues, have a blackened appearance, are dry and generally not painful, and carry the danger of deep infection. Third- and fourth-degree burns may take longer than 1 month to form scar tissue and much longer to heal.

TABLE 1   Depth classification of burns

Type	Tissue affected	Characteristics
First-degree	Epidermis	Erythema, pain, no blistering
Second-degree	Epidermis, some dermis	Erythema, blisters, pain
Third-degree	Full-skin thickness	No blisters, leathery white appearance, less pain
Fourth-degree and char burn	Full-skin thickness and underlying tissue	Blackened appearance, dryness, little pain, danger of deep infection

nitrofurazone can be used (14). The agents work best in patients who have burns on less than 50% of their body surface, and have resulted in improved survival rates of patients with burns involving 50–70% of their body surface. However, when more than 70% of the body surface is affected, studies of these agents have demonstrated no reduction in mortality (13–15). This reduction in mortality is attributed to the control of bacterial flora and the elimination of burn-wound sepsis. If sepsis occurs, systemic antibiotics should also be used.

Sunburn

Sunburn (erythema) is usually self-limiting and does not require treatment by a physician unless the burn is quite severe, becomes infected, or is associated with other serious problems. Energy emissions from the sun include radiation wavelengths ranging from 200 nm to more than 18,000 nm (16). Ultraviolet (UV) radiation is in the 200–400 nm range; this spectrum is subdivided into three bands as follows (17):

- UV-A (320–400 nm) radiation can cause some tanning of the skin, but is weak in causing mild sunburn of the skin. UV-A radiation may contribute about 15% of the erythema produced at noontime.

- UV-B (290–320 nm) radiation causes sunburn reaction, which also stimulates pigmentation (tanning) of the skin. UV-B radiation at 290 nm is 1,000 times more potent in producing erythema than UV-B radiation at 320 nm (11).

- UV-C (200–290 nm) radiation from sunlight does not reach the earth's surface, but artificial ultraviolet sources can emit its radiation. It does not tan the skin, but can burn it.

Other wavelengths of light also are absorbed and, if intense enough, produce erythema and burning. This type of burning differs from sunburn in that it is due to generated heat rather than a photochemical reaction.

The vascular changes that occur secondary to exposure to ultraviolet radiation are biphasic. An immediate erythema reaction, which is a faint, transient reddening of the skin, begins shortly after exposure to ultraviolet radiation and fades within 30 minutes after the exposure ends. A delayed erythema reaction appears after 2–5 hours and peaks 10–24 hours after exposure to ultraviolet radiation. (See *Plate 3–13*.) This erythema gradually subsides over the next 2–4 days. Peeling follows 4–7 days after a moderate to severe sunburn. The mechanisms by which these two types of erythema are produced are not completely understood.

Kinins (18, 19), histamine (20), prostaglandins (21–26), other vasoactive substances (27), hydrolytic enzymes (28), and free radicals (29) have been implicated as mediators (causes) of the erythema caused by sunlight. Although prostaglandins have received much attention in the scientific and lay press, they are not universally accepted as the mediators in sunburn causes.

Clinically, mild sunburn is tender to the touch, and the patient may complain of a hot, drawn feeling of the skin. A patient with a more severe burn may experience intense pain, inability to tolerate contact with clothing, and systemic symptoms of fever, chills, nausea, and prostration. Newborns, young children, and elderly patients are more susceptible to sunburn than adults.

Photosensitization

A photosensitivity reaction should be considered in a patient who experiences sunburn in greater amounts than would be normally expected from exposure to ultraviolet radiation or who develops a rash in areas exposed to the sun. Photosensitivity reactions can occur from topically applied or systemically administered compounds. Photosensitivity reactions require the presence of drug or chemical and light. There are two types of photosensitivity reactions. (See *Plates 3–14* and *3–15*.) The first type is a photoallergic reaction, in which the drug is altered in the presence of sunlight so that it becomes antigenic or acts as a haptene (Figure 3). Photoallergic eruptions require previous exposure to the offending drug and are not dose related. These eruptions may be induced by chemically related drugs and may appear in various forms, such as eczematous, macular, or papular lesions, which may not appear for 24 hours or longer after exposure. Eczematous reactions are the most common type of lesion seen with photoallergic reactions. Acute urticarial lesions may also develop within minutes after exposure to ultraviolet radiation. This eruption is not exclusively localized at sun exposure sites but frequently extends beyond the exposure area. These types of photosensitivity eruptions are usually caused by topical agents but occasionally may be seen with systemically administered drugs. Photoallergic reactions are more commonly seen in adults than children (30). This is probably because adults have taken more drugs than children during their lives and thus have a greater risk of sensitization.

The second type of photosensitivity eruption is known as a phototoxic reaction. In this reaction, the drug is altered by light to a toxic form that damages the skin tissue. It is independent of an allergic response. In contrast to the first type, this eruption can occur on the first exposure to the drug, is dose related, and occurs within several hours of exposure to the sun. There usually is no cross-sensitivity with other drugs with phototoxic reactions (Figure 3). A phototoxic reaction almost always appears as an exaggerated sunburn, with most patients reporting burning or stinging of the skin prior to the appearance of sunburn. Most phototoxic reactions occur between 310 and 420 nm of ultraviolet radiation. In some instances, a drug may produce both photoallergic and phototoxic reactions (photosensitivity) (Table 2) (29–33).

ASSESSMENT

To recommend treatment to the burn patient, the pharmacist must accurately assess the patient and the

Photoallergy	**Phototoxicity**
Drug + UV light	Drug + UV light
⬇	⬇
Photo-altered drug (haptene)	Photo-excited drug
+	⬇
Skin protein	Release of absorbed energy into skin
⬇	⬇
Complete antigen	Potentiated sunburn response
+	
Reexposure to UV light	
⬇	
Photosensitivity reaction	

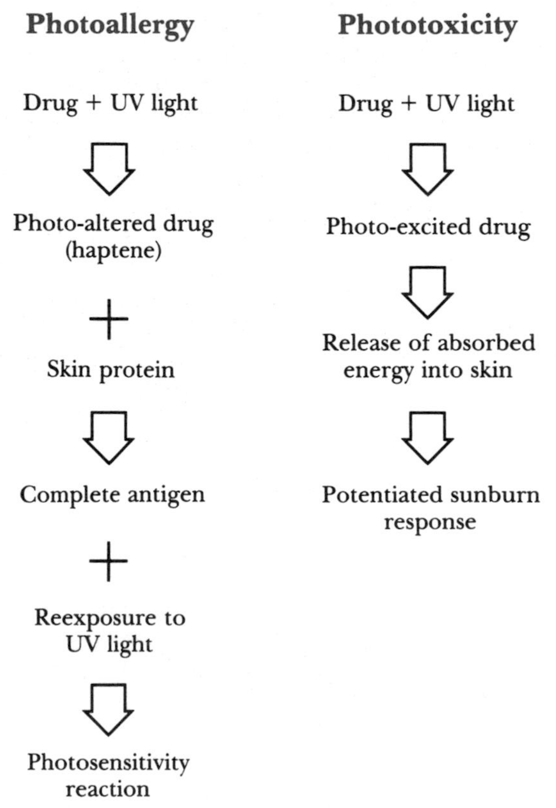

FIGURE 3 Comparison of photoallergy and phototoxicity reactions. Reprinted with permission from *Am. Pharm.*, NS21, 296 (1981).

injury to determine if the burn is amenable to self-treatment or if consultation with or referral to the patient's physician is necessary. The pharmacist should learn the cause of the burn and when it occurred to determine what, if any, self-treatment is appropriate. If necessary, the pharmacist should arrange transportation to a medical facility.

Newborns, young children, and the elderly generally should be referred to a physician because they may poorly tolerate burn trauma. Also, patients in these age groups may complain less about their burn than older children or young adults.

Burn patients with chronic or debilitating conditions (diabetes, obesity, alcoholism, cardiovascular disease, and renal disease) also should be referred to a physician. Individuals with a moderate to severe chronic illness poorly tolerate burn trauma and are more susceptible to complications from burns. The burn trauma may also exacerbate the patient's underlying disease.

Burns of the eye, genitalia, and perineum have more serious consequences and should be evaluated by a physician. Facial burns may be associated with respiratory injuries. Because of the possibility of scarring, burns greater than first degree on the face should be referred to a physician for treatment. Burns of the hands and feet may deserve special attention because healing may be delayed in these areas and because they can be quite painful.

TREATMENT

Initial Care

Thermal Burns

Evidence suggests that the inflammatory process secondary to thermal burns can be reduced and sometimes reversed by cold-water therapy. One study showed that when cold water was applied to a burn, the visible area of redness was reduced in extent and did not reappear later, suggesting an alteration in pathologic state. It has been suggested that the lower skin temperature inhibited capillary engorgement and the resulting loss of fluids. This in turn leads to a lowered metabolic requirement of the already damaged tissues, allowing preservation of such tissues (34). Cold-water therapy includes the following procedures:

TABLE 2   Some drugs that may cause photosensitivity

Anticancer drugs

*Dacarbazine
Fluorouracil
Methotrexate
Procarbazine
Vinblastine

Antidepressants

Amitriptyline
Amoxapine
Desipramine
Doxepin
Imipramine
Isocarboxazid
Maprotiline
Nortriptyline
Protriptyline
Trimipramine

Antihistamines

Cyprohepatidine
Diphenyldramine

Antimicrobials

*Demeclocyline
Doxycycline
Griseofulvin
Methacycline
Minocycline
*Nalidixic acid

Oxytetracycline
Sulfacytine
Sulfadoxine-
pyrimethamine
Sulfamethizole
Sulfamethoxazole
Trimethoprim-
sulfamethoxazole
Sulfasalazine
Sulfathiazole
Sulfisoxazole
Tetracycline

Antiparasitic drugs

*Bithionol
Pyruinium
Quinine

Diuretics

Acetazolamide
Amiloride
Bendroflumethiazide
Benzthiazide
Chlorothiazide
Cyclothiazide
Furosemide
Hydrochlorothiazide
Hydroflumethiazide
Methyclothiazide
Metolazone

Polythiazide
Quinethazone
Trichlormethiazide

Hypoglycemics

Acetohexamide
Chlorpropamide
Glipizide
Glyburide
Tolazamide
Tolbutamide

**Nonsteroidal anti-
inflammatory drugs**

Ketoprofen
Naproxen
Phenylbutazone
Piroxicam
Sulindac

Sunscreens

Benzophenones
Cinnamates
Oxybenzone
Para-aminobenzoic acid
PABA esters

Antipsychotic drugs

Chlorpromazine
Chlorprothixine

Fluphenazine
Haloperidol
Periphenazine
Piperacetazine
Prochlorperazine
Promethazine
Thioridazine
Thiothixine
Trifluoperazine
Triflupromazine
Trimeprazine

Other

*Amiodarone
Benzocaine
*Bergamot oil, oils of
citron, lavender, lime,
sandalwood, cedar (used in
many perfumes and
cometics)
Carbamazepine
*Coal tar
Disopyramide
Gold salts
Hexachlorophene
Isotretinoin
*Methoxsalen
Oral contraceptives
Quinidine sulfate and
gluconate
*Trioxsalen

*Reactions occur more frequently.
Reprinted with permission from *Med. Lett. Drugs Ther., 28 (713)*, 51 (1986).

■ The burned area should be immersed immediately in water drawn from the cold tap.

■ The burned area should be kept in static (nonrunning) water until it is free of pain both in and out of the water; this may require up to 45 minutes.

■ Usually no further treatment is necessary because blisters, which otherwise would appear, do not form; the injury may not even need a dressing.

■ Nothing should be applied to the burn if cold-water therapy is ineffective and the patient wants to consult a physician (35).

One investigator cautions against the use of this technique for the seriously burned child because the time involved may delay the emergency treatment of shock (36).

The public should be made aware of the value of cold water in controlling the intense pain of minor burns (37).

Electrical Burns

Electrical burns may appear to be superficial because the only area that seems to be burned is where the current entered and exited the body. However, there may be extensive damage to underlying nervous and muscle tissue. Only very minor electrical burns should be self-medicated. When in doubt, refer the patient to a physician.

Chemical Burns

Clothing should be removed from the affected area (taking care to avoid further contact with the chemicals). The burn should be flooded with large amounts of water (at least 15 minutes for acids, and until the skin no longer feels soapy for alkalies). Chemical antidotes should not be used because the acid-base reaction heat may cause further damage. For more severe chemical burns, the depth of the injury may be reduced by up to 2–4 hours of washing. If the eye is involved, it should be washed immediately and irrigated with tepid water for 15–30 minutes. The eyelid should be gently opened while irrigating the eye from the nasal corner to the outer corner. The face and eyelids also should be washed, and care should be taken not to wash the chemical into the other eye. The eye should be covered with a clean dressing, and the patient should be transported to a medical facility as soon as possible.

Sunburn

Sunburned patients should protect the burned area from further exposure to UV radiation as soon as possible. Generally, if sunburn on the eyes and genitalia produces second-degree burns or the patient is having severe pain, the patient should be referred to a physician. If the sunburn affects more than 10% of a child's body surface or more than 15–20% of an adult's body surface, the patient should be referred to a physician.

Heat stroke can occur with excessive exposure to sunlight in a hot and/or humid environment. Because of the complications of heat stroke, patients exhibiting hyperpyrexia, confusion, weakness, or convulsions should be referred to their physician or an appropriate medical facility.

Minor Burns

Cleansing

The goals of treating first- and second-degree burns are relieving the pain associated with the burn, protecting the area from air, preventing dryness, and providing a favorable environment for healing that minimizes the chances of infection. After applying cold moisture to the burned area, which stops the progression of the burn injury, reduces local edema, and re-lieves pain, the area should be cleansed with water and a bland soap (38–42). After the burn is cleansed, a non-adherent, hypoallergenic burn dressing may be applied if the area is small, or a skin protectant/lubricant may be applied if the burn is extensive or in an area that cannot be dressed easily. If the burn is weeping, soaking the burn 3–6 times a day for 15–30 minutes will provide a soothing effect and diminish the weeping. Minor burns usually are benign and repair themselves without treatment.

Dressings

Sterile, nonadherent dressings are the most convenient way to treat a small burn on an area of the body that may be easily bandaged, such as the arm or leg.

The following is the recommended sequence for dressing a small burn (normally necessary only with second-degree burns) (43):

- A nonadherent primary layer of sterile, fine-mesh gauze lightly impregnated with sterile petrolatum should be applied over the burn. Petrolatum gauze does not stick to the wound and allows burn exudate to flow freely through the dressing, thus avoiding tissue maceration. Commercially prepared nonadhering petrolatum dressings, such as Xeroflow or Adaptic, incorporate hydrophilic petrolatum into the gauze to aid permeability.

- An absorbent intermediate layer of piled-up gauze should be applied over the petrolatum gauze. This layer draws and stores exudate away from the wound, which guards against maceration. Cotton or paper products should not be used because they often stick to the burn and are painful and difficult to remove. This layer should be applied loosely to accommodate edema, should it occur.

- A supportive layer of rolled gauze bandage should be applied over the primary and intermediate gauze layers to hold these layers in place and mildly restrict movement. Elastic or other expandable bandages that tighten after being applied should not be used because they could restrict circulation if edema develops.

The dressing should be changed every 48 hours. If the dressing sticks to the wound, soaking in warm water will loosen the gauze from the burn with minimal pain and trauma. Also, removing the sticking gauze slowly will protect the regenerating epithelium and minimize pain. The wound should be examined for signs of infection at each dressing change. The earliest signs of infection may be inflamed wound edges, new blistering, or intensification of pain. If the affected skin begins to become macerated (feels or looks wrinkled or fissured), dressing the wound should be temporarily discontinued, and the wound should be exposed to air. Once the pain subsides and healing begins (in 4–10 days), wound dressings may be discontinued.

Soaks

The inflammation from first- and second-degree burns may be reduced by having the patient soak the affected area in water, normal saline, or Burow's solution (diluted 1:20–1:40) for 15–30 minutes 3–6 times a day. All soaking solutions should be freshly prepared. Soaking solutions become concentrated if they are allowed to sit open and can cause irritation if reused. They also could serve as a growth medium for bacteria and could promote infections. Soaking is particularly applicable to weeping lesions because it provides a cooling, soothing treatment that promotes drying. Once weeping subsides, a skin protectant may be applied to the skin. Depending on the burn size and location, the patient may immerse the affected areas directly into the soak, or apply a towel or cloth soaked in the solution (lightly wrung), or draw a bath and soak in it for the prescribed time. The temperature of the soak should be cool to warm (not cold or hot) depending on the patient's preference. If maceration occurs, soaks should be discontinued. When drying the affected areas after the soak, care must be taken not to irritate the burn by rubbing with a towel. The proper technique for drying the burned area (or other irritated areas of the skin) is patting, not rubbing, the area gently with a dry clean towel.

PHARMACOLOGIC AGENTS

As previously mentioned, most minor burns heal by themselves. The purpose of pharmacotherapy is to make the patient more comfortable and allow the skin to heal. Pharmacists should generally limit their recommendations to patients with first- or minor second-degree burns (<1% of body surface). The pharmacist should not recommend a product for extensive or deep second-, third-, or fourth-degree burns because this may cause the patient to delay appropriate treatment by a physician. Additionally, inappropriate applications of topical preparations to severe burns must be removed (usually with considerable discomfort) when the patient seeks medical treatment. The pharmacist should also be aware that damaged skin, secondary to burns, loses some of its barrier function, thus enhancing percutaneous absorption of drugs and chemicals (44). This factor

TABLE 3

Ingredient	Approved concentrations (in %)
Allantoin	0.5–2
Aluminum hydroxyde gel	0.15–5
Calamine	1–25
Cocoa butter	50–100
Dimethicone	1–30
Glycerin	20–45
Kaolin	4–20
Petrolatum	30–100
Shark liver oil	3
White petrolatum	30–100
Zinc acetate	0.1–2
Zinc carbonate	0.2–2
Zinc oxide	1–25

increases the possibility of systemic side effects, especially in patients with large burn areas such as extensive sunburn and in patients who too frequently apply topical medications.

Protectants

Based on recommendations of its over-the-counter (OTC) advisory review panel on skin-protectant drug products, the Food and Drug Administration (FDA) proposed that the agents in Table 3 are safe and effective (Category I) in treating first- and minor second-degree burns (45). Skin protectants benefit patients with minor burns by making the wound area more comfortable. They provide their therapeutic effects by protecting the burn from mechanical irritation caused by friction and rubbing and by preventing drying of the stratum corneum. Rehydrating the stratum corneum relieves the symptoms of irritation and permits normal healing to continue. Skin protectants provide only symptomatic relief and do not stop the underlying burn process.

In selecting a skin protectant for burns, the pharmacist should choose products that prevent dryness and provide lubrication. The FDA panel has proposed classifying bismuth subnitrate, boric acid, sulfur, and tannic acid as not generally recognized as safe and effective or as misbranded when used as skin protectants.

The FDA recently has revised labeling for skin protectants as follows (46):

- "For the temporary protection of minor cuts, scrapes, burns, and sunburn." (See Table 3 for recommended ingredients.)

- "Helps prevent and temporarily protects chafed, chapped, cracked or wind-burned skin and lips." Allantoin, cocoa butter, petrolatum, shark liver oil, dimethicone, and glycerin.

- "Dries the oozing and weeping of poison ivy, poison oak, and poison sumac." Aluminum hydroxide gel, calamine, kaolin, zinc acetate, zinc carbonate, and zinc oxide. (See Chapter 35, *Poison Ivy and Poison Oak Products*.)

Based on the panel's recommendations, the FDA proposed that labeling claims of "cures any irritation" or "prevents formation of blisters" are not generally recognized as safe and effective (Category II). Claims that certain substances (allantoin, live yeast cell derivatives, and zinc acetate) contained in many skin protectants are effective for accelerating wound healing were not recognized by the FDA. There are no controlled studies that conclusively prove that minor wounds amenable to nonprescription treatment can be healed in accelerated fashion.

The provisional FDA-approved skin protectants are both safe and nontoxic. The panel recommended that the restriction preventing use in children under 2 years of age be waived for most skin protectants except for products containing live yeast cell derivatives, shark liver oil, and zinc acetate where the limit applies. An additional exception was made for glycerin and aluminum hydroxide gel. The recommendation for labeling for these two ingredients is "There is no recommended dosage for children under 6 months of age except under the advice and supervision of a physician." The panel made these recommendations on the basis of safety considerations. Generally, the burn patient may apply a skin protectant as often as needed; if the burn has not improved in 7 days or worsens after treatment, the patient should consult a physician (44).

Topical Analgesics

Local Anesthetics

Local anesthetics may be useful for short-term relief of pain associated with minor burns or sunburn. These agents should not be used to treat serious burns because they may cause the patient to delay appropriate treatment by a physician. Based on information submitted to the FDA in response to the panel's report (47), the FDA proposed these ingredients as generally regarded as effective for temporary relief of pain associated with minor burns or sunburn. Table 4 lists the local anesthetics that are safe and effective in relieving pain associated with minor burns (48).

The choice between a product containing benzocaine or lidocaine is difficult. Benzocaine and chemically similar local anesthetics have a higher incidence of sensitization (about 1%) than lidocaine (49), but benzocaine is virtually devoid of systemic toxicities (43). Benzocaine rarely has been reported to induce reversible methemoglobinemia (50, 51). Lidocaine, while having a very low incidence of sensitization, may cause systemic side effects (stimulation or depression of the central nervous system, drowsiness, nervousness, dizziness, blurred vision, nausea, tremors, convulsions, respiratory arrest, myocardial depression, and cardiac arrest) when applied over large areas of damaged skin or used for prolonged periods (47). Systemic toxicity from local

TABLE 4 Local anesthetic ingredients	
Types	**Approved concentrations (in %)**
AMINE AND "CAINE"-TYPE LOCAL ANESTHETICS	
Benzocaine	5–20
Butamben picrate	1
Dibucaine	0.25–1
Dibucaine hydrochloride	0.25–1
Dimethisoquin hydrochloride	0.3–0.5
Dyclonine hydrochloride	0.5–1
Lidocaine	0.5–4
Lidocaine hydrochloride	0.5–4
Pramoxine hydrochloride	0.5–1
Tetracaine	1–2
Tetracaine hydrochloride	1–2
ALCOHOLS AND KETONES	
Benzyl alcohol	10–33
Camphor	0.1–3
Camphor	3–10.8*
Camphorated metacresol	
Camphor	3–10.8
Metacresol	1–5
Juniper tar	1–5
Menthol	0.1–1
Phenol	4.7*
Phenolate sodium	0.5–1.5
Resorcinol	0.5–3
ANTIHISTAMINES	
Diphenhydramine hydrochloride	1–2
Tripelennamine hydrochloride	0.5–2

*When combined in a light mineral oil, USP vehicle.
Adapted from *Federal Register*, *48*, 5867–8 (1984).

anesthetics is rare because short-term use for minor burns generally does not allow elevated toxic blood levels to occur. Cross-sensitization to local anesthetics in different classes is very rare; thus, a patient sensitized to one class usually can use a local anesthetic in another class without problems.

Local anesthetics must penetrate the skin to produce their desired effects, and the degree of penetration is determined by the amount of damage to the skin. In general, lower concentrations of local anesthetics (Table 4) that are effective on severely damaged skin may be ineffective on intact skin or mildly damaged skin. For example, in concentrations below 20%, benzocaine fails to have beneficial effects on intact or mildly sunburned skin (52). In studies on severely damaged skin, however, concentrations as low as 5% are effective. To ensure effectiveness, the pharmacist should select a product containing a local anesthetic in concentrations approaching the upper limits of the FDA-recommended concentrations. Benzocaine is recommended in concentrations of 5–20% applied to the affected area; lidocaine and lidocaine hydrochloride are recommended in concentrations of 0.5–4%. However, no claim for effectiveness is made when the lidocaine hydrochloride is used on intact skin in the available nonprescription concentrations (47).

The FDA recognized the recommendation by the advisory review panel on OTC topical analgesic drug products that products containing local anesthetics should not be applied more than 3 or 4 times a day, should not be used in large quantities, and should not be applied over extensive areas or on raw, blistered, or damaged skin. These recommendations were made to reduce the possibility of systemic side effects. The duration of action of local anesthetics is only 15–45 minutes (45), so it is impossible to provide continuous pain relief. Because of these factors, the pharmacist should recommend that products containing local anesthetics be used only when the pain may be particularly bothersome to the patient, such as at bedtime.

Topical Hydrocortisone

Nonprescription topically applied hydrocortisone is reported to be a safe and effective alternative to the nonprescription anesthetics that are currently used for mild sunburn (e.g., benzocaine, diphenhydramine, menthol, and phenol) (53). Topical hydrocortisone is very beneficial when applied to mild to moderate sunburns (particularly when it is formulated in an ointment vehicle).

Counterirritants

Counterirritant agents relieve pain by stimulating cutaneous neurons to provide a feeling of warmth or coolness. Because counterirritants may irritate the burned tissue and ultimately result in more pain for the patient, they should not be used on burns. (See Chapter 32, *External Analgesic Products*.)

Antimicrobials

The FDA has recognized recommended subclassifications by the advisory review panel (Antimicrobial I) on OTC topical antimicrobial drug ingredients, including quaternary ammonium compounds, iodophors, organic mercurials, and phenols. The panel defined several subclasses of antimicrobial preparations that may be used to prevent infection in minor burns or sunburn (49, 54). These subclasses include:

- Antimicrobial soap—a soap containing an active ingredient with both in vitro and in vivo activity against skin microorganisms;

- Skin antiseptic—a nonirritating antimicrobial-containing preparation that prevents overt skin infections;

- Skin-wound cleanser—a nonirritating liquid preparation (or product to be used with water) that assists in removing foreign material from small superficial wounds, does not delay wound healing, and may contain an antimicrobial ingredient;

- Skin-wound protectant—a nonirritating antimicrobial-containing preparation applied to small cleansed wounds that provides a protective physical barrier and a chemical (antimicrobial) barrier that neither delays healing nor favors microbial growth (54).

As previously mentioned, burn wounds are particularly susceptible to infection. Because the effects of infection can be devastating, any patient with an infected burn should be referred to a physician for evaluation and treatment.

The use of topical antibiotics is covered more fully in Chapter 28, *Topical Anti-infective Products*.

Product Formulation

Rarely will a product that is intended to treat minor burns contain only one ingredient. The FDA advisory review panel on OTC skin-protectant drug products concluded that two or more skin-protectant active ingredients may be combined provided that (47):

- Each is present in sufficient quantity to act additively or by summation to produce the claimed therapeutic effect when the ingredients are within the effective concentration range specified for each ingredient in the monograph;

- The ingredients do not interact with each other and that one or more do not reduce the effectiveness of the other or others by precipitation, change in acidity or alkalinity, or in some other manner that reduces the claimed therapeutic effect;

- The partition of the active ingredients between the skin and the vehicle in which they are incorporated is not impeded and that the therapeutic effectiveness of each remains as claimed or is not decreased.

Additionally, this panel recognized that skin protectants are suitable vehicles for use in delivering active ingredients classified in other categories such as topical analgesics and sunscreens. Under these circumstances, the skin protectant may serve a different purpose and is expected to meet the criteria established for this other purpose (analgesic or sunscreen).

The FDA did not accept recommendations by the advisory review panel dealing with external analgesics, which concluded that combinations of topical analgesics listed in Table 4 may be combined with Category I counterirritants. Because the FDA has required products containing counterirritants to carry a warning label stating that this product should not be applied to wounds or damaged skin, use of these combination products on burns would be inappropriate.

PRODUCT SELECTION GUIDELINES

Once the burn has been cooled and cleansed, the pharmacist should assess the burn, determine whether nonprescription therapy is appropriate, and either refer the patient to a physician or recommend specific therapy. The pharmacist should recommend bandaging the area as previously outlined if the burn wound is small and in a location amenable to bandaging. Petrolatum-impregnated bandages are preferred, but if they are not available, a nonsticking gauze may be used. With nonsticking gauze, a protectant should be applied to the burn or on the gauze to provide a barrier that prevents dryness and reduces the chances of infection.

If bandaging is not possible, the pharmacist should recommend that the patient apply a protectant to prevent dryness and relieve some pain. Protectants are available in cream, lotion, and ointment formulations. Ointments generally provide the best protection from dryness but can be difficult to apply and remove. Creams are easier to apply but provide less protection from dryness. Emulsion lotion vehicles are useful in preventing and treating dryness when large areas are affected. Water-in-oil emulsions provide better efficacy than oil-in-water emulsions because they have greater occlusive properties. Emulsions provide more protection from dryness than creams.

Shake lotions are intended to cool, soothe, and dry. Drying of the wound is not desirable with a burn. These lotions are most useful for eczematous lesions and should not be used when weeping occurs because the powder residue (left after the lotion dries) will cake and become difficult to remove. Additionally, this caked powder can allow bacteria to grow under it, which may result in infection.

The pharmacist should tell the patient that only a thin layer of creams, lotions, or ointments is needed. If, after rubbing in the preparation, the patient can still see it on the skin, too much has been applied. The patient should apply the protectant as often as needed with clean fingers or an applicator. To minimize the chances of contamination, the protectant should not be applied directly from its container.

To treat the pain associated with minor burns, various therapeutic modalities are available. Soaks may be particularly useful if the burn is inflamed or weeping. Protectants also provide some pain relief. Local anesthetics provide some short-term relief and probably are most useful with sunburn.

Aerosol dosage forms have a limited advantage because the patient does not have to apply the local anesthetic mechanically (causing pain). Aerosols generally are not very useful as protectants because oleaginous (occlusive) preparations are difficult to formulate into this dosage form. Aerosols should be shaken well before using, and the patient should be cautioned not to spray the product around the face, where it could get into the eyes or nose or could be inhaled. Generally, the aerosol should be sprayed from about 6 inches above the skin in bursts of 1–3 seconds. Aerosols are costly compared with creams, lotions, and related products. Moreover, when used on large areas of the body, such as the back, aerosols may cause shivering and nausea.

Aspirin and acetaminophen are valuable adjuvants in relieving burn pain. Because aspirin is an inhibitor of prostaglandin synthesis and also an anti-inflammatory agent in high doses, theoretically it should provide greater benefit than acetaminophen (51). Because prostaglandins are believed to be involved in the delayed erythema reaction in sunburn, some authorities recommend that patients take 1,200 mg of aspirin every 4 hours for 1 day after a sunburn has begun to prevent or modify this reaction. If gastrointestinal upset or tinnitus (ringing or buzzing in the ears) occurs, the high-dose aspirin therapy should be discontinued. At this time, no scientific evidence supports or refutes high-dose aspirin therapy. Undoubtedly, high doses of aspirin provide more pain relief than standard doses, but whether aspirin actually modifies the sunburn reaction is unknown. (See Chapter 5, *Internal Analgesic Products*.) Nonprescription sedatives also may be useful for the burn patient because many patients with burns have trouble sleeping. Whatever the pharmacist recommends for the burn patient, the patient should be cautioned that a physician should be contacted if the condition worsens or has not improved within 7 days.

SUMMARY

The pharmacist's understanding of burn and sunburn is important in making an accurate assessment of the burn patient and recommending appropriate treatment. The pharmacist should be able to:

- Understand the etiology and pathophysiology of burns and sunburns;

- Understand the complications associated with burns and sunburns;

- Accurately assess the condition of the burn patient and refer the patient to a physician if necessary;

- Deliver initial care to the patient with a minor burn;

- Recommend appropriate nondrug therapy for the burn patient;

- Recommend appropriate pharmacotherapy for the burn patient.

In addition to providing accurate information and product recommendations to the burn patient, the pharmacist should be able to instruct the patient on how to care for the burn and how to appropriately use medications.

REFERENCES

1 "National Electronic Injury Surveillance System," Vol. 4, No. 2, U.S. Consumer Product Safety Commission, Washington, D.C., 1975, p. 22.

2 C. A. Atrz, *Med. Times*, *104*, 128 (1976).

3 "Health and Vital Statistics," Department of Health, Education, and Welfare, Publication HSM 73–1763, Washington, D.C., 1973, p. 12.

4 D. Dressler et al., "Thermal Injury," C. V. Mosby, St. Louis, Mo., 1988, p. 6.

5 J. A. Boswick, "The Art and Science of Burn Care," Aspen, Rockville, Md., 1987, p. 14.

6 T. Skoog, "The Surgical Treatment of Burns," Almquist and Wiksells, Stockholm, Sweden, 1963, p. 91.

7 C. Artz et al., "Burns, A Team Approach," W. B. Saunders, Philadelphia, Pa., 1979, p. 19.

8 J. R. Hinshaw, *Arch. Surg.*, *87*, 131 (1963).

9 S. A. Order and J. A. Moncrief, "The Burn Wound," Charles C. Thomas, Springfield, Ill., 1965, p. 132.

10 B. E. Zawacki, *Ann. Surg.*, *180*, 98 (1974).

11 T. B. Fitzpatrick et al., "Dermatology in General Medicine," 3rd ed., McGraw-Hill, New York, N.Y., 1987, p. 1425.

12 B. C. Macmillan, *J. Infect. Dis.*, *124* (suppl.), 278 (1971).

13 J. A. Moncrief, *J. Trauma*, *4*, 233 (1964).

14 J. A. Moncrief, *J. Arch. Surg.*, *92*, 558 (1966).

15 J. A. Moncrief, *N. Engl. J. Med.*, *288*, 444 (1973).

16 J. R. Wuest and T. A. Gossel, *Am. Pharm.*, NS21, 46 (1981).

17 *Federal Register*, *43*, 38209 (1978).

18 J. H. Epstein and R. K. Winkelmann, *Arch. Dermatol.*, *95*, 532 (1967).

19 M. W. Greaves and J. Sondergaard, *J. Invest. Dermatol.*, *54*, 365 (1970).

20 E. J. Valtonen, *Acta Derm. Venerol.* [Stockh.], *44*, 269 (1964).

21 G. Logan and D. L. Wilhelm, *Br. J. Exp. Pathol.*, *47*, 300 (1966).

22 P. Crunkhorn and A. L. Willis, *Br. J. Pharmacol.*, *41*, 507 (1971).

23 M. E. Goldyne, *J. Invest. Dermatol.*, *64*, 377 (1975).

24 J. Lord, *Br. J. Dermatol.*, *95*, 397 (1976).

25 D. K. Kurban et al., *J. Invest. Dermatol.*, *66*, 153 (1976).

26 W. L. Morrison, *J. Invest. Dermatol.*, *68*, 130 (1977).

27 G. Logan and D. Wilhelm, *Br. J. Exp. Pathol.*, *47*, 286 (1966).

28 B. E. Johnson and F. Daniels, *J. Invest. Dermatol.*, *53*, 85 (1969).

29 J. H. Epstein and B. U. Wintroub, *Drugs*, *30*, 42, (1985).

30 M. A. Pathak and K. Stratton, *Arch. Biochem. Biophys.*, *123*, 468 (1961).

31 W. P. Coleman, *Med. Clin. N. Amer.*, *51*, 1073 (1967).

32 E. Stempel and R. Stempel, *J. Am. Pharm. Assoc.*, *13*, 200 (1973).

33 J. R. Wuest and T. Gossel, *Am. Pharm.*, *21*, 46 (1981).

34 E. Epstein, *Arch. Dermatol.*, *106*, 741 (1971).

35 A. Shulman, *J. Am. Med. Assoc.*, *173*, 1916 (1980).

36 B. Sorenson, *Mod. Treatment*, *4*, 1199 (1967).

37 J. S. Barnett, *Med. J. Aust.*, *1*, 240 (1968).

38   H. Kravitz, *Clin. Pediatr.*, *9*, 695 (1970).

39   H. Kravitz, *Pediatrics*, *53*, 766 (1974).

40   A. Blumefield, *N. Engl. J. Med.*, *290*, 58 (1974).

41   J. G. Appleyard, *Lancet*, *2*, 1370 (1972).

42   J. Moylan, *Postgrad. Med.*, *59*, 766 (1974).

43   M. F. Epstein and J. D. Crawford, *Pediatrics*, *52*, 430 (1973).

44   *Patient Care*, *1*, 64 (1976).

45   J. Pietsch and J. L. Meakins, *Lancet*, *1*, 280 (1976).

46   *Federal Register*, *48*, 6820–33 (1983).

47   *Federal Register*, *43*, 4110–3 (1978).

48   *Federal Register*, *48*, 5867–9 (1983).

49   *Federal Register*, *43*, 1210–49 (1978).

50   *Federal Register*, *44*, 234 (1979).

51   E. Epstein, *J. Am. Med. Assoc.*, *198*, 517 (1966).

52   E. Gordon-Smith, *Clin. Haematol.*, *9*, 557, (1980).

53   N. Goluboff and D. S. MacFayden, *J. Pediatr.*, *47*, 222 (1955).

54   C. Mueller and D. West, *Am. Pharm.*, *NS21*, 299 (1981).

BURN AND SUNBURN PRODUCT TABLE

Product (Manufacturer)	Dosage Form	Anesthetic	Antimicrobial	Other Ingredients
A and D (Schering)	ointment			vitamins A and D lanolin petrolatum
aeroCaine (Health & Medical Techniques)	aerosol	benzocaine, 13.6%	benzethonium chloride, 0.5%	
aeroTherm (Health & Medical Techniques)	aerosol	benzocaine, 13.6%	benzethonium chloride, 0.5%	
After Burn (Tender Corp.)	gel spray	lidocaine hydrochloride, 0.5%		aloe vera gel, 95.38% triethanolamine, 1.37% germaben, 1% carbomer 940, 0.7% ethoxylan 50, 0.5% polysorbate 60, 0.5% fragrance, 0.05%
After Burn Plus (Tender Corp.)	gel spray	lidocaine hydrochloride, 1%		aloe vera gel, 94.88% triethanolamine, 1.37% germaben, 1% carbomer 940, 0.7% ethoxylan 50, 0.5% polysorbate 60, 0.5% fragrance, 0.05%
Americaine (Pharmacraft)	aerosol ointment	benzocaine, 20%	benzethonium chloride, 0.1% (ointment)	
Bactine First Aid (Miles)	aerosol liquid spray	lidocaine hydrochloride, 2.5%	benzalkonium chloride, 0.13%	alcohol, 3.17%
Balmex (Macsil)	ointment			vitamins A and D balsam Peru zinc oxide bismuth subnitrate silicone
Benzocaine (Various manufacturers)	cream	benzocaine, 5%		
Benzocol (Hauck)	cream	benzocaine, 5%		
Betadine (Purdue Frederick)	aerosol cream ointment		povidone-iodine, 5% (aerosol, cream) 10% (ointment)	aqueous base (aerosol) water-miscible base (cream, ointment)
Bicozene (Sandoz)	cream	benzocaine, 6%		resorcinol, 1.67%
Boric Acid (Various manufacturers)	ointment			boric acid, 10%
Borofax (Burroughs Wellcome)	ointment			boric acid, 5% lanolin
Burn Ointment (Pfeiffer)	ointment	benzocaine, 2%	chloroxylenol, 1%	zinc oxide, 3% pyrilamine maleate polyethylene glycol
Burntame (Otis Clapp)	spray	benzocaine, 20%	8-hydroxyquinoline	

BURN AND SUNBURN PRODUCT TABLE, continued

Product (Manufacturer)	Dosage Form	Anesthetic	Antimicrobial	Other Ingredients
Butesin Picrate (Abbott)	ointment	butamben picrate, 1%		anhydrous lanolin ceresin wax mineral oil mixed triglycerides parabens potassium chloride sodium borate white wax
Caldesene (Pharmacraft)	ointment			vitamins A and D zinc oxide, 15% lanolin petrolatum, 54% talc
Clocream (Upjohn)	cream			vitamins A and D
Comfortine (Dermik)	ointment			vitamins A and D zinc oxide lanolin
Dermacoat (Century)	aerosol	benzocaine	chloroxylenol	menthol propylene glycol
Derme D (Holloway)	cream			vitamins A and D hydrogenated vegetable oil

Dermoplast (Whitehall)	aerosol
	lotion
		benzocaine,
		  20% (aerosol)
		  8% (lotion)
				menthol, 0.5%

Desitin (Leeming)	ointment			vitamins A and D zinc oxide, 40% talc lanolin petrolatum
Dibucaine (Various manufacturers)	ointment	dibucaine, 1%		
E-Vitamin (Forest)	ointment			vitamin E, 30 mg/g
Foille (Blistex)	aerosol ointment	benzocaine, 5%	8-hydroxyquinoline chloroxylenol	vegetable oil
Foille Plus (Blistex)	aerosol cream	benzocaine, 5%	chloroxylenol	water-washable base
Foille Medicated First Aid (Blistex)	aerosol ointment	benzocaine, 5%	chloroxylenol, 0.1%	benzyl alcohol (aerosol)
Gebauer's Tannic Spray (Gebauer)	pump spray	benzocaine, < 1%	chlorobutanol, 1.3%	tannic acid, 4.5% menthol, < 1% ethyl alcohol, 60%
Gordo-Vite E (Gordon)	cream			vitamin E, 50 mg/g
Kreo-Benz (Halsey)	liquid	benzocaine		amyl metacresol myrrh phenol, < 0.5% aromatic oils alcohol, 70%

BURN AND SUNBURN PRODUCT TABLE, continued

Product (Manufacturer)	Dosage Form	Anesthetic	Antimicrobial	Other Ingredients
Lagol (Alvin Last)	ointment	benzocaine, 5%		petrolatum cornstarch allantoin
Lanacane (Combe)	aerosol	benzocaine, 20%	benzethonium chloride, 0.1%	
Lobana Derm-Ade (Ulmer)	cream			vitamins A, D and E moisturizers emollients silicone
Medicone Derma (Medicone)	ointment	benzocaine, 2%	8-hydroxyquinoline sulfate, 1.05%	zinc oxide, 13.7% ichthammol, 1% menthol, 0.48% petrolatum lanolin
Medicone Dressing (Medicone)	cream	benzocaine, 5 mg/g	8-hydroxyquinoline sulfate, 0.5 mg/g	cod liver oil, 125 mg/g zinc oxide, 125 mg/g menthol, 1.8 mg/g petrolatum lanolin paraffin talc perfume
Mediconet (Medicone)	cloth wipe		benzalkonium chloride, 0.02%	hamamelis water, 50% glycerin, 10% ethoxylated lanolin, 0.5% methylparaben, 0.15% alkylaryl polyether perfume
Medi-Quik (Mentholatum)	spray	lidocaine, 2%	benzalkonium chloride, 0.13%	camphor, 0.2% benzyl alcohol BHA isobutaine isopropyl palmitate methyl gluceth-20 sesquistearate methyl glucose sesquistearate phosphoric acid polyglyceryl-6-distearate
Mercurochrome II (Becton Dickinson)	liquid spray	lidocaine hydrochloride	benzalkonium chloride	menthol isopropyl alcohol, 5%
Noxzema (Noxell)	cream		phenol, < 0.5%	menthol camphor clove oil eucalyptus oil water-dispersible base
Nupercainal Cream (Ciba)	cream	dibucaine, 0.5%		acetone sodium bisulfite water-washable base fragrance glycerin potassium hydroxide stearic acid trolamine
Nupercainal Ointment (Ciba)	ointment	dibucaine, 1%		acetone sodium bisulfite lanolin light mineral oil white petrolatum

BURN AND SUNBURN PRODUCT TABLE, continued

Product (Manufacturer)	Dosage Form	Anesthetic	Antimicrobial	Other Ingredients
Obtundia (Otis Clapp)	cream liquid spray		cresol-camphor complex	
Panthoderm (Jones Medical)	cream lotion			dexpanthenol, 2% water-miscible base
Phicon (T.E. Williams)	cream	pramoxine hydro-chloride, 0.5%		vitamin A, 7500 IU/oz aloe vera sorbic acid
Pontocaine (Winthrop)	cream ointment	tetracaine hydro-chloride, 1% (cream) 0.5% (ointment)		methylparaben (cream) sodium bisulfite (cream) menthol, 0.5% (ointment) white petrolatum (ointment) white wax (ointment)
Pramegel (GenDerm)	gel	pramoxine hydro-chloride, 1%		menthol, 0.5%
Prax (Ferndale)	cream lotion	pramoxine hydro-chloride, 1%		hydrophilic base
Primaderm (Arrow Medical)	ointment			vitamins A and D zinc oxide petrolatum lanolin
Pyribenzamine (PBZ) (Ciba)	cream	tripelennamine, 2%		glycerin glyceryl monostearate sodium lauryl sulfate stearyl alcohol white petrolatum
San Cura (Thompson)	ointment	benzocaine	chlorobutanol	chlorothymol benzoic acid salicylic acid benzyl alcohol cod liver oil lanolin petrolatum
Soft 'N Soothe (B.F. Ascher)	cream	benzocaine		menthol natural oat protein lanolin oil mineral oil lanolin alcohol
Solarcaine (Schering-Plough)	cream lotion	benzocaine	triclosan	menthol camphor
Solarcaine Spray (Schering-Plough)	aerosol spray	benzocaine	triclosan	isopropyl alcohol, 24%
Sperti (Whitehall)	ointment			shark liver oil, 3% live yeast cell derivative supplying respiratory factor, 67 units/g
Sting Kill (Kiwi Brands)	swab	benzocaine, 18.9%		menthol, 0.9%
Sting Relief (Pfeiffer)	lotion	benzocaine, 10%	chloroxylenol	propylene glycol camphor eucalyptus oil

BURN AND SUNBURN PRODUCT TABLE, continued

Product (Manufacturer)	Dosage Form	Anesthetic	Antimicrobial	Other Ingredients
Stypt-aid (Pharmakon)	spray	benzocaine, 28.71 mg/ml	methylbenzethonium hydrochloride, 9.95 mg/ml	aluminum chloride hexahydrate, 55.43 mg/ml ethyl alcohol, 70.97% glycerin menthol
Tega Caine (Ortega)	aerosol	benzocaine, 20%	chloroxylenol, 0.51%	benzyl alcohol, 2.3% urea, 5.38% propylene glycol, 71.8%
Tronothane HCl (Abbott)	cream	pramoxine hydrochloride, 1%		cetyl alcohol synthetic spermaceti glycerin sodium lauryl sulfate parabens
Unguentine (Mentholatum)	aerosol ointment spray	benzocaine, 3.3% (spray)	parahydracin (ointment) benzalkonium chloride (spray) chloroxylenol (spray)	phenol, 1% aluminum hydroxide zinc carbonate zinc acetate zinc oxide eucalyptus oil thyme oil metacresol mercuric chloride alcohol, 42% (spray)
Unguentine Plus (Mentholatum)	cream	lidocaine hydrochloride, 2%	chloroxylenol, 2% phenol, 1%	aluminum hydroxide zinc carbonate zinc acetate zinc oxide eucalyptus oil thyme oil menthol eugenol
Vaseline First-Aid Carbolated Petroleum Jelly[a] (Chesebrough Ponds)	ointment		chloroxylenol	petrolatum
Vaseline Pure Petroleum Jelly (Chesebrough Ponds)	gel			white petrolatum, 100%
Vitamin E (Various manufacturers)	cream liquid oil			vitamin E
Vitamins A and D (Various manufacturers)	ointment			vitamins A and D
Vitec (Pharmaceutical Specialties)	cream			vitamin E
Y-Itch (Halsey)	cream	benzocaine dibucaine tetracaine	benzalkonium chloride	
Xylocaine (Astra)	ointment	lidocaine, 2.5%		polyethylene glycols propylene glycol
Zinc Oxide (Various manufacturers)	ointment paste			zinc oxide, 20% (ointment) zinc oxide, 25% (paste) starch, 25% (paste)

[a]Not meant for use over extensive body areas (eg, sunburn).

Edward M. DeSimone II

34

SUNSCREEN AND SUNTAN PRODUCTS

*Q*uestions to ask in patient/consumer counseling

Do you sunburn easily?

Is it difficult for you to tan?

Do you normally spend much time in the sun because of your job or other activities?

Are you currently using a sun protection product?

What products have you used in the past?

Have you ever had a growth on your skin or lip caused by sun exposure?

Have you ever had a reaction to any sunscreen products?

Are you taking any medications such as tetracycline, diuretics, or sulfa drugs?

Will you be using the product while swimming, skiing, participating in strenuous activities, or working?

Sunbathing is a popular recreational activity. However, for some people, extended exposure to the sun is a normal part of their occupation. Sunburn, with its pain, swelling, and tenderness, often occurs whether the exposure is recreational or occupational. The severity of sunburn depends on the responsiveness of the individual's skin type and/or the effectiveness of measures taken to protect the skin.

Many people consider sunburn's effects disagreeable but relatively minor. However, the consequences of continued exposure to the sun can be significant. Long-term exposure even without severe burning causes skin to age prematurely, resulting in loss of elasticity, thinning, wrinkling, and drying. Cumulative exposure from childhood to adulthood may cause precancerous skin conditions; years later skin cancer may follow.

Many sunscreen and suntan products are marketed to help darken the complexion as well as to protect the skin from the harmful effects of exposure to the sun. Applied properly, these products physically or chemically block some or all of the sun's harmful ultraviolet rays. Pharmacists need to be aware of several important factors to properly educate the public on effective use of products.

Sunburn is caused by certain wavelengths of ultraviolet (UV) radiation striking the skin. The UV radiation alters the keratinocytes in the basal layer of the epidermis. A slight alteration results in erythema, and a severe alteration causes the formation of bullae from fluid collected in the epidermis. To produce a suntan, UV radiation stimulates the melanocytes in the germinating layer to generate more melanin and oxidizes melanin already in the epidermis. Both of these processes serve as protective mechanisms by diffusing and absorbing additional UV radiation. The effects of the sun on the skin usually begin to appear anywhere from 1 to 24 hours after exposure and range from mild erythema to tenderness, pain, and edema. Severe reactions to excessive exposure involve the development of vesicles or bullae as well as the constitutional symptoms of fever, chills, weakness, and shock. Shock caused by heat prostration or hyperpyrexia can lead to death (1). (See Chapter 33, *Burn and Sunburn Products*.) In addition, more than 40 different diseases have been associated with sunlight. These include chronically dry, flaky, and itchy skin; malignant melanoma; damage to deoxyribonucleic acid (DNA); and death of living cells (2, 3).

ULTRAVIOLET RADIATION

UV radiation is commonly referred to as ultraviolet "light." However, "light" technically refers only to the visible spectrum. Because the correct terminology is "radiation," this term will be used throughout (4).

The UV spectrum is subdivided into three major bands: UV-A, UV-B, and UV-C (4).

UV-A (Longwave Radiation)

The wavelength of UV-A radiation ranges from 320 to 400 nanometers (nm). Although most of the concerns about the hazards of sunlight exposure to date have focused specifically on UV-B, recent studies and reports have shown a heightened awareness of and increased concerns about the effects of UV-A (5, 6). Recent evidence indicates that UV-A radiation penetrates deeper into the skin than UV-B, causing vascular damage (7). This evidence raises questions of further and more serious damage to the underlying tissue.

Erythemogenic activity (producing redness) is relatively weak at this wavelength, requiring 800 to 1,000 times more UV-A energy than UV-B. The irradiance (intensity of the radiation reaching a surface) of UV-B is most intense from late morning to early afternoon; however, the irradiance of UV-A is considerable and occurs throughout the day (8, 9). In fact, at least 10 times more UV-A reaches the earth's surface than UV-B (10). UV-A radiation can produce an immediate pigment darkening (IPD) reaction followed by delayed tanning (DT) or melanogenesis (11, 12). This leads to the development of a slow natural tan.

UV-A triggers new pigment formation as well as a thickening of the stratum corneum (horny layer) of the epidermis (13). This increase in thickness protects against subsequent UV radiation by increasing the dis-

tance that the radiation must travel. The stratum corneum also absorbs radiation in the 280–300 nm range, further reducing the total amount of energy reaching the basal and suprabasal layers (14). In addition, UV-A represents the range in which most photosensitizing chemicals such as 8-methoxypsoralen are active.

UV-B (Sunburn Radiation)

The wavelength of UV-B is between 290 and 320 nm. This is the most effective UV radiation wavelength for producing erythema, which is why it is called sunburn radiation. Cutaneous UV-B exposure is responsible for vitamin D_3 synthesis. Current consensus suggests this to be the only true therapeutic effect of UV-B (15, 16). For infants in the United States who receive vitamin D fortified milk, vitamin D deficiency does not seem to be a problem. However, vitamin D deficiency may be a problem for elderly individuals who spend little time outdoors (17).

UV-B is also considered to be responsible for inducing skin cancer. The carcinogenic effects of UV-B are believed to be augmented by UV-A (18–20).

UV-C (Germicidal Radiation)

The wavelength of UV-C radiation is within the 200–290 nm band. UV-C radiation from the sun does not reach the surface of the earth. However, UV-C is emitted by artificial ultraviolet sources. Although it will not stimulate tanning, it can cause some erythema (21).

LONG-TERM HAZARDS OF SUNLIGHT

Malignant Changes

Numerous epidemiologic studies have been conducted during the past 40 years demonstrating a strong relationship between sunlight exposure and human skin cancer (22–29). One of the most common skin cancers is squamous cell epithelioma. There is also a significant relationship between sun exposure and the growth of premalignant actinic keratoses, basal cell epitheliomas, squamous cell carcinoma, and keratoacanthomas (30). The relative incidence of actinic keratosis and squamous cell carcinomas increases with increased exposure to damaging solar rays. The relationship between UV radiation and squamous cell cancer is well established. About 80% of both cancers occur on the most exposed areas of the body (31, 32). However, the incidence of basal cell epithelioma appears to be related to factors other than UV radiation alone (33).

Although the evidence linking sun exposure to malignant changes is strong, there are several contributory factors: age, sex, skin pigmentation, and occupation. In a frequently cited study, the incidence of skin cancer in white adults in a rural Tennessee county was found to be a function of both age and sex. The rate ranged from 0.7/100 for males under 44 years of age to 13.6/100 for males between the ages of 65 and 74; for females, the incidence was 0.4/100 and 6.8/100, respectively (34). It has also been shown that the exposed areas of the body (the hands, arms, head, and neck) are most prone to the development of skin cancer. This finding is supported by the relationship between occupation and skin cancer. Some of the more susceptible groups have been identified as farmers, sailors, and construction workers. The three factors of age, sex, and occupation appear to be interrelated. The findings related to age indicate a cumulative effect from UV radiation. The findings regarding sex and occupation seem to be related because, traditionally, fewer women have held these susceptible occupations.

The fourth contributory factor is skin pigmentation. Studies have indicated that skin cancer occurs more frequently in whites than in nonwhites (35–37). These findings support the belief that the darker pigmentation protects against the effects of UV radiation.

Another important factor is the relationship between skin cancer and latitude. It has been shown that the incidence of skin cancer increases steadily in populations closer to the equator. The quantity of harmful radiation that reaches the earth's surface is increased as the angle of the sun to a reference point on earth approaches 90° and the distance of the sun to the earth decreases (28, 33, 38–41). A constant rate of increase in the incidence of skin cancer was found in approaching the equator from north to south; the incidence approximately doubled for every 3°48′ reduction in latitude (42). In the United States, the incidence of skin cancer increases dramatically from north to south.

Premature Aging

Another long-term hazard of UV radiation is premature aging of the skin. As with skin cancer, aging is also genetically determined; whites are more susceptible than blacks. The condition is characterized by wrinkling and yellowing of the skin. It is called premature aging because the obvious physical findings are similar to those seen in natural aging. However, histologic and biochemical differences distinguish these degenerative changes from those associated with normal aging (43). As with normal aging of the skin, solar damage is generally believed to be irreversible. However, there is some preliminary evidence that, in certain cases, sun protection allows for true repair of existing damage (44). Conclusive evidence exists that, in susceptible individuals, prolonged exposure to UV radiation results in elastosis (degeneration of the skin due to breakdown of the skin's elastic fibers) (45). Pronounced drying, thinning, and wrinkling of the skin result (46). Other physical changes include cracking, telangiectasis (spider vessels), solar keratoses (growths), ecchymoses (subcutaneous hemorrhagic lesions), and loss of elasticity (47).

Although the immediate effects of UV radiation may be cosmetically and socially gratifying, the long-term effects are cumulative and potentially serious.

SUNSCREENS

Sunscreen agents exert their effects either through physical or chemical means. A physical sunscreen such as titanium dioxide scatters and reflects UV radiation. The majority of agents such as aminobenzoic acid are chemical sunscreens and absorb UV radiation rather than reflect or scatter it.

Indications

Sunscreens are primarily used to prevent sunburn and to aid in the development of a tan. They also are used to protect exposed areas of the body from the long-term hazards of skin cancer and premature aging. Sunscreens can also be used to protect against drug-related UV-induced photosensitivity.

Photosensitivity

Photosensitivity encompasses two types of conditions: photoallergy and phototoxicity. Drug photoallergy, which is relatively uncommon (48), is an increased reactivity of the skin to UV and/or visible radiation produced by a chemical agent on an immunologic basis. UV radiation (typically UV-A) triggers an antigenic reaction in the skin characterized by urticaria, bullae, and/or sunburn (49). This reaction, which is not dose related, is usually seen after at least one prior exposure to the involved agent.

Phototoxicity is an increased reactivity of the skin to UV and/or visible radiation produced by a chemical agent on a nonimmunologic basis (48). It is often seen upon first exposure to a chemical agent (drug), is dose related, and usually exhibits no cross-sensitivity. It is most likely to appear as a sunburn (50–51). Some of the drugs associated with phototoxicity are tetracyclines (especially demeclocycline), sulfonamides, antineoplastics (e.g., 5-FU), hypoglycemics, thiazides, phenothiazines (especially chlorpromazine), and the psoralens. However, this type of reaction is not limited to drugs. It is also associated with plants, cosmetics, and soaps (52). For a more detailed description of photosensitivity, see Chapter 33, *Burn and Sunburn Products.*

The efficacy of sunscreens in preventing photosensitization has been questioned by some investigators (53). The issue is yet to be resolved; however, it seems reasonable to assume that because UV-A radiation is responsible for triggering a photosensitivity reaction, a sunscreen effective against UV-A would be effective in preventing photosensitivity.

Traditionally, aminobenzoic acid (formerly known as *p*-aminobenzoic acid or PABA) has been used. However, it absorbs only UV-B (290–320 nm) radiation and not UV-A (320–400 nm) radiation. One study compared the efficacy of 5% aminobenzoic acid (ABA) in alcohol with a mixture of the esters of ABA and benzophenone. It was demonstrated that the 5% ABA was ineffective. The ABA and benzophenone ester solution blocked the phototoxic effects of chlorpromazine, 8-methoxypsoralen, and demeclocycline (54). It seems likely that similar wide-spectrum sunscreens that contain sulisobenzone, oxybenzone, dioxybenzone, or butyl methoxydibenzoylmethane (Parsol 1789) could be effective in combination with ABA.

However, ABA is chemically similar to certain other drugs that have been reported to cause photosensitivity reactions in susceptible individuals. These drugs include the thiazide diuretics, sulfonamides, sulfonylureas, furosemide, and carbonic anhydrase inhibitors.

Individuals who have experienced a photosensitivity reaction while taking one of these drugs should not use a sunscreen containing ABA or one of its derivatives such as aminobenzoate, menthyl anthranilate, or padimate A or O. A sunscreen containing oxybenzone or cinoxate may be recommended instead (46).

Photodermatoses

Photodermatoses are idiopathic skin eruptions that are initiated or exacerbated by radiation of varying wavelengths including UV-A or UV-B. The most common of the photodermatoses is polymorphic light eruption (PMLE) (55). It usually manifests itself in a single morphologic form including erythema, vesicles, or plaques on skin exposed to sunlight. It appears to affect approximately 10% of the population with a first occurrence usually before the age of 30. It affects women more often than men and is most often seen in persons of skin types I to IV, as shown in Table 1 (56).

In addition to the various photodermatoses, sunlight can exacerbate many existing dermatologic conditions including psoriasis, herpes simplex, rosacea, lupus erythematosus (and skin lesions of systemic lupus erythematosus), erythema multiforme, chloasma (which affects pregnant women and women taking oral contraceptives), atopic and contact dermatitis, and a variety of solar lesions (57).

Avoidance of sunlight is the best way to prevent the occurrence or exacerbation of photodermatoses. It is generally believed that sunscreens with a wide range of UV absorbance (especially in the UV-A range) (58) may afford some protection.

Sunscreen Efficacy

Minimal Erythemal Dose

It is difficult to ascertain the efficacy of sunscreens on humans because of the great individual variation in responsiveness to UV radiation. One measure that is used is the minimal erythemal dose (MED). This dose is defined as the "least exposure dose at a specified wavelength that will elicit a delayed erythema response. It is a dose of radiation and not a grade of erythema." The MED is indicative not only of the amount of energy reaching the skin but also of the responsiveness of the skin to the radiation. For instance, 2 MEDs will produce a bright erythema, 4 MEDs will produce a painful sunburn, and 8 MEDs will produce a blistering burn. The MED for blacks with heavy pigmentation has been estimated to be up to 33 times higher than that for whites with light pigmentation (59).

Sun Protection Factor

Another important measure is the sun protection factor (SPF). It is derived by dividing the MED of protected skin by the MED of unprotected skin. For example, assume that an individual requires 25 milli-joules/cm^2 (25 units) of UV radiation to experience 1 MED on unprotected skin. If, after application of a given sunscreen, the person requires 250 units of radiation to produce 1 MED, the product would be given an SPF rating of 10. The higher the SPF, the more effective the agent in preventing sunburn. However, as the SPF goes up (and the amount of radiation reaching the melanocytes goes down), the longer it will take for the development of a slow natural tan. Table 1 illustrates the proposed classification and the relationship of skin types to SPF and product category designations (PCD) (56).

With all of these proposed guides, a system should now exist to accurately evaluate not only the relative effectiveness of sunscreens but also the length of time a person using a sunscreen product can spend in the sun before a burn will occur. If it normally takes 30 minutes for someone to experience 1 MED, a sunscreen with an SPF of 6 will allow that individual to stay in the sun six times longer or 3 hours before receiving 1 MED.

Measures of UV-A Protection

With the growing concern about the effects of UV-A, the utility of the SPF value has been questioned. The SPF provides a measure of the relative amount of UV-B striking the skin (i.e., erythemogenic response). On the other hand, UV-A-induced erythema is different in a number of ways from UV-B-induced erythema (60). Therefore, another measure must be used to evaluate the efficacy of substances that block UV-A.

Phototoxic Protection Factor

Several workers employed topical or systemically administered photosensitizers such as 8-methoxypsoralen or anthracene to elicit erythema with small UV-A exposures (61, 62, 63). By comparing the minimal dose of UV-A that causes erythema in sensitized individuals, the minimal phototoxic dose (MPD) can be calculated. By comparing the MPD of sunscreen-protected skin to that of unprotected skin, the phototoxic protection factor (PPF) of a sunscreen can be determined. The PPF has been established for at least one commercial product (Photoplex).

UV-A Protection Factor

UV-A protection in sensitized skin (PPF) creates an artificial state of photosensitivity to certain regions of the UV spectrum (64) and may not provide an accurate index of protection for normal skin in outdoor condi-

TABLE 1 Skin types and recommended sunscreen products

Skin type	Sunburn and tanning history	Recommended sun protection factor (SPF)	Recommended product category designation (PCD)
I	Always burns easily Never tans (sensitive)	8 or more	Maximal, ultra
II	Always burns easily Tans minimally (sensitive)	6–7	Extra
III	Burns moderately Tans gradually (light brown-normal)	4–5	Moderate
IV	Burns minimally Always tans well (moderate brown-normal)	2–3	Minimal
V	Rarely burns Tans profusely (dark brown-insensitive)	2	Minimal
VI	Never burns Deeply pigmented (insensitive)	–	–

Adapted from the *Federal Register, 43,* 38213 (1978).

tions. A method that measures the UV-A protection factor (APF) in unsensitized skin has recently been described (65). This measure of UV-A protection is defined as the sunscreen-protected MED for UV-A divided by the unprotected MED for UV-A, analogous to SPF. However, the APF is not yet being used for commercial products. An APF range of 3–6 is tentatively proposed to provide a full day's protection similar to an SPF of 15 for UV-B.

Ancillary Factors Affecting Efficacy

Several factors affect the efficacy of nonprescription sunscreen products. These all relate to the vehicle/solvent system.

- The partition coefficient relative to the skin should favor passage of the sunscreen to the skin.

- The pH of the solvent can vary the fraction of ionized and nonionized sunscreen agent, thereby rendering it less effective or even ineffective.

- The solvent system should provide a high degree of substantivity.

- The sunscreen must remain stable for the desired period of protection.

Although the pharmacist cannot control the formulation of the various commercially available sunscreen products, a knowledge of the specific active ingredients and their concentrations helps differentiate a good product from a mediocre one.

According to the Food and Drug Administration (FDA) advisory review panel, "An ideal sunscreen vehicle would be stable, neutral, nongreasy, nondegreasing, nonirritating, nondehydrating, nondrying, odorless, and efficient on all kinds of human skin. It should also hold at least 50% water, be easily compounded of known chemicals, and have infinite stability during storage" (66). The panel stated that an ideal vehicle does not exist and recommended that all inactive ingredients be included on product labels. This labeling would allow evaluation by the consumer, pharmacist, and physician for several factors including sensitivity to the agent.

In addition, the vehicle and final dosage form may influence the effectiveness of the active ingredient. One study showed that ABA (5%) in ethanol was superior to ABA dissolved in methanol, propyl alcohol, acetone, *n*-butyl alcohol, and isobutyl alcohol. This study indicated that the increased effectiveness was due to the absorption of ABA by the intact epidermis and partial chemical conjugation of ABA with constituents of the horny layer. This effect prevented transmission of erythemogenic wavelengths to the underlying vulnerable cells of the viable epidermis (67).

The ability of a sunscreen to remain effective under the stress of prolonged exercise, sweating, and swimming is called substantivity. This property appears to be a function of both the absorbing agent and the vehicle. As mentioned, ABA in ethanol is substantive, and studies have suggested that other ABA esters, such as glyceryl ABA, may be more substantive than ABA (68). One investigation into the substantivity of sunscreens placed subjects in a whirlpool bath for 10 minutes as a means of assessing the effects of profuse sweating (69). This study reported that the product offering the best protection included a combination of 3% oxybenzone and 7% padimate O, an ABA derivative. Products with cream-based (water or oil) vehicles may in some cases be more resistant to removal than those in alcohol bases and will reduce desquamation of the skin (70). Oil-based products are the most popular and are the easiest to apply. They also tend to have lower SPF values (71).

Commercial formulas include ingredients such as glycerin, hydroxypropyl cellulose, and fragrances to increase the cosmetic appeal and acceptability. Alcohol, which is also often included, can dry the skin.

PRODUCT SELECTION GUIDELINES

The FDA advisory review panel on over-the-counter (OTC) topical analgesic, antirheumatic, otic, burn, and sunburn prevention and treatment drug products has recommended three definitions for therapeutic sunscreen types (56):

- Sunscreen–sunburn preventive agent—an active ingredient that absorbs 95% or more of the radiation in the UV range at wavelengths from 290 to 320 nm and thereby removes the sunburning rays;

- Sunscreen–suntanning agent—an active ingredient that absorbs at least 85% of the radiation in the UV range at wavelengths from 290 to 320 nm, but transmits UV wavelengths longer than 320 nm (such agents permit tanning in the average individual and also permit some erythema without pain);

- Sunscreen–opaque sunblock agent—an opaque agent that reflects or scatters all radiation in the UV and visible range from 290 to 760 nm and thereby prevents or minimizes suntan and sunburn.

Most of the products on the market contain a combination of the first two types of agents. The primary differences between the preventive agent and the suntanning agent may be only the concentration of the active ingredient.

The FDA advisory review panel on OTC burn and sunburn prevention and treatment drug products has recommended that 21 agents be classified as safe and efficacious for nonprescription use as topical sunscreens. These tentative recommendations are included in Table 2 (72, 73). Those sunscreen agents that have not been judged to be both safe and efficacious are listed in Table 3. Based on recent evidence, the Division of OTC Drug Evaluation intends to recommend that the FDA place padimate A in Category III at concentrations less than 5% and in Category II at concentrations of 5% or more because of the possibility of phototoxicity reactions (74).

TABLE 2 Agents recommended to be safe and effective by the FDA advisory review panel

Sunscreen	Absorbance (nm)	Maximum (nm)	Concentration	Sunscreen	Absorbance (nm)	Maximum (nm)	Concentration
ANTHRANILATES				SALICYLATES			
Methyl anthranilate	260–380[a]	340[a]	3.5–5%	2-Ethylhexyl salicylate	280–320	305	3–5%
				Homosalate	295–315	306	4–15%
BENZOPHENONES				Triethanolamine salicylate	260–320	298	5–12%
Dioxybenzone	260–380[b]	282[b]	3%				
Oxybenzone	270–350	290	2–6%	MISCELLANEOUS			
Sulisobenzone[c]		285	5–10%	Digalloyl trioleate	270–320	300	2–5%
				Lawsone with dihydroxyacetone (DHA)	290–400		0.25% lawsone, 3% DHA
CINNAMATES							
Cinoxate	270–328	310	1–3%	2-Phenylbenzimidazole-5-sulfonic acid	290–320	302	1–4%
Diethanolamine *p*-methoxycinnamate	280–310	290	8–10%				
2-Ethylhexyl 2-cyano-3, 3-diphenylacrylate			7–10%	Red petrolatum[f]			30–100%
				Titanium dioxide[g]			2–25%
Ethylhexyl *p*-methoxycinnamate	290–320	308–310	2–7.5%				
DIBENZOYL-METHANE DERIVATIVES							
Butyl methoxydibenzoylmethane[d,e] (Parsol 1789)	320–400						
ABA AND DERIVATIVES							
Aminobenzoic acid	260–313	288.5	5–15%				
Ethyl 4-[bis(hydroxypropyl)] aminobenzoate	280–330	308–311	1–5%				
Glyceryl *p*-aminobenzoate	264–315	295	3%				
Padimate A	290–315	310	1–5%				
Padimate O	290–315	310	1.4–8%				

[a] Values are for concentrations higher than normally found in nonprescription drugs.

[b] Values available when used in combination with other sunscreens.

[c] Absorbs throughout the entire UV range.

[d] Currently marketed through an NDA.

[e] Commercially available as 3% in combination with 7% padimate O.

[f] A 0.03-mm film absorbs UV radiation below 320 nm. At 334 nm, 16% of radiation is transmitted; at 365 nm, 58% is transmitted.

[g] Scatters radiation from 290 to 700 nm rather than absorbs it.

Adapted from the *Federal Register*, *43*, 38223 (1978), and (with permission) T. A. Gossel, *U.S. Pharmacist*, *14 (5)*, 82 (1989).

Sunscreen Categories

Aminobenzoic Acid and Derivatives

ABA is an effective sunscreen especially when formulated in a hydroalcoholic base (maximum of 50–60% alcohol). The SPF of such formulations increases proportionally as the concentration of ABA increases from 2% to 5%. Some UV-A is also blocked at the 5% level (71). One advantage of ABA is its ability to penetrate the skin and provide lasting protection. The disadvantages of ABA include the development of contact dermatitis (75), photosensitivity (76), stinging and drying of the skin, and yellow staining of clothes upon exposure to the sun (77). A primary advantage of the esters over ABA itself is that they do not stain clothes. However, a cross-sensitivity exists across all ABA derivatives; therefore, they should be avoided by individuals with a known sensitivity to them.

Anthranilates

The anthranilates are ortho-ABA derivatives. Methyl anthranilate is a weak UV-B sunscreen whose maximal absorbance is in the UV-A range. It is usually found in combination with other sunscreen agents to provide broad-spectrum UV coverage (78).

TABLE 3 Agents cited to lack safety and/or efficacy data by the FDA advisory review panel

Agent	Safe	Effective
CATEGORY II		
2-Ethylhexyl 4-phenylbenzophenone-2'-carboxylic acid	Insufficient data	Insufficient data
3-(4-methylbenzylidene) camphor	Insufficient data	No data
Sodium 3,4-dimethyl-phenylglyoxylate	Insufficient data	No data
CATEGORY III		
Allantoin with aminobenzoic acid (AL-PABA)	Safe	Insufficient data
5-(3,3-Dimethyl-2-norboryliden)-3-penten-2-one	Safe	Insufficient data
Dipropylene glycol salicylate	Insufficient data	Insufficient data

Adapted from the *Federal Register*, *43*, 38219-53 (1978).

Benzophenones

Benzophenones are considered to be effective sunscreens for both UV-A and UV-B radiation. Because their coverage extends high into the UV-A range, they are often found in combination with other sunscreens to provide a very broad-spectrum action (79).

Cinnamates

The primary problem with the cinnamates is that they do not adhere well to the skin and must rely on the adhesiveness of the vehicle for their substantivity (80).

Salicylates

Salicylic acid derivatives are weak sunscreens and must be used in high concentrations (81). They do not adhere well to the skin and are easily removed by sweating or swimming (82).

Physical Sunscreens

Physical sunscreens scatter rather than absorb UV-A and visible radiation (290–760 nm). They are most often used by people who cannot limit or control their exposure to the sun (e.g., lifeguards). The nose and tops of the ears are often coated with a white or colored substance such as zinc oxide. Zinc oxide, which was inadvertently skipped when the review panel evaluated the various sunscreen agents, will be added to the list of approved agents when the tentative final monograph is published (83). Unfortunately, transparent agents of similar efficacy are not yet on the market. The effectiveness of such products is related to the thickness with which they are applied. The disadvantages are that they can discolor clothing and can occlude the skin to produce miliaria (prickly heat) and folliculitis (84).

UV-A Sunscreens

A new class of full-spectrum sunscreen agents in the UV-A range has recently been introduced in the United States. The first of these dibenzoylmethane derivatives is butyl methoxydibenzoylmethane (Parsol 1789), which has maximum absorbance at 360 nm (85). Clinical trials have demonstrated that optimal sunscreen protection can be obtained by using a combination of 3% butyl methoxydibenzoylmethane and 7% padimate O. This combination produced the highest PPF when compared to butyl methoxydibenzoylmethane alone; padimate O alone; and a combination of padimate O, oxybenzone, and octyl salicylate (86, 87). The mean PPF for the combination in each study was 4.8 and 4.5 (using artificial light indoors).

Combination Products

The FDA has not recommended any limits for the number of sunscreen agents that may be used together in a nonprescription product. The panel made only two major recommendations:

- Any additional sunscreen agents must contribute to the efficacy of the product and not be just a marketing gimmick (88).

- Any combination of sunscreens with active non-sunscreen agents must meet the requirements for safety and efficacy.

Substantivity

The efficacy of a product is related to its substantivity. Swimming, heat, high humidity, and sweating can reduce the substantivity (or true SPF) of a product.

Proposed labeling guidelines for sunscreen products meeting the specific criteria are (89):

- Sweat-resistant products—protect for up to 30 minutes of continuous heavy perspiration;

- Water-resistant products—protect for up to 40 minutes of continuous water exposure;

- Waterproof products—protect for up to 80 minutes of continuous water exposure.

Sunscreen Application

For sufficient protection, the average person in a bathing suit should apply nine portions (of approximately one-half teaspoon) of sunscreen. The sunscreen should be distributed as follows (59):

- Face and neck—one-half teaspoon;

- Arm and shoulder—one-half teaspoon to each side;

- Torso—one-half teaspoon each to front and back;

- Leg and top of foot—one teaspoon to each side.

One study demonstrated that the effective SPF of commercial products was only 50% of the labeled value when subjects were allowed to apply sunscreen as needed (90). Because of the cost of sunscreen products and the need to apply it often and in sufficient amounts, people may use far less than necessary to provide adequate protection.

SUNTAN PRODUCTS

Low-Efficacy Sunscreens

For cosmetic rather than therapeutic needs, an individual may desire a suntan product. In many cases suntan products differ from sunscreens only by having a lower concentration of the sunscreen agent. The concentration of the active ingredient is an important factor in judging the use and effectiveness of a product. For example, one commercial *suntan* product with an SPF of 4 contains 1.75% cinoxate while a commercial *sunscreen* product contains 4% cinoxate (about twice as much as the suntan product) and 5% menthyl anthranilate, a second sunscreen, giving it an SPF of 8.

The activity of an agent may also be an intrinsic quality unrelated to concentration. A given agent may also work solely by absorbing radiation below 320 nm

and allowing rays above 320 nm to penetrate the skin. ABA almost totally absorbs radiation in the range of 260–313 nm. Radiation above 313 nm is, however, transmitted to the skin (91). This agent will allow a mild short-lived tan but will protect against a burn.

Technically, suntan products do not "promote" a tan. In addition, some suntan products, including cocoa butter and mineral oil alone or with staining materials such as iodine or tannic acid, do not contain a sunscreen agent. They may stain and lubricate the skin but do not impede either the aging process or carcinogenesis caused by UV radiation. The advisory review panel has stated that "claims such as 'promotes tanning' for sunlight protective agents are unsubstantiated" (66).

Pigmenting Agents

Topical Agents

Another type of agent available is a skin-browning agent or dye such as dihydroxyacetone (DHA). For years this has been the major ingredient in products that claim to "tan without the sun." Dihydroxyacetone produces a reddish brown color by binding with specific amino acids in the stratum corneum. The intensity of the "tan" is related to the thickness of the skin. One problem with this product is that if it is not washed off the hands after application, the palms may also develop this "tan." In addition, dry areas such as elbows and kneecaps will absorb the agent more readily, resulting in uneven coloration. The color fades after several weeks with desquamation of the stratum corneum. The FDA advisory panel has recommended that dihydroxyacetone alone is ineffective as a sunscreen and that it should be classified as a cosmetic. However, in combination with lawsone, a major dye component of henna, the product is classified as a sunscreen and not a cosmetic. It should be noted that this combination does not directly affect melanin production and that, in one study, the SPF of such a product was calculated to be less than 2 (92). This combination is recommended as safe and effective as a sunscreen product (Table 2).

Oral Agents

A relatively new type of product is the "oral tanning" compound. Its active ingredients are the dyes canthaxanthin and/or beta-carotene, which are chemically similar to one another. Canthaxanthin is a synthetic dye that the promotional literature describes as "similar to those dyes found naturally in fruits, vegetables and flowers. It has long been used in the food industry *in lower concentration* [author's emphasis] for coloring cheese, ketchup, salad dressing, and other foods.'' The dyes apparently work by coloring the fat cells under the epidermal layer. Because of the variation in fat cells and epidermal thickness, the extent of the tan varies from person to person. Canthaxanthin is dosed by body weight, with a 20-day schedule necessary to achieve pigmentation. This process is followed by maintenance doses of 1–2 capsules a day to maintain the color. The literature cautions the user that if the palms are turning orange, too much of the product is being consumed. Another caution is that a normal reaction is the development of ''brick red feces.''

Any proposed new use of an approved color additive must still be submitted to the FDA for approval according to the 1960 Color Additive Amendment (95). The FDA has not yet approved either compound for whole body coloring. One major concern may be the color of the feces, which could mask any type of gastrointestinal (GI) bleeding. A second concern may be the size of the dose because these compounds are being used in concentrations higher than that normally used as a food dye. There is no evidence for safe use of these agents at a high dose.

Currently, more than 10 agents may have some utility in producing systemic photoprotection. Taken orally, beta-carotene, chloroquine, and the psoralens may have some limited effectiveness when used in certain situations (94). Most of the available data are anecdotal, and no recommendation is made for the use of oral agents.

Tan Accelerators

Tan accelerators are cosmetic products that claim to stimulate a faster and deeper tan. The major ingredient in these products is tyrosine, an amino acid necessary for the production of melanin. Product literature recommends application once daily for at least 3 days before sun exposure. A study that tested two commercial products using indoor UV radiation found no evidence of significant tanning (95).

Tanning Booths and Beds

The availability of tanning booths and beds may prompt questions from patients concerning their safety. The newer type of tanning booth uses a light source composed of over 95% UV-A and less than 5% UV-B, a considerably different mix of UV radiation than that obtained from sunlight (96).

It would appear that UV-A, if used properly, could generate a tan without producing a sunburn. However, there is a concern about UV-B contamination of these lamps. It is believed that even 1% UV-B emission can cause a significant increase in the incidence of skin cancer. In addition, some UV-A lamps produce more than five times as much UV-A per unit of time than does sunlight (97).

UV-A also presents other hazards. UV-A radiation may trigger the eruption of cold sores. In addition, it can produce a photosensitivity reaction in patients who have ingested or applied photosensitizing agents. Because UV-A does not produce the burning of UV-B, patients may become complacent and forego the use of eye goggles. This practice will produce eye burns and an increased risk of developing cataracts. The possibility of long-term hazards related to UV-A has not yet been fully assessed.

PRODUCT SELECTION GUIDELINES

Before recommending a suntan product, the pharmacist should know the identity of the active ingredient, its concentration, the SPF of the product, and the tanning history of the patient. In addition, it should be remembered that the SPFs and product category designations (PCDs) are determined for the specific nonprescription product and are not based on the active ingredient alone.

The identity and concentration of the active ingredients should appear on the label. Without this information, recommendations can be based only on intuition or personal experience. If the information is not supplied by the manufacturer, recommendations should be limited to products that indicate the identity and concentration of the active ingredients.

The most important consideration in selecting a product should be the individual's skin type as defined in Table 1. Once the skin type is identified, a product with the recommended SPF should be selected. In making a recommendation to prevent sunburn, it is important to keep in mind that with a product with an SPF of 15, a tan will develop very slowly. This type of product should be reserved for the person who cannot tan or cannot afford any degree of sunburn. Patients who have a personal or family history of certain dermatologic problems such as excessive dryness and aging, sunburn with short exposure, and skin cancer should use a total blocking agent or a sunscreen with an SPF of 15 or higher when prolonged exposure to sunlight is expected (46). Animal studies have shown that even low protective sunscreens (SPF-2) reduce by 50% the risk of tumorigenesis associated with UV radiation (98). However, some authorities suggest that SPF-4 be the lowest allowable level (99).

Sunscreens and Children

Special consideration is needed when recommending a sunscreen for young children. The consensus is that the absorptive characteristics of human skin in children under 6 months of age are different from those of adult human skin. Related to this is the belief that metabolic and excretory systems of children under 6 months of age are not fully developed to handle any drug absorbed through the skin. Therefore, the FDA advisory panel has recommended that only persons over 6 months of age are considered to have adult human skin.

Because of this, the panel has made two major recommendations regarding the labeling of nonprescription sunscreens with respect to the age of the person using the products (100):

- Sunscreen products should not be used on any children under 6 months of age.

- Products with an SPF as low as 2 or 3 are not to be used on children under 2 years of age.

Products with an SPF of 2 or 3 should not be used in children under 2 years of age because this SPF range does not supply enough protection. It has been estimated that regular use of an SPF-15 product starting after 6 months of age and continuing through 18 years of age will reduce the incidence of tumors over a person's lifetime by 78% (101). In addition, there would also be a reduction in sunburn, reduced risk of premature skin aging, and reduced risk of melanoma.

Use of Sunscreens

If properly applied, products with an SPF of 8–14 allow an individual to stay out in the sun for long periods and slowly develop a tan over several days. It is important to remember, however, that as an individual tans, a natural protection against burning also develops. Therefore, an individual who begins the summer using a product with an SPF of 15 may want to switch to a product with an SPF of 8 as the natural tan progresses. This change will allow a more rapid deepening of the tan. The person can, however, continue to use the product with the SPF of 15; it will simply take longer to achieve the desired tan.

Studies that compare several sunscreen products in humans also serve as a basis for professional judgment. One such study evaluated 17 sunscreen products, using a mean protection factor to evaluate each product (102). Products that contain 5% ABA were shown to be superior to those that contain ABA esters. However, ABA esters are generally used in a concentration of less than 5%. A study showed that alcoholic preparations of 5% ABA were more effective than commercial products tested (103). Another evaluation substantiates this finding in products that contain 5% ABA (104). Several investigators (103, 105) agree that ABA is more effective as a sunscreen than popular proprietary products, but they disagree whether ABA esters are less effective than the parent compound, ABA.

In addition, the sunscreen or suntan agent may damage clothing or other objects. One evaluation of commercial sunscreens found that a number of products puckered vinyl fabric, stained bathing suit material, and damaged and stained fiberglass boat finish (100, 106).

Study findings revealed that none of the product labels suggested how much sunscreen should be used. The amount used by the study participants varied as much as 10-fold. It was decided that a dose of one-half teaspoon (2.5 ml) applied as described previously delivered the FDA standard test rate of 2 $\mu l/cm^2$ (106). Based on the evaluation, the recommendation followed that products within the same SPF rating group showed no advantage over one another. The cost per dose is another factor in the decision of which product to purchase. However, the staining and fabric-damaging properties and cosmetic properties should also be taken into account. All commercial products tested demonstrated an SPF several units higher than the labeled value. There appears to be a margin of safety built into the products. However, it is best to assume that the product provides only the labeled SPF.

Several products are now on the market in "stick" or "lipstick" form. These products prevent burning of the lips (or nose) and carry the same labeling, including the SPF, as the sunscreen lotions. These can also differ in terms of their UV-A and UV-B spectrum. The SPF of these products is at least 15.

Products that dye the skin or fat cells can provide a false sense of security. Although the individual might look tanned and thereby feel protected, these agents provide no sunscreen protection whatsoever and may allow a serious burn to develop.

In regard to product selection, several investigators have suggested using a combination of agents that protect against both UV-A and UV-B (50, 52, 54). There are several explanations for this combination. First, most photosensitive chemicals are active in the UV-A (320-nm) range. However, UV-B can also trigger such reactions. Two reports have provided preliminary evidence that repeated doses of UV-A radiation at doses less than the MED produced enhanced melanogenesis. In addition, these findings indicate that UV-A radiation may be more responsible than UV-B in producing cumulative dermal degenerative changes (aging) (107, 108). These are preliminary reports, but they may have a significant impact on the understanding of cumulative UV radiation damage to the skin. Based on these findings, it should be noted that ABA and its esters are more effective sunscreens in the UV-B range than the wide-spectrum agents (the benzophenones). The combination of ABA or one of its esters with a benzophenone (dioxybenzone, oxybenzone, and sulisobenzone) or a dibenzoylmethane would seem to be a rational and logical choice except when the photosensitizing drug is chemically similar or cross-reacts with ABA. Various products of this type are available.

SUNGLASSES

Recently, some concern has been expressed about the relationship between UV radiation and eye damage such as cataracts (109) or long-term retinal damage. In addition, UV radiation may cause temporary injuries such as photokeratitis (a painful type of snow blindness associated with highly reflective surfaces). This concern is all the more serious because of the general belief that sunglasses screen out UV radiation. In response to this, the FDA has announced a voluntary labeling program for manufacturers of sunglasses. Abbreviated information concerning the UV radiation properties will be directly attached to each pair of sunglasses. In addition, brochures describing the appropriate use of each type of lens will be available at outlets selling sunglasses (110). Based on its UV radiation properties, each pair of sunglasses is placed in one of the following three categories:

- Cosmetic sunglasses block at least 70% of UV-B, 20% of UV-A, and less than 60% of visible light. They are recommended for activities in non-harsh sunlight, such as shopping.

- General purpose sunglasses block at least 95% of UV-B, at least 60% of UV-A, and 60–92% of visible light; their shades range from medium to dark. They are recommended for most activities in sunny environments, such as boating, driving, flying, or hiking.

- Special purpose sunglasses block at least 99% of UV-B, 60% of UV-A, and at least 97% of visible light. They are recommended for activities in very bright environments such as ski slopes and tropical beaches.

PATIENT CONSULTATION

Pharmacists can provide a great service by counseling consumers about the suntanning process and the proper use of sunscreens. In one study of almost 500 persons, a considerable amount of misinformation was found to exist concerning sunscreen use. For example, of the 41% who used sunscreens, one-third thought that they would promote tanning. Fifty-one percent did not know the definition of SPF or its significance, and 26% were not even aware of the existence of sunscreens before the study (111).

The rays of the sun are the most direct and damaging between 10 a.m. and 2 p.m. It is best to avoid sunning during this period, especially at the beginning of the season before any protective tan has developed. Closely related to this is the misconception that one cannot burn on an overcast or cloudy day. Although varying amounts of sunlight may not pass through the cloud cover, very little UV radiation is blocked and most will penetrate. The clouds tend to filter out the infrared radiation that contributes to the sensation of heat. This reduction in heat sensation provides a false sense of security against a burn (112). In addition, the intensity of exposure increases closer to the equator. People in the southern part of the United States are at greater risk to the harmful effects of UV radiation than those in northern areas. Also, the irradiance of UV-B increases by 4% for every 1,000 feet of altitude.

Another problem is that UV radiation reflects off surfaces. Snow will reflect nearly 100% of the light and radiation that strikes it, hence the need for sunglasses while skiing on a sunny day. This reflected light is also why a skier can receive a significant sunburn even on a cloudy day. Therefore, a sunscreen is indicated for the sun-sensitive skier. Sand, while not as effective a reflective surface as snow, reflects about 4% of the radiation striking it. Therefore, a person sitting in the shade of a beach umbrella is still being bombarded by the UV radiation off the sand. This contributes to the overall radiation received, and a severe sunburn may result. Water reflects not more than 5% of the UV radiation and allows the remaining 95% to penetrate and burn the swimmer. Therefore, time in the water, even if the swimmer is completely submerged, should be considered as part of the total time spent in the sun. In addition, although dry clothes reflect almost all UV radiation, wet clothes allow transmission of approximately 50% of the UV radiation. However, if light passes through dry clothing when held up to the light, then UV radiation will also penetrate that clothing.

People should be advised that although tanning and thickening of the skin serve as protective mechanisms against future injury, peeling of the skin removes part of this protection. The amount of exposure to the sun as well as the SPF of the product being used must be reevaluated as tanning and peeling occur.

Other specific information related to the safe and effective use of sunscreen agents has been reviewed by the FDA panel. The panel concluded that two major causes of poor sun protection with sunscreen use are application of inadequate amounts and infrequent re-application. Sunscreens must be liberally applied to all exposed areas of the body. The sunscreen must be reapplied as frequently as the package recommends for maximum effectiveness. These two factors drive up the cost of sunscreen use. However, the long-term benefits of proper sunscreen use far outweigh the costs. The panel recommends that the directions for use state: "Apply liberally before sun exposure and reapply after swimming or after excessive sweating" (113). The panel also recommends that labeling of all sunscreens should contain the following warnings:

- For external use only, not to be swallowed.

- Avoid contact with eyes.

- Discontinue use if signs of irritation or rash appear.

The reapplication of a sunscreen does not extend the amount of time a person can spend in the sun. Outdoor exposure to UV radiation should be within the limits of the SPF value of the sunscreen. Moreover, although some sunscreen products now have an SPF of 50, the use of an SPF over 15 offers little advantage to the average person (114). The best recommendation for providing optimal protection from immediate as well as long-term injury from sun exposure is to use a product with an SPF of 15. This will allow the development of a slow but safe tan. Children should use SPF–15 sunscreens daily whenever they play outdoors, not just when swimming. These recommendations should be emphasized during consultation.

Recently, questions have been raised about the possibility that the substantivity of a sunscreen may affect the temperature-regulating ability of the body (115). One study reported that exercising in hot weather after application of a sunscreen product may cause an increased risk of overheating. Under hot, humid conditions there is increased sweating but poor evaporation. When the humidity is low, overheating during exercise may still occur, possibly because of a blockage of the pores by the oily vehicle of the sunscreen. Therefore, sunbathers should be cautious when exercising in hot weather after the application of a sunscreen product.

Because of widespread use of products containing 5% ABA, the dosage and administration for a particular product will vary. Generally, the instructions are:

Apply liberally and evenly 1 hour before exposure. Allow time for the product to dry before dressing to avoid absorption of the agent into the garment. If used, cosmetics or emollients may usually be applied after application of the product. Mention should be made that aminobenzoic products will stain light-colored fabric and damage and/or stain vinyl and/or fiberglass.

There has been a recent report of individuals ingesting ABA orally in doses up to 1g daily in order to prevent phototoxic reactions (116). In the past, oral use of ABA was associated with a lowered white blood cell count, drug fever, and organ damage. There is no evidence demonstrating the safety or efficacy of ABA when taken orally. Because of its potential hazards, the oral use of ABA should be vigorously discouraged.

SUMMARY

Tanning or burning of the skin can be the result of recreational sunbathing or outdoor activities, such as yard work or sports, or it can be an occupational hazard. Whatever the case, the long-term hazards of exposure to UV radiation are well known to the scientific and medical community and are becoming well documented. However, the public must be educated about the hazards of the sun as well as methods to minimize these hazards.

The key to proper protection is the identification of skin type. Once this is done, a product with the appropriate SPF should be selected. It appears that within SPF rating groups, no difference exists regarding efficacy. Other considerations that may determine the selection are substantivity, ability to damage fabrics, and price.

Once a product is selected, it should be applied at least 30 minutes before exposure to the sun (up to 2 hours with ABA and its esters). The product should be applied frequently, especially after heavy sweating and swimming.

If a patient is taking photosensitizing drugs, a wide-spectrum product is preferred. Most authorities prefer a product containing ABA or its esters in combination with a benzophenone. However, avoidance of unnecessary exposure to UV radiation is the primary preventive measure.

If the individual's ultimate goal is to develop a deep tan, the best approach is slow and cautious. Brief and gradually increasing exposure to the sun and avoidance of peak sun times allow for gradual tanning with minimal burning. This gradual tanning provides natural protection to the skin. With proper use of sunscreen products and judicious tanning, both the short-term and long-term hazards of exposure to the sun may be minimized.

REFERENCES

1   "The Merck Manual," 15th ed., R. Berkow, Ed., Merck, Rahway, N.J., 1987, p. 2348.

2   M. Lane-Brown, *Australian Prescriber*, *9*, 84 (1986).

3   M. A. Pathak et al., in "Dermatology in General Medicine," T. B. Fitzpatrick et al., Eds., McGraw-Hill, New York, N.Y., 1987, p. 254.

4   I. E. Kochevar et al., in "Dermatology in General Medicine," T. B. Fitzpatrick et al., Eds., McGraw-Hill, New York, N.Y., 1987, p. 1443.

5   L. H. Kligman, in "The Biological Effects of UV-A Radiation," F. Urbach and R. W. Gange, Eds., Praeger Publications, New York, N.Y., 1986, p. 98.

6   B. A. Gilchrest et al., *J. Am. Acad. Dermatol.*, *9*, 213 (1983).

7   B. Staberg et al., *J. Invest. Dermatol.*, *79*, 358 (1982).

8   I. E. Kochevar et al., in "Dermatology in General Medicine," T. B. Fitzpatrick et al., Eds., McGraw-Hill, New York, N.Y., 1987, p. 1442.

9   R. W. Gange, in "Dermatology in General Medicine," T. B. Fitzpatrick et al., Eds., McGraw-Hill, New York, N.Y., 1987. p. 1454.

10   M. A. Pathak, in "The Biological Effects of UV-A Radiation," F. Urbach and R. W. Gange, Eds., Praeger Publications, New York, N.Y., 1986, p. 160.

11   M. A. Pathak, in "The Biological Effects of UV-A Radiation," F. Urbach and R. W. Gange, Eds., Praeger Publications, New York, N.Y., 1986, p. 157.

12   G. Plewig and E. Hoelzle, in "The Biological Effects of UV-A Radiation," F. Urback and R. Gange, Eds., Praeger Publications, New York, N.Y., 1986, p. 168.

13   R. W. Gange, in "Dermatology in General Medicine," T. B. Fitzpatrick et al., Eds., McGraw-Hill, New York, N.Y., 1987, p. 1451.

14   M. A. Pathak et al., "Dermatology in General Medicine," T. B. Fitzpatrick et al., Eds., McGraw-Hill, New York, N.Y., 1986, p. 1513.

15   P. D. Forbes et al., in "Photobiology of the Skin and Eye," E. M. Jackson, Ed., Marcel Dekker, New York, N.Y., 1986, p. 68.

16   "Consensus Development Conference Statement on Sunlight, Ultraviolet Radiation, and the Skin," National Institutes of Health, Bethesda, Md., May 8–10, 1989, p. 1.

17   "Consensus Development Conference Statement on Sunlight, Ultraviolet Radiation, and the Skin," National Institutes of Health, Bethesda, Md., May 8–10, 1989, p. 13.

18   B. S. Paul and J. A. Parrish, *J. Invest. Dermatol.*, *78*, 37 (1982).

19   I. Willis et al., *J. Invest. Dermatol.*, *59*, 416 (1973).

20   F. Urbach and P. D. Forbes, in "Dermatology in General Medicine," T. B. Fitzpatrick et al., Eds., McGraw-Hill, New York, N.Y., 1987, p. 1478.

21   J. R. Wuest and T. Gossel, *Am. Pharm.*, *NS21*, 46 (1981).

22   H. F. Blum, "Carcinogenesis by UV Light," Princeton University Press, Princeton, N.J., 1959, pp. 285–305.

23   F. Urbach, *J. Invest. Dermatol.*, *32*, 373 (1959).

24   F. Urbach et al., in "Environment and Cancer," Williams and Wilkins, Baltimore, Md., 1972.

25   E. A. Emmett, *CRC Crit. Rev. Toxicol.*, *2*, 211 (1973).

26   Monograph No. 10, F. Urbach, Ed., U.S. National Cancer Institute, Washington, D.C., 1964.

27   J. F. Dorn, *Public Health Reports*, *59*, 33 (1944).

28   F. Urbach et al., in "Tenth International Cancer Congress" (Abstracts), Lippincott, Philadelphia, Pa., 1970, pp. 109–110.

29   A. G. Glass and R. N. Hoover, *J. Am. Med. Assoc.*, *262*, 2097–2100 (1989).

30   M. A. Pathak et al., in "Dermatology in General Medicine," T. B. Fitzpatrick et al., Eds., McGraw-Hill, New York, N.Y. 1987, p. 256.

31   R. DeVorc, in "Sunbathing and Skin Cancer," *FDA Consumer* (May 1977).

32   W. F. Stanaszek and B. C. Carlstedt, *U.S. Pharmacist*, *11 (6)*, 22 (1986).

33   K. V. Sanderson, in "Comparative Physiology and Pathology of the Skin," A. J. Rook and G. S. Walton, Eds., Davis, Philadelphia, Pa., 1965, p. 637.

34   Z. W. Zagula-Mally et al., *Cancer*, *34*, 345 (1974).

35   D. M. Pillsbury et al., "Dermatology," Saunders, Philadelphia, Pa., 1956, p. 1145.

36   M. Moushovitz and B. Modan, *J. Nat. Cancer Inst.*, *51*, 77 (1973).

37   M. A. Pathak et al., in "Dermatology in General Medicine," T. B. Fitzpatrick et al., Eds., McGraw-Hill, New York, N.Y., 1987, p. 256.

38   M. Segi, Monograph No. 10, U.S. National Cancer Institute, Washington, D.C., 1963, p. 245.

39   J. Belisario, "Cancer of the Skin," Butterworth, London, England, 1959, p. 15.

40   J. A. Elliott and D. G. Welton, *Arch. Dermatol. Syphitol.*, *53*, 307 (1946).

41   V. A. Belinsky and L. N. Guslitzer, in "Tenth International Cancer Congress Abstracts" (Abstracts), Lippincott, Philadelphia, Pa., 1970, p. 109.

42   H. Averbach, *Public Health Reports*, *76*, 345 (1961).

43   L. H. Kligman and A. M. Kligman, in "Dermatology in General Medicine," T. B. Fitzpatrick et al., Eds., McGraw-Hill, New York, N.Y., 1987, p. 1472.

44   "Consensus Conference Statement on Photoaging/Photodamage," American Academy of Dermatology, St. Louis, Mo., March 3–4, 1988, p. 10.

45   A. M. Kligman, *J. Am. Med. Assoc.*, *210*, 2377 (1969).

46   J. R. Wuest and T. A. Gossel, *Am. Pharm.*, *NS21*, 46 (1981).

47   L. H. Kligman and A. M. Kligman, in "Dermatology in General Medicine," T. B. Fitzpatrick et al., Eds., McGraw-Hill, New York, N.Y. 1987, p. 1473.

48   K. Boudreaux and B. Davidson, *U.S. Pharmacist*, 46 (June/July 1977).

49   E. Emmett, *Int. J. Dermatol.*, *17*, 370 (1978).

50   C. A. Bond, in "Applied Therapeutics for Clinical Pharmacists," 3rd ed., M. A. Koda-Kimble et al., Eds., Applied Therapeutics, San Francisco, Calif., 1983, p. 1178.

51 S. Epstein, *Medical Times* (March 1965).

52 D. A. Lopez, *J. Assoc. Military Dermatol.*, *4*, 19 (1979).

53 *Br. Med. J.*, *2*, 494 (1970).

54 F. J. Akin et al., *Toxicol. Appl. Pharmacol.*, *49*, 219 (1979).

55 J. D. Bernhard et al., in "Dermatology in General Medicine," T. B. Fitzpatrick et al., Eds., McGraw-Hill, New York, N.Y., 1987, p. 1481.

56 *Federal Register*, *43*, 38213 (1978).

57 M. W. Hursthouse, *Curr. Ther.*, 18 (November 1973).

58 F. D. Bernhard et al., in "Dermatology in General Medicine," T. B. Fitzpatrick et al., Eds., McGraw-Hill, New York, N.Y., 1987, p. 1484.

59 R. L. Olson et al., *Arch. Dermatol.*, *108*, 541 (1973).

60 R. Breit and L. Endres, in "The Biological Effects of UV-A Radiation," F. Urbach and R. W. Gange, Eds., Praeger Publications, New York, N.Y., 1986, p. 98.

61 R. W. Gange et al., *J. Am. Acad. Dermatol.*, *9*, 496 (1986).

62 N. J. Lowe et al., *J. Am. Acad. Dermatol.*, 226 (1987).

63 K. Kaibey et al., *J. Am. Acad. Dermatol.*, *16*, 346–353 (1987).

64 K. Kaibey et al., *J. Am. Acad. Dermatol.*, *16*, 347 (1987).

65 J. W. Stanfield et al., *J. Am. Acad. Dermatol.*, *20*, 745 (1989).

66 *Federal Register*, *43*, 38218 (1978).

67 M. Pathak et al., *N. Engl. J. Med.*, *280*, 1459 (1969).

68 B. Compelik, *Cosmet. Toiletr.*, *91*, 59 (1976).

69 R. M. Sayre et al., *Arch. Dermatol.*, *115*, 46–49 (1979).

70 R. Sayre et al., *Arch. Dermatol.*, *115* (1979).

71 R. Roelandts et al., *Int. J. Dermatol.*, *22*, 250 (1983).

72 T. A. Gossel, *U.S. Pharmacist*, *14 (5)*, 82 (1989).

73 *Federal Register*, *43*, 38219–38253 (1978).

74 W. E. Gilbertson, (Letter to Howard Iserman, June 6, 1989), Freedom of Information, Comment No. C00058, Docket No. 78N–0038.

75 C. Mathias et al., *Arch. Dermatol.*, *114 (46)*, 1665 (1978).

76 K. H. Kaidberg et al., *Arch. Dermatol.*, *114*, 547 (1978).

77 M. A. Pathak, *J. Am. Acad. Dermatol.*, 7, 301 (1982).

78 R. Roelandts, *Int. J. Dermatol.*, *22*, 251 (1983).

79 M. A. Pathak, *Am. Acad. Dermatol.*, 7, 302 (1982).

80 J. C. Belisario, *Med. J. Aust.*, *1*, 598 (1967).

81 R. Roelandts, *Int. J. Dermatol.*, *22*, 254 (1983).

82 T. A. Gossel, *U.S. Pharmacist*, *14*, 83 (1989).

83 Jean Rippere, FDA OTC Drug Evaluation, personal communication, October 23, 1989.

84 A. A. Fisher, "Contact Dermatitis," Lea and Febiger, Philadelphia, Pa., 1967, p. 151.

85 M. A. Pathak, *J. Dermatol. Surg. Oncol.*, *13*, 744 (1987).

86 R. W. Gange et al., *J. Am. Acad. Dermatol.*, *15*, 497 (1986).

87 N. J. Lowe et al., *J. Am. Acad. Dermatol.*, *17*, 227 (1987).

88 *Federal Register*, *43*, 38216 (1978).

89 *Federal Register*, *43*, 38215 (1978).

90 C. Stenberg and O. Larkö, *Arch. Dermatol.*, *121*, 1401 (1985).

91 S. Rothman and J. Rubin, *J. Invest. Dermatol.*, *5*, 445–454 (1952).

92 M. A. Pathak, *J. Amer. Acad. Dermatol.*, 7, 309 (1982).

93 "Talk Paper," Food and Drug Administration, Rockville, Md., July 6, 1981.

94 M. A. Pathak, *J. Dermatol. Surg. Oncol.*, *13*, 742 (1987).

95 C. Jaworsky et al., *J. Amer. Acad. Dermatol.*, *16*, 771 (1987).

96 *FDA Consumer*, *21* (October 1980).

97 "Consensus Development Conference Statement on Sunlight, Ultraviolet Radiation and the Skin," National Institutes of Health, Bethesda, Md., May 8–10, 1989, p. 6.

98 *J. Am. Acad. Dermatol.*, *3*, 30 (1980).

99 *FDC Reports*, *41*, T and G2 (January 1979).

100 *Federal Register*, *43*, 38217 (1978).

101 R. S. Stern et al., *Arch. Dermatol.*, *122*, 537 (1986).

102 D. J. Cripps and S. Hegedus, *Arch. Dermatol.*, *109*, 202 (1974).

103 M. A. Pathak et al., *N. Engl. J. Med.*, *280*, 1461 (1969).

104 "Summary Minutes of the FDA Advisory Review Panel on OTC Topical Analgesic, Antirheumatic, Otic, Burn, and Sunburn Treatment Drug Products," Meetings 1–6, Rockville, Md., March 1973–January 1975.

105 I. Willis and A. M. Kligman, *Arch. Dermatol.*, *102*, 405 (1970).

106 *Consumer Reports*, *45*, 353 (1980).

107 K. H. Kaidberg and A. M. Kligman, *J. Invest. Dermatol.*, *76*, 356 (1981).

108 J. A. Parrish et al., *J. Invest. Dermatol.*, *76*, 356 (1981).

109 H. R. Taylor et al., *N. Engl. J. Med.*, *319*, 1429–1433 (1988).

110 "HHS NEWS," U.S. Department of Health and Human Services, Washington, D.C., May 15, 1989.

111 E. Y. Johnson and D. P. Lookingbill, *Arch. Dermatol.*, *120*, 727 (1984).

112 M. A. Pathak et al., in "Dermatology in General Medicine," T. B. Fitzpatrick et al., Eds., McGraw-Hill, New York, N.Y., 1987, p. 1521.

113 *Federal Register*, *43*, 38254 (1978).

114 M. Abramowicz et al., *Med. Lett.*, *30*, 63 (1988).

115 T. D. Wells et al., *The Physician and Sportsmedicine*, *12*, 132–142 (1984).

116 *J. Am. Med. Assoc.*, *251*, 2348 (1984).

SUNSCREEN AND SUNTAN PRODUCT TABLE

Product (Manufacturer)	SPF Value	Sunscreen Agent	Other Ingredients
A-Fil Cream (GenDerm)	8-15	methyl anthranilate, 5%	titanium dioxide, 5%
Bain de Soleil Lip Protecteur (Richardson-Vicks)	30	ethylhexyl p-methoxycinnamate oxybenzone 2-ethylhexyl salicylate	oleyl alcohol, petrolatum
Bain de Soleil Protecteur Gentil Body Silkening (Richardson-Vicks)	25	padimate O ethylhexyl p-methoxycinnamate oxybenzone dioxybenzone	
Bain de Soleil Protecteur Gentil Body Silkening Creme (Richardson-Vicks)	25	padimate O ethylhexyl p-methoxycinnamate oxybenzone	benzyl alcohol
Bain de Soleil Protecteur Gentil Body Silkening Spray (Richardson-Vicks)	20	padimate O oxybenzone ethylhexyl p-methoxycinnamate	
Bain de Soleil Protecteur Gentil Face Creme (Richardson-Vicks)	25	padimate O ethylhexyl p-methoxycinnamate oxybenzone	
Bain de Soleil Protecteur Gentil Under Eye Protecteur (Richardson-Vicks)	30	ethylhexyl p-methoxycinnamate oxybenzone 2-ethylhexyl salicylate	
Blistex Lip Conditioner (Blistex)	15	octyl dimethyl PABA, 7.5% oxybenzone, 3.5%	petrolatum, 57%
Blistik Lip Balm (Blistex)	10	padimate O, 6.6% oxybenzone, 2.5%	dimethicone, 2%
Block Out by Sea & Ski (Carter)	15	padimate O octyl methoxycinnamate oxybenzone	
Block Out Clear by Sea & Ski (Carter)	15	padimate O octyl methoxycinnamate octyl salicylate	SD alcohol 40
Bullfrog Gel (Chattem)	9	octyl methoxycinnamate	benzophenone-3 isostearyl alcohol
Bullfrog Gel (Chattem)	18	octyl methoxycinnamate	octocrylene, benzophenone-3, isostearyl alcohol
Bullfrog Gel (Chattem)	36	octyl methoxycinnamate	octocrylene, benzophenone-3, isostearyl alcohol
Bullfrog for Kids (Chattem)	18	octyl methoxycinnamate octyl salicylate	octocrylene
Bullfrog Stick (Chattem)	18	octyl methoxycinnamate	benzophenone-3, isostearyl alcohol
Chap et Sun Ban 15 Lip Conditioner (Stanback)	15	padimate O, 7% oxybenzone, 3%	petrolatum, isopropyl myristate, aloe vera extract, synthetic beeswax, cetyl palmitate, ceresin, flavor
Chap Stick Sunblock (A.H. Robins)	15	padimate O, 7% oxybenzone, 3%	petrolatum, 44%; lanolin, 0.5%; isopropyl myristate, 0.5%; cetyl alcohol, 0.5%
Coppertone Lipkote (Schering-Plough)	15	ethylhexyl p-methoxycinnamate oxybenzone	
Coppertone Lite Lotion (Schering-Plough)	4	ethylhexyl p-methoxycinnamate	
Coppertone Lite Oil (Schering-Plough)	2	2-ethylhexyl salicylate	

SUNSCREEN AND SUNTAN PRODUCT TABLE, continued

Product (Manufacturer)	SPF Value	Sunscreen Agent	Other Ingredients
Coppertone Lotion (Schering-Plough)	4	ethylhexyl p-methoxycinnamate oxybenzone	
Coppertone Oil (Schering-Plough)	2	homosalate	
Coppertone Sunblock Lotion (Schering-Plough)	15	ethylhexyl p-methoxycinnamate oxybenzone	
Coppertone Sunblock Lotion (Schering-Plough)	25, 30	ethylhexyl p-methoxycinnamate 2-ethylhexyl salicylate homosalate oxybenzone	
Coppertone Sunblock Lotion (Schering-Plough)	45	ethylhexyl p-methoxycinnamate 2-ethylhexyl salicylate oxybenzone	octocrylene
Coppertone Sunscreen Lotion (Schering-Plough)	6	ethylhexyl p-methoxycinnamate oxybenzone	
Coppertone Sunscreen Lotion (Schering-Plough)	8	ethylhexyl p-methoxycinnamate oxybenzone	
Daily Conditioning Treatment for Lips (Blistex)	15	padimate O, 7.5% oxybenzone, 3.5%	petrolatum, cetyl alcohol
Eclipse (Eclipse)	NS[a]	glyceryl p-aminobenzoate, 3% padimate O, 3%	alcohol, 5%; oleth-3 phosphate; petrolatum; synthetic spermaceti; glycerin; mineral oil; lanolin alcohol; cetyl stearyl glycol; lanolin oil; triethanolamine; carbomer 934P; benzyl alcohol, 0.5%; perfume
Eclipse, Original Sunscreen Gel (Eclipse)	10	glyceryl p-aminobenzoate, 2.8% padimate O, 3.3%	
Eclipse, Original Sunscreen Moisturizing Lotion (Eclipse)	10	glyceryl p-aminobenzoate, 0.85% padimate O, 4.4%	
Eclipse, Partial Suntan Lotion (Eclipse)	5	padimate O, 2%	
Eclipse, Sunscreen Lip and Face Protectant (Eclipse)	15	padimate O, 7% oxybenzone, 4%	
Eclipse, Total Sunscreen Cooling Alcohol Lotion (Eclipse)	15	glyceryl p-aminobenzoate, 2.8% padimate O, 3.3% oxybenzone, 5.6%	
Eclipse, Total Sunscreen Moisturizing Lotion (Eclipse)	15	padimate O, 7.35% octyl salicylate, 5.25% oxybenzone, 3.15%	
Faces Only Clear Sunscreen (Schering-Plough)	6	ethylhexyl p-methoxycinnamate oxybenzone	
Faces Only Moisturizing Sunblock (Schering-Plough)	15	ethylhexyl p-methoxycinnamate oxybenzone	
Hawaiian Tropic Aloe PABA Sunscreen (Tanning Research)	8	padimate O oxybenzone	aloe

SUNSCREEN AND SUNTAN PRODUCT TABLE, continued

Product (Manufacturer)	SPF Value	Sunscreen Agent	Other Ingredients
Hawaiian Tropic Baby Faces Sunblock (Tanning Research)	25	2-ethylhexyl p-methoxy-cinnamate oxybenzone octyl salicylate methyl anthranilate	
Hawaiian Tropic Dark Tanning with Sunscreen (Tanning Research)	4	2-ethylhexyl p-methoxy-cinnamate methyl anthranilate	
Hawaiian Tropic 15 Plus Sunblock (Tanning Research)	15	2-ethylhexyl p-methoxy-cinnamate oxybenzone methyl anthranilate	
Hawaiian Tropic Protective Tanning (Tanning Research)	6	padimate O oxybenzone	
Hawaiian Tropic Sunscreen (Tanning Research)	10	padimate O oxybenzone	
Johnson's Baby Sunblock (Johnson & Johnson)	15	octyl methoxycinnamate octyl salicylate oxybenzone	titanium dioxide, benzyl alcohol, cetyl alcohol
Johnson's Baby Sunblock (Johnson & Johnson)	30	octyl methoxycinnamate octyl salicylate	benzophenone-3, titanium dioxide
Maxafil Cream (GenDerm)	NS[a]	methyl anthranilate, 5% cinoxate, 4%	
Mentholatum Stick (Mentholatum)	14.7	padimate O	petrolatum, menthol, camphor, essential oils
Noskote Sunblock Creme (Schering-Plough)	15	ethylhexyl p-methoxycinnamate 2-ethylhexyl salicylate oxybenzone	benzyl alcohol
Pabanol (Elder)	14	aminobenzoic acid, 5%	alcohol, 70%
Photoplex Broad Spectrum Sunscreen Lotion (Herbert)	15	avobenzone, 3% padimate O, 7%	benzyl alcohol; carbomer 934P; cetyl esters wax; EDTA; glycerin; imidurea; mineral oil; oleth-3 phosphate; stearyl alcohol; cetereth-20; white petrolatum
Piz Buin Glacier Stick (cream and stick combination) (Johnson & Johnson)	15	octyl methoxycinnamate, 7.5% (cream) 7% (stick) oxybenzone, 2.5% (cream and stick)	titanium dioxide, 5% (stick)
Piz Buin Lotion (Johnson & Johnson)	4	octyl methoxycinnamate, 4% oxybenzone, 1%	
Piz Buin Lotion (Johnson & Johnson)	8	octyl methoxycinnamate, 6.5% oxybenzone, 1.5%	
Piz Buin Lotion (Johnson & Johnson)	15	octyl methoxycinnamate, 7.5% oxybenzone, 2.5%	
Piz Buin Lotion (Johnson & Johnson)	25	octyl methoxycinnamate, 7.5% oxybenzone, 4% octyl salicylate, 1%	titanium dioxide, 2.56%
Piz Buin Lotion (Johnson & Johnson)	30	octyl methoxycinnamate, 7.5% oxybenzone, 4% octyl salicylate, 3%	titanium dioxide, 4.48%

SUNSCREEN AND SUNTAN PRODUCT TABLE, continued

Product (Manufacturer)	SPF Value	Sunscreen Agent	Other Ingredients
PreSun 8 Creamy (Westwood)	8	octyl dimethyl PABA oxybenzone	carbomer 940, cetyl alcohol, DEA cetyl phosphate, diazolidinyl urea, dimethicone, isopropyl myristate, kathon CG, PG dioctanoate perfume, pvp/eicosene copolymer, stearic acid, triethanolamine
PreSun 15 Creamy (Westwood)	15	octyl dimethyl PABA oxybenzone	carbomer 940, cetyl alcohol, DEA cetyl phosphate, diazolidinyl urea, dimethicone, isopropyl myristate, isodecyl neopentanoate, kathon CG, PG dioctanoate, pvp/eicosene copolymer, stearic acid, triethanolamine
PreSun 39 Creamy (Westwood)	39	octyl dimethyl PABA oxybenzone	carbomer 940, cetyl alcohol, DEA cetyl phosphate, diazolidinyl urea, dimethicone, fragrance, isodecyl neopentanoate, isopropyl myristate, kathon CG, PG dioctanoate, pvp/eicosene copolymer, stearic acid, triethanolamine
PreSun 15 Sensitive Skin (Westwood)	15	octyl methoxycinnamate oxybenzone octyl salicylate	carbomer 940, cetyl alcohol, DEA cetyl phosphate, diazolidinyl urea, dimethicone, isopropyl myristate, isodecyl neopentanoate, kathon CG, PG dioctanoate, pvp/eicosene copolymer, stearic acid, triethanolamine
PreSun 29 Sensitive Skin (Westwood)	29	octyl methoxycinnamate oxybenzone octyl salicylate	carbomer 940, cetyl alcohol, DEA cetyl phosphate, diazolidinyl urea, dimethicone, isopropyl myristate, isodecyl neopentanoate, kathon CG, PG dioctanoate, pvp/eicosene copolymer, stearic acid, triethanolamine
PreSun 15 Ultra Sunscreen Lip Protector (Westwood)	15	octyl dimethyl PABA, 8% oxybenzone, 3%	mineral oil, ozokerite, petrolatum, PEG-4-dilaurate, lanolin oil, propylparaben, flavor
Q.T. Quick Tanning Lotion (Schering-Plough)	2	ethylhexyl p-methoxycinnamate	dihydroxyacetone
Ray Block (Del Ray)	15	padimate O, 5%	benzophenone-3, 3% SD alcohol
Ray-Nox (Torch)	NS[a]	PABA	stearyl alcohol cetyl alcohol
RVP (Elder)	4	red petrolatum	hydrocarbon oil, ointment base
RVPaba Stick (Elder)	NS[a]	PABA, 5%	
RVPaque (Elder)	NS[a]	cinoxate red petrolatum	zinc oxide
Sea & Ski Baby Lotion Formula (Carter)	2	padimate O	
Sea & Ski Golden Tan (Carter)	4	padimate O	
Shade UVA/UVB Sunblock Lotion (Schering-Plough)	15	ethylhexyl p-methoxycinnamate oxybenzone	

SUNSCREEN AND SUNTAN PRODUCT TABLE, continued

Product (Manufacturer)	SPF Value	Sunscreen Agent	Other Ingredients
Shade UVA/UVB Sunblock Lotion (Schering-Plough)	30	ethylhexyl p-methoxycinnamate 2-ethylhexyl salicylate homosalate oxybenzone	
Shade UVA/UVB Sunblock Lotion (Schering-Plough)	45	ethylhexyl p-methoxycinnamate oxybenzone 2-ethylhexyl salicylate	octocrylene
Shade UVA/UVB Sunblock Oil-Free Gel (Schering-Plough)	15	ethylhexyl p-methoxycinnamate octyl salicylate oxybenzone	SD alcohol 40, 74%
Shade UVA/UVB Sunblock Oil-Free Gel (Schering-Plough)	25	ethylhexyl p-methoxycinnamate octyl salicylate homosalate oxybenzone	SD alcohol 40, 74%
Shade UVA/UVB Sunblock Stick (Schering-Plough)	30	ethylhexyl p-methoxycinnamate 2-ethylhexyl salicylate oxybenzone	
Snootie by Sea & Ski (Carter)	10	padimate O	
Solar Cream (Doak)	15	PABA, 4%	titanium dioxide, 12%; water-repellent cream base, 84%
Solar Lotion (Doak)	8	octyl methoxycinnamate DEA methoxycinnamate	
Solar Lotion (Doak)	15	PABA	
Solbar PF 15 (Person & Covey)	15	oxybenzone, 5% octyl methoxycinnamate, 7.5%	
Solbar PF Cream PABA Free Waterproof (Person & Covey)	50	oxybenzone octyl methoxycinnamate	octocrylene
Solbar PF Liquid PABA Free (Person & Covey)	15	octyl methoxycinnamate, 7.5% oxybenzone, 6%	SD alcohol 40, 76%
Solbar Plus 15 (Person & Covey)	15	octyl dimethyl PABA, 6% oxybenzone, 4% dioxybenzone, 2%	
Sudden Tan Foam and Lotion by Coppertone (Schering-Plough)	NS[a]	ethylhexyl p-methoxycinnamate	dihydroxyacetone, caramel
SunDare Clear Lotion (Rydelle)	4-6	cinoxate, 1.75%	alcohol, 51.8%
SunDare Creamy Lotion (Rydelle)	4-6	cinoxate, 2%	lanolin derivative
Sundown Lotion, Extra (Johnson & Johnson)	6	padimate O, 3.3% oxybenzone, 1%	
Sundown Lotion, Maximal (Johnson & Johnson)	8	padimate O, 4.75% oxybenzone, 1.75%	
Sundown Lotion, Moderate (Johnson & Johnson)	4	padimate O, 3.3%	
Sundown Lotion, Ultra (Johnson & Johnson)	15	padimate O, 6.5% oxybenzone, 3%	
Sundown Stick, Maximal (Johnson & Johnson)	8	padimate O, 5.3% oxybenzone, 1.75%	

SUNSCREEN AND SUNTAN PRODUCT TABLE, continued

Product (Manufacturer)	SPF Value	Sunscreen Agent	Other Ingredients
Sundown Stick, Ultra (Johnson & Johnson)	15	padimate O, 7% oxybenzone, 3%	
TI• Screen (T/I Pharm)	8	ethylhexyl p-methoxycinnamate, 6% oxybenzone, 2%	
TI• Screen (T/I Pharm)	15	ethylhexyl p-methoxycinnamate, 7.5% oxybenzone, 5%	
Tropical Blend Dark Tanning Lotion (Schering-Plough)	5	ethylhexyl p-methoxycinnamate oxybenzone	
Tropical Blend Dark Tanning Oil - Hawaii Blend (Schering-Plough)	2	homosalate	
Tropical Blend Dark Tanning Oil - Hawaii Blend (Schering-Plough)	4	padimate O oxybenzone	
Tropical Blend Dark Tanning Oil - Jamaica Blend (Schering-Plough)	2	homosalate	
Tropical Blend Dark Tanning Oil - Rio Blend (Schering-Plough)	2	homosalate	
Tropical Blend Gradual Tanning Oil - Hawaii Blend (Schering-Plough)	8	padimate O oxybenzone	
Tropical Blend Gradual Tanning Oil - Hawaii Blend (Schering-Plough)	15	padimate O ethylhexyl p-methoxycinnamate oxybenzone homosalate	
Tropical Blend Sunblock Lotion - Hawaii Blend (Schering-Plough)	30	ethylhexyl p-methoxycinnamate 2-ethylhexyl salicylate homosalate oxybenzone	
Water Babies SPF-15 Sunblock Lotion (Schering-Plough)	15	ethylhexyl p-methoxycinnamate oxybenzone	
Water Babies SPF-25 Sunblock Cream (Schering-Plough)	25	ethylhexyl p-methoxycinnamate 2-ethylhexyl salicylate homosalate oxybenzone	
Water Babies SPF-30 Sunblock Lotion (Schering-Plough)	30	ethylhexyl p-methoxycinnamate 2-ethylhexyl salicylate homosalate oxybenzone	
Water Babies SPF-45 Sunblock Lotion (Schering-Plough)	45	ethylhexyl p-methoxycinnamate 2-ethylhexyl salicylate oxybenzone	octocrylene
Youth Garde Moisturizer Lotion (Whitehall)	4	octyl dimethyl PABA, 3%	aloe vera gel

[a] SPF not specified.

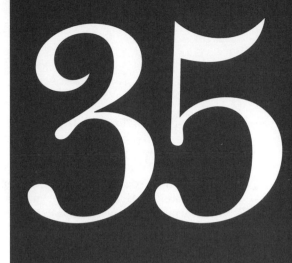

Henry Wormser

POISON IVY AND POISON OAK PRODUCTS

Poison ivy, poison oak, or poison sumac dermatitis is a common, seasonal, allergic contact dermatitis. It may be acute or chronic depending on the extent of exposure and the degree of sensitivity to the allergens. Symptoms range from transient redness to severe swelling and the formation of bullae (blisters); itching and vesiculation usually occur. (See Chapter 30, *Dermatitis, Dry Skin, Dandruff, Seborrheic Dermatitis, and Psoriasis Products.*)

ETIOLOGY

Causative Plants

Various plants and parts of plants may cause allergic reactions in hypersensitive individuals (1). Although more than 60 plants frequently cause contact dermatitis, four species of the Anacardiaceae family are most commonly encountered and cause the more severe lesions: poison ivy *(Toxicodendron radicans)*; western poison oak *(Toxicodendron diversilobum)*; eastern poison oak *(Toxicodendron quercifolium)*; and poison sumac, or poison dogwood *(Toxicodendron vernix)* (2). The Anacardiaceae family has both noxious and useful plants; member plants grow in many parts of the world. Members include the Japanese lacquer tree *(Rhus verniciferum)*, which grows in Japan, China, and Indochina and from which a rich furniture lacquer is obtained; the cashew nut tree *(Anacardium occidentale)*, which grows in India and Pakistan, the East Indies, Africa, and Central and South America; and the mango tree *(Mangifera indica)*, which grows in tropical areas. Cross-sensitivity may occur on skin contact with parts of or products from these plants, such as cashew nut shells, mango rinds, and furniture painted with natural lacquer.

Poison ivy is abundant in the United States and Canada. It grows as either a shrub or a vine and is identified by its characteristic clusters of three lobe-shaped leaflets arranged on stalks; by its white berries that appear in the fall; and by its usual climbing nature (when a vine) (Figure 1). Western poison oak grows along the Pacific Coast from New Mexico to Canada. It commonly grows as an unsupported bush, and the center leaf of the three-leaflet cluster resembles an oak leaf. Eastern poison oak ranges from New Jersey to Florida and from central Texas to Kansas (Figure 2). Poison sumac is a coarse, woody shrub or small tree commonly found in swamps of the southern and eastern United States (3, 4). Its leaves differ by having 7–13 leaflets arranged on each side of the leaf stalk (5) (Figure 3).

Formerly the species were assigned to the genus *Rhus;* hence, the term rhus dermatitis is used to describe the topical reactions caused by exposure to these plants. The lesions of rhus dermatitis are more severe than those of dermatitides caused by other plants. In the United States, poison ivy and poison oak are the main causes of rhus dermatitis. In England and western Europe, primrose dermatitis, caused by the sensitizing agent primulin, is more common than poison ivy dermatitis (6). A few isolated cases of rhus dermatitis have been reported from France and Australia (7–9).

Development of a plant contact dermatitis requires that an individual be sensitized to the toxic agent by a previous exposure; therefore, an allergic reaction does not occur on first contact with the plant. The degree of hypersensitivity to the toxic agent is variable. Dark-skinned people seem less susceptible to the dermatitis. Young people are more susceptible than the elderly, and newborns are readily sensitized if they come in contact with sap from the plants (10). Interestingly, poison ivy and poison oak dermatitis account for the greatest proportion of workman's compensation payments related to outdoor injuries (11).

Irrespective of their origin (poison ivy, poison oak, or poison sumac), the dermatitides and treatments discussed in this chapter generally pertain to reactions to all three plants.

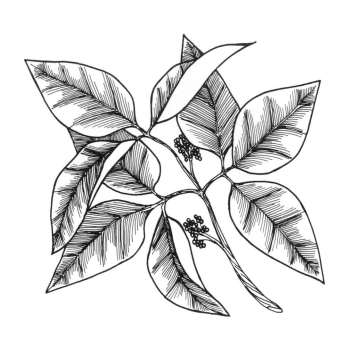

FIGURE 1 Poison ivy.

Allergenic Constituents

Toxicodendrol, a phenolic oily resin, is present in all of the poisonous species and contains a complex active principle, urushiol. Urushiol is distributed widely in the roots, stems, leaves, and fruit of the plant, but not in the flowers, pollen, or epidermis (12). Contact with the intact epidermis of the plant is harmless; dermatitis occurs only after contact with a bruised or injured plant or its sap. Because neither toxicodendrol nor urushiol is volatile, the dermatits cannot be contracted through the air, unless the plants are burned. Smoke from burning plants carries a substantial amount of the oleoresin and may cause serious external and systemic reactions in susceptible individuals.

The chemical structure of poison ivy's allergenic constituents has been identified and elucidated (13–15). Researchers identified four allergens, all of which possess a 1,2-dihydroxybenzene or catechol nucleus with a 15-carbon atom side chain at position 3. The chemical structure of the allergens differs by the degree of unsaturation of the side chain. The four allergens include a saturated component (3-pentadecylcatechol or 3-PDC), a mono-olefin (unsaturated at C-8), a diolefin (unsaturated at C-8 and C-11), and a triolefin (unsaturated at C-8, C-11, and C-14). Certain individ-

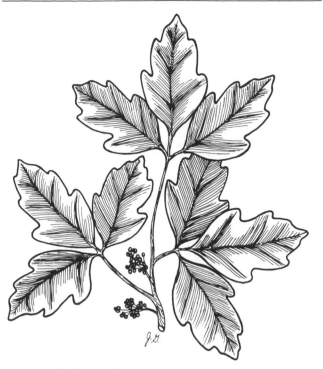

FIGURE 2   Poison oak.

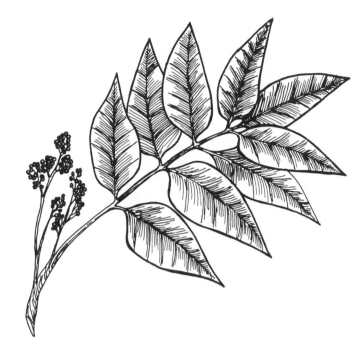

FIGURE 3   Poison sumac.

uals hypersensitive to 3-pentadecylcatechol show cross-reactivity with other compounds such as resorcinol, hexylresorcinol, and the hydroquinones, but not with phenol itself (16).

As little as 1 mcg of crude urushiol causes dermatitis in hypersensitive individuals (17). Direct contact with the plant is not necessary; contact with the allergens may be made from an article that injured the plant or from soot particles that contain allergenic material from the plant. Stroking a pet whose fur is contaminated is also a common source of allergenic material. The oleoresin may be active for months on tools, shoes, and clothing. Contaminated clothing, a frequent source of allergens, is decontaminated by machine washing with laundry detergent (10).

Although the highest incidence of rhus dermatitis occurs in spring and summer when the leaves are young, soft, and easily bruised, it may also occur in autumn and winter (3, 18). In autumn, yellow leaves still have allergenic properties, but they are more resistant to injury. Once they wither and fall, the leaves are much less allergenic. Winter episodes of the dermatitis usually occur around Christmas in tree nursery employees and in people who cut their own trees; contact with the roots or vines of toxicodendron plants growing on the trees causes the reaction.

Mechanism of Contact Dermatitis

Contact dermatitis has two phases: a sensitization phase, during which a specific hypersensitivity to the allergen is acquired, and an elicitation phase, during which subsequent contact with the allergen elicits a visible dermatologic response (19). In the sensitization phase, urushiol components (catechols) are oxidized to the *o*-quinone derivatives, which react readily with human epidermal proteins by nucleophilic addition to form complete antigens (conjugates). Each conjugate leaves the skin through the lymphatic system. The conjugate is then carried to the reticuloendothelial system, where, in response to the antigenic stimulus, special globulins and antibodies are synthesized and lymphocytes are sensitized. In the elicitation phase, repeated contact with the allergen again produces the antigenic conjugate, this time causing a noticeable reaction. The reaction appears to be triggered by the association of specific immunologic elements carried by the blood to the skin.

The interval between contact with the allergen and the appearance of the rash varies with the degree of sensitivity and the amount of allergen contacted. Reaction time, the time between contact of sensitized skin with the allergen and the first sign of reaction, is usually

2 to 3 days, but not less than 12 hours. This interval is characteristic of delayed hypersensitivity reactions involving cell-mediated immunity.

Dermatitic lesions vary from simple macules to vesicles and bullae. Contrary to popular belief, fluid in the vesicles and bullae is not antigenic; accordingly, patch tests with the fluid give negative results. Histologically, nonspecific inflammatory changes occur in the dermis, and spongiosis (edema) followed by intraepidermal vesicles occurs in the epidermis in the acute stage of the disease. Bursting of the vesicles may lead to secondary infection.

SYMPTOMS

Although the limbs, face, and neck are common sites of the dermatitis, all skin areas that come in contact with the sensitizing substance may be affected. Sometimes, distribution of the lesions is bizarre, especially if the antigenic agent is in the clothes or is transferred to various parts of the body by the fingers. The dermatitis may appear early in one area and later in another. Thoroughly washing the skin, cleaning under the fingernails, and laundering clothes remove the oleoresin before it contacts other areas of the body and may prevent the spreading of the dermatitis. Different parts of the body may not have the same sensitivity. Often, parts of the body that are in contact with a heavy concentration of the antigen show more severe reactions and remain hypersensitive for several years.

Poison ivy is specifically an allergic eczematous contact dermatitis. Following exposure to the antigen, the initial reaction is erythema, or rash. The development of raised lesions (erythematous macules and papules) follows, and finally, fluid accumulates in the epidermis, forming vesicles and bullae. (See *Plate 7–30A and B.*) The initial lesions are usually marked by mild to intensive itching and burning. The affected area, often hot and swollen, oozes and eventually dries and crusts (20). Secondary bacterial infections may occur. Chewing poison ivy leaves may result in edematous swelling and pain of the tongue, cheeks, palate, pharynx, and anal region (21). Very rare complications include eosinophilia, kidney damage, urticaria, erythema multiforme, dyshidrosis, marked pigmentation, and leukoderma (loss of melanin pigmentation occurring in patches). Most cases of the dermatitis are self-limiting and disappear in 14–20 days. Again, the duration of the dermatitis depends on the degree of sensitization and frequency of reexposure to the allergen.

Rhus dermatitis may be diagnosed not only from the morphologic appearance of its lesions but also from their distribution: linear streaking is common and occurs naturally as the result of brushing the skin against the poisonous plant. A patient's history of exposure to the causative plants facilitates the diagnosis. Because toxicodendron plants are not photosensitizers, the dermatitis occurs on covered and uncovered parts of the body.

Diagnostic patch testing is a valuable tool in investigating allergic contact dermatitis (22); however, substances used in patch testing may sensitize the patient during testing. Patch testing should be performed only by allergists or other individuals thoroughly familiar with accepted techniques and should never be done during the acute phase of any dermatitis. Patch testing results alone are not diagnostic. To properly interpret the test results, the patient history, physical findings, and the practitioner's clinical experience must also be considered.

TREATMENT

Prophylaxis

Because the poison ivy antigen enters the skin very rapidly, prompt thorough washing of the skin with soap or organic solvents (within 10 minutes of exposure) is necessary to prevent absorption of the antigen. Other topical prophylactic measures include application of barrier creams prior to contact and use of detoxicants (oxidizing and complexing agents that chemically inactivate the antigen) (16). However, many investigators question the effectiveness of these measures (23–25).

Thirty-four barrier preparations were tested over a 2-year period on a group of people highly susceptible to rhus dermatitis (16). The preparations were detoxicants that contained substances such as potassium permanganate, hydrogen peroxide, sodium perborate, iodine, and iron and silver salts. The investigator concluded that none of the preparations could prevent the dermatitis. This conclusion suggests that the antigen reacts rapidly and quite selectively with the skin and that irreversible damage occurs before preventive action can be taken. Although enthusiastic claims have been made for zirconium oxide, an agent used in some nonprescription products, tests found it to be completely ineffective (16). In addition, several researchers found extensive, sarcoid-like granulomas of glabrous skin had developed because of allergic hypersensitivity to insoluble zirconium oxide (26–28). More recently, success has been obtained with some formulations of organoclay (a quaternary ammonium salt of bentonite) (29), polyamine salts of linoleic acid dimer (30), and a product marketed under the name Ivy Shield (31).

The best prevention of allergic contact dermatitis is complete avoidance of the allergen. People should learn to recognize and avoid poison ivy and related plants and to observe and search surrounding terrain carefully before choosing a picnic area or campsite. Susceptible individuals should wear protective clothing, such as long sleeves, long pants, socks, and shoes, when exposure to the offending agents is probable (e.g., on a picnic or hike). These individuals should dispose of or carefully launder their clothing after an outing. They should also wash any object that may have come in contact with the plants to remove the oleoresin, which will remain potent on the object's surface for a considerable time.

A black, enamel-like deposit is frequently present on injured areas of poison ivy, poison oak, and poison sumac plants. This deposit can be reproduced by crushing leaves onto a sheet of paper. The resultant stain should darken on exposure to air if the expressed substance came from a toxicodendron plant (32).

When a poisonous plant is in a garden or cannot be avoided, it should be removed physically or destroyed chemically. Applying herbicides is easier and less dangerous, but there are areas where they cannot be used (e.g., around hedges and shrubbery). In such situations, digging up and pulling up the plants, while wearing gloves, are the only satisfactory methods of removal. The herbicides most effective against poison ivy include amitrole (aminotriazole); ammonium sulfamate; (2,4-dichlorophenoxy) acetic acid (2,4-D); (2,4,5-trichlorophenoxy) acetic acid (2,4,5-T); ammonium thiocyanate; borax; carbon disulfide; coal tar; creosote oils; fuel oil and similar petroleum distillates; sodium chlorate; and sodium arsenite. Individuals using these herbicides should wear appropriate protective gear. Herbicide sprays may be used at any time when poison ivy is in full leaf, but June and July are the best months. Ordinarily, spraying should begin no later than mid-August because poison ivy begins to go dormant then and the herbicides are ineffective. At least three to four sprayings at intervals of 2–8 weeks are necessary to kill all the plants (33).

the original sensitivity returns approximately 6 months after the therapy ends (34, 35). Various forms of the plant antigens, administered either by mouth or by intramuscular (IM) injection, have been used in hyposensitization therapy. For equivalent effects, larger amounts of the oleoresin are required orally than parenterally. When taken orally, the oleoresin may undergo partial inactivation and imperfect absorption. Sustained release is probably the major factor in the superior efficacy of injecting the antigen intramuscularly. Maximal hyposensitization can be achieved with 2–2.5 g IM or 2.5–3 g orally of poison ivy oleoresin antigen. Pure 3-pentadecylcatechol may be administered in doses of 2.5–3 g IM or 3.5–4 g orally (34).

Hyposensitization by administering crude extracts or oleoresins from plants has usually been ineffective because extract potency varies and recommended dosages of the antigens are usually far below those required. Three or four injections cannot provide clinical protection for moderately or extremely hypersensitive persons. Although an alum-precipitated pyridine extract has been used with some success, the availability of intramuscularly administered 3-pentadecylcatechol has improved the outlook for successful hyposensitization. Large doses of this antigen (1–3 g) may be needed in a course of 8–20 injections to provide clinical protection—the greater the person's hypersensitivity, the larger the dose needed. Administering an antigenic substance to hypersensitive individuals involves risk. The exact course of treatment must be individualized and geared to the person's sensitivity level and capacity to tolerate the antigen without serious allergic reactions. If the dermatitis appears during prophylactic treatment, the treatment should be stopped for the duration of the eruption.

Because hyposensitization is temporary, maintenance doses of the antigen should be administered at predetermined intervals. Hyposensitization generally results in milder and shorter reactions and lessens the reaction's tendency to spread to other parts of the body. The dermatitis must be diagnosed by a dermatologist before hyposensitization begins because prophylactic administration of toxicodendron antigens has no effect on contact dermatitis caused by other substances. The only objective proof of successful hyposensitization is a negative or weakly positive reaction to the antigens at a site that previously gave a strong positive reaction.

Hyposensitization Therapy

Specific hyposensitization may be tried by administering repeated doses of toxicodendron antigens, but such prophylaxis is neither complete nor permanent;

Topical Treatment of Dermatitides

The initial symptoms of the dermatitis reaction may be alarming, and the temptation to treat is strong. However, simplicity and safety are keynotes of treatment. Many claims for products used for self-medication take credit for the body's own natural reparative processes; in most cases, the contact dermatitis is self-resolving. The major treatment objectives are:

- To provide protection to the damaged tissue until the acute reaction has subsided;

- To prevent excessive accumulation of debris, resulting from oozing, scaling, and crusting, without disturbing normal tissue;

- To relieve itching and prevent potential scratching and excoriation.

Mild Dermatitis

Linear streaks of papules and vesicles often characterize a mild poison ivy or poison oak dermatitis. These lesions and the accompanying pain and itching can be treated by an antipruritic "shake lotion" such as calamine or zinc oxide. A combination of menthol (1%), equal parts of calamine lotion or zinc oxide lotion, and rubbing alcohol can be soothing (36).

Soaks, baths, or wet dressings can also be effective in soothing pain and itching. Dilute aluminum acetate solution (Burow's solution), saline solution, or sodium bicarbonate solution can be used in this manner for 30 minutes, 3 or 4 times a day. Aluminum acetate solution for topical use is usually a 1:10 or 1:40 dilution of aluminum acetate solution USP in water (37). In addition, the application of either very cold or warm water may provide relief.

Topical preparations containing local anesthetics and/or antihistamines are available; however, their use is controversial because of their sensitizing capabilities. Nonprescription topical steroids, such as hydrocortisone, are also available and have been proven safe and effective for use in mild dermatitis (38).

Greasy ointments should not be used when vesicles are present and oozing.

Moderately Severe Dermatitis

Moderately severe poison ivy dermatitis is characterized by the presence of bullae and edematous swelling of body parts in addition to the papules and vesicles present in milder cases. To reduce discomfort, large bullae may be drained by puncturing their edges with a sterilized needle. The tops of the lesions should be kept intact because they protect the underlying, denuded epidermis of the lesions as they dry. The patient should be reassured that fluid from the lesions will not spread the dermatitis and that the dermatitis is not contagious. Application of cool compresses of aluminum acetate solution (1:10) to edematous areas may be helpful. If the eyelids are affected, cold compresses of boric acid

solution can be used (10). During the healing phase, application of a neutral soothing cream, such as cold cream, helps prevent crusting, scaling, and lichenification (thickening) of the lesions.

Lesions on the face can be treated by applying wet dressings. Lotions should be avoided because they tend to cake, causing discomfort. Men may find that shaving, although uncomfortable, is more comfortable than the accumulation of crust and debris in the beard.

Tub baths using potassium permanganate, oatmeal, or a commercially available colloidal preparation, such as Aveeno, may be soothing and aid drying of lesions. Potassium permanganate is especially effective after vesicles or bullae are opened in drying of the lesions and preventing secondary infection. The patient should be instructed to sit for 15–20 minutes in a tubful of lukewarm water to which 1 tsp of potassium permanganate crystals has been added (10). To avoid skin burns, the crystals should be completely dissolved before the patient gets into the tub.

Colloidal oatmeal baths may be very soothing; however, the patient should be warned that these preparations make the tub very slick and that a nonskid mat should be used.

Severe Dermatitis

When the reaction is spread over the body and/or is associated with major swelling or involvement on or around the eyes, systemic treatment is necessary. The patient should be referred to a physician.

Systemic treatment usually involves prescription drugs such as anti-inflammatory steroids. Corticosteroids commonly are administered orally over 7 days to 3 weeks in a gradually descending dosage schedule. This type of treatment is relatively safe, because it does not lead to hypercorticism or depress adrenal cortical function significantly, as is inevitably the case in more chronic conditions.

Oral antihistamines may be useful for their antipruritic and sedative effects (10, 39).

Topical treatment of severe poison ivy dermatitis is similar to the treatment recommended for moderately severe dermatitis (10).

PHARMACOLOGIC AGENTS

Four major types of pharmacologic agents—local anesthetics, antipruritics, antiseptics, and astringents—are used in topical nonprescription products for poison ivy and poison oak dermatitis.

Local Anesthetics

Local anesthetics affect sensation by interfering with the transmission of impulses along the sensory nerve fiber. Many nerve fibers, specialized endings (receptors), and free nerve endings are in the epidermis. The topically applied anesthetic acts very near the application site. However, whether the agent can reach the nerve endings when applied to unbroken skin is questionable. Benzocaine, diperodon hydrochloride, pramoxine hydrochloride, dibucaine, tetracaine hydrochloride, and cyclomethycaine are the most common agents found in poison ivy/poison oak products. Poorly soluble anesthetics (e.g., benzocaine) are less likely to be absorbed and produce systemic toxicity than soluble anesthetics (e.g., tetracaine hydrochloride). However, the high serum concentrations necessary to cause systemic toxicity are difficult to achieve with nonprescription topical anesthetics. Side effects include dermatitis, characterized by cutaneous lesions, urticaria, and edema; and anaphylactic reactions. Topically applied "caine" anesthetics can be strong sensitizers in susceptible individuals. (See Chapter 33, *Burn and Sunburn Products*.)

Antipruritics

Topically applied antipruritics, including antihistamines, counterirritants, and hydrocortisone, are agents that help to alleviate itching.

Antihistamines

Antihistamines, such as diphenhydramine, pyrilamine, tripelennamine, and phenyltoloxamine, relieve the discomfort of itching by competing with histamine at the H_1 receptor (one of two broad classes of histamine receptors) and also by having a topical anesthetic effect. The topical use of antihistamines does not cause anticholinergic action or systemic toxicity. However, like the "caine" anesthetics, antihistamines may act as sensitizers. Antihistamines are more effective as antipruritics when taken orally, particularly when itching is generalized. For topical products, application of a 1 to 2% concentration of the drugs to the affected area 3 times a day will relieve itching. (See Chapter 36, *Insect Sting and Bite Products*.)

Counterirritants

Counterirritants, such as menthol, phenol, and camphor, produce a sensation of coolness and reduce the irritation of the dermatitis. The sensation is difficult to explain because these chemicals produce local hyperemia. However, low concentrations of counterirritants relieve irritation by the depression of cutaneous receptors. Conversely, applying these agents to damaged skin may cause irritation. (See Chapter 32, *External Analgesic Products*.)

Hydrocortisone

Hydrocortisone is a naturally occurring steroidal hormone manufactured endogenously in the adrenal cortex.

Although useful for a variety of dermatitides, the effectiveness of topical corticosteroids on poison ivy and poison oak dermatitis is disputed. Steroids previously were implicated in the exacerbation of bacterial infections. However, the Food and Drug Administration (FDA) advisory review panel on over-the-counter (OTC) external analgesic drug products reported that there seems to be no danger of exacerbation of cutaneous bacterial, fungal, or viral infections by topical application of 0.5% hydrocortisone. The panel also reported that allergic reactions to hydrocortisone at these concentrations were rare. Additionally, the panel found evidence that prolonged administration of 0.5% hydrocortisone did not appear to cause toxic effects by systemic absorption, even when applied to large areas of damaged or abraded skin (40).

Nonprescription hydrocortisone products approved by the FDA for use on rashes and minor skin irritations must carry the following labeling: "For the temporary relief of minor skin irritations, itching, and rashes due to eczema, dermatitis, insect bites, poison ivy, poison oak, poison sumac, soaps, detergents, cosmetics, and jewelry and for itchy genital and anal areas but not for ophthalmic use."

The dosage for adults and children 2 years of age and above is 0.5% hydrocortisone applied to the affected area 3 or 4 times a day. Children under 2 years of age should be treated only under the advice and supervision of a physician.

Antiseptics

Antiseptics used in poison ivy and poison oak products are intended for prophylaxis against secondary infections, but their effectiveness is questionable. Of the available antiseptics (phenols, alcohols, and oxidizing agents) and quaternary ammonium compounds (e.g., benzalkonium chloride), the quaternary ammonium agents seem to be more effective. Unfortunately, their action is antagonized by anionic compounds such as soaps (8).

Astringents

Astringents are mild protein precipitants that either form a thick coagulum on the surface of lesions or coagulate and remove overlying debris. The astringent action is accompanied by contraction, wrinkling, and blanching of tissue. The cement substance of the capillary endothelium is hardened so that pathologic transcapillary movement of plasma proteins is inhibited, which reduces local edema, inflammation, and exudation. These substances, including aluminum acetate, tannic acid, zinc and iron oxides, and potassium permanganate, are used to stop oozing, reduce inflammation, and promote healing. Astringents also have mild antiseptic properties.

Aluminum acetate solution is generally diluted with 10–40 parts of water and used as a wet dressing 3 or 4 times a day. Therapy may be continued for approximately 5–7 days. Continuous use or prolonged use for extended periods may produce necrosis.

Zinc oxide lotion (15–25%) has mild astringent, protective, and antiseptic actions. Calamine, a mixture of zinc oxide and 1% ferric oxide, is often preferred to plain zinc oxide because of its tan color.

Potassium permanganate is most effective applied as a dilute solution on opened vesicles or bullae; however, it leaves an objectionable purple stain (36).

PRODUCT SELECTION GUIDELINES

Selection of products depends on the severity of the dermatitis. In severe cases of poison ivy dermatitis, a physician should be consulted. Mild to moderately severe cases of poison ivy or poison oak dermatitis can usually be treated with local or topical products. Preparations that contain benzocaine or other local anesthetics should be used with caution, and zirconium oxide products should be avoided. Although hydrocortisone products may be effective, the pharmacist should recommend other treatments first.

Shake lotions, which may contain phenol or menthol, provide immediate relief due to the cooling effect of water evaporation. Phenol and menthol also increase the antipruritic activity. However, the pharmacist should caution against the frequent use of shake lotions, which piles masses of plaster-like material on the skin that are uncomfortable, as well as difficult and painful to remove.

The pharmacist should inform individuals sensitive to toxicodendron plants that certain cosmetics, hair dyes, bleaches, and other commercial products contain compounds related to 3-pentadecylcatechol and could cause cross-sensitivity.

SUMMARY

Every year poison ivy, poison oak, and poison sumac cause contact dermatitides in many people. Prophylaxis and therapy of this allergy are still in the early stages of study, although research is ongoing and progress is being made. A better understanding of the mechanism of the allergic reaction, cross-sensitivity, and hyposensitization will help in formulating products that are more effective in treating and in possibly eradicating this annoying and often serious disorder.

REFERENCES

1 A. A. Fisher, "Contact Dermatitis," 2nd ed., Lea and Febiger, Philadelphia, Pa., 1973, p. 1.

2 M. A. Lesser, *Drug Cosmet. Ind., 70,* 610 (1952).

3 T. A. Gossel, *U.S. Pharmacist, 8,* 22 (1983).

4 N. Vietmeyer, *Smithsonian, 16,* 89 (1985).

5 C. R. Dawson, *Trans. N.Y. Acad. Sci. Sect. Phys. Chem., 18,* 427 (1956).

6 A. Rook and H. T. H. Wilson, *Br. Med. J., 1,* 220 (1965).

7 J. Beurey et al., *Ann. Dermatol. Venerol., 107,* 65 (1980).

8 J. H. Apted, *Austral. J. Dermatol., 19,* 35 (1978).

9 J. H. Apted, *Int. J. Dermatol., 19,* 81 (1980).

10 A. A. Fisher, "Contact Dermatitis," 2nd ed., Lea and Febiger, Philadelphia, Pa., 1973, pp. 260-266.

11 M. F. Goldsmith, *J. Am. Med. Assoc., 251,* 1389 (1984).

12 J. H. Doyle, *Pediatr. Clin. North Am., 8,* 259 (1961).

13 S. V. Sunthankar and C. R. Dawson, *J. Am. Chem. Soc., 76,* 5070 (1954).

14 W. E. Symes and C. R. Dawson, *J. Am. Chem. Soc., 76,* 2959 (1954).

15 B. Love and C. R. Dawson, *J. Am. Chem. Soc., 78,* 1180 (1956).

16 A. M. Kligman, *Arch. Dermatol., 77,* 149 (1958).

17 F. A. Stevens, *J. Am. Med. Assoc., 127,* 192 (1945).

18 T. A. Gossel and J. R. Wuest, *Ohio Pharm. 32,* 192 (1983).

19 A. L. deWeek, in "Dermatology in General Medicine," T. B. Fitzpatrick et al., Eds., McGraw-Hill, New York, N.Y., 1971, p. 669.

20   P. M. Selfon, *Milit. Med., 128,* 895 (1963).

21   S. H. Silvers, *J. Am. Med. Assoc., 116,* 2257 (1941).

22   A. M. Kligman, *J. Invest. Dermatol., 47,* 369, 375, 393 (1966).

23   B. Shelmire, *J. Am. Med. Assoc., 113,* 1085 (1939).

24   O. Gisvold, *J. Am. Pharm. Assoc. Sci. Ed., 30,* 17 (1941).

25   J. B. Howell, *Arch. Dermatol. Syphilol., 48,* 373 (1943).

26   P. J. LoPresti and G. W. Hambrick, Jr., *Arch. Dermatol., 92,* 188 (1965).

27   W. L. Epstein and J. R. Allen, *J. Am. Med. Assoc., 190,* 940 (1963).

28   N. A. Hall, *J. Am. Pharm. Assoc., NS12,* 576 (1972).

29   W. L. Epstein, *Arch. Dermatol, 125,* 499 (1989).

30   S. Orchard et al., *Arch. Dermatol, 122,* 783 (1986).

31   D. Basiliere, Interpro, Inc., Haverhill, Mass., personal communication, 1989.

32   J. D. Guin, *J. Am. Acad. Dermatol., 2,* 332 (1980).

33   D. M. Crooks and L. W. Kephart, "Farmers' Bulletin," Pub. No. 1972, U.S. Department of Agriculture, Washington, D.C., 1951, 30 pp.

34   A. M. Kligman, *Arch. Dermatol., 78,* 47 (1958).

35   A. M. Kligman, *Arch. Dermatol., 78,* 359 (1958).

36   "Current Therapy," H. F. Conn, Ed., W. B. Saunders, Philadelphia, Pa., 1979, p. 588.

37   *Federal Register, 54,* 13489 (1989).

38   A. W. P. du Vivier, *Practitioner, 230,* 897 (1986).

39   "Applied Therapeutics for Clinical Pharmacists," 2nd ed., M. A. Koda-Kimble et al., Eds., Applied Therapeutics, San Francisco, Calif., 1978, p. 860.

40   *Federal Register, 44,* 69822 (1979).

POISON IVY AND POISON OAK PRODUCT TABLE

Product (Manufacturer)	Application Form	Anesthetic	Antipruritic/ Antihistamine	Antiseptic	Astringent	Other Ingredients
Aveeno (Rydelle Labs)	bath					colloidal oatmeal, 100% or colloidal oatmeal, 43% and mineral oil
Aveeno (Rydelle Labs)	lotion					colloidal oatmeal, 1% glycerin distearyldimonium chloride petrolatum isopropyl palmitate cetyl alcohol dimethicone sodium chloride benzyl alcohol
Caladryl (Parke-Davis)	cream lotion		diphenhydramine hydrochloride, 1% camphor		calamine, 8% glycerin (lotion)	cetyl alcohol (cream) cresin white propylene glycol propylparaben polysorbate 60 sorbitan stearate alcohol, 2% (lotion) sodium carboxy-methylcellu-lose (lotion)
Calamatum (Blair)	ointment lotion spray	benzocaine, 3%	camphor	phenol	zinc oxide calamine	
Calamine, Regular and Phenolated (Various manufacturers)	lotion			phenol, 1% (phenolated)	calamine, 8% zinc oxide, 8%	glycerin, 2% bentonite magma calcium hydroxide solution
Calamox (Hauck)	ointment				calamine, 0.17 g/g	
Dalicote (Dalin)	lotion	diperodon hydrochloride, 0.25%	pyrilamine maleate camphor		zinc oxide	dimethyl polysiloxane silicone grease-less base
Dermapax (Recsei)	lotion		pyrilamine maleate, 0.44% chlorpheniramine maleate, 0.06%	chlorobutanol, 1% benzyl alcohol, 1%		isopropyl alcohol, 35%
Di-Delamine (Commerce)	gel spray		tripelennamine hydrochloride, 0.5% diphenhydramine hydrochloride, 1% menthol, 0.1%	benzalkonium chloride, 0.12%		

POISON IVY AND POISON OAK PRODUCT TABLE, continued

Product (Manufacturer)	Application Form	Anesthetic	Antipruritic/ Antihistamine	Antiseptic	Astringent	Other Ingredients
Ivarest (Blistex)	cream lotion	benzocaine, 5%	pyrilamine maleate		calamine, 14%	hydroxyethylcellulose lanolin oil petrolatum polysorbate 60 propylene glycol sorbitan stearate
Ivy Dry Cream (Ivy)	cream	benzocaine, 5 mg/g	menthol, 4 mg/g camphor, 6 mg/g		tannic acid, 80 mg/g	methylparaben, 2.5 mg/g propylparaben, 0.3 mg/g isopropyl alcohol, 7.5%
Ivy Dry liquid (Ivy)	liquid				tannic acid, 100 mg/ml	isopropyl alcohol, 12.5%
Ivy Super Dry (Ivy)	liquid	benzocaine, 5 mg/ml	menthol, 2 mg/ml camphor, 4 mg/ml		tannic acid, 100 mg/ml	isopropyl alcohol, 35% methylparaben, 0.01 mg/ml propylparaben, 0.1 mg/ml
Ivy-Chex (Jones Medical)	non-spray aerosol		methyl salicylate	benzalkonium chloride		SD alcohol, 89.5% polyvinyl-pyrrolidone vinylacetate copolymers
Ivy-Rid (Hauck)	aerosol			benzalkonium chloride		SDA alcohol isopropyl-myristate isobutane methylene chloride polyvinyl-pyrrolidone vinylacetate copolymers
Nupercainal Cream (Ciba)	cream	dibucaine, 0.5%				acetone sodium bisulfite glycerin potassium hydroxide stearic acid trolamine water-washable base
Nupercainal Ointment (Ciba)	ointment	dibucaine, 1%				acetone sodium bisulfite lanolin light mineral oil white petrolatum
Obtundia Calamine Cream (Otis Clapp)	cream			cresol-camphor complex	calamine zinc oxide	

POISON IVY AND POISON OAK PRODUCT TABLE, continued

Product (Manufacturer)	Application Form	Anesthetic	Antipruritic/ Antihistamine	Antiseptic	Astringent	Other Ingredients
Poison Ivy Cream (McKesson)	cream	benzocaine, 2.5%	pyrilamine maleate, 15 mg/g		zirconium oxide, 4% (as carbonated hydrous zirconia)	
Poison Ivy Spray (McKesson)	aerosol	benzocaine, 0.5%	menthol camphor		calamine, 2% zinc oxide, 1%	isopropyl alcohol, 9.44%
Pontocaine (Winthrop)	cream ointment	tetracaine hydrochloride, 1% (cream); 0.5% (ointment)	menthol, 0.5% (ointment)			methylparaben (cream) sodium bisulfite (cream) white petrolatum (ointment) white wax (ointment)
Pyribenzamine (Ciba)	cream ointment		tripelennamine, 2%			water-washable base (cream) petrolatum base (ointment)
Rhuli Cream (Rydelle Labs)	cream	benzocaine, 5%	camphor, 0.3%		calamine, 3%	glycerin distearyldimonium chloride petrolatum isopropyl palmitate cetyl alcohol dimethicone sodium chloride
Rhuli Gel (Rydelle Labs)	gel		menthol, 0.3% camphor, 0.3%	benzyl alcohol, 2%		SD alcohol 23A, 31% propylene glycol carbomer 940 triethanolamine benzophenone-4 EDTA
Rhuli Spray (Rydelle Labs)	spray	benzocaine, 5%	camphor, 0.7%	benzyl alcohol	calamine, 13.8%	hydrated silica isobutane isopropyl alcohol, 70% oleyl alcohol sorbitan trioleate
Surfadil (Lilly)	lotion		diphenhydramine hydrochloride, 1%			benzyl alcohol, 2% carboxymethylcellulose sodium carmel iron oxide sodium lauryl sulfate sorbitol titanium dioxide
Topic (Syntex)	gel		camphor menthol	benzyl alcohol, 5%		isopropyl alcohol, 30% greaseless base

POISON IVY AND POISON OAK PRODUCT TABLE, continued

Product (Manufacturer)	Application Form	Anesthetic	Antipruritic/ Antihistamine	Antiseptic	Astringent	Other Ingredients
Tronothane Hydrochloride (Abbott)	cream	pramoxine hydrochloride, 1%				cetyl alcohol cetyl esters wax glycerin sodium lauryl sulfate parabens
Ziradryl (Parke-Davis)	lotion		diphenhydramine hydrochloride, 1% camphor, 0.1%		zinc oxide, 2%	alcohol, 2% chlorophylline sodium polysorbate glycerin methocel
Zotox (Commerce)	spray				zirconium hydrate, 8.36%	

Farid Sadik and Jeffrey C. Delafuente

INSECT STING AND BITE PRODUCTS

*Q*uestions to ask in patient/consumer counseling

Have you developed hives, excessive swelling, dizziness, vomiting, or difficulty in breathing since being bitten or stung?

———

Do you have a personal or family history of allergic reactions such as hay fever?

———

Have you previously had severe reactions to insect stings or bites?

———

What have you tried so far, if anything, to treat the reaction?

———

How extensive are the stings or bites on your body?

———

If a child, what is the patient's age and approximate weight?

———

Have you ever had adverse reactions to topically applied products?

———

Insect stings and bites are common occurrences, particularly during the summer. Their effects range from the trivial to the lethal: many people die and many more are treated for severe systemic reactions to insect stings. Medical literature is replete with articles on allergic reactions to insect stings and bites.

About 0.4–0.8% of the population is hypersensitive to insect stings, and the allergic reactions can be either systemic reactions or severe local reactions (1). Although accurate statistics are lacking, an estimated 30–50 Americans die annually from systemic reactions to insect stings, and 1–2 million patients are at risk because of severe hypersensitivity to insect stings (2). Estimates based on death certificates may be low because death caused by insect stings may be attributed to other causes, such as heart attacks, strokes, or unknown causes. For example, a 42-year-old man became unconscious 3 minutes after he was stung on the forehead, neck, and underarms by yellow jackets. Five minutes later he was dead. In spite of this, the county coroner reported the death as "natural—cause unknown" (3).

An insect sting or bite is an injury to the skin caused by penetration of the stinging or biting organ of an insect. The reactions are produced mainly by substances contained in the venom of stinging insects or in the saliva of biting insects. Although the pain associated with the skin penetration by stinging or biting is brief, the aftereffects vary according to the degree of exposure and hypersensitivity.

TYPES OF INJURIES

Stinging Insects

More people die each year from insect stings than from scorpion stings, venomous snake bites, and spider bites combined. Stinging insects belonging to the order Hymenoptera (membranous wings) are most frequently responsible for insect sting hypersensitivity. Among the three families commonly involved are the Apidae, including honeybees (genus *Apis*); the Vespidae, including paper wasps (genus *Polistes*), yellow jackets, and hornets (genus *Vespa*); and the Formicidae, including imported fire ants (genus *Solenopsis*) and harvester ants (genus *Pogonomyrmex*). Although they are small, these insects have a venom as potent as that of snakes. Death from an insect sting is the result of an anaphylactic reaction and usually occurs within 5–30 minutes, whereas death from a snake bite usually is not associated with hypersensitivity and occurs within 3 hours to several days.

The stinging insects inject the venom into their victims through a piercing organ (stinger), a modified ovipositor delicately attached to the rear of the female's abdomen. (Males do not have an ovipositor and consequently are stingless.) The stinger consists of two lancets, made of highly chitinous material, separated by the poison canal. The venom flows through the canal from the venom sac attached to the stinger's dorsal section. The tip of the stinger, which is directed posteriorly, has sharp barbs, and the base enlarges into a bulblike structure. Most species of bees and wasps have two types of venom glands under the last abdominal segment. The larger gland secretes an acidic toxin directly into the venom sac; the smaller one, at the base of the sac, secretes a less potent alkaline toxin. The injected venom is usually a mixture of the two toxins.

Honeybees

When the honeybee stings, it attaches firmly to the skin with tiny, sharp claws at the tip of each foot, then arches its abdomen, and immediately jabs the barbed stinger into the skin. The barbs firmly embed the stinger, and when the honeybee pulls away or is brushed off, the entire stinging apparatus (stinger, appendages, venom sac, and glands) is detached from the bee's abdomen. The disemboweled bee later dies. The abandoned stinger, driven deeper into the skin by rhythmic contractions of the venom sac's smooth muscle wall, continues to inject venom. Honeybees are most commonly found in the western and midwestern United States. Wild honeybees usually nest in hollow tree trunks.

Paper Wasps, Hornets, Yellow Jackets, and Bumblebees

The stinging mechanism of these insects resembles that of the honeybee, except that their stingers are not barbed. The stingers can be withdrawn easily after injecting the venom, enabling these insects to survive and sting repeatedly. Paper wasps, hornets, and yellow jackets are more commonly found in the southcentral and southwestern United States. Yellow jackets, considered the most common stinging culprits, usually nest in low places, such as burrows in the ground, cracks in walls, or small shrubs. Paper wasps tend to nest in high places, under eaves of houses, or on branches of high trees, whereas hornets prefer to nest in hollow spaces, especially hollow trees.

Ants

Some ants only bite; others bite and sting simultaneously. Stinging ants (fire ants) use their mandibles to cling to the skin of their prey, then bend their abdomen, sting the flesh, and empty the contents of their poison vesicle into the wound (4). Because they use their mandibles, it is often believed that the bite causes the reaction. Fire ants, commonly found in the southern and western United States, live in underground colonies.

Biting Insects/Arachnids

Insects such as mosquitoes, fleas, lice, and bedbugs, and arachnids such as ticks and chiggers ("red bugs") bite their prey. They insert their biting organs into the skin to feed by sucking blood from their hosts. (See *Plate 2–9.*)

Mosquitoes

Mosquitoes usually attack exposed parts of the body (face, neck, forearms, and legs). They can, however, bite through thin clothing. When a mosquito alights on the skin, it cuts through the skin with its mandibles and maxillae. A fine, hollow, needle-like, flexible structure (proboscis) is introduced into the cut and probes the tissue for a blood vessel. Blood is sucked directly from a capillary lumen or from previously lacerated capillaries with extravasated blood (5). During feeding, the mosquito injects into the wound a salivary secretion containing an anticoagulant and antigenic components, which cause the itching.

Fleas

Fleas are tiny (1.5–4 mm long), bloodsucking, wingless, laterally compressed parasites with strongly developed posterior legs used for leaping. Fleas parasitize a variety of avian and mammalian hosts. Most people are bitten about the legs and ankles. Bites usually are multiple and grouped and cause intense itching. Each lesion is characterized by an erythematous region around the puncture. Fleas not only are annoying but are responsible for transmitting diseases such as bubonic plague and endemic typhus. Fleas are found throughout the world (including arctic regions) but breed best in warm areas with relatively high humidity. They may survive and multiply without food for several weeks. Places that have been vacant for weeks may be heavily infested, partly because of the hatching of eggs, which are usually deposited in floor crevices or on rugs, particularly those on which pets have been sleeping.

Bedbugs

Bedbugs have a short head and a broad, flat body (4 to 5 mm long and 3 mm wide). Their mouth parts consist of two pairs of stylets used to pierce the skin. The outer part has barbs that saw the skin, and the inner part is used to suck blood and to allow salivary secretions to flow into the wound. Depending on the severity of the reaction and subsequent bullous papules, itching and an occasional small dermal hemorrhage are present at the puncture site. These insects usually hide and deposit their eggs in crevices of walls, floors, picture frames, bedding and other furniture. They normally hide during the day, become active at night, and bite their sleeping victims. Persons may also be bitten in subdued light by day while sitting in theaters or other public places. A bedbug can engorge itself with blood within 3–5 minutes, then seeks its hiding place.

Ticks

Ticks are arachnid parasites that feed on the blood of humans and domestic animals. During feeding, the tick's mouth parts are introduced into the skin, enabling it to hold firmly. If the tick is removed, the mouth parts are torn from the tick and remain embedded, causing intense itching and nodules. (See *Plate 2–10.*) If the tick is left attached to the skin, it becomes fully engorged with blood and remains as long as 10 days before it drops off.

Rocky Mountain spotted fever is transmitted to humans by several species of ticks. Deer ticks (*Ixodes dammini*) may transmit Lyme disease, an infectious condition caused by the spirochete *Borrelia burgdorferi*. Lyme disease is characterized by a "bull's-eye" surrounding the bite site, skin rash, fever, arthritis, fatigue, headache, cardiac arrhythmia, and neurologic damage (e.g., facial paralysis and numbness). The name of the disease was coined by Dr. Allen Steere, a rheumatologist who noticed an unusual number of arthritis cases in Lyme, Connecticut. The deer tick lives in wooded areas and parasitizes deer, mice, and other mammals, including humans. (See Figure 1 for the life cycle of the deer tick.) Other common ticks (e.g., dog ticks and lone star ticks) are suspected transmitters of Lyme disease.

Chiggers

Only the chigger larvae, which are nearly microscopic, attack the host by attaching to the skin and sucking blood. Once in contact with the skin, the larvae insert their mouth parts into the skin and secrete a digestive fluid that causes cellular disintegration of the affected area and intense itching. Chiggers do not burrow in the skin; however, as a result of the injected fluid, the skin hardens and a tube is formed. The chigger lies in this tube and continues to feed until engorged, after which it drops off and changes to the adult. Chiggers are prevalent in southern parts of the United States mainly during summer and fall. They usually live in wooded areas, grass, and brush.

Scabies

The mite causing scabies neither bites nor stings. Scabies, commonly called "the itch," is a contagious parasitic skin infestation caused by the arachnid mite *Sarcoptes scabiei*, which burrows beneath the stratum corneum. Characterized by secondary inflammation and intense itching, this infestation is often associated with poor hygiene, crowded conditions, and venereal disease. Scabies is transmitted through bodily contact with an infested host, clothing, or bed linen. An infected person may easily spread the disease to other members of the family. It is also possible to acquire scabies from a toilet seat. The immunology of scabies is interesting because it takes at least a month for the symptoms (primarily itching) to be noted in previously uninfected persons (6). The female mite, which is responsible for causing scabies, is transmitted readily by close personal contact with an infected person. Once on the skin, the impregnated female burrows into the stratum corneum with her jaws and the first two pairs of legs, forming tunnels in which she lays eggs and excretes fecal matter. In a few days, the hatched larvae form their own burrows and develop into adults. The adult mites copulate, and the impregnated females burrow into the stratum corneum to start a new life cycle. The most common infestation sites are the interdigital spaces of the fingers, the flexor surface of the wrists, the external male genitalia, the buttocks, and the ante-

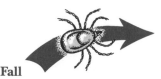

Fall

Nymphs molt and become adult ticks. Adults may feed on dogs, people, and other mammals such as deer.

Fall/Winter/Spring

Adult ticks feed on deer and other large mammals.

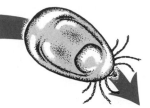

Spring/Summer

Nymphs emerge and feed on small mammals. While taking a blood meal, the tick may inject the Lyme disease bacteria into the small mammal. Later in spring, newly hatched larvae will feed on these animals and become infected with the Lyme disease bacteria. Nymphs are likely to attach to people from May through July, making this the period in which most people acquire infections.

Early spring

Female ticks drop off large mammals and lay eggs.

Late spring/Summer

Larvae hatch from eggs and attach to mice and other small mammals and birds. Larvae may ingest Lyme disease bacteria as they feed. Before larvae find their first host, they are unlikely to carry Lyme disease bacteria.

Late summer/Fall/Winter

Larvae molt and become nymphs. Nymphs overwinter without feeding.

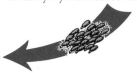

FIGURE 1   Life cycle of the deer tick (*Ixodes dammini*). Reprinted from "Lyme Disease in Wisconsin: An Update," Wisconsin Department of Natural Resources and Department of Health and Social Services, Madison, Wisc., 1989.

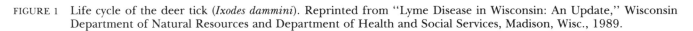

rior axillary folds. (See *Plate 2–11.*) The head and neck are not affected, except in infants.

Lice

Lice are wingless parasites with well-developed legs. Each leg has a claw that helps the louse cling firmly to hair or clothing fibers while sucking blood. Three types of lice attack humans: head lice (*Pediculus humanus capitis*), body lice (*Pediculus humanus humanus*), and pubic lice (*Phthirus pubis*). Head lice usually infest the head and are rarely found on other hairy parts of the body. The female deposits 10–150 eggs (nits), which become glued to the hair and hatch in 5–10 days. Body lice live, hide, and lay their eggs in clothing, particularly in seams and folds of underclothing, and generally infest crowded environments. Pubic lice, commonly called crab lice because of their crablike appearance, may be encountered even in patients with high standards of hygiene. They infest the pubic area, armpits, and occasionally eyelashes, mustaches, beards, and eyebrows.

Lice cause an immediate wheal around the bite in sensitive individuals. A local, delayed papular reaction appears within 24 hours. Itching and scratching result in excoriation or secondary pyogenic infections.

In some regions, head lice infestation has reached near epidemic proportions in classrooms (7). It can be diagnosed by observation with the naked eye. Although both the louse and the nit are visible, diagnosis is made most often by visualization of nits. Adult lice may occasionally be seen moving through the hair. (See *Plate 3–12A* and *B.*)

The nits are immobile, white to gray oval bodies about the size of a grain of salt attached to the hair shaft. The eggs are laid on the shaft close to the scalp. As the hair grows, the nit is moved away from the scalp. Because hair grows at a relatively constant rate, approximately a half-inch per month, the duration of infestation may be estimated by measuring the distance of the nit from the scalp surface.

Head lice infestation often causes itching. Scratching the irritation may result in excoriation of the scalp tissue. In some instances, pyoderma results, characterized by erythema, crusting, and oozing on the scalp and hair margins.

Head lice infestation is especially prevalent among schoolchildren, who are often in close contact with each other and who may share clothing or toilet articles. Lice also can be spread by contact with seats on buses and in theaters. Good personal hygiene and careful grooming unfortunately cannot prevent infestation, only stopping the organism can. Awareness and action by health officials, school authorities, and parents are essential in stopping the spread of lice; pharmacists can be effective in this regard.

Pharmacists can obtain information on safe treatments and preventive measures for head lice from the National Pediculosis Association, a nonprofit health education agency and resource center on head lice located at the following address: National Pediculosis Association, P.O. Box 149, Newton, MA 02161, (617) 449-NITS.

ALLERGIC REACTIONS TO STINGING INSECTS

In the past decade significant progress has been made in understanding the pathogenesis of allergic reactions to the Hymenoptera order of insects. Venoms from these insects have been purified and analyzed. Their mechanisms for causing severe reactions have been investigated, and they are now being used to diagnose and treat allergic reactions to insect stings. Because reactions to stinging insects can be more severe than those to biting insects, reactions to insect stings are discussed in more detail.

Reactions to insect stings range from small local reactions, limited to the sting site, to systemic reactions leading to death. Reactions may be divided into three categories: anaphylactic, local, and unusual.

Anaphylactic Reactions

These reactions are immunologically mediated, usually occurring within 15 minutes after the sting. Most allergic reactions from insect stings are cutaneous. Symptoms include erythema, pruritus, urticaria (hives), or angioedema. The most serious sequelae from stings are systemic anaphylactic reactions. In severe reactions, hypotension, laryngeal edema, bronchospasm, and respiratory distress may occur, leading to a shocklike state. If not treated promptly, death may ensue. Less common anaphylactic reactions may cause nausea, vomiting, or diarrhea. Mechanisms of anaphylaxis are discussed below.

Local Reactions

These reactions occur at the sting site. The manifestations are erythema and varying amounts of pain with symptoms lasting from several hours to several days. Swelling may extend from the sting site, covering an extensive area. Immune mechanisms have been implicated as the cause of the reaction in some patients. However, not all patients studied have evidence of immunologically mediated reactions (8).

Unusual Reactions

Occasionally, unusual reactions follow insect stings. Neurologic reactions, renal involvement, serum sickness reactions, encephalopathy, and delayed hypersensitivity skin reactions have been reported. The mechanisms for these reactions have not been clearly elucidated, but immunologic causes have been implicated in some cases (9, 10).

REACTIONS TO BITING INSECTS

Reactions to biting insects are usually local. The pathogenesis of these reactions has not been well characterized (9). Some species of mosquitoes have agglutinin and anticoagulant agents in their salivary secretions; others have neither (11).

Many attempts have been made to identify the antigenic factors in mosquito bites by studying whole mosquito extracts. Extracts from *Aedes aegypti* were shown by paper chromatography to contain at least four fractions that can produce skin reactions (12). Eluates of each constituent caused positive reactions in sensitized individuals (13). Eighteen amino acids have been identified in the extracts of all species of mosquitoes (14).

Reactions to mosquito bites vary in intensity. Wheal formation, erythema, papular reaction, and itching are characteristic. Hypersensitivity to mosquito bites aggravated by scratching causes papule and nodule formations that may persist and lead to secondary infections such as impetigo, furunculosis, or infectious eczematoid dermatitis. The bite site may influence reaction intensity; bites on the ankles and legs are more severe than elsewhere on the body because of the relative circulatory stasis in the legs. Consequently, the tendency toward vesiculation, hemorrhage, eczematization, and ulceration is greater in these areas (15). Systemic reactions such as fever and malaise also are common.

Intense itching caused by scabies, especially at night, occurs at the infestation site. The burrow (< 1 cm long) is visible to the naked eye and appears as a narrow, slightly raised dark line. Unrestrained scratching may cause secondary bacterial infections, such as impetigo, furuncles, or cellulitis, and excoriation. Scabies diagnosis may be made by identification of the mite under a microscope and by the burrows in the skin.

PATHOGENESIS OF ANAPHYLAXIS

Anaphylactic reactions are mediated by IgE antibodies that bind to the specific antigens (allergens) causing the reaction. The insect sting antigens are proteins and glycoproteins contained in insect venom. After an initial exposure to certain antigens, the body responds by making IgE antibodies against the antigens. These IgE antibodies bind to tissue mast cells and blood basophils. Mast cells are primarily located in lung tissue, bronchial smooth muscle, and vascular endothelium. Once these IgE antibodies are bound to the cells, the person is considered "sensitized."

When sensitized persons are exposed to antigens to which they are sensitive, under the appropriate circumstances, IgE on mast cells or basophils will bind the antigens. When this occurs, IgE receptors on the cells are bridged together and the cells release active substances from their granules (16). Active substances released or immediately generated by degranulation include histamine, serotonin, eosinophil chemotactic factor of anaphylaxis (ECF-A), leukotrienes, and bradykinin.

Histamine is a bioactive amine that increases capillary permeability, contracts bronchial and vascular smooth muscle, and increases nasal and bronchial mucous gland secretion. Serotonin increases vascular permeability in mice, but its role in human anaphylaxis is unknown. Leukotrienes contract smooth muscle. Unlike histamine, which is preformed in the cell granules, leukotrienes are formed after the IgE-antigen interaction occurs and are then released. Antihistamines are ineffective at reversing the effects of leukotrienes, but epinephrine will terminate muscle contractions induced by them. ECF-A is also released by mast cells and causes eosinophils to accumulate in the area of the allergic reaction. Eosinophils can release an enzyme, arylsulfatase B, which inactivates leukotrienes. Bradykinin contracts vascular and bronchial smooth muscle,

increases vascular permeability, increases mucous secretion, and stimulates pain fibers.

The severity and type of anaphylactic reaction depends on the location and number of cells degranulating their mediators. Degranulation in specific target organs produces local anaphylaxis. If the reaction is limited to the gastrointestinal tract, diarrhea may occur; if mast cell mediators are released in the nasal mucosa, rhinorrhea may occur; if the mediators are limited to the skin, hives may be the only prominent sign.

Systemic degranulation of mast cells and basophils leads to severe systemic symptoms and is responsible for shock and death occurring after an insect sting. Release of large amounts of mediators can cause a marked increase in capillary permeability, leading to leakage of intravascular fluids and hypotension. This shocklike state can be further compounded by mediator-induced laryngeal edema and bronchoconstriction, resulting in respiratory distress or failure.

Several theoretical factors may explain why a local reaction occurs in one instance and a systemic reaction in another (17). The dose of venom injected at each sting may vary, thereby varying the amount of antigen entering the body. The location of the sting may also influence the type of reaction. Head and neck stings may cause more laryngeal edema, while stings on extremities may produce only local reactions. A sting that limits the venom to the intradermal space may present as a local reaction; a sting on a capillary or venule would allow for systemic injection of the venom and may present as a systemic reaction.

COMPONENTS OF HYMENOPTERA VENOM

Hymenoptera venom contains a number of allergenic proteins, as well as several pharmacologically active molecules. The contents of venoms vary among different families within the Hymenoptera order. Therefore, venoms will be discussed in general terms.

The major antigenic proteins are the enzymes hyaluronidase and phospholipase A (18, 19). Hyaluronidase breaks down hyaluronic acid, which is a binding agent in connective tissue. By altering tissue structure, hyaluronidase acts as a spreading factor allowing for enhanced penetration of venom substances. Phospholipase A attacks phospholipids in cell membranes. In addition, phospholipase A contracts smooth muscle, causes hypotension, increases vascular permeability, and destroys mast cells.

Studies have shown that 50–100% of individuals with a history of local or systemic reactions to insect stings will have demonstrable IgE antibody to venom constituents (8, 17). The variability among studies in detecting IgE may be due to differences in laboratory techniques and lack of positive identification of the insect eliciting the reaction. Studies further show that the presence of venom-specific IgE in the sera of patients with local reactions correlates with the duration of the reaction (8).

Other venom components include histamine, melitin, apamin, and mast cell degranulating peptide (MCD-peptide) (20, 21). Of these substances, only melitin is antigenic, and not all individuals make antibodies against it (17). While these mediators do not directly contribute to insect sting anaphylaxis, they do affect the rate at which venom antigens become available to the systemic circulation following a sting. These molecules have direct and indirect effects on mast cell mediator release, vascular permeability, and smooth muscle contraction. Table 1 summarizes the pharmacologic actions of the venom constituents.

PREVENTIVE MEASURES

Individuals who are hypersensitive to insect stings should take precautions to avoid exposure to these insects. Foods and odors tend to attract insects; therefore, outdoor activities such as picnicking should be done cautiously. Keeping garbage contained and food covered will help keep insects away. Shoes should always be worn in grass and fields. In addition, perfumes and brightly colored clothes attract stinging insects and should not be worn while outdoors. A commonsense approach will lower the risk of stings and subsequent adverse reactions.

Venom Immunotherapy

Hymenoptera venom is used prophylactically to treat patients who have had reactions to stings. Venom immunotherapy, also known as desensitization, is done by subcutaneous injection of small amounts of venom at regularly scheduled intervals. The dose of the venom is gradually increased over many weeks until a predetermined maintenance dose is reached. The optimal doses, frequency of injections, and duration of maintenance therapy are still being investigated (22–24).

Immunotherapy causes a decrease in venom-specific serum IgE levels, with a rise in venom-specific serum IgG (blocking antibodies) levels. It is believed that production of blocking antibodies offers protection against anaphylactic reactions (18, 24), although unequivocal proof is lacking (23, 25). Blocking antibodies compete with IgE antibodies for binding of venom antigens, preventing the antigens from reacting with mast cell-bound IgE. Other factors may also be responsible for successful immunotherapy.

Lyophilized venom extracts are now available for diagnosis and treatment of hypersensitivity to insect stings. Greater than 95% of patients treated with these venoms in recommended doses and regimens are protected against serious reactions when stung again (23, 25, 26). The remaining 5% are partially protected (25, 26). Before the use of venom extracts, whole-body ex-

TABLE 1 Properties of Hymenoptera venom components

	Histamine	Melitin	Apamin	MCD-peptide	Hyaluronidase	Phospholipase A
Pain production	+	+	?	?	O	?
Increased capillary permeability	+	+	+	+	I	+
Smooth muscle contraction	+	+	O	O	O	+
Histamine release	O	+	O	+	O	+
Cellular damage	O	+	?	+	O	+
Antigenic	O	+	?	?	+	+

+, occurs; O, does not occur; ?, not demonstrated; I, indirectly.

tracts of insects were used for immunotherapy. Whole-body extracts have been shown to be no better than placebo treatment and should not be used (9, 24).

A kit of individual venoms of stinging insects is available to diagnose hypersensitivity by skin testing. The same individual venoms or fixed venoms from yellow jackets and white-faced hornets are used for immunotherapy. Mixed venoms are used because some individuals develop cross-sensitivity among vespids. These injections can be dangerous if improperly administered. Thus, the following warning is stated in the package insert (2):

> **WARNING** Hymenoptera venom preparations should be used only by physicians experienced in administering allergens to the maximum tolerated dose and/or after allergy consultation.

Because of the possibility of severe systemic reactions, the patients should be fully informed by the physician of the risks involved and should be under constant supervision. The venom preparations should be used only in settings where emergency resuscitative equipment and trained personnel are immediately available to treat such reactions. Treatment with Hymenoptera venom preparations should be restricted to patients who have previously experienced a potentially life-threatening systemic reaction following the sting of the honeybee, yellow jacket, hornet, or wasp. In addition, Hymenoptera venom preparations should be given only after venom hypersensitivity has been confirmed by venom skin testing. All patients receiving venom immunotherapy should have instruction on emergency self-injection of subcutaneous epinephrine. These patients should be advised to carry an emergency epinephrine kit during the Hymenoptera season, even while receiving venom immunotherapy. Before administering these venom preparations, physicians should be thoroughly familiar with the information concerning adverse reactions, treatment of overdosage, and precautions for use during pregnancy. After stopping venom immunotherapy, patients may again be at high risk for anaphylaxis following a sting.

Active Treatment

Because of the wide range of reactions to insect stings and bites, treatment usually depends on the symptoms. Nonprescription drugs are of no value in systemic reactions; such cases need prompt medical attention. For local reactions, a nonprescription product that minimizes scratching by relieving discomfort, itching, and pain may be recommended. Prophylactic prod-ucts, such as insect repellents, also are available.

Physician-directed medical treatment (acute or prophylactic) is important in many cases. Because hypersensitive reactions to insect stings and bites occur rapidly and may be severe, the sooner medical attention is given, the better the chances for recovery.

Systemic reactions caused by insect stings and bites are considered emergencies for which aqueous epinephrine (1:1,000; 0.3–0.5 ml) should be injected immediately, either subcutaneously or intramuscularly. Aqueous epinephrine (1:1,000; 0.1–0.3 ml) may also be injected directly into the sting site to delay absorption of the venom. Sublingual isoproterenol should not be administered simultaneously because it may induce serious arrhythmia. Parenteral antihistamines may be used for persistent urticaria, angioedema, or laryngeal edema in patients who do not respond to epinephrine. Pressor agents may be used if shock persists. Parenteral corticosteroids administered through the systemic route may be used for patients with protracted anaphylaxis and delayed reactions (27). Respiratory support should be available if needed; in severe cases, a tracheotomy may be necessary (28).

The pharmacist should advise hypersensitive individuals of the following:

- If symptomatic, the victim must seek medical attention immediately after an insect sting or bite.

- Basic first aid, such as applying ice to the sting and removing the stinger, is generally helpful.

- Emergency kits for insect stings are available by prescription. Kits containing epinephrine are preferable to those containing antihistamines for treating allergic reactions to stings.

- Receiving injections of venom extract for protection against systemic reactions (desensitization) is useful.

- Insect repellents are not effective against stinging insects.

First Aid

Basic first aid is helpful until medical help is available. Prompt application of ice packs to the sting site helps to slow absorption and reduce itching, swelling, and pain (29). Removal of the honeybee's stinger and venom sac, which usually are left in the skin, is another measure that should be offered or explained, particularly to allergic individuals. The stinger should be removed before all venom is injected; it takes approximately 2 to 3 minutes to empty all the contents from the honeybee's venom sac. The sac should not be squeezed; rubbing, scratching, or grasping it releases more venom

(28). Scraping the stinger with tweezers or a fingernail minimizes the venom flow. After the stinger is removed, an antiseptic should be applied.

Emergency Kits (Prescription Only)

Emergency kits for individuals hypersensitive to insect stings are available by prescription. In addition to tweezers for removing the honeybee stinger, the typical kit includes epinephrine hydrochloride and antihistamines. Also, kits containing autoinjectable epinephrine syringes are now available. Emergency kits for insect stings no longer require refrigeration but must be stored in the dark at room temperature. A kit should not be left in the glove compartment of a car. The pharmacist should carefully explain the directions for and the benefits of using an emergency kit for insect stings, emphasizing that epinephrine is the drug of choice for anaphylactic reactions.

Epinephrine Hydrochloride

Because of its potent and rapid action, epinephrine hydrochloride (1:1,000) injection is preferred to counteract the bronchoconstriction associated with anaphylaxis. It should be administered subcutaneously immediately after stinging. Some insect sting emergency kits have a preloaded (0.3 ml) sterile syringe. Generally, a 0.25-ml dose is injected subcutaneously and, after 15 minutes, another dose is injected if necessary. For individuals with cardiovascular disease, diabetes, hypertension, or hyperthyroidism, the injection should be administered with caution.

The Food and Drug Administration (FDA) encourages physicians to prescribe kits containing epinephrine injections for patients who are allergic to insect stings and for individuals responsible for those who may be exposed to insect stings, such as scout leaders, camp counselors, and paramedical personnel. These individuals should be trained to administer epinephrine injections. In some states, specially trained nonphysicians may legally administer epinephrine to individuals suspected of having an anaphylactic reaction to insect stings (localized or generalized urticaria, difficult breathing, wheezing, abdominal pain, weakness, confusion, lowered blood pressure, cyanosis, collapse, and unconsciousness). The FDA opposes the nonprescription sale of epinephrine kits because of possible misuse or deliberate abuse of the material in the kit (30).

Antihistamines

Although they are slow in onset of action and may be ineffective in severe reactions, antihistamines often are used in conjunction with epinephrine hydrochloride. They are administered orally or parenterally.

INGREDIENTS IN NONPRESCRIPTION PRODUCTS

Most nonprescription products used for symptomatic relief of insect stings and bites contain one or more pharmacologic agents, which fall into one of three main categories: external analgesics, skin protectants, and antibacterials.

External Analgesics/Antipruritics

This category is subdivided further into three groups: agents with analgesic activity derived from stimulation of cutaneous sensory receptors (counterirritants), from depression of cutaneous sensory receptors (anesthetics and antihistamines), and from reduction of inflammation (hydrocortisone). These agents are considered safe and effective when used as recommended for adults and children above 2 years of age. These agents are not recommended for children under 2 years of age except under the advice or supervision of a physician.

Insect Bite Neutralizers

Ammonium Hydroxide and Trimethanolamine

Ammonium hydroxide and trimethanolamine have been claimed to have a neutralizing effect on insect bites and stings. The FDA advisory review panel concluded that the submitted data do not fully establish the effectiveness of ammonium hydroxide as an insect bite neutralizer. Therefore, the panel recommends Category III classification for effectiveness of the compound either alone or in combination with other ingredients.

Counterirritants

Counterirritants reduce pain and itching by stimulating cutaneous sensory receptors to provide a feeling of warmth, coolness, or milder pain, which obscures the more severe pain of the injury. The activity of these agents is dependent on the concentration. In low concentrations, they may depress the cutaneous receptors and result in an anesthetic effect. (See Chapter 32, *External Analgesic Products.*)

Camphor At concentrations of 0.1–3%, camphor depresses cutaneous receptors, thereby relieving itching and irritation. At higher concentrations of 3–11%, camphor acts as a counterirritant because it stimulates cutaneous receptors. Camphor is safe and effective for use as an external analgesic at these concentrations when applied to the affected area no more than 3 or 4 times a day.

Camphor-containing products can be very dangerous if ingested. Patients should be warned to keep these (and all drugs) out of the reach of children and to contact a physician or poison control center immediately if ingestion is suspected.

Cresol Camphor complex (camphorated metacresol) is used to reduce pain. The FDA advisory review panel on over-the-counter (OTC) external analgesic drug products concluded that there are insufficient data available to permit final classification of the safety and effectiveness of this drug for use as a nonprescription external analgesic.

Menthol In concentrations of >1.25%, menthol acts as a counterirritant and excites cutaneous sensory receptors. However, in concentrations of <1%, it depresses cutaneous receptors and exerts an analgesic effect. Menthol is considered a safe and effective antipruritic when applied to the affected area in concentrations of 0.1–1%.

Methyl Salicylate Methyl salicylate stimulates cutaneous receptors when used in concentrations of 10–60%.

Peppermint and Clove Oils When applied externally, peppermint and clove oils act as mild counterirritants, causing a sensation of warmth.

Ichthammol Ichthammol has bacteriostatic and irritant properties. However, its effectiveness for insect stings is difficult to assess in concentrations used in nonprescription products.

Local Anesthetics

The FDA advisory review panel on OTC external analgesic drug products concluded that the local anesthetics used in insect sting and bite products, benzocaine and dibucaine, are safe and effective when used according to label directions. Dermatitis resulting from topically applied local anesthetics, including benzo-

caine, has been reported (31). Although adverse reactions from topical applications are often blamed on allergy to local anesthetics, allergy is an infrequent cause of reaction (32). The dermatitis that may occur is caused by frequent contact, and patients should be warned against continued applications for prolonged periods. (See Chapter 33, *Burn and Sunburn Products.*)

Phenol Phenol exerts topical anesthetic action by depressing cutaneous sensory receptors. It is caustic when applied in undiluted form to the skin. Phenol aqueous solutions of >2% are irritating and may cause sloughing and necrosis. Phenol is considered safe and effective as a nonprescription external analgesic when applied to the affected area no more than 3 or 4 times a day in concentrations of 0.5–1.5% for adults and children 2 years of age and older. Nonprescription products that contain phenol should include the following specific warning: "Do not apply this product to extensive areas of the body or under compresses or bandages" (33).

Benzocaine Benzocaine was found to be safe and effective for use by adults and children over 2 years of age when applied to the affected area no more than 3 or 4 times a day. The concentrations of benzocaine available in nonprescription products range from 5 to 20%.

Cyclomethycaine Sulfate The FDA advisory review panel on OTC external analgesic drug products concluded that cyclomethycaine sulfate is safe and effective but that there are insufficient data available to permit final classification of its effectiveness for use as a nonprescription external analgesic.

Dibucaine Dibucaine is another local anesthetic found in insect sting and bite products. Although in the same class as benzocaine, dibucaine products carry specific additional labeling:

WARNING Do not use in large quantities, particularly over raw surfaces or blistered areas.

This is because of the danger of systemic toxicity. Convulsions, myocardial depression, and death have been reported from systemic absorption (34). The recommended dosage for adults and children over 2 years of age is a 0.25–1% solution applied to the affected area no more than 3 or 4 times a day.

Antihistamines

Topical antihistamines are considered to be safe and effective external analgesics. These ingredients relieve pain and itching by depressing cutaneous sensory receptors. Although some absorption occurs through the skin, these ingredients are not absorbed in sufficient quantities to cause systemic side effects even when applied to damaged skin. However, antihistamines are capable of acting as haptenes, producing hypersensitivity reactions.

Continued use of these agents over 3 to 4 weeks increases the possibility of allergic contact dermatitis. In addition, their continued antipruritic action over a period of time is questionable. With this in mind, the FDA advisory review panel on OTC external analgesic drug products recommended that these agents be used for no longer than 7 days except under the advice of a physician. These agents are not recommended for children under 2 years of age.

Diphenhydramine Products containing diphenhydramine in concentrations of 1 to 2% may be applied 3 or 4 times a day.

Tripelennamine Tripelennamine in concentrations of 0.5–2% may be applied 3 or 4 times a day.

Both local anesthetics and antihistamines carry the following labeling as recommended by the FDA advisory review panel: "For the temporary relief of pain and itching due to minor burns, sunburn, minor cuts, abrasions, insect bites, and minor skin irritations."

Hydrocortisone

Hydrocortisone is an anti-inflammatory agent that is capable of preventing or suppressing the development or the regression of edema, capillary dilation, swelling, and tenderness accompanying inflammation. It relieves pain and itching by reducing inflammation. Preparations containing hydrocortisone in concentrations of 0.25–0.5% are considered relatively safe and effective for use as a nonprescription antipruritic. These preparations should be applied 3 or 4 times a day for adults and children 2 years of age and older. Patients should be warned against using topically applied hydrocortisone in the presence of scabies, tinea, bacterial infections, and moniliasis. Not only may the underlying condition be worsened, but hydrocortisone may also mask these disorders, making accurate diagnosis difficult (35).

Products containing hydrocortisone or its acetate salts carry specific labeling as follows: "For the temporary relief of minor skin irritations, itching, and rashes due to eczema, dermatitis, insect bites, poison ivy, poison oak, poison sumac, soaps, detergent, cosmetics, and jewelry, and for itchy genital and anal areas." (See Chapter 35, *Poison Ivy and Poison Oak Products.*)

Aspirin

The topical use of aspirin for insect stings has been reported to be effective in reducing the wheal reaction and its subsequent itching and irritation (36). The FDA advisory review panel on OTC external analgesic drug products concluded that aspirin is safe but there are insufficient data available to permit final classification of its effectiveness for use as a nonprescription external analgesic (37). Aspirin possesses no direct topical anesthetic activity; therefore, it exerts no anesthetic, analgesic, or antipruritic effect on the skin.

Skin Protectants

Zinc Oxide and Calamine

Zinc oxide and calamine are used in lotions, ointments, creams, and sprays for their cooling, slightly astringent, antiseptic, antibacterial, and protective actions. Calamine is a mixture of zinc and ferrous oxide. The ferrous oxide acts only as a coloring agent and is not an active ingredient. Zinc oxide and calamine tend to absorb fluids from weeping rashes. The FDA advisory review panel on OTC skin-protectant drug products concluded that zinc oxide and calamine are safe and effective in the nonprescription concentration range of 1–25% and for use as a nonprescription skin protectant (38). Topical dosage for adults, children, and infants is application of the preparation to the affected areas as needed.

Titanium Dioxide

Titanium dioxide has an action similar to that of zinc oxide. Its safety and effectiveness have not been established.

Aluminum Acetate

Aluminum acetate solutions in concentrations of 2.5–5% are used as an external astringent.

Hamamelis Water

Hamamelis water (witch hazel) possesses astringent properties and may act as a hemostatic for small superficial wounds.

Glycerin

The FDA advisory review panel on OTC skin-protectant drug products concluded that glycerin is safe and effective for nonprescription use as a skin protectant because of its absorbent, demulcent, and emollient properties. In addition, glycerin is widely used for its solvent properties.

Antibacterials

The most commonly used antibacterial agents in nonprescription products for insect stings and bites are benzalkonium chloride, benzethonium chloride, and methylbenzethonium chloride. These medications are included to prevent and treat secondary infection that may result from scratching. These quaternary ammonium compounds are classified as safe and effective for first-aid use. (See Chapter 28, *Topical Anti-infective Products*.)

Chloroxylenol

Chloroxylenol is a bacteriostatic agent that primarily acts against Gram-positive bacteria. Evaluation and safety of chloroxylenol in topical preparations could not be made by the FDA advisory review panel on OTC antimicrobial drug products because of insufficient data.

8-Hydroxyquinoline Sulfate

The 8-hydroxyquinoline sulfate chemical is included in topical preparations for its antibacterial effect.

Chlorothymol

Chlorothymol acts as an antibacterial and antifungal agent. However, it is irritating to mucous membranes.

Cresol

Cresol has a similar action to phenol. It is frequently used as a preservative.

Salicylic Acid

At concentrations ranging from 2 to 20%, salicylic acid acts as a keratolytic. In addition, it exerts a slight antiseptic action.

Scabies and Lice Treatment

Scabies and lice are controlled by using gamma benzene hexachloride; benzyl benzoate is mainly effective against scabies and other mites. Both products are available by prescription only. The patient should bathe, vigorously scrubbing the infested area. Then a 25% emulsion of benzyl benzoate or 0.5–1% cream of gamma benzene hexachloride is applied to the entire body except the face. (Benzyl benzoate may produce marked burning and stinging.) It should remain on the skin for 8–12 hours, after which the patient may bathe. A second application is recommended 1 week after the first one to destroy the hatched eggs. Additional applications should be avoided because contact dermatitis may occur. The concurrent use of a nit comb is recommended for removing nits from scalp hair. If itching, which may last for weeks, is not relieved immediately after treatment, a soothing lotion such as calamine lotion with menthol and camphor may be used.

Most nonprescription products are based on pyrethrums, which are natural pesticides derived from chrysanthemum plants. They are safe and effective as pesticides. According to product claims, pyrethrum-based products are pediculicidal for head, body, and pubic lice (and the nits) on contact. Pyrethrums are active by way of toxicity to the insects' nervous systems. Most pyrethrum-containing products also contain piperonyl butoxide, which blocks detoxification of the pyrethrums by the insect.

Pyrethrum-based products containing piperonyl butoxide have a lower order of toxicity when ingested by mammals. Some pyrethrum-based products are formulated in deodorized kerosene, which has more potential for toxicity when ingested than the active ingredients. These products are irritating to the eyes, and product information includes a warning against permitting contact with mucous membranes. In its tentative final monograph for pediculicide drug products, the FDA recognizes as safe and effective the combination of pyrethrins (0.17–0.33%) with piperonyl butoxide (2–4%) in a nonaerosol dosage formulation (39).

Patients who seek advice concerning treatment of *P. pubis* infestation of the eyelashes may be advised to apply petrolatum ophthalmic ointment thickly to the eyelashes twice daily for 8–10 days, with the remaining nits being mechanically removed (40).

Nonprescription products are more efficacious and safer than many home remedies such as kerosene. Nonprescription products are recommended for active treatment of patients with documented infestations rather than prophylaxis against lice. Duration of effectiveness of nonprescription treatment is related to environmental conditions connected with the possibility for reinfestation as well as physical contact with another infected human.

To prevent subsequent reinfection of lice, washing or dry cleaning all clothing is necessary. Families should conduct routine weekly checks during periods of peak infestation. Animals do not become infested by human head lice; therefore, household pets can be spared treatment.

Insect Repellents

Insect repellents do not kill insects but keep them away from treated areas. When applied to the skin, repellents discourage the approach of insects and, thus, protect the skin against insect bites. Most repellents are volatile, and when they are applied to skin or clothing, their vapor tends to prevent insects from alighting.

Oils of citronella, turpentine, pennyroyal, cedarwood, eucalyptus, and wintergreen were previously used in insect repellent formulations. However, after World War II, investigations showed that these agents were relatively ineffective. Although more than 15,000 compounds have been tested, only a few are effective and safe enough to use on the skin. An insect repellent should be relatively safe. It should have an inoffensive odor, protect for several hours, be effective against as wide a variety of insects as possible, withstand all weather conditions, and have an aesthetic feel and appearance.

The best all-purpose repellent is *N,N*-diethyl-*m*-toluamide (commonly called DEET). Use of products containing DEET is discouraged in children under 2 years of age because of possible toxicity to the central nervous system. Ethohexadiol dimethyl phthalate, dimethyl ethyl hexanediol carbate, and butopyronoxyl are effective repellents, but they are not as effective against as many kinds of insects as *N,N*-diethyl-*m*-toluamide. However, a mixture of two or more of these repellents is more effective against a greater variety of insects than a single repellent. Repellents may be toxic if they are taken internally. People who are sensitive to these chemicals may develop skin reactions such as itching, burning, and swelling. Repellents cause smarting when they are applied to broken skin or mucous membranes. They should be applied carefully around the eyes because they may cause a burning sensation.

The FDA's final rule on insect repellents for OTC oral human use indicates that these products are not generally recognized as safe and effective and that they are misbranded (41). Thiamine hydrochloride (vitamin B₁) has been marketed as an ingredient in nonprescription drug products for oral use as an insect repellent. Oral sulfur tablets have also been suggested. However, lack of adequate data fails to establish the effectiveness of these, or any other, ingredients for nonprescription oral use as a systemic insect repellent. Labeling claims for nonprescription orally administered insect repellents are either false, misleading, or unsupported by scientific data. For example, the following claims have been made for these products: "oral mosquito repellent," "mosquitoes avoid you," "bugs stay away," "keep mosquitoes away for 12 to 24 hours," and "the newest way to fight mosquitoes."

PRODUCT SELECTION GUIDELINES

Medication is often requested after symptoms appear; thus, it is important to determine the nature of symptoms following the sting or bite, how soon the symptoms appeared, the severity of the symptoms, and what other drugs are being used concurrently.

Nonprescription products are of minimal value to hypersensitive individuals. The pharmacist should record all information on hypersensitive individuals and should recommend that the person wear a tag or carry a card showing the nature of the allergy. If the symptoms, such as localized irritation, itching, or swelling, are minor, an appropriate nonprescription product may be recommended. Topical lotions, creams, ointments, and sprays are the main nonprescription products used for symptomatic relief of local reactions to insect stings and bites. The main considerations in product selection are reducing the possibility of additional stings or bites, providing proper protection to the affected skin, preventing secondary infection in the affected area, and relieving itching and irritation. The pharmacist may suggest a number of measures that will relieve itching and irritation:

- Avoid rough and irritating clothing, especially wool, over the affected area.

- Avoid strong soaps, highly perfumed soaps, or harsh detergents.

- After bathing, apply an occlusive skin protectant to the affected area.

- Bathe in cool water (never warm water) for 10–20 minutes.

- Avoid scratching the affected area. Also, keep fingernails trimmed short and filed smooth to minimize possible skin damage of the affected area if scratching occurs.

In spite of being capable of producing topical or systemic adverse reactions, external analgesics and antipruritics are considered to be relatively safe and effective. These nonprescription products are for adults and children 2 years of age and older and should be applied no more than 3 or 4 times a day. For children under 2 years of age, there is no recommended dosage except under the advice and supervision of a physician.

The labels on external analgesic nonprescription products should indicate the ingredients and their concentrations, the manner of usage and frequency of applications, and the indications for use. The FDA advisory review panel on OTC external analgesic drug products recommended that the labels should include the following warnings:

- For external use only.

- Avoid contact with eyes.

- If condition worsens, or if symptoms persist for more than 7 days, discontinue use of this product and consult a physician.

- Do not use for children under 2 years of age except under the advice and supervision of a physician.

SUMMARY

Stings of honeybees, bumblebees, yellow jackets, hornets, wasps, and ants may cause pain, discomfort, illness, and severe local and systemic reactions. In normal individuals, insect stings and bites cause local irritation, inflammation, swelling, and itching that provoke rubbing and scratching. In hypersensitive individuals, anaphylactic reactions may pose serious emergency problems. Papules or nodules from bites or stings may form and persist for months. Potential secondary infections may lead to impetigo, furunculosis, or eczematoid dermatitis. Topical nonprescription products that contain hydrocortisone, calamine, benzocaine, antihistamines, benzalkonium chloride, benzethonium chloride, camphor, and menthol may relieve or prevent these symptoms.

People sensitized to insect venom may react violently when they are stung. They need immediate, active treatment, such as the administration of epinephrine hydrochloride. Partial desensitization may be accomplished by insect venom immunotherapy. The pharmacist can play a significant role by advising hypersensitive individuals on emergency procedures for insect stings and bites.

REFERENCES

1   "Cecil Textbook of Medicine," 16th ed., J. B. Wyngaarden and L. H. Smith, Eds., W. B. Saunders, Philadelphia, Pa., 1982, p. 2239.

2   *FDA Drug Bull., 9* (3), 15 (1979).

3   H. G. Rapaport, *Drug Ther., 23* (1975).

4   N. A. Weber, *Am. J. Trop. Med., 17,* 765 (1937).

5   R. M. Gordan and W. Crewe, *Ann. Trop. Med. Parasitol., 42,* 334 (1948).

6   Y. Felman and J. A. Nikites, *Cutis, 25,* 32 (1980).

7   L. C. Parish and J. A. Witkowski, *Drug Ther., 10,* 145 (1980).

8   A. W. Green et al., *J. Allergy Clin. Immunol., 66,* 186 (1980).

9   R. E. Reisman, in "Allergy and Clinical Immunology," R. F. Lockey, Ed., Medical Examination, Garden City, N.J., 1979.

10   W. C. Light et al., *J. Allergy Clin. Immunol., 59,* 391 (1977).

11   W. R. Horsfall, "Medical Entomology," Ronald Press, New York, N.Y., 1962, p. 182.

12   J. A. McKiel and J. C. Clunie, *Can. J. Zool., 38,* 479 (1960).

13   A. Hudson et al., *Mosq. News, 18,* 249 (1958).

14   D. W. Micks and J. P. Ellis, *Proc. Soc. Exp. Biol. Med., 78,* 69 (1951).

15   H. V. Allington and R. R. Allington, *J. Am. Med. Assoc., 155,* 240 (1954).

16   T. Ishizaka, *J. Allergy Clin. Immunol., 67,* 90 (1981).

17   D. R. Hoffman, *Ann. Allergy, 41,* 278 (1978).

18   A. K. Sobotka et al., *J. Allergy Clin. Immunol., 57,* 29 (1976).

19   B. R. Paull et al., *J. Allergy Clin. Immunol., 59,* 334 (1977).

20   D. R. Hoffman et al., *J. Allergy Clin. Immunol., 59,* 147 (1977).

21   E. Habermann, *Science, 177,* 314 (1972).

22   D. B. K. Golden et al., *J. Allergy Clin. Immunol., 67,* 370 (1981).

23   D. B. K. Golden et al., *J. Allergy Clin. Immunol., 67,* 482 (1981).

24   R. E. Reisman, *J. Allergy Clin. Immunol., 64,* 3 (1979).

25   D. B. K. Golden et al., *Ann. Intern. Med., 92,* 620 (1980).

26   L. M. Lichtenstein et al., *J. Allergy Clin. Immunol., 64,* 5 (1979).

27   J. Parrino and R. Lockey, in "Current Therapy," W. B. Saunders, Philadelphia, Pa., 1980, p. 602.

28   M. D. Ellis, "Dangerous Plants, Snakes, Anthropods and Marine Life of Texas," U.S. Department of Health, Education, and Welfare, Washington, D.C., 1975, p. 175.

29   R. E. Arnold, "What to Do About Bites and Stings of Venomous Animals," Collier Books, New York, N.Y., 1973, p. 9.

30   *FDA Drug Bull., 10* (2), 12 (1980).

31   *Federal Register, 44,* 69833 (1979).

32   H. Wilson, *Practitioner, 197,* 673 (1966).

33   J. Adriani, *J. Am. Med. Assoc., 196,* 119 (1966).

34   *Federal Register, 44,* 69807 (1979).

35   A. Kligman and K. Kaidberg, *Cutis, 2,* 232 (1978).

36   R. J. von Witt, *Lancet, 2,* 1379 (1980).

37   *Federal Register, 44,* 69845 (1979).

38   *Federal Register, 43,* 34641 (1978).

39   *Federal Register, 54,* 13487 (1989).

40   M. Nienhuis and B. Rowles, *U.S. Pharmacist, 9,* 41 (1980).

41   *Federal Register, 50,* 25170 (1985).

INSECT STING AND BITE PRODUCT TABLE

Product (Manufacturer)	Application Form	Ingredients
After-Bite (Tender Corp)	topical applicator	ammonium hydroxide, 3.6%
Americaine (Fisons)	aerosol ointment	aerosol: benzocaine, 20%; butane; isobutane; PEG-200; propane ointment: benzocaine, 20%; benzethonium chloride; PEG-300; PEG-3350
Bactine Antiseptic/Anesthetic First Aid Spray (Miles)	spray liquid spray aerosol	liquid: benzalkonium chloride, 0.13%; EDTA; octoxynol 9; propylene glycol; alcohol, 3.17%; lidocaine, 2.5% aerosol: benzalkonium chloride, 0.13%; dimethyl polysiloxane fluid 1000; edetic acid; isobutane; malic acid; povidone; propylene glycol; sorbitol; lidocaine, 2.5%
BiCozene (Sandoz)	cream	benzocaine, 6%; resorcinol, 1.67%; castor oil; chlorothymol; ethanolamine stearates; glycerin; glyceryl borate; glyceryl stearates; parachlorometaxylenol; polysorbate 80; sodium stearate; triglycerol di-isostearate; perfume
Chiggerex (Scherer)	ointment	benzocaine, 2%; camphor, 0.008%; olive oil, 0.008%; menthol, 0.005%; peppermint oil, 0.005%; methylparaben, 0.002%; clove oil, 0.002%
Chiggertox Liquid (Scherer)	liquid	isopropyl alcohol, 53%; benzyl benzoate, 21.4%; soft soap, 21.4%; benzocaine, 2.1%
Dermoplast (Whitehall)	spray lotion	spray: benzocaine, 20%; menthol, 0.5%; acetylated lanolin alcohol; aloe vera oil; butane; cetyl acetate; hydrofluorocarbon; methylparaben; PEG-8 laurate; polysorbate 85 lotion: benzocaine, 8%; menthol, 0.5%; aloe vera gel; carbomer 934P; ceteth-16; glycerin; glyceryl stearate; laneth-16; oleth-16; parabens; simethicone, steareth-16; triethanolamine
Di-Delamine Double Antihistamine (Commerce)	gel spray	tripelennamine hydrochloride, 0.5%; diphenhydramine hydrochloride, 1%; menthol, 0.1%; benzalkonium chloride, 0.12% (spray)
Medicone Derma (Medicare)	ointment	benzocaine, 2%; 8-hydroxyquinoline sulfate, 1.05%; zinc oxide, 13.73%; ichthammol, 1%; menthol, 0.48%; lavender perfume, 0.08%; petrolatum-lanolin base 79.87%
Mediconet (Medicone)	saturated medical pads	hamamelis water, 50%; glycerin, 10%; ethoxylated lanolin, 0.5%; methylparaben, 0.15%; benzalkonium chloride, 0.02%; alkylaryl polyether; perfume
Nupercainal (Ciba)	cream ointment	cream: dibucaine, 0.5%; acetone sodium bisulfite; water-washable base; glycerin; potassium hydroxide; stearic acid; fragrance; trolamine ointment: dibucaine, 1%; acetone sodium bisulfite; lanolin; light mineral oil; white petrolatum
Obtundia First Aid Cream (Otis Clapp)	cream	cresol-camphor complex
Obtundia Surgical Dressing (Otis Clapp)	liquid spray	cresol-camphor complex
Rhuli Gel (Rydelle)	gel	benzyl alcohol, 2%; menthol, 0.3%; camphor, 0.3%; SD alcohol 23A, 31%; propylene glycol; carbomer 940; triethanolamine; benzophenone-4; EDTA
Rhuli Spray (Rydelle)	spray	calamine, 13.8%; benzocaine, 5%; camphor, 0.7%; benzyl alcohol; hydrated silica; isobutane; isopropyl alcohol, 70% (concentrate); oleyl alcohol; sorbitan trioleate
Rhuli Cream (Rydelle)	cream	benzocaine, 5%; calamine, 3%; camphor 0.3%; glycerin; distearyldimonium chloride; petrolatum; isopropyl palmitate; cetyl alcohol; dimethicone; sodium chloride

INSECT STING AND BITE PRODUCT TABLE, continued

Product (Manufacturer)	Application Form	Ingredients
Skeeter Stik (Triton)	stick	lidocaine, 4%; phenol, 2%; isopropyl alcohol, 45.5%; propylene glycol base
Solarcaine (Schering-Plough)	aerosol cream lotion	aerosol: benzocaine, 20%; triclosan, 0.13%; isopropyl alcohol, 35% cream: benzocaine; triclosan. Medicated cream contains lidocaine lotion: benzocaine; triclosan
Sting-Eze (Wisconsin Pharm)	concentrate	diphenhydramine hydrochloride; camphor; phenol; benzocaine; eucalyptol
Sting Kill (Kiwi Brands)	swabs	benzocaine, 18.9%; menthol, 0.9%
Sting Relief (Pfeiffer)	concentrate lotion	benzocaine, 10%; camphor; chloroxylenol; eucalyptus oil; propylene glycol base
Surfadil (Lilly)	lotion	diphenhydramine hydrochloride, 1%; benzyl alcohol, 2%; carboxymethylcellulose sodium; carmel; iron oxide; sodium lauryl sulfate; sorbitol

PEDICULOCIDE PRODUCT TABLE

Product (Manufacturer)	Application Form	Active Ingredients	Other Ingredients
A-200 Pyrinate (SmithKline Beecham)	gel shampoo	pyrethrins, 0.33% piperonyl butoxide, 4%	benzyl alcohol butyl stearate mineral spirits octoxynol 9 oleic acid oleoresin parsley seed petroleum distillate carbomer 940 (gel) triisopropanolamine (gel)
Barc (Commerce)	gel liquid	pyrethrins, 0.18% piperonyl butoxide, 2.2%	petroleum distillate, 4.8% (gel), 5.52% (liquid)
Lice-Enz (Copley Pharmaceuticals)	foam	pyrethrins, 0.3% piperonyl butoxide, 3%	
Licetrol (Republic)	liquid	pyrethrins, 0.2% piperonyl butoxide, 2%	petroleum distillate, 0.8%
Nix (Burroughs Wellcome)	liquid	permethrin, 1%	
Pronto (Commerce)	shampoo	pyrethrins, 0.33% piperonyl butoxide, 4%	
R & C (Reed & Carnrick)	shampoo	pyrethrins, 0.3% piperonyl butoxide, 3%	petroleum distillate, 1.2%
RID (Leeming)	shampoo	pyrethrins, 0.3% piperonyl butoxide, 3%	petroleum distillate, 1.2% benzyl alcohol, 2.4%
Tisit (Pfeiffer)	liquid	pyrethrins, 0.3% piperonyl butoxide, 2%	
Tisit (Pfeiffer)	shampoo	pyrethrins, 0.3% piperonyl butoxide, 3%	benzyl alcohol, 2.4% petroleum distillate, 1.2%
Tisit Blue (Pfeiffer)	gel	pyrethrins, 0.3% piperonyl butoxide, 3%	petroleum distillate, 1.2%
Triple X (Carter)	shampoo	pyrethrins, 0.3% piperonyl butoxide, 3%	petroleum distillate, 1.2% benzyl alcohol, 2.4%

INSECT REPELLENT PRODUCT TABLE

Product (Manufacturer)	Application Form	Other Ingredients
Insect Repellent (Revco)	aerosol	N-N-diethyl-m-toluamide, 14.25%; other isomers, 0.75%; inert ingredients, 85%
Insect Repellent, Evergreen and Original Formula (Cutter)	aerosol	N-N-diethyl-m-toluamide, 20.9%; other isomers, 1.1%; N-octyl bicycloheptene dicarboximide, 3%; inert ingredients, 74%
Muskol Maximum Strength (Schering-Plough)	spray pump	N-N-diethyl-m-toluamide, 100%
Muskol Ultra (Schering-Plough)	aerosol	N-N-diethyl-m-toluamide, 38%; other isomers, 2%; inert ingredients, 60%
Off (Johnson Wax)	aerosol	N-N-diethyl-m-toluamide, 14.25%; other isomers, 0.75%; inert ingredients, 85%
Off (Johnson Wax)	spray pump	N-N-diethyl-m-toluamide, 19% other isomers, 1%; N-octyl bicycloheptene dicarboximide, 4%; inert ingredients, 75%
Off (Johnson Wax)	spray pump	N-N-diethyl-m-toluamide, 14.25%; other isomers, 0.75%; inert ingredients, 85%
Off Deep Woods Formula (Johnson Wax)	aerosol	N-N-diethyl-m-toluamide, 19%; other isomers, 1%; N-octyl bicycloheptene dicarboximide, 4%; 1%; inert ingredients, 75%
Off Maximum Protection, Deep Woods Formula (Johnson Wax)	spray pump	N-N-diethyl-m-toluamide, 100%
Repel Scented (Wisconsin Pharm.)	aerosol	N-N-diethyl-m-toluamide, 32.25%; other isomers, 1.75%; inert ingredients, 66%
Repel Sportsman Formula (Wisconsin Pharm.)	aerosol	N-N-diethyl-m-toluamide, 38%; other isomers, 2%; inert ingredients, 60%
6-12 Plus (D-Con)	aerosol	2-ethyl-1, 3-hexanediol, 25%; N-N-diethyl-m-toluamide, 4.75%; other isomers, 0.25%; inert ingredients, 70%
Tick Garde (Eclipse)	spray	N-N-diethyl-m-toluamide, 38.35%; other isomers, 25%; N-octyl bicycloheptene dicarboximide, 1.34%; di-N-propyl isocinchomeronate, 1.92%; inert ingredients, 61.65%

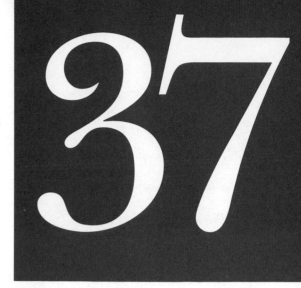

Nicholas G. Popovich

FOOT CARE PRODUCTS

Questions to ask in patient/consumer counseling

General Foot Conditions

Where is the lesion located (on or between the toes or on the sole of the foot)? Is the toenail involved?

Is there any redness, itching, blistering, oozing, scaling, or bleeding from the lesion?

Is a physician treating you for any other medical condition, such as diabetes, heart trouble, or problems with your circulation?

Do you take insulin? What other medications do you take?

Is the condition painful? Is it too uncomfortable to walk?

During which activities is the pain noticed?

Did you see your physician about this problem? If so, what did he or she tell you to do? What have you done? Did it help?

Have you ever had vascular surgery or been treated for circulation problems?

How long have you had the problem?

Have you tried to treat this problem yourself? If so, how?

Did the problem begin with the use of new shoes (sandals or enclosed shoes, jogging or tennis shoes, flat or high heels), socks, or soaps?

Do you have allergies, asthma, or skin problems?

Is there any history of injury to the foot?

Do your feet sweat excessively?

(When appropriate) How often and in what manner do you trim your toenails?

What is your occupation?

Do you participate in a daily exercise program such as jogging or aerobics?

Foot Conditions Related to Running/Jogging

Is the discomfort getting progressively worse?

Has the discomfort plateaued at a level that continues to affect your performance?

Is the discomfort more frequent while running or is it present while not running?

Is the discomfort preventing you from running?

Have attempts at self-treatment (e.g., new shoes, change of running surface or training intensity) failed to relieve the symptoms?

Is the discomfort causing you to compensate and develop additional injuries?

Has the depression, denial, or guilt that you are experiencing been identified to you by your friends?

Orthotic Devices

Is there a symptom that requires treatment?

———

Did the symptom occur gradually?

———

Do you have a history of a fracture, dislocation, or surgery in the legs or feet?

———

Did you wear corrective shoes or braces on the legs or feet as a child?

———

Have you significantly increased repetitive weight-bearing activity? Do you plan to continue this activity?

———

Have attempts at self-treatment with nonprescription inserts failed?

———

A 1988 Gallup survey of family/general practitioners, dermatologists, and podiatrists identified the foot problems most often encountered and how patients deal with them (1). The five most common foot complaints from patients were sore, aching feet, ingrown toenails, corns, warts or plantar warts, and calluses. The survey identified harmful foot practices that patients engaged in, such as scraping or cutting corns and calluses, improper trimming of toenails, opening blisters or removing the skin cover, and inappropriate use of hot water. The survey also identified potentially harmful home remedies for foot problems, including the application of caulk plaster, WD 40 motor oil, Crisco or butter, Clorox or other bleach products, and gasoline or kerosene.

Obviously there is a significant need to educate patients about their feet, including self-care measures; the pharmacist can serve a valuable purpose in doing so. Proper instruction in foot care should begin at an early age when good health habits can be nurtured. The simplest rule is routine daily inspection of the feet to note any signs of early foot problems. Obese or arthritic patients should use a hand-held mirror to inspect the feet.

At birth, a baby's foot has 35 joints, 19 muscles, more than 100 ligaments, and cartilage that will develop into 26 bones. These small components continue to develop and mature until the age of 14–16 for females and 15–21 for males. Men will begin to notice changes in their feet in their 40s, while women will notice changes in their feet in their 30s. The feet tend to broaden and flatten after years of bearing the body's weight, which stretches ligaments and causes bones to shift positions. These changes subject the feet to greater stress, which increases the potential for painful foot conditions. The feet are subject to added stress from prolonged standing. An estimated 40% of the U.S. population spend about 75% of their workday standing.

In the past two decades, society's attitude toward physical fitness and body awareness has changed dramatically. Millions of people exercise every day; most frequently, jogging or running is the method used to remain or to get "in shape." Unfortunately, however, if people do not take adequate precautions, problems can arise, particularly involving the feet. Appropriate footwear, running environment, and running surface are just a few factors that should be addressed by joggers and runners to prevent foot problems.

Although foot conditions are generally not life threatening, except perhaps in diabetics or severely arthritic patients and those with impaired circulation, they may cause a measure of discomfort and impaired mobility—from a limitation of activity to a serious disease condition (2). Corns, calluses, and ingrown toenails are common and may contribute to impairment.

Pain usually is associated with corns and warts. The pain from corns may be severe and sharp (when downward pressure is applied) or dull and discomforting. Calluses usually are asymptomatic, causing pain only when pressure is applied (3). Individuals who suffer from calluses on the sole of the foot frequently compare their discomfort to that of walking with a pebble in the shoe. Another important sign of foot problems is hardening of the skin, which may signal a biomechanical problem and cause abnormal weight distribution in a particular area of the foot. This hardening, which can be identified physically by the physician and the patient, is an objective sign, as opposed to pain, which is subjective. A podiatric examination is warranted to determine whether an imbalance is present.

Human mycotic (fungal) infections that have cutaneous manifestation may be subdivided into five categories based on site of invasion (Table 1) (4). The superficial and cutaneous types usually warrant the pharmacist's advice. (See Chapter 28, *Topical Anti-infective Products*.)

The primary lesions of athlete's foot often consist of macerated tissues, slight scaling, occasional vesiculation, and fissuring between and under the toes (5). Any or all of the interdigital webs of the foot may be affected, although usually the skin beneath the fourth and fifth toes of each foot is involved. A relapse of the disease is inevitable if there is nail involvement (unless treated with griseofulvin or ketoconazole), or if the infection is present on the soles of the feet and treatment has not been adequate (6, 7).

TABLE 1 Classification of mycotic infections that possess cutaneous manifestation according to site of invasion

Mycotic infection type	Site(s) of invasion	Example
Superficial	Outermost layer of skin and appendages	Tinea versicolor (caused by *Malassezia furfur*)
Cutaneous	Skin lesion and/or nail	Tinea pedis (caused by *Trichophyton rubrum*)
Subcutaneous	Cutaneous and subcutaneous tissue	Sporotrichosis (caused by *Sporotrichum schenkii*)
Intermediate	Skin, mucous membranes, internal viscera	Vaginal candidiasis (caused by *Candida albicans*)
Deep systemic	Viscera, bone, nerve, skin	Blastomycosis (caused by *Blastomyces dermatitidis*)

Reprinted with permission from J. Raskin, in "Current Therapy," H. F. Conn, Ed., W. B. Saunders, Philadelphia, Pa., 1976, pp. 611–614.

CORNS AND CALLUSES

Pressure from tight-fitting shoes is the most frequent cause of pain from corns. Narrow-toed or high-heeled shoes crowd toes into the narrow toe box. The most lateral toe, the fifth, experiences the most pressure and friction and is the usual site of a corn. Friction (caused by loose-fitting shoes), walking barefoot, and structural biomechanical problems contribute to the development of calluses. Structural problems include improper weight distribution, pressure, and the development of bunions with age (8). Tight-fitting hosiery and nonlubricated friction in hosiery may cause blisters, calluses, and corns.

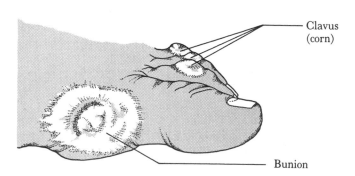

FIGURE 1 Conditions affecting the top of the foot.

Symptoms

Corns and calluses are similar in one respect: each has a marked hyperkeratosis of the stratum corneum. (See Chapter 28, *Topical Anti-infective Products*.) Besides this feature, however, there are marked differences.

A corn (clavus) is a small, sharply demarcated, hyperkeratotic lesion having a central core (Figure 1) (9). It is raised, has a yellowish gray color, and ranges from a few millimeters to 1 cm or more in diameter. The base of the corn is on the skin surface. The apex of the corn points inward and presses on the nerve endings in the dermis, causing pain.

Corns may be either hard or soft. Hard corns occur on the surfaces of the toes and are shiny and polished. Soft corns are whitish thickenings of the skin usually found on the webs between the fourth and fifth toes. Accumulated perspiration macerates the epidermis and gives the corn a soft appearance; soft corns are often mistaken for fungal infections. This situation occurs because the fifth metatarsal is much shorter than the fourth, and the web between these toes is deeper and extends more proximally than the webs between other toes.

Hard corns (usually) and soft corns (less frequently) are caused by underlying bony prominences. A bony spur, or exostosis (a bony tumor in the form of an ossified muscular attachment to the bone surface), nearly always exists between long-lasting hard and soft corns. A lesion located over non-weight-bearing bony prominences or joints, such as metatarsal heads, the bulb of the great toe, the dorsum of the fifth toe, or the tips of the middle toes, is usually a corn (10).

A callus may be broad based or have a central core with sharply circumscribed margins and has more diffuse thickening of the skin (Figure 1) (8, 9). It has indefinite borders and ranges from a few millimeters to several centimeters in diameter. It is usually raised, yellow, and has a normal pattern of skin ridges on its surface. Calluses form on joints and weight-bearing areas, such as the palms of the hands and the sides and soles of the feet. (See *Plate 8–33*.)

During corn or callus development, the cells in the basal cell layer undergo accelerated mitotic division, leading to the migration of maturing cells through the prickle cell (stratum spinosum) and the granular (stratum granulosum) skin layer. The rate is normally equal to the continual surface cellular desquamation. Normal mitotic activity and subsequent desquamation lead to complete replacement of the epidermis in about 1 month (11). In the case of a callus, friction and pressure cause faster mitotic activity of the basal cell layer (11). This activity produces a thicker stratum corneum as more cells reach the outer skin surface. When the friction or pressure is relieved, mitotic activity returns to normal, causing remission and disappearance of the callus.

Treatment

Successful treatment of corns and calluses with nonprescription products depends on eliminating the causes: pressure and friction. This process entails the use of well-fitting, nonbinding footwear that evenly distributes body weight. For anatomical foot deformities, orthopedic corrections must be made. These measures relieve pressure and friction to allow the resumption of normal mitosis of the basal cell layer, the normalization of the stratum corneum after total desquamation of the hyperkeratotic tissue, and the action of efficacious topical products. Before instituting a self-treatment program, it may be wise to secure a medical opinion; this should definitely be done if circulatory problems are present.

In the tentative final monograph for corn and callus remover drug products, the Food and Drug Administration (FDA) adopted the advisory review panel's recommendations that only salicylic acid be categorized as safe and effective for the removal of corns and calluses (12). Further, the FDA indicated that salicylic acid could be used for hard and soft corns. Although a foot-soaking regimen enhances the salicylic acid treatment, the FDA did not believe it necessary to soak the foot before treatment with the product.

Experiments have been made to treat corns by injecting fluid silicone subdermally (13). The injected silicone, at times, seems to augment digital and plantar tissues, using a cushioning effect, reducing pain, and decreasing the need for regular palliative treatment.

BUNIONS

Bunions are swellings of the bursae and/or exostoses, and can be caused by various conditions. Pressure from a tight-fitting shoe over a period of time generally aggravates the condition, but pressure may result from the manner in which a person sits, walks, or stands. Friction on the toes from bone malformations (wide heads or lateral bending) also is a major factor in bunion production.

Symptoms

The hallux, or great toe, along with the inner side of the foot, provides the elasticity and mobility needed to walk or run. Thus, the hallux is a dynamic organ (14). However, this mobility causes several anatomical disorders associated with the foot, such as hallux valgus, the deviation of the great toe toward the lateral (outer) side of the foot (15). Prolonged pressure caused by hallux valgus may result in pressure over the angulation of the metatarsophalangeal joint of the great toe, causing inflammatory swelling of the bursa over the metatarsophalangeal joint (Figure 2A and B). This may result in bunion formation (Figure 1) (16).

Treatment

Corrective steps to alleviate bunions often depend on the degree of discomfort. Bunions are usually asymptomatic but may become quite painful, swollen, and tender. The bunion itself usually is covered by an extensive keratinous overgrowth. Topical nonprescription drugs provide some relief; however, surgery may be indicated.

Bunions are not amenable to topical drug therapy. The patient should correct the etiologic condition by wearing properly fitting shoes or seek the advice of a podiatrist or orthopedist. If the condition is not severe, shielding the bunion with protective pads (moleskin) may be all that is necessary. However, if the manifestation is severe or particularly unsightly, surgical correction is usually indicated.

Larger footwear may be necessary to compensate for the space taken up by the pad; not increasing shoe size may cause pressure in other areas. Also, protective pads should not be used on bunions when the skin is broken or blistered. Abraded skin should receive palliative treatment before pads are applied. If these conditions persist, particularly in diabetic patients, the pharmacist should recommend that the patient see a podiatrist or orthopedist. Surgical treatment may be necessary.

WARTS (VERRUCAE)

Warts, or verrucae, are common viral infections of the skin and mucous membranes, which have been identified since the time of the ancient Greeks and Romans. They are caused by human papillomaviruses (HPVs), which contain deoxyribonucleic acid (DNA) (17). Because inoculation of extracts from common warts and anogenital warts induced warts when injected into a different site, the unitarian theory proposed that all warts were caused by a single agent. However, in the past decade, immunologic techniques in conjunction with DNA purification and restriction endonuclease digestion have identified at least 50 HPV types (18), each with its own characteristic histopathology and cytopathology.

The Latin term "verruca" means "a steep place" and was used because warts resembled small hills on the skin. Papillomavirus particles assemble in the nuclei of upper layer keratinocytes, with subsequent release into the milieu with the stratum corneum. It has been demonstrated that HPVs do not bud from the cell membrane and thus lack a thermosensitive lipid envelope like the herpes viruses and the human retroviruses. It is thought that the presence of this stable protein coat allows the HPV to remain infectious outside of the host cells for substantial periods of time.

Information in humans is based on observation of existing infections because for ethical reasons it is not possible to inoculate human subjects with typical HPV isolates (19). Further, scientific studies with HPVs remain limited because the viruses are species limited and cannot be propagated in vitro. Thus, viral isolates must be obtained from infected individuals. Newer cloning techniques are being attempted to provide insights into the host cell (keratinocyte)–viral interactions. This genetic manipulation may hold the key to identifying why certain HPV types are associated with malignant or benign disease and to identifying compounds that block viral infectivity or inhibit viral proteins.

Past studies had shown that HPV-6 and HPV-11 were responsible for anogenital condylomas, and that

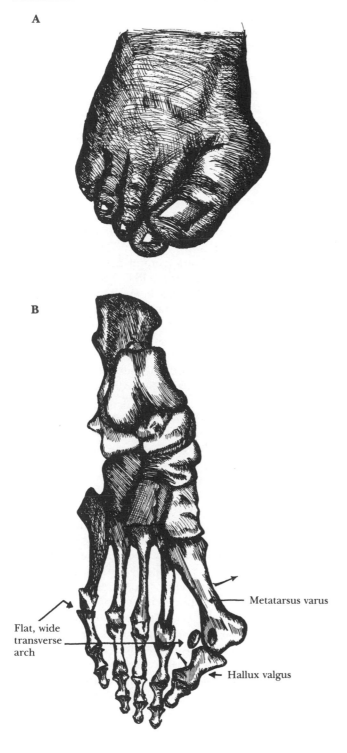

FIGURE 2A and B   Two views of hallux valgus.
A, gross representation of hallux valgus.
B, bone structure of hallux valgus.

Metatarsus varus

Flat, wide transverse arch

Hallux valgus

these strains were different from other HPVs in serologic molecular hybridization (20, 21). This prompted the belief that HPV type dictated the kind of wart and that these viruses were confined to specific body locations. Evidence now suggests that HPV types are not restricted to a specific site, but that, for unknown reasons (perhaps epithelial cell receptor specificity), viral particles function in keratinocytes only in specific locations and will induce warts only in these locations.

Common virogenic warts are defined according to their location. Common warts (verruca vulgaris) are usually located on the hands and fingers, although they may occur on the face. (See *Plate 8–34*.) Periungual and subungual verrucae occur around and underneath the nail beds, especially in nail-biters and cuticle pickers (22).

Juvenile, or flat, warts (verruca plana) usually occur in groups on the face, neck, and dorsa of the hands, wrists, and knees. Venereal warts (condyloma lata and condyloma acuminata) occur near the genitalia and anus. Plantar warts (verruca plantaris) are common on the soles of the feet (23). (See *Plate 8–35*.)

Symptoms

Warts begin as minute, smooth-surfaced, skin-colored lesions that enlarge over time. Repeated irritation causes the wart to continue enlarging. Plantar warts (on the soles of the feet) usually are asymptomatic and may not be noticed. However, if the plantar warts are large or occur on the heel or ball of the foot, the limitation of function and the discomfort may be bothersome to the point where professional advice is sought.

Three criteria must be met for an individual to develop a wart. The papovavirus must be present; there must be an open avenue for the virus to enter through the skin, such as abraded skin; and the individual immune response of the patient must be susceptible to the virus (probably the key reason that certain individuals develop warts and others do not). Indeed, immuno-deficient patients (those maintained on systemic or topical glucocorticoids), once infected, develop widespread and highly resistant warts (24).

Warts are most common in children and young adults and usually appear on exposed areas of the fingers, hands, face, and soles of the feet. The peak incidence of warts occurs between 12 and 16 years of age; as many as 10% of schoolchildren under 16 years of age have one or more warts (22). In addition, the incidence of warts is significantly higher in butchers and meat-cutters than in the general population (25). Whether this is the result of bovine papillomaviruses or human papillomaviruses remains unresolved (25).

Warts may spread by direct person-to-person contact, by autoinoculation to another body area, or indi-rectly through public shower floors or swimming pools. The incubation period after inoculation is 1–20 months, with an average of 3 to 4 months. An increase in plantar warts in England may have been due to an increase in the number and use of swimming pools (26). The hypothesis was that swimming, especially in warm water with a pH greater than 5, produces swelling and softening of the horny skin layer cells on the sole of the foot. The abrasive surface area of the pool and diving board contributes to tissue debridement, and inoculation in the area of heavy foot traffic around the pool (the diving board) is likely, especially when running and springing contribute to stress on the soles of the feet. Scrapings of the horny layer of plantar warts contain virus particles; therefore, it is conceivable that a heavy traffic area of a pool can be easily contaminated by one person with a plantar wart.

Condyloma acuminata (genital and venereal warts) is a sexually transmitted disease (STD) whose incidence between 1966 and 1981 has been estimated to have increased 459% (27). Each year in the United States, an estimated 12 million cases of genital warts (caused by HPV) occur; 750,000 new cases are diagnosed (28). In comparison, it is estimated that there are 20–30 million cases of symptomatic genital herpes infection (herpes simplex virus type 1 or 2), with 500,000 new cases a year (28).

Young adults, particularly those 20–24 years of age, most frequently consult physicians for genital warts. Symptoms include dyspareunia (painful intercourse), rectal pain, and tenesmus (painful, ineffectual straining to defecate or urinate) (27). The incidence of laryngeal papillomas on vocal cords and laryngeal mucosa is increasing at an alarming rate in young children. The epidemiologic observation has been made that infants with laryngeal papillomas are often born to mothers infected with genital condylomas of the birth canal at the time of delivery. This suggests that attempts should be made before delivery to eradicate these maternal lesions. Further, the incidence of papillomatous lesions within the oral cavity (e.g., tongue, gums, palate, and the esophagus) is increasing (29). It has been theorized that some of these infections may have been transmitted through oral–genital sex. However, recent evidence that demonstrates the environmental stability of the virus and the ability of HPVs to infect both genital and nongenital skin imply that this is not necessarily true (30).

Warts are not necessarily permanent; approximately 30% clear spontaneously in 6 months, 65% in 2 years, and most warts in 5 years (31, 32). The mechanism of spontaneous resolution is not fully understood.

It is assumed that wart regression is immune mediated (33). Evidence for this comes in part from frustrating attempts to treat warts in patients who exhibit compromised cellular (not humoral) immunoresponses (e.g., 40% of immunosuppressed renal recipients). Because the skin would be expected to function as an immune organ, it is difficult to understand why a wart can remain for so long in such patients and not simultaneously regress. It has been theorized that warts may be able to avoid immunologic detection by directing the synthesis of only minute quantities of potential protein antigen. Further, it is thought that the physical destruction of the skin epithelium with salicylic acid, podophyllum, or cryotherapy exposes the papillomavirus antigens inside the infected cells, promoting the resolution of the wart. It has also been proposed that leukocyte migration to the site of iatrogenic injury may be critical to resolution or that some viral products may permit the infected cell to avoid detection by inhibiting expression of class I major histocompatibility genes, as occurs in other viral systems (34).

There is a distinct difference between regression of an HPV-induced tumor (such as a wart or genital tumor) and host eradication of the HPV infection. Latent HPV has been demonstrated in laryngeal papilloma patients in remission and in clinically and histologically normal genital skin peripheral to condyloma acuminata (35, 36). Thus, it would appear that the HPV DNA is capable of residing in a host cell nucleoplasm without creating viral replication, and probably without stimulating production of viral antigens on the surface of the epithelial cell. Thus, the HPV genetic material could avoid detection and destruction by a host cellular immune response, persist within the epithelial cell, and theoretically cause wart disease in the future. This may explain why HPV-induced warts appear after eradication of the clinically detectable warts.

Because of the uncertainty of a patient-developed immune response to the HPV and the contagious nature of the warts, many practitioners believe that early and vigorous treatment is best. Prolonged treatment with nonprescription products may increase the chance of autoinoculation. In addition, the urgency for treatment will also include such considerations as the cosmetic effect (facial warts), the number of warts present in an area, the site of the wart (weight-bearing area of the foot), and the age of the patient (37).

Plantar warts, hyperkeratotic lesions resulting from pressure, are more common in older children and adolescents but also occur in adults (33). They may be confined to the weight-bearing areas of the foot (the sole of the heel, the great toe, the areas below the heads of the metatarsal bones, and the ball), or they may occur in non-weight-bearing areas of the sole of the foot (Figure 3). Calluses are also commonly found on weight-bearing areas of the foot, and their smooth keratotic surfaces resemble that of an isolated plantar wart. Therefore, the distinction between a wart and a callus or corn is sometimes unclear. However, unlike a callus, a plantar wart is tender with pressure and interrupts the

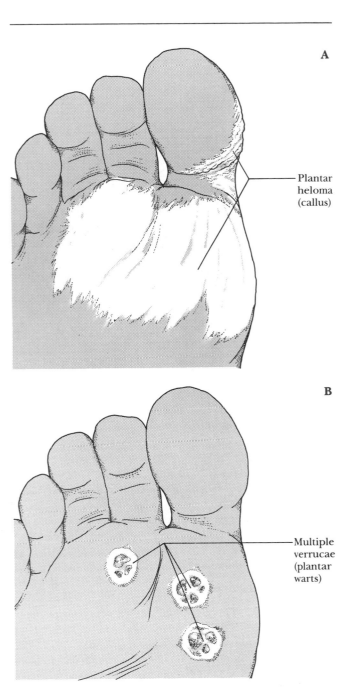

FIGURE 3 Conditions affecting the sole of the foot. A, plantar heloma (callus). B, multiple verrucae (plantar warts).

footprint pattern. Optimally, a podiatrist or dermatologist can make a differential diagnosis. To make the diagnosis, the physician may shave away the outer keratinous surface to expose thrombosed capillaries in the papilloma, which appear as black dots or seeds (33).

Plantar warts, if located on weight-bearing portions of the foot, are under constant pressure and usually are not raised above the skin surface. The wart itself is in the center of the lesion and roughly circular with a diameter of 0.5–3.0 cm. The surface is grayish and friable, and the surrounding skin is thick and heaped. Several warts may coalesce and fuse, giving the appearance of one large wart (mosaic wart) (33).

Common warts are recognized by their rough cauliflower-like appearance. These warts are slightly scaly, rough papules or nodules, alone or grouped; they can be found on any skin surface (33), although they most often occur on the hands. Flat warts are small, slightly elevated and flat-topped papules. Usually they are 2–4 mm in diameter and are found on the face and hands of children (33). Genital warts may resemble common warts or appear as a large mass with a cauliflower-like surface. Genital warts are generally soft and occur on the surface of the perineum, but also may occur in the vagina or the anus (33).

Treatment

Warts are a result of a viral infection. No specific effective medication is available, but topical agents and procedures help in their removal and relief of pain. Treatment is extremely difficult. Because of the latency factor, warts may reappear several months after they have been "cured."

Multiple flat warts, facial warts, painful plantar warts, periungual warts, and venereal warts should all be treated by a physician. Topical therapy might not be indicated. For instance, periungual warts will not be resolved until nail-biting is stopped through behavioral modification. The FDA advisory review panel on over-the-counter (OTC) miscellaneous external drug products recommended that these products be labeled for treating only common and plantar warts (38). This panel excluded the other wart types from self-therapy because of the difficulty in recognizing and treating these warts without the supervision of a physician (38). Indeed, patient referral to a physician is crucial, especially with venereal warts in the female.

Considerable controversy exists about the link between some HPVs and subsequent development of cancer in some patients. Squamous cell carcinoma of the cervix and vulva have been associated with HPV infection, and recent epidemiologic studies indicate a higher incidence of anal carcinoma among homosexual men (39) with anorectal condyloma. Further, immunosuppressed renal recipients demonstrate an increased risk of developing squamous and basal cell carcinomas, especially in sun-exposed areas (40), and the role of HPVs

in the development of malignant tumors of the skin in these patients is currently under investigation. Especially in view of the latency potential of the HPV, this evidence suggests the importance of physician follow-ups over a prolonged period of time for women who are treated for genital warts and for immunosuppressed patients (33).

Simple, localized common or plantar warts may be self-treated with salicylic acid either in a plaster vehicle (disk or pad) or in a collodion-like vehicle (41). Before application, the affected area should be washed and thoroughly dried. A plaster is sized with scissors to fit the wart, applied for 48 hours, and then removed. A collodion-like product is applied one drop at a time to sufficiently cover the wart once or twice a day. Both delivery systems can be used for up to 12 weeks. If the wart is not removed in this time, the patient should consult a physician or podiatrist.

Nonprescription products are not intended for application on moles, birthmarks, or unusual warts with hair growing from them because premalignant and malignant lesions may be mistaken as warts (41). Some patients may develop irregularly shaped pigmented moles (dysplastic nevi) on the skin at any time after birth. These moles are about a quarter of an inch in diameter and can eventually grow and turn into a melanoma. Thus, a patient should observe these moles and note their size and appearance every month, even to the point of actually measuring their size. Further, these moles should be examined by a physician every 6 months and, if they begin to grow, should be surgically removed before becoming melanomas.

EVALUATION OF CORNS, CALLUSES, AND WARTS

Many foot conditions require a physician's attention, especially those accompanying chronic, debilitating diseases such as diabetes mellitus or arteriosclerosis. Without proper supervision, nonprescription products may induce more ulceration and possibly gangrene, particularly in cases of vascular insufficiency in the foot (2). In addition, simple lesions may mask more serious abscesses or ulcerations. If exostoses associated with corns are not excised by a physician, the corns will persist. Sites with many corns, many calluses, or lesions that ooze purulent material (a sign of secondary infection) should be examined by a physician.

Most patients with rheumatoid arthritis eventually have foot involvement (42). Painful metatarsal heads, hallux valgus, and clawfoot are the major forefoot deformities in patients with rheumatoid arthritis. Corrective surgical procedures are often indicated to reduce pain and improve function. There is little evidence of the effectiveness of conventional nonsurgical therapy (orthopedic shoes, metatarsal inserts, conventional arch supports, or metatarsal bars) (42).

The patients' medical histories and medication profiles are extremely valuable, particularly in cases where self-medication has been tried. Warts, calluses, and corns can mask more serious abscesses and ulcerations; if left medically unattended, they may lead to conditions, such as osteomyelitis, requiring hospitalization. Because circulation is impaired in chronic, debilitating diseases, inadvertent injury may easily occur as a result of treatment with nonprescription products. Such injury may heal slowly. Diabetics and patients not properly screened for ischemic changes are susceptible to gangrene. (See Chapter 16, *Diabetes Care Products*.)

The pharmacist must be aware that warts occasionally can be indicators of more serious conditions, such as squamous cell carcinoma and deep fungal infections (43). Squamous cell carcinomas may develop rapidly, attaining a diameter of 1 cm within 2 weeks. The lesion appears as a small, red, conical, hard nodule that quickly ulcerates (44). Subungual verrucae, which occur under the nail plate, may exist in conjunction with periungual verrucae. A long-standing subungual verruca may be difficult to differentiate from a squamous cell carcinoma, especially in elderly patients (43). Condyloma acuminata are venereal warts that are moist and often cauliflower-like in appearance. They must be differentiated from condyloma lata (secondary syphilis), which have a smooth, whitish surface (45). Because of the possible link between this wart type and the development of cervical cancer, the patient must be advised to consult a physician (33).

The medical history and medication profile should include the following:

- Characteristics (particularly oozing and bleeding of warts) and duration of the condition;

- Whether similar problems have occurred in other family members;

- Any medical treatment being given for the problem or other conditions (e.g., immunosuppressive therapy, diabetes mellitus, rheumatoid arthritis);

- Any drug allergies.

Medical referral is indicated if:

- A peripheral circulatory disease, diabetes mellitus, or a condition already under a physician's care exists.

- Hemorrhaging or oozing of purulent material occurs.

- Corns and calluses indicate an anatomical defect or fault in body weight distribution.

- Corns and calluses on the foot are extensive or are painful and debilitating.

- Facial warts, plantar warts on weight-bearing areas, periungual warts, perianal or venereal warts, or extensive warts at one site exist.

- Proper self-medication for warts has been tried for an adequate period without success.

- The patient has a history of rheumatoid arthritis and complains of painful metatarsal heads and/or deviation of the great toe.

Self-treatment is appropriate if:

- Chronic, debilitating diseases do not contraindicate the use of foot care products.

- The patient is not a diabetic.

- The directions for use of the products can be followed with no difficulty.

- No concurrent medication (immunosuppressives) is being taken that contraindicates the use of these products.

- Corns and calluses are minor.

- Predisposing factors (ill-fitting footwear and hosiery) of corns and calluses are removed.

- Neither an anatomical defect nor faulty weight distribution is indicated by corns or calluses.

- Plantar warts are not spread extensively over the sole of the foot.

Pharmacologic Agents

A wide variety of topical drugs can be used to treat corns, calluses, and warts. The respective FDA OTC advisory panels reviewed these drugs; the categorization of these drugs as recommended by these panels appears in Table 2. Salicylic acid was the only drug found to be both safe and effective for the treatment of corns, calluses, or warts.

Several prescription products or nondrug modalities might better serve the patient. For example, injection of a small amount of a corticosteroid beneath a painful corn results in a dramatic relief of symptoms (2). Further, desiccatory curettage or cryotherapy (application of liquid nitrogen) might be advantageous to use for certain wart types.

Agents Used To Treat
Corns, Calluses, and Warts

Glacial Acetic Acid and Lactic Acid   Glacial acetic acid and lactic acid are organic acids included in several legend and nonlegend formulations for corns, calluses, and warts because of their corrosive properties. They should be applied only on the affected area, not on surrounding healthy skin. The FDA advisory panel placed these agents individually and in combination with salicylic acid into Category III for lack of clinical effectiveness data. The panel concluded that there was insufficient evidence to demonstrate that the addition of glacial acetic acid (11%) or lactic acid (5–17%) to salicylic acid increases the effectiveness of the product as a wart remover (46). These acids are contraindicated in cases involving debilitating illness. Overuse may cause skin irritation and ulceration. Used appropriately, these agents are safe for adults and children.

Salicylic Acid   Salicylic acid is the oldest of the keratolytic agents and is formulated in many strengths from 0.5% to 40% depending on its intended use. For self-treatment of corns, calluses, and warts, its concentration is 5–17% in a collodion-like vehicle and 12–40% in a plaster vehicle. It is the only drug adjudged to be safe and effective as a keratolytic agent for the treatment of corns, calluses, common warts, and plantar warts.

The action of salicylic acid on hyperplastic keratin is hypothesized twofold: to decrease keratinocyte adhesion and to increase water binding leading to a hydration of keratin. Because of the latter effect, the presence of moisture was thought to be an important component for the therapeutic efficacy of the drug in topical corn, callus, and wart therapy, and soaking the area in a warm water bath for 5 minutes before application of salicylic acid was recommended. However, recent evidence submitted to the FDA indicated that soaking produced no significant effects for any efficacy parameter assessed (47). Thus, the FDA is proposing to delete recommendations to soak the area before treatment with a salicylic acid product.

Although occlusive vehicles can enhance the percutaneous absorption of salicylic acid, it is doubtful that "salicylism" will result during corn, callus, or wart therapy. One study demonstrated a complete absence of systemic side effects in 3,165 foot clinic patients who had treated themselves with corn removers containing salicylic acid (48). Further, recent studies have demonstrated that it is not necessary to encircle surrounding healthy skin with a film of white petrolatum to protect it from inadvertent salicylic acid application during corn or callus treatment. Thus, the FDA is also proposing to delete this instruction on salicylic acid product packages. Patients with diabetes mellitus or peripheral vascular disease, where acute inflammation or ulcer formation from topical salicylic acid would be difficult to treat, should not use salicylic acid products except under direct physician supervision.

Significant percutaneous absorption should be expected when salicylic acid is applied over large body areas, for example, during therapy for extensive psoriasis on the face, trunk, or extremities. Absorbed salicylic acid is metabolized in the liver to a large degree and is excreted in the urine; patients with impaired liver or kidney function are therefore predisposed to systemic salicylic acid buildup. These patients cannot tolerate absorbed salicylate because toxic serum levels may develop (49, 50).

Most often salicylic acid is applied to the corn, callus, or wart in a collodion or collodion-like vehicle. The patient should thoroughly wash and dry the affected area before applying the product. For corns and calluses the solution is applied once or twice daily as needed for up to 14 days or until the corn or callus is removed. For warts the product is applied once or twice daily as needed for up to 12 weeks or until the wart is removed. For all three conditions, the product is applied one drop at a time to sufficiently cover the affected area. The patient should be advised not to overuse the product.

The liquid dosage form is often the easiest for the patient to apply. However, this modality requires patience and persistence because of the length of time necessary to resolve the problem. It is suggested that the patient keep the adjacent healthy skin dry and clean and that the collodion film be peeled away every 2 or 3 days to remove keratotic debris (22).

Salicylic acid may also be delivered to the skin through the use of a plaster disk or pad. This delivery system provides direct and prolonged contact of the drug with the affected area. Salicylic acid plaster (USP XIX) is a uniform solid or semisolid adhesive mixture of salicylic acid in a suitable base, spread on appropriate backing material (felt, moleskin, cotton, or plastic) which may be applied directly to the affected area. The usual concentration of salicylic acid in the base is 40%. A small piece of the 40% plaster may be cut to the size of the wart and held in place by waterproof tape. More convenient, however, are corn or callus pads that have small salicylic acid disks for direct application to the skin. The patient selects the appropriately sized disk, places it directly on the affected area, and then covers it with the pad.

For corns and calluses, salicylic acid plasters or disks are to be applied and removed within 48 hours with a maximum of five treatments over a 2-week period. For warts, salicylic acid plasters or disks are to be applied and removed every 48 hours with a maximum treatment period not to exceed 12 weeks. If the wart remains, a physician should be consulted.

TABLE 2 FDA OTC advisory review panel outcomes for various classes of nonprescription foot products

FDA OTC panel	Category assignment		
	Category I	Category II	Category III
Topical antifungal drug products; establishment of a monograph (*Federal Register*, 3/23/82)	Haloprogin Clioquinol Miconazole nitrate Nystatin Tolnaftate Undecylenic acid and its salts	Camphor Candicidin Coal tar Menthol Phenolates Resorcinol Tannic acid Thymol Tolindate	Aluminum salts [a] Basic fuchsin Benzethonium Cl Benzoic acid Borates Caprylates Chlorothymol Chloroxylenol Oxyquinolines Povidone–iodine Salicylic acid Triacetin
Topical corn and callus remover products; tentative final monograph, notice of proposed rulemaking (*Federal Register*, 2/20/87)	Salicylic acid	Acetic acid [a] Allantoin Ascorbic acid Ichthammol Methylbenzcthonium chloride Methylsalicylate Vitamin A	Phenoxyacetic acid Zinc chloride
Ingrown toenail relief drug products; tentative final monograph (*Federal Register*, 9/3/82)	None	Chloroxylenol Urea	Sodium sulfide Tannic acid
Wart remover drug products; tentative final monograph; notice of proposed rulemaking (*Federal Register*, 3/27/87)	Salicylic acid	Benzocaine Camphor Castor oil Iodine Menthol	Glacial acetic acid Ascorbic acid Calcium pantothenate Lactic acid SA/LA combination [b] SA/AA combination [b] Ascorbic acid/calcium pantothenate/starch combination

[a] Partial listing only

[b] SA–salicylic acid; AA–acetic acid; LA–lactic acid

Collodions Topical keratolytics used in treating corns, calluses, and warts generally are formulated in flexible collodion-like delivery systems containing pyroxylin, various combinations of volatile solvents, such as ether, acetone, or alcohol, and a plasticizer, usually castor oil. Pyroxylin is a nitrocellulose derivative that, after evaporation of the volatile solvents, remains on the skin as a water-repellent film (51). The advantages of collodions are that they form an adherent flexible or rigid film (52) and prevent moisture evaporation, thus aiding penetration of the active ingredient into the affected tissue, which results in sustained local action of the drug. The systems are water insoluble, as are most of their active ingredients, such as salicylic acid. They are less apt to run than aqueous solutions.

The disadvantages of collodions are that they are extremely flammable and volatile, and they may be mechanically irritating by occluding normal water transport through the skin. Also, the collodion's occlusive nature allows systemic absorption of some drugs. Patients also may abuse these vehicles by sniffing their aromatic odors (53).

Additional Agents Used To Treat Corns and Calluses

Local Anesthetics The FDA advisory panel on corn and callus remover products concluded that the corn and callus remover products concluded that the local anesthetics used with salicylic acid may mask the pain from the keratolytic action of salicylic acid on subcutaneous tissue or developing infections. Thus, the patient might be totally unaware of the potential danger. Subsequently, the panel recommended that combinations of local anesthetics, particularly benzocaine, with salicylic acid be classified as Category II (48).

Zinc Chloride Zinc chloride was combined with salicylic acid in several formulations of topical nonprescription products as an escharotic agent for corns and calluses. However, the FDA advisory panel concluded that there was no evidence to establish that this combination contributed significantly more to corn and callus removal than salicylic acid alone. Thus, it remains classified as a Category III drug and is generally not used on corns and calluses (12).

Agents Used To Treat Warts

Ascorbic Acid Although ascorbic acid is essential to the development of supporting tissue (collagen and intracellular ground substance) and healing, there are insufficient data available to establish its efficacy in topical wart therapy (38). The panel has recommended further study of ascorbic acid before it can be considered effective for nonprescription use (38).

Calcium Pantothenate Application of the alcohol derivative pantothenol in various ulcerative and pyogenic dermatoses stimulates epithelialization and allays itching. There have been no reports of sensitization or allergic reaction to topical therapy with pantothenic acid or its derivatives (54). The use of these drugs in adults and children seems safe. Topical formulations contain 2–5% of the active pantothenic acid derivative. However, there are insufficient data available on the effectiveness of this agent. Thus, the panel classified calcium pantothenate as Category III (38).

Cantharidin Cantharidin is a potent vesicant available by prescription only as an ingredient of Cantharone. For wart therapy, this liquid is applied lightly with a stick or swab, allowed to dry, and then covered by a piece of waterproof adhesive tape slightly larger than the wart (43). Depending on the physician's directions, the bandage is left in place between 24 hours and 1 week and then removed. The drug effects a separation at the dermal–epidermal junction and therefore the removal of the epidermal-residing wart (37). Following the blister formation, minor inflammation can be resolved with tap water soaks (37).

In approximately 7–14 days, the blister, often hemorrhagic, breaks, crusts, and falls off. At this time, the physician debrides the dead material with fine-curved iris scissors. Because the effect of cantharidin is entirely intraepidermal, no scarring ensues.

A disadvantage of cantharidin is that, on occasion, annular warts may develop at the blister periphery (24). In addition, this method is considered dangerous and should be performed only by a physician or podiatrist. However, a successful trial of cantharidin treatment of warts at home has been reported (55). Application of the occlusive tape was omitted from the instruction to simplify the process and produce fewer reactions. This mode proved to be easy, safe, and reasonably effective in treating warts. To facilitate correct application of this product, some investigators advocate that the product be colored with a green food coloring dye (37).

Podophyllum Podophyllum resin (in concentrations of up to 25%) dispensed in compound benzoin tincture or as a solution in alcohol is effective in the treatment of condyloma acuminatum (genital warts). Podophyllum should not be prescribed for inclusion in a flexible collodion vehicle because of the collodion's occlusive nature and the possibility of enhancement of the drug's percutaneous absorption. It is a cytotoxic agent that arrests mitosis in metaphase. This caustic and powerful skin irritant is available only by prescription for short-term use. It may be reapplied every 4–7 days, generally for 2–4 weeks, depending on individual response and any residual chemical irritation (22). Within 24–48 hours of application, lesions become necrotic, and in the following days, begin to slough off and gradually disappear.

The primary toxicologic problem associated with the use of podophyllum resin, aside from its topical irritant qualities, is peripheral neuropathy when it is absorbed percutaneously into the systemic circulation (56). Podophyllum should be applied only in small amounts by the physician. The patient should be instructed to wash off the podophyllum preparation with soap and water within 8–12 hours of its application. Because the usual delivery system is a low-viscosity suspension (compound tincture of benzoin) or tincture (alcohol), the solution tends to run and damage adjacent tissue. This risk may be minimized if white petrolatum or talc is applied to the healthy surrounding skin before the podophyllum preparation is applied to the wart (22, 37).

Podophyllum resin for vulvar warts in pregnant women should be used cautiously, if at all. Podophyllum applied topically five times for 4 hours each from the 23rd to the 29th week of pregnancy was suspected of causing teratogenic effects (57). Because of this adverse effect and to prevent the possible development of laryngeal papillomatosis in the neonate after delivery, the physician should consider using cryosurgery to remove the venereal wart or deliver the neonate by caesarean section (58). Podophyllum should not be used on hemorrhaging skin or where an extensive skin surface area is involved. These conditions increase the possibility of percutaneous absorption. Because podophyllum is a potent corrosive, it should not be used with other keratolytic agents, such as salicylic acid.

Miscellaneous Prescription Drugs Used To Treat Warts Other prescription drugs used fairly successfully in treating warts are the antibiotic bleomycin sulfate (Blenoxane) for recurrent or recalcitrant plantar warts, tretinoin (retinoic acid) for flat warts and plantar warts (59–61), and fluorouracil (62). Although the FDA has not approved bleomycin for wart treatment, evidence indicates that bleomycin's effectiveness is due to the drug's selective inhibition of DNA synthesis. In addition, local injection of bleomycin into the wart results in hemorrhagic necrosis secondary to microthrombosis, which is followed by a gradual reduction and detachment of the wart (63). Theoretical objection to the use of bleomycin for warts stems from its ability to interfere with DNA metabolism and induce skin cancer (64). One report indicated the appearance of nail dystrophy following the injection of bleomycin into a periungual wart (63). Results with tretinoin and fluorouracil therapy are variable; in those cases that do respond, it has not been determined whether the disease is simply taking its natural course (41). Idoxuridine 0.25% ointment demonstrated efficacy in the treatment of six women suffering from condyloma acuminatum (65). The drug was applied twice daily for 1 week. No side effects were observed and there were no recurrences in these women 3 months after follow-up. However, idoxuridine has induced congenital anomalies in animals, and thus its safety for use to treat genital warts during pregnancy remains in doubt.

Adjunctive Therapy

In addition to nonprescription drugs, self-therapy measures include daily soaking of the affected area throughout treatment for at least 5 minutes in very warm (not hot) water to remove dead tissue (24). Dead tissue should be gently removed after normal washing. Skin should not be forcibly removed because further damage could result. Sharp knives or razor blades that have not been properly sterilized should not be used to cut dead tissue because they may cause bacterial infection. A rough towel, callus file, or pumice stone effectively removes dead tissue of corns and calluses. Petroleum jelly need not be applied to healthy skin surrounding the affected area before application of corrosive products. However, this precaution should be suggested to persons with poor eyesight or other condi-

tions that increase the likelihood of misapplication or accidental spillage.

To relieve painful pressure emanating from inflamed underlying tissue and irritated or hypertrophied bones directly underneath a corn or callus, patients may use a pad such as Dr. Scholl's with an aperture for the corn or callus. If the skin can tolerate the pads, they may be used up to 1 week or longer (66). To prevent the pads from adhering to hosiery, patients may wax the pads with paraffin or a candle and powder them daily with a hygienic foot powder or cover them with an adhesive bandage. If, despite these measures, friction causes the pads to peel up at the edge and stick to hosiery, the pharmacist may recommend that patients cover their toes with the forefoot of an old stocking or pantyhose before putting on hosiery (66).

Patients should be advised that if at any time the pad begins to cause itching, burning, or pain, it should be removed and a podiatrist should be consulted. The pharmacist also should advise the patient that these pads will provide only temporary relief and rarely cure a corn or a callus.

To avoid the spread of warts, which are contagious, patients should wash their hands before and after treating or touching wart tissue, and a specific towel should be used only for drying the affected area after cleaning. Patients should not probe or poke the wart tissue. Footwear should be worn in the case of plantar warts. If warts are present on the sole of the foot, patients should not walk in bare feet unless the wart is securely covered.

Product Selection Guidelines

Corns and Calluses

There are no clinical studies to indicate whether prescription-only products are superior to nonprescription products. Conclusions are based only on subjective physician evaluation reports (2, 10). Salicylic acid in a plaster or collodion-like dosage form appears to be the most effective treatment for corns and calluses. Some studies advocate the use of a 50% silver nitrate solution, applied by the physician, followed by weekly applications of 40% salicylic acid plasters for corns (8, 10).

Bunions

If the pharmacist recommends the use of topical adhesive cushioning to alleviate the pressure on a bunion, instructions should be given on proper use. Before the protective pad is applied, the foot should be bathed and thoroughly dried. The pad then is cut into a shape that conforms to the bunion. If the intent is to relieve the pressure from the center of the bunion area, the pad can be cut to surround the bunion. Precut pads are available for immediate patient use. Constant skin contact with adhesive-backed pads should be avoided, unless under the recommendation of a podiatrist or other physician.

Warts

The management of warts depends on the age of the patient, the extent and number of lesions present, the immunologic status of the patient, and the patient's desire for treatment. Opinions vary about the best treatment for elimination of warts. Prescribed treatments and self-care depend on wart type and include intralesional application of fluorouracil, isotretinoin, salicylic acid, nitric acid, cantharidin, and interferon (67, 68). Cryotherapy, which involves the use of liquid nitrogen or dry ice, is commonly used by dermatologists for a number of wart types. Electrodesiccation of venereal warts is effective but requires local anesthesia. Carbon dioxide and argon lasers hold promise to help eradicate resistant warts in the future.

The findings of the FDA advisory review panel on OTC miscellaneous external drug products clarified the effectiveness and safety of these drugs (38, 46). Only common warts and plantar warts may be treated with nonprescription products. Common warts are easily identified by the rough cauliflower-like appearance on the surface of the skin. Plantar warts are identifiable on the bottom of the foot by their tenderness and the interruption of the footprint pattern.

For self-care purposes, collodion-like liquid preparations or plasters of salicylic acid are suitable for most patients. The patient, however, must be educated in the proper application techniques for these dosage forms, and the treatment should not exceed 12 weeks.

Patient Consultation

Remission of corns, calluses, and warts does not happen quickly; it can take several days to several months. Usually nonprescription treatment lasts 14 days for corns and calluses and up to 12 weeks for warts; if the wart remains, a physician should be consulted. Adherence to the dosage regimen and selection of a convenient time to apply the product are important. The pain and lack of mobility associated with corns, calluses, or warts are strict reminders to adhere to the treatment. Topical products should be applied no more than twice daily; the most convenient times are generally in the morning and at bedtime.

The pharmacist should clearly explain how to use the medication. Because many products contain corrosive materials, the product should be applied only to the corn, callus, or wart. If a plaster or pad is used, the process of trimming the pad to follow the contours of the corn or callus should be explained.

If a solution is used, one drop at a time is applied directly to the corn, callus, or wart and is allowed to dry and harden to avoid running; the procedure continues until the entire area is covered. Adjacent areas of normal healthy skin should not come in contact with the product. If the solution touches healthy skin, it should be washed off immediately with soap and water. If the solution is intended for a soft corn between the toes, the toes should be held apart until the solution is applied and allowed to dry. This procedure is followed for 3–6 days. The solution should solidify before a dressing is applied.

A plaster is cut to the size of the lesion, applied to the skin, and covered with adhesive occlusive tape. The next day, the dressing is removed and the foot is soaked in warm water. The macerated, soft white skin of the corn or callus is then removed by scrubbing gently with a rough towel, pumice stone, or callus file, and the plaster is reapplied. Patients must be careful not to debride healthy skin when using a pumice stone or callus file.

A cream should be applied after washing the wart with soap and water. Then an occlusive dressing generally is placed over the wart.

Because nonprescription preparations contain volatile and irritating ingredients, the patient should take precautions in using them. After use, the container should be tightly capped to prevent evaporation and to prevent the active ingredients from assuming a greater concentration. The volatile delivery systems are quite flammable, and the product should be stored in amber or light-resistant containers away from direct sunlight or heat.

The products that contain collodions are poisonous when taken orally, and they should be stored out of children's reach. They have an odor similar to that of airplane glue and may be subject to abuse if the vapors are inhaled (53).

Nonprescription products are not recommended for patients with diabetes or circulatory problems. Contraindications should be pointed out to all patients to avoid inadvertent use of these products by other family members who have such conditions. These products are keratolytic and cause skin tissue to slough off, leaving an unsightly pinkish tinge to the skin; nevertheless, they should continue to be used. They should be discontinued only when a severe inflammatory response (swelling or reddening) or irritation occurs, or when pain occurs immediately upon application.

INGROWN TOENAILS

An ingrown toenail occurs when a section of nail presses into the soft tissue of the nail groove. The nail curves into the flesh of the toe corners and becomes embedded in the surrounding soft tissue of the toe, causing pain. Swelling, inflammation, and ulceration are secondary complications that can arise from this condition.

Etiology

The frequent cause of ingrown toenails is incorrect trimming of the nails. The correct method of cutting the toenail is to cut the nail straight across without tapering the corners in any way. Wearing pointed-toe or tight shoes, as well as wearing hosiery, including elastic hosiery, that is too tight, also has been implicated. In these instances, direct pressure can force the lateral edge of the nail into the soft tissue. Bedridden patients may develop ingrown toenails because tight bed covers press the soft skin tissue against the nails. Those people who have toenails that naturally curl also are predisposed to this malady.

Treatment

Prevention through education is probably the best way to prevent the development of ingrown toenails. In the early stages of development of an ingrown toenail, therapy is directed at providing adequate room for the nail to resume its normal position adjacent to soft tissue. This is accomplished by relieving the external source of pressure and applying medications that will harden the nail groove or help shrink the soft tissue. The patient should be referred to a podiatrist or other physician if the condition is recurrent.

Pharmacologic Agents

The FDA in a tentative final monograph has classified two active ingredients in ingrown toenail products, sodium sulfide and tannic acid, as Category III (Table 2) (69). At present, there are insufficient data to determine their effectiveness for this condition. In theory, sodium sulfide is intended to soften the keratin in the nail and the calloused skin surrounding the nail, thereby providing relief of pressure and pain caused by the embedded nail (70). The claimed effect of tannic acid is that it hardens the skin surrounding the embedded nail and shrinks the soft tissue adjacent to the nail, providing enough room for the nail to resume its normal position adjacent to soft tissue (70).

Ingrown toenail products with these active ingredients should not be used for more than 7 days. If there is no improvement within this time, a podiatrist or other physician should be consulted. These products should not be applied to open sores, and use of the product should be stopped and a physician consulted if swelling and redness increase or if a discharge is present around the nail. Patients with diabetes mellitus and circulatory disease should not use these products without the knowledge of their physician.

To enhance the effectiveness of these products, the panel recommended that the directions for use include the statement, "Cleanse affected toes thoroughly. Place a small piece of cotton in the nail groove (the side of the nail where the pain is) and wet cotton thoroughly with the solution. Repeat several times daily until nail discomfort is relieved but do not use more than 7 days" (70).

To temporarily protect the toe while the ingrown nail is being treated, a patient may use a soft foam toe cap. However, continual use of a toe cap without removing the source of the problem merely delays corrective treatment.

Patients with ingrown toenails frequently fail to realize that they may be helped by oral medication intended to allay pain and inflammation. The pharmacist may recommend aspirin or ibuprofen, two proven analgesics with anti-inflammatory activity, provided there are no contraindications to their use for a particular patient (See Chapter 5, *Internal Analgesic Products*).

FROSTBITE

Frostbite is defined as the actual freezing of tissues by excessive exposure to low temperatures. Frostbite is not amenable to therapy with nonprescription drug products. To maintain normal core temperature in cold weather, the body reduces reflexly the flow of blood to the skin surface and the extremities. Therefore, frostbite usually involves areas of the body that are the farthest from deep organs or large muscles such as the feet, hands, ear lobes, nose, or cheeks (71). Minor frostbite may cause only blanching of the skin; severe frostbite may result in the loss of fingers and toes (71).

Etiology

Predisposing factors to the development of frostbite include the following:

- Low temperatures (especially with high winds);

- Long periods of exposure to cold;

- Lack of proper clothing;

- Wet clothing;

- Poor nutrition, exhaustion, or dehydration;

- Circulatory disease;

- Immobility;

- Direct contact with metal or petroleum products at low temperatures;

- Individual susceptibility to cold.

Treatment

The frostbitten part should be promptly and thoroughly rewarmed in water heated to 104–108°F (45.6–47.8°C) (71). The water should not be hot to a normal hand at room temperature and should not be tested with the frozen part. The container of water should be large enough for the frozen part to be moved freely without bumping against the sides. Rewarming should be continued until a flush returns to the most distal tip of the thawed part (72). This usually takes about 20–30 minutes (71). Dry heat (heating pad) should be avoided because it is difficult to control the temperature and evenly rewarm the part (71). The injured part should be soaked for about 20 minutes in a whirlpool bath once or twice daily until the healing process is complete (75).

The best treatment for frostbite is prevention; there are a few simple rules to follow (77):

- Dress to maintain body warmth, including areas of the face, neck, extremities, and head.

- Avoid exposure to cold during times of sickness or exhaustion.

- Do not exceed your tolerance to cold exposure.

- Avoid tight-fitting garments; dress with layered clothing.

- Wear clothing that allows ventilation and prevents perspiration buildup (water enhances heat loss).

- Wear insulated boots or shoes and socks (preferably wool) that fit snugly but are not tight in spots.

- Wear mittens instead of gloves in severe cold (the thumb should be with the rest of the fingers and not by itself).

- Never touch objects (especially cold metal or petroleum products) that facilitate heat loss.

When given the opportunity, the pharmacist should seek to correct a few misconceptions. It is dangerous to rub the affected limb with ice or snow even though it seems to provide warmth (71). This can result in prolonged contact with the cold and may cause lacerations of the cells from the ice crystals. In addition, persons should refrain from drinking alcohol for antifreeze purposes at least until they are in a warm place. Alcohol can induce a loss of body heat even though it may give the person a feeling of warmth when ingested. Lastly, smoking should be avoided by frostbite victims. Nicotine can induce peripheral vasoconstriction and effect a further decrease of blood supply to the frostbitten extremity (70, 73).

ATHLETE'S FOOT

The most prevalent cutaneous fungal infection in humans is athlete's foot (dermatophytosis of the foot or tinea pedis), the itchy, scaling lesions between the toes. Athlete's foot is more prevalent in males (68.4/1,000) than females (10.7/1,000) (74), probably because fewer women are exposed to environments conducive to the spread of the organism, for example, athletic organizations or the military. When exposure to these environments is equal, the incidence of tinea infections in women approaches that of men (75). Also, women tend to be more thorough when drying their feet and toes after bathing. Men are more apt to only blot the feet and to put the damp feet directly into their socks and shoes. Because ringworm fungi (dermatophytes) generally are the causative or initiating organisms, athlete's foot often is synonymous with a ringworm infection (4).

The clinical spectrum of athlete's foot ranges from mild scaling to a severe, exudative inflammatory process characterized by fissuring and denudation. The prevalent type of athlete's foot, midway between these two extremes, is characterized by maceration, hyperkeratosis, pruritus, malodor, and a stinging sensation of the feet.

Etiology

Tinea pedis is an infection type of relatively recent onset. It was not common until humans began wearing occlusive footwear and was not reported in the medical literature until 1888 (76). Tinea pedis is most commonly caused by *Tricophyton rubrum, Tricophyton mentagrophytes,* or *Epidermophyton floccosum. T. rubrum* often causes a dry, hyperkeratotic, moccasin-like involvement of the feet; *T. mentagrophytes* often produces a blister-like or vesicular pattern. *E. floccosum* is capable of producing both of these patterns.

In addition to specific microorganisms, other predisposing environmental factors contribute to the disease's development. Footwear is a key variable, as illustrated by the incidence of the disease in any population that wears occlusive footwear with little ventilation. Occlusion with a nonporous material increases temperature and hydration of the skin and interferes with the barrier function of the stratum corneum. The climatic conditions of the area and the customs of the resident population also play roles in the location of the dermatophytosis infection. The infection is common in the summer or in tropical or semitropical climates in individuals who customarily wear occlusive footwear that promote overhydration of the skin.

The type of dermatophytosis present also varies with geographic location (75). In Vietnam, U.S. soldiers often acquired a disabling, inflammatory *T. mentagrophytes* infection, but South Vietnamese soldiers did not become infected with the organism. Presumably, this demonstrated that the Vietnamese had acquired a resistance to the infection. In a resident population, dermatophytosis infection is often observed as chronic and noninflammatory, while the same infection in virgin hosts is markedly inflammatory and self-limited (75).

Anthrophilic species of dermatophytes (e.g., *T. rubrum, T. mentagrophytes*) are transmitted either directly by human contact or indirectly by exposure to inanimate objects. It is theorized that this infection is acquired most often by walking barefoot on infected floors (e.g., hotel bathrooms, swimming pools, or locker rooms). It is theorized that the infection is spread within families by exposure to bathroom floors, mats, or rugs. Therefore, tinea pedis is considered to be an exogenously transmitted infection in which cross-infection among susceptible individuals readily occurs (75).

Susceptibility

Although there are many pathogenic fungi in the environment, the overall incidence of actual superficial fungal infections is remarkably low. Many degrees of susceptibility produce a clinical infection—from instantaneous "takes" by a single spore to severe trauma with massive exposure (77). It appears, however, that trauma to the skin, especially blister-producing trauma (from wearing ill-fitting footwear), may be significantly more important to the occurrence of human fungal infections (78) than is simple exposure to the offending pathogens.

Although tinea pedis may occur at all ages, it is more common in adults, presumably because of their increased opportunities for exposure to pathogens. However, tinea pedis should not be ignored as a diagnostic possibility in children because of its infrequent occurrence (79). Individual susceptibility is also affected by other disease processes the patient may have. For example, dermatophytosis infections may be more severe and difficult to ameliorate in patients with diabetes mellitus, lymphoid malignancies, immunologic compromise, and Cushing's syndrome (75).

Pathophysiology

After inoculation into the skin under suitable conditions, the infection progresses through several stages. The stages include periods of incubation and then enlargement, followed by a refractory period and a stage of involution.

During the incubation period, the dermatophyte grows in the stratum corneum, sometimes with minimal signs of infection. The fungal infestation is demonstrated by the presence of the dermatophyte by 10% potassium hydroxide (KOH) microscopic examination of scales scraped from the skin or clippings taken from the nail. The KOH dissolves keratin and permits better visualization of the fungal structures such as hyphae or spores. In dermatophyte infections, only branching hyphae are observed.

After the incubation period and once the infection is established, two factors appear to play a role in determining the size and duration of the lesions. These factors are the growth rate of the organism and the epidermal turnover rate (75). The fungal growth rate must equal or exceed the epidermal turnover rate or the organism will quickly shed.

Dermatophytic infestations remain within the stratum corneum. This resistance to spread of infection seems to involve both immunologic and nonimmunologic mechanisms. For example, the substance "serum inhibitory factor" (SIF) appears to limit the growth of dermatophytes beyond the stratum corneum. SIF is not an antibody but a dialyzable, heat-labile component of fresh sera. It appears that SIF binds to the iron that dermatophytes need for continued growth (75).

Once into the stratum corneum, dermatophytes produce keratinases and other proteolytic enzymes. In Vietnam, U.S. combat personnel demonstrated a particularly inflammatory type of *T. mentagrophytes* infection associated with elastase production. This indicated that enzymes or toxins produced by these microorganisms account for some of the severe clinical reactions. An alpha-$_2$-macroglobulin keratinase inhibitor that has been identified within sera may also play a role in limiting the growth of dermatophytes deeper into the skin.

The major immunologic defense mechanism identified in dermatophyte infections is the type IV delayed hypersensitivity response as illustrated by the course of human experimental infections. It appears that during the host's first exposure to the trichophyton cell wall glycopeptide antigen, the antigen diffuses from the stratum corneum to stimulate sensitized lymphocytes. Inflammatory mediators and lymphokines are produced by these cells and probably act on the host cells rather than the dermatophytes. Because of this response, the epidermal barrier is abrogated and SIF gains access to the otherwise privileged layers of the stratum corneum. SIF is fungistatic and so the cell-mediated immune response typically leads to inhibition but not complete destruction of the dermatophyte. Hence, the organism is still identified in cultures and microscopic KOH preparations of the infected area. This may also explain why about 20% of those afflicted with superficial fungal infections develop a chronic infection. Thus, they seem to have a fungus infection "that comes and goes and that no one can cure" (80). These chronic infections are characterized clinically by relatively long-standing, widespread disease with plantar involvement with little or no associated inflammatory response (75).

Clinically, there are four accepted variants of tinea pedis; two or more of these types may overlap. The most common is the chronic, intertriginous type (75). It is characterized by fissuring, scaling, or maceration in the interdigital spaces. Typically, the infection involves the lateral toe webs, usually between the fourth and fifth or third and fourth toes. From these sites the infection spreads to the sole or instep of the foot but rarely to the dorsum of the foot. Warmth and humidity aggravate this condition. Consequently, hyperhydrosis becomes an underlying problem and must be treated along with the dermatophyte infestation.

It is also known that normal resident aerobic diphtheroids may become involved in the athlete's foot process (5). After initial invasion of the stratum corneum by dermatophytes, enough moisture may accumulate to trigger a bacterial overgrowth. Increased moisture and temperature then lead to bacterial proliferation and release of metabolic products that diffuse easily through the underlying horny layer already damaged by fungal invasion. In the more severe cases, Gram-negative organisms intrude and may exacerbate the condition, causing skin maceration, white hyperkeratosis, or erosions with increased patient symptomatology.

The second variant of athlete's foot is known as the chronic, papulosquamous pattern (75). It is usually found on both feet and characterized by a small amount of inflammation and a diffuse moccasin-like scaling on the soles of the feet. Tinea unguium or onychomycosis of one or more toenails may also be present. It is thought that the toenail involvement may continue to fuel the infection and that, before resolution of the skin can take place, the toenails must first be cured with oral drug therapy, such as griseofulvin or ketoconazole, or removed with surgical avulsion to rid the area of the offending fungus. Surgery is preferred because of the high failure rate associated with oral antifungal therapy.

The third variant of tinea pedis is the vesicular type, usually caused by *T. metagrophytes* var. *interdigitale* (75). Small vesicles or vesicopustules are observed near the instep and on the midanterior plantar surface. Skin scaling is seen on these areas as well as on the toe webs. This variant is symptomatic in the summer and clinically quiescent during the cooler months, that is, "it seems to come and go with the season" (80).

The acute ulcerative variant is the fourth variant of tinea pedis. This variant is frequently associated with macerated, denuded, weeping ulcerations of the sole of the foot. Typically, white hyperkeratosis and a pungent odor are present. This type of infection is complicated by the presence of an overgrowth of opportunistic Gram-negative bacteria such as *Proteus* and *Pseudomonas*. This type has been called dermatophytosis complex or Gram-negative athlete's foot, and may produce an extremely painful, erosive, purulent interspace that can be disabling (81).

Evaluation

The most common complaint of patients suffering from tinea pedis is pruritus. However, if fissures are present, particularly between the toes, painful burning and stinging may also occur. If the foot area is abraded, denuded, or inflamed, weeping or oozing may occur in addition to frank pain. Some patients may merely remark on the bothersome scaling of dry skin, particularly if it has progressed to the soles of the feet. Small vesicular lesions may combine to form a larger bullous eruption marked by pain and irritation. The only symptoms may be brittleness and discoloration of a hypertrophied toenail.

The only true determinant of a fungal foot infection is clinical laboratory evaluation of tissue scrapings from the foot. As mentioned, this process involves a potassium hydroxide mount preparation of the scrapings and cuttings on a special growth medium to show the actual presence and specific identity of fungi (82). The procedure can be ordered and performed only at the direction of a physician. However, microscopic confirmation probably will be possible only in the dry, scaly type. The recovery of fungi for diagnosis decreases as athlete's foot becomes progressively more severe (81). In typical cases of dermatophytosis complex, fungus recovery rates are only about 25–50% (5).

The pharmacist should question the patient thoroughly as to the condition and its characteristics to determine a description of the condition, the extent of disease, previous patient compliance with medications, and any mitigating circumstances, such as diabetes or obesity, that would render the patient susceptible. Diabetics, for example, may present a mixed fungal and monilial infection.

The pharmacist should seek to distinguish tinea pedis from diseases with similar symptoms. Dermatitis, allergic contact dermatitis, and atopic dermatitis also may occur on the feet and should be treated by a podiatrist or other physician. Shoe dermatitis is perhaps the most common form of allergic contact dermatitis from clothing. Typically, lesions are more common than tinea pedis on the dorsum of the foot. In children, peridigital dermatitis or atopic dermatitis is more common than tinea pedis. Recently, an 8-year-old boy developed contact allergy to accelerators, chemical compounds used to speed up the processing of rubber used in sponge-rubber insoles for tennis shoes (83). Since 1950, the increased use of rubber and adhesives in footwear has paralleled the increase in reports of shoe dermatitis in the dermatologic and podiatric literature. In addition to accelerators, antioxidants have frequently been implicated as major chemical allergens; various phenolic resins used in adhesives are also troublesome. A difficulty is that the patient is usually unaware that the footwear may be causing the problem.

Hyperhidrosis of the sole of the foot and infection of toe webs by Gram-negative bacteria are common. In hyperhidrosis, tender vesicles cover the sole of the foot and toes and may be quite painful. The skin generally turns white, erodes, and becomes macerated. This condition is accompanied by a foul foot odor.

Infection by Gram-negative bacteria is characterized by a soggy wetness of the toe webs and immediately adjacent skin (84). The affected tissue is damp, softened, and soggy. The last or next to last (adjacent to the little toe) toe webs are the most common areas of primary or initial involvement (84). The web between the fourth and fifth toes is deeper and extends more proximally than the web between the other toes. Furthermore, a semiocclusive anatomical setting, abundant exocrine sweat glands, and the added occlusion pro-

vided by footwear enhance development of the disease at this site. The pharmacist must be careful not to confuse this condition with soft corns, which also appear between the fourth and fifth toes.

Severe forms of this disease may progress to disintegration and denudation of the affected skin and profuse, serous, or purulent discharge. Denudation may involve all of the toe webs, the dorsal and plantar surfaces of the toes, and an area about 1 cm wide beyond the base of the toes on the plantar surface of the foot. When the disease is out of control, its progression is observed on the dorsum of the foot and the calf in the form of tiny red follicular crusts. This condition paradoxically may be caused by use of reputed germicidal soaps such as pHisoHex, Dial, and Safeguard (84). It was hypothesized that these soaps reduce harmless saprophytes and thus promote resistant pathogens (such as *Pseudomonas aeruginosa* and *Proteus mirabilis*) by removing their competitors.

If the patient has used a nonprescription antifungal product appropriately for several weeks without relief, a disease other than tinea pedis may be involved. Therapeutic failure may be due to Gram-negative athlete's foot; no nonprescription antifungal product will ameliorate the condition. Persons suffering from hyperhidrosis, allergic contact dermatitis, atopic dermatitis, or a possible Gram-negative infection of the toe should see a podiatrist or family physician for treatment.

Treatment

Before self-medication can be effective, the correct type of tinea pedis and correct treatment must be evaluated. Treatment of an acute, superficial tinea foot infection may be effective if certain conditions are met. In acute, inflammatory tinea pedis, characterized by reddened, oozing, and vesicular eruptions, the inflammation must be counteracted before antifungal therapy can be instituted. This step is especially important if the eruptions are caused by a secondary bacterial infection (77).

Hydrocortisone, in conjunction with clioquinol (formerly iodochlorhydroxyquin), demonstrated favorable results toward a resolution of uncomplicated cutaneous fungal infections (tinea cruris, tinea pedis, and moniliasis) (85). Erythema and itching were relieved more with the combination of these two drugs than by either drug itself or the placebo cream. However, with the availability of nonprescription topical hydrocortisone products, it is conceivable that the indiscriminate use of one of these products for the relief of the itching and redness of athlete's foot could complicate and delay appropriate medical care (86). Topical hydrocortisone by itself is contraindicated in the presence of fungal infections.

Self-treatment is effective only if the patient understands the importance of compliance with all facets of the treatment plan. Specific antifungal products must be used appropriately in conjunction with other treatment measures, including general hygienic measures and local drying. Some clinical studies have demonstrated efficacy in the placebo groupings with local hygienic measures alone (74, 87).

The pharmacist should recommend that the patient consult a podiatrist or other physician in the following circumstances:

■ If the toenail is involved, topical treatment is ineffective and does not allay the condition until the disease's primary focus is treated with oral griseofulvin or ketoconazole or until other preventive measures are instituted (surgical avulsion, or tearing away of the nail).

■ If vesicular eruptions are oozing, including purulent material that could indicate a secondary bacterial infection, topical astringent therapy and/or antibiotic therapy may be appropriate.

■ If the interspace between the toes is foul smelling, whitish, painful, very soggy, characterized with erosions, oozing, or serious inflammation, and especially if the condition is disabling, the patient should be referred to a physician. Fortunately, this variety is not common (81).

■ If the foot is seriously inflamed or swollen and a major portion is involved, supportive therapy must be instituted before an antifungal agent may be applied.

■ If the patient is a child who presents with an eczematous eruption of the feet, including that complicated by blisters and/or pyoderma, self-treatment should not be recommended.

■ If the patient is under a physician's supervision for a disease, such as diabetes or asthma, where the normal defense mechanism may be deficient, nonprescription products should not be used.

Pharmacologic Agents

The pharmacologic agents used to treat athlete's foot have been evaluated for safety and efficacy by the FDA advisory review panel on OTC antimicrobial drug products (II) (88). Table 2 lists these agents according to assigned category. The panel concluded that to best serve all consumers, a nonprescription product must provide more than temporary symptomatic relief of athlete's foot, jock itch, and ringworm. Such products must contain a Category I antifungal ingredient capable

of killing the fungus. The panel required each antifungal ingredient to have at least one well-designed clinical trial demonstrating its effectiveness in the treatment of athlete's foot in order to be classified as Category I. The panel also believed that these ingredients used to treat athlete's foot will also be effective for jock itch and ringworm because the infecting organisms of these conditions effect athlete's foot as well. However, the panel recognized that the groin area represented a more sensitive and easily irritated area compared to the feet and recommended that any antifungal products intended to treat jock itch have a low potential for irritation.

Carbolfuchsin Solution Basic fuchsin (NF XIII) dye is a mixture of rosaniline and pararosaniline hydrochlorides. It is used only in superficial fungal foot infections in the form of carbolfuchsin solution (NF XIII) or Castellani's paint. The solution is dark purple but appears red when painted onto the affected area in a fine film. It has local anesthetic, drying, and antimicrobial properties.

The use of carbolfuchsin solution in tinea pedis is indicated in the subacute or chronic stages of infection when there is little or no inflammation. The solution should not be applied to inflamed or denuded skin.

In one study, carbolfuchsin solution demonstrated equivalent efficacy to a 30% aluminum chloride solution for interdigital dermatophytosis (6). The drying and antimicrobial properties of carbolfuchsin are well suited for the ultrasoggy, steaming athlete's foot. However, the medication's staining properties and poisonous nature limit its usefulness.

Before the solution is applied, the affected area should be cleaned thoroughly with soap and water and dried. The solution then is applied to the area with an applicator and reapplied once or twice daily for 1 week. If the condition has not improved after this time, choice of medication as well as assessment of the actual condition should be reevaluated.

The efficacy of carbolfuchsin solution must be questioned, especially if an infected toenail is involved. Because the preparation contains several volatile components, the bottle cap should be securely tightened to avoid evaporation. Otherwise, volatile ingredients escape, causing other nonvolatile components (resorcinol) to become more concentrated, and irritation may result with subsequent applications.

Although carbolfuchsin solution is an effective agent, it should not be applied to an area greater than 10% of the foot or to a severely inflamed foot because of systemic toxicity if percutaneously absorbed. This limitation, its staining properties, and possible patient sensitivity to the product ingredients limit the usefulness of carbolfuchsin solution for tinea pedis. This is unfortunate because carbolfuchsin solution possesses all facets necessary for effective athlete's foot therapy.

The solution suppresses fungi and bacteria and simultaneously produces a local drying or astringent effect. Testimonial evidence indicates that the extemporaneous preparation and use of the paint without the fuchsin dye may be just as effective and more esthetically acceptable (89, 90). The FDA advisory panel on OTC antimicrobial drug products (11) has classified basic fuchsin into Category III (88).

Clioquinol Clioquinol (formerly iodochlorhydroxyquin) has demonstrated efficacy in the treatment of both athlete's foot and jock itch. Based on the review of the literature, the FDA advisory panel classified it as safe and effective for topical nonprescription use in the treatment of athlete's foot and jock itch. Evaluations of clioquinol used alone and in combination with hydrocortisone indicated the following effectiveness, from highest to lowest: clioquinol–hydrocortisone combination > clioquinol alone > hydrocortisone alone > placebo. Clioquinol has a low incidence of side effects; however, itching, redness, and irritation are possible with its use. Even though the possibility of its percutaneous absorption is low, clioquinol may interfere with thyroid function tests. Thus, patients undergoing these tests must be questioned carefully to assess use of clioquinol.

Clioquinol is also used to treat diaper rash; concerns for its safety in this regard have been raised. In 1985, a petition for a ban on clioquinol was submitted to the FDA from the Public Citizen's Health Research Group on the basis of studies performed on five dogs (91). In the experiment, a cream dosage form of clioquinol (3%) was applied twice daily to the skin for 28 days. After application the skin was covered with plastic to simulate conditions with a disposable diaper. During the course of the treatment all dogs lost weight and became lethargic and less responsive to stimuli; one dog developed paralysis of its hind legs. Autopsy demonstrated liver damage in all dogs, and periodic blood levels during the study demonstrated significant blood levels of the clioquinol from percutaneous absorption. Although it is difficult to extrapolate these findings to humans, caution is advised. Those who do use topical clioquinol should be monitored for any signs or symptoms of neurologic toxicity, for example, abdominal pain, weakness or paralysis of the legs, or muscle twitching.

Miconazole Nitrate Miconazole nitrate is an imidazole derivative that demonstrates fungicidal efficacy against *T. mentagrophytes*, *T. rubrum*, and *Candida albicans*. It acts by inhibiting the biosynthesis of ergosterol, a constituent of fungal plasma membranes (92). This inhibition leads to disruption of the plasma membrane and consequential leakage of cellular contents. Its spectrum of activity also includes Gram-positive bacteria. Controlled studies have demonstrated its effectiveness

for jock itch and athlete's foot. Miconazole nitrate would be expected to demonstrate comparable efficacy to tolnaftate and haloprogin for tinea pedis. In the event of primary failure with tolnaftate or haloprogin where patient factors (e.g., compliance, proper foot hygiene program) have been ruled out as a problem, it can be suggested as an alternate retreatment modality. Occasional side effects with its use include burning, irritation, and maceration of tissue.

The FDA advisory panel also recommended that this agent be classified as Category I for the treatment of external feminine itching associated with vaginal yeast (i.e., candidal) infections and superficial infections caused by species of *Candida* (88). It is conceivable that in the future, products with miconazole nitrate and nystatin, both approved by this panel, would be available on a nonprescription basis to treat vaginal yeast infections. Although a woman might not be expected to diagnose vaginal candidiasis the first time she has the infection, some gynecologists believe that women are capable of self-diagnosing recurring vaginal yeast infections.

Tolnaftate Tolnaftate's spectrum of action encompasses typical fungi responsible for tinea pedis, including *T. mentagrophytes* and *T. rubrum*. It is also effective against *E. floccosum* and species of *Microsporum*. Although the exact mechanism of action of tolnaftate has not been reported, it is believed that it distorts the hyphae and stunts the mycelial growth of the fungi species. Tolnaftate is more effective in tinea pedis than in onychomycosis or tinea capitis. For onychomycosis or tinea capitis, concomitant administration of oral griseofulvin or ketoconazole is necessary, unless the condition is superficial.

Tolnaftate is well tolerated when applied to intact or broken skin in either exposed or intertriginous areas. Tolnaftate usually stings slightly when applied. Although there has been one report of a developed delayed hypersensitivity reaction to tolnaftate, there have been no references to hypersensitivity associated with its use (93). As with all topical medications, irritation, sensitization, or worsening of the skin condition warrants discontinuance of the product.

Tolnaftate (1% solution or 1% cream) is applied sparingly twice daily after the affected area is cleaned thoroughly. Effective therapy usually takes 2–4 weeks, although treatment lasting 4–6 weeks may be necessary with some individuals (patients with lesions between the toes or on pressure areas of the foot). When medication is applied to pressure areas of the foot, where the horny skin layer is thicker than normal, concomitant use of a keratolytic agent may be advisable. Neither keratolytic agents nor wet compresses, such as aluminum acetate solution (Burow's solution), which promote the healing of oozing lesions, interfere with the efficacy of tolnaftate. If weeping lesions are present, the inflammation should be treated before tolnaftate is applied.

The cream dosage form of tolnaftate is formulated in a polyethylene glycol 400-propylene glycol vehicle; the solution is formulated in polyethylene glycol 400. The solution may be more effective than the cream. These vehicles are particularly advantageous in superficial antifungal therapy because they are nonocclusive, nontoxic, nonsensitizing, water miscible, anhydrous, easy to apply, and efficient in delivering the drug to the affected area.

High molecular weight polyethylene glycol bases have been reported to form associated complexes with some medications, such as benzoic and salicylic acids. Although diffusion of the medication to the skin is adequate with polyethylene glycol bases, little percutaneous absorption occurs (94, 95). In regard to topical antifungal therapy, however, complex formation seems inconsequential because the role of the vehicle in this instance is to supply drug to the horny skin layer.

Tolnaftate solution solidifies when exposed to cold. However, if the preparation is allowed to warm, it will liquefy with no loss in potency.

The topical powder formulation of tolnaftate uses cornstarch–talc as the vehicle. This vehicle not only is an effective drug delivery system but also offers therapeutic advantage because of the water-retaining nature of the two agents. The topical aerosol formulation of tolnaftate includes talc and the propellant vehicle.

Tolnaftate has demonstrated marked clinical efficacy since its commercial introduction into the United States in 1965, and it has become the standard topical antifungal medication (96, 97). In addition, there has been a consistent absence of irritation and hypersensitivity to tolnaftate in cream, solution, or powder form, thus enabling its approval for nonprescription use.

Tolnaftate is valuable primarily in the dry, scaly type of athlete's foot. Superficial fungal infection relapse has occurred after tolnaftate therapy was discontinued (98). However, the relapse may have been caused by an inadequate treatment time, patient noncompliance with the medication, or the use of tolnaftate where oral griseofulvin or ketoconazole should have been instituted. Because tolnaftate does not possess antibacterial properties, its value must be viewed with skepticism for use in the soggy, macerated type of athlete's foot in which bacteria are involved (5, 81).

Organic Fatty Acids Studies of the antifungal effect of various fatty acids and their salts on dermatophytes reported encouraging clinical results with sodium propionate, a constituent of sweat (99). The sodium salt of caprylic acid (an eight-carbon fatty acid) was more effective than sodium undecylenate in treating dermatophytosis of the foot (100). However, both propionic and undecylenic acids are weakly fungistatic (101).

Whether organic fatty acids are more effective than sulfur and/or iodine preparations in treating superficial fungal infections is questionable. Organic acid preparations should be used, if at all, only for very mild or chronic forms of tinea pedis. The FDA advisory panel placed these agents into Category III (88).

These organic fatty acids and their salts are available in various dosage forms. The cream or ointment form usually is used at bedtime; solutions should be used for their soothing effects after a footbath. The powder usually is sprinkled into the socks and shoes in the morning.

Acetic Acid Acetic acid is delivered to the infected area as triacetin. The fungistatic activity of triacetin is based on the fact that at the neutral or alkaline pH of infected skin, fungal esterase enzymes cleave triacetin into acetic acid and glycerin (102). The acetic acid then effects antifungal activity by lowering the pH at the infection site. As the pH increases after the initial release of acetic acid, more acetic acid is generated by the enzymes, and the process is repeated. The efficacy of products containing triacetin has not been proven by controlled clinical trials (88). Because the ultimate efficacy of triacetin will depend on the presence of moisture for conversion to the active acetic acid, the FDA advisory panel on OTC antimicrobial drug products (II) placed this drug in Category III with the proviso it be recommended and used only for the soggy, wet form of athlete's foot (88).

Used topically, triacetin is relatively colorless and odorless. In the concentrations used, the small amount of acetic acid liberated is nonirritating to the skin in most cases. The corresponding incidence of sensitization also is low. However, the acetic acid formed may damage rayon fabrics, so the treated areas should be covered with a clean bandage. Triacetin must not come into contact with the eyes.

Triacetin is available in a number of topical dosage forms. These should be applied every morning and evening after thorough cleaning of the affected area. The product should be used until the infection has cleared entirely, then once a week as a preventive measure.

Undecylenic Acid–Zinc Undecylenate This combination is widely used and may be effective for various mild superficial fungal infections excluding those involving nails or hairy parts of the body. It is fungistatic and is effective in mild chronic cases of tinea pedis. Compound undecylenic acid ointment (USP XX) contains 5% undecylenic acid and 20% zinc undecylenate in a polyethylene glycol vehicle. It is believed that zinc undecylenate liberates undecylenic acid (the active antifungal entity) on contact with moisture (perspiration). In addition, zinc undecylenate has astringent properties because of the presence of zinc ion (103). This astringent activity decreases the irritation and inflammation of the infection.

Applied to the skin as an ointment, diluted solution, or dusting powder, the combination undecylenic acid–zinc undecylenate, is relatively nonirritating, and hypersensitivity reactions are not common. The undiluted solution, however, may cause transient stinging when applied to broken skin, because of its alcohol content. Caution must be exercised to ensure that these ingredients do not come into contact with the eye or that the powder is not inhaled.

The vehicle in compound undecylenic acid ointment has a water-miscible base, making it nonocclusive, removable with water, and easy to apply. The powder uses talc as its vehicle and absorbent. The aerosol contains menthol, which serves as a counterirritant and antipruritic. The solution contains 10% undecylenic acid in an isopropyl alcohol vehicle with either an applicator or spray pump container. The product is applied twice daily after the affected area is cleansed. The usual period for therapeutic results depends on the patient. However, if improvement does not occur in 2–4 weeks, the condition should be reevaluated and an alternative medication tried.

When the solution is sprayed or applied onto the affected area, the area should be allowed to air-dry. Otherwise, the possibility of water accumulation and further tissue maceration could exist. The relatively high alcohol concentration in these solutions could cause some burning with application. The rancid odor of undecylenic acid may be objectionable to some patients and may promote patient noncompliance.

A comparison study of two 20% zinc undecylenate–2% undecylenic acid powder formulations used in the treatment of tinea pedis demonstrated no difference in clinical efficacy between products (104). However, these two formulations collectively effected clinical and mycologic cures in 53% of the patients treated as compared with 7% of those treated with the talc vehicle or left untreated (using daily foot washings or changes of socks). There was no indication whether patients failing to respond to either formulation possessed the more severe forms of tinea pedis. Another study (105) with a powder containing the same active ingredients reported similar results. In this study, 88% of patients treated with the active powder had negative cultures after 4 weeks compared with 17% of those treated with placebo powder ($p < 0.001$).

Two clinical studies demonstrated the clinical effectiveness of undecylenic acid compared with tolnaftate (87, 106). One study demonstrated indistinguishable clinical and mycologic effects between undecylenic acid ointment and tolnaftate cream (87). Both formulations were superior to placebo (ointment base of the undecylenic acid) although the gross improvement toward erythema, fissuring, and vesiculation was slow. These medications seem best suited for the mild forms of athlete's foot characterized by dry scaling of tissue. In light of the prior studies, undecylenic acid and/or its derivatives (10–25% total undecylenate content) have been classified into Category I by the FDA advisory review panel on OTC antimicrobial drug products (II) for the treatment of athlete's foot (88).

Other preparations, such as ointments, powders, and tinctures, incorporate undecylenic acid (10%) by itself in the vehicle. This concentration has minor irritant effects on the skin.

Phenolic Compounds and Derivatives Phenol and resorcinol have been included in many topical antifungal products for their keratolytic or fungicidal effects. The fungicidal potency of resorcinol is about one-third that of phenol. Phenol is reported to be more effective in aqueous solutions than in glycerin or fats; it is relatively ineffective when incorporated into soaps (107).

Applied to unabraded skin in low concentrations, phenol causes warmth and a tingling sensation. Its irritant qualities usually restrict its effectiveness in athlete's foot remedies. To be fungicidal in these preparations, concentrations irritating to human skin generally must be used.

Resorcinol, in concentrations usually applied topically ($< 10\%$), is nonirritating; higher concentrations may be irritating. Resorcinol rarely produces allergic reactions.

Phenol and resorcinol resemble each other with regard to systemic action, particularly on the central nervous system (CNS). Thus, preparations containing either agent should never be applied to large areas or to irritated or denuded skin because of possible absorption and systemic toxicity. In the future, nonprescription phenol products will be limited to concentrations of 1.5% or less (108). Local and systemic toxicity may occur following the use of phenol-containing products covered with bandages or occlusive dressings. Therefore these products should be used with caution for athlete's foot because occlusive footwear could enhance its absorption. This percutaneous absorption would seem to be more favorable from the top of the foot rather than beneath the foot where the thick outer layer of skin would seem to inhibit any penetration. With the inherent safety problems associated with the use of phenol and the fact that sufficient data were lacking about phenol's efficacy for athlete's foot in concentrations equal to or less than 1.5%, the FDA advisory review panel on OTC antimicrobial drug products (II) classified phenol into Category II (88).

Chloroxylenol, a substituted phenol, is a nonirritating antiseptic agent. Chloroxylenol (0.5% solution) was reported to be effective in treating and preventing athlete's foot (109). It is included in some topical preparations in liquid, cream, and powder forms. Chloroxylenol's limited water solubility makes its efficacy in powder drug delivery systems questionable. If the inert agents of the vehicle are effective in adsorbing moisture, the effect of the chloroxylenol may be diminished. Chloroxylenol causes no cutaneous irritation up to concentrations of 5% (110). It is less toxic than phenol, but eczematous reactions have followed its use (111). Because efficacy data are lacking, chloroxylenol was placed in Category III by the FDA advisory panel on OTC antimicrobial drug products (II) (88).

Salicylic Acid In high concentrations, salicylic acid is a keratolytic agent, causing the keratin layer of the skin to shed, thereby facilitating penetration of other drugs. Lower concentrations (< 2%) are keratoplastic; they aid normal keratinization. Salicylic acid (5–10%) softens the stratum corneum by increasing the endogenous hydration of this layer. This effect probably results from lowering the pH, which causes the cornified epithelium to swell, soften, macerate, and then desquamate (75). If no moisture is present, cornified epithelium is not softened significantly by tolerable amounts of salicylic acid. Because salicylic acid accelerates exfoliation of the infected keratin tissue, its use in conjunction with topical antifungals may be very beneficial in appropriate conditions (98).

Salicylic acid alone has little or no antifungal activity. It usually is applied to the skin as a combination of 3% salicylic acid and 6% benzoic acid in a polyethylene glycol base (Whitfield's ointment). Benzoic acid alone is alleged to have some fungistatic activity, but this claim is debatable. This ointment is available in double strength and half strength. The half-strength formula (1.5% salicylic acid) does not have the keratolytic properties of the regular or double strength and therefore should never be used when keratolytic activity is necessary. The basic criterion for evaluating the efficacy of salicylic acid products as keratolytic agents is the concentration of salicylic acid. Thus, on the basis of current literature, these products should contain concentrations of more than 2% salicylic acid. Because there was insufficient evidence to support either salicylic or benzoic acid for the treatment of athlete's foot, these agents were classified as Category III by the FDA advisory review panel on OTC antimicrobial drug products (II) (88).

The pharmacist should be aware of the irritant properties of topically applied salicylic acid. Many skin irritations have been reported following unsupervised self-medication.

Quaternary Ammonium Compounds Quaternary ammonium compounds (benzethonium chloride and methylbenzethonium chloride) are used in several antifungal aids for their skin antiseptic and detergent properties. Solutions of these agents have emulsifying properties that favor wetting and penetration of surfaces to which they are applied. The fungicidal activity of quaternary ammonium compounds is generally less than their bactericidal activities (112). (See Chapter 28, *Topical Anti-infective Products.*)

The disinfectant action of these compounds may not be as great as expected. Gram-positive microorganisms generally are more susceptible to the effect of quaternary ammonium compounds than are Gram-negative pathogens. A concern with quaternary ammonium compounds is that their misuse or overuse could lead to overgrowth of species of *Pseudomonas* or other Gram-negative pathogens, especially in debilitated patients. This possibility should be kept in mind with nonprescription antifungal products, although this occurrence would be expected to be rare with the use of low concentrations of quaternary ammonium compounds. These agents are cationic and have a chemical incompatibility with anionic compounds such as soaps. Thus, any residual soap or soap film on the skin may inactivate them (113). Patients who are told to clean their feet thoroughly every day also must be instructed to rinse the affected area thoroughly before drying it. Otherwise, if the nonprescription product contains a quaternary ammonium compound, any beneficial effects may be negated. This precaution should also be considered for any formulations of these products that contain anionic compounds (zinc undecylenate and sodium propionate) to prevent the germicide from being rendered ineffective (112).

A tincture delivery system of these cationic compounds is more effective as a skin disinfectant and is less affected by soap than an aqueous solution (114). Accordingly, tincture forms of these agents are used in more dilute concentrations than aqueous solutions.

Therefore, in a liquid form, especially a tincture, quaternary compounds should be effective if appropriate concentrations are used. However, when applied topically in powder form with adsorbent agents included in the formulation, their efficacy is doubtful. If all moisture is removed effectively by the adsorbing material, the quaternary compound may be unable to dissolve and exert its germicidal activity, although these compounds dissolve in a minimal amount of water.

Quaternary ammonium compounds generally are safe when applied topically. However, the assignment of quaternary ammonium compounds (most notably benzethonium chloride) to Category III indicates a need for substantive data relevant to efficacy (88). However, each compound has its own sensitization index and its own ability to produce contact dermatitis resulting from widespread usage and multiple exposures to these chemicals.

Quinoline Derivatives Of 24 quinoline derivatives investigated in vitro, only benzoxiquine (8-hydroxyquinoline benzoate) salt was active in fungistatic and fungicidal testing (115). It has been postulated that the activity of 8-hydroxyquinoline is caused by the chelation of trace metals, essential for the growth of fungi, in either the nutritive media or the cell of the fungus (116). A 3% benzoxiquine preparation in a vanishing cream base was fungicidal in vitro when compared to other antifungal ointments (101). Subsequently, an antifungal preparation containing 2.5% benzoxiquine was used successfully in the treatment of dermatophytosis (117).

Several proprietary powder antifungals use 8-hydroxyquinoline sulfate in their formulations. This compound is fungicidal. Because the sulfate salt is fairly water soluble and forms an acidic solution in the presence of moisture, it may enhance the antifungal effect of 8-hydroxyquinoline. However, there is no clinical evidence to support the hypothesis; these agents have been classified into Category III (88).

Salts of Aluminum Historically, the foremost astringent used for the acute inflammatory stage of tinea pedis and the wet, soggy type of tinea pedis has been aluminum acetate. However, evidence also supports the use of aluminum chloride in treating the wet, soggy type (6).

The action and efficacy of these aluminum salts appear to be two-pronged. First, these compounds act as astringents. Their drying ability probably involves the complexing of the astringent agent with proteins, thereby altering the proteins' ability to swell and hold water (6). These astringents decrease edema, exudation, and inflammation by reducing the cell membrane permeability and hardening the cement substance of the capillary epithelium. Second, aluminum salts in concentrations greater than 20%, aluminum chloride for instance, possess antibacterial activity. Aluminum chloride (20%) may exhibit its antibacterial activity in two ways: by directly killing bacteria and by drying the interspaces (6). Solutions of 20% aluminum acetate and 20% aluminum chloride demonstrated equal in vitro antibacterial efficacy (6).

Aluminum acetate solution for use in tinea pedis generally is diluted with about 10–40 parts of water. Depending on the situation, the patient either immerses the whole foot in the solution for 20 minutes up to 3 times a day (every 6–8 hours) or applies the solution to the area in the form of a wet dressing. In a clinical trial, 10 subjects compared undiluted aluminum acetate solution (5%) to the recommended 1:20 dilution (of the 5% solution) on the macerated, soggy type of athlete's foot (6). After 7 days, the 5% solution produced moderate drying and symptomatic improvement in five subjects; the 1:20 dilution was ineffective.

For patient convenience, aluminum acetate solution (Burow's solution) or modified Burow's solution products are available in a number of dosage forms for immediate use (in solution) or for preparation with water (powder packets, powder, and effervescent tablets). These products are intended for external use only, are not to be ingested, and should be kept away from contact with eyes. Prolonged or continuous use of aluminum acetate solution may produce necrosis (118). In the acute inflammatory stage of the tinea pedis, this solution should be used less than 1 week. The pharmacist should instruct the patient to discontinue use of the solution if extensive inflammatory lesions appear to worsen or if irritation becomes more apparent.

Concentrations of 20–30% aluminum chloride have been the most beneficial for the wet, soggy type of athlete's foot (6). Twice-daily applications of aluminum chloride generally are used until the signs and symptoms, such as odor, wetness, and whiteness, abate. Once-daily applications control the symptoms after that time (119). In hot, humid weather, the original condition returns within 7–10 days after the application is stopped (119).

The application of aluminum salts does not entirely cure athlete's foot. This treatment merely shifts the disease process back to the simple dry type of athlete's foot, which then can be controlled with other agents such as tolnaftate. Safety and efficacy data were submitted for only two aluminum compounds, alcloxa (aluminum chlorhydroxyallantoinate) and aluminum sulfate, to the FDA advisory review panel on OTC antimicrobial drug products (II). Due to a lack of sufficient data available on the effectiveness of these agents, both were classified as Category III (88).

Because aluminum salts penetrate skin poorly, the toxicity of salts like aluminum chloride is rather low. However, one study demonstrated a few cases of irritation in patients where deep fissures were present (6), so that the aluminum salt was able to come in contact with sensitive skin. Thus, a contraindication to the use of concentrated aluminum salt solutions would be severely eroded or deeply fissured skin. In these cases, dilution of the salts to a lower concentration (10% aluminum chloride) is necessary for initial treatment.

Used appropriately, aluminum acetate solution or aluminum chloride solution is valuable in the wet, soggy, macerated form of athlete's foot and in the acute inflammatory stages of athlete's foot. However, each solution has potential for misuse (accidental childhood poisoning by ingesting the solutions or ingesting the solid tablets), and precautions must be taken to prevent this occurrence.

Benzoyl Peroxide A 5% or 10% gel of benzoyl peroxide has been suggested for use in the symptomatic interdigital treatment of athlete's foot (120). The drying or astringent effect of this formulation, coupled with the antimicrobial activity of the benzoyl peroxide, offers the advantage of rapid clinical improvement of this form of tinea pedis. However, this product must be used with caution because it may be irritating, particularly to denuded areas or deep fissures. Prolonged use of benzoyl peroxide on inflamed or ulcerated skin should be avoided because of its strong sensitizing ability. (See Chapter 29, *Acne Products*.)

Other Ingredients and Dosage Forms The primary drug delivery systems used for treatment of tinea pedis are creams, solutions, and powders. Powders, including those in aerosol dosage forms, generally are indicated for adjunctive use with solutions and creams. In very mild conditions, powders may suffice as the only therapy.

Solution and cream forms should be formulated in a vehicle that is:

- Nonocclusive (it should not retain moisture or sweat, which exacerbates the condition);

- Water miscible or water washable (removable with minimal cleansing efforts) because hard scrubbing of the affected area further abrades the skin;

- Anhydrous, because including water in the formulation introduces a variable that is one of the primary causes of the condition;

- Spreadable with minimal effort and without waste;

- Capable of efficient drug delivery (it must not interact with the active ingredient, but allow it to penetrate to the seat of the fungal infection);

- Nonsensitizing and nontoxic when applied to intact or denuded skin, especially if it is absorbed into the systemic circulation.

Most vehicles used to deliver topical solutions and creams are essentially polyethylene glycol and alcohols, which meet these criteria. Polyethylene glycol bases deliver water-insoluble drugs topically more efficiently than water-soluble agents. This feature is an added advantage because most topical antifungal drugs are largely water insoluble (tolnaftate, for example).

Criteria for the powder dosage form (shaker or aerosol) are basically the same as those for creams or solutions. Certain agents in powder forms are therapeutic and also serve as vehicles (talc and cornstarch). Powders inhibit the propagation of fungi by adsorbing moisture and preventing skin maceration. Thus, they actually alter the ecologic conditions of the fungi, but the actual effective agent in these formulations is unknown (96). For example, the adsorbing material within the powder, rather than the intended active ingredient, might be responsible for the remission of the disease.

Many authorities consider cornstarch superior to talc for these formulations because it is virtually free of chemical contamination and does not tend to produce granulomatous reactions in wounds as readily as talc

(121). Moreover, a study comparing adsorbance showed that cornstarch adsorbed 25 times more moisture from moisture-saturated air than talc (122).

Product Selection Guidelines

Patient compliance is influenced by product selection. Therefore, the pharmacist should recommend an appropriate dosage form designed to cause the least interference with daily habits and activities without sacrificing efficacy. Product selection should be geared to the individual patient. For example, elderly patients may require a preparation that is extremely easy to use; obese patients, in whom excessive sweating may contribute to the disease, should use topical talcum powders as adjunctive therapy.

Before recommending a nonprescription product, the pharmacist should review the patient's medical history. For example, diabetics should have their blood glucose levels moderately controlled because increased glucose in sweat may promote fungus growth (109). Patients with allergic dermatitides are extremely sensitive to most oral and topical agents. Such patients usually have a history of asthma, hay fever, or atopic dermatitis, which is indicated on the medication profile. Thus, the pharmacist can distinguish a tinea infection from atopic dermatitis and avoid recommending a product that may cause skin irritation.

The concentration of organic fatty acids and/or their salt forms usually is too low to irritate the skin. Although these products are nonsensitizing, treatment should be discontinued if irritation or sensitivity develops with their use.

The pharmacist should bear in mind that in some cases prescription-only drugs may be more beneficial than nonprescription products (123, 124). In the soggy, macerated athlete's foot complicated by bacterial infection, the broad-spectrum antifungal agents econazole nitrate and clotrimazole are preferable to both tolnaftate and the prescription drug haloprogin (5).

Patient Consultation

The pharmacist should advise patients not to expect dramatic remission of the condition. The onset of symptomatic relief may take several days because generally healing is gradual. Patients should be advised that depending on certain factors (extent of the affected area and patient variability to medication), the medication may have to be used a minimum of 2–4 weeks. The

FDA advisory panel recommended that products used for athlete's foot should effect improvement within 4 weeks (88). For jock itch, the panel recommended that improvement of the condition should be seen within 2 weeks (88). If there is no improvement within these time frames, the patient should consult a physician. The patient should be told of the necessity to adhere to the physician-prescribed dosage regimen or the suggested directions on the product label. Although patient noncompliance is not documented, it probably contributes to the failure of topical products in treating tinea pedis. The pharmacist should advise the patient to continue the medication for a few days beyond the recommended time period to help prevent relapse.

All topical antifungal products may induce various hypersensitivity reactions. Although the incidence of hypersensitivity is small, patients should be advised to discontinue the product if itching, swelling, or exacerbation of the disease occurs. In addition, patients should avoid contact of the product with the eyes. After applying the product, patients should thoroughly wash their hands with soap and water.

The pharmacist should emphasize the need for proper hygiene before effective drug therapy for athlete's foot can be instituted. The feet should be cleaned and thoroughly dried each day. Even though transmission of the disease to other individuals may be rare, patients should have their own washcloths and towels. The affected area should be thoroughly patted dry. After bathing, the feet should be dried last so the towel does not spread the infection to other sites.

General measures should be taken to eliminate the predisposing factors of heat and perspiration. Shoes and light cotton socks that allow ventilation should be worn. Wool and some synthetic fabrics interfere with foot moisture dissipation. Occlusive footwear, including canvas rubber-soled athletic shoes, should not be worn. Shoes should be alternated as often as possible so that the inside can adequately dry. Socks should be changed daily and washed thoroughly after use. Shoes should be dusted with drying powders. Interestingly, there was a mycologic improvement in 25% of the test population that used a topical placebo formulation with preventive hygienic measures (87).

Clothing and towels should be changed frequently and laundered well in hot water. The feet, particularly the area between the toes, should be dusted with a drying powder at every change of socks. Whenever possible, the feet should be aired to prevent moisture buildup. Dr. Scholl's Smooth Touch Pedi-spreads or cotton balls may be placed between the tips of the toes to keep the web spaces open. Pencil erasers have been recommended for this purpose, but they may contain sensitizing accelerators or antioxidants. Nonocclusive protective footwear (e.g., rubber or wooden sandals) should be worn in areas of family or public use such as home bathrooms or community showers.

Individuals whose feet perspire excessively may find odor-controlling insoles (e.g., Odor Attackers, Sneaker Snuffers) useful for casual dress or sports activities. These insoles are useful because they absorb moisture and prevent the growth of odor-causing bacteria. An added advantage is that these insoles also provide some support and cushioning for the feet. Patients must be advised, however, to change insoles routinely.

The pharmacist should inform the patient of the need for protective measures that aid the topical antifungal product in eradicating the fungal infection. However, patients should be cautioned against overzealous cleansing with soap and water and vigorous drying between the toes; this practice may further irritate the area.

Because dermatophytes thrive on moist warm wood, public baths and shower areas should not be constructed with wooden grills (80).

Serious Conditions that Affect the Feet

It is important for the pharmacist to realize that chronic disease states predispose certain patients to foot problems. Most noteworthy is the diabetic patient in whom poor blood circulation and diminished limb sensitivity are complications of this disease process. These factors make the diabetic especially vulnerable to foot problems. Other vulnerable patients include those with peripheral circulatory disease and/or arthritis. The pharmacist can identify these patients by asking appropriate questions about daily medication use or reviewing the patient's drug profile. Typical drugs for these conditions include insulin, oral antidiabetic medications, drugs for circulation (e.g., cyclandelate, isoxsuprine, nylidrin, papaverine, pentoxifylline), and/or drugs for arthritic conditions (e.g., aspirin, nonsteroidal anti-inflammatory drugs).

It has been estimated that 25% of diabetics (12 million nationwide as of 1988) will develop severe foot or leg problems within their lifetimes; 20% of hospitalizations for diabetics are due to foot infections, accounting for more in-hospital days than any other complication of this disease (125). Diabetics are 17 times more likely than nondiabetics to develop gangrene of the extremities; approximately two-thirds of all nontraumatic amputations occur in diabetics, accounting for almost 40,000 amputations a year (125).

The safety of nonprescription products for the feet depends on the absence of any mitigating circumstances that contraindicate their use; therefore, diabetic patients should be under the care of a podiatrist or other physician for their foot care needs. (See Chapter 16, *Diabetes Care Products*.) However, the pharmacist can educate the diabetic about simple foot care guidelines, as follows:

- Inspect the feet every day. If the diabetic's eyesight is poor, a family member should inspect the feet.

- Control the diabetic disease process through diet, exercise, and drug therapy. Tight control is linked to decreasing long-term complications of the disease.

- Prevent cracks and fissures from occurring on the feet through a daily foot bath and application of a skin moisturizer. However, do not apply the moisturizer between the toes because it may promote the development of a bacterial or fungal infection.

- Sprinkle a foot powder into the socks every day if the feet perspire excessively.

- Gradually break in new shoes and limit the time they are worn each day.

- Avoid using nonprescription foot care products without the knowledge of a podiatrist or other physician.

- Avoid using pumice stones to mechanically debride corns or calluses; never use a razor blade to remove a corn, callus, wart, or bunion because of the danger of a resultant infection.

- Wash the foot in mild soap and water every day; use only a mild disinfectant such as ST–37; do not use strong disinfecting agents such as tincture of iodine or phenol.

- Initiate prompt care of the foot for any cuts or scratches and seek medical attention as soon as possible. Apply a clean, sterile dressing to the injured area using paper tape. Never use adhesive tape because it will make the skin soggy and encourage the growth of microorganisms and can be irritating when removed.

- Do not use hot water bottles or heating blankets on the feet because these devices can result in serious injury to the skin.

- When traveling, remember to maintain foot care and inspect the feet often.

Patients with poor circulation of the feet may complain of persistent, unusual feelings of cold, numbness, tingling, burning, or fatigue in the feet and the legs. Other symptoms may include discolored skin, dry skin, absence of hair on the feet or legs, or a cramping or tightness in the leg muscles.

If a review of the patient's medication history does not indicate use of medications intended to relieve these symptoms, the patient with suspected circulatory problems should be advised to consult a physician or podiatrist for evaluation.

A daily foot bath is a simple measure that will assist these patients. After the foot is patted dry, an emollient foot cream can be applied to help the skin of the foot retain moisture and pliability. The foot bath also will soften brittle toenails for clipping and filing. The feet should be kept warm and moderately exercised every day.

Arthritic patients, particularly those with osteoarthritis or rheumatoid arthritis, are also vulnerable to foot problems. See Chapter 5, *Internal Analgesic Products*, for a review of rheumatoid arthritis. Osteoarthritis is a noninflammatory degenerative joint disease that occurs primarily in older people. The degeneration of the articular cartilage and changes in the bone result in a loss of resilience and a decrease in the skeleton's shock absorption capability.

Proper foot care is especially important for arthritics and should include properly cushioning and padding the shoes with insoles to protect feet from the shock of hard surfaces. These patients should wear properly fitted shoes and undergo regular podiatric or medical examinations.

Exercise-Induced Foot Problems

The pharmacist should be aware of the problem of exercise-induced foot injuries, particularly those caused by running or jogging. Frequently, individuals fail to take certain precautions in their rush to recapture physical fitness and dive headlong into a strenuous exercise program that can cause injury. Individuals, especially those over 36 years of age, should consult a physician before embarking on a training program. The physician can provide advice and ensure the individual's capability for such a program. Jogging and running are not without risk; one study demonstrated that several participants have died from heart attacks, specifically coronary heart disease, while jogging (126). In addition, persons whose heavy smoking, prolonged lack of exercise, high blood pressure, or family history of heart disease or diabetes, should check with a physician before starting out. For some of these patients, an exercise test is advisable to determine the capacity of the heart under exercise conditions. Further, the individual should use the most enjoyable form of exercise, such as walking briskly, jogging, or swimming, so that exercise becomes a valuable part of a weight-reduction or fitness program. A vigorous walking program may be a more prudent form of exercise for middle-aged, flabby, unconditioned individuals, and may minimize potential orthopedic problems incurred from the more strenuous forms of exercise, such as jogging (127).

Several characteristics distinguish the jogger from the runner. In general, joggers attempt to maintain physical fitness by jogging about 2–4 miles per day at most, no more than 3–4 days per week. At a pace of 9–12 minutes per mile, joggers enjoy the psychologic pleasures that the sport affords (128). On the other hand, runners continually attempt to improve pace and distance. Usually the runner's mileage exceeds 4 miles per day with a pace under 8 minutes per mile. Runners will usually work out every day and compete either with themselves or others. These individuals enjoy the psychologic aspects of the completion of a hard workout. It has been demonstrated that those individuals who are athletically conditioned exhibit increased levels of beta-endorphins (129). These peptides are thought to have opium-like properties, which cause euphoria and have been linked to the "addiction" to running that many runners exhibit.

Jogging and running occasionally must be interrupted to allow the person to rest an injured leg or foot. Relative rest (that is, avoiding activities that produce the symptoms) is often indicated, but some runners resist this suggestion. The pharmacist should encourage alternative exercise modes, such as swimming, running in water with the aid of a floatation device, or bicycling (stationary or outdoor). This allows the serious runner to maintain aerobic conditioning and minimize guilt about missing regular exercise.

Prevention is the best way to treat foot problems. This entails the use of proper footwear, running environment, and running posture. Most running injuries can be successfully treated with shoe modifications, in-shoe supports, shoe alterations, correction for leg length discrepancies, modification of training methods, ice applications, and stretching exercises.

Many traumatic injuries can be prevented by adoption of commonsense measures, which include running without headphones, running on a roadside toward traffic, running in single file when in a group, and wearing light-colored clothing and reflective gear for high visibility. The latter is very important because drivers often encounter visibility problems caused by sun, snow, or the time of day.

The approximate locations of the more common foot and leg injuries arising from foot shock in exercise-related activities are shown in Figure 4.

Proper Footwear Numerous manufacturers provide a variety of shoes for running. A good running shoe should provide the runner with cushioning, support, and stability (130). At the same time, the shoe should maintain its flexibility, softness, and lightness. Running shoes usually have a waffle tread and a deep toe box area. Basketball shoes, tennis shoes, and base-

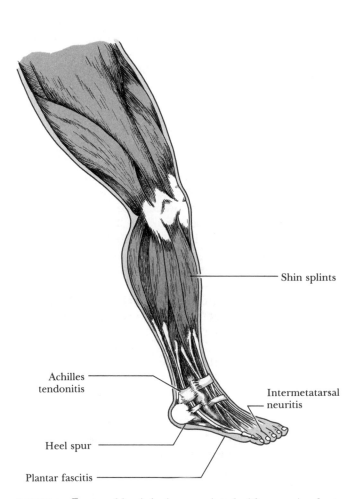

FIGURE 4 Foot and leg injuries associated with excessive foot shock.

ball shoes are not designed for running and should never be worn for this purpose (131). Jogging and running shoes should fit immediately, as opposed to ice skates or ski boots which have to be "worked in." The toes should have ample room, but there should be no slip in the heel. The toes should not feel crunched or squeezed into the toe box. If the shoe is too loose, however, the foot tends to move forward during the foot strike onto the running surface, causing a callus on the plantar surface of the ball of the foot or blood blisters under the toenail.

Buying a fitness shoe can be very confusing. Because there are so many shoes from which to select, the most important step is finding the right store and salesperson. Shoes are an important piece of equipment and they change so frequently that it is important to find a salesperson who is conscientious and knowledgeable and a shoe store that provides good service. A specialty store is more likely to have personnel dedicated to working with the client; an all-purpose sports store or a department store is less likely to have knowledgeable salespeople. A shoe store owned and operated by an active sports enthusiast is probably the best choice.

Pharmacists should advise patients to seek out sales personnel who have experience in the sport in which the patients are participating. Salespeople with little or no experience or those who try to hurry through a sale should be avoided. The buyer should understand that service is as important as the shoe.

Clients should understand that a quality fitness shoe is not inexpensive. A pair of high-quality running shoes may cost between $35 and $100. However, there is no relationship between the best shoe and the most expensive. The buyer should tell the salesperson the price range that can be afforded.

When purchasing a pair of shoes, the client should wear socks of the thickness that will be worn when exercising. It is also helpful if the buyer brings the pair of shoes that is being replaced. Shoe wear patterns will help the salesperson recommend footwear. It is also helpful to shop later in the day because the feet are most swollen at this time; sometimes one foot may actually be larger than the other. The shoes should feel comfortable from the start and should not require ''breaking in.''

When purchasing athletic footwear, the buyer should look at more than one pair of the same shoes because it is not unusual for at least one shoe in the pair to be poorly constructed and put onto the market without proper inspection. The buyer should closely inspect the shoes and watch for defects. If a defect is found, the buyer should ask for another pair of the same model. If no other pairs are available, the buyer should go to another store for the preferred model.

Once joggers or runners find a particular shoe model that works for them, they should repurchase the same model until it is discontinued by the manufacturer. However, they should not continue to wear worn footwear because they cannot find the same model. Many people are unaware that injuries can be prevented by replacing old, worn athletic shoes. Experienced runners will often report that nagging injuries developed because they continued to use worn shoes. Buying a new pair of shoes is an effective method of self-treatment for repetitive use injuries to the lower extremities. Attempting to get a few more miles or days out of a worn-out pair of athletic shoes is not cost effective if it leads to an injury.

The upper part of the shoe provides much of its stability. Cushioning is provided primarily by the shoe's midsole. Unfortunately, many athletes mistakenly assume a shoe is worn out by examining only the outer sole. The outer sole is perhaps the least important in terms of support or cushioning. It is the midsole that wears out first, especially if a person has rigid, high-arched feet.

The midsole is between the outer sole and the upper sole. Its primary function is to provide cushioning. However, the shoe industry has encountered difficulty in finding appropriate material for the midsole. Manufacturers are researching materials, including air bladders, gel packets, and water pockets, in an attempt to improve the midsole's shock absorbency and fatigue characteristics.

Studies of running shoes have demonstrated that they lose 60% of their initial shock absorption capacity after 250–500 miles of use (132). For a runner who runs an average of 20 miles per week, this translates to 3–6 months of shoe wear. It is difficult to determine when the midsole of the shoe becomes worn out. An early sign of fatigue is the development of wrinkles in the material of the midsole. A rule is that the shoe should be replaced when the midsole loses 10% of its original thickness. To determine this, the runner should measure the thickness of the midsole when the shoes are purchased and remeasure periodically to check for loss of thickness. The compression of the midsole typically occurs in a focused area, for example, in the lateral heel, under the ball of the foot.

Another sign of shoe fatigue is the deviation of the heel counter, which cups the heel. To determine this a person can look at the shoe from behind while it is on a flat surface. The shoes should be replaced if the heel counter of either shoe is deviated toward the inside or outside. Further, if the heel counter gives under when squeezed with the fingers, it is fatigued and no longer capable of providing support.

Running Environment A number of runners enjoy the exhilaration of running out of doors, while others retreat to a favorite indoor track. The outdoor runner must be particularly cautious and understand the implications of hazards, such as unfriendly dogs, motorists, and weather (e.g., hot, humid, cold, rainy).

Regardless of the running environment, the runner should carry appropriate identification. Incidents have been reported in which runners have been brought for emergency care without identification; if the patient is unconscious, vital information is usually unobtainable (133). A simple waterproof identification card with basic information is appropriate.

The Running Surface The convenience of the runner often dictates the running surface (e.g., concrete sidewalk, grassy surfaces, dirt shoulder of roads). Hard surfaces encourage intense shock to the legs, feet, and back. These surfaces are ill-advised because they have no give and provide little shock-absorbing capacity. Grassy surfaces are often irregular, and an unsuspecting runner can easily incur a sprained ankle. Running on a sloping or banked surface (e.g., shoulder of a road) may cause the foot on the higher part of the slope to rotate excessively and place additional stress on the tendons and ligaments of the leg and foot (134). Uphill running places a strain on the Achilles tendon and the muscles of the lower back; downhill running places much impact on the heel.

The ideal running surface is relatively smooth, level, and resilient (e.g., dirt track). However, a compromise might have to be made if this is not obtainable. Basically, the runner should minimize running on hard surfaces, running uphill or downhill, and running on banked surfaces.

Warmup Exercises Some type of preliminary physical activity or warmup exercise is believed to be important in physiologically or psychologically preparing for an event, and may reduce the chance of injury to joints and muscles. During the warmup period, the cardiovascular system is put on notice and prepared for the rigor of the workout. The heart increases its rate and volume per beat, ensuring that sufficient amounts of oxygenated blood will be supplied to the working muscles. The warmup period effects a slight rise in muscle and body temperature for an optimal metabolic and physiologic environment (135).

The length of the warmup period depends on the participant. However, it should not be so protracted or rigorous that it depletes muscle glycogen and leaves the person physically fatigued and mentally dull for the workout.

To help soothe aching muscles before a workout, some persons may use a counterirritant (e.g., methyl salicylate). However, there is no conclusive evidence to suggest the effectiveness of this practice. Indeed it is ill-advised to continually use a drug such as this because the aching muscles may indicate a problem in training technique. See Chapter 32, *External Analgesic Products*, for appropriate information and instructions about methyl salicylate and other counterirritants.

Running Posture and Form Using the correct form is thought to be important in allowing the runner to run faster, more efficiently, and with less injury. However, there is insufficient evidence to support this contention or to specify the optimal running form. There is no simple prescription for efficient running because each person is unique (136). Running comes naturally and each person develops an individual running stride. Anyone can read about a correct running stride; however, developing an optimal running form is best performed under the direction of a trained individual who can suggest corrections to obvious faults (137). The pharmacist should be able to refer individuals who need suggestions about proper running form to a knowledgeable individual in the community (e.g., an athletic coach).

Treatment

The pharmacist may play a triage role in the treatment of an exercise-induced injury to the foot (138); that is, the pharmacist may decide whether the person should be referred to a physician or podiatrist, or whether a self-treatment program is advisable. When consulted by the patient for advice about foot injuries resulting from an exercise or jogging program, the pharmacist must ask appropriate questions. These questions are listed at the beginning of the chapter. Based on the individual's responses, the pharmacist can then advise patient referral or some form of nonprescription therapy.

Common causes of foot injuries in runners or joggers can be attributed to a disregard for sound, proper training techniques. Responses to questions may indicate that the person has had a number of continuous days of high-intensity workouts. It is essential that the body be allowed to recuperate after vigorous exercise; continual strenuous workouts cause accumulated fatigue and microtrauma. Some runners believe that the more mileage logged per week, the better their running ability; however, the incidence of acquired injuries among runners increases dramatically after 25–30 miles per week (139). In addition, an increased injury rate is observed in runners who increase mileage too rapidly. Strenuous back-to-back workouts in a short period of time should be avoided. Thus, a good training program entails "hard–easy" days, with extended mileage on 3 or 4 days per week and light, easy workouts (e.g., easy jogging, swimming, bicycling) on the remaining days (140).

If the runner answers yes to one or more of the questions listed earlier, the person should be advised to seek the assistance of a health care professional. It is often difficult for serious runners to recognize or admit that they have been training too hard. These individuals are more likely to heed the advice of a fellow runner; runners rarely accept as a final opinion the advice of a nonrunner health practitioner (141). Even if a fellow runner recommends cutting back on running, the injured runner still must make a personal decision based on the perceived risk-to-benefit ratio. Thus, the pharmacist can help the person arrive at a decision by sharing the risks of continued running or training, for example, rupture of a tendon or development of an overt stress fracture. This decision will usually involve an assessment of the benefit of continued running, for example, the next big race or the enjoyment of daily exercise.

Shin Splints The term "shin splints" is used generically by some to describe all the pain emanating from below the knee and above the ankle. Shin splints are an overuse phenomenon that occurs in runners or walkers who use hard surfaces (142). This condition can occur from running on a banked track or the sloped shoulder of a road, wearing improper footwear, or overstriding.

The typical complaint of a runner with shin splints is pain in the medial lower third of the shin that seems to increase gradually with the training program. The patient may admit that soreness begins after running; with a continual running program, the pain will eventually occur during and after running. Complaints of pain when walking or climbing stairs may indicate a serious case of shin splints, and the person should be advised to consult a physician, podiatrist, or physical therapist (134). If the discomfort is located on the anterior lateral aspect of the skin, is described as a "cramping, burning tightness," and occurs at the same distance or time during a run, the runner should be referred to an appropriate health care individual.

Relative rest and application of ice (e.g., ice bag, cold compression wrap) to the painful area are good initial treatments (143). The cold anesthetizes the area and effects a decrease in pain. Alternating compresses (30 minutes applied, 30 minutes off) is best. If longer application of cold is not tolerable to the patient, 8–10 minutes of application may be preferred. To ensure greater surface area contact, the patient should be advised to use crushed or shaved ice. In addition, aspirin or ibuprofen can be recommended to relieve pain and reduce tissue inflammation if the patient is not allergic to aspirin and can tolerate these drugs. The use of analgesics to suppress pain or increase endurance during a workout is not recommended.

Stress Fracture Stress fracture, also known as march, army, or fatigue fracture, is usually encountered in individuals who participate in endurance sports and is considered part of the leg overuse syndrome. It is not an overt break of the bone but rather an alteration in the architecture of the normal bone after repeated cyclic loading. This injury usually involves the long bones of the foot or the leg. Stress fractures are common in those who run repetitively on hard, inflexible surfaces, which increase the risk of bone fatigue and fracture (144).

The person suffering from a stress fracture will frequently complain of a deep pain in the lower leg with an area of extreme tenderness (145). The onset of pain is insidious and definitely associated with runners who drastically change aspects of their training routine, for example, running surface, speed, or distance. A misconception among runners is that they can "work out" the problem by continuing to jog (145). This can ultimately result in the person's inability to even stand.

These individuals must be instructed that pain is the body's communication mechanism to indicate that enough is enough, and that something is abnormal.

Treatment for stress fractures is complete rest from running, sometimes for 4–6 weeks, or longer if the tibia is involved.

Achilles Tendinitis Achilles tendinitis should be referred to a physician, podiatrist, or physical therapist because the exact cause of the problem is difficult to distinguish. It is not caused solely by running, but may be an early sign of arthritis or rupture of a tendon. By definition, Achilles tendinitis is a painful inflammation about the Achilles tendon. However, it may not show the classic signs of inflammation such as pain, erythema, increased skin temperature, or swelling.

In runners and joggers, hill running, improper footwear, and excessive pronation are common causes of this problem (146). Hill running places a strain on the Achilles tendon as the runner toes-off to go up the hill. Excessive pronation (rolling in of the foot) puts excessive eccentric forces on the tendon, causing a ringing out (clement).

Biomechanical problems, such as tight calf muscles, cavus foot, excessive subtalar varus, can also predispose the runner to the development of this problem. Prevention includes appropriate footwear and a stretching program for the calf muscles.

Runners with this problem will describe a burning pain in the heel, particularly when getting out of bed in the morning or at the start of a run. The runner may mention that this pain is present at the beginning of the run, dissipates a little during the run, and worsens after the run.

The best treatment is prevention, most notably an adequate warmup with stretching and flexing of the Achilles tendon. This is accomplished by having the person lean forward against a wall with the heels flat on the ground with a slow, continuous stretch for 20–30 seconds (147). The runner should also avoid extensive hill running and use a heel lift, an orthotic device, to balance muscle function and development.

Self-treatment for Achilles tendinitis includes the application of ice after running, use of appropriate aspirin or ibuprofen therapy to allay inflammation, stretching exercises for the calf, new shoes, and a temporary heel lift. Severe injury may ultimately dictate surgical intervention.

Blisters Blisters are the most annoying and bothersome injury to the runner. Ill-fitting footwear is frequently the cause, exemplifying the need for a proper fit at the time of purchase. Inappropriate hosiery can also contribute to the development of blisters, especially if the same sock type worn at shoe purchase is not worn during running. Running barefoot can also cause blisters. Some individuals with soft skin will continue to suffer from blisters until their skin toughens enough to withstand the constant friction during running (148).

During running the shoe can place excessive pressure on a specific area on the skin. Fluid quickly accumulates at this site between the stratum corneum and stratum lucidum, frequently on the heel, the ball of the foot, and the ends or tops of the toes.

Again, prevention is the key to treating blisters. Cotton or woolen socks are preferred for running. The runner can wear two pairs of socks with ordinary talcum powder sprinkled between the socks. Application of compound tincture of benzoin or a flexible collodion product (e.g., New Skin) will help toughen the skin.

One study demonstrated the best method to treat a blister. First, the blister and adjacent areas are cleaned with 70% isopropyl alcohol (149). Then the blister is asceptically punctured with a sterilized needle or pin at three or four distinct sites at the bubble–skin interface and allowed to drain. By allowing the blister to remain essentially intact, a natural barrier to infection is for the most part still present. After draining, a triple antibiotic ointment (e.g., bacitracin, neomycin, polymixin) may be applied to the area and a sterile gauze dressing used to cover the area (148).

Ankle Sprains Ankle sprains are not common in runners because the typical mechanism of lateral ligament injury to the ankle is through the rotation of the body over the fixed foot (139). This occurs most often in contact sports where the foot remains stationary while the body is unintentionally rotated. The incidence of this injury during jogging and running is low because runners usually do not take sharp diagonal cuts and because running footwear does not have cleats that can catch in the running surface.

The differential diagnosis of an ankle fracture from a sprained ankle is impossible without an X-ray. Thus, the injured runner should be referred to a physician for this purpose. The immediate treatment of an ankle sprain involves the application of a compressive bandage or wrap, elevation of the ankle, and application of ice. If possible, the ankle should be wrapped with a wet elastic wrap while the cold is being applied. The wet wrap facilitates the transfer of heat so that the ankle benefits from the cold application. The recovery process can be facilitated if the ankle is in a dorsiflexed position (foot toward the nose) when it is wrapped in the elastic bandage. Consistent with all sprains, including those of the neck and lower back, the use of alternating cold applications should continue for 24–72 hours depending on injury severity.

Ice, compression, elevation (I.C.E.) therapy, is well accepted as the most appropriate treatment for an ankle sprain. However, it remains controversial whether cold application without elevation is helpful or harmful (150). Regardless, treatment for a sprained ankle should be initiated as soon as possible. Sometimes an ankle sprain is perceived as a minor problem, even by trained professionals; however, the severity of the ligament damage can vary widely, and an extensive ligament rupture that has been given insufficient treatment could result in a permanently unstable ankle.

Intermetatarsal Neuritis Intermetatarsal neuritis is characterized by an uncomfortable cramping pain between the toes when running, most often within the third interspace. The cause is linked to the foot jamming forward into the running shoe without enough space to accommodate the foot. Nerves become inflamed when compressed or caught in the area between the metatarsal heads and digital bases (151).

The solution for this problem is correct fitting of the running shoe, most often a wider shoe fitted with an orthotic device modified to accommodate the entrapped area of the forefoot. A useful suggestion to alleviate the problem is that the shoe be relaced to eliminate the bottom two eyelets, thereby providing additional room for the ball of the foot (151).

A runner should not "tough out" this problem because severe, persistent cases may result in an inflammation or even an enlargement of the nerve sheath. This can develop into a neuroma which will have to be either surgically removed or treated with corticosteroid injections.

Toenail Loss Toenail loss results from improper care of the toenails. Toenails should be kept trimmed and groomed with straight edges because long toenails can effect excessive rubbing or friction by catching on the sock, particularly during a long run. This friction causes the nail to separate from the nail bed and may cause blood to accumulate under the nail bed. Eventually the nail will fall off. If a runner notices a separation, the nail should be trimmed back so that it is not uncomfortable. The patient should be advised to keep the foot clean to allay infection until the nail grows back. Toenail loss can also be prevented by taping down the nail before running.

Runner's Bunion In runners, a bunion can progressively increase in size and discomfort (152). If a runner describes what appears to be a bunion, the patient should be advised to consult a podiatrist or other physician. When treating bunions in runners, it is very important to determine the etiology of the problem, for example, improperly fitted shoes, excess pronation and hypermobility of the foot, or mechanical deformities.

The first consideration in runner's bunion is proper footwear. The shoe must fit properly and have a toe box that is wide and long enough. If it is determined that the bunion pain is effected by bursitis, supportive padding and anti-inflammatory medication may be prescribed. Sometimes the injection of corticosteroids is helpful; however, surgery may be indicated eventually (147).

Heel Pain   Heel pain in runners is a fairly common and insidious injury. The common diagnosis is plantar fascitis; it is typically symptomatic when getting out of bed in the morning or standing up after sitting. The etiology is often a biomechanical imbalance that becomes significant as the runner increases the stress placed on the plantar fascia. Like Achilles tendinitis, it may be an early sign of an arthritic disease. Therefore, the patient should be referred to the appropriate health care professional for evaluation.

Self-treatment of heel pain involves applying ice after running, using new shoes, using heel lifts or heel cups, stretching the calf and plantar fascia, strapping or taping the arch, resting from running, and using appropriate nonsteroidal anti-inflammatory medication. If the problem becomes chronic, orthotic inserts may be indicated.

There are many kinds of shoe inserts and orthotics; anything placed into the shoe will influence foot function. The choice of shoe inserts should be based on specific treatment objectives. Their properties vary (e.g., flexible, rigid); they can be custom made or purchased off the shelf. Empirically, arch supports are intended to provide buttressing for the foot, and custom-made inserts are designed to account for specific biomechanical abnormalities. An orthotic device appropriately positions the rearfoot and forefoot segments so that the arch supports itself.

The pharmacist should ask several questions of a person seeking information about the necessity of wearing an orthotic. These questions are listed at the beginning of this chapter. If the patient answers "yes" to one or more of these questions, it is appropriate to refer the patient to a health care practitioner who can provide orthotic or shoe therapy.

Patient Consultation

A pharmacist can play an integral role in the education of the exercise enthusiast, especially when consulted about an injury or problem. The pharmacist does not necessarily have to be an enthusiast of the sport to be able to convey information because the basic premise is simply the use of common sense.

Runners and joggers should carry some identification in the event of an accident or injury. The runner should realize that mileage should be increased gradually and be consistent with weather conditions. For example, it might take from 10 days to 6 weeks to acclimate to hot, humid weather. Runners and joggers tend to exceed their capacity at first; patience is the key. Just as it is a rule to avoid sunburn, it is wise for joggers and runners to avoid running outdoors during peak sunlight (i.e., 10 a.m. until 2 p.m.) in hot, humid climates.

Hydration is crucial for joggers and runners especially in the summer when perspiration can effect loss of body water. It is advisable to drink 6–8 oz of water before the workout. If participating in runs of 5K or greater, the runner should drink 6–8 oz of water every 20 minutes or about 2.5 miles of running. In the summer, joggers and runners should not overindulge in fluids, but at least attempt to keep the mouth moist. Runners and joggers should avoid using salt (NaCl only) tablets because they can induce an electrolyte imbalance by increasing potassium loss in perspiration.

Runners and joggers should be advised to wear clothing commensurate with existing conditions. Light-colored, porous clothing is advisable in the summer. Wearing a plastic sweat suit in an effort to lose weight is a dangerous practice; because this type of sweat suit affords no ventilation, it can induce hyperthermia. A white hat with a brim or beak also helps to protect the head; for extended runs in summer, wearing a terrycloth hat soaked in water will help retain moisture. In winter the runner should be advised to wear layers of clothing dependent on the individual's sensitivity to cold, the outdoor temperature, and the wind chill. Thermal underwear, a wool or polypropylene turtleneck sweater, and a nylon or all-weather running outfit should be worn in the coldest weather. In addition, the runner should wear a scarf, a hat, and gloves to protect the neck, the ears and hands from frostbite.

When self-treatment is appropriate, the pharmacist can provide invaluable assistance in selecting nonprescription drugs (e.g., aspirin, ibuprofen, topical antibiotic ointments) and make recommendations for their administration. The pharmacist can also assist in the selection of prescription accessories (e.g., compression ice wrap, ice bags, Ace bandages, arch supports, heel cushions) that will alleviate injuries or problems.

Information and instructions about aspirin and ibuprofen are found elsewhere in this book (see Chapter 5, *Internal Analgesic Products*) as is similar material about topical anti-infective ointments (see Chapter 28, *Topical Anti-infective Products*). However, it is important to review some points about ice bags and cold wraps. If an ice bag is used, the English type, which is identified by its commercial cloth material, is advantageous because the patient does not have to wrap a towel around it to help protect the skin. The ice should be broken into walnut-sized pieces with no jagged edges, and should fill the bag to about one-half to two-thirds capacity. If the bag is overfilled, it will be difficult to apply because the bag will not rest on the counter of the body area. Once the ice has been added and before application, trapped air from the bag should be squeezed out, the outside dried, and the bag checked for leaks. The bag is then applied to the specific body area. Usually, the ice should be replaced every 2–4 hours depending on patient preference. Alternate applications are suggested to avoid tissue damage, (30 minutes applied–30 minutes rest). After use, the patient should be encouraged to drain the bag and allow it to air dry. If possible, the bag should be turned inside out for more efficient drying. After this, the cap should be placed on the bag and the whole accessory stored in a cool, dry place.

Cold wraps are also useful for cold application. These can be either one-use products (e.g., Faultless Instant Cold Pack) or those intended for multiple use. The patient activates the one-use product by squeezing the middle of the pack to burst the bubble, which initiates an endothermic reaction of ammonium nitrate, water, and special additives. Reusable products consist of a cold pack or gel pack that is stored in the freezer and a cloth cover that is kept at room temperature. Once placed in the freezer, the cold pack will reach optimal temperature within 2 hours. The patient removes the cold pack from the freezer, inserts it in the cloth cover, and applies it to the specific body area. The patient should be instructed that the cold pack should not be uncomfortable. If it is, the patient should remove it for a minute or two and then reapply it. After use, the cold packs are stored in the freezer and the cloth cover is kept at room temperature in a cool, dry place. Although some gel packs are nontoxic, all cold packs should be kept out of the reach of children to prevent accidental ingestion.

A difficult decision a pharmacist must make centers around the Ace bandage. An important consideration is whether the patient will understand how to use the bandage in conjunction with ice application so that additional damage is not incurred. Typically, an Ace bandage is used for an ankle sprain or a knee sprain. The patient should be advised to unwind about 12–18 inches of bandage at a time, allow the bandage to relax before wrapping, and to start with the outstretched bandage. After the bandage is unwound it can be soaked in water. When applied with ice, a wet elastic bandage facilitates transfer of cold. The injured area should be wrapped by overlapping the previous layer of bandage by about one-third to one-half its width. The width of bandage needed depends on the injury site. For example, a foot or an ankle requires a 2.5- to 3-inch bandage. At the time of purchase, the pharmacist should review with the patient the correct procedure for wrapping, which is described on the bandage package. The patient should assess the degree of discomfort after wrapping. If the bandage feels tight or uncomfortable it should be removed and rewrapped. After use the bandage should be washed, not scrubbed, in lukewarm, soapy water and thoroughly rinsed. It should be allowed to air dry on a flat surface, then rolled to prevent wrinkles. The bandage should not be ironed.

SUMMARY

The nonprescription drug of choice in the treatment of corns, calluses, and warts is salicyclic acid in a collodion-like vehicle (10%) or plaster dosage form (40%), whichever is more convenient. However, salicyclic acid is ineffective if predisposing factors responsible for corns and calluses are not corrected. (Only surgical excision of corns associated with exostoses prevents development of corns in that area.) The effectiveness of salicylic acid in treating warts is increased if the wart is pared to the point of bleeding or pain. This procedure should be performed only by a podiatrist or other physician. Plantar warts should be treated with a higher concentration (20–40% of salicylic acid); warts on thin epidermis require a lower concentration (10–20%). Because warts are usually self-limiting, treatment should be conservative; vigorous therapy with salicylic acid may scar tissue.

Historically, the nonprescription drug of choice to treat the dry, scaly type of athlete's foot was tolnaftate. However, other agents such as clioquinol, miconazole nitrate, and undecylenic acid and its derivatives would be expected to be just as efficacious for this purpose. The efficacy of these agents will be limited unless the patient eliminates other predisposing factors to tinea pedis. These drugs are effective in all their delivery systems, but the powder form should be reserved only for extremely mild conditions or as adjunctive therapy. When recommended for suspected or actual dermatophytosis of the foot, these drugs should be used twice daily, morning and night. Because the vehicle forms of the solution and cream are spreadable, they should be used sparingly. Treatment should be continued for 2–4 weeks, depending on the symptoms. After this time, the patient and pharmacist should evaluate the effectiveness of the drug.

The value of any topical nonprescription product for the treatment of the soggy, macerated type of athlete's foot is dubious. The complex nature of the topical flora (resident aerobic diphtheroids) superimposed on the fungal infection dictates rigorous therapy with broader-spectrum antifungals (e.g., ciclopiroxolamine, clotrimazole, econazole nitrate). In addition, oral therapy with either griseofulvin or ketoconazole may be indicated. Soaks and compresses of astringent agents (e.g., aluminum chloride) may be used as an adjuvant therapy to dry the soggy, macerated tissue. Once this condition is converted to the dry form, appropriate use can be made of such agents as tolnaftate, miconazole nitrate, and undecylenic acid derivatives.

To minimize noncompliance associated with a product believed to be ineffective, patients should be advised that alleviation of the symptoms does not occur overnight. Patients should also be cautioned that frequent recurrence of any of these problems is indication for consultation with a podiatrist or other physician.

In this era of physical fitness and health awareness, the pharmacist must be prepared to help triage patients who develop athletic injuries. With careful questioning, the pharmacist can assist the patient determine whether the problem can be addressed through self-care or whether the assistance of a physician, podiatrist, or physical therapist should be sought. Most running injuries can be treated with modifications of shoes, in-shoe supports, shoe alterations, correction of leg length discrepancies, modifications of training methods, ice applications, and stretching exercises. It is important that the pharmacist be capable of providing informed recommendations to the sports enthusiast.

REFERENCES

1   J. A. Brown, Scholl, Inc., Memphis, Tenn., personal communication, 1988.

2   S. Rosen, *J. Med. Assoc. St. Ala., 43*, 617 (1974).

3   K. A. Arndt, "Manual of Dermatological Therapeutics," Little, Brown and Co., Boston, Mass., 1974, pp. 23–25.

4   J. Raskin, in "Current Therapy, 1976," H. F. Conn, Ed., W. B. Saunders, Philadelphia, Pa., 1976, pp. 611–614.

5   J. J. Leyden and A. M. Kligman, *Postgrad. Med., 61*, 113 (1977).

6   J. J. Leyden and A. M. Kligman, *Arch. Dermatol., 111*, 1004 (1975).

7   H. T. Behrmann et al., "Common Skin Diseases: Diagnosis and Treatment," 3rd ed., Grune and Stratton, New York, N.Y., 1978, p. 39.

8   A. N. Domonkos, "Andrews' Diseases of the Skin," 6th ed., W. B. Saunders, Philadelphia, Pa., 1971, pp. 54–58.

9   G. K. Potter, *J. Am. Podiatr. Assoc., 63*, 57 (1973).

10   J. W. Burnett and H. M. Robinson, Jr., "Clinical Dermatology for Students and Practitioners," 2nd ed., Yorke, New York, N.Y., p. 143.

11   W. D. Stewart et al., "Dermatology: Diagnosis and Treatment of Cutaneous Disorders," 4th ed., C. V. Mosby, St. Louis, Mo., 1978, p. 129.

12   *Federal Register, 52*, 5412 (1987).

13   S. W. Balkin, *Arch. Dermatol., 111*, 1143 (1975).

14   N. J. Glannestras, "Foot Disorders: Medical and Surgical Management," 2nd ed., Lea and Febiger, Philadelphia, Pa., 1973, pp. 24–26.

15   I. Yale, "Podiatric Medicine," Williams and Wilkins, Baltimore, Md., 1974, pp. 244–246.

16   "DuVries' Surgery of the Foot," 3rd ed., V. T. Inman, Ed., C. V. Mosby, St. Louis, Mo., 1973, pp. 206–223.

17   E. Jawetz et al., "Review of Medical Microbiology," 11th ed., Lange Medical, Los Altos, Calif., 1974, pp. 449–450.

18   J. C. Vance et al., *Arch. Dermatol., 122*, 272 (1986).

19   J. R. Coggin, Jr., and H. zur Hausen, *Cancer Res., 39*, 545 (1979).

20   G. Orth et al., *J. Virol., 24*, 108 (1977).

21   L. Gissmann and H. zur Hausen, *Int. J. Cancer, 25*, 605 (1980).

22   M. Jarratt, *Pediatr. Clin. N. Am., 25*, 339 (1978).

23   "Dermal Pathology," J. H. Graham et al., Eds., Harper and Row, Hagerstown, Md., 1972, pp. 533–535.

24   M. H. Bunney, *Drugs, 13*, 445 (1977).

25   G. Orth et al., *J. Invest. Dermatol., 76*, 97 (1981).

26   J. S. Pegum, *Practitioner, 209*, 453 (1972).

27   MMWR, *J. Am. Med. Assoc., 250*, 336 (1983).

28   Medical News and Perspectives, *J. Am. Med. Assoc., 261*, 3509 (1989).

29   Medical News, *J. Am. Med. Assoc., 251*, 2185 (1984).

30   E. J. Androphy, Editorial, *Arch. Dermatol., 125*, 683 (1989).

31   F. A. Ive, *Br. Med. J., 4*, 475 (1973).

32   K. A. Arndt, "Manual of Dermatological Therapeutics," Little Brown and Co., Boston, Mass., 1974, pp. 167–173.

33   W. D. Stewart et al., "Dermatology: Diagnosis and Treatment of Cutaneous Disorders," 4th ed., C. V. Mosby, St. Louis, Mo., 1978, pp. 316–321.

34   D. R. Lowy and E. J. Androphy, in "Dermatology in General Medicine," 3rd ed., McGraw-Hill, New York, N.Y., 1987, pp. 2355–2364.

35   A. Ferenczy et al., *N. Engl. J. Med., 313*, 784 (1985).

36   B. M. Steinberg et al., *N. Engl. J. Med., 308*, 1261 (1983).

37   W. B. Harwell et al., *J. Tennessee Med. Assoc., 71*, 830 (1978).

38   *Federal Register, 45*, 65609 (1980).

39   A. A. Gal et al., *J. Am. Med. Assoc., 257*, 337 (1987).

40   S. Obalek et al., *Arch. Dermatol., 124*, 930 (1988).

41   *Federal Register, 52*, 9992 (1987).

42   J. P. Barrett, Jr., *J. Am. Med. Assoc., 235*, 1138 (1976).

43   B. B. Sanders, Jr., and G. S. Stretcher, *J. Am. Med. Assoc., 235*, 2859 (1976).

44   R. B. Rees, Jr., in "Current Diagnosis and Treatment," M. A. Krupp and M. J. Chatton, Eds., Lange Medical, Los Altos, Calif., 1979, p. 73.

45   A. S. Wigfield, *Br. Med. J., 3*, 585 (1972).

46   *Federal Register, 47*, 39102 (1982).

47   J. J. Goodman and L. Farris, Scholl Study No. S-82-47, Unpublished Study, Comment No. LET, Docket No. 81N-0122, Docket Mgmt. Branch, Food and Drug Administration, Rockville, Md.

48   *Federal Register, 47*, 522 (1982).

49   "Drug Design," vol. 4, E. J. Ariens, Ed., Academic, New York, N.Y., 1973, p. 178.

50   J. A. Mills, *N. Engl. J. Med., 290*, 781 (1974).

51   "Sprowls' American Pharmacy," 7th ed., L. W. Dittert, Ed., Lippincott, Philadelphia, Pa., 1974, p. 167.

52   H. C. Ansel, "Introduction to Pharmaceutical Dosage Forms," 4th ed., Lea and Febiger, Philadelphia, Pa., 1985, p. 317.

53 E. M. Brecher and Editors of Consumer Reports, "Licit and Illicit Drugs," Little, Brown and Co., Boston, Mass., 1972, pp. 309–320.

54 "AMA Drug Evaluations," 3d ed., Publishing Sciences Group, Acton, Mass., 1977, pp. 188–189.

55 E. W. Rosenberg et al., *Arch. Dermatol.*, *113*, 1134 (1977).

56 H. Bargman, *Arch. Dermatol.*, *124*, 1718 (1988).

57 M. D. Karol et al., *Clinical Toxicology*, *16 (3)*, 282 (1980).

58 M. A. Lutzner, *Arch. Dermatol.*, *119*, 631 (1983).

59 A. L. Hudson, *Arch. Dermatol.*, *112*, 1179 (1976).

60 R. R. M. McLaughlin, *Arch. Dermatol.*, *106*, 129 (1972).

61 R. Lester and D. Rosenthal, *Arch. Dermatol.*, *104*, 330 (1971).

62 M. W. Hursthouse, *Br. J. Dermatol.*, *92*, 93 (1975).

63 R. A. W. Miller, *Arch. Dermatol.*, *120*, 963 (1984).

64 Medical News, *J. Am. Med. Assoc.*, *237*, 940 (1977).

65 K. Hasumi et al., *Lancet*, *1*, 968 (1984).

66 L. Hymes and G. S. Hymes, *J. Am. Podiat. Assoc.*, *65*, 1023 (1975).

67 R. A. Katz, *Arch. Dermatol.*, *122*, 19 (1986).

68 P. Kirby, *J. Am. Med. Assoc.*, *259*, 570 (1988).

69 *Federal Register*, *47*, 39120 (1982).

70 *Federal Register*, *45*, 69128 (1980).

71 *Medical Letter on Drugs and Therapeutics*, *18 (25)*, 105 (1976).

72 W. J. Mills, Jr., *Emergency Med.*, *8*, 134 (1976).

73 T. Schwinghammer, *U.S. Pharmacist*, *3 (#1)*, 48 (1978).

74 E. H. Tschen et al., *Cutis*, *23*, 696 (1979).

75 J. B. Goslen and G. S. Kobayashi, in "Dermatology in General Medicine," 3rd ed., McGraw-Hill, New York, N.Y., 1987, pp. 2193–2248.

76 C. Pellizari, *Giornale Italiano Della Malattie Veneree*, *29*, 8 (1888).

77 W. D. Stewart et al., "Dermatology: Diagnosis and Treatment of Cutaneous Disorders," 4th ed., C. V. Mosby, St. Louis, Mo., 1978, pp. 265–280.

78 R. L. Baer and S. A. Rosenthal, *J. Am. Med. Assoc.*, *197*, 187 (1966).

79 C. M. Caravati, Jr., et al., *Cutis*, *17*, 313 (1976).

80 J. H. S. Pettit, *Drugs*, *10*, 130 (1975).

81 J. J. Leyden and A. M. Kligman, *Arch. Dermatol.*, *114*, 1466 (1978).

82 J. W. Burnett and H. M. Robinson, Jr., "Clinical Dermatology for Students and Practitioners," 2nd ed., Yorke, New York, N.Y., 1978.

83 J. H. Jung et al., *Contact Dermatitis*, *19*, 254 (1988).

84 R. A. Amonette and E. W. Rosenberg, *Arch. Dermatol.*, *107*, 71 (1973).

85 H. I. Maibach, *Arch. Dermatol.*, *114*, 1773 (1978).

86 C. E. Mueller and D. P. West, *Amer. Pharm.*, *NS21*, 299 (1981).

87 J. F. Fuerst et al., *Cutis*, *25*, 544 (1980).

88 *Federal Register*, *47*, 12480 (1982).

89 H. L. Arnold, Jr., *Arch. Dermatol.*, *115*, 1287 (1979).

90 L. M. Field, *Arch. Dermatol.*, *115*, 1287 (1979).

91 *Am. Pharm.*, *NS25*, 597 (1985).

92 J. L. Lesher and J. G. Smith, Jr., *Drug Therapy*, *14 (9)*, 113 (1984).

93 G. A. Gellin et al., *Arch. Dermatol.*, *106*, 715 (1972).

94 J. B. Shelmire, Jr., *J. Invest. Dermatol.*, *26*, 105 (1956).

95 K. H. Kaidbey and A. M. Kligman, *Arch. Dermatol.*, *110*, 868 (1974).

96 E. B. Smith et al., *S. Med. J.*, *67*, 776 (1974).

97 A. H. Gould, *Dermatologica Tropica et Ecologica Geographica*, *3*, 255 (1964).

98 "AMA Drug Evaluations," 4th ed., Publishing Sciences Group, Acton, Mass., 1980, p. 1366.

99 S. M. Peck and H. Rosenfeld, *J. Invest. Dermatol.*, *1*, 237 (1938).

100 E. L. Keeney et al., *Bull. Johns Hopkins Hosp.*, *17*, 422 (1945).

101 M. J. Golden and K. A. Oster, *J. Am. Pharm. Assoc., Sci. Ed.*, *39*, 47 (1950).

102 W. C. Cutting, "Handbook of Pharmacology," 5th ed., Meredith, New York, N.Y., 1972, p. 56.

103 F. Sadik, *PharmIndex*, *15 (7A)*, 5 (1973).

104 E. B. Smith et al., *Int. J. Dermatol.*, *16*, 52 (1977).

105 J. H. Chretien et al., *Int. J. Dermatol.*, *19*, 51 (1980).

106 F. E. Lyddon et al., *Int. J. Dermatol.*, *19*, 24 (1980).

107 "The Pharmacological Basis of Therapeutics," 6th ed., A. G. Gilman et al., Eds., Macmillan, New York, N.Y., 1980, p. 967.

108 *Federal Register*, *43*, 1238 (1978).

109 M. H. Walker, *J. Am. Podiatr. Assoc.*, *52*, 737 (1962).

110 R. E. Gosselin et al., "Clinical Toxicology of Commercial Products, Acute Poisoning," 4th ed., Williams and Wilkins, Baltimore, Md., 1976, Section II, p. 131.

111 J. K. Morgan, *Br. J. Clin. Pract.*, *22*, 261 (1968).

112 *Federal Register*, *3*, 1236 (1978).

113 "Sprowls, American Pharmacy," 7th ed., L. W. Dittert, Ed., Lippincott, Philadelphia, Pa., 1974, p. 49.

114 P. B. Price, *Arch. Surg.*, *61*, 23 (1950).

115 K. A. Oster and M. J. Golden, *J. Am. Pharm. Assoc., Sci. Ed.*, *37*, 429 (1948).

116 G. A. Zentmyer, *Science*, *100*, 294 (1944).

117 K. A. Oster and M. J. Golden, *Exp. Med. Surg.*, *1*, 37 (1949).

118 R. E. Gosselin et al., "Clinical Toxicology of Commercial Products, Acute Poisoning," 4th ed., Williams and Wilkins, Baltimore, Md., 1976, Section II, p. 89.

119 L. Goldman, in "Current Therapy, 1972," H. F. Conn., Ed., W. B. Saunders, Philadelphia, Pa., 1972, p. 585.

120 A. M. Kligman et al., *Int. J. Dermatol.*, *16*, 413 (1977).

121 H. Myllarniemi et al., *Acta Chirurgica Scand.*, *131*, 312 (1966).

122 *Federal Register*, *43*, 34636 (1978).

123 E. B. Smith et al., *S. Med. J.*, *70*, 47 (1977).

124 H. E. Jones et al., *Arch. Dermatol.*, *117*, 129 (1981).

125 D. N. Gerding et al., *Patient Care*, *23*, 102 (1988).

126 P. D. Thompson et al., *J. Am. Med. Assoc.*, *242*, 1265 (1979).

127 W. B. Kannel, Editorial, *J. Am. Med. Assoc.*, *248*, 3143 (1982).

128 W. G. Clancy, Jr., *Am. J. Sports Med.*, *8*, 137 (1980).

129 D. B. Carr et al., *N. Engl. J. Med.*, *305*, 560 (1982).

130 D. Drez, *Am. J. Sports Med.*, *8*, 140 (1980).

131 R. J. Geline, "The Practical Runner," Collier Macmillan Canada, Ltd., New York, N.Y., 1978.

132 S. Cook et al., *Am. J. Sports Med.*, *13*, 248 (1985).

133 M. I. Rossman and R. Carvejal, *N. Engl. J. Med.*, *299*, 424 (1978).

134 D. M. Brody, *Running Injuries*, in "Clinical Symposia," A. Brass, Ed., Ciba-Geigy Corporation, Summit, N.J., 32 (1980).

135 J. Daniels et al., "Conditioning for Distance Running," Wiley and Sons, New York, N.Y., 1978.

136 J. Galloway, "Galloway's Book on Running," Shelter, Bolinas, Calif., 1984.

137 R. Glover and J. Shepard, "The Runner's Handbook," Penguin, New York, N.Y., 1977.

138 N. G. Popovich et al., *US Pharmacist*, *8*, 28 (1983).

139 R. O. Schuster, "Biomechanical Running Problems," in *Sports Med. '79*, R. R. Rinaldi and M. L. Sabla, Eds., Futura, Mount Kisco, N.Y., 43 (1978).

140 S. L. James et al., *Am. J. Sports Med.*, *6*, 40 (1978).

141 T. Noakes, "Lore of Running," Oxford, Cape Town, S. Afr., 1985.

142 D. E. Detmer, *Am. J. Sports Med.*, *8*, 141 (1980).

143 J. W. Pagliano, *Sports Med. '78*, 55 (1978).

144 R. S. Gilbert et al., "Stress Fractures of the Tarsal Talus," in *Sports Med. '80*, R. R. Rinaldi and M. L. Sabia, Eds., Futura, Mount Kisco, N.Y., 133 (1980).

145 S. L. Alchermes et al., "Stress Fracture of the Fibula in a Jogger: Secondary to a Change in Running Surface," in *Sports Med. '80*, R. R. Rinaldi and M. L. Sabia, Eds., Futura, Mount Kisco, N.Y., 133 (1980).

146 S. Curwin and W. Stanish, "Tendonitis: Its Etiology and Treatment," Collamore, Lexington, Mass., 1984.

147 R. E. Leach et al., *Am. J. Sports Med.*, *9*, 93 (1981).

148 J. I. Seder, "Treatment of Blisters in the Running Athlete," in *Sports Med. '78*, R .R. Rinaldi and M. L. Sabia, Eds., Futura, Mount Kisco, N.Y., 29 (1978).

149 S. I. Subotnick, "The Running Foot Director," World Publications, Mt. View, Calif., 1977.

150 D. J. Cote et al., *Physical Therapy J.*, *68*, 1072 (1988).

151 S. I. Subotnick, "Podiatric Sports Medicine," Futura, Mount Kisco, N.Y., 1975.

152 C. Kahn and M. Blazina, Questions and Answers, *J. Am. Med. Assoc.*, *252*, 565 (1984).

CALLUS/CORN/WART PRODUCT TABLE

Product (Manufacturer)	Application Form	Active Ingredients	Other Ingredients
Compound W Wart Remover (Whitehall)	liquid gel	salicylic acid, 17%	ether, 63.5% (liquid)
Corn Fix (Alvin Last)	liquid	phenol	soap turpentine oil
Dr. Scholl's Corn Removers (Scholl)	medicated discs unmedicated pads	salicylic acid, 40% (medicated discs) salicylic acid, 20% (for soft corns)	
Dr. Scholl's Ingrown Toenail Reliever (Scholl)	liquid	tannic acid, 25% chlorobutanol, 5%	isopropyl alcohol, 80%
Dr. Scholl's Liquid Corn Remover (Scholl)	liquid	salicylic acid, 12.6%	alcohol, 15% ether, 0.321g/ml
Dr. Scholl's Wart Remover Kit (Scholl)	liquid	salicylic acid, 17%	ether, 52%
Dr. Scholl's Waterproof Corn Removers (Scholl)	medicated discs unmedicated pads	salicylic acid, 40% (medicated discs)	
Freezone Corn and Callus Remover (Whitehall)	liquid	salicylic acid, 13.6%	alcohol, 20.5% ether, 64.8%
Gets-It Liquid (Oakhurst)	liquid	salicylic acid, 13.9% zinc chloride, 2.7%	ether alcohol collodion
Johnson's Foot Soap (Combe)	powder[a]		borax iodide bran
Mosco (Medtech)	ointment	salicylic acid, 40%	methyl salicylate
Nail-A-Cain (Medtech)	liquid	benzocaine, 15% tannic acid, 4%	isopropyl alcohol, 61% diethyl ether, 20%
Off Ezy Wart Removal Kit (Commerce)	liquid and special skin buffer	salicylic acid, 17%	flexible collodion
Outgro (Whitehall)	liquid	tannic acid, 25% chlorobutanol, 5%	isopropyl alcohol, 83%
Vergo (Daywell)	ointment-cream	calcium pantothenate ascorbic acid	starch
Wart-aid (Republic)	liquid	calcium pantothenate ascorbic acid	starch
Wart Fix (Alvin Last)	liquid	castor oil	
Wart-Off (Leeming)	liquid	salicylic acid, 17%	flexible collodion alcohol ether

[a] Product is diluted or reconstituted and then applied to the skin.

ATHLETE'S FOOT PRODUCT TABLE

Product (Manufacturer)	Application Form	Antifungal	Keratolytic	Other Ingredients
Aftate (Schering-Plough)	gel powder spray liquid spray powder	tolnaftate, 1%		
Blis Foot Bath (Commerce)	powder		salicylic acid, 17%	boric acid, 47.5% epsom salt, 10.7%
Blis-To-Sol (Chattem)	liquid powder	undecylenic acid, 5% benzoic acid, 2%	salicylic acid, 9% (liquid) 2% (powder)	
Bluboro (Herbert)	liquid[a]			aluminum sulfate calcium acetate boric acid
Buro-Sol (Doak)	powder			aluminum acetate, 46.8% sodium diacetate, 48.8% benzethonium chloride, 4.4%
Cruex (Fisons)	powder	calcium undecylenate, 10%		talc
Decylenes (Rugby)	ointment	undecylenic acid zinc undecylenate		
Dermasept Antifungal (Pharmakon)	liquid	tolnaftate, 1% undecylenic acid, 5%	tannic acid, 6%	zinc chloride, 5% benzocaine, 2% methylbenzethonium hydrochloride, 3% ethanol, 58%
Desenex (Pharmacraft)	aerosol powder cream ointment powder soap	zinc undecylenate, 20% (not in soap) NS[b] (cream) undecylenic acid, 5% (ointment) 2% (powder, soap) NS[b] (cream)		
Desenex Antifungal (Pharmacraft)	foam	undecylenic acid, 10%		isopropyl alcohol, 29%
Desenex Liquid (Pharmacraft)	solution	undecylenic acid, 10%		isopropyl alcohol, 40% propylene glycol triethanolamine
Deso-Creme (Columbia Medical)	cream	zinc undecylenate, 20% caprylic acid, 5% sodium propionate, 2%		
Domeboro (Miles)	powder[a] tablet[a]			aluminum sulfate calcium acetate
Dr. Scholl's Athlete's Foot (Scholl)	aerosol powder aerosol spray cream powder	tolnaftate, 1% (all)		alcohol, 36% (aerosol powder) 14% (aerosol spray) talc (powder) cornstarch (powder)
Fungacetin (Blair)	ointment	triacetin, 25%		
Genaspor (Goldline)	cream	tolnaftate, 1%		
Iodochlorhydroxyquin (Various manufacturers)	cream ointment	iodochlorhydroxy-quin, 3%		

ATHLETE'S FOOT PRODUCT TABLE, continued

Product (Manufacturer)	Application Form	Antifungal	Keratolytic	Other Ingredients
Merlenate (Vortech)	ointment	zinc undecylenate, 20% sodium propionate, 2% caprylic acid, 5%		
Micatin (Ortho)	aerosol powder cream powder spray liquid	miconazole nitrate, 2%		alcohol, 10% (aerosol powder) 17% (spray liquid)
NP-27 (Thompson Medical)	cream powder solution spray powder	tolnaftate, 1%		
Quinsana Plus Medicated (Mennen)	powder	zinc undecylenate, 20% undecylenic acid, 2%		talc silica fragrance
Rid-Itch (Thomas & Thompson)	liquid	resorcinol, 1% benzoic acid, 2% chlorothymol, 1%	salicylic acid, 7%	boric acid, 5% alcohol glycerin
Tinactin (Schering)	aerosol liquid aerosol powder cream powder solution	tolnaftate, 1%		PEG-400 (cream, solution) propylene glycol (cream titanium dioxide (cream) cornstarch (powder) talc (aerosol, powder) propellants (aerosol) BHT (aerosol, cream, solution)
Ting (Fisons)	cream powder spray liquid spray powder	tolnaftate, 1%		boric acid zinc oxide alcohol, 16% (cream)
Torofor (Torch)	cream	iodochlorhydroxy-quin, 3%		
Undoguent (Torch)	ointment	undecylenic acid, 5% zinc undecylenate, 20%		
Undecylenic Acid Compound (Various manufacturers)	ointment	undecylenic acid, 5% zinc undecylenate, 20%		
Vioform (Ciba)	cream ointment	iodochlorhydroxy-quin, 3%		
Zeasorb-AF (Stiefel)	powder	tolnaftate, 1%		talc

[a] Product is diluted or reconstituted and then applied to the skin.
[b] Quantity not specified.

Peter P. Lamy

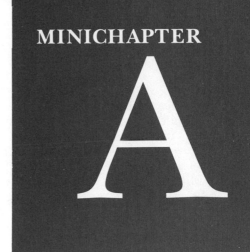

NONPRESCRIPTION DRUGS AND THE ELDERLY

Any elderly person presenting to the emergency department of a hospital with nonspecific signs or symptoms, particularly those of the central nervous system (CNS) or gastrointestinal (GI) system, should be asked for a careful drug history on nonprescription medications. For example, bleeding and GI symptoms may be caused by salicylates. Elderly patients are particularly prone to chronic salicylate intoxication, which presents as tinnitus, respiratory alkalosis, and noncardiogenic pulmonary edema. Salicylates can also displace anticoagulants from their albumin binding sites, inhibit platelet aggregation, inhibit procoagulant factors, and be ulcerogenic. Diphenhydramine, particularly in overdose or if added to a host of other drugs with anticholinergic effects, may contribute to anticholinergic toxicity. An increasing number of drugs with significant anticholinergic activity are now available in nonprescription preparations and may, in acute poisoning, produce central anticholinergic toxicity. This syndrome refers to an acute psychosis of delirium resulting from a primary blockade of cerebral cholinergic inhibitory pathways accompanied by signs of muscarinic blockage.

The fast-growing elderly population is often intent on self-care. If they are to be well served, health care professionals must understand that nonprescription drugs, although safe and effective individually, may be problematic when used in a nondirected manner, that is, in doses exceeding those recommended or within the context of a complex therapeutic regimen.

Nonpharmacologic factors, altered pharmacokinetics, or altered pharmacodynamics, individually or in combination, may be responsible for potential problems with nonprescription drugs.

SPECIAL CONSIDERATIONS

Nonprescription drugs cure acute ailments, prevent diseases, and help patients manage or monitor chronic diseases after professional diagnosis (1). The latter point is important because a number of nonprescription drug products are used to treat symptoms or conditions that are not self-diagnosable (e.g., bronchodilators for asthma, and pancreatic enzymes for pancreatic enzyme deficiency).

Statistics on the use of nonprescription drugs by the elderly are scarce (2). It is estimated that two-thirds of the elderly use nonprescription drugs and that their use generally parallels prescription drug use. It has also been estimated that nonprescription drugs account for 40% of all drugs used in nursing homes and 80% of all drugs used for people in the assisted living sector. A Canadian group reported that almost 60% of the elderly population in its study used nonprescription drugs, with women using them more often than men (3). Many studies have shown that about half of elderly study subjects take self-prescribed vitamins (4); some investigators report an even higher use. Another study found that almost two-thirds of elderly ambulatory patients used nonprescription drugs (5); more than 50% of these drugs were oral analgesics.

As the availability of nonprescription drugs increases, their use will increase. One reason, of course, is the savings in health care expenditures. It has been estimated that nonprescription drug use provides gross savings in health care expenditures that will increase from roughly $24 billion in 1987 to $73 billion in the year 2000; reduced physician visits and reduced use of prescription drugs contribute significantly to these projected savings (6). The increasing use of nonprescription products and the expectation that more powerful drugs will be switched from prescription to nonprescription status (e.g., H_2 blockers) have raised safety and therapeutic management concerns because of the inherent properties of the drugs *per se*, as well as their potential to adversely affect concurrent therapy. These concerns are heightened by the suggestion that perhaps as many as 50% of all chronic care drugs (e.g., cholesterol-lowering drugs) will achieve nonprescription status by the year 2000 (7). Clearly, more and better information on the risks and benefits of these drugs in the elderly will be needed, as will be better information exchange between patient and health care provider, and among health care providers. The need for reliable, understandable, easily accessible information, goes hand-in-hand with self-care and nonprescription drug use; this is an area of need requiring increasing attention and expanded services (1).

ALTERED DRUG ACTION IN THE ELDERLY

The elderly respond differently to drugs (including nonprescription drugs) than do younger people (8). Their physiologic response to drugs is much more scattered, and the predictability of drug action is much less certain (9, 10). This is because biologic (physiologic, primary), pathophysiologic (secondary), and sociogenic (tertiary) age changes exert individual or combined action. For a variety of reasons, both therapeutic response and the incidence of adverse reactions can be affected in the elderly. For example, drugs that affect alertness, coordination, and balance (antihistamines, for example) will likely cause more falls and accidents in the elderly than in younger people. On the other hand, most GI problems in the elderly are neither age nor disease induced, but are behaviorally induced and aggravated by chronic laxative abuse and poor eating habits (11).

Most studies addressing the problem of altered drug action in the elderly have been cross-sectional rather than longitudinal (12); therefore, more is known about age differences in drug action than about changes of drug action with age. Clearly, however, the reasons for altered drug action with age are multifactorial. For example, tissue sensitivity may change, depending on the tissue and the drug used. Genetic fac-

tors play a role (13) that may be increasingly important with advancing age and reduced reserve capacity (14). Several well-established or suspected dietary factors may increasingly influence drug action with advanced age (15). Many patient-related factors, such as dehydration, to which the elderly are more susceptible, can alter drug action (smaller volume of distribution). The physiologic loss of vestibular and cochlear hair cells and ganglia makes the elderly more susceptible to hearing problems when they receive drugs (e.g., aspirin) that can affect their hearing. It is most likely, however, that the failure to achieve the desired symptomatic relief or the appearance of adverse effects is caused by a mixture of nonpharmacologic factors, age-associated pharmacokinetic changes, and age-associated pharmacodynamic changes. The interaction of many factors that cause problems often associated with nonprescription drug use is shown in Table 1, which addresses the reasons for constipation in the elderly (16).

Nonpharmacologic Factors

Perceptions and Misperceptions

The general belief that nonprescription drugs are used most often for symptoms that the elderly interpret as nonthreatening and that elderly persons exhibiting symptoms they associate with a serious condition will consult their physicians must be reassessed in the context of actual nonprescription drug use. Moreover, many physicians (and other health care providers) still do not harmonize the use of nonprescription drugs and prescription drugs (1); this practice must change. Also, misperceptions about the potency of nonprescription drugs still abound. For example, both providers and patients often underestimate the analgesic potency of both aspirin and acetaminophen because these drugs can be obtained without a prescription.

Misperceptions about the active ingredient in nonprescription products are still much too common. For example, many providers and patients underestimate the effect of certain sleep aids, not realizing that, some time ago, the active ingredient in most products was changed from pyrilamine maleate to diphenhydramine hydrochloride. The ethanolamine antihistamines (including diphenhydramine) cause more CNS depression than the ethylenediamines (pyrilamine) (17), and the anticholinergic action of the former is stronger than that of the latter.

Demographics

The number of elderly patients living alone is increasing. The percentage of elderly women living alone

TABLE 1   Multifactorial causes of constipation

Factors	Changes
Primary aging	Change in rectal awareness
	Decreased bowel tone
	Decreased motility
Secondary aging	Endocrine diseases:
	Diabetes mellitus
	Hypothyroidism
	Uremia
	Hypokalemia
	Intrinsic bowel lesions
	Neurogenic/psychiatric problems:
	Organic brain syndrome
	Cerebrovascular accident
	Parkinson's disease
	Severe pulmonary disease
	Severe shortness of breath
Tertiary aging	Excessive use of enemas and laxatives
	Inability to cook
	Inadequate fluid intake
	Lack of physical activity
	Low fiber intake
	Unwillingness to eat alone
Medications	Antacids
	Antidepressants
	Bismuth
	Diuretics
	Iron
	Laxative addiction
	Opiates

Adapted from: B. Yachmetz et al., *Geriatr. Consult.*, *6 (4)*, 20 (1988).

has increased steadily from 29% in 1965, to 36% in 1975, and 39% in 1981. Of nearly 9 million elderly living alone in 1987, 81% were women (18). It has been documented that health care providers, patients, and family caregivers have different perspectives, particularly concerning the adverse effects of drugs on quality of life (19). Recently, it was confirmed that patients, particularly those living alone, may not notice some side effects, such as the lessened self-care capacity of patients with high anticholinergic levels (20); this side effect is much more likely to be noticed by a family caregiver than by the patient.

Physical and Cognitive Changes

Accurate perception (and reporting) of symptoms is vital to the successful use of any drug (21); however, the elderly are believed to confuse at least one-third of their problems with age-associated problems and therefore to misreport their symptoms. In addition, elderly males are often reluctant to share health information with others (22), and female proxies vary in their ability to report common complaints (23).

Loss of visual acuity increases with advancing age (9), which raises doubt about the ability of the elderly to read, much less understand, the information and instructions provided with nonprescription drugs. Furthermore, 15-20% of community-living elderly are thought to be cognitively impaired to varying degrees, making comprehension of directions even more difficult (10). In addition, many of the elderly may not be able to read and understand the English language, even though they may be quite educated in their own native language. However, the ability to read and understand directions is essential for correct nonprescription drug use. For example, acetaminophen must be administered every 4 hours to provide steady-state plasma levels; however, with aspirin, the total daily dose is more important than the amount and administration time of individual doses. The patient's inability to read or understand often leads to uncontrolled and nondirected use of nonprescription drugs, which almost invariably causes problems in the elderly. Adverse drug events, which include patient and provider errors and mishaps and which are often not related to the active drug moiety (24), seem to occur with increased frequency among the elderly, perhaps because directions were not clear, could not be understood, or could not be read (10).

Among problems not related to active drug moiety are reports of chewable antacid tablets that were swallowed whole and, subsequently, had to be surgically removed. Surgical intervention was also necessary in the case of a bulk laxative administered with an insufficient volume of fluids. Chewable vitamin C tablets have caused serious erosion of teeth, and aspirin tablets allowed to dissolve in the mouth have caused painful burns of the oral mucosa.

The necessity for a clear understanding of the directions is demonstrated by nonprescription products containing sympathomimetic amines. This agent is contraindicated in patients with high blood pressure (perhaps as many as 65% of the elderly), in diabetics, and in patients taking antidepressants or thyroid preparations. Numerous case reports have shown that phenylpropanolamine (PPA) can stimulate the CNS, with symptoms ranging from anxiety and hallucinations to grand mal seizures produced by overdoses. PPA in the usual dose can also cause nausea, tremors, dizziness, palpitations, and agitation (25).

Elderly persons with asthma or glaucoma and men with prostate gland enlargement should be advised against using preparations containing the traditional antihistamines.

Furthermore, if nonprescription drug products are taken without a clear understanding of their action within a complex therapeutic regimen, they may contribute considerably to the hazards of drug interactions and subsequent undesirable clinical sequelae, such as gastrotoxicity (26).

The Patient's Nutritional Status

The aging process, as well as many chronic diseases (e.g., decubiti, depression, dementia), can alter a patient's nutritional status (27). The elderly most at risk to undernourishment or malnutrition are homebound patients and nursing home residents; poverty, multiple chronic diseases, multiple drug therapy, or a combination of these factors may cause malnutrition in these patients (28–30). The patient's nutritional status and weight are important because they can alter the pharmacokinetics (31) and the action of drugs (32). Patients weighing 50 kg (110 lb) or less are most at risk of altered drug action.

Dosage Forms

Providers and patients often overlook the problems that a particular dosage form can cause. Some tablets or capsules, particularly aspirin and iron tablets (33, 34), may lodge in the esophagus and cause irritation, ulceration, and stricture. The elderly are most at risk because of age-associated changes in the oral cavity and the esophagus, insufficient fluid intake, and left ventricular hypertrophy. Elderly patients with swallowing difficulties may often crush medications. The literature has identified dosage forms that should not be crushed, including items with pharmacologic activity obtained in the health food store, such as long-acting niacin. Other nonprescription products that should not be crushed include Dulcolax, Ecotrin, and Feosol.

Age-Associated Altered Pharmacokinetics

Kinetics describe the rate per unit time at which a drug is absorbed, distributed, metabolized, and excreted. Pharmacokinetics altered with age have been well described in the literature (35–38). These changes are caused not only by advancing age, but also by the effects of disease states and, often, multiple drug use. For example, antacids may alter the absorption of many drugs, either by chelation, by altering their metabolism, by delaying gastric emptying (as do anticholinergic drugs), or by pH changes. Absorption of most drugs, for example, does not change with altered nutritional intake. Intercurrent diseases may alter the absorption of some drugs. All of these factors may alter the rate of absorption, the extent of absorption, or both (33, 39). The rate of drug disposition is age and disease dependent, and changes lead to altered drug action. The ratio of lean body weight to lipid tissue changes with age: Lean body weight decreases; lipid tissue increases. This change decreases the volume of distribution of water-soluble drugs, possibly leading to more intense action of these drugs. Extracellular fluids and other body fluids also decrease with age, which decreases the volume of distribution of water-soluble drugs. Alpha-l-glycoprotein, a plasma protein, increases with age in healthy elderly patients, altering the binding characteristics of some drugs. In contrast, increased age is directly related to decreased albumin levels (40, 41). Overall, albumin levels decrease by 4% per decade of life. The effect is greater in those 70 years of age and over; there is a high prevalence of abnormally low serum albumin in the very old. Therefore, drugs that are highly protein bound should show altered distribution patterns in elderly patients.

Theoretically, elderly patients should have reduced rates of hepatic drug metabolism because of age-related changes. The weight of the liver is correlated with body weight, which both decrease beginning in the fifth or sixth decade of life. Both hepatic function and blood flow decrease with age, but changes are effected by many other factors, such as smoking and alcohol intake. Nevertheless, it is generally agreed that elderly patients probably have diminished capacity to metabolize drugs, and that it is primarily the oxidative drug metabolizing mechanism that changes with age. Normal age-related changes may be overshadowed by the effects of simultaneously administered drugs on drug metabolism and liver blood flow. For example, cimetidine, which will soon have nonprescription status, is thought to reduce liver blood flow.

Age-related changes in renal function must also be considered. Renal function declines with age but to a variable degree and at a variable rate (42). Little decline is observed in about one-third of the elderly. In the remainder of patients, normal renal function at age 70 may be 40% less than at age 30. The glomerular filtration rate declines with age, even in the absence of cardiovascular, renal, or acute illnesses (43). The decline is more rapid in men than in women. Altered physiologic processes, such as reduced cardiac output, cardiac contractility, total vascular resistance, and hypotension may also reduce the glomerular filtration rate (43). Furthermore, the renal function of older people is more vulnerable to insults imposed by drug therapy and overall stress.

Finally, antacids and diuretics may also alter the excretion profile of drugs by alkalinization of urinary pH, a process that contributes to the increase or decrease of renal tubular secretion of other drugs (39).

The salicylates illustrate the effects of age- and disease-associated altered pharmacokinetics. The salicylates exhibit saturable protein binding (44). Saturable binding of salicylates to albumin depends on the concentrations of both the drug and albumin (45). Thus, as the plasma concentration of a salicylate increases, the proportion of unbound (active) drug increases. It also increases with a decrease of albumin. Thus, per given dose, the fraction of unbound salicylate is higher in the elderly than in younger patients because average serum albumin concentrations are lower in the elderly, even though the concentrations may still be within the "normal" range (46).

Salicylates are also among the drugs with capacity-limited, rather than flow-limited, clearance (44). In other words, salicylates are eliminated in a dose-dependent or, more correctly, in a concentration-dependent manner. At low salicylate concentrations, elimination follows first-order kinetics and the half-life is about 3 hours. Higher concentrations are achieved when the metabolic process becomes saturated. The metabolism of salicylates depends on the intrinsic metabolic capacity of the liver, which may be reduced in the elderly. That means that once capacity is reached, a small increase in dose will produce a large increase in blood levels. At higher concentrations, when the salicylate metabolism becomes saturated, the half-life may be extended to 22 hours, and dose frequency needs to be adjusted. These factors are more important in elderly patients, who have lessened ability to eliminate salicylates (49). Finally, drugs that acidify urine (e.g., ascorbic acid) may decrease the rate of elimination of salicylates, while drugs that increase the urinary pH (e.g., antacids) will increase their elimination.

Age-Associated Pharmacodynamic Changes

When all nonpharmacologic factors and age-associated altered pharmacokinetics are taken into account, the increased toxicity even of some nonprescription drugs cannot be fully explained. For example, elderly patients, particularly those with altered bowel function or severe organ-system disease, are generally very susceptible to the complications of antacid therapy. Aluminum salts can cause constipation and have been much discussed recently because of their possible role in the development of Alzheimer's disease. Magnesium salts can cause diarrhea, dehydration, vitamin and electrolyte depletion, increased risk of digoxin toxicity in patients receiving that drug, neuromuscular and neurologic dysfunction, and potential cardiac compromise

(39). Prolonged and intensive use of antacids containing aluminum can also lead to osteomalacia, particularly in low-weight women. They can also cause intestinal obstruction in bed-bound patients (33). Age- and disease-associated changes in pharmacodynamics often explain these problems.

Physiologic, psychologic, and possible toxic responses (i.e., the pharmacodynamics) are of major interest in the pharmacologic management of the chronic diseases of the elderly (50, 51). The pharmacodynamics of a drug govern the type, intensity, and duration of drug action or, more precisely, the duration of a given concentration of a drug at its site of action. Thus, pharmacodynamics represent the physiologic and psychologic responses to a drug or a combination of drugs. The hypoglycemic effect, the extent and duration of pain relief, and the effect of a drug on heart rate are examples of the pharmacodynamics of a drug. As is the case with pharmacokinetics, pharmacodynamics change with age (and disease), but it is still difficult to differentiate between normal aging effects and pathophysiologic effects and their influence on pharmacodynamics. Advancing age heightens the interplay between the aging processes and chronic diseases, which has made it difficult to clearly identify only age-associated pharmacodynamic changes. In fact, pharmacodynamic changes have not been as intensively studied as pharmacokinetic changes.

Drug–receptor response, defined as the pharmacologic response after a drug–end-organ interaction, may be altered in the elderly. Pharmacodynamic response may be increased or decreased. However, in the absence of pathological changes, the evidence of altered end-organ response to drugs caused exclusively by the aging processes is still controversial (52). One of the reasons for this controversy is that changes occur to significantly varying degrees. These variations preclude clinically useful generalizations (53). Importantly, some variables change with age, but others, such as the hematocrit, do not. Therefore, neither the influence of aging on clinically relevant variables nor the possible effect of normative changes is clear in many instances.

It has been suggested for some time that the elderly appear to be more "sensitive" to some drugs. Neuromuscular blockade is more intense and prolonged with advancing age, and reversal by antagonists is more difficult with advancing age (54), perhaps because the neuromuscular junction is more sensitive to these agents. For example, ganglionic blockade results in decreased GI tone and motility in elderly patients. Drugs whose pharmacodynamic effects in the elderly are most intensively studied include the barbiturates, methyldopa, the benzodiazepines, warfarin, heparin, and morphine.

The increased warfarin efficacy has been ascribed to an increased efficacy of the drug in inhibiting clotting factor synthesis, which is not related to pharmacokinetic parameters in the elderly (55). The heparin effect may not be age-dependent, but may be caused by age-related changes in serum protein concentrations or coagulation factors (56). Few studies have simultaneously investigated both pharmacokinetics and pharmacodynamics (57). In general, drug action altered with age has been ascribed to the elderly's reduced reserve capacity and changes in the autonomic nervous system, brain, CNS, cardiovascular system, drug receptors, and endocrine system (58–61).

Reduced Reserve Capacity and Altered Homeostasis

In the elderly, reserve capacity is significantly decreased. It has also been suggested that 95% of the remaining reserve capacity is needed by the elderly simply to deal with the stresses of daily life. Thus, the elderly are more susceptible to decompensation under stress because of the loss of physiologic reserve (62). The systems that are most limited with increasing age and are most vulnerable (i.e., the CNS, the cardiopulmonary system, and the musculoskeletal system) appear to be affected most often. For example, the perfusion of vital organs is often diminished in the elderly, and small changes in blood flow (perhaps induced by drugs) can endanger organ function because the functional reserve capacity is reduced in the elderly. The body's decreased ability to maintain homeostasis has been well described (63, 64). Older people are less able to regulate blood glucose levels, blood pH, pulse rate, blood pressure, and oxygen consumption. Therefore, it is not unreasonable to assume that drugs can have an adverse effect on the elderly's functional reserve and bring about unanticipated (although not unpredictable) adverse drug effects.

Balance There is evidence that the efficiency of postural stability is reduced with advancing age; the elderly have a greater tendency to sway when standing (65). Any drugs that affect this homeostatic mechanism (e.g., antihistamines, which affect the CNS) can decrease the body's ability to maintain balance, possibly leading to a greater incidence of falls and fractures.

Body Temperature The efficiency of the thermoregulatory mechanism, which controls body temperature, decreases with advancing age (10). Impaired shivering, defective vasoconstriction, and poor appreciation of low temperatures occur with increased prevalence in the elderly (66). Elderly patients taking aspirin chronically or in high doses often complain about "shivering" or "feeling cold" (67). Hypothermia can be induced if aspirin is added to a regimen containing other drugs that adversely affect the thermoregulatory mechanism (e.g., psychotropics). Hypothermia is more pro-

nounced and prolonged in the elderly than in younger patients (68), and is often fatal. As a result of reduced cardiac and pulmonary reserve, the elderly may develop cardiovascular problems during rewarming and may shiver because of increased oxygen consumption. Older patients with hypertension and/or increased vascular resistance may exhibit dysrhythmias or even congestive heart failure.

Inhibition of the normal cooling mechanism is also likely, with resultant hyperthermia. The anticholinergic effect of drugs may prevent heat loss by CNS-induced anhydrosis. Vasoconstriction may increase body temperature by peripheral mechanisms (69).

Bowel and Bladder Function Control of bowel and bladder function is lessened with advancing age, and is therefore less efficient. A further decrease in efficiency is likely with laxative use (direct effect) or by indirect action. Drugs with anticholinergic action and other CNS drugs may lessen neurologic control. The impact of nonprescription drugs is often increased when added to an already existing therapeutic regimen.

Cardiovascular System It is frequently overlooked that agents such as the antihistamines may lower blood pressure, usually because of alpha blockade, thus causing postural hypotension.

Altered Receptor Function

Paracelsus, around 1500 AD, first suggested the existence of receptors. He speculated that drugs might contain barbed hooks (spicula) with which they could become fixed to organisms, thus producing their effect. In 1878, Langley described the receptive substances to which drugs might be bound (70). Around the beginning of the 20th century, Ehrlich suggested that drugs adhered to chemoreceptors in the organism with "haptophoric" groups, while "actophoric" groups were responsible for drug action. It is now known that receptors are macromolecular protein complexes found in mitochondriae, lysozymes, cytoplasmic granules, cell membranes, and other cell sites. When a drug complexes with a receptor, an agonist or antagonist action will result.

A drug has affinity and intrinsic activity in relation to each of its receptors. Affinity is the efficiency with which a drug binds to its receptors, and intrinsic activity is its power to generate a stimulus. Drugs with both affinity and intrinsic activity are defined as agonists. Drugs that have affinity but lack intrinsic activity are defined as antagonists.

Most drugs bind to receptors, and thus initiate their action (71). Perhaps age-related altered drug action is also related to altered receptor–drug interactions. It has been postulated that a given receptor site or drug concentration produces a greater pharmaco-dynamic effect in the elderly than in younger persons. However, generalizations cannot be drawn because the number of receptors is not fixed but is regulated by a number of factors, including certain disease states (ischemia, hypertension, heart failure, cardiac hypertrophy), drugs (glucocorticoids, hormones, adrenergic agonists and antagonists), and the aging processes themselves (71). It is known that certain receptors or their responsiveness change with age, while others, such as the alpha-adrenoceptors, do not (72, 73). There may be receptor changes with age in certain parts of the body, but not in others. The CNS cholinergic receptors decline in the basal ganglia, but probably not in other brain regions. Receptors, in adapting to drug therapy, may also become supersensitive or desensitized (74). For example, alterations in insulin receptors account for some forms of insulin resistance.

Age-related changes have been documented for brain benzodiazepine receptors and for several hormone receptors (75, 76). Most studies, however, have concentrated on the cholinergic, the dopamine, and the beta-adrenergic receptors.

Beta-Receptors There is evidence that beta-receptors change with age. The resistance of older adults to both the adrenergic agonist, isoproterenol (77, 78), and the antagonist drug, propranolol (78, 79), is well-known. Increased age and blood pressure are associated with a progressive reduction in beta-adrenoreceptor sensitivity and/or reactivity. Defective beta-adrenoreceptor-mediated responses may result in unopposed alpha-adrenoreceptor-mediated vasoconstriction and thus contribute to the development of hypertension (72).

It was originally thought that age differences in beta-adrenergic responsiveness were caused by alterations in receptor number and affinity (78, 80), a theory that was also used to explain the positive correlation of age with plasma norepinephrine levels (77) and the positive correlation of age with the resistance of the heart to the chronotropic response of isoproterenol (77). The dose of isoproterenol needed to increase the heart rate by 25 beats per minute is 4–6 times higher in older than in younger persons (78). Later studies partially agreed with these findings (81) or did not confirm them (82). Apparently, even in the absence of a reduced number of beta-receptors, the elderly exhibit decreased beta-receptor sensitivity to both beta-agonists and antagonists, which cannot be explained on the basis of pharmacokinetic changes alone (83).

In the elderly, the proportion of beta-receptors in the "high" versus "low" affinity state is diminished (84). Additionally, the plasma norepinephrine concentration is elevated in older subjects (85). Perhaps the circulating norepinephrine competes with a beta-blocker for occupancy of the beta-receptors, causing an apparent reduction in the affinity of the receptor for the antagonist, resulting in decreased drug sensitivity (82). Other explanations have been offered. The activity of beta-blockers also appears to be related to the activity of the plasma renin-angiotensin-aldosterone system. Plasma renin activity decreases with age. The percentage of patients with low-renin hypertension decreases with age, and beta-blockers are less effective in patients with low-renin hypertension (86). It is also possible that the altered action of beta-adrenergic blockers with age may be caused by lower levels of cyclic adenosine monophosphate (cyclic AMP) and reduced adenylate cyclase activity (87).

Autonomic Nervous System

There is evidence that the beta-agonist effect of bronchodilators is reduced in the elderly (88), possibly to a clinically significant degree. Furthermore, the bladders of elderly patients are often deficient in detrusor strength, which may help to explain the tendency of anticholinergic drugs to cause urinary retention in this age group.

Brain and Central Nervous System

Between 20 and 80 years of age, brain weight is reduced by 20%, and there may be neuronal dropout of up to 25% in some areas of the brain (89, 90). Neuronal loss in the superior frontal and temporal regions and the striatum has been reported (91). Hippocampal pyramidal and granular cells and cerebellar Purkinje's cells decline with age. There is a large decrease in neo-cortical choline acetyltranferase enzyme activity in the frontal and temporal cortex and the hippocampal regions. There is also an age-related decline in dopamine receptor numbers (92). On the other hand, there is no change in brain metabolic function with age, perhaps because of compensatory mechanisms. It is likely, however, that under various stressed states, there would be a different pharmacologic response between younger and older subjects (93, 94).

Evidence indicates that, with advanced age, there is increased conduction time, decreased cerebral blood flow, and, possibly, increased permeability of the blood–brain barrier (9). Both subjective and objective evidence indicates that the elderly have an enhanced CNS sensitivity to drugs, prompting a reduced dose requirement (perhaps as much as 50%) for some drugs (95). In an animal study designed to exclude or account for pharmacokinetic variables and to avoid confounding secondary effects, such as hypothermia and development of functional tolerance, a substantial increase in CNS sensitivity to phenobarbital and alcohol was seen with increasing age (96). Plasma and brain barbiturate concentrations are higher in older than in younger animals. Furthermore, the relative ratio of plasma levels to brain levels has been found to increase in older animals (97); that may be the basis for the increased sensitivity of the elderly to the toxic effects of barbiturates and, perhaps, other CNS drugs.

Increased brain sensitivity and other changes, such as decreased coordination, prolongation of reaction time, and impairment of short-term memory, manifest as increased frequency of confusion, increased number of falls (particularly among elderly women), and increased frequency of urinary incontinence. Drug therapy may exaggerate all of these changes, particularly if drugs are used in the "usual" dose or if multiple drugs are used. Such exaggerated changes also extend to secondary effects of drugs (e.g., anticholinergic effects). What may lead to a minor irritation in the younger patient may lead to debilitation, confusion, dry mouth, oversedation, unsteadiness, fecal impaction, and urinary retention in the elderly. Importantly, the effects may lead to greater memory impairment and to prolonged impairment of standing steadiness (98). The most clear-cut evidence of enhanced brain sensitivity to the action of some drugs and, thus, of altered and age-associated pharmacodynamic drug action exists for the benzodiazepines (99). Confusion, ataxia, immobility and incontinence have been demonstrated when some of these drugs are given in the normal adult dose to elderly patients (100). Impairment of neurologic function in elderly patients prescribed these drugs appears to be the rule rather than the exception, particularly among those at high risk to toxicity and regarding the more subtle aspects of toxicity (101). Compelling evidence that pharmacodynamic changes occur with benzodiazepines is provided by the fact that although pharmacokinetic changes appear to occur with some of these drugs, enhanced sensitivity occurs with all. Postural sway, reaction time, and subjective sedation tend to be more pronounced in elderly than in younger patients, given the usual dose (98).

Other evidence exists for the tricyclic antidepressants. "Subtherapeutic" plasma drug concentrations have produced positive clinical response in depressed elderly women, indicating that the substrate for drug activity may be changed in the elderly (102). However, the delirium that can be induced by anticholinergic drugs, to which the elderly appear more sensitive, is probably caused not only by a higher risk to such toxicity of the aged CNS, but also by pharmacokinetic changes (103). The altered pharmacodynamic response to tricyclics is most apparent in terms of the actual noradrenergic function (i.e., in terms of their altered effect on the cardiovascular system). Even though these drugs may produce a significant elevation of plasma norepinephrine concentrations, there may be no alteration in baseline heart rate and blood pressure, which is normally seen in younger patients. Middle-aged patients would most likely show a rise in supine heart rate (104). The elderly are also especially sensitive to both the intended pharmacologic effects and the undesirable adverse effects of other psychotropic agents (105). Age changes and many other factors increase the risk of adverse effects (106). For example, the use of psychotropic agents, particularly the intermediate- and long-acting benzodiazepines, has been strongly associated with an increased incidence of falling and fractures (107–109).

CNS changes associated with aging also increase the risk of the elderly to tardive dyskinesia, even when neuroleptic doses are small and treatment periods are brief (110).

Cardiovascular System

The action of cardiac drugs in the elderly is assumed to differ from that in younger people because measurements start from a different point. For example, the cardiac index changes with age; the elderly have a higher peripheral resistance and intrinsic heart rate and a lower vagal restraint. Sinus node and atrioventricular node dysfunction increase with age; maximum heart rate decreases. Peak cardiac output at exercise also declines with age. The lower maximum exercise heart rate is largely the result of changes in response to beta-adrenergic stimulation (111). Total left ventricular mass increases, decreasing maximum coronary blood flow. Adaptation of the aging heart to stress is diminished because of a delayed and reduced reaction of the sympathetic nervous system (112). Reduced work performance and oxygen consumption at maximal workload are associated with a lesser capacity to increase heart rate, cardiac output, and ejection fraction.

The maximal response of the myocardium to catecholamines is reduced with aging (113, 114). The decreased response to isoproterenol (a lesser increase in heart rate per unit dosage) has been well demonstrated. Plasma levels of norepinephrine are often higher in the elderly than in younger people, suggesting a defect in responsiveness to catecholamines, not in synthesis (115). On the other hand, cyclic AMP and protein kinase responses to catecholamines are apparently unchanged. As a result of these changes, the heart manifests an increased sensitivity to the toxic effects of some drugs (e.g., digoxin), which is heightened in the presence of hypokalemia, but manifests a lessened increase in contractility to cardiac glycosides (113). Various age changes also account for an increased risk of the elderly to effects associated with antihypertensive drugs (Table 2).

Changes in the cardiovascular system also involve changes in blood vessels (116). Between 20 and 80 years

TABLE 2 Age-related changes and their possible effects on action of antihypertensives

Organ/System	Change with age	Possible effect
Brain	Cerebral blood flow decreased by 25%. Cerebral autoregulation impaired.	Use drugs that preserve cerebral blood flow. Caution: possibility of inducing hyperfusion (?) or stroke (?)
	Increased permeability of blood/brain barrier.	Exaggerated CNS effects by lipid-soluble drugs: clonidine, methyldopa, metopropolol, propranolol.
Cardiovascular	A poor homeostatic system. Impaired control and vascular reactivity. Deterioration of conducting system.	Caution: drugs that interfere with cardiac impulse (beta-blockers).
	Between 20–80 years of age, a 90% loss of vessel elasticity and distensibility.	Greater fall in blood pressure with decrease in blood volume. Increased risk to hypotension, hypovolemia.
	Baroreceptor sensitivity decreased.	Altered compensatory mechanism, drug-induced fall in blood pressure.
	Vascular aging (aortic arch), attenuated beta-adrenergic response, blunted postural reflexes, decreased body water, varicose veins, etc.	Increased risk to drug-induced orthostatic hypotension. Caution: diuretics, ganglionic blockers, vasodilators.

of age, vessel elasticity and distensibility are reduced by 90%, leading to increased arterial blood pressure. In both younger and older subjects, an increase in peripheral resistance is mainly responsible for essential hypertension. In the elderly, hyaline thickening of arterioles may be a contributing factor. In both normotensive and hypertensive elderly patients, plasma renin and aldosterone concentrations decline. Increases in plasma renin activity in response to sodium depletion or diuretics may also be reduced. The elderly generally present with a relatively reduced fluid volume; extracellular volume is decreased to the greatest degree. Therefore, these hemodynamic and fluid volume changes are expected to change the response of elderly to antihypertensive drugs (117–119). Baroreceptors, located in the carotid sinus and aortic arch, function by responding to changes in arterial pressure. Arterial baroreceptor reflexes respond to changes in blood pressure by changes in sympathetic and parasympathetic outflow (56), decreasing arterial pressure via vasodilation and decreasing both the rate and force of cardiac contractility. Altered action of antihypertensive agents in the elderly involves changes in sympathetic and parasympathetic pathways, as well as in the afferent and central connections of the baroreceptor reflex arc, the hypothalamic neural afferent pathways, and the hypothalamo-pituitary effector system (56). Baroreceptor sensitivity is significantly and progressively decreased with age, in both normotensive and hypertensive patients. Reduced baroreceptor sensitivity manifests with a reduced heart rate response to alterations of pressure within the aorta and the carotid arteries (120, 121).

Additionally, the elderly are more likely than younger people to become symptomatically orthostatic even without drugs. Orthostatic hypotension is more common in older people. As many as 5% of elderly patients show a drop in systolic hypertension upon standing; one contributing factor is the reduced sensitivity of the baroreceptor system, which does not allow the elderly to compensate as efficiently for either elevated or reduced blood pressure. Therefore, all drugs that could cause orthostatic hypotension (antihypertensives, antihistamines, psychotropics), particularly if used in combination, should be used cautiously for the elderly (122). The risk of orthostatic hypotension is further increased in elderly patients with volume depletion, caused by salt and/or water depletion, or with circulatory changes, caused by infections or fever (121). Indeed, women receiving antihypertensive drugs report significantly more fainting, dizziness, and "blacking-out" than controls. Similar effects, except blacking-out, have been recorded for men (123). The altered homeostatic system of the elderly patient must also be remembered. If potassium homeostasis is impaired, all currently available potassium-sparing diuretics can induce severe hyperkalemia, which could be asymptomatic until potentially fatal toxicity is manifested.

Endocrine System

Age-related changes in the endocrine system have been documented (124). Specific age-related disturbances in the extrahepatic hormonal regulatory mechanism have also been proposed (125). The reduced availability of hormones results in diminished endocrine regulatory mechanisms with age, as well as deficiencies in hormonal feedback mechanisms. It also leads to decreasing binding affinities and receptor numbers with age (126).

Alterations in pancreatic and adrenal hormone levels result in decreased glucose tolerance with age and an increased susceptibility of the elderly to drug-induced hypoglycemia (9). Some elderly suffer from a decreased release of insulin, while others have a decreased number of insulin receptors and/or postreceptor abnormalities (127). Production of sex hormones also decreases with age (9). In women, reduced estrogen levels have been correlated with a greater incidence of osteoporosis (which, at that stage of life, cannot be addressed with increased calcium intake). Because of these hormonal changes, women are also more susceptible to orthostatic hypotension. Decreased thyroid levels make the elderly more sensitive to the action of digitalis and increase the risk of drug-induced hypothermia (128).

Immune System

Some, but not all, immunologic functions show a gradual decline with age. The thymus probably has less power than the central immunologic organs and the bone marrow to maintain functional levels of peripheral T-lymphoid population.

The immunologic theory of aging, or the so-called "thymus clock" theory, addresses the possible role of the thymus and the cell-mediated immune system in the aging process. With increasing age, the thymus apparently loses its ability to facilitate the differentiation of immature lymphocytes. Consequently, elderly persons have an increased number of immature cells in the thymus and among circulating peripheral T-cells (129).

The T-lymphocytes that initiate cell-mediated immunity recognize foreign substances. They are activated or sensitized, and then either play a central role as helper T-cells, or, as cytotoxic T-cells, directly kill infected host cells. Although there is still no evidence of a change with age in the absolute number of peripheral blood lymphocytes (130), the altered T-cell function is thought to be responsible for a diminished response to mitogens and allogeneic cells (131), a decreased secre-

tion of antibody (132), a diminished expression of delayed hypersensitivity (133), and an increased frequency of autoantibody production (132).

In humoral immunity, the B-lymphocytes first recognize a foreign substance and then differentiate into plasma cells. This process produces cells that secrete antibodies. These antibodies bind to an antigen, triggering complement fixation. Phagocytes then remove the antibody–antigen complex.

No change in the number of circulating B-cells in the elderly has been documented (134). However, these cells apparently do lose their ability to function and respond normally, producing less antibody than younger B-cells. That decline, however, apparently occurs to a lesser degree than the T-cell activity decline (135).

There is still little definitive information regarding age-dependent alterations in the secretory immune system (136). However, it has been suggested that the mucosal surfaces of the GI and respiratory tracts in elderly persons exhibit increased susceptibility to infections (137), which may be caused by an age-related decline in the secretion of the primary immunoglobulin of the secretory immune system (i.e., immunoglobulin A) (138).

The immune function is under a complex regulatory control, and immunologic changes are probably caused by disturbances in that regulatory process. Indeed, age-related changes in immune function reflect several different alterations. Overall, T-cells are diminished in function with age. The deficiency includes most T-cell effector and regulatory functions, with the possible exception of T-suppression. All of these factors combine to decrease cellular immune competence (139, 140). There is no question that infections are more prevalent in the elderly; however, the infections common in older people (influenza, pneumococcal pneumonia) are not usually associated with immune deficiency, as are pneumocystitis and infections caused by opportunistic organisms. It has been suggested that reduced immune competence may mandate the use of bactericidal agents more often than bacteriostatic agents.

Gastrointestinal System

Many prospective and retrospective studies have addressed the possibly heightened risk of the elderly to the gastrotoxic and ulcerogenic effects of aspirin and nonaspirin, nonsteroidal anti-inflammatory drugs (NSAIDs). (A host of other drugs, ranging from reserpine and potassium to ascorbic acid, may be gastrotoxic in the elderly.) Usually, a "highly significant" statistical correlation is reported between perforated peptic ulceration and ingestion of NSAIDs, when age- and sex-matched elderly patients and controls are compared. Apparently, elderly patients who are prescribed

TABLE 3 Changes with age that increase risk of the elderly to the adverse GI effects of NSAIDs

Changes	Possible consequences
PRIMARY AGE CHANGE	
Morphologic: Decreased mucosal thickness	Devitalization of mucosa, atrophic gastritis, greater risk of ulcers.
Motor: Delayed gastric emptying (?)	Longer residence time for gastrotoxic (erosive) drugs. Greater risk to injury.
Secretory: Reduced gastric secretion, altered pH	Less resistance to injury. Increased incidence of ulcers. Injury less rapidly repaired.
SECONDARY AGE CHANGE	
Increased number of intercurrent diseases. Increased drug use (gastrotoxic, gastrokinetic)	Greater risk to injury. May interfere with healing.
TERTIARY AGE CHANGE	
Behavioral changes, anxiety, fear	Increased incidence of GI complaints. Thirty percent of all complaints by elderly are induced by fear and/or anxiety.

NSAIDs (and, who may also take self-prescribed non-prescription products) are at heightened risk of gastric and duodenal ulceration (141, 142). Elderly women, especially those receiving diuretics, appear to be at particular risk.

Primary, secondary, and tertiary age changes heighten the elderly's risk of GI problems, including drug-induced problems (Tables 3, 4). Aging is associated with secretory and morphologic changes in the stomach. Muscular atrophy, thinning of gastric mucosa, and infiltration of the submucosa with elastic fibers are evident in the stomachs of 80% of patients over 50 years of age (143, 144). The cumulative effects of surface injury and repair lead to atrophy of the mucosa. Accelerated and substained cell turnover and shortening of the period of maturity of differentiated cells are responsible for reduced secretion of protective mucus. Intestinal blood flow may be reduced by as much as 50% by age 65, being further diminished by stress, congestive heart failure, hypoxia, and hypovolemia. Ischemia may result, and subsequent arterial occlusion and mesenteric vascular insufficiency may often be related to GI complaints. The influence of psychosomatic and behavioral factors is particularly important to community-living elderly. Tension, fear of disease and death, depressive illness, anxiety, and worry influence stomach motility and secretory function. Chronic gastritis, irritable colon, spastic colitis, heartburn, ulcer-like distress, and nausea can result. In one study of 300 elderly patients, 31% suffered from these problems (11).

Altered Secretory Function Gastric secretion declines with age. Gastric cell function decreases, and gastric pH is elevated. In one study, the secretory volume in patients 61–70 years of age was only 50%, and the concentration of gastric acid only 30%, when compared to people 21–30 years of age. In another study, among those 60 years of age and over, 43% of men and 36% of women exhibited basal achlorhydria. After stimulation, achlorhydria was still observed in 21% of the men and

TABLE 4 Suggested reasons for increased risk* of elderly to the GI side effects of NSAIDs

Intestinal blood flow diminished by 50%. Ischemia and occlusion. Damage in ischemic areas.

Gastric secretory volume may decrease by 50%.

Increased incidence of gastritis and gastric ulcers.

Ulcer disease more virulent in elderly. Gastric hemorrhage from superficial lesions most life-threatening. May present silently. Older female patients receiving diuretics are most at risk.

*Identified risks include:
Complications rising from 31% (60–64 years of age) to 75% (70–79 years of age);
Rebleeding in as many as 40% of elderly;
Mortality: 25% in those 85 years of age and older.

10% of the women. Furthermore, gastric secretion is diminished in diabetes and untreated hyperthyroidism and hypothyroidism. Some elderly people maintain a normal and even high acid secretory function; duodenal ulceration in people older than 70 years of age may occur because acid secretion is high. Indeed, acid suppression may be more important for mucosal protection in the duodenum than in the stomach, where other defense mechanisms may be operative (142).

Altered Motor Function Gastric emptying is about 2.5 times faster in younger than in older persons because gastric emptying is under the control of the CNS, which may lose efficiency with advancing age. Slowing of gastric emptying follows a reduction in gastric acid secretion; gastric emptying is also negatively affected by stress, lack of ambulation, gastric ulcer, intestinal obstruction, myocardial infarct, and diabetes mellitus. Some drugs (e.g., antacids, anticholinergics, ganglionic blockers, isoniazid, lithium, and narcotic analgesics) delay gastric emptying. Fatty meals delay gastric emptying more in elderly than in younger people. A delay in gastric emptying, of course, permits gastrotoxic agents a longer residence time and, therefore, more opportunity to exert their toxic effect.

Other Factors Local ischemia caused by atherosclerosis may predispose elderly to ulcer formation (an effect that may be heightened by the prostaglandin inhibition of NSAIDs), which further reduces gastric mucosal blood flow. Furthermore, estrogens and progestogens increase mucus production in the stomach; postmenopausal women may therefore have lessened mucus production, which could further be reduced by the action of NSAIDs.

Nonsteroidal Anti-inflammatory Drugs The use of NSAIDs increases with age, but their adverse drug effects increase disproportionally with age. One reason, of course, is their possibly inappropriate use in the management of pain of osteoporosis. Another reason may be that they are overprescribed—internists, rheumatologists, family physicians, podiatrists, and dentists all prescribe NSAIDs. Of course, many NSAIDs may also be obtained without a prescription (more NSAIDs will soon have nonprescription status). The potential gastrotoxicity of these drugs may be enhanced by their simultaneous administration with other gastrotoxic drugs, coffee, or alcohol (145, 146). Through inhibition of the protective effects of GI prostaglandins and via local noxious effects, salicylates and NSAIDs can cause superficial gastric and duodenal erosions and ulcer formation, which can then result in GI bleeding and perforations. Decreased platelet aggregation can enhance the potential for bleeding. All NSAIDs can interfere with platelet function and prolong bleeding time, which is generally quickly reversible on withdrawal of the offending drug, except for aspirin. However, the combination of GI irritation and prolonged bleeding time can cause serious GI hemorrhage, especially in the elderly. There is no question that the elderly, particularly the very old, suffer from greater morbidity and mortality from these adverse events (147). Nonspecific ulcerative processes in the small bowel have been described, perhaps because of inhibited mucosal glycoprotein synthesis and increased intestinal permeability to these drugs. About 70% of patients on long-term NSAID therapy have inflammation of the small intestine, with bleeding, protein loss, and ileal dysfunction as major complications (148). Patients occasionally develop strictures. Mucosal lesions of the stomach and duodenum are frequently reported in patients taking NSAIDs. Elderly patients may be especially susceptible to NSAID-associated peptic ulcer perforation (149). In fact, 21% of all adverse drug reactions (ADRs) reported to the spontaneous reporting system of the Food and Drug Administration (FDA) are caused by NSAIDs (150). In the United Kingdom, 17% of all fatalities reported to the Committee on Safety of Medicines were caused by NSAIDs, and about 25% of all ADRs reported there were attributable to these drugs (151). However, only a small percentage of NSAID-induced problems may be reported (152).

Renal System

With advancing age, renal blood and plasma flow decrease, and the kidney's ability to concentrate urine decreases, as does its maximum diluting ability (153, 154) and its ability to compensate for abnormalities of the acid–base balance and electrolytes. The elderly do not conserve sodium efficiently, probably because of lower plasma renin activity and urinary aldosterone excretion. Therefore, both of the broad excretory functions of the kidneys, namely preservation of body fluid volume and maintenance of their composition, are adversely affected by aging.

In the elderly, even those with mild renal impairment and those with underlying intrinsic renal disease, the NSAIDs can exacerbate the severity of renal disease by blocking interrenal cyclo-oxygenase (reduction of renal prostaglandin secretion). This risk is increased in volume-depleted elderly (Table 5). Acute renal failure has been documented in patients with congestive heart failure (CHF), cirrhosis, or nephrotic syndrome, and in patients on diuretic therapy. Among the documented problems are functional acute renal failure, interstitial nephritis, hyponatremia, and hyperkalemia (155). Although most of these problems are reversible on withdrawal of the drug, it is suggested that these problems may not be recognized early enough in the fast-growing and relatively unsupervised sectors of home care and

TABLE 5 NSAIDs: Risk factors for adverse renal effects in the elderly

Factors	Potential outcomes
PRIMARY AGING FACTORS	
Physiologic and functional changes in heart and kidneys	Less perfusion of kidneys, hemodynamic insufficiency. Kidneys may depend critically on endogenous prostaglandins.
Reduced thirst mechanism	Dehydration, volume depletion, hemodynamic insufficiency.
SECONDARY AGING FACTORS	
Increasing number of chronic intercurrent diseases: CHF, hypertension, diabetes	Increased hemodynamic insufficiency, water retention. Increased angiotensin II and adrenergic activity. Increased need for prostaglandins in autoregulation of renal blood flow and GFR.
Management of secondary changes: increased drug use (diuretics), salt restriction	Hypovolemia and salt restriction may lead to potassium excretion. Volume depletion can lead to hyponatremia. Increased risk of nephrotoxicity.
TERTIARY AGING FACTORS	
Altered nutritional intake: elderly (25%) often buy potassium supplements, salt substitutes	Increased risk to hyperkalemia.

assisted living. Anecdotal and unconfirmed reports have raised the question of the danger of NSAIDs when sold without a prescription and when taken in a nondirected and unsupervised manner. Apparently, some otherwise healthy elderly people have been seen in emergency rooms with symptomatology of CHF, which, on differential diagnosis, was ascribed to an overdose of a nonprescription NSAID and subsequent salt and water retention.

SUMMARY

There is no doubt that many age-associated factors alter drug action in the elderly and, therefore, that the elderly are more susceptible to adverse drug reactions and a drug-induced reduction in their quality of life. Among the factors least studied are pharmacodynamic changes with age. Health care providers prescribing, dispensing, and administering drugs and monitoring the therapeutic outcome must become very familiar with these changes because they can significantly alter the action of drugs in the elderly.

REFERENCES

1   F. E. Young, "Self-Care, Self-Medication in America's Future," The Proprietary Association, Washington, D.C., 1988.

2   P. P. Lamy, *Am. Fam. Phys.*, *39*, 175 (1989).

3   A. Chaiton et al., *Can. Med. Assoc. J.*, *114*, 33 (1976).

4   C. S. Rose et al., *Am. J. Clin. Nutr.*, *29*, 847 (1976).

5   D. Guttman, "Medication Management and Education of the Elderly," C. Beber and P. P. Lamy, Eds., Excerpta Medica, Princeton, N.J., 1978.

6   C. H. Kline, "Self-Care, Self-Medication in America's Future," The Proprietary Association, Washington, D.C., 1988.

7   P. P. Lamy, *Maryland Pharm.*, *64 (9)*, 9 (1988).

8   G. E. Schumacher, *Am. J. Hosp. Pharm.*, *37*, 559 (1980).

9   P. P. Lamy, "Prescribing for the Elderly," PSG Publishing, Littleton, Mass., 1980.

10   P. P. Lamy, *Pharm. Internat.*, *7*, 46 (1986).

11   M. Sklar, "Clinical Aspects of Aging," W. Reichel, Ed., Williams & Wilkins, Baltimore, Md., 1983.

12   H. L. Bleich et al., *N. Engl. J. Med.*, *297*, 1332 (1977).

13   B. Gachalyi et al., *Europ. J. Clin. Pharmacol.*, *26*, 43 (1984).

14   J. Beckman et al., *Br. Med. J.*, *297*, 1316 (1988).

15   E. S. Vesel, *Clin. Pharmacol. Ther.*, *36*, 285 (1984).

16 B. Yachmetz et al., *Geriatr. Consult.*, *6 (4)*, 20 (1988).

17 P. P. Gerbino, *J. Am. Geriatr. Soc.*, *30*, S88 (1982).

18 The Commonwealth Fund Commission on Elderly Living Alone, The Commonwealth Fund, Washington, D.C., 1987.

19 S. J. Jachuk et al., *J. R. Coll. Gen. Pract.*, *32*, 103 (1982).

20 B. W. Rovener, et al., *Am. J. Psychiatry*, *145*, 1 (1988).

21 S. E. Levkoff et al., *J. Am. Geriatr. Soc.*, *36*, 622 (1988).

22 T. L. Hickey, *Geriatr. Med. Today*, *7 (6)*, 59 (1988).

23 B. R. Clarridge, *Med. Care*, 27, 352 (1988).

24 R. E. Grymonpre et al., *J. Am. Geriatr. Soc.*, *36*, 1092 (1988).

25 J. S. Walker, *J. Pharm. Sci.*, *78*, 986 (1989).

26 P. P. Lamy, *J. Am. Geriatr. Soc.*, *34*, 586 (1986).

27 A. J. Silver et al., *J. Am. Geriatr. Soc.*, *36*, 487 (1988).

28 L. Davies, *Nutr. Soc.*, *43*, 295 (1984).

29 P. P. Lamy et al., "Oral Health and Aging," A. F. Tryon, Ed., PSG Publishing, Littleton, Mass., 1986.

30 P. P. Lamy, "CRC Handbook of Nutrition in the Aged," R. R. Watson, Ed., CRC Press, Boca Raton, Fla., 1985.

31 P. P. Lamy, *J. Am. Geriatr. Soc.*, *31*, 560 (1983).

32 E. W. Campion et al., *Arch. Intern. Med.*, *147*, 945 (1987).

33 P. P. Lamy, *J. Am. Geriatr. Soc.*, *30*, S69 (1982).

34 A. Herxheimer, *Drug Ther. Bull.*, *19 (9)*, 33 (1981).

35 P. P. Lamy and L. J. Lesko, *Annl. Rep. in Med. Chem.*, *20*, 295 (1985).

36 P. P. Lamy, *J. Am. Geriatr. Soc.*, *30*, S11 (1982).

37 D. J. Greenblatt et al., *N. Engl. J. Med.*, *306*, 1081 (1982).

38 D. L. Schmucker, *Pharmacol. Rev.*, *30*, 445 (1986).

39 P. P. Gerbino and J. A. Gans, *J. Am. Geriatr. Soc.*, *30*, S81 (1982).

40 J. Cooper and C. Gardner, *J. Am. Geriatr. Soc.*, *36*, 660 (1988).

41 E. M. Brown and C. H. Winograd, *J. Am. Geriatr. Soc.*, *36*, 653 (1988).

42 D. L. Schmucker and E. T. Lonergan, *Rev. Biol. Res. Aging*, *3*, 509 (1987).

43 M. E. Tinetti, *J. Am. Geriatr. Soc.*, *31*, 174 (1983).

44 G. R. Wilkinson, *Pharmacol. Rev.*, *39*, 1 (1987).

45 G. M. Rubin et al., *J. Pharm. Pharmacol.*, *35*, 115 (1983).

46 R. K. Verbeek, *J. Rheumatol.*, *15* (suppl. 17), 44 (1988).

47 D. E. Furst et al., *Clin. Pharmacol. Ther.*, *26*, 380 (1979).

48 G. Levy, *J. Pharm. Sci.*, *54*, 959 (1965).

49 P. C. Ho et al., *Br. J. Clin. Pharmacol.*, *19*, 675 (1985).

50 P. P. Lamy, *Meth. Find. Exptl. Clin. Pharmacol.*, *9 (3)*, 13 (1987).

51 P. P. Lamy, *ElderCare News*, *5 (4)*, 25 (1989).

52 J. Crooks, *J. Chron. Dis.*, *36*, 85 (1983).

53 R. E. Vestal, *Drugs*, *16*, 358 (1978).

54 A. P. Kaplan, *J. Allergy Immunol.*, *74*, 573 (1984).

55 B. R. Jones et al., *J. Am. Geriatr. Soc.*, *28*, 10 (1980).

56 J. L. Reid, *Triangle*, *23*, 7 (1984).

57 B. J. Cusack and R. E. Vestal, "The Practice of Geriatrics," E. Calkins et al., Eds., W. B. Saunders, Philadelphia, Pa., 1986.

58 D. M. Bowen and A. N. Davidson, *J. Chron. Dis.*, *36*, 3 (1983).

59 N. W. Shock, *J. Chron. Dis.*, *36*, 137 (1983).

60 T. Mikiten, "Handbook of Physiology of Aging," E. J. Masoro, Ed., CRC Press, Boca Raton, Fla., 1981.

61 E. G. Lakatta, *J. Chron. Dis.*, *36*, 15 (1983).

62 R. B. Hickler, "Emergency Problems in the Elderly," E. P. Hoffer, Ed., Medical Economic Books, Oradel, N.J., 1985.

63 R. R. Kohn, *J. Chron. Dis.*, *16*, 5 (1983).

64 J. Sartin et al., *Fed. Proceed.*, *39*, 3163 (1980).

65 C. G. Swift, *Br. Med. J.*, *296*, 913 (1988).

66 K. J. Collins et al., *Br. Med. J.*, *1*, 353 (1977).

67 R. H. Fox et al., *Br. Med. J.*, *1*, 21 (1973).

68 S. Powell et al., *Am. J. Hosp. Pharm.*, *39*, 1963 (1982).

69 M. F. Laventurier et al., *J. Am. Pharm. Assoc.*, *16*, 77 (1976).

70 J. N. Langley, *J. Physiol.*, *1*, 339 (1978).

71 R. J. Lefkowitz et al., *N. Engl. J. Med.*, *310*, 1570 (1983).

72 O. Bertel et al., *Hypertension*, *2*, 130 (1980).

73 P. J. Scott and J. L. Reid, *Br. J. Clin. Pharmacol.*, *13*, 237 (1982).

74 J. A. Severson, *J. Am. Geriatr. Soc.*, *32*, 24 (1984).

75 R. S. Bar and J. Roth, *Arch. Intern. Med.*, *137*, 474 (1977).

76 M. Memo et al., *J. Pharm. Pharmacol.*, *33 (1)*, 64 (1981).

77 G. M. London et al., *J. Clin. Pharmacol.*, *16*, 174 (1976).

78 R. E. Vestal et al., *Clin. Pharmacol. Ther.*, *26*, 181 (1979).

79 J. Conway et al., *Cardiovasc. Res.*, *5*, 577 (1971).

80 D. D. Schocken and G. S. Roth, *Nature*, *267*, 856 (1977).

81 C. Klein et al., *Clin. Pharmacol. Ther.*, *40*, 161 (1986).

82 L. B. Abbrass and P. J. Scarpace, *J. Gerontol.*, *36*, 298 (1981).

83 G. Hitzenberger et al., *Gerontology*, *28* (suppl. 1), 93 (1982).

84 R. D. Feldman et al., *J. Clin. Invest.*, *72*, 164 (1983).

85 C. R. Lake et al., *N. Engl. J. Med.*, *296*, 208 (1977).

86 R. F. Buehler et al., *Am. J. Cardiol.*, *36*, 653 (1975).

87 J. F. Krall et al., *J. Clin. Endocrinol. Metabol.*, *52*, 863 (1981).

88 M. I. Ullah et al., *Thorax*, *36*, 523 (1981).

89 B. E. Tomlinson and G. Henderson, "Neurobiology of Aging," R. D. Terry and S. Gershon, Eds., Raven Press, New York, N.Y., 1976.

90 J. M. Anderson et al., *J. Neurol. Sci.*, *58*, 235 (1983).

91 M. J. Bell, *Acta Neuropathologia*, *37*, 111 (1977).

92 H. N. Wagner et al., *Science*, *221*, 2164 (1983).

93 R. Duarra et al., *Ann. Neurol.*, *16*, 702 (1984).

94 R. Duarra et al., *Brain*, *106*, 761 (1983).

95 J. C. Scott and D. R. Stanski, *J. Pharmacol. Exptl. Ther.*, *240*, 59 (1987).

96 S. Wanwimilruk and G. Levy, *J. Pharm. Sci.*, *76*, 503 (1987).

97 I. M. Kapetanovic et al., *Drug Metabol. Disp.*, *10*, L586 (1982).

98 C. G. Swift et al., *Br. J. Clin. Pharmacol.*, *20*, 119 (1985).

99 D. L. Schmucker, *Pharmacol. Rev.*, *37*, 133 (1985).

100 J. G. Evans and E. H. Jarvis, *Br. Med. J.*, *4*, 133 (1972).

101 B. R. Meyer, *Med. Clin. North. Am.*, *66*, 1017 (1982).

102 N. R. Cutler et al., *Am. J. Psychiatry*, *138*, 1235 (1983).

103 R. L. Livingston et al., *J. Clin. Psychiatry*, *44*, 173 (1983).

104 R. C. Veith et al., *Clin. Pharmacol. Ther.*, *33*, 763 (1983).

105 D. E. Everitt and J. Avorn, *Arch. Intern. Med.*, *146*, 293 (1986).

106 E. H. Rubin, *Hosp. Pract.*, *21*, 95 (1986).

107 E. B. Larson et al., *Ann. Intern. Med.*, *107*, 169 (1987).

108 W. A. Ray et al., *N. Engl. J. Med.*, *3316*, 363 (1987).

109 C. Cooper et al., *Br. Med. J.*, *295*, 13 (1987).

110 T. L. Thompson II et al., *N. Engl. J. Med.*, *308*, 194 (1983).

111 J. B. Schwartz and D. R. Abernethy, *Geriatrics*, *21*, 349 (1987).

112 F. Bend, *Ztg. Kardiol.*, *74* (suppl. 1), 49 (1985).

113 E. G. Lakatta et al., *Circ. Res.*, *36*, 262 (1975).

114 T. Guarnieri et al., *Am. J. Physiol.*, *239*, H501 (1980).

115 J. W. Rowe and B. R. Troen, *Endocr. Rev.*, *1*, 167 (1980).

116 J. H. Fleisch, *Pharmacol. Therap.*, *8*, 477 (1980).

117 J. D. Swales, *Age Ageing*, *8*, 104 (1981).

118 M. Esler, *Clin. Sci.*, *60*, 217 (1981).

119 R. B. Hickler, *J. Am. Geriatr. Soc.*, *31*, 421 (1983).

120 A. D. Norris et al., *Circulation, 8*, 521 (1953).

121 F. I. Caird et al., *Br. Heart J., 35*, 527 (1973).

122 B. Gribbin et al., *Circ. Res., 29*, 424 (1971).

123 W. D. Hale et al., *J. Am. Geriatr. Soc., 32*, 5 (1984).

124 R. Andres and J. D. Tobin, "Handbook of Aging," C. E. Finch and L. Hayflick, Eds., Van Norstrand Reinhold, New York, N.Y., 1977.

125 R. C. Adelman, *Fed. Proceed., 38*, 1968 (1979).

126 S. H. Snyder, *N. Engl. J. Med., 300*, 465 (1979).

127 M. B. Davidson, *Metabolism, 28*, 688 (1979).

128 P. Orlander and D. G. Johnson, *Otolaryngol. Clin. North Am., 15*, 439 (1982).

129 I. M. Smith, *Hosp. Pract., 17*, 69 (1982).

130 M. A. Cobliegh et al., *Clin. Immunol. Immunopathol., 15*, 162 (1980).

131 M. E. Weksler and T. M. Hutteroth, *J. Clin. Invest., 53*, 99 (1974).

132 M. J. Rowley et al., *Lancet, 2*, 24 (1968).

133 D. S. Waldorf et al., *J. Am. Med. Assoc., 203*, 831 (1968).

134 J. L. Ceuppens and J. S. Goodwin, *J. Immunol., 128*, 2429 (1982).

135 L. J. Greenberg and E. J. Yunis, *Fed. Proceed., 37*, 128 (1978).

136 I. D. Gardner, *Rev. Infect. Dis., 2*, 801 (1980).

137 D. L. Schmucker and C. K. Daniels, *J. Am. Geriatr. Soc., 34*, 377 (1986).

138 I. R. Mackay, *Gerontologia, 18*, 285 (1972).

139 T. Makinodan and M. M. B. Kay, *Adv. Immunol., 29*, 287 (1980).

140 G. B. Price and T. Makindon, *J. Immunol., 108*, 302 (1972).

141 F. Lanza et al., *Am. J. Gastroenterol., 75*, 17 (1981).

142 M. G. Robinson et al., *Dig. Dis. Sci., 34*, 424 (1989).

143 P. P. Lamy, *Geriatr. Med. Today., 7 (4)*, 30 (1988).

144 P. P. Lamy, "Side Effects of Anti-inflammatory Drugs," K. D. Rainsford and G. P. Velo, Eds., MTP Press, Ltd, Lancaster, England, 1986.

145 K. Goulson and A. R. Cooke, *Br. Med. J., 14*, 664 (1968).

146 P. P. Lamy, *Generations, 12 (4)*, 9 (1988).

147 K. Beard et al., *Arch. Intern. Med., 147*, 1621 (1987).

148 T. I. Bjarnason, *SCRIP, 1208 (9)*, 30 (1987).

149 D. St. J. Collier and J. A. Pain, *Gut, 26*, 359 (1985).

150 A. C. Rossi et al., *Br. Med. J., 294*, 147 (1987).

151 K. D. Rainsford and G. P. Velo, "Side Effects of Anti-inflammatory/Analgesic Drugs," Raven Press, New York, N.Y., 1983.

152 Committee on Safety of Medicines, *Br. Med. J., 292*, 614 (1986).

153 J. W. Rowe et al., *Nephron, 17*, 270 (1976).

154 M. Epstein and N. K. Hollenberg, *J. Laborat. Clin. Med., 87*, 411 (1976).

155 P. P. Lamy, *J. Am. Geriatr. Soc., 34*, 361 (1986).

Mark W. Veerman and Miriam L. Marcadis

MINICHAPTER

B

NONPRESCRIPTION DRUG USE IN CHILDREN

When asked to recommend a product for a young child, pharmacists often find that products contain no specific labeling recommendations for that age group. Statements such as "Consult your physician for children less than 12 years old," or "Not recommended for infants or children, consult your physician," often appear on the product. Dosage guidelines are not always available for a medication that may potentially benefit an important medical consumer, the pediatric patient. Many of the drugs available in the United States (both prescription and nonprescription) are not approved by the Food and Drug Administration (FDA) for use in pediatric patients. The Kefauver-Harris Act of 1962 stated that a drug must be shown safe and effective in a specific population before it can be indicated in that population; drug companies, however, do not perform the necessary research and testing of many drugs for pediatric patients. The lack of FDA approval does not prevent the use of a drug in that patient age group; however, lack of dosage guidelines often makes drug selection very difficult. In recommending such an "unapproved" drug, the physician or pharmacist must use the same judgment and prudence as with any "approved" drug and could be held accountable for any untoward problem. Therefore, it is important to understand that pediatric patients are not just small adults.

In considering nonprescription drug products for the pediatric age group, certain important differences and problems must be considered: pharmacokinetic dif-

ferences between pediatric and adult patients, effects of disease states on selection of nonprescription products, and the most appropriate method to administer medications. Special consideration should be given to the drug classes commonly used with pediatric patients and to the dosage guidelines relevant to use of these drugs in the pediatric age group. It is important for the practicing pharmacist to understand the principles of nonprescription pediatric drug selection, know when and how to recommend nonprescription medication, and when it is beyond practice limitations to recommend a nonprescription medication for pediatric patients.

Terms frequently used in the professional literature to describe relatively distinctive pediatric age periods may be arbitrarily defined as follows:

- Preterm neonate = gestational age less than 37 weeks;

- Full-term neonate = gestational age 37–41 weeks;

- Neonate = first postnatal month of life;

- Infant = 1–12 months;

- Toddler/schoolage = 1–12 years;

- Adolescent = 12–18 years;

- Adult = over 18 years.

PHARMACOKINETIC DIFFERENCES BETWEEN PEDIATRIC AND ADULT PATIENTS

One of the major differences between pediatric and adult patients is the change in the pharmacokinetic parameters: absorption, distribution, metabolism, and elimination. Significant changes occur in the neonate and infant, followed by gradual changes until adult values are reached. Over time, these changes affect the selection and dosing of prescription drugs and, to a lesser extent, nonprescription medications. Nonprescription medications are not affected as much because of their wider therapeutic index, which increases the margin of safety.

Absorption

The gastrointestinal (GI) absorption of drugs is influenced by many factors, including gastric pH, gastric emptying time, motility of the GI tract, enzymatic activity, blood flow/perfusion of the GI mucosa, permeability and maturation of the mucosal membrane, and any concurrent disease process (1–3). Significant changes in these factors, occurring during the first few years of life, affect both nonprescription and prescription drugs.

The pH of the stomach changes significantly during the first few months of life. At birth, the pH is basic, ranging from 6 to 8. The pH decreases rapidly to 1–3 within a few days, but then slowly increases during the next few weeks to reach about 5 (4). The frequent feedings of milk during the early months of life may explain the high pH during infancy (5–7). The gastric acidity then falls slowly until adult values are reached at about 2 or 3 years of age (2, 5, 8, 9).

Gastric emptying in both the neonate and infant is prolonged and reaches adult values after 6–8 months (10, 11). Intestinal transit time is initially prolonged in the neonate, but intestinal motility increases within several months, leading to variable and unpredictable drug absorption. The pH changes and gastric and intestinal emptying times have a complex effect on drug absorption. Medications undergoing hydrolysis in the stomach have higher bioavailability because of a decrease in breakdown of the medication (12). Changes in pH also affect the absorption of drugs that are weak acids and weak bases. Because drugs are more completely absorbed as un-ionized compounds, weak acids have a decreased absorption in neonates and infants because of their higher pH (13, 14). Drugs such as acetaminophen have decreased bioavailability. The opposite is true of weak bases in the same situation. Delayed intestinal motility can lead to increased drug bioavailability because of an increased residence time available for absorption in the intestinal tract.

Both bile acids and pancreatic enzymes are reduced in the newborn infant. The effect is most noticeable in the absorption of lipid-soluble drugs such as vitamins D and E (15, 16).

Disease states can also have a pronounced effect on drug absorption. Pediatric patients with previous GI surgery may have shortened intestinal length, which results in decreased bioavailability of a drug. Infantile diarrhea and gastroenteritis also decrease transit time, leading to lower absorption of drugs (17, 18).

Distribution

The distribution of a drug in the body is most often expressed in terms of its volume of distribution (Vd). A higher Vd means more drug is concentrated in other areas of the body (e.g., fat, muscle, body water) relative to the concentration in the blood. Several differences in pediatric age groups affect the distribution of drugs when compared with adults (19).

One of the major factors determining the distribution of water-soluble drugs is total body water (TBW). TBW represents the relationship of body water to total body weight. In adults, water comprises about 55% of total body weight. However, neonates have a much higher Vd because their TBW is about 75%. This decreases rapidly in the first year of life; adult values are reached by about 12 years of age (20). A water-soluble drug has a lower serum concentration for a given milligram per kilogram dose in a neonate or infant than for the same milligram per kilogram dose in an adult (21).

The changes in body fat with age are just the opposite. A full-term infant will have an average of 12% body fat (22). The percentage of body fat increases with age to about 21% and 33%, respectively, in adult males and females (19).

Plasma protein binding is also an important parameter in the Vd of a drug. The higher the amount of drug bound to plasma proteins, the lower the amount of "free" drug available to have a pharmacologic action. Drugs administered to neonates and infants have a lower protein binding than adults; adult values occur at about 1 year of age (1, 4, 23, 24). Lowered protein binding is a result of decreased serum proteins and a decreased drug affinity for binding to proteins (23–25). Drugs that have a high degree of protein binding exert a greater effect in the younger age group because of the relatively low quantities of binding proteins.

Metabolism and Elimination

The elimination of drugs in pediatric patients also changes significantly between birth and adulthood. The metabolism of drugs is primarily the responsibility of the liver. The liver handles drugs in one of two ways: by changing the structure of the drug through oxidation, reduction, demethylation, or hydrolysis (phase I reactions); or by conjugating the drug molecule to make it more water soluble (phase II reactions) (2, 11, 26, 27). Phase I reactions are primarily the function of mixed function oxidase systems (cytochrome P-450). The activity of these reactions remains low in the neonate, and each hepatic metabolic process matures at a different rate. This delayed maturation of metabolic processes makes it difficult to characterize elimination of drugs undergoing Phase I biotransformations, but they begin in the neonate at 20–40% of the adult activity level (27). Phase II reactions are even more variable and probably slower to mature in the developing neonate and infant. Glucuronidation does not approach adult values until about 70 days of life (28, 29).

Once the metabolic function of the liver matures, it may actually exceed the adult capacity to metabolize drugs on a mg/kg per day basis. This increased capacity probably occurs because the percent weight of the liver in children exceeds that of adults, creating a higher relative metabolic surface area (30).

Excretion

Excretion or elimination is primarily the function of the kidneys; the elimination processes also undergo significant age-related changes. At birth, the glomerular filtration rate (GFR) is approximately 30% or less than that of adults (31). GFR increases significantly in the first 2 weeks of life and reaches adult values by 1 year of age (31–33). Therefore, drugs eliminated primarily by glomerular filtration require special dosage considerations during this period of time. In addition, renal tubular secretion and reabsorption also mature with age; the renal tubular reabsorption process matures slightly slower than the GFR (11, 33).

Summary of Pharmacokinetic Developmental Changes

Developmental aspects of preterm and full-term infants through adulthood significantly affect the pharmacokinetic properties of almost all medications. Al-
though these changes have the greatest effect on drugs with narrow therapeutic ranges (prescription medications), they can also influence the use of nonprescription medications. Table 1 summarizes these pharmacokinetic differences.

The pharmacist must estimate the extent of gastrointestinal activity, renal function, and liver function before making an appropriate dosage recommendation. These parameters can be estimated from a child's age, weight, or height. Generally, nonprescription labeling uses age-based guidelines for determining dosages. This method is convenient but may be the least reliable because of the wide variation between age and the degree of organ system development. Some clinicians suggest using height rather than weight to determine medication doses because it correlates better with lean body mass. Body surface area may be the best measure because it correlates well with all the body parameters, but body surface area is not easily determined. Because nonprescription medications have a wide therapeutic index (the ratio of the toxic dose to the therapeutic dose), safe doses may be determined by weight. Currently, the FDA advisory review panel on over-the-counter (OTC) cold, cough, allergy, bronchodilator, and asthmatic drug products is developing a uniform dosing schedule based on weight and age (34, 35).

A pharmacist familiar with general pediatric pharmacokinetics will help both the pediatric patient and the physician in the proper use of nonprescription medications.

PEDIATRIC DOSAGE ADMINISTRATION

Once the correct drug and dose are chosen, the child must receive the medication to gain any therapeutic benefit. The pharmacist should understand and be able to explain to the parents proper and helpful administrative techniques.

Liquids are relatively easy to administer, and the dose can be titrated to the patient's weight; therefore, liquid medications are frequently used in pediatrics. Because elixirs and syrups can have a high alcohol and sugar content, respectively, these forms of liquid medications are less desirable than suspensions and solutions. A suspension can also cover the disagreeable taste of a drug and is more chemically stable than solutions. When two similar drugs are available in different forms, the pharmacist should help parents choose the most appropriate form.

One problem associated with liquid medications is proper measuring of the dose. Studies have shown the

TABLE 1 Pediatric pharmacokinetic developmental changes		
Pharmacokinetic parameter	**Effect of change on drug disposition**	**Age group**
ABSORPTION		
Decreased gastric acidity	Increased absorption of basic drugs Decreased hydrolysis of drugs Decreased absorption of acidic drugs	Neonates, infants, children 2 to 3 years of age
Delayed gastric/intestinal motility	Variable bioavailability (see text)	Neonates, infants
DISTRIBUTION		
Increased total body water	Increased volume of distribution of drug (decreased blood concentration)	Neonates, infants
METABOLISM		
Decreased enzyme quantity/maturation	Decreased clearance of drugs ($\uparrow$ t½)	Neonates, infants
Increased enzyme quantity/activity	Increased clearance of drugs ($\downarrow$ t½)	Toddlers, older children
ELIMINATION		
Decreased glomerular filtration rate	Decreased renal elimination of drugs	Neonates, infants
Increased glomerular filtration rate	Increased renal elimination of drugs	Toddlers, older children
Decreased renal tubular reabsorption	Decreased renal elimination of drugs	Neonates, infants

volume delivered by household teaspoons ranges from 2.5 to 7.8 ml, and the volume varies greatly when the same spoon is used by different individuals (36, 37). The American Academy of Pediatrics Committee on Drugs highly recommends the use of appropriate liquid administration devices (38). Ease of administration and accuracy should be considered when choosing one of the dosing devices, which include the medication cup, cylindrical dosing spoon, oral dropper, and oral syringe. Potent liquid medications such as digoxin, theophylline, and phenobarbital should be administered with an oral syringe to ensure the correct dose is given. The pharmacist should briefly explain to patients or parents how to use and read an oral syringe. Plastic medication cups are fairly accurate for volumes of 5 ml or exact multiples of 5 ml (i.e., 5 ml, 10 ml, 15 ml). With high viscosity liquids, the oral syringe is preferable to the other oral dosing devices because the syringes completely expel the total measured dose. However, drawing up the dose in the oral syringe requires more dexterity. The use of oral dosing devices helps ensure adequate therapeutic response by reducing the incidence of underdoses and should eliminate adverse drug effects from potential overdoses. They may also enhance acceptance of medications by infants and children (39).

Tablets or capsules can usually be swallowed by a child over 4 years of age. Tablets that are not sustained-release or enteric-coated formulations may be crushed; most capsules may be opened. The contents should be sprinkled on small amounts of food (applesauce, jelly,

pudding) to ensure that all the drug is taken. The child may be more cooperative if allowed to choose what flavored drink to use and which medication to take first if multiple drugs are prescribed (40). Table 2 summarizes the guidelines for administering medications to pediatric patients.

NONPRESCRIPTION DRUG CLASSES AND DOSAGES

Table 3 lists dosage recommendations for some common nonprescription products. Doses were determined using a mg/kg per dose calculation. This guide is not intended as an all-inclusive list of nonprescription products, but as a listing of representative products within each class. Usually, in products containing more than one drug entity (e.g., Dimetapp) the concentration of each individual ingredient is the same as the concentration in products with only one ingredient.

For many of the young age groups, package labeling advises use only under the direction of a physician. Similarly, the doses listed in Table 3 should be used only for informational purposes, not for a pharmacist's recommendation without a physician's involvement. For example, this guide may be used to verify correct doses on a prescription for a nonprescription medication

TABLE 2 Medication administration guidelines

Infants

Use a calibrated dropper or oral syringe.
Support the infant's head while holding the infant in your lap.
Give small amounts of medication to prevent choking.
Place medication to the back and side of the infant's mouth.
Nonenteric coated or slow-release tablets may be crushed to a powder and sprinkled on small amounts of food.
Physical comforting while administering medications will calm the infant.

Toddlers

Allow the child to choose a position to take medication.
Follow routine home feeding.
Taste of medication may be disguised with a small volume of flavored drink or small amounts of food. A rinse with a flavored drink or water will help remove an unpleasant aftertaste.
Use simple commands in the toddler's jargon to obtain cooperation.
Allow toddler to choose which of several medications to take first.
Provide immediate verbal and tactile responses to promote cooperative taking of medication.
Allow toddler to become familiar with the oral dosing device.
Relate the benefit of taking medication to the immediate physical needs or wants of the toddler.

Preschool children

If possible, a tablet or capsule should be placed near the back of the tongue and swallowed with water or flavored drink.
If child's teeth are loose, do not use chewable tablets.
Use a straw to administer medications that could stain teeth.
A follow-up rinse with a flavored drink will help minimize unpleasant medication aftertaste.
Allow child to make decisions about dosage formulation, place of administration, which medication first, and the type of flavored drink to use.

Reprinted from *Am. Drug.*, *183 (6)*, 82–86 (1987).

written by a physician. This guide may also be used to make a recommendation regarding a nonprescription product and a dose if a physician has been consulted. Children who are small for their age should receive a conservative dose, but large children may require doses recommended for the next age bracket. Some pharmacists may make a dosage recommendation for children when no package labeling exists, while others may not. The important point is that the pharmacist is comfortable with the recommendation.

Keeping in mind the general principles discussed to this point, several nonprescription drug classes will now be examined to see how those principles apply with specific reference to pediatric patients. The reader should refer to the other chapters cited for more detailed discussions on the general pharmacology of the drug classes.

COMMON CLASSES OF NONPRESCRIPTION DRUGS

Cold and Allergy Medications

Young infants are obligate nose-breathers; they do not know to breathe through the mouth if the nose is obstructed. Therefore, the nasal stuffiness of a cold can interfere with a young infant's ability to sleep and eat. The treatment of choice is the use of normal saline nose drops. The infant or child is placed in the supine position with the neck hyperextended and 2 or 3 drops are placed in each nostril. After several minutes the secretions are removed with an ear or nose type suction bulb (for an infant) or by blowing the nose (for a child). If saline drops do not work, 1:1 or 1:2 dilutions of nonprescription topical decongestants may be tried.

Antihistamines are relatively safe because they have a high therapeutic index. The toxicity associated with an overdose is primarily caused by the anticholinergic activity of these drugs, resulting in excitement, ataxia, incoordination, muscular twitching, and respiratory depression. Although most adults suffer from drowsiness when taking an antihistamine, children can experience a paradoxical central nervous system (CNS) stimulation with insomnia, nervousness, and irritability (41, 42). Neonates and young infants are especially susceptible to these adverse reactions. Caution should be taken when the patient is an asthmatic because the potential drying effect on respiratory secretions may worsen asthmatic symptoms.

TABLE 3 Dosage recommendations for some common nonprescription drugs

	Age Weight (lb) Weight (kg)	0-3 mo 7-12 3-6	4-11 mo 13-22 7-10	12-24 mo 23-28 11-13	2-3 yr 29-32 14-16
ANTIPYRETICS					
Acetaminophen 10-15mg/kg/dose		40mg	80mg	120mg	160mg
Tylenol Drops 80mg/0.8ml		0.4ml	0.8ml	1.2ml	1.6ml
Tylenol Elixir 160mg/5ml		1.25ml	2.5ml	3.75ml	5.0ml
Tylenol Chew Tabs 80mg		—	1 tab	1½ tab	2 tabs
		Q4-6H	Q4-6H	Q4-6H	Q4-6H
Acetylsalicylic Acid 10-15mg/kg/dose[a]		30-60mg[b]	60-90mg[b]	120mg	160mg
St. Joseph's/Bayer 81mg		—	1 tab	1½ tab	2 tabs
		Q4H	Q4H	Q4H	Q4H
Ibuprofen 5-10mg/kg/dose		20mg[b]	25-50mg[b]	50-100mg	75-150mg
Advil/Nuprin Tabs 200mg		—	—	—	—
PediaProfen Susp 100mg/5ml (Rx only)		1ml	1.25-2.5ml	2.5-5ml	3.75-7.5ml
		Q6-8H	Q6-8H	Q6-8H	Q6-8H
ANTIHISTAMINES					
Brompheniramine 0.125mg/kg/dose		0.41mg[b]	0.82mg[b]	1.64mg[b]	2.0mg[b]
Dimetane Elixir 2mg/5ml		1.25ml	2.5ml	3.75ml	5ml
Dimetane Tabs 4mg		—	—	—	½ tab
		Q6H	Q6H	Q6H	Q6H
Chlorpheniramine 0.0875mg/kg/dose		0.5mg[b]	0.5mg[b]	1.0mg[b]	1.0mg[b]
Chlortrimeton Allergy Syrup 2mg/5ml		1.25ml	1.25ml	2.5ml	2.5ml
Chlortrimeton Chew Tabs 2 mg		—	¼ tab	½ tab	½ tab
		Q6H	Q6H	Q6H	Q6H
COUGH AND COLD PRODUCTS					
Diphenhydramine 0.83mg/kg/dose		2.5mg[b]	5mg[b]	5mg[b]	6.25mg[b]
Benylin Cough Syrup 12.5mg/5ml		1ml	2ml	2ml	2.5ml
		Q4H	Q4H	Q4H	Q4H
Pseudoephedrine 1mg/kg/dose		3-6mg[b]	7.5mg[b]	7.5mg[b]	15mg
Children's Sudafed Syrup 30mg/5ml		0.5-1.0ml	1.25ml	1.25ml	2.5ml
Sudafed Tabs 30mg		—	—	—	—
		Q6H	Q6H	Q6H	Q6H
Guaifenesin 2mg/kg/dose		10mg[b]	20mg[b]	25mg[b]	50-100mg
Robitussin (Regular) Syrup 100mg/5ml		0.5ml	1ml	1.25ml	2.5-5.0ml
		Q6H	Q6H	Q6H	Q4-6H
Dextromethorphan 0.25-0.5mg/kg/dose		1-3mg[b]	3-5mg[b]	5mg[b]	5mg
Benylin DM 2mg/ml		0.5-1.5ml	1.5-2.5ml	2.5ml	2.5ml
Delsym 6mg/ml		0.5ml	0.5-1ml	1ml	1ml
		Q6-8H	Q6-8H	Q6-8H	Q4-6H
Guaifenesin + dextromethorphan					
Robitussin DM		0.5ml[b]	1.0ml[b]	1.25ml[b]	2.5ml
Vick's Children's Cough Syrup		1.0ml[b]	2.0ml[b]	2.5ml[b]	5.0ml
		Q8H	Q8H	Q6-8H	Q6-8H
Pseudoephedrine + chlorpheniramine 0.15ml/kg/dose					
Sudafed Plus Syrup		0.5-1.0ml[b]	1.25ml[b]	1.25ml[b]	2.5ml[b]
Sudafed Plus Tabs		—	—	—	—
		Q6H	Q6H	Q6H	Q6H

TABLE 3 *continued*

	Age Weight (lb) Weight (kg)	0-3 mo 7-12 3-6	4-11 mo 13-22 7-10	12-24 mo 23-28 11-13	2-3 yr 29-32 14-16
Brompheniramine + phenylpropanolamine					
Dimetapp Elixir		1.25ml[b]	1.25-2.5ml[b]	2.5ml[b]	3.75ml[b]
Dimetapp Tabs		—	—	—	—
		TID	TID-QID	TID-QID	TID-QID
Phenylephrine 5mg/5ml + chlorpheniramine					
2mg/5ml Novahistine Elixir		1.25ml[b]	1.25ml[b]	2.5ml[b]	2.5ml[b]
		Q4H	Q4H	Q4H	Q4H
Pseudoephedrine 30mg/5ml + dextromethorphan 10mg/ 5ml + guaifenesin 100mg/5ml					
Novahistine DMX Syrup		0.5-1.0ml[b]	1.25ml[b]	1.25ml[b]	2.5ml
		Q6H	Q6H	Q6H	Q4-6H
Pseudoephedrine 30mg/5ml + dextromethorphan 10mg/ 5ml + chlorpheniramine 2mg/5ml					
Novahistine Cough & Cold Formula Liquid		0.5-1.0ml[b]	1.25ml[b]	1.25ml[b]	2.5ml
		Q6H	Q6H	Q6H	Q4-6H
Phenylpropanolamine 12.5mg/5ml + chlorpheniramine 2mg/5ml 0.4ml/kg/dose					
Triaminic Cold Syrup		1.0-2.0ml[b]	2.5ml[b]	2.5ml[b]	2.5ml
+ dextromethorphan 10mg/5ml 0.4ml/kg/dose					
Triaminic DM Liquid		1.0-2.0ml[b]	2.5ml[b]	2.5ml[b]	2.5ml
+ guaifenesin 100mg/5ml 0.4ml/kg/dose					
Triaminic Expectorant		1.0-2.0ml[b]	2.5ml[b]	2.5ml[b] No more than 10ml/ 24 hrs	2.5ml No more than 10ml/ 24hrs
		Q6H	Q6H	Q4H	Q4H
ANTIDIARRHEALS					
Calcium Polycarbophil					
Mitrolan Tabs		—	—	—	500mg 1 tab BID
Attapulgite					
Diasorb Tabs 750mg		—	—	—	750mg 1 tab
Kaopectate Tabs 750mg		—	—	—	1 tab
Kaopectate Liquid 600mg/15ml		—	—	—	15ml TID
Kaolin + pectin					
Kapectolin Suspension		—	—	—	15ml PRN
Loperamide 0.04-0.08mg/kg/dose					
Imodium AD 1mg/5ml		—	—	—	1mg 5ml BID-TID

[a]Aspirin has been associated with Reye's syndrome especially in the presence of a viral illness. Caution must be used when aspirin is recommended for a patient.

[b]Package labeling recommends use of these products in these age groups only under the direction of a physician. Doses for these age groups included in this table are for your use if the physician asks for a dosage. In some cases, the mg/kg/dose calculation for a young infant may exceed the dosage recommended on the product label for an older infant because the doses on the table are maximum daily doses while the manufacturer gives conservative doses for OTC labeling.

TABLE 3 *continued*

	Age	0-3 mo	4-11 mo	12-24 mo	2-3 yr
	Weight (lb)	7-12	13-22	23-28	29-32
	Weight (kg)	3-6	7-10	11-13	14-16

LAXATIVES

		0-3 mo	4-11 mo	12-24 mo	2-3 yr
Bisacodyl 0.3mg/kg/dose		5mg	5mg	10mg	10mg
Dulcolax Suppository 10mg		½ suppos	½ suppos	1 suppos	1 suppos
Dulcolax Tablets 5mg		—	—	—	—
		QD	QD	QD	QD
Docusate		12.5mg	12.5mg	25mg	25mg
Colace Solution 10mg/ml		1.25ml	1.25ml	2.5ml	2.5ml
Colace Capsules 50mg		—	—	—	—
		QD	QD	QD	QD
Magnesium hydroxide 0.5ml/kg/dose					
Phillip's MOM		2.5ml[b]	5ml[b]	5ml[b]	7.5ml
		QD	QD	QD	QD

	Age	4-5 yrs	6-8 yrs	9-10 yrs	11-12 yrs
	Weight (lb)	33-40	41-60	61-72	73-87
	Weight (kg)	17-19	20-27	28-33	34-39

ANTIPYRETICS

		4-5 yrs	6-8 yrs	9-10 yrs	11-12 yrs
Acetaminophen 10-15mg/kg/dose		200mg	240mg	320mg	400mg
Tylenol Drops 80mg/0.8ml		2.0ml	2.4ml	3.2ml	4.0ml
Tylenol Elixir 160mg/5ml		6.25ml	7.5ml	10ml	12.5ml
Tylenol Chew Tabs 80mg		2½ tabs	3 tabs	4 tabs	5 tabs
		Q4-6H	Q4-6H	Q4-6H	Q4-6H
Acetylsalicylic Acid 10-15mg/kg/dose[a]		200mg	240mg	320mg	400mg
St. Joseph's/Bayer 81mg		2½ tabs	3 tabs	4 tabs	5 tabs
		Q4H	Q4H	Q4H	Q4H
Ibuprofen 5-10mg/kg/dose		100-200mg	125-250mg	150-300mg	200-400mg
Advil/Nuprin Tabs 200mg		1 tab	1 tab	1 tab	1-2 tabs
PediaProfen Susp 100mg/5ml (Rx only)		5-10ml	6.25-12.5ml	7.5-15ml	10-20ml
		Q6-8H	Q6-8H	Q6-8H	Q6-8H

ANTIHISTAMINES

		4-5 yrs	6-8 yrs	9-10 yrs	11-12 yrs
Brompheniramine 0.125mg/kg/dose		2.0mg[b]	4.0mg	4.0mg	4.0mg
Dimetane Elixir 2mg/5ml		5ml	10ml	10ml	10ml
Dimetane Tabs 4mg		½ tab	1 tab	1 tab	1 tab
		Q6H	Q6H	Q6H	Q6H
Chlorpheniramine 0.0875mg/kg/dose		1.0mg[b]	2mg	2mg	2mg
Chlortrimeton Allergy Syrup 2mg/5ml		2.5ml	5ml	5ml	5ml
Chlortrimeton Chew Tabs 2 mg		½ tab	1 tab	1 tab	1 tab
		Q6H	Q4-6H	Q4-6H	Q4-6H

COUGH AND COLD PRODUCTS

		4-5 yrs	6-8 yrs	9-10 yrs	11-12 yrs
Diphenhydramine 0.83mg/kg/dose		6.25mg	12.5mg	12.5mg	12.5mg
Benylin Cough Syrup 12.5mg/5ml		2.5ml	5ml	5ml	5ml
		Q4H	Q4H	Q4H	Q4H

TABLE 3 *continued*

	Age	4-5 yrs	6-8 yrs	9-10 yrs	11-12 yrs
	Weight (lb)	33-40	41-60	61-72	73-87
	Weight (kg)	17-19	20-27	28-33	34-39
Pseudoephedrine 1mg/kg/dose		15mg	30mg	30mg	30mg
Children's Sudafed Syrup 30mg/5ml		2.5ml	5ml	5ml	5ml
Sudafed Tabs 30mg		—	1 tab	1 tab	1 tab
		Q6H	Q6H	Q6H	Q6H
Guaifenesin 2mg/kg/dose		50-100mg	100-200mg	100-200mg	100-200mg
Robitussin (Regular) Syrup 100mg/5ml		2.5-5.0ml	5-10ml	5-10ml	5-10ml
		Q4-6H	Q4-6H	Q4-6H	Q4-6H
Dextromethorphan 0.25-0.5mg/kg/dose		5mg	10mg	10mg	10mg
Benylin DM 2mg/ml		2.5ml	5ml	5ml	5ml
Delsym 6mg/ml		1ml	2ml	2ml	2ml
		Q4-6H	Q4-6H	Q4-6H	Q4-6H
Guaifenesin + dextromethorphan					
Robitussin DM		2.5ml	5.0ml	5.0ml	5.0ml
Vick's Children's Cough Syrup		5.0ml	10.0ml	10.0ml	10.0ml
		Q6-8H	Q6-8H	Q6-8H	Q6-8H
Pseudoephedrine + chlorpheniramine 0.15ml/kg/dose					
Sudafed Plus Syrup		2.5ml[b]	5.0ml	5.0ml	5.0ml
Sudafed Plus Tabs		—	½ tab	½ tab	½ tab
		Q6H	Q6H	Q6H	Q6H
Brompheniramine + phenylpropanolamine					
Dimetapp Elixir		3.75ml[b]	5ml	5ml	5ml
Dimetapp Tabs		—	½ tab	½ tab	½ tab
		TID-QID	TID-QID	TID-QID	TID-QID
Phenylephrine 5mg/5ml + chlorpheniramine 2mg/5ml					
Novahistine Elixir		2.5ml[b]	5ml	5ml	5ml
		Q4H	Q4H	Q4H	Q4H
Pseudoephedrine 30mg/5ml + dextromethorphan 10mg/5ml + guaifenesin 100mg/5ml					
Novahistine DMX Syrup		2.5ml	5ml	5ml	5ml
		Q4-6H	Q4-6H	Q4-6H	Q4-6H
Pseudoephedrine 30mg/5ml + dextromethorphan 10mg/5ml + chlorpheniramine 2mg/5ml					
Novahistine Cough & Cold Formula Liquid		2.5ml	5ml	5ml	5ml
		Q4-6H	Q4-6H	Q4-6H	Q4-6H
Phenylpropanolamine 12.5mg/5ml + chlorpheniramine 2mg/5ml 0.4ml/kg/dose					
Triaminic Cold Syrup		2.5ml	5ml	5ml	5ml
+ dextromethorphan 10mg/5ml 0.4ml/kg/dose					
Triaminic DM Liquid		2.5ml	5ml	5ml	5ml
+ guaifenesin 100mg/5ml 0.4ml/kg/dose					
Triaminic Expectorant		2.5ml	5ml	5ml	5ml
		No more than 10ml/ 24hrs	No more than 20ml/ 24 hrs	No more than 20ml/ 24 hrs	No more than 20ml/ 24 hrs
		Q4H	Q4H	Q4H	Q4H

TABLE 3 *continued*

Age	4-5 yrs	6-8 yrs	9-10 yrs	11-12 yrs
Weight (lb)	33-40	41-60	61-72	73-87
Weight (kg)	17-19	20-27	28-33	34-39
ANTIDIARRHEALS				
Calcium Polycarbophil	500mg	500mg	500mg	500mg
Mitrolan Tabs	1 tab	1 tab	1 tab	1 tab
	BID	TID	TID	TID
Attapulgite	750mg	1500mg	1500mg	1500mg
Diasorb Tabs 750mg	1 tab	2 tabs	2 tabs	2 tabs
Kaopectate Tabs 750mg	1 tab	2 tabs	2 tabs	2 tabs
Kaopectate Liquid 600mg/15ml	15ml	30ml	30ml	30ml
	TID	TID	TID	TID
Kaolin + pectin				
Kapectolin Suspension	15-30ml	30-60ml	30-60ml	30-60ml
	PRN	PRN	PRN	PRN
Loperamide 0.04-0.08mg/kg/dose	1mg	1.5mg	2mg	2mg
Imodium AD 1mg/5ml	5ml	7.5ml	10ml	10ml
	BID-TID	BID-TID	BID-TID	BID-TID
LAXATIVES				
Bisacodyl 0.3mg/kg/dose	10mg	10mg	10mg	10mg
Dulcolax Suppository 10mg	1 suppos	1 suppos	1 suppos	1 suppos
Dulcolax Tablets 5mg	—	1-2 tabs	1-2 tabs	1-2 tabs
	QD	QD	QD	QD
Docusate	50mg	75mg	75mg	100mg
Colace Solution 10mg/ml	5ml	7.5ml	7.5ml	10ml
Colace Capsules 50mg	1 cap	—	—	2 caps
	QD	QD	QD	QD
Magnesium Hydroxide 0.5ml/kg/dose				
Phillip's MOM	10ml	15ml	20ml	30ml
	QD	QD	QD	QD

Antipyretics

Acetaminophen and aspirin inhibit prostaglandin synthesis, preventing pyrogens from resetting the hypothalamic thermoregulatory center (43). Aspirin has been discouraged for children with viral illnesses because of its association with the development of Reye's syndrome; however, the exact role of aspirin in the pathogenesis of Reye's syndrome has not been determined. If an antipyretic agent is needed for children or teenagers, acetaminophen is generally preferred unless otherwise directed by a physician. Both acetaminophen and aspirin ingestion can result in acute or chronic toxicity. Side effects are rare with acetaminophen in therapeutic doses. Manifestations of toxic doses include nausea, vomiting, anorexia, and diaphoresis.

Ibuprofen is an alternative antipyretic approved for use in children 6 months of age or older. Comparative studies show ibuprofen to be as effective as acetaminophen in reducing fever (44). In pediatric clinical trials, no serious or significant adverse effects were reported. In adults, the most common adverse effects with ibuprofen are gastrointestinal and include nausea, epigastric pain, and heartburn (45). Ibuprofen 100 mg/5 ml suspension is now available, but only by prescription. Tablets containing 200 mg of ibuprofen are available without a prescription and can be used in children who can swallow tablets.

Antidiarrheals

Diarrhea can quickly dehydrate infants and young children. Therefore, patients under 2 years of age who have diarrhea should be referred to a physician. Fluid intake should be maximized (46), and an antidiarrheal product considered. The most frequently used drug class is adsorbents, including bismuth salts (e.g., PeptoBismol), kaolin and pectin (Kaopectate), and attapulgite (Diasorb). These drugs are relatively inert and nontoxic and are relatively safe for nonprescription use in children.

Belladonna alkaloids (e.g., hyoscyamine, hyoscine, atropine) have an anticholinergic action and are theoretically effective in decreasing diarrhea if the cause is increased intestinal tone and peristalsis. However, doses high enough to decrease GI motility often cause side effects such as restlessness, blurred vision, flushed skin, tachycardia, and palpitations (47).

Opiates also relieve diarrhea by inhibiting peristalsis. This drug class includes paregoric, which is available in some states only in combination as a schedule 5 (e.g., Parepectolin), and loperamide, which is now available without prescription (e.g., Imodium A/D). Opiates are CNS depressants; sedation may be a problem in some patients.

The newest class of antidiarrheal compounds is absorbents, such as calcium polycarbophil. Calcium polycarbophil is a synthetic polyacrylic resin, absorbing 60 times its weight in water. Because of this mechanism of action, it can be used to treat diarrhea or constipation. Because calcium polycarbophil is inert, it does not demonstrate any systemic toxicities and is also considered safe for nonprescription use in children.

Laxatives

Constipation in a pediatric patient can be difficult to manage, especially because many factors can contribute to the problem, including a change in environment, diet, and febrile illness. Increasing the bulk content and amount of fluid in the child's diet is the preferred management. Stimulants such as bisacodyl suppositories should be avoided because of their harsh action on the intestine. Bulk-forming laxatives are not absorbed and are free from systemic side effects; therefore, this class of drugs is a good choice for use in infants and children. Glycerin suppositories may be used to initiate the defecation reflex for acute constipation (see Chapter 15, *Laxative Products*).

Topicals

The skin provides a barrier to prevent the entry of pathogenic organisms and toxic chemicals into the body. Infants have a limited stratum corneum, allowing easier penetration of substances through the skin (48). The skin of premature neonates is more fragile and more permeable than that of a mature infant and can easily be irritated or manifest a skin reaction. Because a child's skin is more permeable and because a child has a greater surface area to volume ratio compared with adults (48), medications applied topically can produce systemic drug levels resulting in acute toxicity or unwanted systemic effects. For example, boric acid soaks are no longer recommended because significant absorption can occur and toxicity can develop, with GI symptoms, renal or hepatic failure, cardiovascular collapse, and CNS stimulation or depression. Another example is the potential for topical corticosteroid applications to cause adrenal suppression. In general, topical medications should be applied sparingly two or three times a day to a clean surface area.

NONPRESCRIPTION DRUGS IN CHRONICALLY ILL CHILDREN

Another problem that may confront pharmacists is the use of nonprescription drugs in infants and children with chronic illnesses. The advancements of medical care in treating previously fatal conditions (e.g., congenital heart defects) have increased the likelihood that the pharmacist will be asked to recommend a nonprescription drug and dose for chronically ill patients. The pharmacist should ask the parents about the child's medical history, including questions about current or recent illnesses, medications the child is taking or has recently taken for a chronic problem, and medications that are avoided on the advice of a physician. The use of nonprescription drugs in patients with cardiac disease, epilepsy, asthma, cancer, and chronic renal disease requires careful consideration to prevent additional problems. For example, patients with chronic renal disease often have hypertension, so it is important to avoid sympathomimetic drugs such as pseudoephridrine. Patients with chronic renal failure should avoid laxatives containing magnesium. Patients with cardiac disease should avoid nonprescription sympathomimetic drugs unless indicated by the physician. In many of these circumstances, it would probably be best and safer to refer these patients to a physician for drug therapy. Physicians are not necessarily more knowledgeable about nonprescription drug selection, but may have patient information that is not available to the pharmacist. Pharmacists should refer patients to a physician when they lack the necessary background information to make appropriate nonprescription recommendations.

SUMMARY

This chapter provides considerations for dosing nonprescription medications in infants and children. Selection of the appropriate medication depends on many factors and is beyond the scope of this chapter. The choice of the correct medication for a specific pediatric patient should be based on the judgment of the pharmacist and, in some situations, the physician. Table 3 provides dose recommendations, including doses for young infants. This table may be used when a physician asks the appropriate dose or to check the dose on a prescription. Nonprescription products are considered to be safe for self-medication. However, if used improperly, they may be harmful. Pharmacists should ensure that parents know how to correctly administer these medications to their children in order to maximize efficacy and minimize adverse effects.

REFERENCES

1   L. O. Boreus, "Principles of Pediatric Clinical Pharmacology," Churchill, Livingstone, New York, N.Y., 1982.

2   S. L. Young, *J. Pharm. Practice*, 2, 13–20 (1989).

3   W. F. Balistreri, in "Nutrition During Infancy," R. S. Tsang and B. L. Nichols, Eds., C. V. Mosby, Philadelphia, Pa., 1988, pp. 35–57.

4   P. L. Morselli, *Clin. Pharmcokinet.*, 1, 81–98 (1976).

5   D. M. Hilligoss, in "Applied Pharmacokinetics," W. E. Evans et al., Eds., Applied Therapeutics, San Francisco, Calif., 1980, pp. 76–94.

6   R. L. Milsap and S. J. Szfler, in "Applied Pharmacokinetics," W. E. Evans et al., Eds., Applied Therapeutics of America, Spokane, Wash., 1986, pp. 295–330.

7   P. E. Hyman et al., *J. Pediatr.*, 106, 467–471 (1985).

8   G. B. Avery et al., *Pediatrics*, 37, 1005–1007 (1966).

9   M. Agarod et al., *Am. J. Dig. Dis.*, 14, 400–414 (1969).

10   E. Signer and R. Fridrich, *Acta Pediatric. Scand.*, 64, 525–530 (1975).

11   P. L. Morselli et al., *Clin. Pharmacokinet.*, 5, 485–527 (1980).

12   J. Silverio and J. W. Poole, *Pediatrics*, 51, 578–580 (1973).

13   B. L. Mirkin, *Pediatr. Ann.*, 542–557 (Sept. 1976).

14   G. C. Cupit and V. A. Serrano, *J. Cont. Educ. Pharmacy*, 55–67 (Jan.-Mar. 1979).

15   L. Lebenthal et al., *J. Pediatr.*, 13, 879–886 (1972).

16   L. W. Matthews and D. Drotar, *Pediatr. Clin. N. Am.*, 31, 133–152 (1984).

17   J. D. Nelson et al., *Clin. Pharmacol. Ther.*, 13, 879–886 (1972).

18   H. L. Greene et al., *J. Pediatr.*, 87, 695–704 (1975).

19   B. Friis-Hansen, *Pediatrics*, 47, 264–274 (1971).

20   B. Friis-Hansen, *Pediatrics*, 28, 169–181 (1961).

21   G. R. Siber et al., *J. Infect. Dis.*, 78 (suppl.), 959–982 (1975).

22   E. M. Widdowson and C. M. Spray, *Arch. Dis. Child.*, 26, 205–214 (1951).

23   P. G. Dayton et al., *Ann. N.Y. Acad. Sci.*, 226, 172–194 (1973).

24   H. Kurz et al., *Eur. J. Clin. Pharmacol.*, 11, 463–467 (1977).

25   M. Ehrnebo et al., *Eur. J. Clin. Pharmacol.*, 3, 189–193 (1971).

26   A. K. Brown et al., *J. Clin. Invest.*, 37, 332–340 (1958).

27   A. H. Neims et al., *Ann. Rev. Pharmacol. Toxicol.*, 16, 426–445 (1976).

28   G. B. Odell et al., in "Care of the High-Risk Neonate," M. H. Klaus and A. A. Fanaroff, Eds., W. B. Saunders, Philadelphia, Pa., 1973, pp. 183–204.

29   G. J. Datton, *Ann. Dev. Pharmacol. Ther.*, 18, 17–36 (1978).

30   T. J. Haley, *Drug Metabol. Rev.*, 14, 295–335 (1983).

31   J. M. H. Loggie et al., *J. Pediatr.*, 86, 485–496 (1975).

32   J. P. Guignard et al., *J. Pediatr.*, 87, 268–272 (1975).

33   B. S. Arant, *J. Pediatr.*, 92, 705–712 (1978).

34   *FDC Reports*, 50 (36), 9, 10 (1988).

35   *FDC Reports*, 50 (51, 52), 13, 14 (1988).

36   H. V. Arny, *Am. Pharm. Assoc. J.*, 6, 1056 (1917).

37   W. I. Wilbert, *Am. J. Pharm.*, 74, 120 (1902).

38   American Academy of Pediatrics Committee on Drugs, *Pediatrics*, 56, 327–328 (1975).

39   M. McKenzie, *U.S. Pharmacist*, 55, 66 (1981).

40   R. P. Iafrate, *Am. Drug.*, 195 (6), 82–86 (1987).

41   E. M. Mandel et al., *N. Engl. J. Med.*, 316, 432–437 (1987).

42   E. I. Cantekin et al., *N. Engl. J. Med.*, 308, 297–301 (1983).

43   "The Pharmacological Basis of Therapeutics," 7th ed., A. G. Gilman et al., Eds., Macmillan Publishing, New York, N.Y., 1985, pp. 674–688.

44   P. D. Watson et al., *Clin. Pharmacol. Ther.*, 46, 9–17 (1989).

45   Pediaprofen product information, McNeil Laboratories, Fort Washington, Pa., 1989.

46   "Nelson Textbook of Pediatrics," 13th ed., W. E. Nelson et al., Eds., W. B. Saunders, Philadelphia, Pa., 1987, pp. 199–202.

47   "The Pharmacological Basis of Therapeutics," 7th ed., A. G. Gilman et al., Eds., Macmillan Publishing, New York, N.Y., 1985, pp. 130–144.

48   L. B. Howry et al., "Pediatric Medications," J. B. Lippincott, Philadelphia, Pa., 1981.

49   W. E. Benitz and D. S. Tatro, "Pediatric Drug Handbook," 2nd ed., Yearbook Medical, Chicago, Ill., 1988.

50   H. R. Silver et al., "Handbook of Pediatrics," 15th ed., Appleton and Lange, Norwalk, Conn., 1987.

51   "Problems in Pediatric Drug Therapy," 2nd ed., L. A. Pagliaro and A. M. Pagliaro, Eds., Hamilton Press, Hamilton, Ill., 1987.

52   "Harriet Lane Handbook," 11th ed., P. C. Rowe, Ed., Yearbook Medical, Chicago, Ill., 1987.

53   S. M. Maclead and I. C. Radde, "Textbook of Pediatric Clinical Pharmacology," PSG, Littleton, Mass., 1985.

54   G. M. Maxwell, "Principles of Pediatric Pharmacology," Croom Helm, Philadelphia, Pa., 1984.

55   "Pediatric Therapy," 6th ed., H. C. Shirkey, Ed., C. V. Mosby, St. Louis, Mo., 1980.

COLOR PLATES

PLATE 1

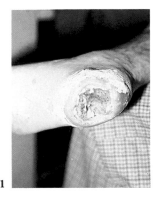

1-1 **Gangrene** of the foot is a serious and common complication of diabetes caused by trauma that has gone unrecognized due to neuropathy (loss of sensation) or to vascular lesions. Eventually, trauma may lead to gangrene when the dead (necrotic) skin is removed and ulceration results (as shown). (See Chapter 16, *Diabetes Care Products*.)

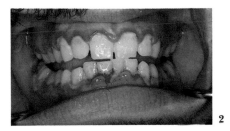

1-2 **Chronic gingivitis**, an early stage of periodontitis, is an asymptomatic inflammation of the gingivae (gums) at the necks of the teeth. The gingivae are erythematous and may have areas that appear swollen and glossy. There may be mild hemorrhage when the teeth are brushed. Gingivitis is usually caused by poor oral hygiene. (See Chapter 23, *Oral Health Products*.)

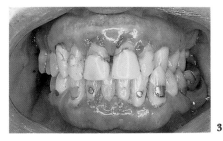

1-3 **Chronic periodontitis (pyorrhea)** is an inflammation of the tissues surrounding the teeth, including the gingivae, periodontal ligaments, alveolar bone, and the cementum (bony material covering the root of a tooth). It is caused by plaque accumulation resulting from poor oral hygiene. The gingivae may be erythematous and swollen and may recede from the necks of the teeth. It is not painful and usually is accompanied by halitosis, loosening of the teeth, and mild hemorrhage when the teeth are brushed. (See Chapter 23, *Oral Health Products*.)

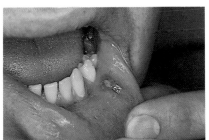

1-4 **Aphthous ulcers (canker sores)** are recurrent, painful, single or multiple ulcerations of bacterial origin. The central ulceration is sharply demarcated, often has a yellow to white surface of necrotic debris, and is surrounded by an erythematous margin. (See Chapter 23, *Oral Health Products*.)

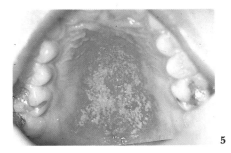

1-5 **Candidiasis (candidosis, moniliasis, thrush)** is an infection caused by overgrowth of *Candida albicans*. This condition tends to occur in people with debilitating or chronic systemic disease or those on long-term antibiotic therapy. It commonly appears as a whitish-gray to yellowish, soft, slightly elevated pseudomembrane-like plaque on the oral mucosa (often described as having a "curdled-milk" appearance). A dull burning pain often is present. If the membrane is stripped away, a raw bleeding surface remains. (See Chapter 23, *Oral Health Products*.)

PLATE 2

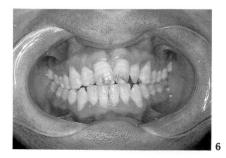

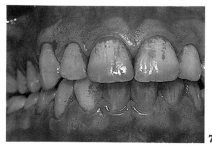

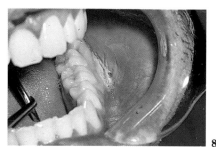

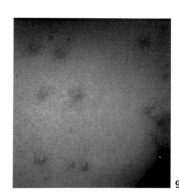

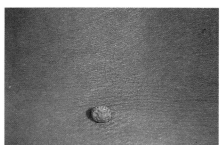

2-6 **Dental fluorosis (mottled enamel)** is caused by the long-term ingestion of drinking water containing fluoride at greater than 1 ppm concentration during the time of tooth formation. The appearance of the teeth varies, depending upon the level of fluoride in the water, and ranges from white flecks or spots to brownish stains, small pits, or deep irregular pits that are dark brown in color. (See Chapter 23, *Oral Health Products*.)

2-7 **Disclosing agents**, which stain mucinous film and plaque on teeth, are helpful to the patient in evaluation of the effectiveness of their brushing and flossing efforts. These agents, such as erythrosin (FD&C Red No. 3), will reveal the presence and extent of deposits on the teeth, which otherwise appear clean. (See Chapter 23, *Oral Health Products*.)

2-8 **Aspirin burn** results from the topical use of aspirin to relieve toothache. An aspirin tablet is placed against the tooth where it is held in place by pressure from the buccal (cheek) mucosa. The mucosa becomes necrotic and is characterized by a white slough that rubs away revealing a painful ulceration. (See Chapter 23, *Oral Health Products*.)

2-9 **Insect bites** are often characterized as itchy red papules in small clusters. A small overlying superficial vesicle may be present. (See Chapter 36, *Insect Sting and Bite Products*.)

2-10 **Ticks** can attach to human skin and burrow into superficial layers. The back of the organism is usually visible on the surface with careful examination. Ticks are vectors of several systemic diseases. (See Chapter 36, *Insect Sting and Bite Products*.)

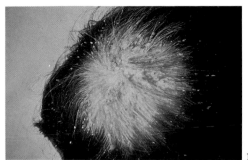

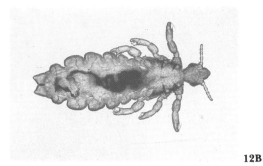

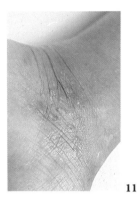

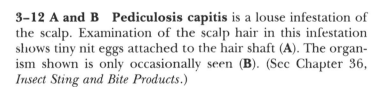

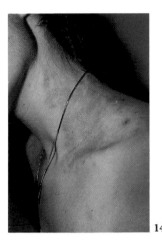

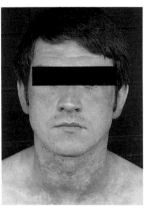

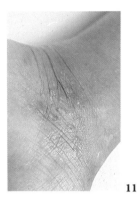

PLATE 3

12A

12B

11

13

14

15

3–11 Scabies is caused by a small mite that burrows under the superficial layers of the skin. Small linear blisters, which cause intense itching, can be seen between the finger webs, inner wrists, axilla, around the areola (nipple) of the breast, and on the genitalia. (See Chapter 36, *Insect Sting and Bite Products.*)

3–12 A and B Pediculosis capitis is a louse infestation of the scalp. Examination of the scalp hair in this infestation shows tiny nit eggs attached to the hair shaft (**A**). The organism shown is only occasionally seen (**B**). (See Chapter 36, *Insect Sting and Bite Products.*)

3–13 Sunburn presents as erythema (redness), reaching a peak 4–6 hours after excessive sun exposure. Severe burns can result in large blister formation. Photoprotection can be achieved for susceptible patients by proper sunscreen application. (See Chapter 33, *Burn and Sunburn Products.*)

3–14 Cosmetic-induced photosensitivity can be caused by ingredients in certain topical colognes and perfumes. They produce erythema (redness) locally, which leaves characteristic postinflammatory pigmentation. (See Chapter 33, *Burn and Sunburn Products.*)

3–15 Drug-induced photosensitivity is a reaction that occurs on sun-exposed surfaces of the head, neck, and dorsum (back) of the hands. The erythema (redness) spares photoprotected areas (under the nose and chin, behind the ears, and between the fingers). (See Chapter 33, *Burn and Sunburn Products.*)

PLATE 4

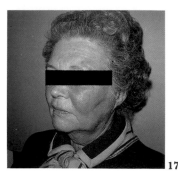
17

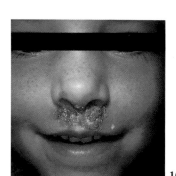
16

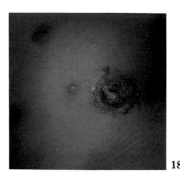
18

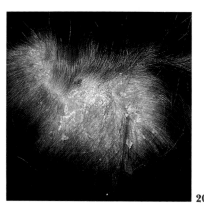
20

19

4–16 **Impetigo** is a bacterial infection identified by honey-comb crusts on erythematous bases. A bullous (blistering) form can also be seen. (See Chapter 28, *Topical Anti-infective Products.*)

4–17 **Erysipelas** is a streptococcal infection often involving the face or extremities. The infected area is red and raised with local warmth and edema. The margins are rapidly changing, often in serpiginous (irregular) patterns. (See Chapter 28, *Topical Anti-infective Products.*)

4–18 **Infections of the hair follicles** can be superficial (folliculitis). Deeper involvement is called a furuncle (small boil). A carbuncle forms when adjacent hair follicles are involved. They are usually caused by staphylococcal or streptococcal organisms. (See Chapter 28, *Topical Anti-infective Products.*)

4–19 **Paronychia** is caused by overexposure of the nails to water, causing cuticle loss and inflammation around the nail folds. About 50% of cases have candidal infection. (See Chapter 28, *Topical Anti-infective Products.*)

4–20 **Tinea capitis** is a fungal infection of the scalp. There is scale on the scalp with local breaking or loss of hair; erythema (redness) is usually not observed. (See Chapter 28, *Topical Anti-infective Products.*)

PLATE 5

5–21A and B   Tinea versicolor is caused by a yeast organism that overgrows locally, resulting in hyperpigmentation or hypopigmentation (**A**). These mildly scaling eruptions characteristically occur on the chest, upper back, and arms (**B**). (See Chapter 28, *Topical Anti-infective Products.*)

5–22   Herpes simplex lesions of the mouth and the eye usually start as a small cluster of vesicles (tiny blisters) that subsequently heal over with a serosanguinous (blood-tinged) crust. Local stinging, burning, and pain often herald the onset of lesions. Eye involvement should always be referred to an ophthalmologist. (See Chapter 28, *Topical Anti-infective Products.*)

5–23A and B   Herpes zoster is a reactivation of previous chickenpox virus that has remained latent in the nerve roots. Pain precedes small clusters of vesicles (blisters) on an erythematous base along the distribution of the infected nerve (**A**). It characteristically stops in the midline (**B**). (See Chapter 28, *Topical Anti-infective Products.*)

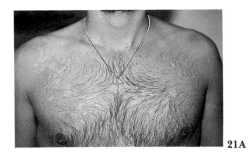

21A

21B

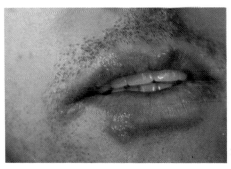

22

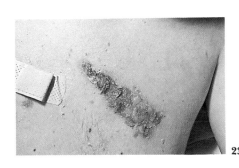

23A

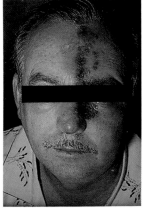

23B

PLATE 6

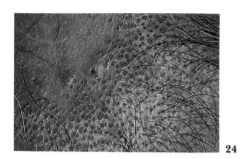

6-24 Comedonic acne (noninflammatory) occurs when follicles become plugged with sebum, forming a comedone on the surface. The black color is caused by oxidation of lipid and melanin, and not dirt, as is commonly believed. (See Chapter 29, *Acne Products*.)

6-25 Pustular acne (inflammatory) presents as inflamed papules, which are formed when a superficial hair follicle is plugged and ruptures at a deeper level. Superficial inflammation results in pustules. Deep lesions cause large cysts to form, resulting in scars. (See Chapter 29, *Acne Products*.)

6-26 Fixed drug reaction is an adverse reaction that can appear as erythematous (red) oval patches, which recur in the same site on reexposure to the causative drug. The patches resolve with characteristic tan-brown pigmentation. (See Chapter 30, *Dermatitis, Dry-Skin, Dandruff, Seborrhea, and Psoriasis Products*.)

6-27A, B, and C Atopic dermatitis (eczema) is an itchy condition that occurs on the outer aspect (extensor) surface of the elbows and knees (**A**) during the first year of life and then involves predominantly the flexors (**B**). The hands, feet, and face are often involved as well as with erythema, scale, increased skin surface markings, small blisters, and crusting (**C**). Secondary infection is common. (See Chapter 30, *Dermatitis, Dry Skin, Dandruff, Seborrheic Dermatitis, and Psoriasis Products*.)

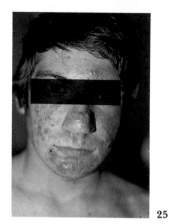

24

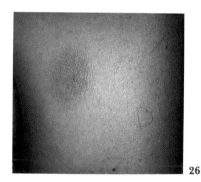

25

26

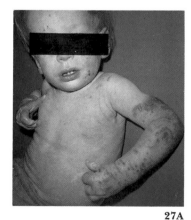

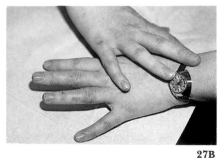

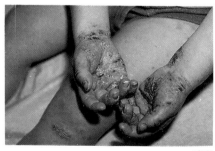

27A

27B

27C

PLATE 7

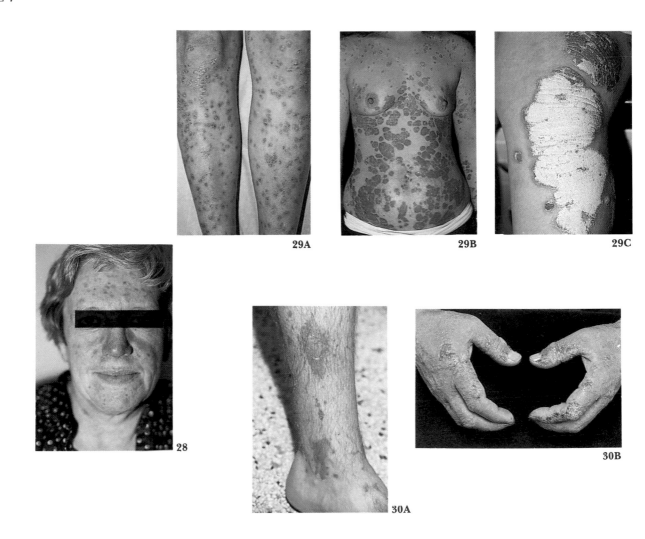

29A   29B   29C

28   30A   30B

7–28   Seborrhea (seborrheic dermatitis) is a red scaling condition of the scalp, midface, and upper midchest of adults. Characteristic greasy yellow scale is seen in the eyebrows and around the folds of the nose. (See Chapter 30, *Dermatitis, Dry Skin, Dandruff, Seborrheic Dermatitis, and Psoriasis Products.*)

7–29 A, B, and C   Psoriasis is a scaling condition in which erythematous plaques (red raised areas) are covered by a thick adherent scale. The borders of the lesions are well defined and vary from guttate (very small plaques) to large plaque types: (**A**) guttate (small drop size); (**B**) medium-sized plaques; (**C**) large plaques. (See Chapter 30, *Dermatitis, Dry Skin, Dandruff, Seborrheic Dermatitis, and Psoriasis Products.*)

7–30 A and B   Poison ivy causes a linear erythema that can develop large blisters (**A, B**). Similar reactions can also be caused by poison oak and poison sumac. (See Chapter 35, *Poison Ivy and Poison Oak Products.*)

PLATE 8

8–31 Diaper dermatitis presents as erythema of the groin (crease area around the genitals) and is common in infants. This case was caused by a contact allergen. Contact irritants such as urine and feces along with bacterial and yeast infection may also cause problems in this area. (See Chapter 31, *Diaper Rash and Prickly Heat Products*.)

8–32 Miliaria rubra (heat rash) is an obstruction of sweat glands. Superficial involvement results in only a tiny vesicle (blister) on the skin surface (miliaria crystallina). When deeper inflammation is also present, the surrounding erythema (redness) is characteristic of miliaria rubra. (See Chapter 31, *Diaper Rash and Prickly Heat Products*.)

8–33 Calluses are thickened scales often found over pressure areas. This callus appears on the plantar surface of the foot. (See Chapter 37, *Foot Care Products*.)

8–34 Common warts are lesions caused by a virus. The lesions are localized rough accumulations of keratin (hyperkeratosis) containing many tiny furrows. If the surface is pared, small bleeding points can be seen. (See Chapter 37, *Foot Care Products*.)

8–35 Plantar warts, caused by a viral infection, can often be found on the plantar surface of the foot and present with hard localized accumulations of keratin. The punctate bleeding points seen when the lesions are pared are not found in calluses. (See Chapter 37, *Foot Care Products*.)

8–36 Tinea pedis infection of the toes characteristically starts between the fourth and fifth web space and spreads proximally. Scaling can progress to maceration with resultant small fissures. (See Chapter 37, *Foot Care Products*.)

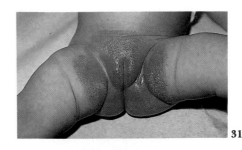

31

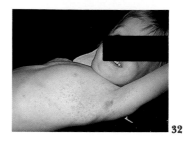

32

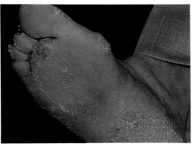

33

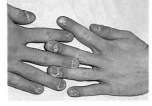

34

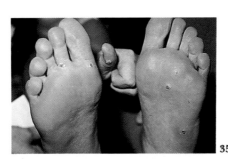

35

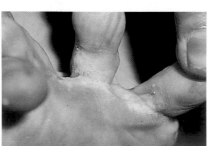

36

APPENDIX

APPENDIX

MAJOR NONPRESCRIPTION DRUG MANUFACTURERS

A

Abbott Laboratories
Department 355, AP30
Abbott Park
North Chicago, IL 60064-3500
312-937-6100

Adria Laboratories, Inc.
(*also* Warren-Teed)
P.O. Box 16529
Columbus, OH 43216-6529
614-764-8100

Advanced Care Products
(see Ortho Pharmaceutical
 Corporation)

Alberto-Culver Company
2525 Armitage Avenue
Melrose Park, IL 60160
312-450-3000

Alcon Laboratories, Inc.
P.O. Box 6600
Fort Worth, TX 76101

Allercreme
(see Owen Laboratories)

Allergan Pharmaceuticals Inc.
2525 Dupont Drive
Irvine, CA 92713
714-752-4500

Alval/Amco Pharmacal Company Inc.
6625 North Avondale
Chicago, IL 60631

American Critical Care
(see Du Pont Critical Care)

American Foundation for the Blind
15 West 16th Street
New York, NY 10011

American Pharmaceutical Company
245 Fourth Street
P.O. Box 448
Passaic, NJ 07055
201-779-5300

Ames Division Miles Laboratories, Inc.
P.O. Box 40
Elkhart, IN 46515
219-264-8111

Anabolic Laboratories, Inc.
17802 Gillete Avenue
Irvine, CA 92714
714-863-0340

Ansell-Americas, Inc.
78 Apple Street
Tinton Falls, NJ 07724

Arch Laboratories
319 South 4th Street
St. Louis, MO 63102

Armour Pharmaceutical Company
920A Harvest Drive
Suite 200
Blue Bell, PA 19422

B.F. Ascher & Company, Inc.
P.O. Box 717
Shawnee Mission, KA 66201-0717
913-888-1880

Astra Pharmaceutical Products, Inc.
50 Otis Street
Westborough, MA 01581
508-366-1100
800-225-6333 (Outside Massachusetts)
800-922-8584 (Massachusetts only)

Atlantic Surgical Company, Inc.
5200 Northeast 12th Avenue
Ft. Lauderdale, FL 33334

Auto Syringe Division
Baxter Healthcare Corporation
198 Londonderry Turnpike
Hooksett, NH 03106
603-669-9805
800-258-3591

A.V.P. Pharmaceuticals Inc.
9829 Main Street
P.O. Box N
Clarence, NY 14031

Ayerst Laboratories
Division of American Home Products
 Corporation
685 Third Avenue
New York, NY 10017-4071
212-878-5000

B

Baker/Cummins
4400 Biscayne Boulevard
Miami, FL 33137
305-652-2276
800-327-9054

Barnes-Hind Pharmaceuticals, Inc.
895 Kifer Road
Sunnyvale, CA 94086
408-736-5462

Bausch & Lomb Pharmaceuticals, Inc.
11300 49th Street North
Clearwater, FL 34622-4807
813-572-4040
800-832-6393 (Customer service,
 extension 240)

Becton Dickinson Consumer Products
One Becton Drive
Franklin Lakes, NJ 07417
201-848-7100

Beecham Laboratories
Division of Beecham Products USA
501 Fifth Street
Bristol, TN 37620
615-764-5141
800-251-0271 (8 a.m.–4:30 p.m. EST)

Beecham Products USA
P.O. Box 1467
100 Beecham Drive
Pittsburgh, PA 15230
412-928-1000

Berlex Laboratories, Inc.
110 East Hanover Avenue
Cedar Knolls, NJ 07927
201-694-4100

Betatron II
Division of CPI/Lilly
  Ambulatory Infusion
P.O. Box 64079
St. Paul, MN 55164-0079

Biomerica, Inc.
1533 Monrovia Avenue
Newport Beach, CA 92663
714-645-2111

Blaine Company, Inc.
2700 Dixie Highway
Ft. Mitchell, KY 41017
606-341-9437

Blair Laboratories, Inc.
100 Connecticut Avenue
Norwalk, CT 06856
203-853-0123

Blairex Laboratories, Inc.
P.O. Box 15190
Evansville, IN 47716
812-476-8077
800-252-4739

Blistex, Inc.
(*also* Carbisulphiol)
1800 Swift Drive
Oak Brook, IL 60521
312-571-2870
800-837-1800

Block Drug Company, Inc.
257 Cornelison Avenue
Jersey City, NJ 07302
201-434-3000

Boehringer Ingelheim
Pharmaceuticals, Inc.
90 East Ridge
P.O. Box 368
Ridgefield, CT 06877
203-798-9988

Boehringer Mannheim Diagnostics
P.O. Box 50100
9115 Hague Road
Indianapolis, IN 46250
800-858-8072

John H. Breck, Inc.
Berdan Avenue
P.O. Box 325
Wayne, NJ 07470

Breon Laboratories, Inc.
Subsidiary of Sterling Drug, Inc.
90 Park Avenue
New York, NY 10016
212-907-2000

Bristol-Myers Company
345 Park Avenue
New York, NY 10154
212-546-4453

Bristol-Myers USPNG
2400 West Lloyd Expressway
Evansville, IN 47721
812-429-5000

Buffington Division
Otis Clapp & Son, Inc.
115 Shawmut Road
Canton, MA 02021
617-821-5400

Burroughs Wellcome Company
3030 Cornwallis Road
Research Triangle Park, NC 27709
919-248-3000
800-443-6763 (Health professionals)
800-722-9292 (Consumers)

C

C & M Pharmacal, Inc.
1519 E. Eight Mile Road
Hazel Park, MI 48030-2696
313-548-7846
800-423-5173 (Except Michigan)

Carbisulphiol
(see Blistex, Inc.)

Carnation Company
5045 Wilshire Boulevard
Los Angeles, CA 90036

Carnrick Laboratories, Inc.
65 Horse Hill Road
Cedar Knolls, NJ 07927
201-267-2670

Carter Products
Division of Carter-Wallace, Inc.
1345 Avenue of the Americas
New York, NY 10105

Carter-Wallace, Inc.
767 Fifth Avenue
New York, NY 10153
212-758-4500

Cemco Pharmacal, Inc.
6121 Pebble Beach
Memphis, TN 38115

H.R. Cenci Laboratories, Inc.
152 North Broadway
Fresno, CA 93701
209-237-3346

Central Pharmaceuticals, Inc.
120 East Third Street
Seymour, IN 47274
812-522-3915

Century Pharmaceuticals, Inc.
10377 Hague Road
Indianapolis, IN 46256
317-849-4210

Char-Mag of Glendale
6026 North Appleblossom Lane
Milwaukee, WI 53217

Chattem Consumer Products
Division of Chattem Drug
  & Chemical Company
1715 West 38th Street
Chattanooga, TN 37409
615-821-4571

Chesebrough-Pond's, Inc.
33 Benedict Place
Greenwich, CT 06830
203-625-1000

Church & Dwight Company, Inc.
469 North Harrison Street
Princeton, NJ 08540
609-683-5900

Ciba Consumer Pharmaceuticals
Division of Ciba-Geigy
  Pharmaceuticals
Raritan Plaza III
Raritan Center
Edison, NJ 08837
201-906-6000

Otis Clapp & Son, Inc.
115 Shawmut Road
Canton, MA 02021
617-821-5400

Clairol Inc.
(see Sea Breeze Laboratories)

CMC Pharmaceuticals
195 East Main Street
Brewster, NY 10509

Colgate-Hoyt Laboratories
575 University Avenue
Norwood, MA 02062
617-821-2880

Colgate-Palmolive Company
300 Park Avenue
New York, NY 10022
212-310-2000

Columbia Laboratories, Inc.
16400 Northwest Second Avenue
Miami, FL 33169
305-944-3666

Combe, Inc.
1101 Westchester Avenue
White Plains, NY 10604
914-694-5454

Commerce Drug Company, Inc.
Division of Del Laboratories, Inc.
565 Broad Hollow Road
Farmingdale, NY 11735
516-293-7070

Cooper Laboratories, Inc.
455 East Middlefield Road
Mountain View, CA 94039
415-969-9030

CooperVision, Inc.
3145 Porter Drive
Palo Alto, CA 94304
415-856-5000

CooperVision Pharmaceuticals, Inc.
(see Cooper Laboratories, Inc.)

Copley Pharmaceuticals Inc.
25 John Road
Canton Commerce Center
Canton, MA 02021
617-821-6111

Creomulsion Company
P.O. Box 1214
345 Glen Iris Drive, N.E.
Atlanta, GA 30301
404-524-5434

Cunningham Distributors
P.O. Box 863
1222 Vilsmeier Road
Lansdale, PA 19446

Cutter Biological
Division of Miles Inc.
2200 Powell Street
Emery, CA 94662

 D

Dalin Pharmaceuticals, Inc.
74-80 Marine Street
Farmingdale, NY 11735

Davol, Inc.
Box D
Providence, RI 02901

Daywell Laboratories Corp.
78 Unquowa Place
Fairfield, CT 06430
203-255-3154
800-243-4141

C.S. Dent & Company
Division of Grandpa Brands Company
317-321 East 8th Street
Cincinnati, OH 45202
513-241-1677

Derata Corporation
7380 32nd Avenue North
Minneapolis, MN 55427

Dermik Laboratories, Inc.
920A Harvest Drive
Blue Bell, PA 19422
215-540-8300
800-523-6674

Dewitt International Corporation
5 North Watson Road
Taylors, SC 29687
803-244-8521

Diabetes Association of Cleveland
2022 Lee Road
Cleveland, OH 44118
216-371-3301

The E.E. Dickinson Company
Two Enterprise Drive
Shelton, CT 06484
203-929-1197

Doak Pharmacal Company, Inc.
700 Shames Drive
Westbury, NY 11590
516-333-7222

Dolcin Corporation
381 Broadway
Westwood, NJ 07675

Dorsey Laboratories
(see Sandoz Pharmaceuticals
  Corporation)

Dover Pharmaceutical, Inc.
P.O. Box 809
Islington, MA 02090
617-821-5400

Doyle Pharmaceutical Company
5320 West 23rd Street
Minneapolis, MN 55416

Drackett Products Company
Division of Mead Johnson Nutritionals
201 East 4th Street
Cincinnati, OH 45201

Du Pont Critical Care
(*formerly* American Critical Care)
Division of American Hospital
  Supply Corporation
1600 Waukegan Road
McGaw Park, IL 60085
312-473-3000

Du Pont Pharmaceuticals
(*also* Endo)
Barley Mill Plaza
Gilpin Mill Building
Wilmington, DE 19898
302-774-1000

 E

Elder Pharmaceuticals
3300 Hyland Avenue
Costa Mesa, CA 92626
714-545-0100
800-556-1937

Endo Laboratories, Inc.
(see Du Pont Pharmaceuticals)

Extar Company
Routes 100 and 401
P.O. Box 593
Chester Springs, PA 19425

 F

Ferndale Laboratories, Inc.
780 West Eight Mile Road
Ferndale, MI 48220
313-548-0900

Fisons Corporation
Pharmaceutical Division
Two Preston Court
Bedford, MA 01730
617-275-1000

Flanders, Inc.
P.O. Box 39143
Northbridge Station
Charleston, SC 29407
803-571-6768

C.B. Fleet Company, Inc.
4615 Murray Place
P.O. Box 11349
Lynchburg, VA 24506
804-528-4000

Fleming & Company
1600 Fenpark Drive
Fenton, MO 63026
314-343-8200

Forest Pharmaceuticals, Inc.
2510 Metro Boulevard
Maryland Heights, MO 63043-9979
314-569-3610
800-325-1605

E. Fougera & Company
Division of Altana Inc.
60 Baylis Road
Melville, NY 11747
516-454-6996
800-645-9833

Fox Pharmacal, Inc.
1750 West McNab Road
P.O. Box 8668
Ft. Lauderdale, FL 33310
305-971-4100

Freshlabs, Inc.
7047 Murthum Avenue
Warren, MI 48092
313-939-0220
800-521-2393

Furst-McNess Company
120 East Clark Street
Freeport, IL 61032
815-235-6151

G

G & W Laboratories, Inc.
111 Coolidge Street
South Plainfield, NJ 07080
201-753-2000
800-922-1038

Gebauer Chemical Company
9410 St. Catherine Avenue
Cleveland, OH 44104
216-271-5252
800-321-9348

GenDerm Corporation
425 Huehl Road
Northbrook, IL 60062
312-564-5435
800-533-3376

Geneva Generics, Inc.
2599 West Midway Boulevard
Broomfield, CO 80020
303-466-8841

Glaxo, Inc.
5 Moore Drive
P.O. Box 13960
Research Triangle Park, NC 27709
919-248-2100

Glenbrook Laboratories
Division of Sterling Drug, Inc.
90 Park Avenue
New York, NY 10016
212-907-2000

H. Clay Glover Company, Inc.
1140 Franklin Avenue
Garden City, NY 11530

Goldline Laboratories
Division of Generix Drug Company
1900 W. Commercial
Ft. Lauderdale, FL 33309

Goody's Manufacturing Corporation
436 Salt Street
P.O. Box 10518
Winston-Salem, NC 27108
919-723-1831
800-322-6639

Greater Detroit Society for the Blind
16625 Grand River
Detroit, MI 48227
313-272-3900

Gricks
Division of "Q-T" Products, Inc.
202-11 Jamaica Avenue
Hollis, NY 11423

Guardian Chemical
Division of United Guardian, Inc.
230 Marcus Boulevard
Hauppauge, NY 11788
516-273-0900
800-645-5566

H

Halsey Drug Company Inc.
187 Pacific Street
Brooklyn, NY 11233
718-467-7500

G.C. Hanford Manufacturing
 Company
P.O. Box 1017
304 Oneida Street
Syracuse, NY 13201
315-476-7418

Harvard Apparatus, Inc.
Medical Division
150 Dover Road
Millis, MA 02054

W.E. Hauck Inc.
P.O. Box 1065
Alphretta, GA 30239-1065
404-475-4758

Healthcheck
150 Sandbank Road
Cheshire, CT 06410
203-271-1120

Helena Laboratories
P.O. Box 752
1530 Lindbergh Drive
Beaumont, TX 77704-0752
409-842-3714

Herbert Laboratories
1202 East Wakeham Avenue
Santa Ana, CA 92705
714-955-6200
800-347-4500

Hoechst-Roussel Pharmaceuticals, Inc.
Route 202-206 North
Somerville, NJ 08876
201-231-2000

Holland-Rantos Company, Inc.
Enterprise Avenue
P.O. Box 5147
Trenton, NJ 08638

Hollister Inc.
2000 Hollister Drive
P.O. Box 250
Libertyville, IL 60048

Humphrey's Pharmacal, Inc.
63 Meadow Road
Rutherford, NJ 07070

Hydrosal Company
Division of Merchandise, Inc.
P.O. Box 8
5929 State Route 128
Miamitown, OH 45041
513-353-2200

Hygeia Sciences
330 Nevada Street
Newton, MA 02160-1432
617-964-0200

Hynson, Westcott & Dunning
Division of Becton Dickinson
P.O. Box 243
Cockeysville, MD 21030
301-771-0100

Hyrex Pharmaceuticals
3494 Democrat Road
P.O. Box 18385
Memphis, TN 38118
901-794-9050
800-238-5282

I

ICI Pharmaceuticals Group
A Business Unit of ICI Americas Inc.
Wilmington, DE 19897
302-886-3000
800-456-3669

I.C.N. Pharmaceuticals
5040 Lester Road
Cincinnati, OH 45213
714-545-0100

Ingram Pharmaceuticals
Subsidiary of Syntex Laboratories
3401 Hillview Avenue
Stanford Industrial Park
Palo Alto, CA 94304
415-855-5050

IOLAB Pharmaceuticals
500 IOLAB Drive
Claremont, CA 91711
714-624-2020

Ives Laboratories, Inc.
685 3rd Avenue
New York, NY 10017
212-878-6200

Ivy Corporation
23 Fairfield Place
West Caldwell, NJ 07006
201-575-1990
800-443-8856

J

Jayco Pharmaceuticals
895 Poplar Church Road
Camp Hill, PA 17011
717-763-7687

Jeffrey Martin, Inc.
419 Claremont Terrace
Union, NJ 07083

JMI-Cantos Pharmaceuticals
Subsidiary of Jones Medical
 Industries, Inc.
11710 Lackland Industrial Drive
St. Louis, MO 63146
314-432-7557
800-525-8466

Johnson & Johnson Baby
 Products Company
Grandview Road
Skillman, NJ 08558
201-874-1000

Johnson & Johnson Health
 Care Company
501 George Street
New Brunswick, NJ 08903
201-524-0400

Jones Medical Industries, Inc.
(see JMI-Cantos Pharmaceuticals)

K

Keystone Laboratories, Inc.
1103 Kansas Street
Memphis, TN 38106
901-774-8860
800-772-8860

K.I.K. Company
Box 256
Bethlehem, PA 18016

Kinney & Company, Inc.
1307 12th Street
P.O. Box 307
Columbus, IN 47201

Kiwi Brands Inc.
Route 662 North
Douglassville, PA 19518
215-385-3041

Knoll Pharmaceuticals
30 North Jefferson Road
Whippany, NJ 07981
201-887-8300
800-526-0221

L

Lactona Products
(see Warner Lambert Company)

Lakeside Pharmaceuticals
Division of Merrell Dow
 Pharmaceuticals Inc.
10123 Alliance Road
Cincinnati, OH 45242
513-948-9111
800-552-3656

The Lannett Company, Inc.
9000 State Road
Philadelphia, PA 19136
215-333-9000

Alvin Last, Inc.
19 Babcock Place
Yonkers, NY 10701
914-376-1000

Lavoptik Company, Inc.
661 Western Avenue, North
St. Paul, MN 55103
612-489-1351

Lederle Laboratories
Division of American
 Cyanamid Company
Onc Cyanamid Plaza
Wayne, NJ 07470
201-831-2000

Leeming/Pacquin
Division of Pfizer, Inc.
235 East 42nd Street
New York, NY 10017
212-573-3600

Lehn & Fink Products Group
Division of Sterling Drug, Inc.
225 Summit Avenue
Montvale, NJ 07645
201-573-5300

Lever Brothers Company
390 Park Avenue
New York, NY 10022
212-688-6000

Eli Lilly & Company
Lilly Corporate Center
Indianapolis, IN 42865
317-276-2000

Loma Linda Food Company
11503 Pierce Street
Riverside, CA 92505
714-687-7800
800-932-5525

Lorvic Corporation
8810 Frost Avenue
St. Louis, MO 63134
314-524-7444

Lumiscope Company, Inc.
400 Raritan Center Parkway
Edison, NJ 08837
201-225-5533

M

Macsil, Inc.
1326 Frankford Avenue
Philadelphia, PA 19125
215-739-7300

Major Pharmaceutical Corporation
8330 Arjons Drive
San Diego, CA 92126

Mallard, Inc.
3021 Wabash Avenue
Detroit, MI 48216
313-964-3910
800-824-8877

Mallinckrodt, Inc.
675 McDonnell Boulevard
P.O. Box 5840
St. Louis, MO 63147
314-895-2000

Marion Merrell Dow Inc.
(*formerly* Marion Laboratories, Inc.)
10236 Bunker Ridge Road
P.O. Box 9627
Kansas City, MO 64134
816-966-5000

Dr. J.H. McLean Medicine Company
3000 Hempstead Turnpike
Levittown, NY 11756
516-731-5380

McNeil Consumer Products Company
Camp Hill Road
Fort Washington, PA 19034
215-233-7000

Meade Johnson Nutritional Group
(see Bristol-Myers USPNG)

Medicone Company
225 Varick Street
New York, NY 10014
212-924-5166

Meditec, Inc.
9485 East Orchard Drive
Englewood, CO 80111
303-771-4863

Medtech Laboratories, Inc.
P.O. Box 1108
3510 North Lake Creek Drive
Jackson, WY 83001
307-733-1680
800-443-4908

Menley & James Laboratories
(see SmithKline Consumer Products)

The Mennen Company
Hanover Avenue
Morristown, NJ 07960
201-631-9000

The Mentholatum Company
1360 Niagara Street
Buffalo, NY 14213
716-882-7660

Merrell Dow Pharmaceuticals, Inc.
(see Lakeside Pharmaceuticals)

Merrell-National Laboratories
(see Lakeside Pharmaceuticals)

Merrick Medicine Company
P.O. Box 1489
Waco, TX 76703
817-753-3461

MiLance Laboratories, Inc.
P.O. Box 39
Maplewood, NJ 07040

Miles Incorporated
Consumer Healthcare Division
P.O. Box 40
1127 Myrtle Street
Elkhart, IN 46515
219-264-8111

Miles Pharmaceuticals
Division of Miles Laboratories
400 Morgan Lane
West Haven, CT 06516
203-934-9221

Milroy Laboratories
Division of Milton Roy Company
P.O. Drawer 849
Sarasota, FL 33578

Mission Pharmacal Company
1328 E. Durango Street
San Antonio, TX 78296

Mizzy, Inc.
Cliftondale Park
Clifton Forge, VA 24422

Modern Products, Inc.
P.O. Box 09398
3015 West Vera Avenue
Milwaukee, WI 53209
414-352-3333

Monoclonal Antibodies, Inc.
2319 Charleston Road
Mountain View, CA 94043
408-739-2700

Monoject
(see Sherwood Medical)

Monticello Drug Company
45 Broad Street Viaduct
Jacksonville, FL 32202
904-355-3666

Moss Chemical Company Inc.
183 St. Paul Street
Rochester, NY 14604

Muro Pharmaceutical, Inc.
890 East Street
Tewksbury, MA 01876
617-851-5981

N

Neutrogena Dermatologics, Inc.
Division of Neutrogena Corporation
5755 West 96th Street
Los Angeles, CA 90045
213-642-1150

Nion Corporation
11581 Federal Drive
El Monte, CA 91731

Norwich-Eaton Pharmaceutical, Inc.
17 Eaton Avenue
P.O. Box 191
Norwich, NY 13815
607-335-2111

Novo-Nordisk Pharmaceuticals Inc.
100 Overlook Center, Suite 200
Princeton, NJ 08540
609-987-5800
800-223-0872

Noxell Corporation
11050 York Road
Hunt Valley, MD 21030
301-785-7300

Nu-Hope Laboratories, Inc.
P.O. Box 39348
Los Angeles, CA 90039-0348
213-666-5248

O

O'Connor Pharmaceuticals
Subsidiary of Columbia
    Laboratories, Inc.
P.O. Box 693530
Miami, FL 33269-9998
305-944-3666
800-521-9522

Ogilvie-Tussy, Inc.
225 Summit Avenue
Montvale, NJ 07645

O'Neal Jones & Feldman, Inc.
Division of Forest
    Pharmaceuticals Inc.
2510 Metro Boulevard
Maryland Heights, MO 63043-9979
314-569-3610
800-325-1605

Oral-B Laboratories
A Gillette Company
One Lagoon Drive
Redwood City, CA 94065
415-598-5000
800-446-7252

Organon, Inc.
375 Mt. Pleasant Avenue
West Orange, NJ 07052

Ortega Pharmaceutical Company
P.O. Box 6212
586 South Edgewood Avenue
Jacksonville, FL 32205

Ortho Pharmaceutical Corporation
Advanced Care Products Division
U.S. Route 202
Raritan, NJ 08869
201-524-0400

Owen Laboratories
(*also* Allercreme)
6201 South Freeway, Box 6600
Ft. Worth, TX 76115
817-293-0450

P

Paddock Laboratories
3101 Louisiana Avenue
P.O. Box 27286
Minneapolis, MN 55427
612-546-4676
800-328-5113

Parke-Davis Consumer Health
 Products Group
Division of Warner-Lambert Company
201 Tabor Road
Morris Plains, NJ 07950
201-540-2000
800-562-6451

Pascal Company, Inc.
P.O. Box 1478
2929 Northeast Northrup Way
Bellevue, WA 98009
206-827-4694

Pennwalt Corporation
Pharmaceutical Consumer
 Products Division
755 Jefferson Road
Rochester, NY 14623
716-475-9000

L. Perrigo Company
117 Water Street
Allegan, MI 49010
616-673-8451

Person & Covey, Inc.
Box 3000
616 Allen Avenue
Glendale, CA 91201
818-240-1030

Personal Laboratories
Division of C.B. Fleet Company, Inc.
P.O. Box 11349
4615 Murray Place
Lynchburg, VA 24506

Peterson Ointment Company
257 Franklin Street
P.O. Box 1565, Ellicott Station
Buffalo, NY 14202
716-854-3787

Pfeiffer Pharmaceuticals Inc.
P.O. Box 100
Wilkes-Barre, PA 18773
717-826-9000

Pfizer Inc.
235 East 42nd Street
New York, NY 10017
212-573-2323

Pharmacraft
Division of Pennwalt Corporation
P.O. Box 1212
Rochester, NY 14603
716-475-9000

Pharmaseal
1015 Grandview Avenue
P.O. Box 1300
Glendale, CA 91209

Pharmex, Inc.
2113 Lincoln Street
P.O. Box 151
Hollywood, FL 33022
305-923-2821

Plough, Inc.
Personal Care Group
P.O. Box 377
Memphis, TN 38151
901-320-2386

Poythress Laboratories, Inc.
16 North 22nd Street
Box 26946
Richmond, VA 23261
804-644-8591

The Procter & Gamble Company
P.O. Box 599
One Procter & Gamble Plaza
Cincinnati, OH 45201
513-983-1100

The Purdue Frederick Company
100 Connecticut Avenue
Norwalk, CT 06854
203-853-0123
800-877-0123

Purepac Pharmaceutical
200 Elmora Avenue
Elizabeth, NJ 07207
201-527-9100

R

Recsei Laboratories
330 South Kellog Avenue
Building M
Goleta, CA 93117
805-964-2912

Reed & Carnrick
One New England Avenue
Piscataway, NJ 08854
201-981-0070

Reid-Rowell, Inc.
901 Sawyer Road
Marietta, GA 30062
404-578-9000

Republic Drug Company, Inc.
175 Great Arrow Avenue
Buffalo, NY 14207

Requa Inc.
1 Seneca Place
P.O. Box 4008
Greenwich, CT 06830
203-869-2445

Rexall Drug Company
3901 North Kings Highway
St. Louis, MO 63115
314-946-6606

Richardson-Vicks USA
Ten Westport Road
Wilton, CT 06897
203-925-6000

Riker Laboratories, Inc.
19901 Nordhoff Street
Northridge, CA 91324
612-736-5968

Roberts Laboratories
2086 R.D. J 25
Austin, CO 81410

A.H. Robins Company
Consumer Products Division
P.O. Box 6235
3800 Cutshaw Avenue
Richmond, VA 23230
804-257-2000

Roche Laboratories
Division of Hoffmann-LaRoche, Inc.
340 Kingsland Street
Nutley, NJ 07110
201-235-5000

Rorer Consumer Pharmaceuticals
500 Virginia Drive
Fort Washington, PA 19034
215-628-6541

Ross Laboratories
625 Cleveland Avenue
Columbus, OH 43216
614-227-3333

Rowell Laboratories, Inc.
(see Reid-Rowell, Inc.)

Roxane Laboratories, Inc.
330 Oak Street
Columbus, OH 43216

Rugby Laboratories, Inc.
100 Banks Avenue
Rockville Center, NY 11570

Rydelle Laboratories
Subsidiary of S.C. Johnson
  and Son, Inc.
1525 Howe Street
Racine, WI 53403-5011
414-631-4000

Rystan Company, Inc.
47 Center Avenue
P.O. Box 214
Little Falls, NJ 07424-0214
201-256-3737

S

Sandoz Pharmaceuticals Corporation
(*formerly* Dorsey Laboratories)
Route 10
East Hanover, NJ 07936
201-503-7500
800-631-8184

Henry Schein Inc.
5 Harbor Park Drive
Port Washington, NY 11050
516-621-4300

Scherer Laboratories, Inc.
14335 Gillis Road
Dallas, TX 75244

Schering Corporation
(see Schering-Plough Corporation)

Schering-Plough Corporation
Galloping Hill Road
Kenilworth, NJ 07033
201-822-7000

Schmid Laboratories, Inc.
Route 46 West
Little Falls, NJ 07424
201-256-5500

Scholl, Inc.
Personal Care Group
Schering-Plough Corporation
3030 Jackson Avenue
Memphis, TN 38151
901-320-4766

Scrip Inc.
101 South Street
Peoria, IL 61602
309-674-3488
800-322-4248 (Illinois only)
800-343-5097 (Outside Illinois)

Sea Breeze Laboratories
Division of Clairol Inc.
345 Park Avenue
New York, NY 10022

Seabee Corporation
Insulin Aid Division
P.O. Box 457
602 South Federal Street
Hampton, IA 50441

Searle Consumer Products
Division of Searle Pharmaceuticals Inc.
P.O. Box 5110
Chicago, IL 60680
312-982-7000

Shaklee Corporation
444 Market Street
San Francisco, CA 94111
415-954-2080

Sherwood Medical
Subsidiary of American Home
  Products Corporation
Monoject Division
1831 Olive Street
St. Louis, MO 63103
314-621-7788

Smith & Nephew United, Inc.
11775 Starkey Road
Largo, FL 34643
813-392-1261

SmithKline & French Laboratories
Division of SmithKline Beckman
  Corporation
1500 Spring Garden Street
Philadelphia, PA 19101
215-751-4000
800-366-8900

SmithKline Beecham
(see SmithKline Consumer Products)

SmithKline Consumer Products
(*formerly* Menley & James Laboratories)
A SmithKline Beckman Company
One Franklin Plaza
P.O. Box 8082
Philadelphia, PA 19101
215-751-4000

Spirt & Company
Subsidiary of Hyrex Pharmaceuticals
3494 Democrat Road
P.O. Box 18385
Memphis, TN 38118
901-794-9050

Squibb Mark
P.O. Box 4000
Princeton, NJ 08543
609-987-6800
800-332-2056

Squibb-Novo, Inc.
211 Carnegie Center
Princeton, NJ 08540-6213
609-987-5800
800-727-6500

S.S.S. Company
71 University Avenue, S.W.
Box 4447
Atlanta, GA 30302
404-521-0857

Stanback Company, Ltd.
P.O. Box 1669
1500 South Main Street
Salisbury, NC 28144
704-633-9231

Stiefel Laboratories, Inc.
2801 Ponce de Leon Boulevard
Coral Gables, FL 33134-6988

Stuart Pharmaceuticals
Division of ICI Pharmaceuticals Group
P.O. Box 751
Wilmington, DE 19897
302-575-3000

Summers Laboratories, Inc.
P.O. Box 162
Fort Washington, PA 19034
215-643-9777
800-533-SKIN (Customer service only)

Support Systems
P.O. Box 88687
Atlanta, GA 30338

Syntex Laboratories, Inc.
3401 Hillview Avenue
P.O. Box 10850
Palo Alto, CA 94304
415-855-5050

T

Tender Corporation
P.O. Box 290
Littleton Industrial Park
Littleton, NH 03561
603-444-5464
800-258-4696

Texas Pharmacal
Subsidiary of Alcon Laboratories, Inc.
6201 South Freeway
Box 1959
Ft. Worth, TX 76101
817-293-0450

Theon Inc.
203 Hawthorn Street
New Bedford, MA 02740
508-994-9400

Thomas & Thompson Company
3927 Falls Road
Baltimore, MD 21211
301-889-2960

Thompson Medical Company, Inc.
919 3rd Avenue
New York, NY 10022
212-688-4420

3M Company
Consumer Products Group
3M Center
St. Paul, MN 55144
612-733-2330

Dr. G.H. Tichenor Antiseptic
  Company
P.O. Box 53374
New Orleans, LA 70153

U

Ulmer Pharmacal Company
2440 Fernbrook Lane
Plymouth, MN 55441
800-328-7157

Ulster Scientific, Inc.
P.O. Box 902
Highland, NY 12528

United Division
Pfizer Hospital Products Group
(see Smith & Nephew United, Inc.)

The Upjohn Company
7000 Portage Road
Unit 9023-TB3-1
Kalamazoo, MI 49001
616-323-4000

USV Laboratories
(see Rorer Consumer Pharmaceuticals)

V

The Vale Chemical Company, Inc.
1201 Liberty Street
Allentown, PA 18102
215-433-7579

Vicks Health Care Products
Division of Richardson Vicks, Inc.
One Far Mill Crossing
Shelton, CT 06484
203-929-2500

Vipont Pharmaceutical, Inc.
P.O. Box 460
Fort Collins, CO 80522
303-482-3126

Vitarine Pharmaceuticals, Inc.
227-15 North Conduit Avenue
Springfield Gardens, NY 11413

Vortech Pharmaceuticals, Ltd.
6851 Chase Road
P.O. Box 189
Dearborn, MI 48126
313-584-4088
800-521-4686

W

Walker Corporation & Company Inc.
P.O. Box 1320
Syracuse, NY 13201
315-463-4511

Wallace Laboratories
(see Carter-Wallace, Inc.)

Warner-Lambert Company
Consumer Health Products Division
201 Tabor Road
Morris Plains, NJ 07950
201-540-2000
(see products for toll-free numbers)

Warren-Teed
(see Adria Laboratories, Inc.)

The Wellspring Enterprise, Ltd.
One Franklin Plaza
Philadelphia, PA 19102
215-561-7540

Westwood Pharmaceuticals
100 Forest Avenue
Buffalo, NY 14213
716-887-3400
800-333-0950

Whitehall Laboratories
Division of American Home
  Products Corporation
685 Third Avenue
New York, NY 10017-4076
212-878-5000

Winthrop Pharmaceuticals
90 Park Avenue
New York, NY 10016
212-907-2577

Wyeth Laboratories
Box 8299
Philadelphia, PA 19101
215-688-4400

Y

Yager Drug Company
430 West Mulberry Street
Baltimore, MD 21201
301-685-8542

W.F. Young, Inc.
111 Lyman Street
Springfield, MA 01103
413-737-0201

Youngs Corporation
580 Bryant Street
San Francisco, CA 94107

Youngs Drug Products Corporation
Subsidiary of Holland-Rantos
P.O. Box 385
865 Centennial Avenue
Piscataway, NJ 08854
609-655-6000

INDEX

INDEX

Chapter title subjects and chapter opening pages are in red boldface.
Product table titles are in red italics.
Major subject entries are in black boldface.
Subhead subject entries are in black type.
Product trade names are in black italics.

NOTES

NOTES

NOTES

NOTES

NOTES

NOTES

NOTES

NOTES